Willard and Spackman's
Occupational Therapy

Willard and Spackman's Occupational Therapy *Sixth Edition*

Edited by

Helen L. Hopkins, *Ed.D., O.T.R., F.A.O.T.A.*

Professor and Chairman of Occupational Therapy
College of Allied Health Professions
Temple University
Philadelphia, Pennsylvania

Helen D. Smith, *M.O.T., O.T.R., F.A.O.T.A.*

Associate Professor of Occupational Therapy
Tufts University—Boston School of Occupational Therapy
Medford, Massachusetts

33 Contributors

J. B. Lippincott Company
Philadelphia
London   Mexico City   New York
St. Louis   São Paulo   Sydney

Sponsoring Editor: Eleanor Faven, Paul Hill
Indexer: Sue Reilly
Art Director: Tracy Baldwin
Designer: William Boehm
Production Supervisor: N. Carol Kerr
Production Assistant: J. Corey Gray
Compositor: Bi-Comp, Incorporated
Printer/Binder: The Murray Printing Company

6th Edition

Library of Congress Cataloging in Publication Data
Main entry under title:

Willard and Spackman's Occupational therapy.

   Bibliography: p.
   Includes index.
   1. Occupational therapy.   I. Hopkins, Helen L.
II. Smith, Helen D.   III. Title: Occupational therapy.
[DNLM: 1. Occupational therapy. 2. Rehabilitation.
WB 555 W692]
RM735.W54   1983   615.8'515   82-20352
ISBN 0-397-54361-1

TO HELEN WILLARD, B.A., O.T.R., F.A.O.T.A.

Occupational Therapy pioneer, educator,
leader, advocate, our teacher and friend

Give a man a fish, and you feed him for a day. Teach a man to fish, and you feed him for a lifetime. Chinese Proverb

CONTRIBUTORS

Abby Abildness, M.S., O.T.R.
Adjunct Instructor of Behavioral Science
Milton S. Hershey Medical Center
Pennsylvania State University
  Hershey, Pennsylvania, and
Occupational Therapist and Biofeedback Counselor
Talbot Place Alcoholic Rehabilitation Center
Hershey, Pennsylvania

Bonnie Sherry Almasy, B.S.
Rehabilitation Home Economist
Harmarville Rehabilitation Center
Pittsburgh, Pennsylvania

Carolyn Manville Baum, M.A., O.T.R., F.A.O.T.A.
Clinical Director
Occupational Therapy Services
Washington University School of Medicine
Irene Walter Johnson Institute of Rehabilitation
St. Louis, Missouri

Marianne Rozycka Dahl, B.S., O.T.R.
Assistant Director
Occupational Therapy Department
Moss Rehabilitation Hospital
Philadelphia, Pennsylvania

Mary Margaret Daub, Ed.M., O.T.R.
Associate Professor of Occupational Therapy
College of Allied Health Professions
Temple University
Philadelphia, Pennsylvania

Elizabeth B. Devereaux, M.S.W., A.C.S.W.,
  O.T.R./L., F.A.O.T.A.
Assistant Professor of Psychiatry
Marshall University School of Medicine
Department of Psychiatry
Huntington, West Virginia

Elnora M. Gilfoyle, D.S.C. (honorary), B.S., O.T.R.,
  F.A.O.T.A.
Associate Professor of Occupational Therapy
Colorado State University
Boulder, Colorado

Ann P. Grady, B.A., O.T.R., F.A.O.T.A.
Director of Occupational Therapy
The Children's Hospital
Denver, Colorado

Carole Hays, M.A., O.T.R., F.A.O.T.A.
Director
Professional Development Division
American Occupational Therapy Association
Rockville, Maryland

L. Irene Hollis, B.S., O.T.R., F.A.O.T.A.
Chapel Hill, North Carolina

Helen L. Hopkins, Ed.D., O.T.R., F.A.O.T.A.
Professor and Chairman of Occupational Therapy
College of Allied Health Professions
Temple University
Philadelphia, Pennsylvania

Margaret V. Howison, B.S., O.T.R.
Director of Occupational Therapy
Elizabethtown Hospital for Children and Youth
Instructor of Occupational Therapy
Elizabethtown College
Elizabethtown, Pennsylvania

A. Joy Huss, M.S., O.T.R., R.P.T., F.A.O.T.A.
Associate Professor
Course in Occupational Therapy
University of Minnesota
Minneapolis, Minnesota

Linda A. Johnson, B.A., O.T.R.
Private Practice
Newport, Oregon

Nancy Allen Kaufmann, Ed.M., O.T.R.
Staff Occupational Therapist
Crozer Chester Medical Center
Chester, Pennsylvania

Dorothy L. Kester, O.T.R.
Senior Research Assistant
Delaware Curative Workshop
Wilmington, Delaware

Gary Kielhofner, M.A., Dr.P.H., O.T.R.
Assistant Professor
Department of Occupational Therapy
Medical College of Virginia
Virginia Commonwealth University
Richmond, Virginia

Ruth Levine, Ed.D., O.T.R.
Program Planning Consultant
Department of Occupational Therapy
College of Allied Health Professions
Thomas Jefferson University
Philadelphia, Pennsylvania

Maude H. Malick, B.S., O.T.R.
Administrative Director of Occupational Therapy
    Services
Harmarville Rehabilitation Center
Pittsburgh, Pennsylvania

Sandra J. Malone, B.S., O.T.R.
Occupational Therapy Consultant
Maryland State Dept. of Health & Mental Hygiene
Baltimore, Maryland

Janice Matsutsuyu, M.A., O.T.R., F.A.O.T.A.
Chief of Rehabilitation Services
Clinical Associate Professor
Dept. of Occupational Therapy
University of Southern California
University of California, Los Angeles
Neuropsychiatric Institute
Center for the Health Sciences
Los Angeles, California

Tina Olson, B.S., O.T.R., F.A.O.T.A.
Regional Director
Cooperative Services
Stormont–Vail Regional Medical Center
Topeka, Kansas

Patricia C. Ostrow, M.A., O.T.R.
Director of Quality Review Division
American Occupational Therapy Association
Rockville, Maryland

Patricia Ann Ramm, M.A., O.T.R., F.A.O.T.A.
Private Practice
Austin, Texas

Reba M. Sebelist, M.S., O.T.R.
Instructor in Occupational Therapy
Elizabethtown College
Elizabethtown, Pennsylvania

Mary Silberzahn, M.A., O.T.R.
Sensory Integrative Specialist
Faculty Member of Center for the Study of Sensory
    Integrative Dysfunction
Los Angeles, California

Helen D. Smith, M.O.T., O.T.R., F.A.O.T.A.
Associate Professor of Occupational Therapy
Tufts University–Boston School of Occupational
    Therapy
Medford, Massachusetts

Elinor Anne Spencer, B.A., O.T.R., F.A.O.T.A.
Director of Occupational Therapy
Harmarville Rehabilitation Center
Pittsburgh, Pennsylvania

Sallie Elizabeth Taylor, M.Ed., O.T.R.
Clinical Specialist
Washington University School of Medicine
Irene Walter Johnson Institute of Rehabilitation
Department of Preventive Medicine
St. Louis, Missouri

Elizabeth Gordon Tiffany, M.Ed., O.T.R.,
  F.A.O.T.A.
Associate Professor of Occupational Therapy
College of Allied Health Professions
Temple University
Philadelphia, Pennsylvania

Gail Tower, M.S., L.P.T.
Associate Professor of Physical Therapy
College of Allied Health Professions
Temple University
Philadelphia, Pennsylvania

Ann Starnes Wade, M.S., O.T.R.
Occupational Therapist
Colerain School
Columbus, Ohio

Elizabeth June Yerxa, Ed.D., O.T.R., F.A.O.T.A.
Chairperson
Department of Occupational Therapy
University of Southern California
Downey, California

FOREWORD
to the Fifth Edition

When thirty-two years ago we agreed to edit what was then called *Principles of Occupational Therapy* it never occurred to us that in 1976 we should at last be passing on the editorship of *Occupational Therapy*. It is with pleasure that we give this task to two of our coworkers and friends—Helen L. Hopkins and Helen D. Smith—who have accepted the responsibility of editing the fifth edition while we become editors emeriti.

Forty-two authors have contributed to the first four editions. To them go our warmest thanks and appreciation. The third and fourth editions have been translated into Japanese and the fourth into Spanish.

During this time our field has changed and grown immeasurably. The present edition reflects recent changes and will add much to the knowledge and understanding of occupational therapy today.

Clare S. Spackman
Helen S. Willard

PREFACE

Willard and Spackman's Occupational Therapy has, over the years, been a textbook written primarily for occupational therapy students. With this in mind, questionnaires were sent to all professional and technical occupational therapy schools during the summer of 1980 in an attempt to evaluate the usefulness of this textbook for students. Detailed comments and constructive criticism were received from numerous faculty members. As a result of the information received changes have been made in the sixth edition. Chapters have been added on Occupation, Biofeedback, Uniform Reporting of Occupational Therapy Data, Strategy Planning, Health-Care Marketing, and Assuring Quality Service Delivery. The chapters on Occupational Behavior, Occupational Therapy with Children, and Management have been expanded. All other chapters have been updated. The Occupational Therapy Standards of Practice, Uniform Terminology for Reporting Occupational Therapy Services, Occupational Therapy Product Output Reporting System, and Uniform Occupational Therapy Evaluation Checklist have been added to the Appendix.

The sixth edition has been divided into eight parts: (1) history, (2) theory and philosophy, (3) occupational therapy approaches for intervention, (4) evaluation process and procedure, (5) treatment process and procedures, (6) implementation of occupational therapy, (7) managing occupational therapy services, and (8) research.

Part 1 gives an historical perspective on the profession, discussing its genesis and development from ancient origins to the present time. A section entitled *Into the Eighties* has been added to this chapter.

Part 2 deals with the bases for theory and philosophy in occupational therapy. Occupational therapy appears to be based in two broad areas—human growth and development and occupation.

Part 3 discusses the occupational therapy process as one that uses problem-solving procedures. Four approaches currently used in occupational therapy practice are identified as developmental, sensorimotor, occupational behavior, and rehabilitation. An overview of each of the approaches is given. Each approach allows for varying frames of reference to be used as the rationale for treatment planning and treatment implementation; these depend upon the type of patients or clients and the philosophy, preferences, biases, and expertise of the therapist, as well as the goals and interests of the patients or clients. Four elements are identified as the organizing principles that give occupational therapy its essence; these are the patient or client, the therapist and therapeutic relationship, the activity, and the context or setting for treatment. The six phases of the occupational therapy process described include initial evaluation, development of treatment objectives, treatment planning, treatment implementation, ongoing evaluation, and termination of treatment.

Part 4 describes the evaluation process and specific occupational therapy evaluation procedures that are used in practice. *Part 5* describes the treatment process and general treatment procedures used in practice. These procedures include therapeutic application of activity, activities of daily living, homemaking, prevocational training, and biofeedback.

Part 6 identifies general and specialized areas of practice. These include psychiatry and mental health; mental retardation; functional restoration, which includes neurologic and orthopedic conditions, human sexuality, upper-extremity orthotics, hand rehabilitation, burns, and amputations; problems with special senses (blindness and deafness); occupational therapy with children (general pediatrics, cerebral palsy, occupational therapy in the school setting); gerontology; general medicine and surgery; and community home health care in both urban and rural settings.

Part 7 deals with the management of occupational therapy services. Included are a systems perspective; financial management; communication; personnel; resources; documentation; uniform reporting of occupational therapy data; strategy planning; health-care marketing; and quality assurance. This section has been expanded in order to meet the needs of the entry-level therapist as a manager. *Part 8* discusses the role of the occupational therapist as a researcher.

Our attempt to provide comprehensive coverage of the profession is evident in our choice of 33 authors with expertise in their areas. Thirty-one are practicing occupational therapists, one is a practicing physical therapist, and one is a rehabilitation home economist. The authors represent nine universities and numerous clinics, community settings, and private practice in fifteen states.

We thank the authors for their excellent contributions and for their assistance in providing a comprehensive overview of the profession. Special thanks are due our friends Theresa McCoy, for typing and support, and Jennifer Tiffany for editorial assistance. Special appreciation is expressed to Elizabeth Tiffany for suggestions, collaboration, and support in the planning, development, and execution of an enormous task.

Helen L. Hopkins, Ed.D., O.T.R., F.A.O.T.A.
Helen D. Smith, M.O.T., O.T.R., F.A.O.T.A.

CONTENTS

Willard and Spackman's
Occupational Therapy

PART 1

History

An Historical Perspective on Occupational Therapy *Helen L. Hopkins*

The term *occupation* has long been recognized as a requirement for survival and, to varying degrees, as a source of pleasure. The term *occupational therapy* may seem to indicate use of "work" as treatment, but those pioneers who fashioned the profession believed that the health of individuals was influenced by "the use of muscles and mind together in games, exercise and handicraft" as well as in work.[1] This, then, is the basis for the use of work, exercise, and play as modalities of treatment in occupational therapy.

In order to obtain a perspective of the profession of occupational therapy it is necessary to trace the history of the use of "occupation" from its ancient origins until the present time. The origin and development of the profession will be traced through the description of the foci of those persons within the field upon whose efforts and ideas occupational therapy practice has been based.

Ancient Origins of Occupation for Treatment

Evidence can be found that the healing qualities of work, exercise, and play were recognized and utilized thousands of years ago. The interrelationship of these three aspects of occupational therapy was also recognized early in the history of civilization.

Exercise (Physical Training)

There is evidence that as early as 2600 BC the Chinese taught that disease was caused by organic inactivity and thus used physical training for the promotion of health. They came to utilize a series of medical gymnastics called *Cong Fu*, which they felt could not only prolong life but would ensure immortality of the soul.[2]

The ancient Persians realized the beneficial effects of physical training and about 1000 BC utilized it to fit their youth for military duty. They used a systematic course of physical training, which began at age 6 and continued through adult years. This resulted in the production of an army of physically fit, able-bodied fighters.

Among the ancient Greeks, physical training was developed to a high degree. Socrates (400 BC) and Plato (347 BC) understood the relationship between physical status and mental health, and Aristotle (340 BC) felt that the "education of the body must precede that of the intellect."[3] The Athenians used physical training for its cultural and social aspects whereas the Spartans used it to build military manpower.

Hippocrates, the father of medicine (359 BC), and Galen, his successor (200 AD), recommended that their patients exercise in the gymnasiums as a means of recovering from illness. The Roman Asclepiades (100 BC) advocated massage, therapeutic baths, and exercises for improving diseased conditions. Scientific medicine is indebted to the interest of the early Greeks and Romans in physical training.[4]

Recreation (Play)

Play, games, and pastimes were a part of the life of all primitive people as is evidenced by the toys, drawings, and sculptures found in excavations of ancient Egypt, Babylonia, and China as well as in the cultural remains of the Aztecs and Incas of the Western Hemisphere. The ancient Egyptians' inscriptions on stone depict the game of draughts, stately dances, the playing of the harp and lute, and children playing with balls, dolls, and jumping jacks.

The Egyptians in 2000 BC and the Greeks in 420 BC described diversion and recreation as a means of treating the sick.[5] One hundred years before Christ, Asclepiades, the Roman, recommended activity treatment for patients with mental diseases. This included diversions and entertainment, but only the diversional value was recognized.

In the fifth century AD Caelius Aurelius of Sicca (Africa) recommended a careful regimen for convalescents that included walks, reading, theater performances, and throwing the discus. Traveling, especially sea voyages, was described as useful for treatment.

During the Dark Ages play was frowned upon by the Church and was regarded as evil, but its mental and physical influences were again recognized during the Renaissance period.

Work

Records from 3400 BC indicate that in Egypt even men of leisure were involved in outdoor work and did not spend their days in idleness. The typical nobleman is pictured as being fond of nature and of working in his garden planting trees, "laying out arbors, excavating a pool, lining it with masonry, and filling it with fish."

The writings of the ancient Hebrews make reference to the beneficial effects of work on the body and mind. The ancient Greeks also recognized the value of work. Socrates said, "A man should inure himself to voluntary labor, and not give up to indulgence and pleasure, as they beget no good constitution of body nor knowledge of mind."

In 17 AD Livy, the historian, wrote "Toil and pleasure in their nature opposites are linked together in a kind of necessary connection." The value of alternating work and play was stressed by Phaedra, a writer of the first century, who said "The mind ought sometimes to be diverted that it may return the better to thinking." Thus, the interrelatedness of work, exercise, and play was recognized 2,000 years ago.[6]

Therapy and Medicine in the Eighteenth and Nineteenth Centuries

Occupational therapy is intimately related to humane treatment. It was not until the last quarter of the eighteenth century, when people on both sides of the Atlantic began to regard others as equals, and fought for this equality, that the practical application of occupational therapy was begun.[7] It was in the midst of the French Revolution (1786) that *Philippe Pinel* introduced work treatment in the Bicêtre Asylum for the Insane near Paris. In his book published in 1801, he describes his methods as "prescribed physical exercises and manual occupations." He said these should be employed in all mental hospitals because "rigorous executed manual labor is the best method of securing good morale and discipline. The return of convalescent patients to their previous interests, to the practice of their profession, to industriousness and perseverance have always been for me the best omen of final recovery."[8] This is the first reference in the literature to medically prescribed use of work for remediation.

On the other side of the Atlantic, where colonists were striving for equality and independence, the first hospital in the colonies, the Pennsylvania Hospital, was established in Philadelphia in 1752. Benjamin Franklin had been involved in drafting the petition for establishing this hospital, and it was probably at his suggestion that inmates who were able were provided with the light manual labor of spinning and carding wool and flax. In 1798 *Benjamin Rush, M.D.*, one of the signers of the Declaration of Independence, advocated work as a remedial measure for patients in this hospital.[9] In an address to the Board of the Pennsylvania Hospital in 1810 Rush advised that "certain kinds of labor, exercise, and amusements be contrived for them, which should act at the same time, upon their bodies and minds. The advantages of labor have been evidenced in foreign hospitals as well as our own, in a greater number of recoveries taking place."[10]

In Germany *Johann Christian Reil* recommended the use of work for treatment of the insane and also suggested the use of exercise and a special hospital gymnasium along with patient participation in dramatic productions and fine arts. Reil's writings give evidence of what was probably the first use of psychodrama in the treatment of the insane.[11]

In the early 1800s *Samuel Tuke*, an English Quaker, established Retreat Asylum for the Insane at York, England. He used work or occupation therapy as Pinel did but placed special emphasis on humane treatment or treating of patients as rational beings who have capability of self-restraint. He called it *moral treatment*. Neither chains nor corporal punishment were used and all patients wore clothes and were induced "to adopt orderly habits" and "participate in exercise and labour."[12]

In 1840 *F. Leuret* wrote a book *On the Moral Treatment of Insanity*. He said all psychiatrists recommend diversions and work to prevent the effects of idleness and boredom. He stressed the improvement of habits and the development of a consciousness of society. He utilized exercise, drama, music, and reading along with manual labor.[13] Moral treatment was virtually synonymous with the principles and practice of occupational therapy; this was probably the first book entirely devoted to occupation therapy.

Many Americans visited Europe following the Revolutionary War and observed the treatment of the insane at European hospitals. *Thomas Scattergood*, a Quaker minister who visited Retreat, brought back to America the principles of "occupation and nonrestraint." These principles were used at Friends Asylum for the Insane in Philadelphia, a hospital that he had helped to establish. The hospital was opened in May 1817 and continues to serve the mentally ill today. *Thomas Eddy* was another visitor to Retreat. A New York merchant and a member of the Society of Friends, he was so impressed with the improved care of the insane that he submitted suggestions for the "moral management" of the insane to the Governors of the Lunatic Asylum of the New York Hospital. As a result of his suggestions, the Bloomingdale Asylum was opened in 1821 in New York City and began moral management including occupation therapy. This hospital continues today as the Westchester Division of the New York Hospital. In 1818 McLean Asylum opened near Boston under the supervision of *Rufus Wyman, M.D.* He established, and was probably the first physician in this country to supervise, a program of occupation therapy.[14]

Around 1843, an innovation, regular classroom instruction, was introduced as a part of the care of the mentally ill in hospitals in both Europe and the United States. In 1844 *Amariah Brigham*, superintendent of the Utica State Hospital in New York, stated that "employment to be of benefit to the patient should not consider the question of gainful occupation, but should divert the patient from his morbid fancies, engage his attention, stimulate his interest, and lead him to resume natural and healthy methods of thought and occupation."[15] The idea that only the therapeutic value to the patient should be considered in selecting the activity was a new and important advance toward the more scientific use of occupation as therapy.

The period of maximum use of occupation therapy in the United States occurred during the lifetime of *Thomas Story Kirkbride, M.D.* He became superintendent of the Pennsylvania Hospital in 1840 and began a program of mental care that stressed occupation therapy. He said the value of occupational therapy cannot be measured in dollars and cents but must be judged in regard to the restoration of comfort to the inmates of the hospital. Crafts, amusements, and hospital occupations were used therapeutically. Kirkbride helped to organize the Association of Asylum Medical Superintendents, which later became the American Psychiatric Association. Through this association, Kirkbride influenced its members regarding the value of occupation therapy.[16]

During the eighteenth and nineteenth centuries work or occupation therapy was utilized primarily in the care of the mentally ill patients. The only mention in the literature of occupation therapy for the physically disabled was in a book published in 1780 in which a physician in the French Cavalry, *Clement-Joseph Tissot*, gave detailed instructions for the use of crafts and recreational activities for disabilities of muscles and joints following disease or injury.[17]

The effective development of work or occupation therapy continued in the United States through 1860. Then it declined suddenly and its emphasis on the therapeutic value of work was lost for more than a quarter of a century. There seem to be several causes for this period of disuse. Physicians became too busy with increasing responsibilities to take sufficient personal interest in work or occupation therapy. There was a lack of public interest and insight and an underestimation of the therapeutic value of occupation as well as "the real returns as compared to the incidental returns or possible economic proceeds from the treatment."[18] The economic pressures felt in all hospitals during and after the Civil War were also a cause for the decline of occupation therapy.

Genesis of the Occupational Therapy Profession in the United States

Forerunner of the Profession— Adolf Meyer's Philosophy

Toward the end of the nineteenth century, work as a therapeutic agent was again utilized in the treatment of the mentally ill in the United States. In a paper presented in December 1892, Adolf Meyer, a psychiatrist, reported that "the proper use of time in some helpful and gratifying activity appeared to be a fundamental issue in the treatment of the neuropsychiatric patient."[19] In 1895 Meyer's wife, Mary Potter Brooks Meyer, a social worker, introduced a systematic type of activity into the wards of a state institution in Worcester, Massachusetts. She was also the first social worker to provide a systematic program to help patients, their families, and the physician.

Meyer's philosophy of treatment and of occupational therapy had a marked impact on the philosophy and history of the profession. His philosophy as stated in the first volume of the first official organ of the profession, published in 1922, was

> Our conception of man is that of an organism that maintains and balances itself in the world of reality and actuality by being in active life and active use, i.e. using and living and acting its time in harmony with its own nature and the nature about it. It is the use that we make of ourselves that gives the ultimate stamp to our every organ.[20]

Meyer described rhythms of life that must be kept in balance even under difficulty. These were work and play, rest and sleep. He said balance was attained by actual doing and practice, with a program of wholesome living as the basis for wholesome thinking, feeling, and interest. He felt that personality was fundamentally determined by performance.[21]

Meyer described mental illness as "a problem of living" and not merely as a disease of structure and function or of a toxic nature. He said because there was habit deterioration, systematic use of time and interest became both an obligation and a necessity. His statement from the yearbook of the Chicago School of Civics and Philanthropy (1908–1911) is the first reference in the literature that indicates that conflicts occur through poor adaptation and that occupation may influence and enhance human adaptiveness:

> During the last decade, we have come to realize more than ever that while some mental disorders are due to toxic conditions, others are rather due to conflicts through poor adaptation. In these conditions a training

in normal activities and a culturation of fruitful interests are the sanest and only efficient point of attack.[22]

Thus Meyer felt that the treatment of the mentally ill must be a blending of work and pleasure that included both recreation and productive activity. He said "the pleasure in achievement, a real pleasure in the use of one's hands and muscles and a happy appreciation of time" should be used as incentives in the management of patients and should replace the use of repressive rules. The goal for patients was to create an "orderly rhythm and sense of a day simply and naturally spent."[23]

Meyer said the philosophy of the occupational therapy worker should be "an awakening to the full meaning of time as the biggest wonder and asset of our lives and the valuation of opportunity and performance as the greatest measure of time."[24] Patients must have the realization of reality and a full sense of actuality. This was to be accomplished by providing opportunities rather than prescriptions, opportunities "to do, to plan and to create."[25]

Interpersonal relationships were also an important part of Meyer's philosophy of occupational therapy, for he felt that personal contact with instructors and helpers brought out an interchange of experiences and resources. Instructors had to be resourceful and respect the native capacities and interests of their patients.[26]

Adolf Meyer had thus provided the profession of occupational therapy with a philosophy upon which it could build.

Founders of the Profession

Susan E. Tracy

Susan E. Tracy probably can be called the first occupational therapist because, in 1905, during her training as a nurse, she noticed the benefits of occupation in relieving nervous tension and making bedrest more tolerable for patients. In working with orthopedic bedfast patients she felt occupation was important because "happiness and contentment will certainly prove conducive to rest, and absolute rest is the foremost condition of recovery." She saw occupation as an important adjunct to drug treatment and also felt that instruction in self-help was important. Tracy believed that wholesome interests could be substituted for morbid ones and could carry over into the patient's life after discharge from the hospital. She also saw interpersonal relationships between the teacher or nurse and the patient as an important factor in the success of occupation treatment.[27]

Tracy began her work with the mentally ill when she became director of the Training School for Nurses at the Adams Nervine Asylum in Boston. It was here that in 1906 she developed the first systematic training course in occupation to prepare instructors for teaching patient activities. Up until this time it was felt that craftsmen were probably the best teachers of patients in craft activities. Since limitations were imposed on patients because of illness or disease, it was determined that persons with medical training would be better qualified because they would recognize signs of fatigue or eyestrain and know the limitations caused by various diseases or injury. Thus the nurse seemed to be the most qualified person to teach occupation to patients. Tracy felt "Kindergarteners" (teachers of small children) could also qualify but would have to become nurses first. She also cautioned that the variety in activity choices must be great in order to meet individual patient requirements.

In 1910 the first book on occupations, *Studies in Invalid Occupations, A Manual for Nurse and Attendants*, was published.[28] This was a compilation of Tracy's lectures with an illustrated guide for the use of activities with patients. The book was primarily a craft book, giving methods of teaching and explaining the rationale for use of specific activities for many patient diagnoses in different types of settings (bed, ward, workshop, home). In this book Tracy describes her concept of occupation by using a quote from John Dewey:

> By occupation is not meant any kind of "busy work" or exercise that may be given to a child to keep him out of mischief or idleness when seated at his desk. By occupation I mean a mode of activity on the part of the child which reproduces or runs parallel to some form of work carried on in the social life . . . The fundamental point of the psychology of an occupation is that it maintains a balance between the intellectual and the practical phases of experience.[29]

Tracy felt that occupations chosen can help retain connections with social life and provide tangible relations between the individual and other people and their needs, and thus "self-respect is preserved and ambition fostered."[30]

Tracy encouraged the use of occupation for treatment by conducting numerous training courses. In 1911, she conducted the first course in occupation at a general hospital, Massachusetts General Hospital Training School for Nurses. In 1914, as director of the Experiment Station for the Study of Invalid Occupations in Jamaica Plains, Massachusetts, she provided instruction for three classes of students: "(1) To invalids, whether inside or out of institutions, (2) To pupil nurses, in order to enlarge their practical equipment and (3) To Graduate Nurses who have felt the need of the work and may become teachers."[31] The course description from a flier on the course is as follows:

Each patient is considered in light of his threefold personality—body, mind and spirit.

The Aim is likewise threefold:
1. The patient's physical improvement
2. His educational advancement
3. His financial betterment

The Method is based upon a threefold principle:
1. The realization of resources
2. The ability to initiate activities
3. The participation in such activities of both sick and well subjects[31]

Through her training courses Tracy did much to disseminate knowledge in regard to use of occupation for treatment of both physically and mentally ill patients.

Herbert J. Hall

In 1904 Herbert J. Hall began to prescribe occupation for his patients as medicine to regulate life and direct interest. He called this the "work cure."[32]

In 1906 Harvard University became interested in work as a form of treatment and gave Hall a grant of one thousand dollars "to assist in the study of the treatment of neurasthenia by progressive and graded manual occupation." Hall established a workshop in Marblehead, Massachusetts, where he used, as treatment, the crafts of handweaving, woodcarving, metalwork, and pottery "because of their universal appeal and the normalizing effect of suitable manual work." He said, "Suitable occupation of hand and mind is a very potent factor in the maintenance of the physical, mental and moral health in the individual and the community."[33]

Hall felt that nurses and social service workers should be trained in the use of work as treatment. Therefore he began a training program for young women at Devereaux Mansion in Marblehead, Massachusetts, around 1908. In 1915 Hall published *The Work of Our Hands—A Study of Occupations for Invalids*.[34] He divided invalid occupation into "diversional" occupation for those patients in advanced stages of incurable diseases and "remedial" occupation for those patients for whom there was therapeutic and economic value in remedial work.

Eleanor Clarke Slagle

In 1908 a training course in occupations for hospital attendants was given at the Chicago School of Civics and Philanthropy, which was directed by Graham Taylor. Jane Addams, the director of Hull House, along with Julia Lanthrop and Taylor, influenced the development of a number of courses to meet the needs of the community. Lanthrop developed the course for hospital attendants with the purpose of substituting "the educational for the custodial idea in the daily care of the mentally unsound." "Attendants learned games, arts, crafts, and hobbies which they could use to reach their patients." The philosophy of the program was that the work of the attendant was educational and the "methods were those used by the best teachers of little children—teaching the use of muscles and mind together in games, exercises and handicraft."[35] These concepts were reinforced by Adolf Meyer who worked with Addams and Lanthrop and supported their work for the improvement of the care of the mentally ill in state hospitals in Illinois.

Up until this point in the development of occupational therapy, the persons most qualified to be occupation workers had fallen into three categories of social workers, nurses, and kindergarten or crafts teachers. There were those who believed that nurses had the most desirable background because they had medical training and thus had higher qualifications for working with the sick and disabled. Lanthrop, however, believed that "occupational treatment was to have a large future in hospital treatment and that this service should be carried on by persons specifically educated for it."[36] This controversy continued for many years as courses designed for nurses or teachers were developed throughout the United States.

Eleanor Clarke Slagle, a social work student in the Chicago School of Civics and Philanthropy, became concerned about the detrimental effects of idleness on the patients at Kankakee State Hospital. Consequently she enrolled in Miss Lanthrop's first course in "curative occupations and recreations" for attendants and nurses in institutions for the insane given at the Chicago School of Civics and Philanthropy. Following her completion of the course in July 1911, she conducted a similar course at the State Hospital in Newberry, Michigan. She then went to Phipps Psychiatric Clinic in Johns Hopkins Hospital in Baltimore under Meyer where she was the director of the Occupational Therapy Department for two years and conducted classes for nurses in "handiwork for dispensary patients."[37] In 1915 Slagle organized the first professional school for occupational therapists, the Henry B. Favill School of Occupations, in Chicago. She served as the director of this school from 1918 to 1922. At this school, Slagle used her background in social work. Special instruction was given in invalid occupations along with experience in working with mentally ill patients in order to develop the "habit training" method of treatment, based on the use of occupation. She based this method on the concept that "for the most part, our lives are made up of habit reactions" and "occupation usually remedially serves to overcome some habits, to modify others and to construct new ones to the end that habit reactions will be favorable to the restoration and maintenance of health."[38] Remedial occupation implied training in conduct, in habit training, and in the art of doing things in a socially acceptable manner. This method stressed the interdependence of mental and physical components; the need to build on the habit of attention; the need to analyze occupations; and the need to grade activity from simple to complex, to go from the known to the unknown, and to provide tasks that are of increasing interest and require increasing degrees of concentration. Included in the program were craft activities and preindustrial and vocational work as well as games, folk dancing, gymnastics, and playground activities. This type of rehabilitation program attempted to create a balanced program of work, rest, and play for mentally ill patients.

Slagle, in the development of her habit training program, built on the philosophy of Meyer and provided a model of treatment that was utilized in occupational therapy for mentally ill patients until the early 1950s.

William Rush Dunton, Jr.—Father of the Profession

William Rush Dunton, Jr.'s endeavors on behalf of occupational therapy, as a practitioner, as a theoretician, as a philosopher, and as an officer of the national group, ensured him the title of "father of occupational therapy." He was involved in the use of occupational therapy as treatment of mental patients as early as 1895. When he was staff psychiatrist at Sheppard and Enoch Pratt Asylum in Baltimore in 1895, a metalworking shop was fitted for treatment of patients. Later other crafts were added and, in 1908, a teacher in arts and crafts was engaged to instruct patients.[39] As Dunton observed his patients as they were engaged in occupations, he noted how important it was to have someone trained to direct their activities, and he became aware of the care required to place a patient in the right activity. Thus, in 1911, after studying Tracy's book on invalid occupations, he undertook the responsibility of conducting a series of classes on occupations and recreation for nurses at Sheppard and Enoch Pratt Asylum. In 1912 he was placed in charge of the occupations and recreation program at the hospital, and his classes for nurses became an ongoing process.[40]

In 1915 the first complete textbook on occupational therapy, *Occupational Therapy—A Manual for Nurses*,[41] written by Dunton, was published. This book outlined the basic tenets or cardinal rules in applying occupation therapy. He said occupation's primary purpose was "to divert the patient's attention from unpleasant subjects, to keep the patient's train of thought in more healthy channels, to control attention, to secure rest, to train in mental processes by educating hands, eyes, muscles, etc., serve as a safety valve, to provide a new vocation."[42] The greatest part of this book dealt with simple activities that the nurse could use or adapt to treatment of patients.

George Edward Barton

Up until this time, the use of activity for therapy had been called by many titles such as moral treatment, work treatment, work therapy, occupation treatment, occupational reeducation, and ergotherapy. It was not until December 1914, at a meeting in Boston of hospital workers and the Massachusetts State Board of Insanity, that the term *occupational therapy* was introduced by a layman, George Edward Barton. Barton, an architect, became an advocate of this treatment after his own illness, during which he experienced the beneficial effects of directed occupation. He consequently organized an institution called Consolation House in Clifton Springs, New York, where, by means of occupations, people could be retrained or adjusted to gainful living. Barton described the purposes of occupational therapy as "to divert the patient's mind, to exercise some particular set of muscles or a limb, or perhaps merely to relieve the tedium of convalescence." He felt that "these activities may have little if any practical value beyond the immediate purpose they serve. . . . the idea is to give that sort [of activity] which will be preliminary to and dovetailed with the real vocational education which is to begin as soon as the patient is able to go farther along." He felt that the fundamental principle upon which occupational therapy rested was "not making of an object but the making of a man." He defined occupational therapy as the "science of instructing and encouraging the sick in such labors as will involve those energies and activities producing a beneficial therapeutic effect."[43]

Founding of the National Society for the Promotion of Occupational Therapy

Shortly before the United States entered World War I, a number of persons who were actively interested in providing occupation for patients decided that an association of workers to exchange views would be advantageous. Thus, in March 1917 at a meeting held at Consolation House, the National Society for the Promotion of Occupational Therapy was formed, incorporated, and chartered under the laws of the District of Columbia. The objectives of the association as noted in its constitution were "the advancement of occupation as a therapeutic measure, the study of the effects of occupation upon the human being, and the dissemination of scientific knowledge of this subject."[44] The title of the organization gives some indication of its character, for its membership included medical doctors, social workers, teachers, nurses, and artists whose main interests were in other areas. They did, however, recognize an inadequacy in the care of the sick and disabled that they felt might be filled by the technique called occupational therapy. The charter members of this society were George E. Barton, Eleanor Clarke Slagle, William Rush Dunton, Jr., Susan C. Johnson (occupational therapist at Montefiore Hospital in New York), Isabel G. Newton (Barton's secretary), and Thomas B. Kidner (vocational secretary of the Military Hospital Commission of Canada). Susan B. Tracy was unable to attend the meeting but was elected as an active member and incorporator of the society. A total of 14 active, 7 associate, and 26 sustaining members were elected to the society of which Barton became the first president.

The first annual meeting of the society was held in September 1917 in New York City.[45] The presentations at this conference were centered on the theme "The Reconstruction of the Mentally and Physically Disabled." Dunton spoke and proposed a system of vocational education whereby the convalescent, while still in the hospital, could be evaluated and taught useful occupations that would be meaningful and useful on discharge.[46] His plan included a plan for community action and canvassing of local businesses to determine if they would hire handicapped but trained persons.

Dunton was elected president of the society at this meeting, a post he held for two years. While he was president it became apparent that there was a need for local organizations for exchange of ideas and concepts. Dunton began organizing a cohesive group in the state of Maryland. Soon other states followed this lead, and a pattern of local organizations becoming affiliated with the national organization was established. This basic pattern remains today.[47]

This marked the beginning of the professional organization of occupational therapy in the United States. In 1923, the name was changed to its present title, the American Occupational Therapy Association.

In 1918, at the second annual meeting of the National Society for the Promotion of Occupational Therapy, Dunton delivered nine cardinal rules to guide practice. These were expanded to fifteen principles by a committee of therapists. Out of these fifteen principles came the first universal definition of occupational therapy: "A method of treatment by means of instruction and employment in productive occupation." The objectives were "To arouse interest, courage and confidence; to exercise the mind and body in healthy activities; to overcome functional disability; and to re-establish a capacity for industrial and social usefulness."[48]

In a second book, *Reconstruction Therapy*, published in 1919, Dunton further delineated the basic tenet upon which the profession of occupational therapy is based in the Credo for occupational therapists:

> That occupation is as necessary to life as food and drink.
> That every human being should have both physical and mental occupation.
> That all should have occupations which they enjoy, or hobbies. These are the more necessary when the vocation is dull or distasteful. Every individual should have at least two hobbies, one outdoor and one indoor. A greater number will create wider interests, a broader intelligence.
> That sick minds, sick bodies, sick souls may be healed through occupation.[49]

The Maryland Psychiatric Quarterly, edited by Dunton, from its inception in 1911, published articles relating to occupations and amusement. This journal became the official organ of the National Society for the Promotion of Occupational Therapy when it was founded in 1917. In 1922, the *Archives of Occupational Therapy* was first published and became the official organ of the American Occupational Therapy Association. In 1925, the title of this journal was changed to *Occupational Therapy and Rehabilitation*. This was the official organ of the Association until 1947 when the American Occupational Therapy Association assumed the total responsibility for publication of its own organ and entitled it *American Journal of Occupational Therapy*.

Expansion During World War I

Shortly after the entrance of the United States into World War I, the nation was faced with wounded men in need of rehabilitation. Slagle approached the armed forces and pleaded the cause of therapy as a means of treating the wounded. After initial opposition, Surgeon General Gorgas of the Army authorized the appointment of Reconstruction Aides to serve in Army hospitals.[50] The National Committee for Mental Hygiene initially recruited four aides to serve in European-based hospitals of the American Expeditionary Forces. The success of this small group was such that in September 1917 General John J. Pershing cabled to Washington from Paris requesting 200 young women to serve in Army hospitals overseas.[51] Thus, directives from the Medical Department of the Army, dated January 1918 (Class 1) and March 1918 (Class 2), established training programs for two groups of reconstruction aides (Class 1, physiotherapy, and Class 2, occupational therapy).

The physiotherapy aides were to be trained "to give massage and exercise and other remedial treatment to the returned soldiers," while the occupational therapy aides were to be trained "to furnish forms of occupation to convalescents in long illnesses and to give to patients the therapeutic benefit of activity." Rigid criteria were established for applicants including at least a high school education with experience in some profession such as social work or library science. Applicants had to be at least 25 years old, be citizens of the United States or one of its allies, and have theoretical knowledge and practical experience in various crafts. Initial intensive courses were given at the Henry B. Favill School in Chicago under Slagle and at the Teachers College of Columbia University in New York and the Boston School of Occupational Therapy (the Franklin Union) in Boston. The courses ranged from 6 to 12 weeks in length and included lectures on psychology of the handicapped, fatigue and the work cure, personal hygiene, anatomy, kinesiology, ethics, and hospital administration. Classes in the use and application of crafts included woodwork, weaving, cordwork, beadwork, basketry, and ceramics. Field work and practice in local hospitals were also a vital part of the training program.[52,53]

As requests for reconstruction aides increased, other emergency war courses were established throughout the country. Between April 1918 and July 1921, 25 schools had graduated 1685 reconstruction aides, of whom 460 served overseas.[54] Reconstruction aides were civilian employees who worked with patients in orthopedic and surgical wards as well as working with those suffering from nervous or mental disorders.

Occupational therapy for the treatment of physical dysfunction gained impetus during this period, and the scientific approach to the treatment of physical disabilities was begun.

Bird T. Baldwin

In the *Army Manual on Occupational Therapy*, Bird T. Baldwin, a psychologist and director of Walter Reed General Hospital's Occupational Therapy Department, gives this explanation of occupational therapy:

> Occupational therapy is based on the principle that the best type of remedial exercise is that which requires a series of specific voluntary movements involved in the ordinary trades and occupations, physical training, play or the daily routine activities of life. Our curative

shops are now being organized and graduated on the principle which will enable us ultimately to isolate, classify, repeat and, to a limited degree, standardize and control the type of movements involved in the particular occupational and recreational operations. The patient's attention is repeatedly called to the particular remedial movements involved; at the same time the movements have the advantage of being initiated by the patient and of forming an integral and necessary part of the larger and more complex series of coordinated movements. The purposive nature of the movements and the end product of the work offer a direct incentive for sustained effort; the periodic measurement of the increase in range and strength of movement makes it possible for the patient to watch his recovery from day to day. . . . The records also enable the examiner to determine which mode of treatment leads to the greatest and most consistent gains in a particular case. . . .[55]

It was during this period that devices were developed to measure range of motion and strength; thus more scientific recording was made possible. The kinesiological analysis of activities begun during the war allowed activities to be chosen based on specific physical limitation. Adapted pieces of equipment were devised. They provided specific motions for increasing range of motion and strength, and their use was then applied for the remediation of selected disabilities.

By the end of World War I thousands of soldiers in the United States had received some form of occupational therapy, and the profession was beginning to gain public support.

Baldwin made a valuable contribution through the development of evaluation and treatment procedures for restoration of physical function and dissemination of these by publication in the *Army Manual*.

Post–World War I to World War II

Many of the schools for training reconstruction aides closed permanently following World War I. The demand for trained occupational therapists in civilian hospitals caused the reopening of the Boston School of Occupational Therapy in the fall of 1919, followed shortly by the opening of the Philadelphia School of Occupational Therapy and the St. Louis School of Occupational Therapy. Two of these schools continue to function today. The Boston School is now located in Tufts University, and the St. Louis School is located in Washington University. The Philadelphia School (at the University of Pennsylvania) was phased out in 1981.

The American Occupational Therapy Association established "Minimum Standards for Courses of Training in Occupational Therapy" in 1923.[56] At this time several war emergency schools were disbanded because of their inability to meet requirements. The minimum standards included a prerequisite of a high school education and a 12-month course of not less than 8 months of theoretical work and 3 months in practice. The establishment of standards did much to raise the status of the profession. However, the schools of occupational therapy trained therapists as teachers of crafts, or occupations, which would help individuals move from acute illness to vocational training. Many therapists gained knowledge of anatomy, kinesiology, and medical conditions through postgraduate courses and developed principles of specific treatment to restore physical function on an empirical basis.[57]

The caliber of publications in the official journal of the Association, however, did not reflect a scientific basis for the profession. Articles generally were undocumented, unscientific, and inconclusive and fell into three categories: (1) description of occupational therapy as it was practiced at various hospitals, (2) helpful hints on crafts, and (3) the relationship of occupational therapy to other medical services.[57] Ethel Bowman, Associate Professor of Psychology at Goucher College, described the problem of the profession in 1922 as follows:

> Literally there is no psychology of occupational therapy today. Although there is abundant material for such, it is, at present, unorganized. In speaking of the psychology of a subject, we may mean that the known facts of scientific psychology have been given practical application, or that the peculiarly psychological aspects of the subject have been singled out and subjected to specific study by the methods which psychology has found applicable in its problems of pure science. In neither of these meanings have we a psychology of occupational therapy.[58]

In spite of the lack of scientific approach, occupational therapy was being utilized in both civilian and military hospitals throughout the United States. After their experiences during the war, physicians recognized the value of occupational therapy and established units in many general and children's hospitals. Treatment was based on the principles advocated by Dunton in 1915. These principles advocated that treatment be prescribed and administered under constant medical supervision and correlated with other treatment of the patient; treatment should be directed to individual needs; treatment should arouse interest, courage, and confidence; treatment should exercise mind and body in healthy activity; treatment should overcome disability and reestablish capacity for industrial and social usefulness; occupation should be regulated and graded as a patient's strength and capabilities increased; employment in groups is advisable to provide opportunity for social adaptation; and the only reliable measure of the treatment is the effect on the patient.[59]

In 1923 the Federal Industrial Rehabilitation Act made it a requirement that every general hospital dealing with industrial accidents or illness provide occupational therapy as an integral part of its treatment. There was a demand for graduates of accredited schools, in spite of budget cuts in hospitals during the Depression, demonstrating an increasing recognition of the necessity for constructive occupation in the maintenance of mental and physical health.[60,61]

By 1928 there were six schools of occupational therapy. In addition to the Boston, Philadelphia, and St. Louis Schools of Occupational Therapy, Milwaukee Downer College, the University of Minnesota, and the University of Toronto in Canada had accredited programs. Each of these met the minimum standard of nine months' didactic and three months' clinical preparation. Each gave a diploma in occupational therapy, with the University of Minnesota giving a bachelor's degree as well. The Minnesota program was discontinued in 1931 because of low enrollment and the resignation of the director.[62]

In 1927 Everett Elwood recommended that the American Occupational Therapy Association safeguard the profession and maintain high standards by requiring all practitioners to be licensed and by utilizing a national examination to qualify graduates of the accredited schools.[63]

In 1931 a National Registry of all qualified occupational therapists was established "for the protection of hospitals and institutions from unqualified persons posing as occupational therapists." When the Association issued its first registry in 1932, 318 therapists were listed, all qualified by a rigid set of standards.[64] Registration required that therapists have one year of active practice under an experienced therapist and be recommended by that therapist.

In March 1931 the American Occupational Therapy Association requested that the American Medical Association undertake inspection and approval of the occupational therapy schools. Because the American Medical Association had experience in medical education and had investigated medical schools and teaching hospitals, the Council on Medical Education and Hospitals agreed to undertake the survey. The inspection began in November 1933. Following the inspection, meetings were held with representatives from the American Occupational Therapy Association, the Council on Physical Medicine, and the Council on Medical Education and Hospitals. The result of these meetings was the drafting of the "Essentials of an Acceptable School of Occupational Therapy." The "Essentials" were adopted by the Council on Medical Education and Hospitals in February 1935 and were ratified the following June by the House of Delegates of the American Medical Association at its Annual Meeting.[65]

The thirteen schools of occupational therapy in operation were evaluated in 1938, and only five schools met the essentials and were approved. They were the Boston, Philadelphia, and St. Louis Schools of Occupational Therapy and Milwaukee Downer College and the University of Toronto in Canada. Kalamazoo State Hospital School of Occupational Therapy received tentative approval. The "Essentials" increased the length of the program to 25 calendar months plus an additional 9 months of hospital practice training. The requirements expanded the theoretical basis of the profession by adding emphasis in biological and social sciences and clinical medicine. Clinical practice was expanded to include experience in mental, tuberculosis, children's, and orthopedic hospitals. Although degree courses were available at Milwaukee Downer and Kalamazoo, few students took advantage of this offering because a degree did not seem necessary. Therefore, most students received highly specialized training with no liberal arts input and received a diploma in occupational therapy in three years. Beginning in 1932, certificate programs for persons with bachelor's degrees were given at Boston, Philadelphia, and St. Louis. These courses required 1-year didactic preparation plus 9 months of hospital practice. Graduates of the certificate program were permitted to become registered occupational therapists. There was no thought of graduate degrees in the field at this time and there seemed to be no desire on the part of practitioners to write or publish literature for the field.[66] These schools graduated a total of 100 qualified therapists per year.

By 1938, 13% of the hospitals approved by the American Medical Association had qualified occupational therapists on their staffs. The majority of therapists were employed in mental hospitals.[67] The impetus given to the treatment of physical dysfunction through occupational therapy by World War I had diminished. The profession had been from its inception primarily one for women, and only one school, the St. Louis School of Occupational Therapy, accepted male students. Thus, only about 2½% of qualified therapists were men, and they were employed primarily in mental institutions, tuberculosis sanitoria, and penal institutions.[68,69] A few occupational therapists were in private practice in 1939 and five cities—Philadelphia, Hartford, Detroit, Milwaukee, and St. Louis—had visiting therapists, similar to visiting nurses, working with the homebound.[70]

In 1939 the first formal subjective registration examination developed by a committee of therapists was given. Those who failed were permitted to register on the basis of experience. About 1944, examinations were developed by each school and submitted for approval to the Registration Committee of the American Occupational Therapy Association.

During World War II and Immediately Following

World War I had given impetus to the new field of occupational therapy, but its development after the war was slow. After World War I, occupational therapy programs and personnel in all Army hospitals had been reduced to a minimum. There were five permanent Army general hospitals, only three of which had an occupational therapist employed.[71] At the beginning of World War II the total number of practicing occupational therapists in the United States was less than was needed by the military hospitals alone.[72]

Because of the need for therapists in both military and civilian hospitals, a number of new schools were organized. The number of approved schools increased from 5 in 1940 to 18 in 1945. At the request of the Surgeon General's Office, war emergency courses were started in a number of schools and prepared over 500 qualified therapists for duty in the Army hospitals. These schools met American Medical Association minimum standards since they were intensive 1-year courses for college graduates who had basic psychology and at least 20 semester hours of fine, applied, or industrial arts, or home economics. The course consisted of 4 months of theory in the civilian occupational therapy schools and 8 months of practical application and training under registered occupational therapists in Army hospitals.[73] Registration was acquired through passing of the Registration Examination approved by the American Occupational Therapy Association.

The critical personnel needs of the armed forces and war industries demanded maximum conservation of manpower. Thus a reconditioning program in the Armed Forces was established to

> accelerate the return to duty of convalescent patients in the highest state of physical and mental efficiency consistent with the capabilities and the type of duty to which they are being returned . . . or to provide for their return to civilian life in the highest possible degree of physical fitness, well oriented in the responsibilities of citizenship and prepared to adjust successfully to social and vocational pursuits.[74]

The reconditioning program included a coordinated program of educational reconditioning, physical reconditioning, and occupational therapy. Occupa-

tional therapists were civilians appointed to Army hospitals by the Surgeon General's Office. They supervised both the treatment programs and the volunteer Red Cross Arts and Skills, Recreational, and Diversional Programs.

By the end of World War II over a thousand occupational therapists were providing services in the military hospitals in the United States and abroad. Occupational therapists had to be prepared to work with persons having psychological and psychiatric problems as well as those having orthopedic and neurological problems. Techniques were developed for rapid total rehabilitation of patients in order to return them physically and mentally fit for service or work. The war had expanded the techniques and knowledge in occupational therapy, especially in the area of the treatment of the physically disabled.

In February 1947 the first National Objective Registration Examination was given. Very few men worked in the profession of occupational therapy so it was looked upon as a woman's field. From 1941 to 1946 the number of registered occupational therapists almost doubled, going from 1144 to 2265,[75] but the number of men in the profession remained at about 2½% of the total, or about 50 men.

Clare S. Spackman—Restoration of Physical Function

Because of increase in medical knowledge, discovery of new drugs, and improved medical care after World War II, the population of patients to be treated changed and increased. This placed new demands on therapists and required that new treatment procedures be developed. Other specialties were developed to satisfy unmet needs (*i.e.*, recreational therapy, educational therapy, and corrective therapy). Occupational therapists became specialized in treatment of certain types of disabilities such as peripheral nerve injuries and amputations. This added to the base of knowledge and improved treatment techniques for these areas of practice.[76]

Occupational therapists had to be skilled in using constructive activities for treatment and also were required to utilize as treatment activities of daily living (ADL), work simplification, rehabilitation techniques for the handicapped homemaker, and training in the use of upper extremity prostheses. This expansion in techniques and knowledge in the area of physical dysfunction required extensive reorganization in the curricula of the accredited schools of occupational therapy. In order to assist schools in providing this new information to students, the first textbook in the United States on occupational therapy written primarily by occupational therapists, edited by Helen S. Willard and Clare S. Spackman, was published in 1947.[77] Spackman provided detailed information in this volume on the evaluation and treatment of patients with physical dysfunction.

Spackman felt that the exact function of occupational therapy in the treatment of physical dysfunction should be specifically defined. In an article in which she traced the history of occupational therapy practice for restoration of physical function she says

> Occupational therapy treats the patient by the use of constructive activity in a simulated, normal living and/or working situation. This is and always has been our function. Constructive activity is the Keynote of occupational therapy. . . . True occupational therapy cannot be used until the patient is capable not only of performing a given motion but of utilizing it to carry out a constructive activity. Occupational therapy's value lies in teaching the patient by use of constructive activities to transfer the motions and strength gained by corrective exercise in physical therapy into coordinated activity which will enable the patient to become personally independent and economically self-suficient.[78]

Spackman made an impact on the treatment of patients physically disabled by disease or injury through publication of the book on occupational therapy and by the education of students utilizing the principles of evaluation and treatment.

Spackman represented the United States when the World Federation of Occupational Therapists was founded in 1954. She was elected to the position of Assistant Secretary-Treasurer at its first meeting, served as President of the organization from 1957 to 1962, and was Secretary-Treasurer from 1964 to 1972. Her interest and involvement with the World Federation did much to develop good relationships with member countries and encouraged expansion of the profession into many underdeveloped countries.

Formation of the World Federation of Occupational Therapists

The aftermath of World War II led to the rapid growth of allied medical services in many countries throughout the world. There was a need for exchange of information in regard to new methods of treatment and many foreign therapists were seeking admission to take the registration examination of the American Occupational Therapy Association. The International Society for the Rehabilitation of the Disabled, concerned with the establishment of rehabilitation programs throughout the world, encouraged the formation of an International Association of Occupational Therapists, which would establish international standards for education and practice. In April 1952 representatives of six countries met in Liverpool, England, and drafted a constitution including qualifications of member associations and proposed "Mini-

mum Educational Standards for Occupational Therapists" (revised in 1963). The American Occupational Therapy Association became one of the ten founding members of the World Federation of Occupational Therapists. The six countries represented at the founders' meeting were Canada, Denmark, Great Britain (England and Scotland), South Africa, Sweden, and the United States. Australia, New Zealand, Israel, and India were represented by written opinion and thus were included as founding members.

The first congress met in Edinburgh, Scotland, in 1954. Four hundred representatives from ten countries attended. The organization continued to grow and by its second congress in 1958 there were 750 representatives from 38 countries.[79] In 1959 the World Federation of Occupational Therapists joined the World Health Organization and established a roster of expert advisors to work with countries trying to establish or develop their own occupational therapy programs. This roster has been maintained and continues to be used when therapists are needed to assist developing programs.

In 1960 the World Federation of Occupational Therapists formulated a code of "Ethics for Occupational Therapists" and "Functions of Occupational Therapy" (revised in 1962). The American Occupational Therapy Association also worked with the World Rehabilitation Fund, the Peace Corps, and the International Cooperation Administration. By the early 1960s there was an active exchange of therapists among countries. Many American therapists worked abroad, and therapists from member countries worked in the United States. Members from countries meeting World Federation of Occupational Therapists standards were permitted to take the registration examination of the American Occupational Therapy Association.[80]

Move Toward an "Exact" Science

The 1950s saw an increase in the development of rehabilitation techniques in physical dysfunction. The use of more exact methods of measuring physical function initiated a movement to make occupational therapy a more exact science. Advances were made in medical science for the control of diseases including poliomyelitis and tuberculosis. This caused a shift in emphasis in occupational therapy of physical dysfunction to the chronic conditions of arthritis, heart disease, stroke, traumatic injuries, and congenital defects. Federal legislation and the interest of insurance carriers and federal and state rehabilitation agencies gave added stimulus to the growth of occupational therapy in the treatment of physical dysfunction.

New techniques were developed by therapists and biomedical engineers, and these new techniques influenced the procedures used in occupational therapy. The emphasis of treatment was to reduce defects related to the patient's pathological condition and to allow the individual to function at the highest level of which he or she was capable.[81] The occupational therapist functioned as a member of a team dedicated to the rehabilitation of the disabled.

During this period the treatment of the psychiatric patient was also being examined by occupational therapists, with an increasing emphasis being made on the social adaptation of the patient or client and the individual's return to functioning in family and community. The concept of the "therapeutic use of self" became the primary focus of treatment and utilized psychotherapeutic techniques. This concept used social interactions as the tool for helping patients or clients to deal with their emotional responses and with both the human and nonhuman environment.[82]

Gail S. Fidler—Psychiatric Occupational Therapy

The first comprehensive book on psychiatric occupational therapy was published in 1954. This book, *Introduction to Psychiatric Occupational Therapy*, by Gail S. Fidler and Jay W. Fidler, M.D., gave impetus to the psychodynamic approach to occupational therapy.[83] The Fidlers presented occupational therapy as a collaborative effort between the occupational therapist and the psychiatrist. Occupational therapy was the laboratory in which the patient or client could experiment in handling emotions and developing living skills through the use of productive activity. Guidelines for detailed activity analysis were developed. The book presented a process in which groups could be used to facilitate treatment; it also encouraged the study of projective techniques. In 1963, a second textbook on psychiatric occupational therapy was published by the Fidlers, *Occupational Therapy—A Communication Process in Psychiatry*. This book presented occupational therapy as an important communication tool because activities could provide a means for understanding individuals through nonverbal communications during the activity process.[84]

From 1963 to 1964 Gail Fidler presented graduate courses in Occupational Therapy Supervision in Psychiatry at Columbia University. In 1967 she developed the master's program in Psychiatric Occupational Therapy at New York University, where she encouraged use of the scientific method in occupational therapy. Some of the leaders in the practice of psychiatric occupational therapy today are graduates of these programs.

Fidler has continued to be involved in clinical, academic, and administrative affairs of the profession because she sees importance in maintaining competence as an occupational therapist in all of these areas.

New Levels in Occupational Therapy Education

In spite of the fact that there was an increase in the number of occupational therapy schools, there continued to be a lack of qualified occupational therapists to fill the vacancies in both psychiatry and physical disability therapy. By 1960 there were 24 accredited schools of occupational therapy, all located in university settings giving bachelor's degrees in conformance with the "Essentials" as revised in 1949.

With the dearth of qualified personnel, employers began to utilize persons trained in other fields to fill vacancies, thereby giving impetus to the expansion of related therapeutic groups such as recreational therapy, art therapy, music therapy, vocational rehabilitation counselors, manual arts therapists, and educational therapists. Development in these fields and the overlapping of roles caused some occupational therapists to question whether the profession was operating without a theoretical base.[85,86]

In 1947 the first program leading to a master's degree in occupational therapy was established at the University of Southern California. This course was for those persons who were registered occupational therapists who had bachelor's degrees. Later in the same year New York University began a similar graduate program. These programs were developed for therapists desiring advanced work in clinical specialty areas such as clinical psychopathology, physical disabilities, vocational rehabilitation, and special education.[87] It was hoped that graduate study on the part of occupational therapists would promote research, which was recognized as essential for increasing the knowledge and theoretical base of the profession.

At this same time the profession began to examine the possibility of training a technical-level person to work as an assistant to the occupational therapist, thereby providing for the lack of manpower in the field.[88] Criteria for the educational programs were determined and standards for training assistants for general practice were implemented in October 1960.[89]

Changes in Focus—1960s and 1970s

During the 1960s psychiatric occupational therapists began to examine their role and function. Grant-funded consultants were hired by the American

Occupational Therapy Association to help these therapists look at the impact of their treatment. Workshops were conducted throughout the country in group techniques and object relations. These workshops led psychiatric occupational therapists to examine neurobehavioral orientation to treatment, thus adding the dimension of perception to psychiatric treatment, which had previously had only a social and emotional base.[90]

During this same period the basic master's program was introduced as a means of educating persons with bachelor's degrees in other fields to the basics of occupational therapy with advanced level work in research methodology for the profession. The first program was a 2-year course conducted at the University of Southern California in 1964. Shortly thereafter basic master's programs were begun at other universities: Boston University and Virginia Commonwealth University. These courses encouraged students to conduct research in the profession and to publish the results. This caused a gradual change in the articles published in the *American Journal of Occupational Therapy* and encouraged therapists to become involved in clinical research.

A. Jean Ayres—Neurobehavioral Orientation

A. Jean Ayres became interested in neurophysiological and developmental approaches to occupational therapy through her contacts with Margaret S. Rood, an occupational therapist and physical therapist who had investigated literature in these areas and developed the following basic principles:

1. Motor output is dependent upon sensory input. Thus sensory stimuli are utilized to activate and/or inhibit motor response.
2. Activation of motor response follows a normal developmental sequence. . . .
3. Since there is interaction within the nervous system between somatic, psychic and autonomic functions stimuli can be used to influence one or more directly or indirectly.[91]

In the early 1960s A. Jean Ayres began conducting research that laid the foundation for a neurobehavioral orientation to occupational therapy. The basis of her work "is the recapitulation of the sequence of development."[92] This orientation was consequently termed "sensory integrative therapy" and accepted developmental stage concepts. Ayres proposed that the "principles that determined the direction of evolutionary development are manifested in the principles that govern the development of the capacity to perceive and learn by each child today." Therapy is based on the premise that the brain is a "self-organizing system" that integrates or coordinates "two or more functions or processes in a manner which enhances the adaptiveness of the brain's responses" and the fact that "one of the most powerful organizers of sensory input is movement which is adaptive to the organism." Treatment is based upon purposeful movement that causes the individual to respond adaptively and requires a response that represents a "more mature or integrated action than previous performance."[93]

Mary Reilly—Occupational Behavior Orientation

In the 1960s Mary Reilly suggested that the concern of occupational therapy should be patient achievement, since we are dealing with behavior that is subject to maturation and regression of illness. She suggests that we use the work–play continuum because "the play of childhood . . . contains a critical ability to transmit the adaptive skills necessary for complex work technology and urban living of today."[94] Thus, it would seem that Reilly is reemphasizing the need for habit training along with reduction of incapacity.

Reilly's orientation indicates recommitment to Meyer's and Slagle's philosophy of occupational therapy. Reilly stresses the importance of "examining the various life roles of the population relative to community adaptation, to identify the various skills that support these roles, and to create an environment where the relevant behavior could be evoked and practiced."[95] The occupational therapist's role is to facilitate achievement of competence. Emphasis is placed on the patient's or client's ability to cope with the community and with changes in life situations. Interpersonal relationships are essential factors in this process.

Wilma West—Prevention and Community Occupational Therapy

In 1966 Wilma West stated that the shift from medical to health concerns had implications for occupational therapy. She said that the profession must be involved in the new emphasis of "maintaining optimum health rather than an intermittent treatment of acute disease and disability" and that "health and medical care in the future . . . will emphasize human development by programs designed to promote better adaptation, rather than technologically oriented programs offering specific solutions to specific difficulties.[96] She described four emerging roles for the occupational therapist that would create new dimensions of function. These were evaluator, consultant, supervisor, and researcher. She suggested that the occupational therapist, to fulfill these roles in the prevention of disease, must move into and work in community settings.

Anne Cronin Mosey—Frames of Reference for Psychiatric Occupational Therapy

In 1970 Anne Mosey said that occupational therapy in psychiatry appeared to be functioning on the basis of intuition and without a theoretical base. She felt there should be a "conscious use of theoretical frames of reference as the basis for the treatment of psychosocial dysfunction." She categorized the three frames of reference available as analytical, acquisitional, and developmental. She said the *analytical* base "describes man as striving for need fulfillment, expression of primitive impulses or control of inherent drives." She described dysfunction as "symptom-producing unconscious content." Therapy attempts to bring the symptom-producing unconscious content to consciousness and integrate it with conscious content.

The *acquisitional* base "focuses upon the various skills or abilities which the individual needs for adequate and satisfactory interaction in the environment." Human abilities are viewed as qualitative and nonstage specific. Dysfunction is described in terms of what behavior must be eliminated and what must be added in order for an individual to function in a normal environment.

The *developmental* base is similar to the acquisitional in that it specifies the various skills and abilities which the individual needs for satisfactory interaction in the community. However, the abilities are considered to be interdependent, qualitative, and stage specific. The developmental base "assumes that the individual must go through incompleted stages in order to function in a mature manner." The individual's current adaptive skill, learning, and the expected environment must all be evaluated.[97] Mosey's developmental base is drawn from the theoretical formulations developed by Ayres.

In 1974 Mosey proposed an orientation to occupational therapy as an alternative to the medical and health model. She called it the "biopsychosocial model." She said this model "directs attention to the body, mind and environment of the client. It takes these facets into consideration without any sense of wellness or sickness on the part of the client." This model focuses on the individual as a "biological entity; a thinking and feeling person and a member of a community of others."[98] Although this model is described as an alternative, it seems to have been drawn from all previous orientations to occupational therapy.

Changes Within the Association—1960s and 1970s

During the 1960s the American Occupational Therapy Association was called upon by its members to perform new functions such as providing administrative guidelines, suggesting treatment and consultative rates, and sponsoring a lobbyist for health legislation. These activities endangered the status of the professional organization as one established for "charitable, scientific, literary and educational nature." Therefore in 1965 the American Occupational Therapy Foundation was established under the laws of the state of Delaware as a philanthropic organization "to administer programs of a charitable, scientific, literary and educational nature." Its work aimed at "advancing the science of occupational therapy, supporting the education and research of its practitioners and increasing the public knowledge and understanding of the profession." This move then allowed the American Occupational Therapy Association to serve as a "business league" and to perform the requested noneducational activities.[99]

The emphasis on accountability to consumers caused the Association to develop new standards for education and practice. In 1970 "Standards and Guidelines for an Occupational Therapy Affiliation Program" were drawn up.[100] In 1972 a new definition and statement of function was developed for the profession.[101] In 1973 "Standards for Occupational Therapists Providing Direct Service" were developed and published in the official journal of the Association.[102] That same year the revised "Essentials of the Accredited Educational Programs for the Occupational Therapist" were adopted by the American Occupational Therapy Association and the House of Delegates of the American Medical Association.[103] These "Essentials" were approved by the Representative Assembly of the American Occupational Therapy Association in 1977.

The "Essentials of an Approved Educational Program for the Occupational Therapy Assistant" were developed and adopted by the Council of Education of the American Occupational Therapy Association in 1975.[104] These were adopted by the Representative Assembly in 1977.

Since 1972 the Association has adopted numerous position papers, including ones on consumer involvement,[105] aging,[106] national system of certification for allied health personnel,[107] and national health issues.[108]

In October 1975 the Delegate Assembly adopted a resolution authorizing the development of a certification examination for occupational therapy assistants.[109] In April 1976 the Assembly passed a resolution authorizing the use of the certification examination as a partial fulfillment for certification of occupational therapy assistants.[110] The first certification examination was given in June 1977.

In September 1976 new bylaws were adopted by the Association; they became effective in November 1976.[111] These bylaws made many changes in the structure and organization of the total Association. They identify the Representative Assembly as the policy-making body, which elects its own officers. Representatives from each state, the Association officers, the first alternate delegate of the World Federation of Occupational Therapists, and the president of the Student Association are voting members of the Assembly. The Executive Board became the management body, with Association officers, Representative Assembly officers, the World Federation Delegate, and the president of the Association of Affiliate Presidents as members. The purpose of changes in the bylaws was to make the Association more responsive to the membership's needs and concerns.

In April 1977, the Representative Assembly adopted a "Definition of Occupational Therapy" for the purpose of licensure. The Assembly adopted a revised version of the definition in March 1981. This is to be used as a legal document and not as a philosophical definition for the profession (see Appendix A). At the same meeting, the Representative Assembly adopted the "Principles of Occupational Therapy Ethics." The Ethics Statements are to be used as guidelines for the profession and its practitioners but are not to be used as standards of expected care. Guidelines for Ethics Statements were developed and adopted by the Representative Assembly in April 1980[112] (see Appendix B).

Into the 1980s

With the adoption of the bylaws in 1976, the Association was committed to an advocacy position that included increased participation and involvement of members in Association activities. In order to obtain input from members, the *Occupational Therapy Newspaper* printed resolutions and other policy items along with a reply sheet for members to send opinions and comments to their representatives on the issues and resolutions that would establish policy for the Association. In 1978, Mae Hightower Vandamm, president of the Association, introduced a plan whereby local task groups, chaired by members of the Executive Board, examined management issues and made recommendations for Executive Board decisions.[113] All meetings sponsored by the American Occupational Therapy Association were opened for membership audit except when material of confidential nature was under discussion.[114] The Association

was thereby providing for as much membership participation and involvement as possible.

Because of changes occurring both within the Association and in society, the Representative Assembly, at their meeting in San Diego, California, in May 1978, authorized a Special Session of the Representative Assembly to examine the status of the Association and the field as a whole. Concerns were identified relating to four areas within occupational therapy: *the philosophical base, practice, education,* and *credentialing.* Leaders from the field were invited to present papers and participate in this meeting.[115] This special session will probably "be recorded in the annals of the history of occupational therapy as one of the events that changed the future of our profession."[116] As a result of this meeting, the Association, for the first time, adopted a statement identifying the philosophical base of occupational therapy[117] and affirmed "occupation" as the common core of occupational therapy,[118] thereby providing the field with parameters within which to develop and grow.

There was increased support of research by the membership because of the need to validate our skills and substantiate the role of occupational therapy in health care. This support was evidenced by establishment of a Committee on Research within the Association, approval of a position of Research Coordinator in the National Office under the American Occupational Therapy Foundation (AOTF), and financial support for research activities within the field.[119] In April 1981 the AOTF published The Occupational Therapy *Journal of Research* for the first time.

In the examination of practice it was evident that there was much diversity within the field; the roles and functions of occupational therapists and occupational therapy assistants were unclear, and new areas of practice were being developed while some of our traditional areas of practice were being eroded. Because of the need for a unified identity and more uniform practice in the field, standards of practice were adopted by the Representative Assembly for Physical Disabilities, Mental Health, Developmental Disabilities and Home Health Care in 1978, and for practice in schools in 1980[120,121] (see Appendix C).

There was also a concern that all practitioners were not operating from the same baseline and that they were not using similar terminology and systems of evaluating and reporting progress. To assure more uniformity in communication, the document "Uniform Terminology System for Reporting OT Services" was developed and adopted by the Representative Assembly in 1979[122] (see Appendix D). This document identifies and describes the services that fall within the domain of occupational therapy, thereby placing some constraints on the field. There was also a need to place some type of value on our services in order to provide guidelines for determining fees for service; therefore another document entitled "Occupational Therapy Product Output Reporting System" was developed and adopted by the Representative Assembly in 1980[123] (see Appendix E). This document provides guidelines for placing relative values on specific services provided by occupational therapists. In order to further clarify the role of occupational therapists in the health-care system, a generic guide for gathering baseline data was developed entitled "Uniform Occupational Therapy Evaluation Checklist,"[124] and this was adopted by the Representative Assembly in March 1981 (see Appendix F). This document was based on the Uniform Terminology document and indicates that all evaluation procedures used should reflect the philosophical base of occupational therapy. These three documents provide practicing therapists with guidance for their practice and give educational programs guidance for education of students.

The roles and functions of the occupational therapist and occupational therapy assistant had been examined for a number of years; however, there had been no consensus regarding differentiation in these roles and functions. An Entry Level/Role Delineation Committee was established by the Representative Assembly. The committee was charged with examining all previously developed documents concerned with roles and functions within occupational therapy and with developing a document that considered the concerns presented in all of the previous documents. A document entitled "Entry Level Role Delineation for OTRs and COTAs" was developed and adopted by the Representative Assembly in March 1981.[125] This was intended to assist members in their practice, to assist in the development of entry-level educational essentials and programs, and to assist in the development of certification criteria.

Occupational therapists seemed to be working in new areas of practice while abandoning some other areas of practice where occupational therapy skills were traditionally used and valued. In order to verify our commitment to some of these areas of practice, position papers were adopted by the Representative Assembly which identified the various contributions of occupational therapy. Position papers were adopted on the role of occupational therapy, in promotion of health and prevention of disability,[126] in the vocational rehabilitation process,[127] in independent living or alternate living situations,[128] as a related education service,[129] and in home health care.[130] Additional areas of practice were being identified in such contexts as correctional institutions. In order to encourage and support the development of new areas of practice, the Commission on Practice was charged with identifying areas of occupational therapy prac-

tice that are in need of standards and guidelines, developing needed standards, and continuing to monitor ongoing and new parameters of practice.[131]

The concern for maintaining competency of practitioners was addressed by the Association in several ways. Support was given to continuing education institutes which were to be conducted throughout the country to meet the educational needs of practicing therapists.[132] A guide to graduate education in occupational therapy leading to a master's degree was endorsed.[133] Also, the process of recertification as a means of assuring competency for OTRs and COTAs was adopted.[134] Pilot studies were conducted to determine the most flexible, the most relevant to all areas of practice, and the most cost-effective ways for carrying out the process of recertification. Following the studies, two options were developed and submitted to the Representative Assembly. They were then submitted for membership vote. Action will be taken on a recertification process at the 1982 meeting of the Representative Assembly.

The response of therapists to the need for further education in order to retain competency and advancement in the field is manifested by the fact that there are now 21 master's level graduate programs for occupational therapists and two doctoral programs in occupational therapy.

Occupational therapists working in school systems were given the opportunity to develop their competence through a research and pilot training project called TOTEMS (Training: Occupational Therapy Educational Management in Schools).[135] Through this project, many therapists working in school systems throughout the country were given a special course for improving the quality of treatment in the school setting.

Support was given to students for development of a student organization in 1977.[136] Since that time, a student organization called the American Student Occupational Therapy Alliance has been founded.

In addition to changes occurring within occupational therapy, changes taking place in society and in the government are affecting occupational therapy practice. The Government and Legal Affairs Division (GLAD) of the National Office has been very active in keeping members informed and in soliciting help for passage of legislation through the publication of the *Federal Report* and the *GLAD Bulletin*. Through the efforts of this division and with membership support, the Medicare Bill was amended to increase occupational therapy coverage by allowing home health therapists to continue to provide service even though they were the only health-care practitioners involved on the case. Occupational therapists cannot, however, initiate or open a case. The amendment allowing free-standing rehabilitation centers to be reimbursed for occupational therapy services was passed also, but to date the regulations have not been issued, thus making this program nonfunctional.

Accountability to health-care consumers has been of concern to all practitioners for many years. However, occupational therapists have not been involved in quality assurance projects until recently. The National Office Division of Quality Assurance has conducted pilot projects in this area that have demonstrated the need for and value of the involvement of occupational therapy departments in an ongoing quality assurance process (see Chap. 43).

Two other projects undertaken by the Association indicate we are coming of age. A Written History Committee was appointed in 1978 to produce a written history for the Association. Help was solicited from the membership for this project. An Archives Committee was also established in 1978 to develop criteria and to process material for the archives and to find suitable storage for the historical documents of the Association.[137]

In July of 1980, the American Occupational Therapy Association moved into its first permanent home. Previously, the Association rented space for their national headquarters. In February 1980, an office building was purchased in Rockville, Maryland as headquarters for the National Office. This was made possible through establishment of a Housing Reserve Account in 1974, which provided sufficient funds to allow the Association to purchase the building.

New bylaws were adopted by the membership of the Association in February 1981. These bylaws were written in outline format for easier use but did not change the overall organization of the Association. All policies of the Association were put into a standard format and collected into a policy manual. A committee is presently in the process of developing a procedural guide for the Association.

Many of the issues and concerns discussed at the landmark meeting of the Representative Assembly in 1978 have been addressed. A philosophical base has been adopted; research is being conducted to verify practice; theoretical positions are being proposed; and practice is being conducted in new arenas. However, many issues and concerns remain to be addressed. The Long-Range Plan of the Association will be used as a tool for monitoring and working for achievement of the long-range goals of the Association.

Summary

Although the focus within occupational therapy has changed, it is evident that there are at least four common propositions that have characterized the profession throughout its history:

1. The use of occupation or purposeful activity can influence the state of health of an individual.
2. Individuals and their adaptation and total functioning must be viewed with respect to their own environment, and remediation must take into consideration all the physical, psychological, and social factors.
3. Interpersonal relationships are an important factor in the occupational therapy process.
4. Occupational therapy is an adjunct to, and has its roots in, medicine and must work in cooperation with medical professionals and other persons involved as health-care providers to ensure maximum benefits for clients.

Being founded on the principles and practices of moral treatment that valued the quality of the daily life of disabled people, occupational therapy from its beginning has focused on health, adaptation, and function.

References

1. Wade, L. C.: Pioneer for Social Justice, 1851–1938; Graham Taylor. Chicago: University of Chicago Press, 1964, p. 170.
2. Levin, H. L.: Occupational and recreational therapy among the ancients. Occup. Ther. Rehabil. 17:311–316, 1938.
3. Ibid., p. 312.
4. Licht, S.: Occupational Therapy Source Book. Baltimore: Williams & Wilkins Co., 1948, p. 1.
5. Haas, L. J.: Practical Occupational Therapy. Milwaukee: Bruce Publishing Company, 1944, p. 6.
6. Levin: Occupational and recreational therapy among the ancients, pp. 311–316.
7. Licht: Source Book, p. v.
8. Pinel, P.: Medical philosophical treatise on mental alienation, Paris, 1801. In Licht: Source Book, p. 19.
9. Dunton, W. R., Jr.: Reconstruction Therapy. Philadelphia: W. B. Saunders Co., 1919, p. 20.
10. Licht: Source Book, p. 8.
11. Reil, J. C.: Rhapsodies on the psychic treatment of the insane, Halle, 1803. In Licht: Source Book, pp. 25 and 27.
12. Tuke, S.: Description of the Retreat, an institution near York, for insane persons, York, 1816. In Licht: Source Book, pp. 41–56.
13. Leuret, F.: On the moral treatment of insanity, Paris, 1840. In Licht: Source Book, p. 63.
14. Ibid., p. 9.
15. Haas: Practical Occupational Therapy, p. 11.
16. Kirkbride, T. S.: Report of the Pennsylvania Hospital for the Insane for the years 1841, 1842, and 1843, Philadelphia. Published by order of the Board of Managers, Pennsylvania Hospital, 1841, 1842, 1843.
17. Dunton, W. R., Jr., and Licht, S.: Occupational Therapy, Principles and Practice, ed. 2. Springfield IL: Charles C Thomas, 1957, p. 11.

18. Haas: Practical Occupational Therapy, p. 13.
19. Meyer, A.: The philosophy of occupational therapy. Arch. Occup. Ther. 1:1–10, 1922.
20. Ibid., p. 5.
21. Haas: Practical Occupational Therapy, p. 11.
22. Chicago School of Civics and Philanthropy Yearbook and Bulletin. August 1908–July 1911, p. 98.
23. Meyer: The philosophy of occupational therapy, p. 9.
24. Ibid., p. 6.
25. Ibid., p. 7.
26. Ibid., pp. 1–10.
27. Tracy, S. E.: Studies in Invalid Occupations—A Manual for Nurses and Attendants. Boston: Whitcomb and Barrows, 1910.
28. Ibid.
29. Dewey, J.: The School and Society. Chicago: University of Chicago Press, 1900. Paperback ed. 1956, pp. 132–133.
30. Tracy: Studies in Invalid Occupations.
31. Tracy, S. E.: Flier on occupation course offered at Experiment Station for the Study of Invalid Occupations, Jamaica Plains MA, 1914.
32. Hall, H. J.: Occupational Therapy, A New Profession. Concord: The Rumford Press, 1923.
33. Hall, H. J.: Work cure, a report of five years experience at an institution devoted to the therapeutic application of manual work. J.A.M.A. 54:12, 1910.
34. Hall, H. J., and Buck, Mertice, M. C.: The Work of Our Hands—A Study of Occupations for Invalids. New York: Moffat, Yard and Co., 1915.
35. Loomis, B., and Wade, B. D.: Chicago. Occupational Therapy Beginnings: Hull House, The Henry B. Favill School of Occupations and Eleanor Clark Slagle. Special Improvement Grant, U.S. Public Health Services, Allied Health 50579-01, 1973, p. 2.
36. Slagle, E. C.: Occupational therapy. Trained Nurse Hosp. Rev. April 1938, p. 380.
37. Experience of Eleanor Clark Slagle, 1910–1922. Document from Archives, American Occupational Therapy Association, Bethesda MD.
38. Slagle, E. C.: Training Aides for Mental Patients. Papers on occupational therapy. Utica NY: State Hospital Press, 1922, p. 40.
39. Slagle, E. C., and Robeson, H. A.: Syllabus for Training of Nurses in Occupational Therapy. Utica NY: State Hospital Press, 1933, p. 10.
40. Bing, R.: William Rush Dunton, Jr.—American Psychiatrist, a Study in Self. Unpublished doctoral dissertation, University of Maryland, 1961.
41. Dunton, W. R., Jr.: Occupational Therapy—A Manual for Nurses. Philadelphia: W. B. Saunders Co., 1915.
42. Ibid.
43. Barton, G. E.: Teaching the Sick, A Manual of Occupational Therapy as Re-education. Philadelphia: W. B. Saunders Co., 1919, p. 60.
44. Constitution of the National Society for the Promotion of Occupational Therapy. Baltimore: Sheppard Hospital Press, 1917, p. 1.
45. Historical Documents and Letters, Archives, American Occupational Therapy Association, Bethesda MD.
46. Proceedings of the National Society for the Promotion of Occupational Therapy: First Annual Meeting. Catonsville MD: Spring Grove State Hospital, 1917.
47. Bing: William Rush Dunton, Jr., Ibid.
48. Dunton, W. R., Jr.: Occupational therapy. In Barr, D. P.: Barr's Modern Medical Therapy in General Practice, Vol. 1. Baltimore: Williams & Wilkins Co., 1940, p. 697.
49. Dunton, W. R., Jr.: Credo. In Reconstruction Therapy. Philadelphia: W. B. Saunders Co., 1919, p. 10.
50. Then and Now, 1917–1967. American Occupational Therapy Association, 1967.
51. History. Occup. Ther. Rehabil. 19:32, 1940.
52. Circulation of information concerning employment of reconstruction aides. Washington: Medical Department, U.S. Army, January 22, 1918–March 27, 1918.
53. Subjects and lectures for the first class (Reconstruction aides) April 24, 1918 to July 13, 1918. Historical documents from Archives, Boston School of Occupational Therapy, Boston, 1918.
54. Historical documents from Archives, American Occupational Therapy Association, Bethesda MD.
55. Baldwin, B. T.: Occupational Therapy Applied to Restoration of Function of Disabled Joints. Washington DC: Walter Reed Monograph, April 1919, pp. 5–6.
56. Minimum standards for courses of training in occupational therapy. Arch. Occup. Ther. 3:295–298, 1924.
57. Greenman, N. B.: The influence of the university setting on occupational therapy education. Unpublished master's thesis, Tufts College, Boston, 1953.
58. Bowman, E.: Psychology of occupational therapy. Arch. Occup. Ther. 1:172, 1922.
59. Principles of Occupational Therapy. AOTA Bulletin No. 4, 1923.
60. Stern, E. M.: The work cure. Survey Graphic April 1939, pp. 1–4.
61. Personal discussion with Clare S. Spackman and Helen S. Willard.
62. Report of the Committee on Teaching Methods. Occup. Ther. Rehabil. 7:287, 1928.
63. Elwood, E. S.: The National Board of Medical Examiners and medical education and the possible effect of the Board's program on the spread of occupational therapy. Occup. Ther. Rehabil. 6:341–348, 1927.
64. Then and Now: Ibid.
65. J.A.M.A. 104:1632–1633, 1935; 105:690–691, 1935; 107:683–684, 1936.
66. Greenman: The influence of the university setting on occupational therapy education, Ibid.
67. Stern: The work cure, pp. 1–4.
68. Fish, M.: Occupational therapy in American colleges. J. Am. Assoc. Collegiate Registrars, October 1945, pp. 21–32.
69. Historical documents from Archives, American Occupational Therapy Association, Bethesda MD.
70. Stern: The work cure, pp. 1–4.
71. Kahmann, W. C., and West, W.: Occupational therapy in the United States Army hospital, World War II. In Willard, H. S., and Spackman, C. S. (eds.): Principles of Occupational Therapy. Philadelphia: J. B. Lippincott Co., 1947, p. 330.

72. Barton, W. E.: The challenge to occupational therapy. Occup. Ther. Rehabil. 22:262, 1943.

73. Barton, W. E.: Training programs for occupational therapists in the U.S. Army. Occup. Ther. Rehabil. 23:282, 1944.

74. Occupational Therapy. War Department Training Manual 8-291. Washington DC: U.S. Government Printing Office, 1944, p. 1.

75. Cobb, M. R.: Report of the Executive Secretary to the twenty-sixth Annual Meeting of the American Occupational Therapy Association, August, 1946. Occup. Ther. Rehabil. 25:259, 1946.

76. Spackman, C. S.: A history of the practice of occupational therapy for restoration of physical function: 1917–1967. Am. J. Occup. Ther. 22:68–71, 1968.

77. Willard, H. S., and Spackman, C. S. (eds.): Principles of Occupational Therapy. Philadelphia: J. B. Lippincott Co., 1947.

78. Spackman: A history of the practice of occupational therapy for restoration of physical function: 1917–1967, pp. 68–71.

79. Spackman, C. S.: The World Federation of Occupational Therapists 1952–1967. Am. J. Occup. Ther. 21:301–309, 1967.

80. Ibid.

81. Spackman: A history of the practice of occupational therapy for restoration of physical function: 1917–1967, pp. 68–71.

82. Semrad, E. V.: The emotional needs of the disabled person. Proceedings of the Occupational Therapy Institute, New York. American Occupational Therapy Association, 1956, pp. 28–38.

83. Fidler, G. S., and Fidler, J. W.: Introduction to Psychiatric Occupational Therapy. New York: Macmillan Publishing Co., 1954.

84. Fidler, G. S., and Fidler, J. W.: Occupational Therapy—A Communication Process in Psychiatry. New York: Macmillan Publishing Co., 1963.

85. Gilette, N. R.: Changing methods in the treatment of psychosocial dysfunction. Am. J. Occup. Ther. 21:230, 1967.

86. West, W.: Professional responsibility in times of change. Am. J. Occup. Ther. 22:9, 1968.

87. Greenman: The influence of the university setting on occupational therapy education, Ibid.

88. Final Report, Project Committee on Recognition of Occupational Therapy Assistants. Am. J. Occup. Ther. 13:269, 1958.

89. Crampton, M. W.: Educational upheaval for occupational therapy assistants. Am. J. Occup. Ther. 21:317, 1967.

90. Mazer, J.: The occupational therapist as consultant. Am. J. Occup. Ther. 23:417–421, 1969.

91. Willard, H. S., and Spackman, C. S. (eds.): Occupational Therapy, ed. 4. Philadelphia: J. B. Lippincott Co., 1971, p. 380.

92. Ayres, A. J.: The development of perceptual motor abilities: a theoretical basis for treatment of dysfunction. Eleanor Clarke Slagel Lecture presented at AOTA Conference, October 1963, St. Louis. Am. J. Occup. Ther. 17:221, 1963.

93. Ayres, A. J.: Sensory Integration and Learning Disorders. Los Angeles: Western Psychological Services, 1972, p. 8.

94. Reilly, M.: The educational process. Am. J. Occup. Ther. 23:303, 1969.

95. Laukaran, V. H.: Toward a model of occupational therapy for community health. Am. J. Occup. Ther. 31:71, 1977.

96. West, W.: The occupational therapist's changing responsibility to the community. Am. J. Occup. Ther. 21:312, 1967.

97. Mosey, A. C.: Three Frames of Reference for Mental Health. Thorofare NJ: Charles B. Slack, 1970, pp. v., 15–17.

98. Mosey, A. C.: An alternative: the biopsychosocial model. Am. J. Occup. Ther. 23:140, 1974.

99. American Occupational Therapy Foundation—The First Decade 1965–1975, Am. J. Occup. Ther. 29:636, 1975.

100. Standards and guidelines on occupational therapy affiliation program. AOTA Committee on Basic Professional Education. Am. J. Occup. Ther. 25:314–316, 1971.

101. Occupational therapy: its definition and functions. Am. J. Occup. Ther. 26:204–205, 1972.

102. Standards for occupational therapists providing direct service. Am. J. Occup. Ther. 28:237, 1974.

103. Essentials of an accredited educational program for the occupational therapist. Am. J. Occup. Ther. 29:485–496, 1975.

104. Essentials of an approved educational program for the occupational therapy assistant. Am. J. Occup. Ther. 30:245–261, 1976.

105. Position paper on consumer involvement. Am. J. Occup. Ther. 27:48, 1972.

106. Position paper on aging. Am. J. Occup. Ther. 28:564, 1974.

107. National system of certification of allied health personnel. Am. J. Occup. Ther. 30:50, 1976.

108. Policy statement on national health issues. Delegate Assembly minutes. Am. J. Occup. Ther. 31:110, 1977.

109. Resolution 465-75: Delegate Assembly minutes. Am. J. Occup. Ther. 30:177, 1976.

110. Resolution 471-76: Delegate Assembly minutes. Am. J. Occup. Ther. 30:587, 1976.

111. AOTA bylaws. Am. J. Occup. Ther. 31:111–118, 1977.

112. Principles of occupational therapy ethics with guidelines. Am. J. Occup. Ther. 34:900–905, 1980.

113. Hightower-Vandamm, M.: Nationally speaking: Ah, faint glow of sunshine. Am. J. Occup. Ther. 33:219–220, 1979.

114. Minutes of Representative Assembly Meeting, May 1978, San Diego, California. Am. J. Occup. Ther. 32:664, 1978.

115. Occupational Therapy 2001, Rockville, Maryland. American Occupational Therapy Association, 1979.

116. Hightower-Vandamm, M.: Nationally speaking: Participation-treatment for survival. Am. J. Occup. Ther. 33:627–628, 1979.

117. Resolution 531-79: Minutes of Representative Assembly, Detroit, Michigan, April 1979. Am. J. Occup. Ther. 33:785, 1979.

118. Resolution 536-79: Minutes of Representative Assembly, Detroit, Michigan, April 1979. Am. J. Occup. Ther. 33:785, 1979.
119. Minutes of Representative Assembly Meeting, May 1978, San Diego, California. Am. J. Occup. Ther. 32:665, 1978; and Resolution 562-80: Minutes of Representative Assembly Meeting, April 1980, Denver, Colorado. Am. J. Occup. Ther. 34:859, 1980.
120. Resolution 525-78: Standards of practice for mental health, developmental disabilities, physical disabilities and home health—Minutes of Representative Assembly, San Diego, California, May 1978. Am. J. Occup. Ther. 32:666, 1978.
121. Resolution 561-80: Standards of practice in schools. Am. J. Occup. Ther. 34:854–857, 1980.
122. Uniform terminology system for reporting occupational therapy services. Representative Assembly minutes, April 1979, Detroit, Michigan. Am. J. Occup. Ther. 33:805, 1979.
123. Occupational therapy product output reporting system. Representative Assembly Minutes, April 1980, Denver, Colorado. Am. J. Occup. Ther. 34:865, 1980.
124. Uniform occupational therapy evaluation checklist. Occupational Therapy Newspaper 35:11, 1981.
125. Entry level role delineation for OTR's and COTA's. Occupational Therapy Newspaper 35:8–13, 1981.
126. Position paper on the role of occupational therapy in promotion of health and prevention of disabilities. Am. J. Occup. Ther. 33:50–51, 1979.
127. Position paper on the role of occupational therapy in the vocational rehabilitation process. Am. J. Occup. Ther. 34:881–883, 1980.
128. Position paper on the Role of Occupational Therapy in independent living or Alternate Living Situations. Am. J. Occu. Ther. 35:812–814, 1981.
129. Position paper on the Role of Occupational Therapy as a Related Education Service. Am. J. Occup. Ther. 35:811, 1981.
130. Position paper on the Role of Occupational Therapy in Home Health Care. Am. J. Occup. Ther. 35:809–810, 1981.
131. Resolution 556-79: New areas of occupational therapy practice—identification and guidelines. Representative assembly minutes, April 1979, Detroit, Michigan. Am. J. Occup. Ther. 33:806–807, 1979.
132. Resolution 544-79: Delineation of the responsibilities of the AOTA continuing education program. Representative assembly minutes, April 1979, Detroit, Michigan. Am. J. Occup. Ther. 33:796, 1979.
133. Guide to graduate education leading to a master's degree. Adopted by Representative Assembly, May 1978. Am. J. Occup. Ther. 32:653, 1978.
134. Resolution 540-79: Recertification as a means of assuring continuing competency for OTR's and COTA's. Representative Assembly Minutes, April 1979, Detroit, Michigan. Am. J. Occup. Ther. 33:793–794, 1979.
135. Gilfoyle, E.: Training Occupational Therapy Educational Management in Schools. American Occupational Therapy Association, Rockville, Maryland, 1980.
136. Resolution 516-77: Formation of a task force to establish guidelines for an occupational therapy student organization. Representative assembly minutes, October 1977, Puerto Rico. Am. J. Occup. Ther. 32:251, 1978.
137. Resolution 526-78: Establishment of an archives task force of the AOTA. Representative Assembly Minutes, May 1978, San Diego, California. Am. J. Occup. Ther. 32:661, 1978.

PART 2

Theory and Philosophy

Current Basis for Theory and Philosophy of Occupational Therapy *Helen L. Hopkins*

Definition of Occupational Therapy

Occupational therapy is the art and science of directing man's participation in selected tasks to restore, reinforce and enhance performance, facilitate learning of those skills and functions essential for adaptation and productivity, diminish or correct pathology, and to promote and maintain health. Its fundamental concern is the capacity, throughout the life span, to perform with satisfaction to self and others those tasks and roles essential to productive living and to the mastery of self and the environment.*

Philosophical Base of Occupational Therapy

Man is an active being whose development is influenced by the use of purposeful activity. Using their capacity for intrinsic motivation, human beings are able to influence their physical and mental health and their social and physical environment through purposeful activity. Human life includes a process of continuous adaptation. Adaptation is a change in function that promotes survival and self-actualization. Biological, psychological, and environmental factors may interrupt the adaptation process at any time throughout the life cycle. Dysfunction may occur when adaptation is impaired. Purposeful activity facilitates the adaptive process.

Occupational therapy is based on the belief that purposeful activity (occupation), including its interpersonal and environmental components, may be used to prevent and mediate dysfunction, and to elicit maximum adaptation. Activity as used by the occupational therapist includes both an intrinsic and a therapeutic purpose.†

The Philosophical Base of Occupational Therapy adopted in 1979 provides a foundation for the theory and practice of occupational therapy. As a further guide to education and practice, in April 1979 the Representative Assembly affirmed

that there be a universal acceptance and implementation of the common core of occupational therapy as

---

* Occupational Therapy: Its definition and function. Am. J. Occup. Ther. 26:204, 1972.

† Adopted by the Representative Assembly—April, 1979, Detroit, Michigan.

active participation of the patient/client in occupation for purposes of improving performance. The use of facilitating procedures is only acceptable as occupational therapy when used to prepare the patient/client for better performance and prevention of disability, through self-participation in occupation. . . . Increased emphasis should be placed "on more creative involvement of the patient/client in purposeful, motivating and constructive occupation based on individual behavioral evaluations and treatment."[1]

The definition of occupational therapy, the philosophical base statement, and the affirmation of occupation as the common core of occupational therapy place parameters on the scope of occupational therapy. They provide guidance for education and practice and for the development and validation of theoretical propositions through research.

Throughout its history the focus of the occupational therapy profession has been on the nature of the individual in relation to society and the world in which the person lives. The body of knowledge in occupational therapy is drawn from several broad scientific areas, including biological and behavioral sciences, sociology, and anthropology. Knowledge in these areas is continually expanding and being modified, making it mandatory that occupational therapy be responsive and change. Occupational therapy uses the broad knowledge areas as its theoretical underpinnings and can be effective only in proportion to the accuracy of these knowledge bases. Theoretical propositions presently are being built upon these broad knowledge areas to form the beginning of occupational therapy's unique body of knowledge.

Occupational therapy's concern is for the health and function of each individual within his or her own environment. It is committed to the uniqueness of the individual and fosters the growth and development of each person. It is concerned "with assisting individuals to develop adaptive skills: those learned patterns of behavior which enable man to satisfy human needs and meet environmental demands."[2] Using both medical and social vantage points, the occupational therapist is committed to providing for development and maintenance of the highest potential in the biological, psychological, and social functioning of each individual.

Because occupational therapy is concerned with both human function throughout the life span and the uniqueness of the individual, it is essential that practice be based on the normal development process. The nature of the individual and the function-dysfunction continuum, along with pathological processes that may impinge on function, must be understood so that appropriate occupational therapy intervention procedures may be determined. The impact of occupation or purposeful activity on the human organism must be understood so that age-appropriate activities may be utilized in the intervention process.

There are numerous theoretical vantage points that are being used as guides for practice; however, no single theoretical proposition has been accepted by the total profession. Clark[3] has identified and analyzed four theoretical frameworks for occupational therapy: *adaptive performance* as integrated from the work of Fidler[4] and Mosey[5]; *biodevelopment,* which integrates sensory-integrative, neurodevelopmental, neurobehavioral, and kinesiological vantage points proposed by Ayres[6], King[7], and Moore[8]; *facilitating growth and development* as proposed by Llorens[9]; and *occupational behavior* as proposed by Reilly[10] (see Table 1 in Chap. 6). All four theoretical frameworks have their bases in human development; however, there is no other unifying concept and there is no consensus among the advocates of the various viewpoints.

There is a need for a theoretical proposition in occupational therapy that would provide a systematic way of thinking about data and that could explain, control, and predict behaviors. Reed and Sanderson have indicated that any theory of occupational therapy should be concerned with the relationship of occupation or activities to human beings. They further state that occupation enables a person to adapt in order to fulfill needs for self-care, work, and play or leisure.[11] Clark suggests a theoretical proposition she calls *Human Development through Occupation,* which she feels unites the human development construct with occupation, both of which comprise the common core of occupational therapy. She suggests that activity analysis and adaptation are the two processes that are generic to occupational therapy.[12] Occupational therapy has now accepted a philosophical base statement that indicates that the process of adaptation through the use of purposeful activity (occupation) is required for human development. This appears to be a perspective that can be accepted by the total profession. Both occupation and human development, including the adaptive process, are basic to the development of a unifying theory of occupational therapy; therefore, the following two chapters in this section will examine occupation and the human development process in depth.

References

1. Resolution #532-79: Occupation or the common core of occupational therapy. Representative Assembly minutes, April 1979, Detroit, Michigan. Am. J. Occup. Ther. 33:785, 1979.
2. Mosey, A. C.: Occupational Therapy: Theory and Practice. Medford, Mass.: Pothier Bros., Inc., 1968.

3. Clark, P. N.: Theoretical frameworks in contemporary occupational therapy practice, Part 1. Am. J. Occup. Ther. 33:509, 1979.

4. Fidler, G., Fidler, J.: Doing and becoming: Purposeful action and self actualization. Am. J. Occup. Ther. 32:305–310, 1978.

5. Mosey, A. C.: Recapitulation of ontogenesis: A theory for the practice of occupational therapy. Am. J. Occup. Ther. 22:426–438, 1968.

6. Ayres, A. J.: Sensory Integration and Learning Disorders. Los Angeles: Western Psychological Services, 1972.

7. King, L. J.: A sensory-integrative approach to schizophrenia. Am. J. Occup. Ther. 28:529–536, 1974.

8. Moore, J. C.: Behavior, bias and the limbic system. Am. J. Occup. Ther. 30:11–19, 1976.

9. Llorens, L. J.: Facilitating growth and development: The promise of occupational therapy. Am. J. Occup. Ther. 24:1–9, 1970.

10. Reilly, M.: Occupational therapy can be one of the great ideas of 20th century medicine. Am. J. Occup. Ther. 16:1–9, 1962.

11. Reed, K., Sanderson, S. R.: Concepts of Occupational Therapy. Baltimore: Williams & Wilkins, 1980.

12. Clark, P. N.: Human development through occupation: A philosophy and conceptual model for practice, Part II. Am. J. Occup. Ther. 33:577–585, 1979.

CHAPTER 3

Occupation *Gary Kielhofner*

In 1910 occupational therapy was defined as the "science of healing by occupation."[1] Though many other definitions have since been proposed to elaborate this simple theme and to reflect growing knowledge in occupational therapy, it still stands as the best reminder of what the occupational therapist is—an expert in the use of occupation as a health-giving art.

Early occupational therapists saw the necessity of having a strong theory of occupation to support their therapy.[2] However, this conviction, and the commitment to theory building it implied, went dormant for many years.[3]

A great deal of knowledge has been accumulated in occupational therapy to explain the effects of activity on damaged minds and bodies. However, the field has done less to advance its knowledge of occupation per se. Most efforts have been devoted to integrating medical knowledge into occupational therapy.[2] More recently, occupational therapists have begun to recognize the necessity of having a clearer and deeper understanding of occupation.[4-6] In the 1960s Reilly and many of her students began developing the thesis that successful application of occupation as a therapeutic medium required a thorough understanding of its nature.[4,7-13] That theme continues in this chapter; accordingly, knowledge that has been accumulated in various fields to explain human occupation will be organized around the following proposed definition of occupation:

> Occupation is the dominant activity of human beings that includes serious, productive pursuits and playful, creative, and festive behaviors. It is the result of evolutionary processes culminating in a biological, psychological, and social need for ludic and productive activity.

This definition is proposed only to point out some characteristics of occupation and to open possibilities for further elaboration. It is unlikely that any single definition of occupation will ever capture its total essence. As knowledge grows, the definition should expand and become more comprehensive and integrated.

Occupation as the Major Activity of Human Beings

Occupation refers to human activity; however, not all activity is occupation. Human beings engage in survival, sexual, spiritual, and social activities in addition to those activities that are specifically occupational in nature. Survival and sexual activities are rooted in the biological requirements of the individual and the species. Survival functions are those that preserve the basic integrity of the organism; they include such activities as eating and avoiding pain and danger. Sexual activities ensure the perpetuation of the species. Social activities refer to the forms of interaction and relations between individuals, and their patterned order.[14] The social characteristic of human beings involves the affiliative or affective bond between members of the species, their ability to share meanings, and their capacity for integration of action. Social activities have their genesis in the requirement of a group for coordinated activities between members.[15,16] Language is probably the most important dimension of social activity, as it is the medium for most human interaction.[17] Spiritual activities are also a fundamental part of human existence. Every civilization has some expression of human belief in an incomprehensible and ultimate dimension. Religions and other forms of spiritual activity usually involve contemplative and ritualistic-expressive activities.

It would be incorrect to suggest that one could clearly categorize all human activities. Social relations and sexuality overlap, spiritual activities involve coordinated human interaction, and social processes are often quite infused with the spirituality of the cultural group. However, just as one can observe human activities that fulfill certain needs and that are primarily or uniquely spiritual, social, or sexual in nature, there are those that are recognizably occupational. Occupation can be seen to fulfill the basic need of human beings, individually and collectively, to explore and master their world.[13]

In everyday life, occupation is often interrelated with sexual, survival, social, and spiritual activities. On the other hand, many work, play, and self-care activities, while they may indirectly serve survival or other needs, are primarily occupational in nature. Further, human beings clearly work and play far beyond immediate demands for survival. Such activities, done for their own sake, serve a basic urge for exploration and mastery. Thus, one can speak of activities that have an occupational dimension and of activities that are solely or primarily occupational in nature.

The statement that occupation is a major human activity is not meant to suggest it is more important than other areas of human behavior, but rather to denote that it ordinarily entails the majority of human time. Most waking hours are spent in play, self-care, and work.[18,19] For all their other characteristics, human beings are most definitely occupational creatures.

Forms of Occupation

Serious study of occupation requires identification and classification of different forms of occupation. A system of classifying and defining occupational forms would be useful, not only for basic theory in the field, but for clinical application. As Rogers notes, occupational therapy will eventually need to develop its own system of classifying occupational dysfunctions to guide treatment.[20] Such a classification of dysfunction could be built upon a previous classification of healthy occupational forms. The concept of a patient having a work or play dysfunction implies that work and play are defined behaviors for which one can posit criteria of adaptive or maladaptive functioning.

In occupational therapy, the concerns of clinical practice have generally focused on the three areas of occupation: work, play, and self-care.[21] Upon examination, these three areas appear to have a great deal of inherent validity, and they will serve as a starting place for defining different forms of occupational behavior. What these behaviors have in common is that they allow individuals to act on their urge to explore and master the world. These behaviors also form an interrelated gestalt. For example, work and play exist in an important dynamic balance throughout life.[18] Further, self-care is a necessary part of having a work role, and adult leisure is earned through work. These examples demonstrate the interrelatedness of these behaviors, and they support the argument that they form a common domain of behavior.

Work

The concept of work should include all forms of productive activities, whether or not they are reimbursed.[22] Productive activities are those that provide a service or commodity needed by another or that add new abilities, ideas, knowledge, artistic objects, or performances to the cultural tradition. The productive activity of work thus maintains and advances society. When an activity is considered to be one's work, it is generally organized into a major life role. Life roles are positions in life recognized by the social environment and by the role incumbent.[23] Thus, activities engaged in to fulfill one's duties as a student, housewife, volunteer, serious hobbyist, or amateur, and that are part of one's identity, can be considered work. According to this definition, work is not limited to adults; it extends to school-age children. Such a broad definition of work is relevant to occupational therapy, since many of the field's clients and patients do not have access to marketplace labor.

Daily Living Tasks

The area of self-care is expanded here to encompass a larger collection of daily living tasks. They include self-care, chores, maintenance of one's living space, and those behaviors required for access to resources (traveling, shopping, and so forth). Daily living tasks are expected of all capable members of the social group; however, they rarely form a major part of one's identity. Unlike work, daily living tasks do not contribute directly to the services or commodities of the social group, and they are not publicly valued like work. But, when an individual cannot perform them, the productivity of another social member (for example, a family member or a caretaker) is required. Thus, daily living tasks are indirectly productive for the social group.

Play

The whole range of ludic behaviors from childhood to old age constitute play. In youth, play predominates in daily life and involves exploratory, creative, and game-like behaviors. In adolescence and adulthood, it decreases in amount and transforms into hobbies, social recreation, sports, cultural celebration, and ritual. In old age, play once again becomes a predominant occupational behavior; it is generally referred to as leisure—a way of life earned through the labor of adulthood.

Continua of Occupational Behaviors

Occupational behaviors can be conceptualized as existing along continua that help differentiate them. For instance, occupational behaviors range from serious to frivolous, from overtly productive to apparently useless, from private to public, and from formal to informal. On the one end of the continua, we find playful behaviors that are typically perceived as frivolous, private, and apparently not productive (though it will be shown later that they serve a very important utility for individuals and social groups). On the other end of the continua, we find the more serious, overtly useful, and public behaviors of work. Daily living tasks fall somewhere in between (Fig. 3-1). While this schema reveals something about the differences in these occupations, it also demonstrates that their characteristics may overlap. Some forms of play are public, whereas some work is private. This points out the difficulty in establishing clear criteria to differentiate these behaviors. However, it is possible to speak of general or typical characteristics of work, play, and daily living tasks. Further, such a schema can reveal a great deal about individuals,

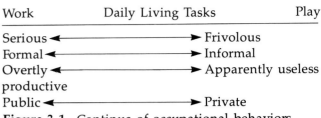

Work	Daily Living Tasks	Play
Serious ◄——————————► Frivolous		
Formal ◄——————————► Informal		
Overtly productive ◄——————————► Apparently useless		
Public ◄——————————► Private		

Figure 3-1. Continua of occupational behaviors.

their occupational styles, and their balance of occupation. The range of serious and frivolous activities, and the formal and informal aspects of occupation can be a useful indication of someone's occupational adaptation. For instance, a person whose work is formal, serious, and highly productive may require play of the opposite character to counterbalance it. Research in this area would be particularly revealing and would contribute not only to further understanding of occupation but to occupational therapy's potential to offer relevant services.

Understanding more about the forms that occupations take would enhance the ability of therapists to deal with the occupational problems of clients and patients as well as their ability to use occupation therapeutically. Further theory and research are needed to augment the field's understanding of occupation through the life span, its various forms in culture, and the overall dynamics of occupation in an individual's life.

Occupation as an Evolutionary Trait

Human behavior is a product of a long period of biological and social-technical evolution.[15,24] Early in the evolutionary process, action formed the basis for the continued existence of all living things; even the simplest organism is fundamentally spontaneous and active.[18] The process of evolution, as reflected in the phylogenetic scale, demonstrates a progressive increase in the organisms' requirements and capacities for more and more complex action.[25] As species acquired advanced nervous systems, they experienced a concomitant increase in the amounts and diversity of action needed. This need first appears in the young where spontaneous playful action is a means of learning basic skills that are biologically transmitted to members of lower, simpler species.[26] As the nervous system of a species advances to a more complex and adaptable form, the rigidity of biologically encoded ability is progressively left behind. Thus, behavior that is innate in simpler species' members must be learned by the individuals of higher species. Animals that have very specialized behavior acquire much of it through genetic inheritance. More complex animals that adapt through their behavioral variability are less endowed with inherent programming; however, they have brains with a greater capacity to organize the information from experience. Many theorists agree that play is the prerequisite for learning this flexible behavior. The play of the young of these more adaptable species is characterized by a greater urge to use capacity and an exploratory urge that arises from the nervous system's requirement for experience as a learning process.[27] Most mammals, in their immature period, romp, jump, run, engage in rough and tumble play, explore objects and places, all with no apparent motive except the playing itself. Studies have supported the hypothesis that these animals must learn to use their bodies and to deal with their environment through this early form of play.[28]

In primate species and in humans, play is more elaborate and includes social acts, fine motor manipulation, tool use, and imitation.[29] In these play forms, the individual learns complex behaviors that are part of the retinue of skills making up its species' typical approach to adaptation. Play enables this learning because it is a nonserious practice in which the organism can make mistakes, engage in trial and error, and try out new behaviors without serious consequences.[29]

Human beings are at the apex of the evolutionary trend toward adaptation through flexible rather than specialized behaviors. The evolution of flexibility in human activity requires a highly plastic nervous system in the young, a behavioral mechanism to provide experience, a social system that supports and protects the young, and a process for storing the collective experience of members to provide a pool of information for the young to acquire.

The route to generalization (that is, adaptation through flexibility rather than specialization) that human beings followed in evolution is also reflected in the highly adaptive human hand and its intimate relationship with the brain. Together with the visual sense, they form a complex that greatly enhances the ability of the organism to explore and master its environment.[24] The human hand is morphologically suited, and it is used for extensive manipulation and exploration of objects in the environment.[30] Consequently, there is a greatly enhanced capacity for gaining technological control over the environment by using and elaborating this eye-hand-brain complex. This is first represented in the emergence of tool use and later in tool making. Tools are primarily extensions of the hand,[24] and they represent elaboration of the urge to explore and to have effects on the world. While many species exhibit some primitive kinds of tool use, human beings alone are spontaneous and

extensive tool makers and inventors.[30] The invention of tools, which is a central component of the tremendous growth of technology characterizing human work throughout history, is, almost parodoxically, an outgrowth or product of play.[29] Behavioral flexibility that is gained in play[26] includes the production of extensions of biological equipment (that is, tool production).

Observations on semidomesticated monkeys provide a model for how play was responsible for the evolution of tool making in human life.[31] In free-ranging monkey troups that have a sufficient food supply provided by caretakers (hence the term, semidomesticated), play becomes more prevalent in the young. From this play emerges a plethora of new behavior forms. Most are idiosyncratic and eventually die out. However, some of these behaviors, which include forms of tool use, prove adaptive. Older monkeys learn the new behavior by imitating it, and eventually the behavior is spread through the monkey troup and is learned by successive generations in their play as they imitate older monkeys. This is a primitive version of the evolutionary complex of humans (including a plastic nervous system, a behavioral mechanism for learning, a pressure-free social group, and imitation as a means of spreading and preserving individual experience in the group). In addition to these primate studies, investigations of children have found evidence that play with objects is an important precursor to the inventive use of objects as tools.[32,33] Thus, play is centrally important for the technological abilities of both individual members and the entire social group.

Play, tool use, the human hand, and brain are all important and interrelated factors in human evolution where both behavior and physical morphology are changed in concert. Each interrelates with and influences the selective advantage of the other. Bruner[29] and Washburn[24] propose the following explanation for how human evolution took place. As prehominids left the jungle for the savannas, they gained adaptive advantage by standing upright on the tall grassy plains. Eventually, they relinquished brachiation for ambulation as a mode of locomotion with the result that the species acquired a stockier pelvis. Simultaneously the pressures of hunting and life on the savanna required coordinated group effort, and individuals with more complex brains to select and interpret the communications of their peers had adaptive advantage. This evolving animal with a larger brain, however, had to be born through the smaller birth canal of the ambulator's stockier pelvis. Thus, the projeny of the changing prehominid were born more immature, with brains that would grow and mature substantially after birth. This more immature brain was, consequently, more plastic and suited to learning. Concurrently, the growing complexity of the social group included a division of labor with some individuals serving as caretakers of helpless infants. This created an ideal environment for the emergence of more and more elaborate play forms. Young prehominids, protected by their mothers and having survival needs met by the work of the troup, were freed to engage in whatever nonserious pursuits they wished. Unlike the young of other species, who had to learn locomotion and other adult skills soon after birth or in a very short period of development, these individuals remained immature for years, during which they played and acquired more and more behavioral flexibility. In time, this youthful play produced a more creative and inventive adult likely to contribute technical or social advancement to the group. Since group members could readily communicate, they could also acquire and proliferate it.

The end results of this evolutionary trend are the creative, aesthetic, and playful characteristics of the human being and the flexible behavior that characterizes the species. Human beings play more than any other animal. In addition, human beings have the unusual characteristic of elaborating their behavior far beyond that required by survival. For instance, hunting and gathering societies that require only about 18 hours of weekly labor for food gathering and other survival needs, manage a long week spent in ritual and festive behaviors that require substantial energy and investment. By evolving a more complex culture, and thereby requiring members to acquire it, human societies are constantly advancing the demands on individuals for adaptation. This is poignantly demonstrated when persons who manage to fulfill their basic survival needs, but violate social norms of conduct, are judged to be maladaptive.

Not only has the human brain evolved to be able to learn these cultural behaviors, but its very structure and processes are intimately interrelated with these varied behavior forms. The human being must acquire the complex behavior of culture to function at all.[34] In the course of evolution the brain was programmed for exploration and mastery; individuals must engage in a wide range of occupational activities, especially early play, to use their biological inheritance properly.

As human culture becomes more and more elaborate, its demands for all forms of occupation increase. Accumulated technology and knowledge make the requirement for learning to work ever more demanding. In human history, simple imitation was replaced with apprenticeship. More recently the explosion of human knowledge and technique expanded apprenticeship to a long period of public tutelage beginning with common knowledge and culminating (sometimes twenty or more years later) in specialized

training. This process continues; just as mathematics and reading have become, in a few generations, almost essential for self-care and work, computer fluency will likely emerge as the new requirement for coming generations.

Thus, it can be seen that the process of human evolution has intimately involved occupation. Through evolution the demands for both play and work have increased. Changes in the organism thrust the human species more and more toward both the capacity and the need for occupation. The human trait of occupation emerged in this evolutionary concatenation of a nervous system of growing complexity, increased playfulness, tool use, an increasing urge for action, and technical-social change and growth. The occupational nature of human beings is reflected throughout the modern human situation. Newborn individuals arrive on the scene, begin their role as players, go through a long period of preparation for productivity, enter worker roles, and eventually return to a play-dominated phase in retirement.[18] This simple schema of daily human life has its origins in a complex interrelated set of factors that have unfolded over eons. It is not by chance that human beings work, play, and care for themselves; it is biologically and socially encoded in the species.

Because occupation has been a central feature of human evolution, it fills an important place in the adaptive capacity of the human species and its individual members. Without occupational activities, individuals would be regressed and disorganized, if they survived at all. Without the playful and productive contributions of members, social and cultural life would cease to continue. Occupation is so central to adaptation that when it is absent or distorted in the individual or culture, there is great cause for alarm. Importantly, the role of the occupational therapists centers on situations where individuals or groups have lost their occupational capabilities.

Occupation and the Biological Dimension

The complex nervous system of human beings requires rich and varied stimuli achievable only through active engagement of the world.[7] Occupation is centrally important in the development of biological features in childhood and their maintenance in adulthood. The nervous and musculoskeletal system of the child receives constant use through the childhood occupation of play. Play is an important arena for the neurological "programming" that the child's developing nervous system requires. Development is not just a predetermined change in the structures of the body, but it includes the effects of experiences that become imprinted into those biological structures.[25,35] All those neurological and musculoskeletal features that make possible such functions as coordinated movement and perception have much of their genesis in play.

In adulthood and in old age, occupation is important for maintaining biological functions. For instance, a severe restriction of occupational activities is associated with the impairment of strength, endurance, mobility, cardiovascular function, metabolism, and nervous system function.[36] Stress has long been recognized to be a major etiological factor in many biological problems.[37] It has also been recognized that boredom (or a lack of satisfying and meaningful occupations) produces severe stress and thus ranks as a physiological threat.[38] Along these same lines longevity and health in old age are related to maintaining meaningful work and leisure throughout adulthood and old age.[39] It is not atypical for an older person upon retirement or upon being forced to give up a lifelong meaningful occupation to suddenly degenerate toward disability and death.

The mechanism by which occupation maintains healthy biological functioning is complex; only a little is understood about it. It is known that exercise has positive effects on the muscles, circulation, and so forth. However, new relationships between occupation and biological well-being are constantly being discovered. Recently it was noted that running seemed to have a positive effect on depressed persons. Later it was discovered that such physical exertion is a catalyst for the release of catecholamines in the brain, which are the organism's natural antidepressants.[40]

It is theorized that the conscious functions of human beings engaged in the purposeful activity of occupation have direct controlling effects on the brain's physiology.[41,42] Such proposals, which attempt to bridge the mind-body dichotomy of Western thinking, are paving the way to a deeper understanding of how a human being's "goal directed use of time and energy" reverberates throughout the organism and how it has positive effects on basic biological processes. When a human being engages in meaningful occupation, the entire mind and body functions in an integrated and resonating manner. Thus, occupation plays a role in maintaining the biologic organization of the organism.

The Psychological Dimension of Occupation

There is also an intimate relationship between occupation and the psychological dimension of human beings. For the present discussion the psychological aspect of human beings will be defined as the symbolic (that is, temporal, meaningful, and purposive) and affective experience of the self and the world.

Childhood play is an extremely important determinant of children's growing sense of control over their world and their destiny; it is critical for the children's positive affect, their feeling of well-being. Children become aware of the effects they can have on the world, and they begin to develop a sense of personal causation—the belief that they have skills, can control events, and will succeed.[40] Poor play experiences can result in the opposite; a failure of play can mean that this all-important image of personal competence will not develop.

Play is also central to children's symbolic development.[35] Their growing awareness of time and its role in structuring activities and their growing sense of meaning or purpose, which can define positive existence, all accrue from play experience.[43,44]

In childhood play, children learn the basic symbolic skills that enable them to deal with motion, objects, people, and events. These have been referred to as the rules that children internalize about their actions and their environment.[44] These rules form an internal map of external reality and its potentials for action. Children deprived of play experiences are poorer practical problem solvers, are less creative, have less information about their environment, and exhibit less flexible and adaptive approaches to their environment.[32,33,45] In play, children learn a growing sense of time as they sequence events, take turns, and compartmentalize activities into meaningful episodes. Eventually, as the child's sense of time grows, there is an increasing future orientation.[46–48] Children, in their fantasy, begin to bridge the transition to the future and, in so doing, create purposes and meanings for themselves about their own existence. The simple dramatic play of a child serves a deep purpose of allowing the child to experience some of the meaning of being a parent, firefighter, nurse, or other adult figure. Paradoxically, the fantasy of childhood is an important process for developing a healthy sense of reality and of how one can competently face and master the requirements of life.[49]

As the child develops, the growing necessity of being productive slowly emerges. The child first learns tasks of self-care, advances to chores, and by adolescence begins entry into work situations. The less serious productive roles that children and adolescents perform in the home are important precursors of competence in adult life.[50] In the transition from childhood to adulthood, the individual also undergoes an important process of occupational choice.[51] The combined experiences of dramatic play, childhood activities yielding interests, a growing sense of meaning and value, and realistic experiences of older childhood and adolescence culminate in the consequential choice to enter or begin preparation for a kind of work. As might be expected, children with poor play experiences and little opportunity for chores and recognition by adults may fail in this occupational choice process, and they may enter into a vicious cycle of dissatisfaction and failure in their adult work careers.[52]

Daily living tasks and work are critical adult activities. For most individuals they are a means of earning a living and contributing to the maintenance of a household. The work role is valued by society, so that working is often the primary source of self-esteem and feelings of control and competence.[53] Work is a means of pursuing personal interests and of developing personal abilities.[54] Many persons who find they cannot meet these needs in work will seek to do so in their recreation or in a more serious amateur pursuit.[55] This reflects the fact that human beings have a need for occupation far beyond that dictated by sheer survival.

Work is a major factor in the structuring of time throughout adult life.[18] Daily and weekly routines are often dictated by the work schedule. The work career may imply a structured sequence of years defining advancement through steps or positions in a given line of work.[56] Individuals measure their own growth, and they progress by their advancement in time through a series of jobs, positions, or work titles. Failure to meet socially normative patterns of advancement can result in a loss of self-esteem and a sense of being out of control.[56]

Satisfaction in work ordinarily requires that the person be able to exercise and develop skills he or she values, to find work interesting, and to see tangible results of his or her efforts.[53,54] The satisfaction and sense of personal mastery that comes from work of whatever type is an important source of mental health in the adult. When persons begin to fail in their work roles, or when they cannot meet their need for satisfaction in work, they can become candidates for mental illness.[57] The stress of not being able to find meaning in one's existence is being recognized more and more as a major etiological factor in mental illness.[58] The growing trend in modern industrial societies toward impersonal, mechanized, and noncreative work has already begun to result in an epidemic of persons who exhibit maladaptive lifestyles.[59,60] As people become disengaged from the meaning of work and its potential for self-satisfaction, they become alienated from society, they demonstrate deviant behaviors, and they lead unhappy and often disorganized lives. As this trend continues, occupational therapy will have to address a whole new area of health problems that come directly from the disintegration of normal occupation. Such a demand will require occupational therapists to compel and encourage institutions and workplaces to make changes that would restore the health of individuals.[61]

Although adult life is still largely dominated by work, there has been a growing trend toward more and more leisure in modern society.[62] Today the leisure or recreational period of an adult's life is likely to be substantial and to have a large impact on life-satisfaction. Vacations, weekends, and retirement are life spaces that the individual literally earns through work. A person in our culture does not experience true leisure in adult life unless it is earned by some kind of productive activity.[63] This is based in part on the proposition that adult life involves a dynamic balance of work, play, and sleep patterns. If balance is not preserved, the individual may have a dysfunction of his or her occupational life with other consequences, such as a loss of life satisfaction and erosion of competence.[18,57]

Old age in modern society is marked by a major transition from working to enjoying leisure. This is often a period of adjustment; persons who have a well-developed leisure role before retirement (those who have hobbies, or other avocational interests) generally have less difficulty adjusting to retirement.[64] However, for many elderly persons, physical problems, lack of resources, and environmental constraints limit their opportunities for engaging in sufficient occupational activities; when this is true, life satisfaction is less.[65]

The Social Dimension of Occupation

The role of occupation in social life can be described in terms of the contributions of both work and play. As already noted, play was a central mechanism in the evolution of the human species. It was responsible for the elaboration and creation of new behaviors that eventually entered the cultural repertoire of the social group. It also served to initiate the immature into the demands of the physical and social environment. In modern society, play still serves the role of preparing the young for adult life in a particular social group. The special beliefs, values, ways of interacting, and technology of the social group are reflected in the play of the young who are thereby inducted into a way of living. For instance, social groups that stress competition in adult interaction have young who play competitive games. On the other hand, social groups that stress cooperation in social interaction have a remarkable absence of such games in childhood[66]; rather, children play to maximize everyone's status instead of competing to have a single team or player that is the winner. In primitive tribes, children play with bows and arrows and the artifacts of that group; children in modern societies play with toy trucks, stoves, and the implements of modern culture. Play also keeps pace with the changes in the culture's technology. For instance, the appearance of electronic games in the play of today's young is an important precurser of a new generation for whom computer fluency will be highly desirable in adult adaptation. The games of each culture reflect its requirements so that the young learn how to participate in the culture through their play.[67] The simple and seemingly unimportant play activities of children serve a vital function of maintaining the continuity of social knowledge and of bringing to the young the technology of the social system.

In human social life, play serves a vital role well beyond the childhood years. Adult play is important for reaffirming the culture's values.[68] Play is a way of stepping back and of affirming the fundamental tenets of a culture.[69] For instance, the football game has been analyzed as a metaphor for the competition, teamwork, and technical precision that characterizes American work.[70] Adult players and spectators become intensely involved in the emotion and meaning of the game at a symbolic level; this serves in subtle ways to cement their commitment to the way of life of their social group. The celebrative or festive and ritual forms of adult play are critical for the maintenance of social life.[69,71] Graduation ceremonies, the Fourth of July, religious rituals, Thanksgiving dinner, and other forms of celebration allow the individual to take account of accomplishments, worthwhile things in life, and central values. These forms of play are critical to the spirit of the culture.

When adult play forms begin to change, it may signal that cultural change is on the way.[72] When such play becomes disrupted or when members of a group lose their affinity to such play forms, a culture may be in deep trouble. It is notable that individuals who find themselves alienated from social life (for example, the mentally ill) often find holidays intolerable, and they have difficulty celebrating. Despite its often frivolous and unproductive facade, the play of adult life is an important process in social life. It is a dynamic that maintains the morale, commitment, and value structure of the social group. Though its contributions to the social group are less apparent than work, it should never be construed as less important.

Work is a basic fact of all social groups. Human societies are characterized by a division in labor in which individuals take on specialized functions. Rarely do individual human beings perform the whole range of labor necessary for self-preservation. Rather, tasks are traditionally divided according to age, sex, social position, and aptitude. Each worker

depends in some important way on the contributions of others. In modern society there is greater specialization of work than in any other time.[73] The network of productive contributions in American society is almost unfathomable. From the perspective of social life, important contributions extend beyond paid labor. In fact, marketplace waged productivity is only a small portion of the actual work that keeps a society functioning.[22] Everything from the household chores done by the young, volunteer work, homemaking, mutual assistance in families and neighborhoods, to the leadership jobs in government are necessary for the ongoing maintenance of social life.

It is for this reason that societies value the productive contributions of their members. The young are inducted into an ethic which defines social expectations for their work. In response, adults feel a sense of self-worth and affiliation with the social group by virtue of making productive contributions. Some trends in modern life raise questions about the future of work in society. The substitution of mechanical and electronic processes for human labor and thinking, as well as economic processes that do not demand everyone's contribution, may have ill effects for both the group and the individual.[74] The social group not only needs the work of its members, but it owes them the opportunity to work. The reciprocity of the individual and the social group in productive exchange is a central feature of human life. Without work, neither the social group nor the individual is adaptive.

One possibility for modern society is the emergence of new valued and valuable work forms. Volunteerism is an important factor in social life today, and it serves both individual and group needs. Hobbies have often been turned into productive pursuits that benefit others. In a society with increasing numbers of disabled, elderly, and unemployed individuals, such nontraditional emerging work forms may well be a useful answer. However, to function, they must become part of the cultural fabric; thus, social change is required. For occupational therapists the implication is involvement in social action as well as individual assistance. Functions such as organizing volunteer groups of disabled persons, or running hobby shops for the elderly, could be important types of socially-based occupational therapy in the future.

Occupation and Therapy

The previous sections examine several facets of the proposed definition of occupation. This final part will discuss the consequences of these characteristics of occupation for therapy. Basically there are two implications: (1) since occupation is so central to human adaptation, its absence or disruption (irrespective of any other medical or social problem) is a threat to health, and (2) when illness, trauma, or social conditions have affected the biological or psychological health of an individual, occupation is an effective means for reorganizing behavior.

While these two statements separate disruption of occupation from medical illness for conceptual clarity, it should be realized that many clients seen by occupational therapists show a complex of interrelated problems involving both a medical problem and a loss or disruption of occupation. Often the picture is complicated when the disorder is a developmental or long-standing one. For instance, children with minimal brain dysfunction may be poor players because of the damaged equipment they have for play. The paucity of play, in turn, slows the developmental process, exacerbating the original medical problem. Another example is the elderly person whose waning physical abilities force confinement to an institution where there are no opportunities to pursue some lifelong occupation; the latter may cause a loss of morale with consequent physical deterioration.

Sometimes a medical problem may not be involved initially, as when a person loses an occupation by virtue of social circumstances (for instance, loss of a job or rearing in an environment that failed to nurture play). However, such disruption of occupation can lead to psychological and biological dysfunctions. Depression, physiological correlates of the stress of boredom, and manifold other medical problems may have their etiology in the loss of normal occupation.

Occupational therapists intervene by replacing the lost occupation with carefully guided and organized activities. These occupational activities often influence both the occupational dysfunction and any extant medical problem. Since the two are likely to be intermingled to begin with, the use of occupation as therapy is an especially efficacious approach. To use the previous examples, engagement of children in more rich and varied play will not only allow them to acquire normal play behaviors, but it will have an organizing and maturing effect on the damaged nervous systems. Providing opportunities to elderly persons to pursue valued occupations will not only restore morale, but it will provide exercise of their physical capacities.

As the organizing influence of occupation is more fully understood, occupational therapists will become increasingly able to expand its therapeutic use. This will require careful study and the development of theories that explain the dynamics and characteristic of occupation. We must have a thorough understanding of any tool to use it effectively. Since an occupational therapist's unique and powerful tool is occupation, it behooves the field and the individual therapist to achieve a deep and penetrating understanding of it.

References

1. Training Teachers for Occupational Therapy for the Rehabilitation of Disabled Soldiers and Sailors. Federal Board for Vocations Education Bulletin No. 6, Government Printing Office, 1918, p. 13.
2. Kielhofner, G. and Burke, J.: Occupational therapy after 60 years: An account of changing identity and knowledge. Am. J. Occup. Ther. 31:675–689, 1977.
3. Johnson, J.: Old values—new directions: Competence, adaptation, integration. Am. J. Occup. Ther. 35:589–598, 1981.
4. Reilly, M.: Occupational therapy—a historical perspective: The modernization of occupational therapy. Am. J. Occup. Ther. 25:243–246, 1971.
5. Finn, G.: The occupational therapist in prevention programs. Am. J. Occup. Ther. 31:658–659, 1977.
6. Weimer, R.: Traditional and Nontraditional Practice Arenas in Occupational Therapy: 2001 A.D. Rockville, MD: American Occupational Therapy Association, 1979, p. 42–53.
7. Reilly, M.: Occupational therapy can be one of the great ideas of 20th century medicine. Am. J. Occup. Ther. 16:1–9, 1962.
8. Matsutsuyu, J.: Occupational behavior—a perspective on work and play. Am. J. Occup. Ther. 25:291–294, 1971.
9. Florey, L.: Intrinsic motivation: The dynamics of occupational therapy theory. Am. J. Occup. Ther. 23:319–322, 1969.
10. Shannon, P.: The work-play model: A basis for occupational therapy programming. Am. J. Occup. Ther. 24:215–218, 1970.
11. Watanabe, S.: Four concepts basic to the occupational therapy process. Am. J. Occup. Ther. 22:339–344, 1968.
12. Woodside, H.: Dimensions of the occupational behavior model. Can. J. Occup. Ther. 43:11–14, 1976.
13. Kielhofner, G. and Burke, J.: A model of human occupation, Part one. Framework and content. Am. J. Occup. Ther. 34:572–581, 1980.
14. Blumer, H.: Symbolic interactionism. Englewood Cliffs, NJ: Prentice-Hall, 1979.
15. Reynolds, V.: The biology of human action. San Francisco: W. H. Freeman and Co., 1976.
16. Tiger, L.: Men in Groups. New York: Random House, 1969.
17. Spier, M.: How to Observe Face-to-Face Communication: A Sociological Introduction. Pacific Palisades, CA: Goodyear Publishing Co., 1973.
18. Kielhofner, G.: Temporal adaptation: A conceptual framework for occupational therapy. Am. J. Occup. Ther. 31:235–242, 1977.
19. Berk, R. and Berk, S.: Labor and Leisure at Home: Content and Organization of the Household Day. Beverly Hills: Sage Publications, 1979.

20. Rogers, R.: Order and disorder in occupational therapy and in medicine. Am. J. Occup. Ther. 36:29–35, 1982.
21. Meyer, A.: The philosophy of occupational therapy. Am. J. Occup. Ther. 31:639–643, 1977.
22. Chapple, E.: Rehabilitation: Dynamic of Change. Ithica, NY: Center for Research in Education, Cornell University, 1970.
23. Heard, C.: Occupational role acquisition: A perspective on the chronically disabled. Am. J. Occup. Ther. 31:243–247, 1977.
24. Washburn, S.: Tools and evolution. Scientific American 203:63–75, 1960.
25. vonBertalanffy, L.: General systems theory and psychiatry. In Arieti, S. (ed): American Handbook of Psychiatry, Vol. 3. New York: Basic Books, 1969.
26. Vandenberg, B. and Kielhofner, G.: Play in evolution, culture, and individual adaptation: Implications for therapy. Am. J. Occup. Ther. 36:20–28, 1982.
27. White, R.: Motivation reconsidered: The concept of competence. Psychological Review 66:313–324, 1959.
28. Cherfas, J. and Lewin, R.: Not Work Alone: A Cross-Cultural View of Activities Superfluous to Survival. Beverly Hills: Sage Publications, 1980.
29. Bruner, J.: Nature and uses of immaturity. Am. Psychol. 27:687–708, 1972.
30. Campbell, B.: The evolution of the human hand. In Cohen, Y. (ed): Man in Adaptation: The Biosocial Background. Chicago: Aldine, 1968.
31. Kawai, M.: Newly acquired pre-cultural behavior of the natural troup of Japanese monkeys on the Koshima Islet. Primates 6:1–30, 1956.
32. Sylva, K., Bruner, J. and Genova, P.: The role of play in the problem-solving of children 3–5 years old. In Bruner, Jolly, and Sylva (eds): Play—Its Role in Development and Evolution. New York: Basic Books, 1976.
33. Dansky, J. and Silverman, I.: Effects of play on associate fluency in preschool children. In Bruner, Jolly, and Sylva (eds): Play—Its Role in Development and Evolution. New York: Basic Books, 1976.
34. Geertz, C.: The interpretation of cultures. London: Hutchinson, 1975.
35. Bruner, J.: The organization of early skilled action. Child Dev. 44:1–11, 1973.
36. Kottke, F.: The effects of limitation of activity upon the human body. J.A.M.A. 196:825–830, 1966.
37. Selye, H.: The Stress of Life. New York: McGraw-Hill, 1955.
38. Dubos, R.: The Mirage of Health. New York: Harper & Row, 1959.
39. Cousins, N.: Anatomy of an Illness. New York: Bantam, 1981.
40. Leer, F.: Running as an adjunct to psychotherapy. Social Work. January:20–25, 1980.
41. Sperry, R.: An objective approach to subjective experience: Further explanation of a hypothesis. Psychol. Rev. 77:585–590, 1970.
42. Furst, C.: Origins of the Mind: Mind-Brain Connections. Englewood Cliffs NJ: Prentice-Hall, 1979.
43. Reilly, M.: Play as Exploratory Learning. Beverly Hills: Sage Publications, 1974.
44. Robinson, A.: Play: The arena for the acquisition of rules of competent behavior. Am. J. Occup. Ther. 31:248–253, 1977.
45. Hutt, C. and Bhavnani, R.: Predictions from play. In Brunner, Jolly, and Sylva (eds): Play: Its Role in Development and Evolution. New York: Basic Books, 1976.
46. DeCharms, R.: Personal Causation. New York: Academic Press, 1968.
47. Cottle, T.: Time's Children. Boston: Little, Brown & Co., 1971.
48. Cottle, T. and Klineberg, S.: The Present of Things Future. New York: The Free Press, 1974.
49. Erickson, E.: Childhood and Society. New York: Norton, 1963.
50. Kielhofner, G.: A model of human occupation, Part 2. Ontogenesis from the perspective of temporal adaptation. Am. J. Occup. Ther. 34:657–663, 1980.
51. Webster, P. S.: Occupational role development in the young adult with mild mental retardation. Am. J. Occup. Ther. 34:13–18, 1980.
52. de Renne-Stephen, C.: Imitation: A mechanism of play behavior. Amer. J. Occup. Ther. 34:95–101, 1980.
53. Neff, W.: Work and Human Behavior. New York: Atherton Press, 1968.
54. Herzberg, F.: The Motivation to Work. New York: John Wiley & Sons, 1959.
55. Stebbins, R.: Amateurs: On the Margin Between Work and Leisure. Beverly Hills: Sage, 1979.
56. Lyman, S. and Scott, M.: A Sociology of the Absurd. New York: Appleton-Century-Crofts, 1970.
57. Shannon, P.: Work-play theory and the occupational therapy process. Am. J. Occup. Ther. 26:169–172, 1972.
58. Frankl, V.: Man's Search for Meaning: An Introduction to Logotherapy. New York: Washington Square Press, 1982.
59. Dubos, R. and Escande J.: Quest: Reflections on Medicine, Science, and Humanity. New York: Harcourt, Brace Jovanovich, 1979.
60. Goodman, P.: Growing Up Absurd. New York: Vintage Books, 1956.
61. Johnson, J. and Kielhofner, G.: The role of occupational therapy in the health care system of the future. In Kielhofner, G. (ed): Health Through Occupation: Theory and Practice in Occupational Therapy. Philadelphia: F. A. Davis, in Press.
62. Haworth, J. T. and Smith, M. A. (eds): Work and Leisure. Princeton NJ: Princeton Book Company, 1976.
63. Reilly, M.: A psychiatric occupational therapy program as a teaching model. Am. J. Occup. Ther. 20:61–67, 1966.
64. Kalish, R.: The Later Years: Social Applications of Gerontology. Monterey: Brooks-Cole, 1977.
65. Gregory, M.: Occupational behavior and life satisfaction among retirees. Unpublished Master's Project, Department of Occupational Therapy, Virginia Commonwealth University, 1981.
66. Cherfas, J.: It's only a game. In Cherfas, Lewin: Not Work Alone: A Cross-Cultural View of Activities Superfluous to Survival. Beverly Hills: Sage Publications, 1980.

67. Mead, G. H.: Mind, Self and Society. Chicago: University of Chicago Press, 1934.
68. Duthie, J.: Athletics: The ritual of a technological society? In Schwartzman H. B. (ed): Play and Culture. West Point NY: Leisure Press, 1980.
69. Cox, H.: The Feast of Fools. New York: Harper and Row, 1969.
70. Arens, W.: Playing with agression. In Cherfas, Lewin: Not Work Alone: A Cross-Cultural View of Activities Superfluous to Survival. Beverly Hills: Sage Publications, 1980.
71. Huizinga, J.: Homo Ludens. Boston: Beacon Press, 1955.
72. Lavenda, R.: From festival of progress to masque of degradation: Carnival in Carcas as a changing metaphor for social reality. In Schwartzman H. B. (ed): Play and Culture. West Point, New York: Leisure Press, 1980.
73. Berger, P.: The Human Shape of Work. Chicago: Henry Regnery Co., 1964.
74. Henry, J.: Culture Against Man. New York: Vintage Books, 1965.

CHAPTER 4

The Human Development Process *Mary Margaret Daub*

What Is Human Development?

Human beings grow and mature, fulfilling their needs and striving to interact with their environment. They gain competence from this process of interaction and adaptation, gradually building a realistic sense of self-worth. Thus, each person becomes a unique individual with the potential of self-actualization.

Human development can be defined as changes in the structure, thought, or behavior of a person that occur as a function of both biological and environmental influences.[1] These changes may be quantitative or qualitative. Quantitative changes, such as height, physical skills, and vocabulary are easily understood and measured. Qualitative changes are not so easily measured, because they include a subjective element; there is no scale on which to weigh the influence of social interactions, the significance of dreams, or the level of a child's self-awareness.

This quantitative and qualitative development involves an ongoing, orderly process that continues from conception to death.

How Is Human Development Studied?

Human development can be studied from many perspectives. Biologists, psychologists, epistemologists, anthropologists, and others investigate the principles and processes of human development but from varied points of view.

Methods of study also differ. We can study and experiment with animal behavior and draw implications concerning human behavior. We can study human behavior in an experimental setting and draw conclusions from controlled situations. We can do a longitudinal study (observation of the same individual over an extended period of time) or a cross-sectional study of behavior (observation of different individuals of different ages at one time). We can follow a specific trait or pattern of behavior in various cultures and construct cross-cultural hypotheses concerning development.

For our immediate purposes, we will view the following developmental aspects of a person that contribute and interrelate to make him or her such a miraculous and complex entity: physical, sensory, perceptual, emotional, cognitive, cultural, and social. As the individual grows, these aspects mature and expand along a developmental continuum. Although the aspects are distinct from each other at one level, they are dynamically interrelated and interdependent.

Why Study Human Development?

Occupational therapists work with individuals who have had an interruption in one or more areas of development somewhere along the life continuum. In order to provide a meaningful service to these individuals, the therapist must understand the underlying principles of man's growth and function and the sequences of growth and behavior that are somewhat predictable for normal human development. (For our purposes, normal is determined by that wide range of data collected for a particular population within a given time and culture, referring to a specific area or segment of development.)

The occupational therapist is an agent of change. The client, often against severe odds, must change and adapt within his or her life situation. The therapist can directly influence the quality of that change. Therefore, the therapist must know the range and potential for change available and must have a working knowledge of those concepts of change and adaptation inherent in the study of human development.

The primary motivation is pragmatic; the normal must be learned in order to assist clients with a disruption in the normal pattern of development. But a second motivation inevitably lures us—the age-old curiosity about who we are, how we began, and how we can grow and change. The study of development sheds light on these questions.

Factors that Influence Human Development

Biological and environmental influences act upon each individual making up that individual's unique gestalt. Biological influences include stages of growth, maturation, and aging. Growth is increase in size, function, or complexity up to some point of optimal maturity. Maturation is the emergence of an organism's genetic potential; it consists of a series of preprogrammed changes which comprise alterations not only in the organism's structure and form but also in its complexity, integration, organization, and function. Aging is biological evolution beyond the point of optimal maturity.[2]

Environmental influences touch everyone at each moment of the day. Sensory input and interpersonal interactions within the home and community can create physiological and emotional stress or comfort. These major influences will be studied further as they relate to learning and the developmental process.

General Principles of Human Development

There are some general principles and issues of human growth and development that must be understood before looking closer at specific areas of normal human growth.

1. *Development is orderly, predictable, sequential, and cumulative.* Even though each individual is unique, he or she possesses particular patterns of behavior following a definite sequence. For example, a child is capable of rolling over before sitting, sitting before standing, and standing before walking. With maturation, development expands by building on previous acquisitions. Developed behaviors continue to influence the future functioning of the emerging being. Since development is cumulative, a child's experiences may have definitive effects on his behavior in adult life.

2. *Each child develops at a different pace.* There is a wide range of individual differences along the normal continuum. Normative data show, for example, that by 26 months a child should be able to combine two words. In reality, some children are speaking by that time, some are not. For example, at two years, Megan is happily combining words into phrases and short sentences: "Me go store," "Mommy give candy." However, Megan's friend Mike speaks only when his need is pressing and then only the short effective word or syllable: "wawa" when he wants a drink, "bye" when he would like to go outside. This does not necessarily mean that Mike has a developmental problem. Other operant factors may be (1) the amount of stimulation in the home environment and (2) the amount and intensity of physical or psychological stress he may be encountering. These factors may cause only a temporary delay in the development of a particular function. Perhaps Mike's assumed hesitant speech follows a recent bout with measles. Once his health and confidence are restored, he may quickly return to a more age-appropriate pattern of speech.

3. *The expectation of others affects a child's behavior.* Mike's parents, for example, may value verbal expression and expect Mike to be more verbal than he is. On the other hand, his sister and brother (siblings) anticipate his needs and often do not allow Mike the opportunity to verbalize his requests.

4. *At any one stage of development a child might be placing particular emphasis on one aspect at the expense of another.* For example, a 3-year-old may be developing gross motor skills in play and doing little in the area of fine motor skills. This emphasis may be a function of maturation, the desire to learn a specific skill, or a result of environmental/cultural influences.

Chess proposes eight areas[3] in which individual differences are most conspicuous:

Activity level. Children vary in their level of movement and activity (even when asleep).

Regularity. Children have different "biological clocks" in terms of self-imposed schedules and their daily demands of themselves and others.

Adaptability to routine changes. Some children readily accept changes in schedules; others bitterly resist the new and different.

Level of sensory threshold. Some children can sleep through a thunderstorm while others awake at the slightest noise.

Positive or negative mood. Some children appear either happy or sad no matter what the situation.

Intensity of response. Some children's responses are always noisy, bellowing, and active (high energy level); some have mild responses even when angry (low energy level).

Distractibility. Some children study with radio and television blaring; some require almost absolute quiet in order to study effectively.

Persistency. Some children just sit for hours and refuse to give up until the task is finished or solved. Some leave trails of unfinished tasks and are always looking for something new.

5. *The behavior of a child does not consistently "improve"; it seems to alternate between periods of equilibrium (a good balance) and disequilibrium (less balance).* The level of balance a child reaches is dependent on his/her stage of maturation and on effective interaction within the environment.

The question then arises: How do I know when a child has a developmental delay?

1. Be a keen observer. Observational skills can be learned. Train yourself to become more aware of your human and nonhuman environment.
2. Know the normal sequences of maturation and the resultant behaviors.
3. Know the extremes of the normative scales, since they may be indicators of a delay or dysfunction.
4. Look at the child as a *total* being.

A person's action or reaction is not a function of any one aspect of human development; rather, it is a function of the relationships of all areas of development at any given point in his or her life span.

Principles of Maturation

There are certain principles of maturation that tend to be relatively independent of environmental influences. They are listed:

1. *Cephalocaudal Pattern of Development.* Muscular development, control, and coordination progress from the head to the feet. Head control precedes

that of the trunk and lower extremities. A child must have good head control if he is to develop other *effective* motor skills.

2. *Proximal–Distal and Medial(Rostral)–Lateral Patterns of Development.* Parts of the body closest (proximal) to the spine tend to be controlled in a coordinated manner before the parts farthest (distal) away from it. Coordination of shoulder musculature, for example, precedes that of the hand and fingers. Muscle coordination also follows a medial–lateral course of development: it proceeds from the mid-point of the body outward (anatomical position). A child is able to grasp first with the ulnar side of his hand, and he gradually develops control from the radial side.

3. *Mass to Specific Pattern of Development.* Initially much of the motor activity of the infant consists of whole body movement. With maturity, these undifferentiated and generalized mass responses become more specific. At first the neonate moves his arms freely in no specific pattern; in a few months he will be able to grasp an object.

4. *Gross Motor to Fine Motor Pattern of Development.* Since control of proximal musculature precedes that of distal musculature, it follows that mastery of the larger muscles precedes mastery of the smaller muscles. This mastery must then become even more refined and definitive to allow for the acquisition of skills.

These four principles governing growth are not static but are continuously influencing motor development.

Theoretical Foundations
Learning Theory

Learning is the basic developmental process by which an individual's behavior is changed by the environment. Learning is a relatively permanent change in behavior or in the capacity for behavior resulting from either experience or practice.[4] This change occurs through experience and repetition. Psychologists have developed theories and paradigms to account for an individual's ability to adapt within his or her life space. Their theories serve as a framework for understanding varied aspects of human development.

Behavioral Theory

Some learning theorists view the individual as a purely responsive being, a mechanistic result of present and past environments. They observe the individual making responses to stimuli but give little regard to interpreting underlying reasons for those responses. Learning theorists view mankind within narrow parameters, assuming that behavior is a function of immediate stimuli. For them, learning takes place via respondent (classical) and/or operant conditioning.

In *classical* conditioning (1) two stimuli are presented *at the same time.* One is reinforcing (*e.g.,* food); the other is irrelevant (*e.g.,* sound of refrigerator door). This leads to (2) the expectation of reinforcement, and concomitant automatic response (*e.g.,* salivation), associated with the irrelevant stimulus (*Learning has taken place.*) Thus (3) the irrelevant stimulus is presented without the reinforcing stimulus, and there is a response.

In *operant conditioning* (1) reinforcement (*e.g.,* praise or candy) is presented *following* behavior. Therefore (2) reinforcement is associated with the behavior. (*Learning has taken place.*) Thus (3) behavior is repeated.

For the learning theorists, learning is a direct result of one or the other of these processes. In reality, even within the limitations of this theory, most learning would probably combine the two processes.

Social Learning Theory

The social learning theory is an outgrowth of learning theory. The proponents of social learning theory believe that most learning takes place through observing behavior and the effects of behavior. They attempt to explain why mankind uses models to learn social traits and how a socially acceptable repertoire of behaviors is developed. Research in this area proves to be very interesting. In 1963 Bandura, Ross, and Ross[5] showed children films that demonstrated levels of aggressive behavior. One group saw this behavior rewarded, another saw it punished, another saw nonaggressive play, and still another saw no film. Results indicated that children who saw aggressive behavior rewarded were more aggressive in play, while those who saw it punished tended to avoid aggressive play.

Although the learning theorists have given developmentalists volumes of empirically-based research explaining human behavior, the types of behavior that lend themselves to experimental methods are limited. These theorists cannot explain complex qualitative behaviors such as emotions or individual differences. Thus the social learning theory is best applied to specific behaviors rather than to the total area of development.

Psychoanalytical Theory

Sigmund Freud, Erik Erikson, and other NeoFreudians, deal primarily with emotional and personality development.

Sigmund Freud

Freud looks at the unconscious biological drives as the primary forces behind human behavior. Personality development, according to Freud, occurs in five psychosexual stages. The first three, *oral stage, anal stage,* and *phallic stage,* center around areas of the body that at each stage become a center for pleasure. These stages are followed by the *latency* and *genital stages,* during which the personality is influenced by degrees of sexual interest, socialization, and an evolving focus on life goals. Freud sets the stage for the explanation of development of an individual's unconscious mind and its relationship to the ability to function.

Erik Erikson

A NeoFreudian, Erikson expands Freud's theory to include the societal environment. He focuses on human psychosocial development. Erikson sees personality development as progressively unfolding throughout the life cycle. He does not place paramount importance on childhood experiences as Freud does. His eight stages of development are delineated by eight emotional crises or issues that must be resolved by the person (Table 4-1).

The resolution of these issues is the balance between the negative and positive poles of each stage. This resolution and its importance at any one point in life is a function of the individual's relationship to his place in his social and cultural environment. How a person resolves a crisis directly affects the quality of his or her ability to deal with a subsequent developmental issue. Further, Erikson believes that these crises may emerge throughout life.

The basic strength of theorists such as Freud and Erikson is their willingness to look at the whole person and at the conscious and unconscious factors of emotional development. They deal with interpersonal relationships, particularly as they relate to childhood experiences.

Table 4-1 *Erikson's Eight Emotional Issues.*

Stages	Ages
Trust—Mistrust	0–1
Autonomy—Shame	1–3
Initiative—Guilt	4–5
Industry—Inferiority	6–11
Identity—Role Diffusion	12–18
Intimacy—Isolation	young adult
Generativity—Stagnation	middle age
Ego Integrity—Despair	aging

The weakness of psychoanalytical theory lies in the difficulty of defining parameters of development and of validating research. Most data are gleaned from adults whose subjective reconstruction of their childhood experiences may lead to invalid or vague conclusions.

Cognitive Theory

Jean Piaget

Piaget, biologist–epistemologist, investigates the origin, nature, methods, and limits of human knowledge (Table 4-2).

In contrast to the learning theorists, Piaget sees the human being as active, alert, and capable. A person processes information rather than merely receiv-

ing it. He does more than respond to stimuli; he gives structure and meaning to stimuli. Piaget postulates that until a certain age, children form judgments via their perceptual world rather than via principles of logic: "What you see is what you get." If the child's perceptions and experiences (schemata—methods of processing information) fit a structure within his mind, they are assimilated or understood. If the information received does not fit existing structure, the mind must change in order to accommodate the new experience. The schemata of a child expand as he/she grows. A person continuously adjusts his or her schemata in order to assimilate and accommodate new information. The human mind seeks equilibrium between assimilation and accommodation just as the human body seeks biological homeostasis.

As the child grows, his structural abilities to accommodate new information grow also. Piaget sees

Table 4-2 *The Continuum of Cognitive Development.*

Modality of Intelligence	Phases	Stages	Approximate Chronological Age
Sensorimotor intelligence	Sensorimotor Phase	1. Use of reflexes	0 to 1 month
		2. First habits and primary circular reactions	1 to 4½ months
		3. Coordination of vision and prehension, secondary circular reactions	4½ to 9 months
		4. Coordination of secondary schemata and their application to new situations	9 to 12 months
		5. Differentiation of action schemata through tertiary circular reactions, discovery of new means	12 to 18 months
		6. First internalization of schemata and solution of some problems by deduction	18 to 24 months
Representative intelligence by means of concrete operations	Preconceptual Phase	1. Appearance of symbolic function and the beginning of internalized actions accompanied by representation	2 to 4 years
	Intuitive Thought Phase	2. Representational organizations based on either static configurations or on assimilation to one's own action	4 to 5½ years
		3. Articulated representational regulations	5½ to 7 years
	Concrete Operational Phase	1. Simple operations (classifications, seriations, term-by-term correspondences, etc.)	7 to 9 years
		2. Whole systems (Euclidian coordinates, projective concepts, simultaneity)	9 to 11 years
Representative intelligence by means of formal operations	Formal Operational Phase	1. Hypothetico-deductive logic and combinatorial operations	11 to 14 years
		2. Structure of "lattice" and the group of 4 transformations	14 years—on

From Maier, H. W. (ed.): *Three Theories of Child Development: The Contributions of Erik H. Erikson, Jean Piaget and Robert R. Sears,* revised ed. New York: Harper & Row, 1969, p. 155. Reprinted with permission. The source was Piaget's paper: Les Stades du Developpement intellectuel de l'Enfant et de l'Adolescent (1956). Adapted from Table 1, Intelligence is an ultimate goal, in Décarié, T. G.: *Intelligence and Affectivity in Early Childhood.* New York: International Universities Press, 1965, p. 15. Reprinted with permission.

this as occurring in four major steps. The steps and mode of learning for each follow:

1. Sensorimotor Period—body and movement
2. Preoperational Period—imagery
3. Concrete Operational Period—concrete human/ nonhuman environment
4. Formal Operational Period—abstraction

Jerome Bruner

Bruner, also a cognitive theorist, investigates the individual as an artist (aesthetic being) and as a scientist (problem solver). Like Piaget, he sees the qualitative changes in the cognitive structures corresponding to biological growth. Both see the mind developing in stages. Bruner describes three stages and the modes of learning:

1. Enactive Stage—the infant learns through action
2. Iconic Stage—the use and development of imagery
3. Symbolic Stage—the use of language to relate

Piaget and Bruner differ on the role of language in development. Piaget views thought as preceding language skill while Bruner sees language as a causative factor in acquiring problem-solving ability.

Unlike learning theorists, cognitive theorists attempt to explain that the individual is motivated by his or her own basic competence and not merely by a stimulus-response reaction.[6] They also account for the role of such things as values, beliefs, and attitudes.

The major concern of cognitive theory is intellectual development; it does not explain all of human behavior (for example, social, emotional, and personality development). However, some of its proponents are now investigating these areas.

Humanistic Self-Theory of Self-Development

Humanistic psychologists react to the environmental determinism of learning and psychoanalytic theorists. Their primary focus is the individual's concept of *self*. They see man as self-determining and creative. Their aim is to maximize human potential. These theorists view each individual optimistically as a function of the individual's self. "Man experiences himself as well as others as spontaneously self-determining and creatively striving toward a goal."[7]

Abraham Maslow

Maslow stresses that each person has an innate need for self-actualization. It is possible to attain this in-nate goal only when a well-integrated individual has satisfied "lower needs" such as safety, love, food, and shelter.

Carl Rogers

Rogers, another humanist, is concerned with helping each individual realize his/her own potential by creating an interpersonal climate for growth with characteristics such as empathy, unconditional willingness to accept a person as he or she is, and a genuine involvement in the person's growth. The strength of this relatively new approach to human development is its concern with real-life situations. Humanistic theory is becoming an important consideration in educational programs for children, although its primary concern is adult adjustment. It does not, however, incorporate a method for achieving self-actualization.

Ethology

Ethologists study humans and animals in their natural environments and view them as having evolved similar behavior traits. They think it possible that humans, like other animals, have inherited behavior patterns. Ethologists do not ignore the history and the situation of behavior patterns, but essentially they are looking at behavior in terms of preserving the individual or the species within the evolution of civilization.

Confronted with the situation of a child crying, an ethologist considers four components: *immediate cause*—hunger; *historical cause*—child was fed when she cried in the past; *adaptive cause*—cry triggers an alarm for the mother to get food; *evolutionary cause*—child is immobile, she cannot run to her mother, and so crying is a dominant response.

Ethology is an interesting and relatively new way of studying human behavior. It presupposes that animal behavior is a valid indicator of human behavior. A growing interest in its methods and principles indicates that ethology will pay an increasing role in the study of human development.

Maturational Theory

Arnold Gesell

Gesell purports that the baby's behavior is modified as a consequence of physiological maturation. He feels that the child requires only general support and attention from the outside environment in order to develop normally. Gesell emphasizes the stability and conservatism of growth. "All things considered, the inevitableness and surety of maturation are the most impressive characteristics of his early development. It is the hereditary ballast which conserves and stabilizes the growth of each individual infant."[8]

Gesell developed normative data about a child's gross motor, fine motor, adaptive skill, language, and social development as they relate to maturation of the central nervous system. He provides actual chronological scales for the parameters of normal development against which possible developmental delays can be detected. Such scales may serve the occupational therapist as a base line for setting occupational therapy goals and plans. Data collected from a large population of children evaluated by such scales may serve as a basis for research in child development.

Normative data are and must be updated continually. Scales must be used cautiously. A therapist has to know the type of population on which the scale was standardized and when it was developed. Many scales are not done cross-culturally and may be invalid for certain groups of children.

Why Theories of Human Development Are Important to the Occupational Therapist

1. Theories serve as an organizing mechanism. They attempt to sort out some of the complex factors in development.
2. Theories provide a basis for frames of reference from which one can develop therapeutic program objectives and treatment.
3. Theories are a basis for the generation of research that is needed in the field of occupational therapy.
4. Knowledge of different theories extends insight into human behavior, presenting alternative explanations of behavior on which to base treatment goals.
5. Theories provide the bases for justification and accountability. In essence, a theory becomes the rationale for our treatment process.

In adhering to a single theory to the exclusion of others the therapist must keep the following in mind.
1. No one theory accounts for each and every aspect of the developmental process; therefore, the therapist must fully understand the parameters of any chosen theory.
2. The therapist must be able to translate the theory effectively into occupational therapy application.
3. Strict adherence to just one theory does not always allow for individual differences.
4. A single-theory approach may narrow a therapist's perspective and limit professional growth potential.

On the other hand, when a therapist chooses an eclectic approach, that is, bases a rationale on varied sources or theories, caution is advised because:
1. In order to be truly eclectic, the therapist must be thoroughly versed in each theory. "A little knowledge" here can be truly dangerous.
2. The therapist must know the advantages and limitations of these theories so as to present a clearly defined rationale for client treatment.

No matter which approach is chosen, it is imperative that everyone involved in the treatment process (1) know what rationale is being used, (2) understand how the rationale can be translated into occupational therapy practice, (3) be clear about how this treatment can be adapted to the individual client's needs, and (4) concur with the adoption of this rationale as a basis for treatment.

Prenatal Development

Aristotle observed the growth of the chick embryo. He surmised that the embryo was a mixture of seminal fluid and menstrual blood and that the embryo carried in the female was stimulated into growth by the male. Five hundred years later Galen purported a different theory. He believed that a miniature baby was encased in the egg, to be "uncased" by the male before growth could begin. This imaginative theory dominated scientific thought for 1500 years.

In 1677 Van Leewenhoek observed the movement of the male sperm. This discovery led to two major theories of prenatal development in the 17th and 18th centuries. The *ovists* believed that a prefabricated baby was contained in the mother's egg, to be stimulated into growth by the sperm. The *homunculists* believed that a baby was formed in the tip of the sperm, the womb serving as the incubator environment for growth.

These theories prevailed until 1759 when Wolff postulated that both the male and female contributed equally to the growth of the human organism. Approximately 50 years later the human ovum was seen under the microscope. It was not until 1930, however, that the ripened human egg and sperm were observed. Finally, in 1944, scientists witnessed the union of the egg and sperm. Since that time a myriad of knowledge about prenatal development has been accumulated, so that now we have a clear picture of human development from a single cell to a person.

Periods of Prenatal Development

Following fertilization of the ovum, there is a gestation period of 266 days (with a grace period of 11 days). The first phase (2 weeks) of prenatal growth is the *germinal period.* This is primarily a time of cell division and differentiation. Once the growing cell is fully implanted in the wall of the uterus, the *embryonic period* begins. During the embryonic period (8 weeks), structures and organs are formed and differentiated. Approximately 12 weeks following conception the *fetal period* begins: the first bone cells are developed, and growth continues until birth.

These first several weeks of development are marked by the emergence of physical characteristics. Approximately 26 days following conception a body form is evolving, and there is the beginning of arm and leg buds. Two days later the arms are developing at a greater rate than the legs. By the end of the first month, the details of the head with rudimentary eyes, ears, mouth, and brain are seen faintly. The brain already shows primitive specialization. There is also a primitive heart and umbilical cord as well as such organs as the liver, kidney, and stomach. The primitive embryo is now ¼ to ½ inch long, the size of half a pea. In one month's time the embryo is 10,000 times larger than the fertilized egg.[9]

By the end of the second month the embryo has familiar features: face, eyes, ears, nose, lips, tongue, muscles, and finally skin covering. Flanagan states that the developing arms are no bigger than exclamation points, but they have discernible fingers and thumbs. The legs have knees, ankles, and toes. All organs in the body are formed. The brain sends out impulses, the muscles and nerves are working together, and the heart is beating regularly and steadily. The endocrine system is functioning and so are the stomach, liver, and kidneys. Even isolated reflexes can be elicited. In several months these primitive systems will be truly functional.

The third month after conception traditionally marks the beginning of the fetal period. By the end of this month the fetus has become active. It can kick, turn, close fingers, move its thumb into opposition, and open its mouth, although its eyelids are still closed. This period is marked by refinements of facial and extremity features. The palate and lips are formed and fused. Sexual differentiation is beginning.

The fourth month is a period of growth in which the lower body parts develop more rapidly. The fetus weighs approximately 4 ounces and is 6 inches long. Its muscles and reflexive capabilities are maturing. The mother can now feel a "quickening" movement.

The fifth month is a stage of continued refinement. There is an increase in spontaneous activity. Fetal movements are markedly perceived by the mother. The fetus sleeps and wakes. However, its respiratory system is still too immature for life outside the uterus.

In the sixth month the eyelids of the fetus open.

Its eyes are formed and capable of movements (lateral and vertical). Taste buds have developed, as have eyelashes and brows. The fetus has a marked grasp reflex. It now weighs approximately 1½ pounds and is 12 to 14 inches long. But its breathing patterns are irregular; it can usually survive for only 24 hours outside the womb.

During the seventh month the cerebral hemispheres cover almost all the brain, and the organism can make specialized responses. If born now, the child can survive in a sheltered environment.

The eighth and ninth months are periods of refinement of function. The immune system of the fetus matures, enabling it to sustain independent life more safely when it is born.

During gestation, the fetus has grown from 1 to 200 million cells, and its weight at birth is 600 billion times greater than its conceptual weight.[10] (If we were to continue to grow at our prenatal rate until adulthood, we would be 20 feet tall and our weight would exceed the earth's weight by many million times.)

Given this brief account of normal prenatal activity, we must consider those factors of heredity and environment which may affect and/or alter normal growth and development.

Inherited and Environmental Influences

Although the uterus is a relatively safe and stable environment, it is not immune to environmental factors. The seriousness of the effect of these factors depends on (1) the type of influence, (2) the intensity of the influence, and (3) the time the influence was introduced.

Since the germinal and embryonic stages are formation and differentiation periods, this first trimester of pregnancy (first 12 weeks) is critical in development. If normal growth is interrupted during this time, defects can originate. Major environmental influences include:
1. Ingestion of certain agents or drugs.
2. Factors in maternal health and nutrition such as vitamin deficiency or excess, endocrine levels, exposure to roentgen rays, exposure to virus and bacteria, emotional state of the mother (brings about chemical changes that may cross the placental barrier), Rh factor, composite factors, and cultural influences.

Hereditary factors also contribute to the integrity of the growing organism. It is imperative that the therapist understand (1) the basis of genetic functioning, (2) implications of genetic malfunctioning on the developing organism, and (3) those dysfunctions that are a direct result of genetic inheritance.

Scientists have researched DNA (deoxyribonucleic acid), the complex molecules which make up the genes. They have shown how the information transmitted by the genes determines the functions of the body. The increased knowledge in this area has shed light on those developmental traits that have specific hereditary components. These components are dependent on one's autosomal, dominant, and recessive inheritance, sex-linked inheritance, and chromosomal integrity. Genetic make-up delineates the parameters for development. Environmental factors influence the quality and extent to which heredity affects the potential for growth.

The nature/nurture controversy or the relationship and extent of hereditary and environmental factors on the individual continues. In a classic article on the nature/nurture question, Anastasi says "the nature and extent of the influence of each type of factor depends on the contribution of the others."[11]

The Developmental Continuum

Fifteen or twenty years ago an infant was considered a dependent creature who could not see, hear, or interact within the environment. Today we know that the infant and growing child possess a vast repertoire of capabilities.

This section presents an overview and appreciation of a normal child's development from birth to adulthood, based on major developmental aspects (Fig. 4-1). Not all aspects will be considered at each milestone of growth, only those considered most significant for that stage. Table 4-7 at the end of the chapter presents several of these major areas in continuity.

To enliven this study, we will observe an imaginary child, Leslie, with her family and friends. Leslie, the typical child, is a prototype of any normal child traversing the developmental continuum.

Infancy

The Neonate

Early one morning, Leslie abandons the warm, dark, comfortable womb of her mother and struggles her way into a cool, bright, noisy, and expectant world. Her lusty protests elicit smiles of relief from her waiting audience but add little to her red, scrunched-up, cheese-coated natural beauty.

The difficult trip down the birth canal leaves most neonates looking a little the worse for wear. The head may be somewhat misshapen as a result of pressure and/or forceps delivery. Face and eyes are usually puffy and the limbs, particularly the feet, may be in an awkward position. The newborn must adjust to several drastic changes in lifestyle: a drop in body temperature, an external mode of nourishment, a different metabolic system, and a redirection of oxygen flow. (Adjustment to change in oxygen concentration is as great as that experienced by a mountain-climber descending from Mt. Everest to Katmandu.)

Leslie is a full-term neonate; she measures 20 inches and weighs 7 pounds. (Normal range: 19 to 22 inches; 5½ to 9½ pounds.) Before she is five minutes old, her general health is evaluated by the Apgar Test (see Table 4-3). Other similar tests may be used. Special attention is given to general reflex response, heart rate, muscle tone, and color. A score of 7 or more indicates that her health is within normal limits.[12]

Leslie can see within an 8 to 12 inch range and soon after birth prefers complex patterns to simple ones. She may show a preference for the human face and for clear rather than blurred images.

Fantz, among others, has made marvelous discoveries about the visual ability of infants. In one test he presented simple pattern stimuli to infants and found there was significant preference for the complex pattern. He also presented three different oval images to 49 infants ranging in age from 4 days to 6 months. The images included (1) a stylized human face, (2) the same features of the stylized face in a scrambled pattern, and (3) an oval with a solid dark patch at one end. All the infants tested showed a definite preference for the human face. Further studies found that the infants selectively focus on the eye region of the face before encompassing the entire face.[13]

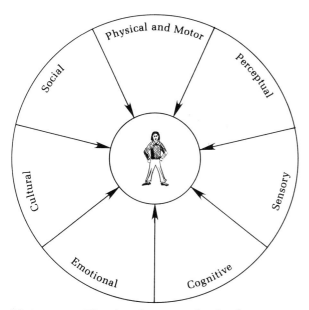

Figure 4-1. The developmental wheel.

Table 4-3 *Apgar Test—An Objective Test for Evaluating a Newborn's Health.*

Test	Scores 0	1	2
Heart rate	Absent	Less than 100	More than 100
Breathing	Absent	Slow (irregular)	Strong cry
Muscle tone	Decreased (floppy)	Some flexion of extremities	Active movement
Reflex response	Absent	Grimace	Vigorous cry
Color (Nonwhite child alternative test of mucous membranes, palms, and soles are used)	Blue, pale	Body pink, extremities blue	Completely pink

Adapted from Apgar, V.: Proposal for a new method of evaluating the newborn infant. Anesth. Analg. 32:260–267, 1953.

Leslie can detect changes in temperature and distinguish tastes. Even as early as the third or fourth day she demonstrates a preference for sweet and a dislike for bitter flavors.[14]

Leslie can also smell and discriminate between odors. Lipsitt has shown that newborns can distinguish between two smells, and that they may actually despise foul odors.[15] He also discovered that infants as little as 55 hours old can differentiate smells with no rehearsals. When introduced to a strong odor, the babies startle and cry. As they grow older, the babies tend to get used to the strong odors if provided in small doses.

Leslie seems to have an amazing auditory ability. She demonstrates preference for certain sounds and volume as well as an ability to localize those sounds. An experiment by Lipsitt and Siqueland[16] demonstrated the 1-day-old infant's ability to hear and learn. They paired (1) the sound of a bell and a bottle on the child's right side and (2) the sound of a buzzer and a bottle on the child's left side. Infants tested were able to distinguish the buzzer from the bell, right from left, and most important, they understood the contingency between the sound and reward. Scientists have also found that infants seem to prefer high-pitched sounds to low-pitched sounds. This poses an interesting question: Since the mother's voice is usually higher pitched, is there an inborn preference for her voice? Other studies have already confirmed the soothing effect of the mother's heartbeat on the infant.

Leslie responds favorably to rocking and bottom-patting. Her contemporary in another culture is content when completely swaddled. No matter which system is employed, babies react favorably to the combination of light touch, warmth, and pressure, and mothers rely heavily on the touch system for peace in the nursery. Touch has been called the communication system of infants, and more and more studies are emphasizing the importance of tactile stimulation in the neonatal period. Frank's studies[17] with institutionalized babies indicate that infrequent handling can lead to delayed development.

Leslie's motor development at this period is primarily reflexive (see reflex development, Table 12-1); *her nonreflexive motor activity is gross and random.* She responds with total body movements to sudden changes within her environment. She typically lies on her tummy in a flexed position with fisted hands, but she has a variety of both fine and gross motor movements.

In observing the neonate, it is important to consider the state of consciousness or *state* of the infant. Reactions to stimuli must be interpreted within the context of the presenting state of consciousness, since reactions may vary markedly as the infant passes from one state to another. State depends on physiological variables such as hunger, nutrition, degree of hydration, and the time within the wake–sleep cycle of the infant. The pattern of states and the movement from one state to another appear to be important characteristics of infants in the neonatal period. This kind of evaluation may be the best predictor of the infant's receptivity and ability to respond to stimuli in a cognitive sense.[18] In addition, the neonate's use of a state to maintain control of reactions to environmental and internal stimuli is an important mechanism and reflects the neonate's potential for organization.[19]

An example of a sleep state would be "deep sleep, with regular breathing, eyes closed, no spontaneous activity except startle or jerky movements at quite regular intervals; external stimuli produce startles with some delay; suppression of startle is rapid, and state changes are less likely from other states; no eye movement."[20]

During the first month of life, Leslie displays undifferentiated crying. Early crying is a reflexive form of communication. Although we often think of it as a reaction to discomfort, we cannot determine anything definite about it at this stage.

Leslie assimilates her environment according to her organic demands, building confidence in it as these demands are met.

To Piaget, the first phase of cognitive development is the sensorimotor phase and the first stage of intelligence is via the use of reflexes (birth to 3 months). By their very nature, a child's reflexes (the spontaneous repetition resulting from internal or external stimulation) provide the necessary experience for future sequential function. Repetition and experience produce regularity, order, and rhythm. Piaget feels that repetitive use of reflexes, combined with neurological and physical maturation, tend to form habits. Repetition and accident lead to new experiences, and these new experiences allow for continued adaptation (assimilation and accommodation) with the environment. For example, Leslie possesses a repertoire of reflexes that support her survival. Her rooting and sucking reflexes meet the need for nourishment. Initially, she does not recognize the breast as the source of nourishment, but with time and repetitive use of the two reflexes, she learns to go right to the source.

Erikson's view of personality development in the infant period centers around acquiring a sense of *trust versus mistrust* (birth to 12 months). This first phase is the foundation for subsequent psychosocial development. For the neonate a sense of trust requires a feeling of physical comfort. If this feeling is given to the child she will extend it to new experiences. If it is not given, the child will have a sense of mistrust arising from unfulfilled physical and psychological needs. Leslie as an infant has her needs met through loving care and attention. Her later outlook on the world will reflect the sense of trust formed in this first stage of development. When an issue relating to trust emerges later in the developmental process, she will resolve it because of her previous positive experience.

According to Freud, a child is in the oral stage of development from birth to 12 to 18 months; her id is striving for immediate gratification of her oral needs. During this stage Leslie gains gratification from sucking, most obviously during feeding. This stage has two substages: (1) oral dependent, when a child can do nothing more assertive than cry to be fed, and (2) oral aggressive, when a child is teething and can achieve gratification by biting as well as sucking.

Behavioral theorists look beyond maturation and environment in order to explain the competency of the infant. Through experimentation with newborns, they conclude that the infant learns through two processes: reward and deprivation. Researchers Kalnins and Bruner[21] wanted to know if infants could control sucking when they were rewarded with something other than food. Pacifiers were wired to slide projec-tors. When the infants sucked the slide was brought into focus; when they did not suck the picture was blurry. The infants were also able to learn to focus the picture if the process for focusing it was reversed. Their only reward was a clear rather than blurred picture.

Behaviorists believe that once the child has learned a specific response to a particular stimulus via reinforcement, he or she can become accustomed to the stimulus and no longer respond to it. This demonstrates another learning phenomenon—*habituation.* Papousek[22] taught infants to turn on a light by movement of the head to the left. The infants turned on the light several times in a short period. Then they stopped, as if they were bored with it all. When the process was reversed (light activated from the right) interest was revived, only to be short lived. This supported not only the competency rather than reward theory of learning, but it indicated that infants (3 weeks old) could habituate. Behaviorists infer from this experiment that infants' sensory capabilities and perceptual processes are more highly developed than was previously thought. It may even imply that children learn best from moderately novel events!

In 1937 an ethologist, Lorenz,[23] described *imprinting*, the process by which animals develop a social attachment for a particular object. Later studies of imprinting imply that the innate instinctual rapid form of learning social behavior common to animals seems evident in human infant/mother relationships as well. Harlow's monkey study[24] is a classical example of imprinting research.

Harlow delineated a number of factors that seem to be important in forming the essential bond between mother and child. He separated baby monkeys from their mothers 6 to 12 hours following birth and raised them with surrogate mothers: one was a terry-cloth-covered mother, the other was a wire-mesh mother. The babies were fed by a bottle attached to each mother. When the monkeys were allowed to spend time with either mother, the babies clung to the cloth mother even if they had been fed by the wire mother. When the baby monkeys were placed in an unfamiliar environment, those babies raised by the cloth mother showed more interest in exploring the surroundings. Following a separation from the mothers for one year, those babies raised by cloth mothers remembered and related to the cloth surrogate, and those raised by the wire mother showed virtually no interest in the wire surrogate.

More recent studies of infant-mother bonding by Klaus and Kennell[25] corroborate our understanding of this very important aspect of development. They expound on maternal and paternal behavior in human beings, extrapolating and expanding observations made on a wide range of animal species. This area of study is interesting, and it may be relevant to extrapolate animal studies to human behavior. However, it must be remembered that human beings rely less on instinctual behavior than do lower animals.

Leslie initiates a social interaction formed with her mother from birth. A social attachment refers to an active, affectionate, reciprocal relationship between two persons as distinguished from all other persons. The interaction between the two individuals continues to strengthen their underlying social bond. The bond between Leslie and her mother seems to be a function of the quality and reciprocity of their initial interaction.

Leslie is also affected, right from the start, by cultural and societal influences. They would include such factors as (1) mothering styles, (2) the role of the father in child rearing, (3) feeding schedules, (4) bottle versus breast feeding, and (5) differences in treatment of male and female infants.

There are many interesting cross-cultural and subcultural studies regarding racial differences and motoric behavior in infants.[26-29] It appears that black babies may be more advanced in motor development, at least during the first 15 months of life. Further study is indicated in order to discover more about the interrelationship between hereditary and environmental influences relating to racial differences in motor development.

Leslie at 1 Month

Leslie is a child of movement and continues to demonstrate reflex postures. She may lift her head briefly but, when unsupported, she still shows definite head lag. When supported in sitting, she may hold her head in line with her back (Fig. 4-2).

Leslie's visual acuity, coordination, and perceptions are evolving. Her eye coordination is better developed. She fixates on her mother's face in response to a smile, and she stares at Mommy for a long time, especially during feeding. She follows a toy from the side to the center of her body. She focuses on objects as long as they are in her direct line of vision. When she sees a person or toy, she gets excited and responds with total body movement. Leslie prefers visual patterns to any kind of color or brightness. She cries deliberately when needing assistance, and she makes small throaty sounds. Leslie now recognizes her parents' voices.

Her physiological state is more stable. According to Dr. Peter H. Wolff, a month-old baby sleeps more than he or she is active and divides the short time awake between drowsiness and alertness.[30]

Leslie expects feedings at certain times, although her daily routine is still somewhat disorganized.

Cultural influences that dominate now include parenting style, schedules and routine, breast or bottle feeding, and amount of handling.

Leslie at 3 Months

Leslie now has an increased capacity to show delight in her world with vocalization, smiling, and increased responsiveness. She is gaining motor function; reflexive postures are decreasing. When picked up, Leslie shows good body alignment. On her tummy (prone), she lifts her head and may be able to maintain that position for a few minutes.

When sitting with support she can assist in holding that position with little head bobbing. Her hands begin to swipe at objects, but they often do not reach the target. Usually Leslie attempts to reach for an object with arms starting at her side and closing in front of her.

Her language is a delight; her vocabulary consists of one-syllable vowel sounds (ooh, ah, ee). She squeals, gurgles, whimpers, and coos in response to someone's voice or smile.

Visually Leslie is able to follow a toy past the midline. Her facial expression toward the toy may be evident. She may also stare at a picture or toy, glancing from one to another. She prefers three-dimensional to two-dimensional pictures. She looks at the rattle in her hand and may accidentally play with it. She explores her face, eyes, and mouth with her hand and repeats an action for its own sake. She virtually searches for a sound and may even stop sucking to search for it. Leslie combines movement and vision more actively within her environment. These behaviors are the precursors of adaptive behavior. According to Piaget,[31] learning now takes place via primary circular responses (1 to 4 months).

A *primary circular response* is an active effort to reproduce a response that was first achieved by accident. The response is repeated purely for the pleasure of the action. This is the beginning of the coordination of sensory information. Leslie, for example, has had the sucking reflex since birth, then one day purely by accident she puts her thumb in her mouth. She sucks her thumb and enjoys it.

Leslie at 7 Months

Leslie moves from a period of total dependence on gravity to a period of emerging control against gravity which ultimately results in postural stability. She sits for several minutes without support, her hands free to hold an object. She can hold two blocks (one in each hand) and can transfer (shift) a block from one hand to the other. She enjoys banging objects.

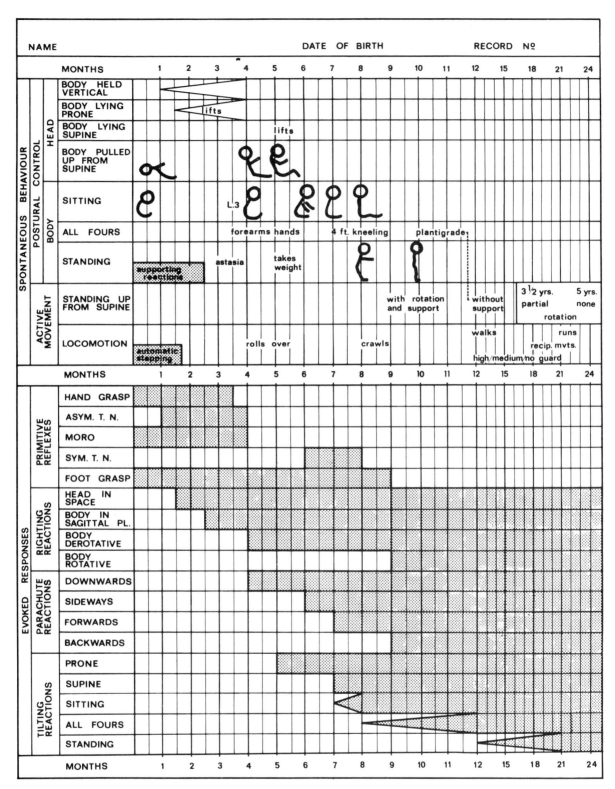

Figure 4-2. Developmental chart. Reprinted with permission from Milani Comparetti A., and Gidoni, E. A.: Routine developmental examination in normal and retarded children. Dev. Med. Child Neurol., 9:766, 1967.

Her creeping is improving, and she goes forward most of the time. She now begins to practice crawling. Leslie puts weight on the palms of her hands and knees, and she rocks back and forth for hours, never quite "getting off." Her 7-month-old friend Andrew demonstrates a variation on this theme. He crawls around using one arm for pulling and one leg for pushing (army crawl). He is very active and even tries pulling himself to standing. In play, both Leslie and Andrew are usually seen with a toy or block in one hand or the other. They love to play with such things as a bunch of keys—shaking, rattling, and mouthing them. They usually prefer larger to smaller objects, and they can pick up toys with thumb and first finger (thumb opposition).

With her increased dexterity and movement, Leslie loves to explore. She scoots around mouthing, poking, and peering at everything. This sudden new freedom of movement exposes her to increased stimulation, and she may have difficulty adapting. She may even experience a period of disequilibrium, temporarily becoming more dependent and fearful of separation, particularly from Mommy. She enjoys interaction, she is delighted with her own image in the mirror, and she displays a delightful sense of humor. Grown up enough to join the family for dinner, she happily finger feeds in her high chair.

Leslie now attempts to imitate sounds. She often puts her favorites together in one breath (for example, ma-mu-di-ba), fooling her vulnerable parents into believing they really hear ma-ma, da-da.

According to Piaget,[32] the child at this age is learning via *secondary circular reactions*. Although new patterns of behavior continue to occur accidentally during random movements, Leslie now repeats them in order to see what results they will bring. She becomes interested in her effect on external objects and events. This stage is the beginning of intentional action.

This stage is also important because it ushers in the beginning of *object permanence*. This concept tells us that objects exist outside of perceptual experience; they are separate entities and continue to exist even if they cannot be seen. Piaget conducted the following experiment to see if his 7-month-old son, Laurent, had the schema of the permanent object:

> At the time of his feeding I show him the bottle, he extends his hand to take it, but, at that moment, I hide it behind my arm. If he sees one end sticking out he kicks and screams and gives every indication of wanting to have it. If, however, the bottle is completely hidden and nothing sticks out, he stops crying and acts for all we know as if the bottle no longer existed, as if it had been dissolved and absorbed into my arm.[33]

Mothers all over the world play peek-a-boo with their infants, who find the game delightful. This activity focuses on the emergence of object permanence.

Leslie at 10 Months

Leslie's struggle against gravity continues; she has gained control of her head, trunk, and arms and is now getting her legs underneath her for support. She is attempting to stand and hesitantly cruises (holds on to objects while walking) around a room. She gets down from a chair or stair now but is cautious of distances, distrusting her visual cues. She carries two small objects in one hand, and she is beginning to differentiate use of her hands. For example, she can hold with one while manipulating with the other.

Socially, Leslie begins to show moods and emotions as she becomes more aware of herself and others. Social approval and imitation are emerging as important facets of behavior. Imitative behavior centers around previous experiences. (For example, Leslie attempts to feed others at the dinner table.) She shows delight when others imitate her posture or movements. Memory of past behavior and objects out of sight (representational memory) and the understanding of distance and depth help Leslie imitate and understand the nature of objects. In play Leslie reaches for toys behind her without seeing them. She continues to learn about properties of objects. Leslie enjoys shaking boxes, listening to a watch tick. She will look into a container and grasp small objects. If she cannot obtain a small object, she usually will poke at it with extended index finger. If she has seen a toy hidden, she will search for it. If the toy is hidden several times in different places, Leslie will continue to return to the first hiding place.

While playing, Leslie jabbers away. She has learned the relationship of certain words and appropriate gestures (for example, "no"—shakes head; "bye"—waves). She says one or two words besides ma-ma and da-da, and she can understand and obey simple commands (for example, "give it to me").

Leslie at 1 Year

Leslie is ready to forge ahead in the world; she has overcome the bondage of gravity. She has been standing and walking with assistance. Now, with increased trunk rotation and eye-hand coordination, Leslie takes her first unsteady steps forward. She walks with her hands raised and a wide-base gait. She meanders forward, looking like a somewhat clumsy, baggy-legged sailor, supremely pleased with her accomplishment. However, when visiting unfamiliar places, Leslie still prefers to crawl.

Her hand control and dexterity is improving. She loves to pick up both small and large objects, and she can hold many toys at one time. At Harvard's Center for Cognitive Studies, visiting infants showed their end-of-the-year dexterity by pushing up and holding a sliding see-through door with one hand and retrieving a toy with the other.[34]

Leslie's conversation has intonation patterns, and she produces sounds specific to her parents' language. She practices her words (two to eight words) such as "bye," "ma-ma," "da-da," "no," "hi." She can imitate sounds of objects ("bow-wow"). (See Sequences of Language Development.[35-37])

Sequences of Language Development

Prelinguistic Speech

Before a child says his first real word, he goes through the following six, and perhaps seven, stages of speech:

1. *Undifferentiated crying.* With "no language but a cry," babies come into this world. Early crying is a reflexive reaction to the environment produced by the expiration of breath.

2. *Differentiated crying.* After the first month of life (and of crying), the close listener can often discriminate a difference between a baby's cries and their causes.

3. *Cooing.* At about six weeks, chance movements of the child's mechanisms produce a variety of simple sounds called cooing. These squeals, gurgles, and bleats are usually emitted when he is happy and contented. The first sounds are vowels, and the first consonant is h.

4. *Babbling.* These vocal gymnastics begin at about three or four months, as a child playfully repeats a variety of sounds. Again, he is most likely to babble when he is contented and when he is alone. As he lies in his crib or sits in his infant seat, he loquaciously, and often loudly, spouts forth a variety of simple consonant and vowel sounds: "ma-ma-ma-ma-ma," "da-da-da-da-da," "bi-bi-bi-bi-bi-bi," and so forth. While most children babble, a few seem to skip this stage. Deaf children babble normally for the first few months of life, but then appear to lose interest when they cannot hear themselves.

5. *Lallation or imperfect imitation.* Some time during the second half of the first year, a child seems to become more aware of the sounds around him. He will become quiet as he listens to some sound. When it stops, he babbles in excitement, accidentally repeating the sounds and syllables he has heard. Then he imitates his own sounds.

6. *Echolalia or imitation of the sounds of others.* At about the age of nine or ten months, a child seems to consciously imitate the sounds made by others, even though he still does not understand them.

7. *Expressive jargon.* During the second year, many children use *expressive jargon.* This term, coined by Gesell, refers to a string of utterances that *sound* like sentences, with pauses, inflections, and rhythms. However, speech is not yet communicated verbally on a consistent basis.

Linguistic Speech

1. *One-word sentence (holophrase).* At about a year, a child points to a cracker, a toy, a pacifier, and says "da." His parents correctly interpret the command as "Give me that" or "I want that." He points to the door and says, "out." His single word thus expresses a complete thought, even though his listeners may not always be able to divine what that complete thought may be.

2. *Multiword sentence.* Some time about the age of two, a child strings together two or more words to make a sentence. When he wants to feed himself with no interference, he says imperiously, "Mommy 'way."

The child may develop a combination of sounds that mean something to him but may not necessarily be understood by the listener. Usually this communication style occurs at the time the child is learning nouns. The sounds or syllables are attached to the newly learned nouns.

The earliest multiword sentences are combinations of nouns and verbs. Other parts of speech, such as articles, prepositions, and adjectives, are lacking. Although these sentences are far from grammatical, they do communicate. This is *telegraphic speech;* it contains only words that carry meaning.

3. *Grammatically correct verbal utterances.* At about the age of three, the child has an impressive command of the language. He now has a vocabulary of some 900 words; he speaks in longer sentences that include all the parts of speech; and he has a good grasp of grammatical principles. His grammar is not the same one used by adults because he makes little allowance for exceptions to the linguistic rules he has assimilated. So, he says, "We goed to the store."

Adapted from: Eisenson, J., et al.: The Psychology of Communication. New York: Appleton-Century-Crofts, 1963; Lenneberg, E. H.: Biological Function of Language. New York: John Wiley & Sons, 1967; Clifton, C.: Language acquisition. In Spencer, T. D., and Kass, N. (eds.): Perspectives in Child Psychology: Research & Review. New York: McGraw-Hill, 1970.

With her peers she engages in parallel play, but while she is on her own Leslie loves to investigate objects. She has the concept of container and contained. She shakes toys, puts blocks in and out of a box, unwraps toys, and delights in looking for a hidden toy, even if she did not see it hidden.

Cognitively, during the first year the child begins to differentiate and generalize experiences. Each experience has signs which evoke a different set of action sequences. Once the child can perceive actions beyond his sensorimotor capabilities, intelligence emerges. The discovery of objects as objects introduces the awareness of spatial relationships. For example, Leslie is putting blocks in a box. She turns them, examines their shapes, and then puts them in the box. For her they occupy space and have dimension. Leslie is also beginning to realize that *she* is doing something, so she is the determiner of some of the events in her environment.

Leslie begins to experience by observation. She lets things happen and observes results. This discovery of new means through active experimentation is referred to by Piaget[38] as *tertiary circular reactions.*

Cultural and societal influences become more diverse. From now on Leslie's learning experiences will be affected more by such cultural factors as:

1. parental attitudes toward activity and their willingness and ability to provide varied learning experiences;
2. schedules and routine;
3. an opportunity for movement and exploration;
4. sexual differences and parental attitudes about them;
5. the type and quality of toys and play the child is allowed to experience.

Preschool Years

Leslie's friends Kim (18 months), Billy (2 years), and Joan (3 years) demonstrate the preschool milestones of behavior.

Kim at 18 Months

Kim is entering the toddler phase—a period of harrowing impulsiveness. He is walking along as most of his peers are, continuing a wide stance gait that lacks a true sense of balance. He may be able to take a few steps backward, but as yet he is unable to kick a ball forward or climb stairs in a smooth, coordinated manner. This is due primarily to his immature equilibrium responses and maturation. He enhances his support system by holding onto objects, and he enjoys pushing and pulling toys. He concentrates on and practices his new-found abilities. For example, Kim has just mastered climbing over the front door-

sill and, much to his mother's chagrin, he keeps going in and out of the door.

In fine motor development, he scribbles spontaneously with a crayon, builds a tower with blocks (two to four blocks), and is able to handle small objects.

At home he is able to bring a cup to his mouth and drink. He can fill his spoon but has difficulty inserting it into his mouth; there is considerable spilling. He attempts to do simple undressing, proudly taking off his hat and socks.

Socially he enjoys other children, but his play is still parallel play. Each child does his/her own thing.

Play at this age is still largely gross motor. The child likes to pull little carts and wagons or carry a favorite doll, teddy bear, or blanket around with him all day. Sensory play is important at this age (for example, sand and water play, pounding and banging pots and pans).

With an increased tone, range, and vocal pitch, Kim enjoys humming and dancing with his whole body. He also enjoys listening to short catchy rhymes, especially if they are action-oriented.

He interacts freely within his environment. Since he is emerging from a relatively dependent phase, Kim cannot always differentiate between what he should and should not do. He forges ahead with great abandon toward autonomy. His feelings about his parents are evolving. His loving attachment continues, but he is beginning to feel and see them as restrictive and frustrating. For the first time Kim encounters a myriad of external limitations.

Kim's vocabulary consists of approximately three words other than "ma-ma" and "da-da." he still communicates primarily by gestures.

According to Erikson,[39] the child is entering Crisis II: *autonomy versus shame* (18 months to 3 years). This stage corresponds to Freud's Anal Period. With the establishment of a sense of trust in his mother and in the world, Kim is developing a sense of self. At the same time, he realizes the limits impinging on him as he begins to assert himself. This push to autonomy is partly maturational. His new-found motor and functional capabilities coupled with increased ability to express desires impel Kim to expand the boundaries of his world. If he is thwarted in this expansion, he may begin to doubt his ability to become autonomous, eventually developing a sense of shame and doubt; however, if he is encouraged to explore (with secure limits or under supervision), his competence will evolve and with it a positive sense of self-worth.

According to Piaget,[40] Kim continues in the Sensorimotor Period (18 months to 2 years), inventing new means through mental combinations. He now has the ability to picture events in his mind; experimentation is not necessary. In effect, he can try out new solutions in his mind and discard solutions that do not work. For example, Kim picks up the plug to the vacuum and toddles over to the socket. Then he remembers (mentally pictures) his mother saying "hot, don't touch." He sits, plug in hand, seriously repeating the warning, "hot, hot, hot." He is also able to imitate actions even when his model is no longer in front of him. The concept of object permanence is fully developed.

Kim now understands visible and invisible displacements. When he looks for a toy that has been hidden in several consecutive places, he will now look for it in the last hiding place. This is an improvement over the previous ability to search for a toy in its first hiding place.

Billy at 2 Years

At 2 years of age, Billy is just beginning to break through into new skill areas and accomplishments. He walks, runs, jumps in place, and climbs stairs. He crawls into, under, around, and over objects. In play he can kick forward and throw a ball overhand.

In fine motor development, he is capable of building a tower of four to eight cubes, and he can make a horizontal bridge of three blocks. His spontaneous block play shows matching of simple shapes and symmetry.

Billy's sensory and perceptual abilities are improving. He is beginning to have good color sense, and by approximately 30 months he will be able to match primary colors. His visual focus is good, and he can recognize objects 8 mm in diameter; but his visual-motor coordination is still rudimentary.

Billy's auditory acuity is double that of a year-old child, and his auditory discrimination has improved.

With increased postural integration, his equilibrium improves and his sense of position in space becomes more accurate.

Emotionally, Billy must learn to deal with a host of feelings such as joy, affection, anger, fear, and frustration. All of these feelings are just as real to a 2-year-old as they are to an adult. He must cope with his new autonomy, with its advantages and limitations.

Autonomy, mastery, and competence refer to slightly different drives, but they are all part of the same motivational and behavioral complex which plays an important part in determining actions throughout life.[41-43]

The "terrible twos" are a time of manifestation of autonomy. Billy must constantly test his new self-image and his hitherto undreamed of powers, sometimes to the destruction of family tranquility.

In play Billy enjoys rhythmical activities. He dances with *great* movement—bouncing, swaying, and tapping his feet. He likes to fill containers with things such as stones and dirt.

At bath time you can hardly see Billy for the boats and toys, and he loves to play in the water. When wielding a crayon he gingerly experiments with vertical, horizontal, and circular motions, but he tends to extend his colorful patterns to his hands, clothes, table, and wall. This is partly due to his lack of fine motor control and partly to his easy distractibility.

Billy also likes to engage in imaginative play, particularly when it involves imitating (playing house, Mommy, Daddy).

At home, Billy can now drink from a small glass. He continues to need supervision when eating and shows definite food preferences. Billy helps dress himself, usually by thrusting his arms into arm holes. He tries to wash and dry his hands but often fails miserably.

"No" becomes his favorite word. He can now combine two words and asks questions such as "What's that?" Billy can verbalize immediate experiences and can talk and play at the same time. He refers to himself "Me Billy."

Between the ages of 2 and 3 (in contemporary American culture) Billy is probably introduced to toilet training. His control of elimination relies on maturational readiness, but he must learn a great deal before training can be initiated. He must know what is expected of him and have some concept of his own capabilities.

Much controversy has raged regarding when and how toilet training should be initiated. Two points must be emphasized: (1) the child must be maturationally ready, and (2) whatever method is chosen, it must be carried out in a clear and consistent manner.

To Freud, the child now enters the Anal Period (12/18 months to 3 years). He obtains pleasure from the ability to control his bowels. Freud feels that the way in which toilet training is handled determines the effective resolution of this stage of development.[44]

Societal and cultural influences are of paramount importance to the child at this time, including:

1. Toilet training. There are cross-cultural attitudes and methods for this training. Parental attitudes, particularly in relationship to punishment, may have a marked influence on the child.
2. Parenting style. There are definite cross-cultural and subcultural differences in "mothering" styles.
3. The father's role in childrearing. Rebelsky and Hanks[45] made 24-hour tapes of father–baby interaction for a group of ten lower–middle class to upper–middle class fathers of infants. The average father in the group spent 37.7 seconds per day doing things with or for his baby; the most devoted spent less than 10 minutes a day with his baby. Initially these men spent more time talking

to their infant daughters, but by the time the babies were 3 months old, the sons were getting more attention. By the end of the study, the fathers were spending less time talking to their babies than they had in the beginning, especially their baby daughters. Other studies have found this to be the reverse of mother-baby interactions.

4. Absence of either the mother or father in child-rearing.
5. Presence of/and relationship to other siblings.
6. Reaction to peers and strangers.

Joan at 3 Years

She has grown 4 inches taller in the last year, and her motor skills have definitely improved. One minute she is standing on one foot (momentarily) in dancing school; the next she is running, turning, climbing, and riding her tricycle. Her eye-hand coordination has also improved. She can copy a circle with a crayon, pour milk from a pitcher, and button and unbutton clothes.

Imitation and dramatic play are an important part of the 3-year-old's play repertoire. If you were to observe Joan in school she would still be engaged in parallel play. Each child in Joan's group continues to show egocentric behavior. Let's listen to a typical conversation between Joan and her playmate Jon as they play house.

Joan: I am pretty like my mommy.
Jon: I like cookies. I want them.
Joan: I have pink toe shoes.
Jon: I want coffee and cookies.

In preschool activities, the "threes" happily engage in many activities: building blocks, puzzles, finger painting, clay, puppets, dolls, simple musical games. They love "grown-up" projects like making vegetable soup with the help of their teacher, who bravely issues plastic knives, carrots, potatoes, and onions to her energetic helpers.

Of greatest delight, however, is gross motor play—jungle gyms, sliding boards, swings, sandbox, and the baby pool.

At home Joan does uncomplicated dressing and undressing, although she has a tendency to look a bit disheveled. She may also develop wardrobe favorites and be hard to dissuade from her favorite Wonder Woman T-shirt. Toilet training is complete with rare accidents at night.

Joan helps with simple chores such as picking up toys, dusting, or working in the garden, mostly when the activity has some special appeal (like "helping daddy").

Emotionally, Joan is learning to control her drives and to develop socially acceptable behaviors (subli-

mation). Her parents, family, and teacher are setting new limits, which she cannot always comprehend or obey.

All these new experiences may put Joan, by 3½, in a state of temporary disequilibrium. Her delightful sense of joy, affection, and curiosity may dissolve quickly into periods of irritability, anger, and sometimes even temper tantrums. For example, Joan comes running into the house with a rock she found while playing. She quizzes her mother about where it came from and what it was made of. She plays with it, giving it magical properties. Then suddenly reality rears its head; dinner is ready and her mother asks her to wash her hands. Joan does not seem to hear her. After some prodding, she retorts with an angry "No!" and throws the rock on the floor.

Joan cannot yet accurately differentiate between reality and fantasy. She thinks and learns by recalling "reality sequences in her head just as she might do overt action."[46] For example, Joan spends a day at the zoo. When asked later what she saw, she recalls only one or two highlights. It is difficult to relive a whole day in her mind!

Joan cannot at this time grasp the concept of reversibility. For instance, if you ask if she has a sister she replies "yes," but if you ask her if her sister has a sister she says "no."

The 3-year-old's concepts are preconcepts. They are active and concrete. They do not allow the child to recognize[47] objects and/or persons in certain circumstances,[48] such as:

1. an object and/or person under different circumstances. For example, Joan may not recognize her mother who is wearing huge *new* sunglasses, but once the glasses are removed, she exclaims, "There's my mommy!"
2. different objects and/or persons of the same type as anything but one and the same. For example, Joan sees a butterfly and calls it *the* butterfly. She thinks that each butterfly she sees is *the* original butterfly.

The child goes from one particular of a situation to another rather than from a particular to the whole (centering). It will be another 3 or 4 years before Joan will have the ability to think in a more sophisticated manner. As a preoperational child, Joan still focuses on successive states and cannot make transformations from one state to another. For example, when equal amounts of water are poured into two different containers (one tall and thin, one short and wide) she invariably says that the taller one has more water because of its height (concept of conservation). When asked who is older, mommy or daddy, she says daddy because he is taller. Because of centering, Joan cannot accommodate to transformations. This type of associative thought process is known in piagetian terms as *transductive reasoning*.

School Years

Sam at 5 Years

For Sam, just entering kindergarten, 5 is a golden age. In general, Sam is self-contained and friendly, both at home and at school. He is just barely discovering the actual world. The 5-year-old gives the impression of competency and stability. He is not overly assertive, and he enjoys small responsibilities as opposed to hard challenges. Sam likes to fit into his culture; he is eager to please others and to conform to social boundaries. This period of calm and conformity does not mean he is highly socialized. He does engage in cooperative play, usually in small groups (one to three peers). But even in group play he is primarily concerned with his own activity.

In his gross motor activities, Sam displays excellent equilibrium on the balance beam, he skips well, and he plays a fair game of ball. His fine motor activity has markedly improved. Sam is now definitely right-handed. He can draw recognizable objects from memory, including a fair representation of a man. He can also copy a square as well as some capital letters. Sam can handle small objects fairly dexterously. He uses children's scissors competently, and he performs most of his activities of daily living. He now dresses and undresses with little or no assistance, although it might be a while before he ties his shoelaces.

Sam likes to finish what he starts. He enjoys most of the kindergarten play materials: paints, crayons, blocks, workbooks, tracing figures, and basic math games. Outdoor play consists of tree climbing, jumping, and acrobatics. Imitative play is becoming more reality-oriented. Kindergarteners play house, doctor, school, and so forth. This type of accurate imitation yields a more extensive comprehension of cultural mores and values.

By the middle of his kindergarten year, Sam tends to gravitate to all-boy play groups. The unspoken patterns of sex-role behavior are becoming more evident. Sam's new-found chauvinism is much more vociferous (girls are yukky) when bolstered by his pals. Alone, he may forget it entirely and enjoy playing with his girlfriend next door.

Five-year-olds have already spent several years acquiring behaviors and attitudes regarded by their culture as characteristically masculine or feminine (sex typing.)[48] The extent to which male and female behavior is biologically or culturally determined continues to be a great controversy. Despite evolving traditional male–female roles, most children develop specific sex-appropriate behavior. Recent studies confirm this. Greenberg and Peck showed 120 preschool children (3 to 6 years) pictures of boys and girls and asked which of the picture-children would grow up to be a teacher, doctor, and so forth. The children were also tested for IQ. All the children gave stereotyped responses: the brightest giving the most traditional answers—boys seen as doctors, girls as teachers, and so forth.[49,50]

Sam's communication has expanded; he now has a 2000 word vocabulary, and he has abandoned most of his infantile speech. He employs egocentric speech, and he often uses words without fully understanding their meaning.

According to Erikson, the preschool child (3 to 6 years) is in Crisis III, *initiative versus guilt.* Sam is turning from total attachment to his parents to identification with them. He is eager to plan and execute activities, but he is limited partly by the Oedipal complex and partly by a developing conscience (superego). Guilt arises if rules and regulations are perceived as too restrictive. The child's own superego may be harder on him than his parents in a given situation (Table 4-4).[51] He must learn to regulate these two parts of his personality so that he will develop a balance between a sense of moral responsibility and joie de vivre.

Jim at 7 Years

Jim, a second grader, takes in more of his environment than he gives back, mulling over his new impressions in a kind of reflective fantasy. Although he has a tendency for self-absorption, Jim is interested in others (parents, teacher, and friends) and is increasingly sensitive to their attitudes. He is becoming more detached from mother, developing new attachments outside the home.

Jim is prone to sudden bursts of active behavior. His strength is increasing, and he is learning to inhibit his motor activity. He repeats activities over and over in order to master them. In school, Jim is writing less painstakingly. His letters are becoming more uniform, and his drawings of a man are more accurate in relation to size. Usually a good listener, he loves a story, though his own reading abilities are still in the labored phonetic stage.

Jim is eager to please his teacher, and with her support he grows more confident of his abilities. The teacher realizes that her children need speech to clarify their thoughts and develop their social contacts. By establishing empathetic two-way relationships, she can foster self-reliance and encourage independence.

Language at this age is increasingly interposed between thought and action. *When* verbal mediation comes into play is much debated, partly as a corollary

Table 4-4 *A Child's View of Rules.*

Practice of Rules	*Thinking About Rules*
Stage I: Motor Activity A child manipulates objects in an individual way to see what he/she can do with them.	*Stage I: Absolutism* (from 4 to 7) Rules are considered as interesting examples, but not reality. A child considers rules sacred, although in practice the child is willing to accept changes in the rules because he/she recognizes them as changes.
Stage II: Egocentrism (from 2 to 5) The child has a general idea of rules and believes he/she is playing by the rules. Actually the child engages in play via idiosyncratic systems and changes the rules to fit his/her needs.	*Stage II: Morality of Constraint* (from 7 to 10) The child is limited by respect for adults and older peers. Authority is absolute; the child refuses to accept any change in rules.
Stage III: Incipient Cooperation (about 7 or 8) The child tries to win and wants to play by a set of rules. Ideas are vague, and each child playing the game will give an individual or different account of the rules.	*Stage III: Morality of Cooperation* (from 10 on) The child sees rules as laws resulting from mutual consent. Most children no longer accept parents and others as the authority figures without question. They see themselves as equals; since people make the rules, people can change them.
Stage IV: Codification (about 11 or 12) The child knows every detail of procedure. The group knows and plays by the same rules.	

Adapted from Papalia, D., and Olds, S.: A Child's World: Infancy Through Adolescence. New York: McGraw-Hill, 1975, p. 427. Original source Piaget (1932).

to the question of whether language must precede the formulation of certain cognitive concepts. Verbal mediation involves the use of verbal links between the overt stimulus and the final result[52] (Jim thinks before he acts).

Jim is gradually developing a sense of time and space orientation. In preschool and kindergarten he had the notion of "before and after"; he understood time differences in relationship to spatial distances. Now he is becoming more independent of sequential and perceptual data. He can read the clock, tell you the month, and identify seasons of the year. Jim will not fully understand the time concept until he can coordinate the concepts of equal distance and speed. By the time he is a young adolescent he will be able to explain that time has equal duration regardless of the content of that time.[53]

Jim's cognitive growth may be indicated by the increasing predictability of his adult IQ (see Chapt. 33). While there is only minimal correlation between a person's IQ at 2 years and his adult IQ, there is a highly significant correlation between his test scores at 7 years and his adult IQ.[54] Psychologists dispute the underlying causes of cognitive changes, but generally they believe that the 7-year-old increasingly resorts to rule-controlled thought, although simple association remains an important part of his mental process. His thought tends to be deliberate and reflective rather than impulsive.

Piaget characterizes the 4-year-old to 7-year-old age span as the Intuitive Phase. The intuitive child relies heavily on immediate perception and on direct experience rather than on logical operation. He centers on one dimension or feature at a time (centering), he views the world from his own point of view (egocentric), and he tends to be static and irreversible in his thinking. Toward the end of this stage, the rigid, static, and irreversible qualities of intuitive thought begin to "thaw out," becoming more reversible and flexible. This emerging ability to go beyond the immediate self with mental leaps and bounds is the precursor of systematic reasoning.

Jim is now emerging into what Piaget terms the Concrete Operational Phase (7 to 9½ years), determining relations through a process of trial and error. He can now coordinate inverse relations as well as understand the concept of conservation. His inner and outer world are going through complex change. At home, he not only handles his own self-care activities, but he is expected to meet increasing household demands and responsibilities. In school, he is learning more complex concepts, and he is becoming more aware of structure and rules.

At play, Jim is inclined to be obsessive in his interests. For instance, he develops a passion for models often to the exclusion of other activities. In gross motor activities, he is cautious but not fearful. He enjoys his bike and rides it on the sidewalk, he climbs trees, he likes to play ball (although he is better at batting than catching). Jim is also taking an interest in swimming and skating. The group games he now enjoys are much better defined and realistic. He gradually abandons the concepts of animism and artificialism and becomes interested in cooperation and competition. His ability to cooperate and compete is tentative. When playing a game, he knows the rules but still likes to add his own—and he loves to win.

In Kohlberg's opinion, a child's moral reasoning is predictable and develops sequentially as does his or her view of rules (Table 4-4).[55]

Summary of Kohlberg's Six Stages of Moral Reasoning

Level I

Pre-Moral (4–10 yrs.). Primary emphasis is on external control and ideas of others. These standards are followed either to avoid punishment or gain reward.

Type I—Punishment and obedience. The child obeys to avoid punishment.

Type II—Naive instrumental hedonism. Conformity to rules is out of self-interest.

Level II

Morality of Conventional Role Conformity (10–13 yrs.). The child wishes to please others and internalizes some of the standards of those persons deemed important to him or her. The child now decides if some action is good by his or her standards.

Type III—Maintaining approval of others. The child judges the intentions of others and yields an opinion.

Type IV—Authority maintaining morality. The child shows respect for authority and maintenance of social order.

Level III

Morality of Self-Accepted Moral Principles (13 to adulthood). True morality. The individual recognizes the possible conflict between standards. He/she realizes that conduct and reasoning about right and wrong are a result of internal control.

Type V—Morality of contract, of individual rights, and of accepted democratic law. People think in logical terms, valuing the will of society as a whole. These values are for the most part substantiated by obeying the law.

Type VI—Morality of individual principles of conscience. The individual does what he/she thinks is right as a result of his/her internalized values.

Adapted from Kohlberg, L.: The child as a moral philosopher. Psychol. Today 2:25–30, 1968.

Freud views personality development of the school-age child as part of the Latency Period. By 6, the child has a functioning superego that allows him to internalize the morals and ethics of society. He has resolved his Oedipal conflicts and sex role, and he now turns his attention to the acquisition of facts, skill, and cultural attitudes. (This does not imply that sexual interest is absent.) It is also during his school-age years that a child develops defense mechanisms to uphold the strength and integrity of his ego and self-concept.

Erikson sees the school-age child as entering Crisis IV, *industry versus inferiority*. This is the age when productivity is important. The school years are critical for the development of self-esteem, because the child must gain a sense of mastery over the tools of his culture and society. If he perceives himself as failing, he may feel hopelessly inadequate.

Maier explains Erikson's view of the school-age child as follows:

> The latent child continues to invest as much of himself and libidinal energy as he did before, and works incessantly on his bodily, muscular and perceptive skills as well as on his growing knowledge of the world which becomes increasingly important to him. Above all, he concentrates on his capacity to relate to and to communicate with individuals who are most significant to him—his peers. A sense of accomplishment for having done well, being the strongest, best, wittiest or fastest are the successes toward which he strives. The child wards off failure at almost any price. As long as ego tasks are mastered within the sphere of his age group, the id and the superego remain unchallenged and within safe boundaries . . . He senses that if he proves his skills within the area of his best competence, his successful future will be assured.[56]

Cultural influences are of paramount importance in the early school years, including:
1. parenting style; for example, permissive versus authoritarian;
2. type of school program;
3. differentiation of sex roles and/or sex typing;
4. emphasis and types of play available.

Laura at 10 Years

Laura refines her skills: she thoroughly enjoys her friends and family and experiences a period of relative equilibrium as she stands on the threshold of adolescence. Her individuality is well defined. Still in the phase of concrete operations, her industry is directed at refining the skills she has mastered. Since her energies and motor functions are better organized and executed, she is freer to interact within her environment. This new relaxed attitude makes Laura more responsive to social influences. She is beginning to make comparative judgments based on her own observations of home, school, family, and peers as well as on her developing sense of fairness.

Laura's peer group is the testing ground for parent-derived attitudes as well as a forum for development of social skills. As a group member, she is learning to adjust to the needs and desires of others. Peer groups at this age tend to be homogeneous according to sex, race, economic status, and general interest. Laura, for example, belongs to a club, The Butterflies. Members share common interests such as hiking and playing ball. They have special meetings, and they enjoy sharing secret experiences.

Bronfenbrenner made a study of American and Russian 12-year-olds and their responsiveness to peer and adult influences. Dramatic cultural differences were displayed:

> The children were confronted with thirty hypothetical situations involving their readiness to cheat, steal, play a practical joke on a teacher, neglect homework, and go against parental wishes in several specific ways. Some children were told that their classmates would see their answers, some that parents and teachers would see them, and some that no one but the researchers would see them. Both Russian and American children gave more socially approved responses when they thought adults would see their answers, although the Russian children were influenced more by adults and the Americans more by peers. Furthermore, the effects of peer-group pressures took different directions for the two groups of children. In Russia, peer-group pressure influenced children toward adult standards of behavior, while just the opposite held true in the United States. American children who thought their friends would see their answers were more likely to show a willingness to go against adult-approved standards.[57]

Child's Play

As a child progresses from infant to adult, his/her major focus of activity evolves along a play–work continuum. At each developmental period the balance between play and work shifts. For the preschool child, play is the central activity. The structure of the early school years teaches the child to balance work and play activities. As a child approaches adolescence, he/she becomes increasingly more involved in structured and work-oriented activity. This work focus increases through the teen years. For adults, work and career development are balanced with either active or passive leisure time activities.

Over the years, educators and developmentalists have developed many definitions for the word *play*. But inherent in all of these definitions is the common concept that play is an activity voluntarily engaged in for pleasure. This activity is significant because it assists the child to adapt within his/her environment or

culture. Through play, the child learns to explore, develop, and master physical and social skills.

A child's play develops through several stages from passive observation to cooperative, purposeful activity.[58]

Functions of Play

Social

During play, the young child tests family roles, adult roles, and gender roles at his/her own pace, free from

---

Play Behavior

Unoccupied Play Behavior. The child seems not to be playing but watches momentarily activity in the environment. When not attending, the child plays with his/her body, engages in gross motor behavior (*e.g.*, climbing up or down from chairs, following people around) or just sits looking around the room.

Onlooker Play. The child watches others play and engages in conversation with those playing. He/she definitely is observing the children rather than events, although he/she does not engage in actual play.

Solitary Independent Play. The child pursues play activities alone and independently from the other children playing. Although the child often positions himself close to others, he/she makes no reference to what they are doing.

Parallel Play. The child plays with toys similar to those used by other children near him/her, but the child plays beside rather than with the children.

Associative Play. The child plays with others. There is no organization of play activities in his/her peer group, no division of labor, and no product. Each child acts individually; his/her interest focusing on the association rather than the play activity.

Cooperative or Organized Supplementary Play. The child plays with other children in an organized manner for a purpose (*e.g.*, making something, formal games). There is a marked sense of belonging to the group, which is now directed by one or two leaders. Each child finds some role in the new organization, his efforts augmented by the other members of the group.

Adapted from Parten, M. B.: Social play among preschool children. J. Abnorm. Soc. Psychol. 27:243–269, 1932.

the limits of the adult world. Play teaches a child to relate to others, first as an observer, and later as a participant in cooperative and/or competitive and group endeavors. Play provides a means by which the child gains an insight into the mores of his/her culture. As the child comes to an understanding of what is "acceptable" and what is "not acceptable," the child begins to develop a sense of social morality.

Physical/Sensory/Perceptual

Children love to repeat activity. They will engage in seemingly endless repetition of both gross and fine motor skills for the pure joy of mastery. As his/her skills proliferate, a child can integrate more complex and coordinated activities. Sensory and motor activity teach the child the physical realities of the world as well as the capabilities and limitations of his/her own body. Play also provides a release for excess energy which restores body equilibrium, freeing the child for new endeavors. It heightens a child's perceptual ability: events or objects in the play environment allow the child to perceive forms, and spatial and temporal relationships. He/she begins to classify objects and relate them to other objects, forming the basis for logical thought.

Emotional

Play allows the child to discover a sense of self, an internal stability. The child begins to trust the constancy and consistency of the environment. This trust forms the basis for ego identity. Play lets a child test the reality of inner and outer worlds. It enables him to express feelings without fear of punishment and, conversely, helps him learn to control his frustrations and impulses. This control provides the basis for ego strength, self-confidence, and potential adaptation to future needs. Play is fun—it opens to the child a world of joy, humor, and creativity.

Cognitive

Play activities are closely related to the child's level of cognitive development. Through play, the child learns to manipulate events and objects in the internal and external environment. This manipulation and combination of novel events lay the foundation for problem solving. Representational thought emerges as the child engages in symbolic and dramatic play; abstract thought has its basis in activities that allow for classification and problem-solving ability. The concrete experiences of play allow the child to make a more accurate assessment of the environment and his/her role in it.

Content and Structure of Play

To gain a real insight into a child's world, we must look intently at his/her play. The classifications which follow are descriptive rather than theoretical.

Elizabeth Hurlock delineates four general stages of play:

1. *The exploratory stage* (infant). During the first few months of life, the child inspects the world visually and via random movements. Once he attains control of his upper extremities, the infant can more determinedly explore his body and the objects within his environment.
2. *The toy stage* (1 to 7–8 years). From the time a child begins to toddle in his new world, he engages in many kinds of make-believe and dramatic play. These two delights of childhood continue into the early school years (peaking at approximately 5½). Constructive play begins at 3 years and culminates in the development of hobbies. During the school years, hobbies and collections serve as social and status agents.
3. *The play stage*. This occurs during the school years and overlaps with Stages 2 and 4. In this period the development of productive construction, games, and sports occurs.
4. *Adolescent play/work stage*. Preadolescent play and work activities become more complex. The young person begins to project future goals and activity plans into his/her creative endeavors. The elements of introspection and daydreaming reach a peak during this stage.[59]

Sara Smilansky focuses only on dramatic play, defining four specific types:

1. *Functional play*. This includes all simple verbal and behavioral play, the focus of which is manipulation of forms. This type of play allows the child to explore the immediate environment.
2. *Constructive play*. At about 2 years of age a child begins to demonstrate dramatic skill. "Making believe" in reality-oriented play helps the child make the link between his/her world and the adult world.
3. *Dramatic play*. According to Smilansky, the two main elements of dramatic play are (a) imitation of an adult (the real world) and (b) a "pretend" situation (the unreal world). The highest level of dramatic play is socio-dramatic play, in which at least two children engage in play-acting activity, imitating the real speech and gestures of others in an imaginary situation. The make-believe element of this socio-dramatic play relies heavily on verbalization. Socio-dramatic play stage has six elements: (1) imitation of a role, (2) use of make-believe objects, (3) use of make-believe actions

and situations, (4) persistence for at least 10 minutes, (5) interaction between two or more children, and (6) the use of verbal communication related to the plot.
4. *Games with rules.* This stage begins during the school years and culminates in adulthood. In order to participate in group games with rules, an individual must be able to control his/her reactions and behavior.

Piaget identified the structure of play according to the cognitive complexity of activities:[60,61]

Practice Games

Practice games appear first. This is any activity that the child repeats for pure pleasure and that can include:
1. pure sensorimotor practice
   (a) mere practice
   (b) "accidentally-produced" combinations
   (c) intentional combinations
2. mental exercise
   (a) mere practice (for example, "Why?")
   (b) fortuitous combinations (putting words together)
   (c) intentional combinations (making up stories).

These practice games appear in Piaget's Substage 2 of the sensorimotor period.

Symbolic Games

Symbolic games appear in Substage 6 of the sensorimotor period. Symbolic games are difficult to differentiate from practice games. The main difference between the two is the introduction of make-believe. The child subjectively interprets his environment (that is, an empty chair is inhabited by a magical friend; a stick becomes a wand).

Games With Rules

As the child grows and interacts with peers, sensorimotor and/or symbolic games become "games with rules." These games require mental organization and operations.

Constructional Games

This fourth category is identified by Piaget, although he specifies that it does not occupy its own space. Constructional games are found in all three structural types, but they occupy space "half-way between play and intelligent work, or between play and imitation" (for example, hobbies, competition, dramatic presentation).[62]

Theories of Play

Erik Erikson discusses play as a sequential unfolding of psychosocial relationships.[63]

Stage 1—the Auto-Cosmic Stage

From birth to 15 months the child focuses on his own body. During the first phase of this stage, the self is the center of exploration. Kinesthetic sensations and sensual perceptions are repeated. In the second phase the child starts to explore other people or objects. Although the focus of his/her actions is still sensual pleasure, the actions may now be directed to cause and effect (for example, crying for attention).

Stage 2—the Microcosmic Stage

From 15 months to 3 years the child uses small toys and objects to play out themes, and he begins to master the environment.

Stage 3—the Macrosphere Stage

From nursery school to 7 years the child's play revolves around other children. This interaction begins with minimal communication. Initially, a child may view other children as objects, but as his experiences increase, the child learns to participate in cooperative role taking.

Stage 4—Industry versus Inferiority

From 7 years to preadolescence the school-age child learns the skills and tools of his/her culture. Mastery of tasks and the development of competency are intrinsic rewards.

Stage 5—Identity versus Role Confusion

During the adolescent years the focus of play and activities is role identification. Work-oriented tasks play a major role in the child's life situation.[64]

To Anna Freud, the ability to work is related to the pleasure of achievement, which has a basis in early play activity. A person's ability to work is related to his/her ego development and ability to (a) control and modify impulses, (b) delay gratification, (c) carry out preconceived plans even when frustration intervenes, (d) neutralize energies of instinctual drives through sublimated pleasures, and (e) be governed by a reality principle rather than a pleasure principle.[65,66]

Piaget believes that activity and/or play may be an end product for a child. What is play at one stage may be work at another. Once the child learns an activity,

Table 4-5 *Piaget's View of the Evolution of Play Activities*

Types of Games	Average Age Range	Activities
Practice games		
Substage I Pure reflex adaptations	0–1 mo.	No differentiation between assimilation and accommodation. Exercising reflex schemas does not constitute "real play"
Substage II Primary circular reactions	1–4 mo.	Slight differentiation between assimilation and accommodation. Repetition of schemata and self-imitation, especially vocal and visual
Substage III Secondary circular reactions	4–8 mo.	Differentiation between assimilation and accommodation, both still overlap. Repeating action on things to prolong an interesting spectacle
Substage IV Coordination of secondary schemata	8–12 mo.	Clear differentiation between assimilation and accommodation. Application of known schema to new situation. Schemata follow one another without apparent aim. Ritualism of activity for play—means becomes an end in itself
Substage V Tertiary circular reactions	12–18 mo.	Ritualistic repetition of chance schema combinations. Accentuating and elaborating rituals, experimenting to see the result
Substage VI Invention of new means through mental combinations	12–24 mo.	Beginning of pretense by application of schema to inadequate object. A symbol is mentally evoked and imitated in make-believe. Reproduction of behavior—primitive symbolic play. Symbolic schema is reproduced outside of context; transition between practice play and symbolic play proper
Symbolic games		
Stage I	2–4 yr.	
Type I		Generalizing symbolic schemata (isolated imitations of schemata)
Subtype A		Projection of symbolic schemata onto new objects
Subtype B		Projection of imitative schemata onto new objects
Type II		Symbolic games (assimilation of one schema to another)
Subtype A		Simple identification of one object with another
Subtype B		Identification of the child's body with that of other people or with things
Type III		
Subtype A	3–4 yr.	Symbolic combinations (construction of whole scenes) Simple combinations (includes imaginary friends). Reconstruction combined with imaginary elements
Subtype B		Compensatory combinations (materializing fears). Reconstruction with compensatory transpositions
Subtype C		Liquidating combinations (intensifying powers, subordinate threat) in pure reconstruction of situations
Subtype D		Anticipatory symbolic combinations (questioning, orders, and advice). Reproduction of reality with exaggerated anticipation of consequences
Stage II	4–7 yr.	Increased orderliness; more exact imitation of reality; use of collective symbolism
Stage III	7–12 yr.	Decline in symbolism; rise in games with rules and symbolic constructions
Games with rules		
Stage I	2–4 yr.	Rare
Stage II	4–7 yr.	Some
Stage III	7–11 yr.	Peak
Adulthood		Continue to develop
Constructional games	2–adult	Imitation of reality or new combinations. Gradually becomes more complex and unique to the individual

From Schuster, C. L. S., and Asburn, S. S.: *The Process of Human Development—A Holistic Approach.* Boston: Little, Brown & Co., 1980, p. 306.

it is repeated for the sherr joy of mastery. Piaget defines play as pure assimilation—the repetition of a behavior or a scheme solely for the pleasure of conquering a skill.[67]

He feels that the types and evolution of play activities a child chooses reflect the child's level of cognitive development (Table 4-5). To Piaget, play and cognitive development are parallel and interdependent. Play fosters the child's ability to master and to become competent within his/her world.

Adolescence

Adolescence is derived from a Latin word meaning *to come to maturity*. It begins at pubescence, a period of about 2 years prior to the onset of puberty. Pubescence is a time of physiological changes: a growth spurt, a synchronous growth of body systems, and increased hormonal activity which triggers the emergence of primary and secondary sex characteristics[68] (Table 4-6). Pubescence culminates at puberty, when sexual maturity and reproductive capacity are complete.

It is not as easy to determine when adolescence ends and adulthood begins. This depends on a combination of physical, emotional, social, legal, and cultural determinants.

Theories of Adolescence

Anthropologist Margaret Mead believes that physiological factors underlie adolescent changes, but that cultural factors determine the quality of these changes. If a society decrees a smooth transition from one developmental period to another, the adolescent experiences little or no conflict.

Freud's view of adolescence centers on the *genital*

Table 4-6 *Emergence of Sex Characteristics.*

Girls	Boys
Primary Sex Characteristics	
ovaries	testes
fallopian tubes	penis
uterus	organs that transmit sperm from
vagina	testes to penis
Secondary Sex Characteristics	
breasts	facial hair
pubic hair	pubic hair
axillary hair	axillary hair
increased width and depth of pelvis	body hair
	voice change

stage, that point of mature adult sexuality when reawakened sexual urges are directed in socially approved channels. Although his theory of adolescent behavior is sketchier than his explanations of earlier development, he does emphasize achievement of identity in respect to career choice, cultural values, and ethics.

Erikson sees adolescence as Crisis V, *identity versus role confusion.* The adolescent's rapid physical maturation implies that adulthood is approaching, and an adult role must soon be assumed. Establishing an identity in his or her life career as well as establishing meaningful psychosocial relationships help the adolescent define and clarify his adult role.

Puberty sees the full development of a system of cognitive thought. Inhelder and Piaget[69] characterize the adolescent's formal operational thought process as follows:

1. The capability of dealing logically with many factors at once.
2. The ability to utilize a secondary system, for example, trigonometry. The ability to manipulate symbols makes the adolescent's thought processes more flexible. He is now able to introspect and reflect upon his own mental capacities.
3. The ability to construct ideal or contrary-to-fact situations.
4. The ability to deal with the possible as well as the real.

These components comprise the basis for hypothetical problem solving, a necessary adult tool.

In *pre- and early adolescence,* physiological changes coupled with emerging cognitive abilities lay the foundation for the establishment of identity. This tumultuous period often finds the adolescent moody, sensitive, and ambivalent about identity and role.

Mid-adolescence centers around a struggle for autonomy and a continued search for self and vocational identity. Pressure to make a vocational choice is mounting. From a developmental point of view, the choice of a career has been going on since childhood, beginning with parental modeling and identification. Besides his parents' values, a child's own needs for creativity, sharing, and self-expression provide a further base for assuming various role behaviors. He explores future vocational aspirations through play activities. During youth and adolescence exposure to "real" jobs allows the young person a pragmatic testing ground for such things as sex-peer group interaction, specific interests and capabilities, attitudes, and patterns of work behaviors.

Despite the ability to conceptualize, the mid-adolescent may manifest lingering egocentrism. He realizes that other people have their own thoughts and perceptions, but his self-preoccupation persuades him that their thoughts are focused on him. Elkind[70] describes manifestations of this egocentrism as follows:

1. *Imaginary audience.* The adolescent is constructing or reacting to an imagined audience. For example, when the student catches the eye of the teacher he wonders what the teacher is thinking about him at that moment.
2. *Personal fable.* The adolescent imagines that because so many people are interested in him, he must be very special. For example, the adolescent knows that "no one ever has felt the way I do."
3. *Pseudostupidity.* The adolescent tends to interpret situations at a more complex level than is warranted. The obvious tends to elude him. For example, he may look for a lost sock, shoe, or book in the places he is least likely to find it.

These phenomena are also a result of the young person's inability to control his/her new-found mental capabilities (*i.e.*, formal operational thought).[71]

Issues in Adolescence

Need for and Development of Independence

The adolescent's need for and development of independence is often manifested in parent–child conflict. Elkind interprets this conflict as a function of the age of the adolescent and the maturity of the parent.* He states that conflicts arise as a result of three kinds of arrangements: bargains, agreements, and contracts.

The *bargain* occurs when the parent offers a reward or rescinds a punishment in exchange for compliance of behavior.

The *agreement* is more complex: the parent and child agree to abide by certain rules over a period of time. Agreements predominate over bargains during adolescence.

The *contract* is the process whereby parent and child interact with each other on the basis of mutual expectation. The contract is usually implicit and unspoken. It becomes known only when it is violated.[72]

For Elkind, the parent–adolescent conflict is a stage in the process of self-differentiation. He hypothesizes that each arrangement has three complementary "invariant clauses" whose content vary with age level.

---

* In this section, *parent* is often used as a generic term indicating the primary caretaker, usually the mother.

Responsibility–freedom. The parent demands that the adolescent fulfill certain social responsibilities in return for complementary freedoms. The content of this clause changes with age. A parent may, for example, ask a young person to take responsibility for social control, money management, and motor vehicles; the adolescent, in turn, may insist on increased freedom in "hour" accountability, spending, and dating privileges.

Achievement–support. This clause functions in the development of a sense of competence: in the adolescent's ability to meet social and academic standards and in the parent's ability to instruct, supervise, and reinforce his/her accomplishments.

Loyalty–commitment. This clause is closely related to the development of a value system. The parent expects the adolescent to give primary allegiance to the family, and the young person expects the parent to support him and make a commitment to his values and beliefs.

Elkind's theory of interpersonal relationships (based on implicit and temporal contracts, accountability, competence, and commitment clauses) highlights how the resolution of parent–child tensions paves the road to a child's independence.[73]

Group interactions and peer relationships provide the transient feedback necessary for the adolescent's development of social independence and self-worth. Peer interaction teaches the adolescent the norms of society, as well as how to contribute to and establish group goals. In peer relationships he tests and begins to understand various social roles while reinforcing his own identity.

The development of independence is often an arduous process which evolves from the feeling of self-worth established through peer and family interaction. It is not the adolescent who "cuts the apron strings." It is the parent, through a process of support and reinforcement, who cuts the strings and launches his or her child on a unique and independent life.

Awakening of Sexuality—Need for and Development of Intimacy

Physical changes in the young adolescent force him/her to face or identify his concept of sexuality and body image. Sexuality is the totality of the individual's attitudes, values, goals, and behaviors (both internal and external) based on, or determined by, his perception of his gender.[74]

Sexual awareness begins in and develops from early childhood. But adolescence brings a heightened, often acute, awareness of gender difference, erotic sensations, sexual relationships, potential adult roles, and the need for intimacy.

Young adolescents (10–13 years) are confronted by rapid physical changes which may confuse and alter their concept about acceptance on a physical and concrete level.

Erikson states that the early adolescent's concept of *love* varies significantly from that of the later adolescent. The younger adolescent enters relationships to test his or her own sexual identity. The partner is used as a mirror of the adolescent's needs and desires. The older adolescent has a more stable self-concept and increased cognitive abilities which allow him or her to see another's viewpoints and needs in a more mature manner. He or she searches for the beginning of intimacy and for more adult relationships.

Problems may arise when young adolescents are involved too soon in intimate relationships. These problems are reflected in the young person's difficulty or inability to identify appropriately with family or peers. In our society the trend toward early sexual intimacy brings with it potential difficulties for the adolescent who may not be mature enough to effectively deal with it. Permissiveness in sexual attitudes seems to be accelerating more among young adolescents than among any other age group. For four decades Udry, Bowman, and Morris conducted a study concerning trends in premarital coitus according to age. The results of this study of black and white women living in 16 cites showed a proportionate increase in premarital coitus between ages 15 to 20 years for each decade.[75]

Though there is no significant intellectual difference between a male and female adolescent, there are cultural and social pressures which may influence his/her self-concept. A young man, for example, may feel that physical strength is more valuable than academic acumen. As a result, his studies suffer. This concept of sexuality will not affect his IQ, but it may prevent him from improving his cognitive potential. This observation is consistent with Kohlberg's cognitive development theory: the young person chooses to expand/repress those attributes which he views as consistent/inconsistent with his concept of sexuality.[76]

Emotionally, adolescents must attempt to come to terms with both their ideal and their real selves. They are forced to evaluate their masculine/feminine roles, reviewing their gender identity, orientation, and gender preference.

As the young person successfully resolves the issues of the adolescent period, a feeling of well-being and self-identity emerges. This process of identity formation does not evolve smoothly for all adolescents. If the crisis is not resolved, role diffusion results. The young person is unable to respond to the demands of various role expectations. The youth beset by role diffusion wanders from one goal to another. Instead of constructive experimentation with options, this adolescent makes aimless and vague attempts at problem solving. The young man Biff in Arthur Miller's *Death of a Salesman* demonstrated a classic example of role diffusion when he states, "I just can't take hold, Mom. I can't take hold of some kind of life."[77]

Socially, adolescents spend more time with peers than with family and/or adults. In this predominantly peer environment, charged with sexual curiosity, they confront two major types of relationships: homosexual and heterosexual.

Evidence suggests that a homosexual relationship is not uncommon in adolescence. Possibly this stems from the adolescent's sexual insecurity—the need to compare himself/herself with someone nonthreatening and sexually similar. The encounter, conducted in a "safe" and comfortable environment, may be his first extrafamilial attachment.

The development of a meaningful heterosexual relationship is based on both physical and psychosocial intimacy. In order to develop true intimacy, the adolescent must be aware of his/her abilities and be able to share himself with others. It is critical that his internal identity be secure in order to prevent identity diffusion and stress on his sexuality.

Development of a Philosophy of Life, a Value System, and a Humanistic Attitude

According to Piaget, the adolescent (12+ years) develops a "morality of reciprocity." When a child reaches formal operational thought, he/she is able to engage in the abstract thinking and introspection which help him to develop an internally monitored value system. The adolescent's ability to interpret and internalize rules enables him to "discover the boundaries that separate his self from the other person, but (he) will learn to understand the other person and be understood by him."[78] Through this process the adolescent begins to develop an empathetic attitude toward others.

Usually the adolescent internalizes the values of his parents and peers, with whom he identifies. Shaefer states that, "In the fullest sense the process of identifying with an object is unconscious, though it may also have prominent and significant pre-conscious and conscious components: in this process the subject modifies his motives and behavior patterns, and the self representations corresponding to them, in such a way as to experience being like, the same as, and merged with one or more representations of that object; through identification, the subject both represents as his own one or more regulatory influences or characteristics of the object that have become important to him and continues his tie to the object."[79]

Many factors influence the development of an ideology—parents, peers, significant others, religious training, and cultural and social background. Some theorists speculate that from the time of adolescence the person is dealing with the "child of the past"; that each early experience in the child's social life and culture directly and indirectly affect his/her development of a philosophy of life. This philosophy comes about, finally, as a result of the interaction between the individual's society and culture and his internal learned responses.

Consistency of attitude is the most valuable commodity a parent can transmit to a child in order to help him form an intact value system. High self-esteem, internalization of expectations, and self-discipline are linked with parental style and are crucial for the formation of adult moral standards.[80,81]

Peers and significant others (family members, teachers, friends) provide an avenue by which the adolescent can identify and test his capabilities and ideas. Through testing, he will eventually crystalize his self-image and value system. Religious training and experience add another dimension to the young person's ability to internalize and reinforce value systems. Religious exposure seems to be most effective when both parents follow similar standards and reinforce their value system.

Different cultures produce different value orientations. There are differences in values both within a culture and between cultures. The expectations of the individual are determined by the way people in a given culture view life roles. Some of the issues around which individual roles are determined include:
1. responsibility versus nonresponsibility,
2. authority figures versus nonauthority figures,
3. dominance versus submission.

The development of a philosophy of life—the result of an internalized value system—is not a light task for the young adolescent. "A person must learn that he is involved with other people, that he has a responsibility to other people, and that he must at times subordinate his wishes for the good of the majority. He cannot pursue his own happiness without concern for other people, even though he believes he is seeking self fulfillment. His own wishes are no unerring guide to morality."[82]

Development of a Career Choice

From approximately 15 through 65 years of age, work occupies a large part of a person's life. The vocational decisions an adolescent makes affect his future social relationships, leisure-time activities, material gains, and marital and child-rearing attitudes.

Prior to World War II, the majority of youth were employed, or were homemakers, by the time they were 16 to 20 years old. Since 1945, urbanization, child labor laws, certification and apprenticeship requirements, and the decrease of available jobs have made the adolescent's transition from home/school to the work force increasingly difficult. Today, the average youth makes this transition between the ages of 16 and 24; at least one-fourth to one-half of the younger people in this age bracket (16–18 years) are either unemployed or employed in only part-time positions. The number of 16 to 24 year olds in the work force was approximately 23.8 million in 1980. This figure is expected to decrease 350,000 per year to about 22.2 million in 1985 and 20.3 million in 1990.[83]

Major influences on career choice include ability, gender, community (rural vs. urban), parental occupation, expectations, and occupational attractiveness.

Planning for work is difficult for a young person, whose aspirations tend to be more idealistic than realistic. Asten notes that "career changes that take place during high school result partly from greater self-awareness and recognition by students of aptitudes and skills that are necessary to educational and occupational success."[84] The merging of vocational interest and personal abilities probably occurs during later high school years.[85] With increased maturity, the adolescent gains a more realistic view of career choice and his/her abilities and needs.

One might surmise that minority students, who sometimes encounter stiff barriers and resistance as they move toward status roles, would tend to lower their career expectations. However, studies have proven that the opposite is true.[86,87] This increase in vocational aspiration may reflect three attitudes: (1) their efforts to conform to the American cultural emphasis on occupational success and status; (2) their substitution of future projections for their inability to move ahead in a success-oriented society; or (3) their exaggerated perception of the new horizons open to minority groups.

Gender also plays an important role in career decisions. In the last few years the feminist movement has had a strong impact on society's view of women's career options. Introduced early in the socialization process, these new attitudes toward female career possibilities can extend a girl's job scope. Even a girl with traditional expectations should take the time to explore her real career potential.

Datta notes that during the last 50 years women have made little progress in regard to salary and occupational status.[88] Although their participation in the work force has more than doubled, their distribution in traditionally masculine and status positions has remained relatively unchanged.

Further studies indicate that rural youth tend to aspire to lower prestige and lower-paying jobs than urban youth.[89,90] Adolescents also tend to want careers that parallel their parents' career choices and level of achievement.[91]

Brief summaries of three theories concerning career choice and development are listed:

Self-Concept Theory (Super). Super purports that as a person grows, he or she must integrate self-images into a self-concept which prevails in all daily activities, including his or her job. Occupational experiences culminate in work roles and career patterns that are consistent with the maturation of this self-concept. Super identifies five vocational developmental tasks:

1. *Crystallization of vocational preference (14–18 years)*. As their self-concept matures, adolescents develop ideas about work, and they begin to make educational decisions based on these ideas.

2. *Specification of vocational program (18–21 years)*. Detailed vocational plans are set forth.

3. *Implementation of vocational preferences (21–24 years)*. The young adult has completed his initial training phase and has secured a job.

4. *Stabilization of career (25–35 years)*. The individual enhances his/her talents, narrows his field of interest, and finds personal satisfaction in his work.

5. *Consolidation of career role (35 upward)*. The person develops expertise, strengthens his/her skills, and acquires status.[92]

This developmental theory is valid only in that there is a progression of vocational tasks. The age range varies with socioeconomic conditions.

Cognitive Social Theory (Ginsberg). Ginsberg feels that vocational choice is related to a developmental process of decision making. A person makes continuous choices "between career preparation and goals and the reality of the world of work."[93] This process is open-ended and is continuous throughout life; it is not confined to the adolescent and young adult.

Life Style Orientation (Holland). Holland focuses on the relationship between personality characteristics and vocational choice (a trait-factor theory). He believes that job choice is a reflection of personality—that a person chooses work environments that foster his/her personal orientation. In his typology, there are patterns of personal orientation that relate to six types of work orientation.[94]

Choosing a career is a vital task for the adolescent. It is a developmental process which lays the foundation for success and potential achievement in his/her adult years.

The Development of Ego Integrity and Individuality

Adolescence is largely concerned with the development of a stable ego identity. Erikson states that a youth is confronted with an internal physiological revolution that threatens his/her body image and ego concept. The adolescent must re-establish ego identity in light of early life experiences and accept bodily changes and libidinal feelings as part of himself. If ego identity is not satisfactorily established, confusion and role diffusion will endanger future emotional development.

Some role diffusion does exist in early adolescence, when young persons often over identify with heroes, teachers, etc. A young adolescent strongly identifies with his/her peer group.[95] His clannishness and occasional intolerance is a defense against possible self-diffusion. His revolt against parental influences may be a necessary part of his development of a separate self-identity.

During late adolescence, a young person becomes less dependent on his peer group and develops a more realistic approach to his vocational choice. With increased cognitive ability, he/she is better able to view alternatives, and he can more easily evaluate himself in relation to his goals.

As adolescence comes to a close, the young person, forced to adapt to the realities of adult life, begins to engage in productive work. He also reassesses the adult world as well as his own limitations, and he becomes more accepting of both.

Adult Life

Developmental progression reaches its height in adulthood. As the individual grows beyond childhood, he refines his self-image, develops sexual and psychosocial intimacy, becomes productive and effective in the world of work and family, and finally reaches an integrity and a sense of fulfillment which affirms his life as a meaningful adventure.

The complexity of the modern world, society, and culture inhibit the smooth resolution of many issues of adulthood. There is no ideal. But as Horace (Epistles) said, "He has half the deed done, who has made a beginning."

Young Adulthood

Psychological Issues

Our society designates young adulthood (the ages between 20 and 40) as prime time—when life is most satisfying and rewarding. Adolescents look ahead with anticipation and older persons look back with nostalgia on this relatively short period of time.

In fact, a study by Cameron[96] indicates that there are no significant differences among various age groups with respect to "fun and happiness," though young adults claim a greater desire for pleasure than others. And those persons considered "happiest" by others are the middle-aged! Cameron concludes that happiness is not determined by, or closely related to, age as such; it is relatively constant across the life span.

In another study Lowenthal also concludes that neither age nor life stage is relevant in measuring life satisfaction, although the sense of well-being is different for men than for women. Women tend to express more complex states of feelings. The "happiest" women in the study are those who have both positive and negative experiences, especially in the recent past; the "happiest" men relate only positive experiences in the recent past.[97]

Erikson feels that young adults are involved in working toward the development of intimacy with others as opposed to isolation from them. This intimacy includes a sense of commitment to concrete affiliations and partnerships, the ability to abide by such commitments, and the experience of cooperating and sharing with others even when this necessitates sacrifice and compromise.[98] A person who is unable to develop a sense of intimacy lives in a world apart, absorbed by himself.

Stress is one factor that does seem relative to age and stage in adult life. Young newlyweds, for example, reported 2½ times the number of stressful situations compared to middle-aged and older adults, though again the type of stress encountered varies with sex. For men, stress is usually related to occupation; for women, it stems more often from health issues (their own and others) and interpersonal conflicts. Middle-aged and older adults seem to experience less stress than the young. Apparently our "youth" cliches are misleading.[99] The influence of age or life stage on psychological well-being can best be understood in the context of a person's lifestyle and the type of environment and/or experiences he/she encounters.

Physical Issues

In early adulthood most of the growth processes have run their course. But the body never remains static: the bright-eyed and sharp-eared young adult is already undergoing decremental changes in vision and hearing.

The earliest change is in visual accommodation ability, which peaks in grade school and begins to decline even before a person's "prime." Other aspects of vision tend to remain unchanged.

The ability to hear high frequency sounds begins to diminish in adolescence, while pitch discrimina-tion (high tones) begins to decline in the midtwenties. These slight negative changes in early adulthood usually have little or no effect on the daily functioning of the young adult.

Cognitive Issues

Intellectual development peaks in the early adult years. Catell proposes two levels of mental ability: fluid and crystallized intelligence. *Fluid intelligence* refers to capabilities such as associative memory, inductive reasoning, and figural relationships. *Crystallized intelligence* refers to skills such as verbal comprehension and the handling of word relationships. The former skills are closely aligned to innate intellect; the latter are more dependent on learning and experience. Horn presented evidence which suggests that fluid intelligence may diminish slightly following adolescence, while crystallized intelligence increases with advancing age.[100]

Creativity seems to peak in the early thirties. In a historical study of thousands of creative men and women, Lehman found that the peak years of most people's creative ventures have been in their thirties. For example, the mean years for symphony writing were 30–34 years of age. Dennis found that creative persons usually continue to produce creative endeavors throughout their lives. However, their most unique and original works were produced in early adulthood.[101]

In Piaget's description of cognitive development, formal operational thought is acquired unevenly during adolescence and early adulthood. The ability to use interpropositional thought, combinational analysis, and hypothetical deductive reasoning are a result of innate intelligence, education, and life experiences. Some adults never attain formal operational thought. When this level of cognitive development is reached in early adulthood, the young adult relies heavily on it in all areas of life.[102]

Vocational and Life Goal Issues

Career choice remains a paramount issue in the twenties. A high school graduate usually experiments with several jobs before settling into stable employment. Those young persons who choose careers that require further education tend to remain on the job longer and feel more secure in their commitment.

Most employment in our culture involves some level of on-the-job training. The process of establishing a career involves the development of job skills and interpersonal working relationships between employer and other employees. Job changes are most frequent during the early adult years. The average duration of employment for the young adult is two years.

There are vast differences in how people view their work. Job satisfaction comes from a feeling of commitment based on a number of personal and interpersonal goals that are being met in a particular job.[103] Research indicates that job satisfaction occurs on many levels, depending on a variety of contributory factors. It is influenced by expectations from family, friends, and employers as well as by personal goals and needs.

By and large, in our society, the twenties are a time of work preparation, job exploration, and settling in, while the thirties are years of work advancement.[104]

Life Style Issues

As the young person enters adulthood, he/she usually leaves his family of origin and establishes his own nuclear family. In the United States, according to 1976 census reports, young women marry at about 21 and young men at about 23 years of age.

Blood suggests five prerequisites for a successful marriage: compatibility, skill, effort, commitment, and support.[105] Folkman and Clatworthy add two more characteristics: flexibility and love.[106] Americans tend to choose mates with similar backgrounds. Studies indicate that race is the most critical factor in this choice, followed by social class, educational group, religious affiliation, and ethnic origin.[107]

Most cultures incorporate some form of courtship ritual. This provides a means of testing compatibility and observing the prospective partner in a variety of situations.

Alternatives to marriage began to emerge in the 1960s and 1970s. More permissive sexual attitudes and greater social acceptance coupled with the advent of the feminist movement brought about an increase in the practice of cohabitation.[108] In many ways, "live-in" relationships appear to be similar to marriage. However, the marriage license seems to have a subtle psychological effect on such a commitment.

The types of cohabitation seem to parallel the types of marriage delineated by Cuber[109]: intrinsic (20% of all marriages) and utilitarian (80% of all marriages). In an intrinsic marriage (or cohabitation) the couple and their relationship is the focus of their living together. In a utilitarian marriage, the interpersonal relationship is not the sole directing force. This type of marriage serves a definite purpose. The purpose may vary—from pure physical pleasure to raising a family and meeting social needs with a minimum of tension.

Many individuals are choosing single life as an alternative to marriage. From 1960 to 1974, according to U.S. census figures, the number of young adults (ages 20–34) living in the single state had quadrupled to 12.7 million. A primary reason for remaining single in our society is career development. Single persons have the advantage of freedom in decision making, though they often spend a large amount of time seeking companions and nurturing relationships.[110]

Other types of relationships, including homosexual bonding, communal living, and being a "swinging single" exist as alternatives to traditional life styles. Choosing the direction of one's personal life pattern is a major decision of early adulthood.

Another major issue in the young adult's life is parenthood. Both cultural and personal influences affect this decision. The reasons for choosing parenthood are as varied as the couples involved in the choice. Children may be viewed as another outlet for one's creativity, as an opportunity to fulfill a life goal, or as another opportunity to share oneself with others. A growing number of young couples are opting not to become parents. Some reasons cited include complete fulfillment with a mate, career development, and socioeconomic factors. Maternal instinct is a myth. Not all women experience loving and protective feelings toward children. Yarrow *et al* found that women who have good self-concepts and who enjoy their roles in life are more apt to be good mothers than those who are dissatisfied with what they are doing.[111] Children can be enriching and exciting additions to the young adult's life when he or she is ready for the responsibility of rearing them.

Social Issues

During adolescence, a person uses the peer group as a sounding board for developing a self-concept. Once this concept becomes stable, the young adult usually develops a few meaningful relationships—friends who usually have parallel interests and who compliment his/her uniqueness and need system.

When the young adult leaves home, the relationship with his family of origin may weaken or grow stronger. The direction this relationship takes strongly depends on his/her ability to understand and react to other value systems and life styles.

Many young adults today have a variety of options available that were not available to their parents and grandparents—more vocational opportunities, more leisure time, and many more life choice possibilities.

Today's young adults are conscious of the need for a balance in the work–play continuum, and they establish meaningful life goals that balance their physical and psychosocial needs.

Mid-Adulthood

Physical Issues

There are vast differences among people in mid-adulthood (the ages between 40 and 60) in terms of physical changes. After a person is 40 years of age, physiological changes occur in all body systems, but the extent of their manifestation depends a great deal on individual genetic and environmental influences.

Menopause refers to all the physiological changes which occur when a woman's monthly menstrual function ceases. The female reproductive system changes with advancing age, and childbearing usually ceases during the late thirties or forties. American women reach menopause at approximately 40 to 54 years of age.[112] As the levels of estrogen decrease, some women experience vasomotor and other physical changes. The psychological changes associated with menopause are often exaggerated. Neugarten *et al* found that about 75% of the women studied felt that menopause did not change them in any important way and that only 50% felt that menopause was an unpleasant experience.[113]

There is a great deal of debate about whether males undergo a parallel experience (the male climacteric). Most social scientists feel that men do experience a transition period. The time of onset is variable and the period may be accompanied by both physical and psychological changes.

Cognitive Issues

As mentioned previously, fluid intelligence may diminish gradually from middle to later years, while crystallized intelligence may increase. Cross-sectional studies comparing people of different ages show generational differences in intelligence. Recent generations tend to be taller, heavier, stronger, and more intelligent.[114] This generational shift is known as the secular trend. Other studies indicate that intellectual ability peaks during the middle years and that it remains stable throughout this period and into the beginning of old age.[115]

Psychological Issues

Erikson sees midlife as a crisis of *generativity versus stagnation*. Unless a person continues to grow and change, he/she stagnates and regresses emotionally. This growth is evidenced in his creativity, interest in others, and concern with the next generation. Generativity is fostered through positive reciprocal contacts with the younger generation.

Social Issues

Certain social issues are paramount during middle age. Havinghurst identifies seven developmental tasks with this period:
1. achieving adult civic and social responsibility,
2. establishing and maintaining an economic standard of living,
3. assisting young people to become responsible adults,
4. developing leisure time activities,
5. relating to one's spouse as a person,
6. accepting the physiological changes of middle age,
7. adjusting to aging parents.[116]

Levinson and Gould find significant differences between the developmental adjustments of the forties versus the fifties. The forties are often years of unrest. Toward 50, adults settle down again.[117]

During his/her forties, a person may experience many transitions. Parents who are undergoing physiological and psychological changes themselves may be confronted by children in the throes of adolescent conflict. Reaching a psychological half-way point sets off reflection on past achievements and concern for future goals. The stress of this midlife transition can be an impetus for developmental growth and change, or it can cause a crisis of discontent.

Midlife is often a time when people redefine relationships with parents. Researchers indicate that the middle-aged adult seems to become more empathetic and/or sympathetic toward his aging parents. He begins to feel that he understands his parents' life situation. But when aging parents become physically or economically dependent on their children, problems may arise.

Gould found that there is an increased interest in social activities during the forties and fifties.[118] Participation in civic and political groups also increases. (This may be related to changing work roles).

For women, midlife may be the beginning of a second career, an exciting renewal. For men, midlife is often the time of highest financial security. Their career power and prestige is usually at a peak. Men seldom make radical shifts or impulsive moves at this life stage. Generally they remain in the same job until retirement. Usually the years between 50 and 65 are the most satisfying of a man's career.

Leisure activities expand during midlife. It is common for adults to pursue activities that they had established in their early adult life. Newgarten notes an interesting change in the concept of leisure in America. A hundred years ago, the higher one's education and income, the more leisure one had. Now, the best educated and most skilled professionals put in 60 to 80-hour work weeks, and it is the blue collar workers who have the most leisure time.[119]

The postparental period for some couples is a time to enjoy the fruits of the hard work of earlier years. These couples find a new pleasure in marriage and a new intensity in their relationship.[120] But while marital happiness increases for some, it evaporates for others. Some couples seek divorce soon after their children leave home, though they have long since lost contact with each other.

When children leave home, one or both parents may experience the empty nest phenomenon—a feeling of loss. This syndrome usually coincides with the marriage (or a comparable declaration of independence) of the last child at home. The crisis is usually resolved through expanding nurturing experiences (parents, pets, etc.). But the "empty nest" can lead, eventually, to sexual problems or divorce.

As their children establish new nuclear families, parents take on new roles as grandparents and in-laws. These new roles bring to midlife another potential for satisfaction and happiness or frustration and despair.

The middle years do more than reflect the accomplishments of earlier years. They are characterized by development and change. The physical and psychological crises which occur hold out tremendous potential for growth. Middle age rings with productivity, generativity, and a high satisfaction with life. See Chapter 34 for information on aging.

Table 4-7 *Definitions of Activities.*

Activity of Daily Living	Developmental Sequence Yr. Mo.	Definition of Task
Bed		
1. Supine position	Birth	Ability to lie on back
2. Prone position	Birth	Ability to lie on stomach
3. Roll to side	1–4 wk.	Ability to roll from back to side lying, reflexive
4. Roll prone to supine	0.6	Ability to roll from stomach to back; deliberate rolling
5. Roll supine to prone	0.7	Ability to roll from back to stomach; deliberate rolling
6. Sit up	0.10	Ability to attain sitting position
7. Propped sitting	0.6	Ability to sit with trunk erect, head and chin lifted, back supported
8. Sitting/hands props	0.7	Ability to sit alone passively without support, hands acting as accessory props
9. Sitting unsupported	0.10–0.12	Ability to sit unsupported indefinitely, hands and arms freed for manipulatory duty, eyes elevated
Reaching		
10. To midline	0.5	Ability to bring hands together at center of body and grasp object with two-handed approach from supine position
11. To mouth and face	0.6	Ability to grasp and bring object to mouth or face in sitting position
12. Above head	—	Ability to reach above head with both arms alternately, maintaining trunk stability in sitting position
13. Behind head	—	Ability to reach behind head with both arms alternately, maintaining trunk stability, hands together for manipulatory duty in sitting position
14. Behind back	—	Ability to reach behind back with both arms alternately, maintaining trunk stability, hands brought together for manipulatory duty
15. To toes	—	Ability to reach forward with both hands alternately when sitting to touch toes, hands free for manipulatory duty; may lean forward on elbows

Table 4-7   *(continued)*

Activity of Daily Living	Developmental Sequence Yr. Mo.	Definition of Task
Feeding		
16. Swallow (liquids)	Birth	Ability to gather up food, squeeze it to back wall of throat, thereby stimulating swallowing reflex
17. Drooling under control	1.0	
18. Suck and use straw	2.0	
19. Chew (semi-solids, solids)	1.6	Ability to masticate solids by well-defined chewing
20. Finger foods	0.10	Ability to reach, grasp, and bring finger food to mouth
Utensils		
21. Bottle	0.10	Ability to grasp utensil, fill with food, and raise it to mouth without spilling
22. Spoon	3.0	
23. Cup	1.6	
24. Glass	2.0	
25. Fork	3.0	
26. Knife	6.0–7.0	
Toileting		
27. Bowel control	1.6	Ability to regulate bowels so elimination occurs when seated on toilet
28. Bladder control	2.0	Ability to maintain sphincter control, remaining dry day and night
29. Sit on toilet	2.9	Ability to climb on lavatory seat unaided
30. Arrange clothing	4.0	Ability to manage fastenings, gets pants up and down, hold dress away from buttocks
31. Cleanse self	5.0	
32. Flush toilet	3.3–5.0	
Hygiene		
33. Turn faucets on/off	3.0	
34. Wash/dry hands/face	4.9	Ability to wash and dry hands and face efficiently without reminder of technique
35. Wash ears	8.0	
36. Bathing	8.0	Ability to care for all needs when bathing
37. Deodorant	12.0	
38. Care for teeth	4.9	Ability to combine all operations—prepare, brush, rinse
39. Care for nose	6.0	Ability to blow nose without assistance
40. Care for hair	7.6	Ability to comb and brush, check style with mirror
41. Care for nails	8.0	Ability to scrub and file nails
42. Feminine hygiene	Puberty	
Undressing		
Lower body		
43. Untie shoe bow	2.0–3.0	
44. Remove shoes	2.0–3.0	Ability to untie shoe bow and remove shoes
45. Remove socks	1.6	
46. Remove pull-down garment	2.6	
Upper body		
47. Remove pullover garment	4.0	

Table 4-7 (continued)

Activity of Daily Living	Developmental Sequence Yr. Mo.	Definition of Task
Dressing		
Lower body		
48. Put on socks	4.0	
49. Put on pull-down garment	4.0	Ability to put on garment, right side out, front and back correctly placed
50. Put on shoe	4.0	Ability to put shoe on correct foot
51. Lace shoe	5.0	
52. Tie bow	6.0	
Upper body		
53. Put on pullover garment	5.0	
Fasteners		
Unfastening		
Button		
54. Front	3.0	
55. Side	3.0	
56. Back	5.6	
Zipper		
57. Front	3.3	
58. Separating front	3.6	
59. Back	4.9	
Buckle		
60. Belt	3.9	
61. Shoe	3.9	
Tie		
62. Back sash	5.0	
Fastening		
Button		
63. Large front	2.6	
64. Series of three	3.6	
65. Back	6.3	
Zipper		
66. Front, lock tab	4.0	
67. Separating	4.6	
68. Back	5.6	
Buckle		
69. Belt	4.0	
70. Shoe	4.0	
71. Insert belt in loops	4.6	
Tie		
72. Front	6.0	
73. Back	8.0	
74. Necktie	10.0	
Snaps		
75. Front	3.0	
76. Back	6.0	

From Coley, Ida Lou: Pediatric Assessment of Self-care Activities. St. Louis: C. V. Mosby, 1978.
Inquiries on the Activities of Daily Living Assessment forms should be directed to the Occupational Therapy Department, Children's Hospital at Stanford, Palo Alto, CA 94304.

References

1. Craig, G. J.: Human Development, Englewood Cliffs, NJ: Prentice-Hall, 1976, p. 11.
2. Ibid., p. 11.
3. Ames, L. B.: Child Care and Development. Philadelphia: J. B. Lippincott, 1970, pp. 15–17.
4. Craig: Human Development, p. 12.
5. Bandura, A., Ross, D., and Ross, S. A.: Vicarious reinforcement and imitative learning. J. Abnorm. Soc. Psych. 66:601–607, 1963.
6. Craig: Human Development, p. 32.
7. Severin, F. T.: What Humanistic Psychology is About. Newsletter Feature Supplement. San Francisco: Association of Humanistic Psychology, 1974.
8. Gesell, A., and Thompson, S.: The Psychology of Early Growth. New York: Macmillan Publishing Co., 1938, p. 198.
9. Flanagan, C.: The First Nine Months of Life. New York: Simon & Schuster, 1960, p. 34–36.
10. Ibid, p. 81.
11. Anastasi, A.: Heredity, environment and the question of "how?" Psychol. Rev. 65:197–208, 1958.
12. Apgar, V.: Proposal for a new method of evaluating the newborn infant. Anesth. Analg. 32:260–267, 1953.
13. Fantz, R.: The origin of form perception. Scientif. Am. May 1961, pp. 66–72.
14. Pratt, K. C., Nelson, A. K., and Sun, K. H.: The Behavior of the Newborn Infant. Columbus: Ohio State University Press, 1930.
15. Lipsitt, L. P., Engen, T., and Kaye, H.: Developmental changes in the olfactory threshold of the neonate. Child Develop. 34:371–376, 1963.
16. Lipsitt, L. P., and Siqueland, E. R.: Conditioned head turning in human infants. J. Exper. Psychol. 3:356–376, 1966.
17. Frank, L.: On the Importance of Infancy. New York: Random House, 1966.
18. Brazelton, T. B.: Neonatal Behavior Assessment Scale. Philadelphia: J. B. Lippincott, 1973, p. 5.
19. Brazelton, T. B.: Psychophysiologic reactions in the neonate. I. The value of observation of the neonate. J. Pediatr. 58:508, 1961.
20. Brazelton: Neonatal Scale, p. 5.
21. Kalnins, J. V., and Bruner, J. S.: The coordination of visual observation and instrumental behavior in early infancy. Perception 1974.
22. Papousek, H.: Conditioned head rotation reflexes in infants in the first months of life. Acta Paed. Scand. 50:565–576, 1961.
23. Lorenz, K.: The companion in the birds' world. Auk 54:247–273, 1937.
24. Harlow and Zimmerman: Affectional responses in infant monkeys. Science 1959.
25. Klaus, M. H., and Kennell, J. H.: Maternal-Infant Bonding. St. Louis: C. V. Mosby, 1976.
26. Mead, M.: Sex and Temperament in Three Primitive Societies. New York: Morrow, 1935.
27. Bayley, N.: Comparisons of mental and motor test scores for age 1–15 months by sex, birthorder, race, geographic location and education of parents. Child Develop. 36:379–411, 1965.
28. Geber, M., and Dean, R. F. A.: The state of development of newborn African children. Lancet 1:1216–1219, 1957.
29. Tronick, E., Koslowski, B., and Brazelton, T. B.: Neonatal Behavior among Urban Zambians and Americans. Presented at the Biennial Meeting of the Society for Research in Child Development, Minneapolis MN, April 1971.
30. Caplan, F.: The First Twelve Months of Life. New York: Grosset and Dunlap, 1973, p. 132.
31. Maier, H.: Three Theories of Child Development. New York: Harper & Row, 1969, pp. 105–107.
32. Ibid., pp. 107–112.
33. Piaget, J.: The Construction of Reality in the Child. New York: Basic Books, 1954, p. 32.
34. Caplan, F.: First Twelve Months, p. 241.
35. Eisenson, J., et al.: The Psychology of Communication. New York: Appleton-Century-Crofts, 1963.
36. Lenneberg, E. H.: Biological Function of Language. New York: John Wiley & Sons, 1967.
37. Clifton, C.: Language acquisition. In Spencer, T. D., and Kass, N. (eds.): Perspectives in Child Psychology: Research & Review. New York: McGraw-Hill, 1970.
38. Maier: Three Theories, pp. 112–115.
39. Erikson, E.: Childhood and Society. New York: W. W. Norton & Co., 1963, pp. 251–254.
40. Maier: Three Theories, pp. 115–118.
41. Erikson, E.: Childhood and Society, pp. 255–257.
42. Murphy, L. B.: The Widening Mastery World of Childhood: Paths Toward Mastery. New York: Basic Books, 1962.
43. White, B.: Motivation reconsidered: the concept of competence. Psychol. Rev. 66:297–333, 1959.
44. Papalia, D., and Olds, S.: A Child's World: Infancy Through Adolescence. New York: McGraw-Hill, 1975, p. 224.
45. Rebelsky, F., and Hanks, C.: Fathers' verbal interaction with infants in the first three months of life. Child Develop. 42:63–68, 1972.
46. Flavell, J.: The Developmental Psychology of Jean Piaget. New York: Van Nostrand Co., 1963.
47. Papalia and Olds: Child's World, p. 280.
48. Ibid., p. 343.
49. Ibid., p. 351.
50. Kirchner, E. and Vondracek, S.: What do you want to be when you grow up? Vocational choice in children aged three to six. Paper presented at the Biennial Meeting of the Society for Research in Child Development, 1973.
51. Papalia and Olds, p. 427.
52. Craig: Human Development, p. 298.
53. Maier: Three Theories, p. 141.
54. Bayley, N.: Consistency and variability in the growth of intelligence from birth to eighteen years. J. Genet. Psychol. 75:165–196, 1949.
55. Kohlberg, L.: The child as a moral philosopher. Psychol. Today 2:25–30, 1968.
56. Maier: Three Theories, p. 54–55.
57. Bronfenbrenner, U.: Responses to pressure from peers versus adults among Soviet and American school children. In Papalia and Olds: Child's World.

58. Parten, M. B.: Social play among pre-school children. J. Abnorm. Soc. Psychol. 27:243–269, 1932.

59. Shuster, C. and Ashburn S.: The Process of Human Development: A Holistic Approach. Boston: Little Brown & Co., 1981, p. 291.

60. Smilanski, G.: The Effect of Sociodramatic Play on Disadvantaged Youth. New York: John Wiley & Sons, 1968, chapters 1–3.

61. Ringler, N. M., Trouse M., and Klaus M.: Mother's speech to her 2 year old; and its effect on speech and language at 5 years. Pediatr. Res. 10:307, 1976.

62. Piaget, J.: The Origins of Intelligence. Cook (trans): New York: International Universities Press, 1953, p. 68.

63. Schuster, C. and Ashburn, S.: The Process of Human Development; A Holistic Approach. Boston: Little, Brown & Co., 1980, p. 299.

64. Ibid.

65. Freud, A.: The concept of developmental lines. In Freud, A.: Normality and Pathology in Childhood: Assessment of Development. New York: International Universities Press, 1965.

66. Schuster: The Process of Human Development, p. 309.

67. Piaget, J.: Play, Dreams, and Imitation in Childhood. Gatteango, C., and Hudson, F. M. (trans): New York: W. W. Norton Press, 1965, p. 6.

68. Papalia and Olds: Child's World, p. 538.

69. Inhelder, B., and Piaget, J.: The Growth of Logical Thinking from Childhood to Adolescence. New York: Basic Books, 1958.

70. Elkind, D.: Egocentrism in adolescence. Child Develop. 38:1025–1034, 1967.

71. Elkind, D.: Understanding the young adolescent. Adolescence 1978, pp. 127–132.

72. Exploration of the Generational Conflict. Unpublished Manuscript. Paper presented at the meeting of A.P.A. San Francisco, 1968, p. 3.

73. Ibid., pp. 3–4.

74. Grender, R.: Adolescence, 2nd ed. New York: John Wiley & Sons, 1978, pp. 242–243.

75. Udry, J., and Bauman, K.: Changes in premarital coital experience in recent decade of birth cohorts of urban American women. J. Marriage and Family 37:783–787, 1975.

76. Schuster, C., and Ashburn, S.: The Process of Human Development: A Holistic Approach. Boston: Little Brown & Co., 1980, p. 512.

77. Miller, A.: Death of a Salesman: Certain Conversations in Two Acts and a Requiem. New York: Viking, 1949.

78. Piaget, J. P.: The Moral Judgement of the Child. Gaban, M. (trans): Glencoe IL: Free Press, 1948.

79. Schafer, R.: Aspects of Internalization. New York: International Press, 1968.

80. Coopersmith, S.: The Antecedents of Self Esteem. San Francisco: Freeman, 1967.

81. Berkowitz, L.: The Development of Motives and Values in the Child. New York: Basic Books, 1964.

82. Havinghurst, R. J., and Gottlib, D.: Youth and the meaning of work. In Havinghurst, and Dreyer, P. H. (eds): Youth—Seventy Fourth Yearbook of the National Society for the Study of Education. Chicago: University of Chicago Press, 1975, pp. 145–160.

83. Chick, J. M.: Implications for counselor education. Vocational Guidance Quarterly 22:108–111, 1973. Part of Project TALENT (Vocational Guidance Quarterly 22:92–96, 1973).

84. Astin: Stability and change in career plans of ninth grade girls. Personnel Guidance Journal 46:961–966, 1968.

85. Cooley, W.: Interaction among interests, abilities, and career plans. J. Appl. Psychol. 51:1–16, 1965.

86. Cosby, A.: Occupational expectations and the hypothesis of increasing realism of choice. J. Vocational Behavior 5:53–65, 1974.

87. Kuvlesky, W., Wright, D., and Juarez, R.: Status projections and ethnicity: A comparison of Mexican American, Negro, and Anglo youth. J. Vocational Behavior 1:137–151, 1971.

88. Datta, L-E., Foreword. In Diamond, E. E.: Issues of sex bias and sex fairness in career interest measurements. Washington, D.C.: Department of Health Education and Welfare, 1975.

89. Sewell, W.: The Educational and Occupational Perspectives of Rural Youth (paper prepared for National Conference on Problems of Rural Youth in a Changing Environment), 1963.

90. Sewell, W., and Orenstein, A.: Community of residence and occupational choice. Am. J. Sociol. 70:551–563, 1965.

91. Hewer, V.: Vocational interest of college freshman and the social origin. J. Appl. Psychol. 49:407–411, 1965.

92. Super, D.: Vocational development in adolescence and early childhood: Tasks and behaviors. In Super, D., Starishevsky, R., and Matlin, J. (eds): Career Development: Self Concept Theory. New York: College Examination Board, 1963.

93. Ginsberg, E.: Toward a theory of occupational choice as a restatement. Vocational Guidance Quarterly 20:169–176, 1972.

94. Isaacson, L.: Career Information in Counseling and Teaching. Boston: Allyn & Bacon, 1968, pp. 36–38.

95. Erickson, E. H.: Childhood and Society, 2nd ed. New York: W. W. Norton, 1967, p. 226.

96. Cameron, P.: Stereotypes about generational fun and happiness versus self appraised fun and happiness. Gerontologist 12:120–123, 1972.

97. Lowenthal, M. T.: Four Stages of Life. San Francisco: Jassey and Bass, Inc., 1975, p. 100.

98. Kastenbaum, R.: Humans Developing: A Life Span Perspective. Boston: Allyn, Bacon, Inc., 1972, pp. 518–522.

99. Freeberg, K.: Human Development. North Scituate MA: Duxbury Press, 1979, p. 296.

100. Horn, J.: Organization of data on life span development of human abilities. In Goulet, L., and Baltes, P. (eds.): Life Span Developmental Psychology. New York: Academic Press, 1970.

101. Dennis, W.: Creative productivity between the ages of twenty and eighty years. J. Gerontol. 21:1, 1966.

102. Piaget, J.: The Origins of Intelligence. Cook (trans): New York: International Universities Press, 1953, p. 150.

103. Quinn, R., et al. Job satisfaction: Is there a trend? U.S. Department of Labor, Manpower Research, Monograph #30. Washington, D.C.: U.S. Government Printing Office.
104. Sheehy, G.: Passages—Predictable Crises of Adult Life. New York: E. P. Dutton & Co. Inc., 1976.
105. Blood, R. O.: Marriage, 3rd ed. New York: Free Press, 1978, p. 40.
106. Folkman, J. D., and Clatworthy, N. M.: Marriage Has Many Faces. Columbus OH: Merrill, 1970, p. 80.
107. Schuster, C. S., and Ashburn, S.: The Process of Human Development: A Holistic Approach. Boston: Little, Brown & Co., 1980, p. 622.
108. Krantz, J.: Living together is a rotten idea. Cosmopolitan. October 1976, p. 218.
109. Cuber, J. F., and Harroff, P. B.: The Significant Americans: A Study of Sexual Behavior Among the Affluent. New York: Appleton-Century-Croft, 1965, p. 25.
110. Schuster, C. S., Ashburn, S.: The Process of Human Development: A Holistic Approach, p. 623–624.
111. Freiberg, K.: Human Development: A Life Span Approach, pp. 359–360.
112. Ibid., p. 361.
113. Neugarten, B., Wood, R., Fraines, R., and Loomis, B.: Women's attitude toward menopause," Vita Humana, 1963, p. 125.
114. Schuster, C., and Ashburn, S.: The Process of Human Development: A Holistic Approach, p. 772.
115. Ibid., p. 773.
116. Havinghurst, R.: Developmental Tasks and Education, 3rd ed. New York: McKay Publishers, 1972.
117. Levinson, D.: The psychological development of man in early adulthood and midlife transition. In Ricks, D., Thomas, A., and Roff, M. (eds.): Life History Research in Psychopathology III. Minneapolis: University of Minnesota Press, 1974, p. 254.
118. Gould, R.: The phases of adult life: A study of adult life. Am. J. Psychiatry 5:129, 1972.
119. Neugarten, B.: The roles we play. Quality of Life: The Middle Years. Acton, Mass.: Publishing Sciences Group, Inc., 1974, Chapter 5.
120. Kieren, D., Henton, J. M.: His and Hers: A Problem Solving Approach to Marriage. Hinsdale IL: Dryden Press, 1973, p. 257.

Bibliography
Prenatal

Developmental Psychology Today. Del Mar CA: CRM Books, 1982.
Flanagan, G.: The First Nine Months of Life. Philadelphia: International Ideas. New York: Simon & Schuster, 1962. Reprinted, 1978.
Fraser, F. C., and Nora, J.: Genetics of Man. Philadelphia: Lea & Febiger, 1975.
Hooker, D.: The Pre-Natal Origin of Behavior. New York: Hafner Press, 1969. (Classic text—out of print.)
Ingleman-Sundberg, A., and Wirsen, C.: A Child is Born: The Drama of Life Before Birth. New York: Dell Publishing Co., 1981.
Langman, J.: Medical Embryology: Human Development—Normal and Abnormal, 3rd ed. Baltimore: Williams & Wilkins, 1975.
Lowrey, G.: Growth and Development of Children, 7th ed. Chicago: Year Book, 1978.
Rugh, R., and Shettles, L. B.: From Conception to Birth: The Drama of Life's Beginnings. New York: Harper & Row, 1971.

Infancy and Childhood

Appleton, T., Clifton, R., and Goldberg, S.: The development of behavioral competence in infancy. In Horowitz, F. D. (ed.): Review of Research in Child Development, Vol. 4. Chicago: University of Chicago Press, 1975.
Arenas, S.: Bilingual/bicultural programs for pre-school children. Children Today, July–August 1978, pp. 2–6.
Beadle, M.: A Child's Mind. Garden City NY: Anchor Books, Doubleday & Co., 1971.
Bettelheim, B.: The Children of the Dream. New York: Macmillan, 1971.
Bloom, L., and Lahey, M.: Language Development and Language Disorders. New York: John Wiley and Sons, 1978.
Borstein, M. H., and Kessen, W.: Psychological Development from Infancy: Image to Intention. New York: John Wiley & Sons, 1979.
Bolwlby, J.: Attachment. New York: Basic Books, 1969. (Classic)
Bowlby, J.: Attachment and Loss, Vol. 2, Separation: Anxiety and Anger. New York: Basic Books, 1973.
Brazelton, T. B.: Infants and Mothers: Individual Differences in Development. New York: Dell Publishing Co., 1979.
Brazelton, T. B.: Neonatal Behavioral Assessment Scale. Philadelphia: J. B. Lippincott, 1973.
Caplan, F. (ed.): The First Twelve Months of Life: Your Baby's Growth Month by Month. New York: Grossett and Dunlap, 1978.
Castle, P., Held, R., and White, B. L.: Observations on the development of visually directed reaching. Child Develop. 35:349–364, 1964.
Coley: Pediatric Assessment of Self Care Activities. St. Louis: C. V. Mosby, 1978.
Connolly, K. J. (ed.): The Growth of Competence. New York: Academic Press, 1974.
Costello, A.: Pre-Verbal Communication. Child Psychol Psychiatry 17:351–353, 1976.
Cottle, T. J.: Time's Children: Impressions of Youth. Boston: Little, Brown & Co., 1971.
Cratty, B. J.: Perceptual and Motor Development in Infants, 2nd ed. Englewood Cliffs NJ: Prentice Hall, 1979.
Elkin, R., and Handel, G.: The Child and Society: The Process of Socialization. 3rd ed. New York: Random House, 1978.
Elkind, D.: Children and Adolescents, Interpretive Essays on Jean Piaget, ed. 2. New York: Oxford University Press, 1974.
Elkind, D.: A Sympathetic Understanding of the Child: Birth to Sixteen, 2nd ed. Boston: Allyn & Bacon, 1978.

Elkind, D., and Weinert: Development of the Child. New York: John Wiley & Sons, 1978.

Frailberg, S.: The Magic Years. New York: Charles Scribner's Sons, 1968.

Furth, H. G., and Wachs, H.: Thinking Goes to School: Piaget's Theory in Practice. New York: Oxford University Press, 1975.

Gesell, A.: The First Five Years of Life. New York: Harper & Row, 1940. (Classic)

Gesell, A., and Ilg, F. L.: The Child from Five to Ten. New York: Harper & Row, 1946. (Classic—out of print)

Gesell, A.: Youth: From Ten to Sixteen. New York: Harper & Row, 1956.

Henderson, R. W., and Bergan, J. R.: The Cultural Context of Childhood. Columbus OH: Charles E. Merrill, 1976.

Hopper, R., and Haremore, R.: Children's Speech. New York: Harper & Row, 1973.

Illingworth, R. S.: The Normal Child: and Some Problems of Early Years and Treatment, 7th ed. New York: Churchill-Livingstone, 1979.

Inhelder, B., and Piaget, J.: The growth of logical thinking from childhood to adolescence. New York: Basic Books, 1958. (Classic)

Ivanans, T.: Effects of maternal education and ethnic background on infant development. Arch. Dis. Child. 50:454–457, 1975.

Kagan, J.: The Growth of The Child. New York: W. W. Norton & Co. Inc., 1978.

Kennell, J., and Klaus, M. H.: Maternal Infant Bonding. St. Louis: C. V. Mosby, 1981.

Krown, S.: Threes and Fours Go to School. Englewood Cliffs NJ: Prentice Hall, 1974.

Lewis, M., and Rosenblum, L. A.: The Child and Its Family. New York: Plenum Press, 1979.

Lipsett, L. P.: Developmental Psychology. The Significance of Infancy. New York: John Wiley & Sons, 1976.

Lowrey, G. H.: Growth and Development of Children, 7th ed. Chicago: Year Book Medical Publishers.

McGraw, M.: The Neuromuscular Maturation of the Infant. New York: Hafner Press, 1963.

MacKeith, R., and Wood, C.: Infant Feeding and Feeding Difficulties. New York: Churchill-Livingstone, 1977.

Mahler, M., Pine, R., and Bergman, A.: The Psychology of Birth of The Human Infant: Symbiosis and Individuation. New York: Basic Books, 1975.

Mead, M., and Wolfstein, M.: Childhood in Contemporary Cultures. Chicago: University of Chicago Press, 1955. (Classic reference)

Morris, S. E.: Pre-Speech Assessment Scale. Unpublished experimental edition. C. P. Project, Curative Rehabilitation Center, 1980.

Nelson, K.: Children's Language, Vol. 2. New York: John Wiley & Sons, 1979.

Palmer, S.: Normal nutrition, growth, and development. In Palmer, S., and Ekvall, S. (eds): Pediatr. Nutrition Developmental Disorders. Springfield IL: Charles C. Thomas, 1978, pp. 3–20.

Papalia, D., and Olds, S.: A Child's World: Infancy throughout Adolescence, 2nd ed. New York: McGraw-Hill, 1979.

Peiper, A.: Cerebral Function in Infancy and Childhood. New York: Plenum Publishing Corp., 1964.

Prechtl, H.: A Neurological Examination of the Full Term Newborn Infant. London: Spastics International Medical Publishers, 1965.

Smith, D. W., and Bierman, E. L. (eds.): The Biologic Ages of Man: From Conception Through Old Age, 2nd ed. Philadelphia: W. B. Saunders, 1978.

Stone, J., et al: The Competent Infant: Research and Commentary. New York: Basic Books, 1974.

Stone, L., and Church, J.: Childhood & Adolescence: A Psychology of the Growing Person, 4th ed. New York: Random House, 1979.

Talbot, T.: The World of the Child: Clinical and Cultural Studies from Birth to Adolescence. New York: Jason Aronson, 1974.

Touwen, B.: Neurological Development in Infancy, Clin. Dev. Med. #58, Philadelphia: J. B. Lippincott, 1976.

Touwen, B.: Examination of Child with Minor Neurological Dysfunction. New York: Harper & Row, 1979.

Uzgiris, I., and Hunt, J.: Assessment in Infancy: Ordinal Scales of Psychological Development. Urbana, IL: University of Illinois Press, 1975.

Watson, R. L.: Psychology of the Child, 4th ed. New York: John Wiley & Sons, 1979.

Wechsler, D.: Manual for the Wechsler Intelligence Scale for Children, rev ed. New York: The Psychological Corporation, 1974.

Wesley, F.: Childrearing Psychology. New York: Behavioral Publications, 1971.

Werner, E. E.: Cross-Cultural Child Development, A View From Planet Earth. Monterey: Books/Cole Publishing Co., 1979.

White, B. L.: The First Three Years of Life. Englewood Cliffs, NJ: Prentice Hall, 1975.

Wyke, B.: The neurological basis of movement: A developmental review. Movement and Child Development, Clin. Dev. Med., #55, Philadelphia: J. B. Lippincott, 1975.

Zigler, E. F., and Child, I. L.: Socialization and Personality Development. Reading MA: Addison-Wesley Publishing Co., 1973.

Play

Ackerman, J.: Play, the Perceptual Motor Way. Seattle WA: Special Child Publications, 1975.

Behrmann, P.: Activities for Developing Auditory Perception. San Rafael CA: Academic Therapy Publishing, 1977.

Bingham, J. T.: Working Together. Tucson AZ: Communication Skill Builders, 1977.

Blake, J.: The Great Perceptual Learning Machine. Boston: Little, Brown & Co., 1976.

Bowden, and Munger: Beyond Peek-a-Boo and Pat-a-Cake. Chicago: Follett Pub., 1982.

Braga, J.: Children and Adults: Activities for Growing Together. Englewood Cliffs NJ: Prentice Hall, 1976.

Broad, L. B.: The Playgroup Handbook. New York: St. Martins Press, 1974.

Brown, S. D.: Developing Programing for Infants and Young Children Stimulation Activities. Ann Arbor MI: University of Michigan Press, 1977.

Caney, S.: Play Book. New York: Workman Publishing Company, 1975.

Cherry, C.: Creative Movement for the Developing Child: A Nursery School Handbook for Nonmusicians. Belmont CA: Fearon Pub., 1971.

Croft, D.: An Activities Handbook for Teachers of Young Children. Boston: Houghton Mifflin, 1975.

deRenne-Stephan, C.: Imitation: A mechanism of play behavior. Am. J. Occup. Ther. 34:95–102, 1980.

Fluegelman, A. (ed.): The New Games Book. Garden City: Doubleday & Co., 1976.

Goldberg, S.: Teaching with Toys: Making Your own Educational Toys. Michigan: University of Michigan Press, 1981.

Gordon, I.: Child Learning through Child's Play. New York: St. Martins Press, 1970.

Gordon, I. Baby Learning through Baby Play. New York: St. Martins Press, 1970.

Hagstrum, J.: More Games Babies Play: Fun with Baby From Birth to First Birthday. New York: A & W Visual Library, A & W Pub., 1981.

Hartley, R., and Goldenson, R.: The Complete Book of Children's Play. New York: Thomas Crowell Co., 1963.

Jenks, W.: Teacher's Handbook of Children's Games: A Guide to Developing Perceptual Motor Skills. New York: Parker Pub., 1976.

Kaplan: A Young Child Experiences. Pacific Palisades: Goodyear Publisher, 1975.

Koch, J.: Total Baby Development. New York: Wallaby Pocket Books, 1978.

Kohl, M., and Young, F.: Games for Children. New York: Cornerstone Library Publishers, 1976.

Largo, R. H., and Howard, J. A.: Development progression in play behavior of children between nine and thirty months. Dev. Med. Child Neurol., 21:299–309, 1979.

Lehane, S.: Help Your Baby Learn. Englewood NJ: Prentice Hall, 1976.

McCready Hurff, J.: A play skills inventory: A competency monitoring tool for the 10 year old. Am. J. Occup. Ther., 34:651–656, 1980.

McCoy, E.: Incredible Year Round Playbook. New York: Random House, 1979.

Malehorn, H.: Encyclopedia of Activities for Teaching Grades K–3. West Nyeck NY: Parker Publishers, 1975.

Margolla, J.: Super Tot. New York: Harper Colophon, 1977.

Meir, J., and Malone, P.: Facilitating Children's Development: Infant and Toddler. Baltimore MD: University Park Press, 1979.

Meir, J., and Malone, P.: Learning Episodes for Older Preschoolers. Baltimore MD: University Park Press, 1979.

Milberg, A.: Street Games. New York: McGraw-Hill, 1976.

Millman, J. B.: Parents as Playmates: A Game Approach to the Pre-School Years. New York: Human Sciences Press, 1979.

Orlick, T.: The Cooperative Sports and Games Book. New York: Patheon Books, 1975.

Painter, G.: Teach Your Baby. New York: Simon & Schuster, 1971.

Reilly, M.: Play as Exploratory Learning. Beverly Hills: Sage Publications, 1974.

Richardson, H.: Games for Elementary School Grades. Minneapolis MN: Burgess Publishing Company, 1976.

Round, S.: Teaching the Young Child. New York: Agathon Press, 1977.

Schaefer, C. (ed.): The Therapeutic Use of Child's Play. New York: Jason Aronson, 1975.

Short, P. D.: Ideas and Activities for Teaching Children 5–8. California: Goodyear Publishing, 1980.

Sparkman, B. S.: Preparing Your Preschooler for Reading: A Book of Games. New York: Schocken Books, 1977.

Sparting, J., and Lewis, I.: Learning Games for the First Three Years: A Guide to Parent Child Play. New York: Walker and Co., 1979.

Stein, L.: Three-Four Open the Door: Creative Fun for Young Child. Chicago IL: Follet Pub., 1971.

Tarbert, M.: Follow Me—A Handbook of Movement Activities for Children. Englewood Cliffs NJ: Prentice Hall, 1980.

Wedemeyer, A., and Cejka, J.: Creative Ideas for Teaching Exceptional Children. Denver CO: Love Publishing Co., 1975.

Weininger, O.: Play and Education. Springfield IL: Charles C. Thomas, 1979.

Witsen: Perceptual Training Activities Handbook. New York: New York Teacher's College, 1973.

Wood, C., and Goddard, G.: The Complete Book of Games. Garden City NY: Doubleday Publishing Co.

Yerian, C. M.: Funtime Games for One, Two or More, Funtime Group Games. Chicago: Childrens Press, 1975.

Yerian, C. M.: Funtime Competitive Games. Chicago: Childrens' Press, 1975.

Adolescent

Adams, J.: Understanding Adolescence, 2nd ed. Boston: Allyn & Bacon, 1973.

Alexander, T.: Children and Adolescence. New York: Atherton Press, 1969.

Angus, D. L., and Winder, A. E.: Adolescence, Contemporary Studies. New York: Van Nostrand Reinhold Co., 1968.

Barrow, J., and Hayashi, J.: Shyness clinic: A social development program for adolescents and young adults. Personnal Guidance J. September, 1980, pp. 58–61.

Bronfenbrenner, U.: Two Worlds of Childhood: US and USSR, Touchstone ed. New York: Simon and Schuster, 1972.

Cantwell, Z., and Suajiaw (eds.): Adolescence Studies in Development. Itasca IL: Peacock, 1974.

Caplan, G., and Lebovici, S. (eds.): Adolescence: Psychosocial Perspectives. New York: Basic Books, 1965.

Conger, J.: Adolescence and Youth. New York: Harper & Row, 1973.

Cottle, T. J., Melchione, J.: Adolescence voices, trying on adult masks. Psychol. Today, February 1979, p. 40.

Dragastin, S., Elder, G. (eds.): Adolescence in the Life Cycle. New York: John Wiley & Sons, 1975.

Elkind, D.: Children and Adolescence: Interpretive Studies of Jean Piaget, 2nd ed., New York: Oxford University Press, 1974.

Fernstein, S., and Giouacchini, P. (eds.): Adolescent Psychiatry, Vol 4. New York: Jason Aronson, 1975.

Friedenberg, E.: Coming of Age in America. New York: Vintage Books, 1963.

Garrison, D. C., and Garrison, K. C. Jr.: Psychology of Adolescence, 7th ed. Englewood Cliffs NJ: Prentice-Hall, 1975.

Grinder, R. (ed.): Studies in Adolescence, 3rd ed. New York: MacMillan, 1975.

Hanks, M., and Eckland, B. K.: Adult voluntary associations and adolescent socialization. Sociol. Quart. 19:481–490, 1978.

Horrocks, J. E.: Psychology of Adolescence. Boston: Houghton-Mifflin, 1976.

Inhelder, B., and Piaget, J.: The Growth of Logical Thinking from Childhood to Adolescence. New York: Basic Books, 1958.

Keniston, K.: Youth and Dissent. New York: Harcourt-Brace-Jovanovich, Inc., 1971.

James, and Jongeward: Born to Win, Reading MA: Addison Wesley Publishing Co., 1971.

Kohen, R. R.: The Child From 9 to 13, London: Aldone-Atherton, 1971.

Mead, M.: Culture and Commitment: A Study of the Generation Gap. Garden City NJ: Natural History Press-Doubleday, 1970.

Murphy, J. M., and Gilligan, C.: Moral development in late adolescence and adulthood, a critique and reconstruction of Kohlberg's theory. Human Develop. 23: 1980.

Muuss, R. E.: Theories of Adolescence. New York: Random House, 1975.

Samsie, S. J.: Youth Problems and Approaches. Philadelphia: Lea and Febiger, 1972.

Adult

Alafat, I.: Drinking behavior in college and young adult groups. Free Inquiry Creative Sociol. 7:87–98, 1979.

Anshel, M.: Effect of aging on acquisition and short term retention of motor skills. Percept. Mot. Skills, 47:993–998, 1978.

Armentano, M.: Growing up at 30. New Physician, June: 29–31, 1980.

Bardwick, J. M.: Middle age and a sense of future. Merill-Palmar Quart. Behavior Develop. 24:129–138, 1978.

Beauvoir, S. de: The Coming of Age. O'Brien, P. (trans): New York: G. P. Putman's Sons, 1972.

BelGeddes, J.: How to Parent Alone: A Guide for Single Parents. New York: Seabury Press, 1974.

Birdwick, J. M.: Middle age and a sense of future. Merill-Palmar Quart. Behavior Develop. 24:129–138, 1978.

Botwinick, J.: Aging and Behavior. New York: Springer Publishing Co., Inc., 1978, pp. 59–86.

Bowlby, J.: Separation. New York: Basic Books, 1973. (Children and Adult).

Brain, R.: Friends and Lovers. New York: Basic Books, 1976.

Brenton, M.: Friendship. New York: Stein and Day Publishers, 1975.

Bukstel, L. H., Roeder, D., Kilmann, P., and Laughlin, J.: Projected extramarital sexual involvement in unmarried college students. J. Marriage Family, August:320–327, 1978.

Calderone, M. S.: Sexuality and Human Values. New York: Association Press Publishers, 1974.

Calhoun, J. F., and Acocella, J. R.: Child rearing. Psychol. Adjustment Human Relationships. New York: Random House, 1978, pp. 324–328.

Comfort, A.: Middle age. A Good Age. New York: Crown Publishers, 1976.

Corroles, B.: The Theory and Techniques of Family Therapy. Springfield IL: Charles C. Thomas, 1979.

Davitz, J., and Davitz, L.: The question of identity, Chapter 3. Making it From 40 to 50. New York: Random House, 1976.

Duvall, E.: Family Development, 4th ed. Philadelphia: J. B. Lippincott, 1971.

Erdwins, C., Small, A., and Gross, R.: The relationship of sex roles to self-concept. Clin. Psychol., 36, 1980.

Feldman, S. S., and Nash, S. C.: Interest in babies during young adulthood. Child Dev. 49:617–622, 1978.

Freeman, H.: Sex role sterotypes, Self concepts, and measured personality characteristics in college men and women. Sex Roles 5:99–103. 1979.

Gaston, S. K.: Death and midlife crises. J. Psychiatr. Nurs. 18:31–35, 1980.

Gaylin, J.: Single father is doing well. *Psychol. Today,* April:36, 38, 1977.

Goldberg, S. R., and Deutsch, F.: Life Span Individual and Family Development, Monterey CA: Brooks/Cole Publishing Co., Inc., 1977.

Goodman, F. S.: Religious motivation and midlife. J. Gerontol. 34:106–115, 1979.

Goldstein, D., Larner, K., Zuckerman, S. G.: The Dance Away Lover and Other Roles We Play in Love, Sex, and Marriage. New York: William Morrow and Co., Inc., 1977.

Gray, M.: Love after 40. The Changing Years. New York: Doubleday & Co., 1967. Chapter 13.

Harris, W. M.: Black Community Development. San Francisco: R and E Research Associates, 1976.

Heiss, J.: The Case of the Black Family. New York: Columbia University Press, 1975.

Herman and Coyne: Mental manipulation of spatial information in young and elderly adults. Dev. Psychol. 16:537–538, 1978.

Hiltner, S.: Personal values in the middle years. The Middle Years. Acton, MA: Publishing Sciences Group, Inc., 1974, pp. 27–35.

Hunt, B., and Hunt, M.: Prime Time—A Guide to the Pleasure and Opportunities of the New Middle Age. New York: Stein and Day Publishers, 1974.

Huston, T. L.: Foundations of Interpersonal Attraction. New York: Academic Press, 1974.

Jacobs, L., and Gossman, M. D.: Three primitive reflexes in normal adults. Neurology 30, 1980, p. 117–123.

Jacques, J. M., and Chason, K. J.: Cohabitation: Its impact on marital success. Family Coordinator 28:1979.

Kimmel, D. C.: Adulthood and Aging. New York: John Wiley & Sons, 1974.

Kivett, V. R.: Religious motivation in middle age: Correlates and implications. J. Gerontol. January:106–115, 1979.

Klein, C.: The Single Parent Experience. New York: Walker Publishing Co., 1973.

Kummerow, J. M.: Adult development: Life stage and

age-group characteristics of a sample of adults ages 23–38. Dissertation Abstraces International 38:7154–7155, 1978.

LaShan, E.: The Wonderful Crisis of Middle Age. New York: David McKay, Inc., 1973.

Leary, T. J., and Erskine, S. W.: Economics and Aging in America, 1978.

Leon, G. R., Gillum, B., Gillum, R., and Gouze, M.: Personality stability and change over a 30 year period—middle age to old age. Consult. Clin. Psychol. 47:517–524, 1979.

Levine, J.: Parent passage. Psychol. Today, November:105–112, 1980.

Levinsen, D., Klein, L., and McKee: Periods in the adult development of man: Ages 18–46. Counseling Adults. Monterey CA: Brooks/Cole Publishing Co., 1977.

Levinson, D.: The Seasons of a Man's Life. New York: Alfred Knopf, 1978.

Levinson, D. J.: The midlife transition: A period of adult psychosocial development. Psychiatry, 40:1977.

Lewis, R., Csato, R., Aguilino, W., and McGuffin, N.: Developmental transitions in male sexuality. Counsel. Psychol. 7:15–18, 1978.

Lidtz: The Person His and Her Development Throughout the Life Cycle, 2nd ed. New York: Basic Books, 1976.

Lowenthal, M., Thurnher, M., and Chiriboga, D.: The Four Stages of Life. London: Jossey-Bass Publishers, 1975.

Masters, W. H., and Johnson, V. E.: Emotional poverty: A marriage crisis of the middle years. The Middle Years. Acton MA: Publishing Science Group, Inc., by the AMA, 1974, pp. 101–108.

McCoy, V. R.: Adult life cycle research, but where are the women?. Paper presented at National Conference on Issues and Trends in Continuing Education Programs for Women, Ohio State University, May 12, 1978.

McFadden, M.: Bachelor Fatherhood. New York: Walker and Co., 1974.

Nadelson, P., and Mathews: Marriage and midlife: The impact of social change. J. Clin. Psychiatry. July:292–298, 1979.

Neugarten, B. L.: Dynamics of transition of middle age to old age. J. Geriatr. Psychiatry 4: p. 176, 1970.

Neugarten, B. L. (ed.): Middle Age and Aging. Chicago: University of Chicago Press, 1968.

Neugarten, B. L.: The roles we play, The Middle Years. Acton MA: Publishing Sciences Group, Inc., by the AMA 1974, pp. 35–39.

Neugarten, B. L., et al.: Personality in Middle and Late Life. New York: Prentice-Hall, 1964, pp. 105–113.

Neugarten, B. L., and Doroty, N.: The middle years. In Areiti, S. (ed.): American Handbook of Psychiatry. March 3, 1972, (1), pt. 3.

Newman, B., and Newman, P.: Development Through Life: A Psychosocial Approach. Illinois: The Dorsey-Press, 1975.

Nicholson, J.: Is there really a mid-life crisis? New Society. August:27–28, 1980.

Nicholson, J.: Kicking down the door into adulthood. New Society. August:303–305, 1980.

Notman, M.: Midlife concerns of women: Implications of the menopause. Am. J. Psychiatry 136:207–211, 1979.

Perry, J. S., and Slemp: Differences between three adult age groups in their attitudes towards self and others. J. Genet. Psychol. 136:275–279, 1980.

Pruchaska, J., and Coyle, J.: Choosing parenthood: A needed family life educational group. Soc. Casework 60:289–295, 1979.

Ross, H.: Time of transition. The Growth of Families Headed by Women. Washington, D.C.: Urban Institute, 1975.

Samuel, D.: Love, Liberation and Marriage. New York: Funk and Wagnals Publishers, 1976.

Schlesinger, B.: The One-Parent Family, 4th ed. Toronto: University of Toronto Press, 1978.

Schlossberg, N. K.: Five propositions about male development, J. College Student Personnel. January 1978.

Schlossberg, N. K.: Perspectives on Counseling Adults: Issues and Skills. Monterey: Brooks/Cole Publishing Co., 1978.

Schneider, S. J., and Gordon, F. S.: Retirement in American Society. London: Cornell University Press, 1971.

Sears, R., and Feldman, S. (eds.): The Seven Ages of Man. Los Altos CA: W. Kaufman, 1973.

Sheehy, G.: Passages: Predictable Crises in Adult Life. New York: Bantom Books. 1976.

Stafford, L. M.: One Man's Family. New York: Random House, 1978.

Stevenson, J. S.: Issues and Crises During Midadolescence. New York: Appelton-Century-Crofts, 1977, pp. 135–151.

Stockard, J., and Johnson, M. M.: Strains in your adulthood. Sex Roles. New Jersey: Prentice-Hall, 1980, pp. 262–263.

Talbot, N. B.: Raising Children in Modern America. Boston: Little, Brown & Company, 1976.

Turner, J. S., and Helms, D. B.: Contemporary Adulthood. Philadelphia: W. B. Saunders and Co., 1979, pp. 25–29.

White, R.: The Enterprise of Living. New York: Holt, Rinehart and Winston, 1972.

Windel, C. H.: Ethnic Families in America. New York: Elesuier North Holander, 1976.

Wyne, M.: The Black Self. New Jersey: Prentice-Hall, 1974.

Zarit, S. H. (ed.): Menopause. Readings in Aging and Death: Contemporary Perspectives. New York: Harper & Row, 1977, pp. 156–164.

Work and Leisure

Argle, M.: The Social Psychology of Work. New York: Taplinger, 1972.

Bachman, J. G., and O'Maller, P. M.: Self-esteem in young men: A longitudinal analysis of the impact of education and occupational attainment. J. Pers. Soc. Psychol. 35:365–388, 1977.

Bedeian, A. G., and Marbert, L. D.: Individual differences in self-perception and the job–life satisfaction relationship. J. Soc. Psychol. 109:111–118, 1979.

Bischof, L.: Vocation. Adult Psychology. New York: Harper & Row, 1976.

Bolton, E. B.: A conceptual analysis of the mentor relationship in the career development of women. Adult Educ. 30:195–207, 1980.

Cherlin, A.: Postponing marriage: The influence of young womens' work expectations. J. Marriage Family 42: 355–365, 1980.

Clayre, A.: Work and Play. New York: Harper & Row, 1974.

Cohn, R. M.: Age and the satisfaction for work. J. Gerontol. 34:264–272, 1979.

Ginzberg, E.: Youth unemployment. Scientif. Am. 242: 43–49, 1980.

Kafry, D., and Pines, A.: The experiance tedium in life and work. Hum. Relations 33:477–503, 1980.

Kelleher, C. A., and Quirk, D. A.: Age functional capacity and work: An annotated bibliography. Industr. Gerontol. No. 19, Fall 1973.

Kielhofner, G., and Burke, J. P.: A model of human occupation, Part 1. Conceptual framework and content. Am. J. Occup. Ther. 34:572–581, 1980.

Kielhofner, G.: A model of human occupation, Part 2. Ontogenesis from the perspective of temporal adaptation. Am. J. Occup. Ther. 34:657–663, 1980.

Kielhofner, G.: A model of human occupation, Part 3. Benign and vicious cycles. Am. Occup. Ther. 34:731–737, 1980.

Kielhofner, G., Burke, J. P., and Igi, C. H.: A model of human occupation, Part 4. Assessment and intervention. Am. J. Occup. Ther. 34:777–788, 1980.

Klaus, R. G.: Recreation Today—Program Planning and Leadership. Santa Monica CA: Goodyear Publishing Co., Inc., 1977.

Klaus, R.: Recreation and Leisure in Modern Society. Santa Monica CA: Goodyear Publishing Co., Inc., 1978.

Neulinger, J.: The Psychology of Leisure-Research Approaches to the Study of Leisure. Springfield IL: Charles C. Thomas, 1974.

Parker, S.: The Future of Work and Leisure. London: Mac-Gibbon and Kee, 1971.

Pursell, D. E., and Torrence, W. D.: The older woman and her search for employment. Aging and Work. Spring:121–128, 1980.

Terkel, S.: Working. New York: Pantheon Books, 1972.

Thomas: Mid-career changes: Self-selected or externally mandated? Vocational Guidance Quart. June:320–328, 1977.

General

Ambion, S.: Child Development. New York: Holt, Rinehart, and Winston Co., 1978.

Ames, L. B.: Child Care and Development. Philadelphia: J. B. Lippincott, 1979.

Babcock: Introduction to Growth and Development and Family Life. Philadelphia: F. A. Davis, 1979.

Bernard, H. W.: Human Development in Western Culture, 5th ed. Boston: Allyn & Bacon, 1978.

Biehler, R. F.: Child Development and Introduction. Boston: Houghton-Mifflin, 1981.

Craig, G. J.: Human Development. Englewood Cliffs NJ: Prentice-Hall, 1980.

Developmental Psychology Today. Del Mar CA: CRM Books, 1971.

Erikson, E. H.: Eight ages of man. Life the Continuous Process. New York: Alfred A. Knopf. Inc., 1975.

Gesell, A., and Armatruda, C.: Developmental Diagnosis. New York: Harper & Row, 1974.

Hurlock, E. B.: Developmental Psychology, 5th ed. New York: McGraw-Hill, 1980.

Kaluger, G., and Kaluger, M. F.: Human Development: The Span of Life, 2nd ed. St. Louis: C. V. Mosby, 1979.

Kopp, C. B. (ed.): Reading in Early Development: For Occupational and Physical Therapy Students. Springfield IL: Charles C. Thomas, 1971.

Lovell, K., and Elkind, D.: An Introduction to Human Development. Glenview IL: Scott, Foresman and Co., 1971 (paperback).

McConnell, J. V.: Understanding Human Behavior, 3rd ed. New York: Holt, Rinehart, and Winston, 1980.

Mussen, P. H. (ed.): Carmichael's Manual of Child Psychology, 3rd ed, Vol. I. New York: John Wiley & Sons, 1970.

Mussen, P. H., and Conger, J. J.: Child Development and Personality, 5th ed. New York: Harper & Row, 1979.

Nelson, K.: Children's Language, Vol. II. New York: John Wiley & Sons, 1979.

Peiper, A.: Cerebral Function in Infancy and Childhood. New York: Plenum Publishing Corp., 1964.

Piaget, J.: Construction of Reality in the Child. New York: Basic Books, 1954.

Piaget, J.: Play, Dreams and Imitation in Childhood. New York: W. W. Norton & Co., 1951.

Piaget, J.: The Moral Judgement of the Child. New York: Macmillan, 1932.

Piaget, J.: The Origins of Intelligence in Children. New York: International Universities Press, 1966.

Piaget, J., and Inhelder, B.: The Psychology of the Child. New York: Basic Books, 1969.

Schuster, C., and Ashburn, S.: The Process of Human Development, A Holastic Approach. Boston: Little, Brown & Co., 1980.

Sears, R., and Feldman, S. (eds.): The Seven Ages of Man. Los Altos CA: W. Kaufman, 1973.

Smith, D. W., and Bierman, E. L. (eds.): The Biologic Ages of Man: From Conception Through Old Age. Philadelphia: W. B. Saunders, 1973.

Spitz, R. A.: The first year of life. New York: International Universities Press, 1965 (Classic).

Stone, J., et al.: The Competent Infant: Research and Commentary. New York: Basic Books, 1974.

Talbot, T.: The World of the Child: Clinical and Cultural Studies from Birth to Adolescence. New York: Jason Aronson, 1967.

Uzgeris, I. C., and Hunt, J. M.: Assessment in Infancy. Ordinal Scales of Psychological Development. Chicago: University of Illinois Press, 1975.

Wesley, F., and Sullivan, E.: Human Growth and Development: A Psychological Approach. New York: Human Sciences Press, Inc., 1980.

White, B.: Human Infants: Experience and Psychological Development. Englewood Cliffs NJ: Prentice-Hall, 1971.

White, B. L.: The Origins of Human Behavior. Lexington, MA: Heath & Co., 1979.

PART 3

Occupational Therapy Approaches for Intervention

CHAPTER 5

Occupational Therapy— A Problem-Solving Process

Helen L. Hopkins and Elizabeth G. Tiffany

The drawing together of the client, the therapist, and the activity represents an exceedingly complex and dynamic situation. When confronted with providing valid and effective treatment for the disabled client, the occupational therapist must address a number of questions: On what basis do I understand this person? How do I conceptualize human personality, human behavior, physical function, and the ways in which human beings learn, grow, and change? How do I understand pathology or the disease process? What about its etiological factors and its prognosis? What do I know about the external factors which now impinge upon this person? What about the social and work worlds in which he or she must function now and in the future? What do I know about the methods of treatment or frames of reference for treatment currently being used with this person? How can I best communicate with this person so that we build a mutual understanding of reality that is as clear as possible?

The occupational therapy process is a problem-solving process. Skill in problem solving is basic to the therapist's success in carrying out the essential purpose of occupational therapy, that is, helping individuals who have problems in their adaptive functioning to reach their highest potential. If this purpose is to be accomplished, the therapist must approach each situation as an opportunity to find meaningful solutions to the problems that patients face.

Problem solving in a clinical situation is a complex process, requiring consideration of several dimensions at each step along the way. Occupational therapists must become skilled in problem identification, using observation and the many evaluation procedures available to them. In this way, a data base can be established which will identify the real problems. The recognition, definition, and analysis of the problem areas, and the collection of data related to those areas, lead to a clarification of goals and objectives toward which therapeutic intervention can be directed realistically. Alternative approaches for solving the problems must be identified, and a plan of action which seems promising for problem resolution must be chosen.

It is important for the patient or client to be involved in the process of problem identification so that the assets as well as liabilities of the situation may be determined. The goals that are established, the alternative chosen, and the plan of action must reflect what is desired by and acceptable to the patient or client. In order to be successful, moreover, the plan of action and the approach chosen must be compatible with those of other professionals working with the individual. The values and lifestyle of the client's family should also be taken into consideration.

Each plan of action must be examined for its probable value and the potential outcomes of treatment or intervention. If the plan appears to be feasible, and if it offers a promising solution, it can be implemented. Short-term goals with manageable elements contribute to the achievement of long-term goals. The therapist needs to be clear about the relationship between the long-term and short-term goals and their sequencing. There must be periodic reevaluation to determine progress, goals reached, and problems solved. It may be necessary to make modifications or to adapt goals and plans as changes occur. There are occasions when abandonment of an unsuccessful plan is necessary, requiring a determination of another course of action from the alternatives available. As new knowledge develops and as new viewpoints evolve, new alternatives arise that provide different approaches for intervention in occupational therapy.

Use of the problem solving process in occupational therapy requires creativity and imagination on the part of the therapist. The therapist must use knowledge, skills, and good professional judgment in order to find the best possible solution for each client.[1,2]

Approaches to Intervention

In occupational therapy today there are several alternative approaches to intervention that may be chosen by practicing therapists, depending on their orientation and their rationale for treatment. Each approach has a specific knowledge base, each is built on stated concepts, and each utilizes a rationale which places constraints on the occupational therapy program by specifying the type of activities appropriate for occupational therapy intervention.

Among the currently identified approaches to treatment are rehabilitation/habilitation[3]; acquisitional or behavioral; developmental (including a variety of special foci, such as neurodevelopmental, adaptive skills, and sensori-integration)[4-6]; psychoanalytic[7]; and occupational behavior.[8] While these approaches overlap in some areas, their importance lies in the fact that they provide the therapist with specific guidelines within which to apply knowledge and skills. The experience, values, sociocultural assumptions, individual points of view,

and the concept of reality inherent in an agency's philosophy promote the choice of a specific frame of reference.[9] For example, within the developmental approach, one occupational therapist, a group of therapists, or agency may favor a neurodevelopmental perspective for treatment of children with cerebral palsy and may choose to utilize the Bobath frame of reference. Others may favor a neurophysiological perspective and may choose to utilize a Rood frame of reference. Some agencies may use more than one approach to intervention, depending on the type of clients as well as on the preferences, biases, and expertise of the therapists. This increases the potential number and variety of frames of reference that may be used. The rationale and basis for choosing an approach and frame of reference as well as the knowledge base and concepts inherent in that approach, must be understood by the therapist.

The occupational therapy intervention process will differ according to the approach and frame of reference chosen, but the overall goals of the process can be described as *prevention* of conditions causing or resulting in loss of function; *remediation, treatment,* or *rehabilitation* for restoration of function and performance; and *maintenance* of health and the ability to function in all aspects of living. Depending upon the conditions and problems involved, any or all of these goals may be appropriate in the intervention process for a patient or client at any time along the developmental continuum.

The need has been recognized for occupational therapy to enunciate clearly its unifying concepts. These are elements that define the uniqueness of occupational therapy and that are common to all of the legitimate approaches to intervention.[10-13] At this point it is possible to say that the following are common to current practice: concern for adaptation; the use of purposeful activity[14]; and the use of problem-solving skills.

Basis for Treatment Approaches
The Four Elements

Occupational therapists are concerned with maintaining, improving, and restoring clients' abilities to function in their own worlds. They are aware, with varying degrees of interest and sophistication, that human beings are complex and whole. Therapists' work has been based on four components: the *patient or client,* the *therapist and therapeutic relationship,* the *activity,* and the *context or setting for treatment.* The therapeutic process, carried out formally or informally, is one of *evaluation, treatment planning,* and *treatment implementation.*

The Patient or Client

Problems in a client's ability to adapt and function are multifaceted. It is, of course, critical to understand as much as possible about the specific motor, cognitive, emotional, or social difficulties which the individual may be experiencing. Clinical diagnoses or clinical impressions are only a starting point in this understanding; it must be couched in a broader sense of the human and nonhuman factors which are involved. There are a great many ways in which human personality and behavior may be conceptualized. For the purpose of establishing a baseline, we will consider here a few of the factors which are especially important in the occupational therapy process. These are in no way exclusive, and the reader is referred to the bibliography and is encouraged to search the literatures of the social and biological sciences for other perspectives.

Stress

Any consideration of disability or dysfunction must include attention to the role that stress plays in the development and exacerbation of problems. In 1956 Hans Selye wrote *The Stress of Life*[15] in which he described the interrelationships of the body systems and the extensive effects of stress upon the whole. In the years which have followed the publication of Selye's work, interest in the nature of stress has spurred a great deal of research as well as much public speculation. During the 1960s and 1970s we have seen a proliferation of popular movements and literature dealing with methods of coping with stress and tension. Stress is often viewed in the context of technological advances and ideational changes such as those described by Toffler in *Future Shock*.[16]

Coleman broadly defines stress as the "adjustive demands made upon the individual." He points out[17] that stress may occur on physiological or psychological levels. On the physiological level, examples of stressors which make adjustive demands upon the individual are a broken limb, invasion by a virus, ingestion of poison, blood sugar imbalance, or an arthritic condition. On the psychological level, stressors may be the loss of a loved one, failure in an important test, the necessity of making a choice between two highly desirable (or undesirable) alternatives, or bombardment with too many things to do. The effects of stress, regardless of the original stressful event, are felt in varying degrees throughout the system. Data on autonomic system responses, cortical changes, muscle tension, and subjective experience have been collected and measured. These data indicate clearly that mind, emotions, and body are inseparably involved in their reactions to stress.

Coleman further points out that the severity of stress depends upon three factors: (1) the characteristics of the adjustive demand; (2) the characteristics of the individual; and (3) the external resources and supports available to the individual. Adjustive demands may be brief or long in duration. The threat to the individual's actual survival may in reality be great or small. The stressful event may occur alone or may occur in combination with a number of other stressful factors. Stressful reactions may predispose an individual to further negative stress reactions.

According to Coleman, the longer stress continues, the more severe it becomes. Many small stresses occurring together at the same time may subject the individual to stress overload, and the gradual building up of insignificant events over a long period of time may add up to greater stress than a single severe incident.

On the other hand, stress, as "the adjustive demands made upon the individual," may be viewed as having the potential for positive effects. It is in the second two factors mentioned by Coleman—the characteristics of the individual and the external resources and supports available—that there exist possibilities for change, growth, and strengthening of coping mechanisms to deal with inevitable future life stresses. A crisis may combine danger with opportunity. Recognition of these possibilities is important in occupational therapy.

Characteristics of the individual include genetic predispositions; intelligence; temperament; body type; structural strengths and weaknesses of the body systems; basic environmental influences such as nutrition, clothing, and housing; parental nurturance; discipline; the cumulative effects of interactions with significant people in school, church, and the neighborhood; and the mores and cultural factors that impinge upon the development of personality. The individual is a total being, a composite of physical, sensory, perceptual, emotional, cognitive, social, and cultural behaviors and skills. The extent to which this composite is elastic (able to rebound), flexible (able to bend, compromise, and change), and strong (able to stand firm) is significant in determining the extent to which individuals can meet the adjustive demands made upon them. The characteristics of the individual, although basically determined by adulthood, may be considered as dynamic and alterable in some measure throughout life. If this were not so there would be no reason for therapy.

External resources for coping with stress are multidimensional. They include factors such as the family, the neighborhood, the church, friends, money, educational opportunities, the possibility of a vacation, and even the climate.

The therapeutic process is inherently a process of

change. It is hoped that occupational therapy intervention will lead the client to new and more effective ways of functioning. Sometimes change can be frightening, and the therapist must be conscious of this as an additional element or stressor in the problem-solving process. For example, independence and a sense of autonomy are not cheaply gained. Often, though highly desired, they pose a sense of risk for individuals whose physical or emotional difficulties have rendered them dependent for a period of time. Within the problem-solving process the therapist must be able to address the question of risk vs. gain. Clients sometimes need reassurance with regard to the efforts they are investing in the therapeutic process. Sometimes they may *feel they are losing more than they are gaining by giving up dysfunction.* This can become a significant consideration, if not a determinant, in the therapeutic outcome. One problem for the therapist is the fact that change as a stressor is frequently not recognized, even by the client.

For the health professional whose commitment is to facilitate competence on the part of the dysfunctional, the careful consideration of Coleman's three aspects is essential. It is important to be sensitive to the possibility that stress, regardless of its nature, may be responsible for regression and a lessened ability to perceive realistically or to behave adaptively. This in itself contributes to further stress and further regression, and a vicious downward spiral has been started. On the other hand, true coping behavior in which an individual is able to feel competent and to experience success or mastery seems to lead to further strengths, more adaptive skills, and successes.

Motivation

The key to success in a program of occupational therapy often lies in the extent to which the patient or client may be motivated to participate in it. Human motivation has been a much studied personality variable, and motivation seems to be one of the most important areas to which the occupational therapist should give attention. Motivation may be defined as an arousal to action, initiating, molding, and sustaining specific action patterns.[18] The task of the occupational therapist requires that the client be motivated, first to participate in treatment, and second to sustain the healthy patterns hopefully established in the process.

One may consider that behavior is motivated by principles of drive-reduction, need satisfaction, and the pleasure principle. The role of reinforcement as a basic motivator has been much studied, and one needs to look carefully at the many aspects of reinforcement and aversive conditioning approaches to achieving motivation. Other theories suggest that behavior, beyond those aspects related to survival, is motivated in addition by innate curiosity and in a need to interact with the environment.[19]

The examination of the range of "normal" behavior reveals that people are motivated by many factors, for example, novelty, complexity, surprise, competition, and cooperation. Personality types have been characterized in terms of dominant social motivational patterns: (1) *affiliation*—liking people; (2) *aggression*—moving against people; (3) *dominance*—trying to dominate people; and (4) *cognizance*—exploring and asking questions.

McClelland has studied factors related to "need for achievement." This is defined as the extent to which a person could enjoy competition against a standard of excellence. Individuals may be characterized as falling somewhere along a continuum with regard to this variable. At the low end the individual tends to prefer to be involved in no risk situations where competition is minimal. This personality variable appears to be dynamic and powerful and seems to be set at a very early age.[20]

Related to achievement motivation as a personality factor is the issue of field dependence. Some people demonstrate unique, integrated, individual, internal schemes; those who do tend to be less conforming to social pressure and who seem to behave more in conformity to standards which are internalized and personal. Such individuals are characterized as field-independent. Those individuals who seem to be highly motivated to conform to standards or pressures which are external are characterized as field-dependent.[21]

Another related and powerful factor is locus of control. Locus of control refers to the extent to which individuals perceive that the events and situations of their lives are controlled by themselves or by chance or luck. This variable is, again, measured on a continuum that goes from an extreme internal locus of control to an extreme external locus of control. Internals perceive themselves as responsible and as able to direct and control their life situations, while externals see themselves as the recipients or victims of fate. Extremes in either direction, obviously, are unrealistic.[22-24]

Two factors may be critical in determining the nature of an individual's orientation with regard to achievement motivation, field dependence, and locus of control. First, there are the quality and quantity of experiences that the individual had as a child, and the extent to which they were pleasurable, reinforcing, or satisfying. Second, and perhaps more basic, is the consideration of the individual's ability to process the information that is received from the world. Both of these considerations appear to be of great importance. There is need for continuing research into their complex relationships with human motivation and basic self-concept.

Piaget[25] and White[26] have spoken eloquently of the importance of the experience of success in promoting feelings of efficacy and providing motivation for further performance. What seems to be of great importance is that the individual clearly understands, experiences, and owns the behaviors and their effects. Those situational variables that are not, in fact, related to an individual's behavior or control need to be understood as such.

Another factor, which is very powerful in determining motivation, is anxiety. Anxiety may be a strong motivator for performance up to a point, a factor that varies from individual to individual and with situations. Beyond that point, anxiety becomes an inhibitor to motivation, tends to render the individual rigid and unable to adapt to new situations, and results in a decrease in integrative mechanisms.

All of these considerations are of great importance to the occupational therapist because of the need to elicit the active cooperation and participation of the patient or client. The results of illness and disability may be perceived differently by different individuals with regard to their sense of responsibility and efficacy. The extent to which standards of achievement must be internalized to be motivating to an individual varies. Clarity of feedback, awareness of anxiety levels, and the ability to identify what may be uniquely reinforcing to an individual may be critical to determining the success or failure of a treatment program.

The Nonhuman World

From the moment of birth, human beings become part of a world of things to be experienced—to be seen, felt, heard, smelled, tasted, feared, and enjoyed.

For infants and growing children, the human and nonhuman objects of their worlds are crucial in determining the kinds of people they will become. For the occupational therapist, understanding the ways in which a person interacts with the nonhuman world is important. Harold Searles, in his book *The Nonhuman Environment*,[27] explores in depth the kinds and qualities of meanings that human beings invest in their worlds of things, places, and spaces. He refers to kinds of relationships that characterize human interactions with their nonhuman worlds as they grow up. People are able to use the nonhuman world to gain a sense of stability and continuity, to practice skills in relating, to assuage strong feelings, to foster self-realization, to deepen the awareness of reality, and to foster appreciation and acceptance of fellow human beings.

The healthy adult has learned to live in some degree of adaptation with the things and places of his or her world. What is the range of feelings inherent in the experiences of the nonhuman world? There are experiences of pleasure in fixing the engine of a car, pride in baking a cake, excitement in riding a roller coaster, frustration in coping with a machine that will not work, discomfort of being wet and cold in a storm, power in moving a heavy object, helplessness in not being able to move a heavy object, catharsis in housecleaning, wholeness in being beside the ocean, or comfort in a warm bed on a cold night.

The things and places of the world offer sources of pleasure and pain, opportunities to practice skills and to express ourselves, challenges to survive, and chances to live well. There is a continual and intimate relatedness with the nonhuman world.

The arts and artifacts that human beings come to treasure become symbolically invested with the values of the people who produce and use them. This goes far beyond things like dishes, vases, furniture, books, toys, and paintings. It goes into the uses of space and the kinds of personal privacy that may be fostered and the extent to which the world of nature is regarded and incorporated into an individual's living space.

What does all this mean to the occupational therapist? It has everything to do with attention to the potential meanings of the tools and materials of the activities used in treatment and the kinds of environments in which the therapist practices. It means the therapist can help the patient or client develop ways of trusting and *using* the nonhuman worlds; that this may have primary importance all by itself. The use of the nonhuman world is significant in providing a bridge for human relationships. It means the articles used and treasured by a person give clues not only to that person's private gestalt but also to the culture of the society in which he or she lives. It means that when a patient or client has permitted himself to invest in creating or producing something tangible or ideational in occupational therapy, the therapist needs to respect the person's ownership of that product.

Cultural Implications

Much is said about the need to understand the family and community to which each patient or client belongs. The rich literatures of sociology and anthropology on the subject of cultural influences are worth studying. There is little doubt that social systems are a powerful, although often subtle, influence on basic ways of perceiving, thinking, feeling, and behaving. Learning begins at conception and continues through interactions with both human and nonhuman environments; therefore, cultural values, biases, and customs are powerful in the formation of personalities. The kinds of toys, games, foods, and other objects that are presented, the kinds of music and stories, the humor, the behavior that is encouraged and the behavior that is discouraged, the quality and quantity of parenting experienced, and the amount of touching and closeness between people are just some of the ways in which children are influenced by the culture of their families. Cultural influences are deep. As Edward Hall says,

> Most of culture lies hidden and is outside voluntary control, making up the warp and weft of human existence. Even when small fragments of culture are elevated to awareness, they are difficult to change, not only because they are so personally experienced but because people cannot act or interact at all in any meaningful way except through the medium of culture.[28]

Both the therapist's perceptions and behavior and the client's perceptions and behavior are filtered through the screen of culture.

The occupational therapist must be concerned about values. Values determine how individuals feel about people, ideas, and things and how they act toward them. Value conflicts, both within self and between individuals and groups, are responsible for many of the difficulties which are part of everyone's living experience. In today's society, with rapid mass communication and mobility, the potential for value conflicts seems to be increasing.

Among the daily behaviors to be considered are the ways in which a client views and manages time, space (personal distance and territory), objects, dress, daily self-care activities, money, work, play, and study. How does the client respond to pain, loss, illness, and death? What is considered rude? How important is the family? What constitutes friendship? What about religious beliefs, rituals, and observances? Is anxiety handled by laughing and talking or by withdrawing? What is the significance of food and mealtimes? How is anger dealt with? What are the characteristic support systems of the group? Certain oriental groups laugh when they are confronted with danger. Some groups consider manual occupations degrading. The average American is more scheduled and time-bound than individuals from most cultural groups.

In a culturally heterogeneous population there will be a wide range of behaviors and lifestyles which may be considered normal. To help the client function within his or her own world, the therapist needs to understand that world.

The Therapist

The therapist in a treatment setting is, by definition, a helper. The roles a therapist assumes may vary. The therapist may legitimately be a teacher or a facilitator who brings knowledge and skills to the client's unique situation.

The most important prerequisite to being an effective helper is self-knowledge. The helper needs to be aware of his or her own needs, perceptual biases, and capabilities.

The relationship that is established between the therapist and the client may well determine the success or failure of the treatment plan. The establishment of effective and clear communication both ways is the first essential part of the relationship. Sensitivity to the level and mode of communication that will work with a given client and skill in using this knowledge may be the critical factor. For example, if a patient is functioning on a preverbal level of understanding, one must think of nonverbal ways of communicating meaning. If a patient thinks in concrete terms and understands only tangible things, one must think of concrete and tangible ways to explain feelings, meanings, and actions. With a patient who is severely regressed, it may be important to use the process of *naming* and showing, as the purposes and processes of the activities are explained.

Frank has pointed out that one must be aware, also, that in any encounter between two people, there may be at least six selves who are communicating; each party possesses an idealized self, a self perceived by the other person, and the actual self.[29] The transactional analysis model describes the parent self, child self, and adult self. Discrepancies between the individuals' perceptions of one another lead to complex distortions. Transference and countertransference phenomena may also be encountered. When one is working within the psychoanalytic frame of reference, these phenomena are recognized and are used as part of the therapeutic process. Most other frames of reference used in the occupational therapy process, however, tend to deemphasize transference when it occurs and instead work toward the conscious perception of the therapist as a new person, different from past significant persons. The therapist can accomplish this by acting as a "total, reacting, feeling person."[30]

Without the establishment of trust between the client and therapist, it is unlikely that a truly collaborative effort will be possible. For some people, the trust issue may be powerful, and the establishment of trust may take a long time. The therapist's own self-confidence, the therapist's ability to be honest and open in the relationship, and the extent to which the therapist is able to communicate "unconditional positive regard" and empathy for the client will affect the client's ability to invest trust in the relationship.[31]

Purtilo[32] has identified some of the issues and factors which are vital in the therapeutic relationship:

The Personal-Professional Self

He decides whether to use the first or last name of each new patient; he is cautious knowing the casual use of the first name may be harmful; he is relaxed in using the last names of patients.

He incorporates actions that communicate caring into the patient-health professional interaction; he recognizes efficiency as a trait which can express caring when it does not impose rigid limits on the interaction.

He recognizes that wearing a uniform does not necessarily make a patient feel *less* cared for nor does the more casual appearance of street clothes make a patient feel *more* cared for.

He combines a pleasant approach with professional competence.

He is interested in the patient as a person with values, needs, and beliefs, but does not encourage a relationship that will lead to over-dependence (detrimental dependence).

He is respected by the patient who recognizes his integrity. He acknowledges that complete, open, mutual sharing with each other is not conducive to the functioning of a public-sector relationship.

He maintains a balance between sound health care and effective patient-health professional interaction.

He does not need to overprotect himself or to take unnecessary risks; he knows his limits.

From Purtilo, R.: *The Allied Health Professional and the Patient* © 1973 by W. B. Saunders Co., Philadelphia PA. Reprinted with permission.

Interpersonal issues such as dependency, aggressiveness or passivity, and personal need gratification or control are often challenges to the therapeutic relationship. They need to be identified for what they are and resolved as realistically and honestly as possible. When these kinds of behaviors emerge they are usually manifestations of the maladaptive modes of thinking, feeling, and acting which have interfered with the person's ability to function. If efforts between the therapist and client to identify and change what may be occurring are unsuccessful, the therapist may wish to find another professional with whom to discuss and objectify the situation.

One of the ways of conceptualizing the progress of a therapeutic relationship is to think in terms of phases. The first phase is an affective one in which the therapist elicits the trust of the client by demonstrating empathy or understanding for his or her feelings and plight. This, depending on the client's need state, or pathology, may be accomplished in a few words, a nod, or touch of the hand. It may, however, take a long time.

The second phase is one of gathering facts and information, identifying the problems to be solved, and sorting out the realistic levels of solution that may be worked toward.

In the third phase, the period of developing an action plan to work on resolving the problems, some form of contract or agreement is made with the patient or client. This is implicit in what has been, on some level at least, a cooperative effort. The contract is an understanding on the part of both the therapist and the client of what the process will be and of what expectations each person may have of the other.

In the fourth phase, the period of implementation of the plan, the conditions of the contract are tested. The issues of trust may emerge again, and it is important for the therapist to meet his or her responsibilities as planned and to communicate clearly the expectation that the client will follow through in meeting his or her responsibilities also.

In the final phase, the termination period, when separation becomes imminent, new issues may arise. If the therapeutic relationship has been important and helpful, the termination of the relationship may feel difficult to both the therapist and the client. On the other hand, all of the focus of treatment in occupational therapy has been directed toward increasingly independent functioning and, thus, the termination of treatment may evoke celebrative feelings.

The Activity

Activities are used as facilitators for transactions between people. The focus on doing, not merely talking, is useful in both one-to-one and group interactions. It allows for nonverbal communication, confrontations around interpersonal issues, and safe withdrawal when needed.

The activities with which occupational therapy is primarily concerned are those that help to promote competence and achievement in the client's ability to function in his or her own world. The three categories of self-care, work, and play, and the maintenance of a healthy balance in the individual's activity life, provide important foci for occupational therapy. This emphasis requires consideration of the client's developmental levels of functioning and of demands placed on the client by daily activities.

Activities used as treatment are limited only by constraints of the treatment context, which includes time, space, cost, the support of other team members, and the preferences and skills of the therapist.

Achieving a scientific understanding of the nature of activities, and their ability to promote performance, is a monumental task and continues to be a major challenge to occupational therapy. We have intuitive notions about activities and have experienced some degree of empirical success in their use through the years. However, hard, scientific research data still are lacking. The importance of understanding the elements of activity cannot be overemphasized.

Choice of Activities

The art of occupational therapy is in finding and using activities that are relevant to meeting the treatment objectives and that have meaning to the patient or client. It seems a simple, almost glib, statement to say that one matches the activity (which has been carefully analyzed) with the needs of the client (who has been carefully evaluated). This process is far from simple. The choice of activity, within the scope and limitations of a program, remains crucial to the success of the treatment. Decisions need to be made centering around whether the activity should be done on a one-to-one basis or in a group. How important is the process and how important is an end product? How much of the activity should rely on verbal communication? How much physical or sensory involvement should be planned? What is the range within which time requirements may be graded? In what ways will the patient experience exploration, mastery, and achievement?

To use crafts or not to use crafts? The early occupational therapists used a wide range of activities of which crafts were an important part. In recent times, except in some segments of the population, crafts became less well respected and less frequently used. The basket-weaver image of the occupational therapist is a ludicrous one which ignores the possibilities for learning and growth which are inherent in crafts. It ignores very basic anthropological and physiological data relating hand use with cognitive functioning. From the perspective of modern mechanistic achievement and production-oriented society, simple handcrafts are viewed as quaint, childish, or primitive. This attitude is a pervasive one

and affects how both the therapist and the client may feel about a given craft activity. Crafts, however, offer a highly flexible, easily controlled modality through which an individual may explore, practice, and develop a wide range of basic physical, perceptual, and cognitive skills. One experiences the tools and materials through the senses. One also experiences the effects of one's actions on something that is visible and tangible. For the patient or client who is unable to cope with many social variables or verbal interactions, the craft still may be the modality of choice.

The Context

When we speak of the context for treatment, we mean much more than merely the setting in which treatment is to take place. Context here has a dimension of time: today with an awareness of yesterday and a deliberate plan for tomorrow. In terms of place, it designates all those areas which a treatment plan utilizes, for example, a shop, a ward, a home, a work setting, Main Street, and the baseball diamond. It also includes some sense of the overall treatment objectives and plan, and the efforts and thinking of all of the people engaged in the helping process. The context for treatment has parts that are controllable and parts that are not controllable. In proceeding with treatment, we may wish to move from a highly controlled context (*e.g.*, the hospital, with a professional team, planned treatment procedures, set schedules) to a gradually less controlled and more realistic context (*e.g.*, the community where the client experiences semiautonomy or the home where the client is autonomous). In modern occupational therapy, contexts for treatment have become highly varied and far more complex than they were when occupational therapy began.

Factors which are considered in identifying contexts for treatment include:
1. The client population—their issues, needs, and objectives.
2. The kind of setting and its means of support.
3. Frames of reference for treatment and the nature of the treatment team.
4. Kinds of evaluative procedures that are used.
5. Kinds of treatment objectives that are set.
6. Kinds of treatment plans that are developed.
7. Kinds of records and reports that are made—to whom the treatment team is accountable and how this is accomplished.

Developing Objectives

When initial evaluation has been concluded, the therapist should have a clear picture of the client, of his or her assets and limitations, and of realistic expectations for future performance. In the evaluation process, there should have been certain basic ingredients contributing to setting both long-term and short-term goals for treatment.

1. *The client's needs and personal goals.* However obliquely they may be communicated, the wishes and needs of the client are there. Unless the goals of treatment are mutually understood by therapist and client on some level, they probably cannot be achieved.
2. *The treatment goals, the treatment approach, and frame of reference for treatment of the total team.* Again, coherence between the client's own goals and those of the team is important. The goals of occupational therapy must fit with both.
3. *Knowledge of the individual's disease process and the possible residual physical or psychological limitations.*
4. *Knowledge of the treatment methods and approaches being used.* What medications is the client receiving?
5. *Knowledge about the world in which the client may be expected to live.* What skills are needed to cope with the demands of life at home, in the community, at work, at play, or in the institution?
6. *Knowledge about the client's value system and what is important to him/her.*

The therapist takes the evaluation data and analyzes its many pieces in the light of the potential situation for treatment in occupational therapy. What does the therapist know about the prognosis for recovery or maintenance of function for people diagnosed as having a specific disease? Who are the other members of the treatment team and what is the potential for collaborative efforts among them? Can the therapist expect professional and/or community support for efforts made in occupational therapy? What are the realistic limits of the occupational therapy setting? To what extent will it be possible to manipulate objects and the environment to provide the best opportunities for the patient to grow and function to maximum capabilities? In what ways can we measure the success of the plan? These are hard, but vital, questions that must be faced in the process of setting objectives and planning treatment.

Long-term objectives in occupational therapy usually represent a part of the long-term treatment objectives of the team. A long-term objective may be stated, "the patient will be able to function well enough to go back to his job." A long-term objective related to this in occupational therapy might be stated, "the patient will be able to organize his thoughts and actions to carry out a task from beginning to end." Short-term objectives are designed to contribute to the achievement of long-term objec-

tives. A short-term objective related to the above might be stated, "the patient will be able to maintain attention to a given task for 15 minutes." Short-term objectives then represent the steps of achievement which will facilitate the ultimate attainment of the long-term objective.

Depending upon the treatment situation and the pathology of the client, there may be either multiple or single sets of objectives for treatment. The results of the evaluation may also indicate that occupational therapy is not needed or relevant for a client at a given time. If viable treatment objectives for occupational therapy cannot be determined, it is probably not appropriate for the client to be referred to occupational therapy.

The Treatment Plan

A description of the methods that are used to meet the treatment objectives constitutes the treatment plan. Just as the treatment objectives represent an action-oriented summary of the client's evaluation, the treatment plan represents a synthesis of the therapist's knowledge of the potential of activities and relationships as facilitators of growth and performance. It is a "nuts and bolts" statement of such things as the tools, materials, and equipment, the kinds of direction or guidance, the structure of the activity, the times and places in which the activity will take place, whether treatment will be accomplished individually or in a group, and the extent to which the family or the community are to be involved. A treatment plan is first stated in reference to each short-term objective, and it needs to be flexible enough to permit changes if re-evaluation suggests that the plan is not working.

It is probably in the development of a treatment plan that the therapist is most often faced with the responsibility for sound professional judgment. The plan needs to be reasonable and possible and to show a clear relationship to the objectives of treatment.

Implementation of Treatment

Implementation of treatment consists of three distinct phases: (1) the orientation phase when the therapist and client define the parameters and expectations of the activities that will be used, and the therapist may describe or demonstrate the procedures that are involved; (2) the development phase during which the therapist guides the client through exploration or practice in doing the activities; and (3) the termination phase when the client has completed the plan, re-evaluation takes place, and the need for further objective setting is considered.

During the development phase there should be a process of ongoing evaluation to check the effectiveness of the plan and the relevance of the objectives. During this time it is likely that new objectives and new treatment plans will evolve.

In reality, the termination phase is not always achieved. Clients may be discharged before objectives are met. In some situations, particularly with chronically ill patients, the treatment goal is maintenance of function, and therefore, short-term objectives are so numerous that the occupational therapy process may continue for a long period of time. In other situations the occupational therapy process is limited to evaluation only. The total occupational therapy process is outlined in Table 5-1.

As occupational therapists move increasingly in the direction of home and community treatment, it becomes increasingly important to conceptualize ways for treatment plans to be implemented in contexts other than the setting where evaluation took place.

Other Problem Solving in Occupational Therapy

The problem-solving process as used in occupational therapy is, of course, not confined to clinical treatment. Other issues, such as scheduling, budget considerations, the establishment of new procedures, or interdisciplinary relationships may present problems to be solved. The problem-solving elements, then, can include the individuals involved, the activities or issues, and their contexts. The same process (problem identification, data collection, data management, goal setting, looking for alternate solutions, choosing and implementing one alternative, reassessing progress) provides a useful, objectifying approach.

References

1. Marshall, E.: A problem solving method of learning, measured against a rote memory method. Am. J. Occup. Ther. 19:60–64, 1965.

Table 5-1 *Occupational Therapy as a Problem-Solving Process*

Problem solving

Problem Identification	Solution Development	Plan of Action	Implementation	Reassessment
Identify and specify problems, analyze elements and components	Explore alternatives for solution. Choose one alternative.	Set goals.	Carry out plan.	Assess results. If indicated, try another alternative or start the process over.

Data collection and management

Initial assessment	Treatment objectives	Treatment plan	Implementation of plan	Periodic or ongoing evaluation	Treatment termination
DESCRIBE client through objective data: skills, history, developmental level, social and cultural world, value systems, as well as pathology and its effect on the client's life.	NAME reasonable predicted outcomes of the occupational therapy process. STATE long-term and short-term goals that can be realistically attained in occupational therapy and that can be measured and/or observed. ESTABLISH contract or mutual understanding between client and therapist.	DESCRIBE the ways in which long-term and short-term goals can be accomplished, the activities to be used, therapeutic relationship, and context for treatment.	CONNECT action and performance of activities with meeting the goals of treatment. ACT upon the implicit contract between therapist and client.	ASSESS the efficacy of the treatment plan and process. DETERMINE the need for changes of approach. DETERMINE when treatment may be terminated.	AFFIRM the success (or failure) of the occupational therapy process in helping the client meet goals.

Adapted from May, B. J. and Newman, J.: Developing competence in problem solving: A behavioral model. Phys. Ther. 60:1140, 1980.

2. Parnes, S. J.: Creative Behavior Guidebook. New York: Charles Scribner's Sons, 1967.
3. Hopkins, H. L., and Smith, H. (eds.): Willard and Spackman's Occupational Therapy, 5th ed. Philadelphia: J. B. Lippincott, 1978, p. 110.
4. Mosey, A.: Three Frames of Reference for Mental Health. Thorofare, N.J.: Charles B. Slack, 1971.
5. Huss, A. J.: Sensorimotor approaches. In Hopkins, H. L., and Smith, H. (eds.): Willard and Spackman's Occupational Therapy, 5th ed. Philadelphia: J. B. Lippincott, 1978, pp. 125–134.
6. King, L. J.: A sensori-integrative approach to schizophrenia. Am. J. Occup. Ther. 28:529–536, 1974.
7. Mosey, A.: Three Frames of Reference for Mental Health.
8. Reilly, M.: Occupational therapy can be one of the greatest ideas of twentieth century medicine. Am. J. Occup. Ther. 16:1, 1962.
9. Conte, J. R., and Conte, W. R.: The use of conceptual models in occupational therapy. Am. J. Occup. Ther. 31:262–265, 1977.
10. Clark, P. N.: Theoretical frameworks in contemporary occupational therapy practice: Part I. Am. J. Occup. Ther. 33:505–514, 1979.
11. Clark, P. N.: Human development through occupation: A philosophy and conceptual model for practice: Part II. Am. J. Occup. Ther. 33:577–585, 1979.
12. American Occupational Therapy Association, Representative Assembly: The philosophical base of occupational therapy. Am. J. Occup. Ther. 33:785, 1979.
13. Fidler, G. S.: From crafts to competence. Am. J. Occup. Ther. 35:568–573, 1981.
14. Fidler, G. S.: Doing and becoming: Purposeful action and self-actualization. Am. J. Occup. Ther. 32:305–310, 1978.
15. Selye, H.: The Stress of Life. New York: McGraw-Hill, 1956.
16. Toffler, A.: Future Shock. New York: Random House, 1970.
17. Coleman, J. C.: Life stress and maladaptive behavior. Am. J. Occup. Ther. 27:169–179, 1973.
18. Cratty, B. J.: Movement Behavior and Motor Learning. Philadelphia: Lea & Febiger, 1967.
19. Piaget, J.: The Origins of Intelligence in Children. New York: International Universities Press, 1966.
20. McClelland, D.: The Achieving Society. New York: Free Press, 1967.
21. Rotter, J. B.: Clinical Psychology. Englewood Cliffs, NJ: Prentice-Hall, 1971.
22. Ibid.
23. Ducette, J., and Wolk, S.: Cognitive and motivational correlates of generalized expectancies for control. J. Pers. Soc. Psychol. 26:420–426, 1973.
24. Wolk, S., and Ducette, J.: The motivating effect of locus of control on achievement motivation. J. Pers. 41:59–70, 1973.
25. Piaget, J.: The Origins of Intelligence in Children.
26. White, R. W.: The urge towards competence. Am J. Occup. Ther. 25:271, 1971.
27. Searles, H.: The Nonhuman Environment. New York: International Universities Press, 1960, pp. 78–120.
28. Hall, E. T.: The Hidden Dimension. Garden City, NY: Doubleday & Co., 1966, p. 188.
29. Frank, J.: The therapeutic use of self. Am. J. Occup. Ther. 12:215, 1958.
30. Mosey, A. C.: Three Frames of Reference for Mental Health.
31. Rogers, C.: Client Centered Therapy. Boston: Houghton Mifflin Co., 1951.
32. Purtilo, R.: The Allied Health Professional and the Patient. Philadelphia: W. B. Saunders Co., 1973.

CHAPTER 6

Developmental Approaches *Elizabeth G. Tiffany*

The Developmental Treatment Approach

Development must be a concern in all aspects of health care services; it influences the focus and goals of both assessment and the treatment process itself. The therapist needs to consider developmental aspects from at least three vantage points: (1) the client's unique levels of functioning and adaptation; (2) the level of function that can be reasonably expected at the client's level of development; and (3) the age-specific crises and vulnerabilities the client might be subject to.

Theorists and spokespeople for the significance of human development include Piaget,[1] Maslow,[2] Erikson,[3] Freud,[4] Arieti,[5] and Searles,[6] among others. Their contribution has included the definition of stages and structures that relate to the unfolding of the human personality. While each of these theorists has chosen to view development from a unique perspective, there is fundamental agreement on certain points regarding the directions and growth of human capacities for functioning. Human feelings and human behavior are the products of exceedingly complex interactions between both internal and external factors. Internal factors include physiological, anatomical, sensory, and perceptual structures and functions, human biochemistry, metabolism, response to pain, the experiences of joy, balance, and remembering, as well as associating and integrating those experiences. External factors include the people, places, and things of life; the kinds of stimuli which impinge upon the senses; the nuances of interpersonal experiences; and the subtle, intangible, but pervasive ambience of the nonhuman environment. Growth and development occur within the limits and horizons effected in the dynamic interplay between an individual's basic equipment and the external world. Human potential is profoundly influenced and shaped by this interplay. It is from this perspective that a developmental approach to occupational therapy has evolved.

Many occupational therapists have chosen to focus primarily upon the developmental process as a base upon which to build treatment. Some, like Llorens,[7,8] have studied and written extensively, describing a broad and comprehensive approach to occupational therapy as a process through which positive human growth can be fostered. King[9] and Mosey[10,11] are among those who have clearly ac-

Table 6-1 *Analysis of Four Theoretical Frameworks for Occupational Therapy*

	Art of Occupational Therapy				Science of Occupational Therapy
Theory	*Focus of Intervention*	*State of Function*	*State of Dysfunction*	*Actions*	*Research Validation*
Adaptive Performance	Adaptive skills of doing Self-care Intrinsic gratification Service to others	Balance between skills and subskills Promotes competence and efficacy	Imbalance due to influence of internal processes or external environment Causes subskill deficits and problems of doing	Identify levels of functions in skills and subskills Provide shared learning experiences in life–work situations Promote subskill development	Descriptive Analytical Criterion-referenced measurements Program plans
Biodevelopment	Developmental sequence of human biological processes	Integrative use of biological processes Promotes adaptive skills Conceptualization Manipulation Socialization	Impairment of ability to process and act upon information received from the environment	Identify process deficits Use developmentally sequenced sensory motor activities, special techniques, and equipment to normalize biological processes	
Facilitating Growth and Development	Physical, social, and psychological parameters of human life roles, tasks, and relationships	Mastery of tasks and relationships necessary to engage in life roles	Stress, trauma, or disease affect performance or achievement of necessary behaviors	Role of change agent Controlled use of purposeful activity to stimulate role behaviors Developmental analysis of problems	Quasi-experimental Descriptive/Analytical Criterion-referenced measurements Standardized measurements Program plans Program modalities
	Acquisition and performance of work and play behaviors	Self-directed achievement of role requirements	Internal and/or external forces impair capacity for participation and adaptation	Promote exploration and competency of role requirements through identification and development of functions, habits, skills, and task performance	Descriptive/Analytical Criterion-referenced measurements Program plans

Clark, P. N.: Human development through occupational therapy. Am. J. Occup. Ther. 33:8, 1979. Reprinted with permission.

Seven Adaptive Skills

1. Perceptual-Motor Skill: The ability to receive, integrate, and organize sensory stimuli in a manner which allows for the planning of purposeful movement.

   The subskills required are the abilities
   a. to integrate primitive postural reflexes, to react appropriately to vestibular stimuli, to maintain a balance between the tactile subsystems, to perceive form, and to be aware of auditory stimuli.
   b. to control extraocular musculature, to integrate the two sides of the body, and to focus on auditory stimuli.
   c. to perceive visual and auditory figure-ground, to be aware of body parts and their relationships, and to plan gross motor movements.
   d. to perceive space, to plan fine motor movements, and to discriminate auditory stimuli.
   e. to discriminate between right and left and to remember auditory stimuli.
   f. to use abstract concepts, to scan, integrate, and synthesize auditory stimuli, and to give auditory feedback.

2. Cognitive Skill: The ability to perceive, represent, and organize objects, events, and their relationships in a manner that is considered appropriate by one's cultural group.

   The subskills required are the abilities
   a. to use inherent behavioral patterns for environmental interaction.
   b. to interrelate visual, manual, auditory, and oral responses.
   c. to attend to the environmental consequence of actions with interest, to represent objects in an exoceptual manner, to experience objects, to act on the bases of egocentric causality, and to seriate events in which the self is involved.
   d. to establish a goal and intentionally carry out means, to recognize the independent existence of objects, to interpret signs, to imitate new behavior, to apprehend the influence of space, and to perceive other objects as partially causal.
   e. to use trial-and-error problem solving, to

   use tools, to perceive variability in spatial positions, to seriate events in which the self is not involved, and to perceive the causality of other objects.
   f. to represent objects in an image manner, to make believe, to infer a cause given its effect, to act on the bases of combined spatial relations, to attribute omnipotence to others, and to perceive objects as permanent in time and space.
   g. to represent objects in an endoceptual manner, to differentiate between thought and action, and to recognize the need for causal sources.
   h. to represent objects in a denotative manner, to perceive the viewpoint of others, and to decenter.
   i. to represent objects in a connotative manner, to use formal logic, and to work in the realm of the hypothetical.

3. Drive-Object Skill: The ability to control drives and select objects in such a manner as to ensure adequate need satisfaction.

   The subskills required are the abilities
   a. to form a discontinuous, libidinal object relationship.
   b. to form a continuous, part-libidinal object relationship.
   c. to invest aggressive drive in an external object.
   d. to transfer libidinal drive to objects other than the primary object.
   e. to invest libidinal energy in appropriate abstract objects and to control aggressive drive.
   f. to engage in total and diffuse libidinal object relationships.

4. Dyadic Interaction Skill: The ability to participate in a variety of dyadic relationships.

   The subskills required are the abilities
   a. to enter into association relationships.
   b. to interact in an authority relationship.
   c. to interact in a chum relationship.
   d. to enter into a peer–authority relationship.
   e. to enter into an intimate relationship.
   f. to engage in a nurturing relationship.

5. Group Interaction Skill: The ability to be a productive member of a variety of primary groups.

(*continued*)

The subskills required are the abilities
a. to participate in a parallel group.
b. to participate in a project group.
c. to participate in an egocentric-cooperative group.
d. to participate in a cooperative group.
e. to participate in a mature group.
6. Self-Identity Skill: The ability to perceive the self as an autonomous, whole, and acceptable person with permanence and continuity.

The subskills required are the abilities
a. to perceive the self as a worthy object.
b. to perceive the assets and limitations of the self.
c. to perceive the self as self-directed.
d. to perceive the self as a productive, contributing member of a social system.

e. to perceive the self.
f. to perceive the aging process of the self in a rational manner.
7. Sexual Identity Skill: The ability to perceive one's sexual nature as good and to participate in a sexual relationship that is oriented to the mutual satisfaction of sexual needs.

The subskills required are the abilities
a. to accept and act upon the bases of one's pregenital sexual nature.
b. to accept sexual maturation as a positive growth experience.
c. to give and receive sexual gratification.
d. to enter into a sustained sexual relationship.
e. to accept physiological and psychological changes that occur at the time of the climacteric.

Adapted from Mosey, A. C.: *Three Frames of Reference for Mental Health.* Thorofare, NJ: Charles B. Slack, 1970.

knowledged the importance of recognizing the individual's levels of adaptation and functioning in the performance of life tasks and in human relationships as the starting points for occupational therapy intervention. Some, like Allen,[12] have chosen specific aspects of development as pivotal concerns, with implications for functioning in all other areas. Clark[13,14] proposed a synthesis of occupational therapy theory and practice based on human development (see Table 6-1).

Briefly described, the developmental approach is based on the following premises:
1. Human beings normally develop in a sequential way;
2. Each new gain in structure (physical or mental) enables the individual to gain in function;
3. Each new gain in functional ability makes further development and adaptation possible;
4. Physical, sensory, perceptual, cognitive, social, and emotional aspects of the individual are intimately connected and affect the developmental state of the *whole* individual;
5. Conditions of stress cause the stressed individual to regress to earlier levels of adaptation;
6. Successful experiences foster a sense of wholeness and competence.

Human beings tend to be facilitated toward positive development or reintegration of their adaptive abilities when their experiences are successful ones.

In 1968 Mosey described seven adaptive skills (see accompanying chart) in their developmental se-

quence. She defined them as learned abilities that enable human beings to satisfy their needs and to meet environmental demands. The subskill components which make up each of the adaptive skills are listed hierarchically. Mosey postulates that each subskill must be learned in proper sequence before mastery of the next subskill may be achieved. The learning of several subskills within one adaptive skill may, however, occur simultaneously. An individual may also be working on the achievement of mastery in more than one adaptive skill at any given time. Failure to master any part of an adaptive skill results in difficulty when the individual attempts to undertake a task at a higher level. Treatment then is aimed at helping the individual to experience personal, social, and task demands that will facilitate mastery of each subskill.

The developmental approach to treatment requires that the therapist assess and understand the levels of adaptation on which the client is functioning, and, as much as possible, the conditions which tend to make the client function at the highest and at the lowest levels. The therapist then needs to think in terms of providing opportunities for the client to have experiences that (1) provide success experiences by meeting his/her levels of adaptation; (2) encourage "safe" exploration and practice as the client is enabled to move to more mature levels of adaptation; and (3) provide opportunities for challenge, surprise, and novelty when the client is ready.

This approach may be applied in a number of therapeutic situations: with infants and children where there is evidence of delay or interruption in the normal process of development; with psychiatrically ill clients whose behaviors show regression to earlier stages of adaptation; with the mentally retarded; and with any clients who, because of the stress of physical pain, illness, loss of function, or some disabling condition, may be unable to think, feel, or act at a normal level.

The reader is referred to Chapter 4—The Human Development Process—for important background and further resource suggestions.

References

1. Piaget, J.: Origins of Intelligence in Children. New York: International Universities Press, 1952.
2. Maslow, A.: Toward a Psychology of Being. Princeton, NJ: Van Nostrand, 1962.
3. Erikson, E.: Identity and Psychosocial Development of the Child. In Discussions on Child Development, Vol. 30. New York: International Universities Press, 1958.
4. Brill, A. A. (ed.): Basic Writings of Sigmund Freud. New York: Modern Library, 1958.
5. Arieti, S.: The Intrapsychic Self. New York: Basic Books, 1967.
6. Searles, H.: The Nonhuman Environment. New York: International Universities Press, 1960.
7. Llorens, L.: Facilitating growth and development. Am. J. Occup. Ther. 24:93–101, 1970.
8. Llorens, L.: Application of a Developmental Theory for Health and Rehabilitation. Rockville, MD: American Occupational Therapy Association, Inc. 1976.
9. King, L. J.: Toward a science of adaptive responses. Am. J. Occup. Ther. 32:429–437, 1979.
10. Mosey, A. C.: Three Frames of Reference for Mental Health. Thorofare, NJ: Charles B. Slack, 1970.
11. Mosey, A. C.: An alternative: The biopsychosocial model. Am. J. Occup. Ther. 26:137–140, 1974.
12. Allen, C.: Assessment in Mental Health. Workshop proceedings. Philadelphia: Friends Hospital, 1981.
13. Clark, P. N.: Human development through occupational therapy: Theoretical Frameworks in occupational therapy practice: Part 1. Am. J. Occup. Ther. 33:8, 1979.
14. Clark, P. N.: Human development through occupational therapy: A philosophy and conceptual model for practice: Part 2. Am. J. Occup. Ther. 33:9, 1979.

CHAPTER 7

Sensorimotor Approaches

SECTION 1
Basis for Sensorimotor
Approaches—Neuroanatomy and
Neurophysiology *A. Joy Huss*

In order to understand human behavior and function it is necessary to have a basic knowledge of the structure and function of the nervous system. This system is responsible for control not only of the skeletal and smooth muscles but also of the emotions, memory, and intellect. Thus it becomes important for the occupational therapist, regardless of specialty area, to have a basic understanding of the nervous system. Since knowledge of the nervous system is not yet complete, it is the professional's responsibility to stay abreast of current information.

Basic Concepts

The nervous system is divided arbitrarily into three divisions: the central nervous system (CNS); the peripheral nervous system (PNS); and the autonomic

nervous system (ANS) which in turn has two subdivisions, the sympathetic (SNS) and parasympathetic (PSNS).

The CNS consists of those structures located inside the skull and vertebral column: the brain and spinal cord. The PNS structures are located outside of the bony cavities and carry sensory and motor information from and to the peripheral structures and sensory information from smooth and cardiac muscles and glands to the CNS.

The ANS is an efferent (motor) system supplying information to the smooth muscles, cardiac muscle, and glands. The SNS (thoracolumbar system) is located at spinal cord levels T_1 to L_2. The PSNS anatomically surrounds the SNS being found in cranial nerves, 3, 7, 9, and 10 and in sacral levels 2, 3, and 4 (craniosacral system). The SNS supplies both axial and appendicular structures, while the PSNS supplies only axial structures. Thus axially the two systems work synergistically. The SNS provides an adrenalin response which is a generalized, fast-acting, excitatory reaction. The PSNS is a specific, slower-acting system which tends to conserve energy. In the appendicular areas the SNS provides its own synergistic action. For example, it can either increase or decrease the blood flow to the extremities depending on the needs of the organism.

Functionally all three divisions (CNS, PNS, ANS) are interrelated and cannot be isolated. What occurs in one division will have an effect on the other divisions. Even though a given treatment approach may be said to affect a certain part of the system, it will ultimately have an effect, either positive or negative, on the entire system and thus on the individual's behavior, because the nervous system functions holistically.

The CNS contains more than 20 billion plus neurons of varying sizes, cell body sizes and shapes, and degrees of axonal myelination. Generally, the larger the axon diameter the more heavily myelinated it becomes with nervous system maturation, and the faster it will conduct an impulse. Conversely, the smaller the axonal diameter, the less myelin and the slower the conduction rate will be. Neurons can thus be classified according to axon diameter and myelin covering (Table 7-1).[1,2] Although the smallest fibers are classified as nonmyelinated, a single Schwann cell may envelop several of these fibers with a single layer of myelin. The heavier the myelin sheath, the

Table 7-1 *Nerve Fiber Classification in Descending Order of Myelin Thickness and Conduction Velocity*

General Classification	Dorsal Root Classification	Ventral Root Classification	
A. Large axonal diameter with heaviest myelin wrap	I. 70–120 m/sec Ia—primary sensory ending from neuromuscular spindle Ib—from Golgi tendon organ II. 30–70 m/sec Encapsulated receptors Secondary sensory ending from neuromuscular spindle cutaneous touch pressure joint receptors dermal receptors	alpha (α)	Motoneurons to extrafusal somatic muscles 15–120 m/sec
		beta (β)	Few in number. Innervate both extrafusal and intrafusal fibers.
		gamma (γ)	Motoneurons to intrafusal fibers of neuromuscular spindles 10–45 m/sec
	III. delta (δ) 12–30 m/sec Nonencapsulated nerve endings mechanoreceptors cold sensitive thermoreceptors some nociceptors		
B. Intermediate axonal diameter and myelin wrap	Visceral afferents 3–15 m/sec		Preganglionic autonomic fibers. 3–15 m/sec
C. Small axonal diameter and essentially unmyelinated	IV. Free nerve endings. Probably serve all sensory modalities. 0.6–2 m/sec Sometimes referred to as d.r.C or dorsal root C fibers		Postganglionic sympathetic axons of ANS. 0.7–2.3 m/sec Sometimes referred to as s.C or sympathetic C fibers.

Adapted from Barr, M. L.: The Human Nervous System: An Anatomic Viewpoint, ed 2. Hagerstown: Harper & Row, 1979, pp. 25–36; and Noback, C. R., and Demarest, R. J.: The Human Nervous System: Basic Principles of Neurobiology, ed. 3. New York: McGraw-Hill, 1981, pp. 165–169.

longer it takes to develop. Therefore it may be years before full functional capacity is reached. Generally, the larger fibers process the more discriminative, exploratory, or epicritic functions, while the intermediate size fibers process the protective or protopathic functions, and the smaller fibers process the more primitive functions of the ANS and reticular formation.

In the spinal cord the A fibers (largest) are found predominately in the dorsolateral portion and will cross over in the medulla. These include such functions as conscious proprioception, discriminatory tactile, two-point discrimination, vibratory sense, and voluntary motor activity. The B fibers (intermediate) are found predominately in the ventro-lateral portion of the spinal cord, and they cross at spinal levels. Functions served include pain, temperature, light touch, vibratory sense, and nonvoluntary motor activity. The C fibers (smallest) are generally found in the area surrounding the gray matter of the cord, and they will have a bilateral effect.

Phylogenetically, the nervous system has developed from the most primitive, bilateral functions such as ANS and reticular, referred to as *archi,* to intermediate protective functions known as *paleo,* to the discriminative functions called *neo.* The neo functions, because they involve larger cell bodies and nerve fibers that require more oxygen, are thus more vulnerable to trauma while the archi systems are the least vulnerable. Although it depends to some degree on the location and nature of the trauma, the nervous system tends to protect the archi systems the longest. This, then, has implications for rehabilitation. If the system has been damaged one should first integrate the archi systems, progress through the paleo functions, and finally attempt to rehabilitate the neo functions such as speech and fine manipulation. It is extremely difficult, for example, to use the hands for fine control if the background base of postural stability is deficient.

At birth the individual operates on an excitatory basis. The slightest stimulus sets off a mass reaction. At this time the nervous system is essentially immature. With maturity of the system a base of inhibition is laid down because of the myelination of higher centers that tend to be inhibitory in function. Normal functioning is dependent on a balance of excitatory and inhibitory influences on the lower motoneurons of the spinal cord and cranial nerves. In order for excitation and inhibition to be mediated by the CNS there are two basic types of neurons: excitatory and inhibitory. Histologically, the two are similar. The difference is the chemical secreted at the synapse and the effect of that chemical on the postsynaptic neuron. Since a given neuron can have synaptic input from 1000 to 100,000 other neurons, whether or not the firing threshold is reached for propagation of

an impulse depends on the total balance between excitatory and inhibitory synapses. For example, if the ratio is 2:1 inhibitory/facilitory, then the excitatory impulse will be blocked. If the total system balance is more towards excitation, then the clinical picture may be one of hyperactivity or hypertonicity. If the balance is more towards inhibition, then the clinical picture will be hypotonicity. Depending on the area of trauma and the moment-to-moment state of the individual, which is based in part on the amount and type of sensory input being received and processed, the tonal picture may fluctuate. One can see such fluctuations even in the normal individual.

Excitation and inhibition within the CNS is a complex interaction of presynaptic and postsynaptic inhibition via interneurons and inhibitory centers. For a more thorough understanding of this process, two of the better references are Noback[3] and Williams and Warwick.[4]

The balance of excitation and inhibition ultimately affects the threshold levels of postsynaptic neurons within the CNS and the lower motoneurons. Generally speaking, the normal resting threshold is -70 mV and the firing potential is -50 mV. With repeated excitation the resting potential may shift toward a -60 mV which means that a lesser amount of additional excitation is needed to reach firing potential. On the other hand, if the system is receiving more inhibitory overlay the resting potential may be close to -80 mV so that additional excitation is needed to reach the firing potential. The hypertonic or hyperactive individual may have an overall balance of too much excitation, so that resting potentials are very close to firing potentials, while conversely the hypotonic individual may have a greater discrepancy between resting and firing potentials. The aim of treatment thus becomes an *appropriate* use of sensory input to change the overall balance of the system toward a more normal range of -70 mV resting potential.

One way this can be accomplished is through the use of the sensory receptors. *Exteroceptors* are located in the skin, eyes, and ears. They respond to changes in the external environment such as the general senses of pain, temperature, light touch or light pressure, tactile or touch pressure, and the special senses of vision and hearing. *Proprioceptors* are concerned with vibration, deep pressure, and the position and movements of the body. These receptors are located in the muscles (neuromuscular spindles), tendons (Golgi tendon organs), fascia, joint capsules, ligaments, and the vestibular or equilibrium mechanisms of the inner ear. *Interoceptors,* also called visceroceptors, mediate sensations from the viscera. They play a role in digestion, control of blood pressure, cardiac function, respiration, and so forth. The sensations of fullness of stomach and bladder or pain from excessive distention are the result of stimulation of these receptors. Visceral sensations are diffuse and poorly localized. The sensations of olfaction and taste have been variously classified as exteroceptors or interoceptors.

Since the nervous system acts as a sensorimotor-sensory feedback system with integration provided by the CNS, various treatment approaches, discussed later in this book, have been developed to excite or dampen these sensory receptors which in turn will have an effect on motor control. If the system is deprived of appropriate sensory input and its integration, disorganized behaviors will result. Sensory deprivation affects synaptic growth and development as well as delaying myelination. An enriched environment will have the opposite effect. Appropriate input includes not only stimulation of the suitable receptors, whether they be exteroceptors, proprioceptors, and/or interoceptors, but it also must be meaningful to the individual's system, be of correct intensity and duration, and be applied with tender loving care (TLC) for concurrent emotional integration.

Each of us is bombarded constantly with a multiplicity of sensory input, most of which does not evoke a response at a conscious level but is filtered by the reticular system and integrated subcortically. The reticular system extends throughout the spinal cord, brainstem, and diencephalic nuclei of the thalamus and hypothalamus with indirect connections with the cerebral cortex and limbic system.[5] The entire system is polysynaptic.

The reticular activating system (RAS), or ascending portion, provides a generalized bombardment of the cerebral cortex for the purposes of providing the level of consciousness or "awakeness" and the level of alertness to that which is most important in the environment. Olfactory and cutaneous stimuli have a profound effect on the level of consciousness. Psychic, auditory, and visual stimuli affect the level of alertness and attention. Damage to this system may result in prolonged coma.[6]

The descending fibers of the reticular system, having received information from the motor centers of the cortex, basal ganglia, and cerebellum, play a major role in influencing the threshold levels of both alpha and gamma motoneurons of the spinal cord and cranial nerves. Since the nuclear centers of this system in the brainstem consist of both excitatory and inhibitory centers, the effect on the motoneurons can be either facilitory or inhibitory. Control centers of the ANS of the brainstem are also affected by this system with effects on respiration, circulation, and heart rate.[7,8,9]

Thus, this entire reticular system has implications for treatment not only of the individual with CNS dysfunction, but also for those with other types of problems, as well as for dealings with students, peers, and others. The type and amount of stimuli being received in relation to the individual's present state will have an effect on his/her responses to the environment and his/her ability to learn.

The limbic system consists of structures found on the medial surfaces of the cerebral hemispheres such as the cingulate, hippocampal, and parahippocampal gyri, the mammillary bodies of the hypothalamus, the fornix, the uncus, and amygdala, and the medial aspect of the thalamus. According to Moore,[10] the limbic system, because of its location and structures involved, serves to integrate the older sensorimotor, visceral, and reticular systems with the newer, higher level cognitive functions. In lower animals these structures serve the olfactory functions.

Moore indicates that in human beings the limbic system is that which drives us to act for survival as individuals and as a species. She uses the mnemonic word *MOVE* to outline the functions. The *M* stands for *memory*. Although memory is probably stored in many areas of the CNS, certain parts of the limbic system such as the hippocampus and mammillary bodies appear to be a necessary part of the circuitry for both long-term and short-term memory.

The *O* stands for *olfaction*. Although human beings no longer depend on the sense of smell for survival, it still has an influence on the sense of taste, recall of past experiences, emotional responses, and visceral functions.

The *V* stands for *visceral* functions related to behavior in conjunction with sensorimotor, cognitive, and emotional responses. The system helps to maintain the homeostatic balance. Excessive emotional or physical stress may disturb this balance with resultant alerting of the SNS for "fight or flight" responses. If continued for too long, the response to fear may disturb the entire balance of the nervous system, leading to disintegration of the individual's behavior.

The *E* stands for the individual's basic *emotional* tone or drive. These have been referred to as the "3 Fs" or feeding, fighting, and reproduction.[11] The feeding drive consists not only of the necessity of food, water, and air for physical survival, but also, and probably even more important, of the need for love or TLC or, as Broadbent[12] has called it, the "belonging instinct." This drive must be met in order to assure the survival of the individual and the species.[13,14,15]

Since the limbic system is so complex, made up of fiber connections not only within the system itself but also with adjacent areas including the reticular system, any stimulation causes long-lasting afterdischarges. Many of its pathways are circular in nature as well as reciprocal. Thus stimulation of one area has an effect on all other areas, which then give feedback both directly and indirectly to the site of original stimulation. Emotional learning thus has strong reinforcement. We are all familiar with an event or song that continually replays itself within our own mind, and with the patient with a cerebrovascular accident who still retains emotional language such as swearing, singing, laughter, and crying although the higher cortical functions of language are lost.[16] Therefore as therapists we cannot ignore the effects of what we do on the limbic system and the implications for affecting the entire balance of the client.

The corticobulbar system, which innervates the motor nuclei of the cranial nerves, and the corticospinal system, both of which are commonly referred to as the pyramidal system, originate in several areas of the cortex. The figures vary from author to author,[17,18,19] but, contrary to popular belief, this system does not originate in only Brodmann's area 4 or motor strip of the frontal lobe. Noback[20] indicates that approximately 60% of the fibers originate in areas 4 and 6 of the frontal lobe, while the remaining 40% come from areas 3, 1, 2, and 5 of the parietal lobe. Barr[21] indicates that 40% are from area 4; 20% from 3, 1, and 2; and the remainder are predominantly from 6 and 8 of the frontal lobe and the rest from areas 5 and 7 of the parietal lobe.[22] Approximately 90% of the fibers in this system are small fibers with 2% to 3% being the large fibers from the Betz cells of area 4. Of the more than one million fibers making up the corticospinal system, 85% to 90% cross over in the medullary pyramidal decussation to form the lateral corticospinal tract. Most of the remaining fibers, which do not cross over, make up the anterior corticospinal tract while a few enter the ipsilateral lateral corticospinal tract. Most of these uncrossed fibers, however, do cross in the spinal cord at their level of function. The lateral corticospinal tracts extend throughout the spinal cord. Approximately 50% of the fibers terminate in the cervical region, 20% in the thoracic area, with the remaining 30% extending to the lumbosacral segments.[23] Barr's figures are 55%, 20%, and 25% respectively.[24] The anterior corticospinal tracts terminate primarily in the cervical area.

Both the corticobulbar and corticospinal fibers traverse the posterior portion of the internal capsule that is supplied primarily by branches of the middle cerebral artery. This is probably the most common area of occlusion in a cerebral vascular accident. Also traversing this area of the internal capsule are sensory projection fibers from the thalamus to the parietal lobe and fibers from the optic and auditory radiations.

At spinal cord levels it is estimated that at least 90% of the corticospinal fibers synapse with interneurons before exerting their influence on both alpha and gamma motoneurons. Some fibers may synapse directly on alpha motoneurons, especially for fine control of the digits. The remainder of the fibers synapse via interneurons in the sensory relay nuclei of the posterior horn of the spinal cord and the brainstem nuclei for the pathways of conscious proprioception.[25,26]

Thus the pyramidal system which was once thought to be *the* direct, monosynaptic pathway for voluntary control of all musculature is now thought by some observers to be a system for control of speed and agility of voluntary movement and especially significant in the ability to use the digits independently for fine skill.[27]

The extrapyramidal system includes all of the motor systems other than the corticobulbar and corticospinal (pyramidal) system. The extrapyramidal system originates from the same cortical areas as well as the basal ganglia of the telencephalon, red nucleus, reticular system, substantia nigra of the brainstem, and certain thalamic nuclei of the diencephalon. There is considerable interaction between the pyramidal and extrapyramidal systems via collaterals and feedback circuits. Thus the extrapyramidal system also plays a role in voluntary movement as well as possibly providing the background base necessary for postural control.[28,29] With a pure lesion of the pyramidal system, which is relatively rare, there will be flaccidity. However, if any extrapyramidal areas are also involved, there will be hypertonicity. The automatic components of movement and posture are controlled subcortically, while the volitional component is controlled primarily at the cortical level. It is difficult, if not impossible, to control on a cortical level more than one act at a time. Therefore, it is necessary for these two systems to act together in order that one may perform a skilled activity on a solid postural base. For example, one can consciously direct the necessary finger movements to perform a Beethoven sonata, but the necessary wrist, forearm, arm, shoulder, trunk, and lower extremity movements are directed simultaneously by subcortical extrapyramidal centers. It is probable that more than 90% of the activities that one performs daily are subcortically controlled.

The circuitry is extremely complex, and a breakdown in one area will affect the functioning of other areas. Thus, the clinical picture will vary considerably from one individual to another. This also makes it extremely difficult to localize the exact area of trauma based on the clinical picture.

The connections and pathways of the vestibulocochlear system are many and very intricate. Any of the newer neuroanatomy texts review this information. At one time the vestibular or equilibrium mechanisms were considered to be separate from the cochlear or auditory processes. The newer evidence from both the clinical and laboratory research areas now indicates that there are many interactions between these two senses. Enhancement of one will affect the other. Input to this total system has been shown to assist in the integration of brainstem functions,[30] which then releases the higher centers to more adequately perform their functions. Vestibular therapy is now an accepted method of treatment. However, its various methods and effects, both positive and negative, should be understood by the clinician before being used with any client. Ayres is an excellent reference for this understanding.[31] Basically any movement that is done slowly and repetitively will dampen the system, while movement that is rapid will enhance the system. Many techniques based on this premise are discussed in the following section.

As research continues into the structure and function of the neuromuscular spindle and the neurotendinous organ (Golgi tendon organ, GTO), these sensory receptors become more complex and thus more difficult to understand. Moore[32] updated this complexity. At the present time it appears that the primary sensory ending of the neuromuscular spindle is highly sensitive to vibration, which is why vibrators are being used in treatment. Bishop[33–35] has written three articles on this subject. Noback, Nolte, and Barr[36–38] provide an understanding of the structure and possible functions of both of these sensory receptors.

It is important to remember that stimulation of these sensory organs is only *one* way to provide input to the CNS and *may* be an appropriate treatment technique if used in conjunction with other types of input. Used in isolation it may not be appropriate.

Basic information at this time seems to indicate that the neuromuscular spindle provides autogenic excitation, while the neurotendinous organ provides autogenic inhibition. These two structures work closely together and are influenced by higher CNS structures as well as the present state of the individual.

References

1. Barr, M. L.: The Human Nervous System: An Anatomic Viewpoint, ed 2. Hagerstown: Harper & Row, 1979, pp. 25–36.
2. Noback, C. R., and Demarest, R. J.: The Human Nervous System: Basic Principles of Neurobiology, ed. 3. New York: McGraw-Hill, 1981, pp. 165–169.
3. Ibid., pp. 99–101, 119–123, 444.
4. Williams, P. L., and Warwick, R.: Functional Neuroanatomy of Man. Philadelphia: W. B. Saunders, 1975, pp. 750, 751, 768, 775, 832.
5. Ibid, pp. 888–890.
6. Barr: Human Nervous System, p. 124.
7. Ibid., p. 125.
8. Noback: Human Nervous System, p. 292.
9. Williams and Warwick: Functional Neuroanatomy, p. 890.
10. Moore, J. C.: Behavior, bias, and the limbic system. Am. J. Occup. Ther. 30:11–19, 1976.
11. MacLean, P. D.: The limbic system with respect to self-preservation and the preservation of the species. J. Nerv. Ment. Dis. 127:1–11, 1958.
12. Broadbent, W. W.: How To Be Loved. Englewood Cliffs NJ: Prentice-Hall, 1976, pp. 175–184.
13. Ibid.
14. Moore: Behavior, bias, and the limbic system.
15. Huss, A. J.: Touch with care or a caring touch? Am. J. Occup. Ther. 31:11–18, 1977.
16. Moore: Behavior, bias, and the limbic system.
17. Noback: Human Nervous System, p. 197.
18. Barr: Human Nervous System, p. 269.
19. Clark, R. G.: Manter and Gatz's Essentials of Clinical Neuroanatomy and Neurophysiology, ed. 5. Philadelphia, F. A. Davis, 1975, p. 20.
20. Noback: Human Nervous System, p. 197.
21. Barr: Human Nervous System, pp. 268–269.
22. Ibid.
23. Noback: Human Nervous System, p. 197.
24. Barr: Human Nervous System, p. 271.
25. Ibid.
26. Noback: Human Nervous System, p. 198.
27. Nolte, J.: The Human Brain: An Introduction to its Functional Anatomy. St. Louis: C. V. Mosby, 1981, pp. 216–217.
28. Barr: Human Nervous System, pp. 276–277.
29. Noback: Human Nervous System, p. 447.
30. Ayres, A. J.: Sensory Integration and Learning Disorders. Los Angeles: Western Psychological Services, 1972, p. 57.
31. Ibid.
32. Moore, J. C.: The Golgi tendon organ and the muscle spindle. Am. J. Occup. Ther. 28:415–420, 1974.
33. Bishop, B.: Vibratory stimulation I. J. Am. Phys. Ther. 54:1273–1282, 1974.
34. Bishop, B.: Vibratory stimulation II. J. Am. Phys. Ther. 55:28–34, 1975.
35. Bishop, B.: Vibratory stimulation III. J. Am. Phys. Ther. 55:139–143, 1975.
36. Noback: Human Nervous System, pp. 81–83, 187–194.
37. Nolte: The Human Brain, pp. 75–78.
38. Barr: The Human Nervous System, pp. 29–31, 117.

Bibliography

Andrew, B. L. (ed.): Control and Innervation of Skeletal Muscle, Dundee, Scotland: D.C. Thomson & Co., 1966.
Angel, R. W., and Eppler, W. G.: Synergy of contralateral muscles in normal subjects and patients with neurological disease. Arch. Phys. Med. 48:233–239, 1967.
Ashworth, B., Grimby, L., and Kugelberg, E.: Comparison of voluntary and reflex activation of motor units. J. Neurol. Neurosurg. Psychiat. 30:91–98, 1967.

Banker, R. J., et al. (eds.): Research in Muscle Development and the Muscle Spindle. Amsterdam: Excerpta Med. Found. 1972.

Basmajian, J. V.: Control and training of individual motor units. Science, 1963.

Bekesy, G. von: Sensory Inhibition. Princeton NJ: Princeton University Press, 1967.

Brooks, V. B., and Stoney, S. D.: Motor mechanisms: The role of the pyramidal system in motor control. Ann. Rev. Physiol. 33:337–392, 1971.

Calne, D. B., and Pallis, C. A.: Vibratory sense: A critical review. Brain 89:723–746, 1966.

Campbell, S. K.: Neural control of oral somatic motor function. Phys. Ther. 61:16–22, 1981.

Carmon, A.: Disturbances of tactile sensitivity in patients with unilateral cerebral lesions. Cortex 7:83–97, 1971.

Chase, M. H., et al.: Somatic reflex response—reversal of reticular origin. Exp. Neurol. 50:561–567, 1976.

Cook, W. A., and Gangiano, A.: Presynaptic and postsynaptic inhibition of spinal motoneurons. J. Neurophysiol. 35:389–403, 1972.

Crosby, E. C., et al.: The alterations of tonus and movements through the interplay between the cerebral hemispheres and the cerebellum. J. Comp. Neurol. Suppl. 1:1–91, 1966.

Crutchfield, C. A., and Barnes, M. R.: The Neurophysiological Basis of Patient Treatment, Vol. 1. The Muscle Spindle, ed. 2. Morgantown WV: Stokesville Publishing Co., 1975.

Curry, E. L., and Clelland, J. A.: Effects of the asymmetric tonic neck reflex and high-frequency muscle vibration on isometric wrist extension strength in normal adults. Phys. Ther. 61:487–495, 1981.

Denny-Brown, D.: The Cerebral Control of Movement. Liverpool: Liverpool University Press, 1966.

Denslow, J. S., and Gutensohn, O. R.: Neuromuscular reflexes in response to gravity. J. Appl. Physiol. 23:2:243–247, 1967.

Dimitrijevic, M. R., and Nathan, P. W.: Studies of spasticity in man. 3. Analysis of reflex activity evoked by noxious cutaneous stimulation. Brain 91:349–368, 1968.

Engberg, I., Lundberg, A., and Ryall, R. W.: Reticulospinal inhibition of transmission in reflex pathways. J. Physiol. (Lond.) 194:201–223, 1968.

Engberg, I.: Reticulospinal inhibition of interneurons. J. Physiol. (Lond.) 194:225–236, 1968.

Ermolaeva, V. Y., and Ermolenko, S. F.: Reciprocal connections between the first and second somatosensory cortical areas and the caudate nucleus. Neuroscience Behav. Physiol. 6:325–331, 1973.

Farber, S. D.: Olfaction in health and disease. Am. J. Occup. Ther. 32:155–160, 1978.

Gellhorn, E.: Principles of Autonomic-Somatic Integrations. Minneapolis: University of Minnesota Press, 1967.

Gordon, B.: The superior colliculus of the brain. Scientif. Amer. 227:72–82, 1972.

Granit, R. (ed.): Nobel Symposium I—Muscular Afferents and Motor Control. New York: John Wiley & Sons, 1966.

Granit, R.: Receptors and Sensory Perception. New Haven CN: Yale University Press, 1955.

Granit, R.: The functional role of the muscle spindles—facts and hypotheses. Brain 98:531–556, 1975.

Grimby, L., and Hannerz, J.: Recruitment order of motor units in voluntary contraction: Changes induced by proprioceptive afferent activity. J. Neurol. Neurosurg. Psychiatr. 1968.

Grimby, L., et al.: Disturbances of voluntary recruitment order of low and high frequency motor units on blockades of proprioceptive afferent activity. Acta Physiol. Scand. 96:207–216, 1976.

Hagbarth, K. E., et al.: Effects of the Jendrassik manoeuvre on muscle spindle activity in man. J. Neurol. Neurosurg. Psych. 38:1143–1153, 1975.

Hall, V. E. (ed.): Annual Review of Physiology. Palo Alto: Annual Reviews, Inc., published yearly.

Harris, F. A.: The brain is a distributed information center. Am. J. Occup. Ther. 24:264–268, 1970.

Hinoki, M., et al.: Optic organ and cervical proprioceptors in maintenance of body equilibrium. Acta Otolaryngol. (Supp.) 330:164–184, 1975.

Houk, J., and Simon, W.: Responses of Golgi tendon organs to forces applied to muscle tendon. J. Neurophysiol. 30:6, 1967.

Howard, I. P., and Templeton, W. B.: Human Spatial Orientation. New York: John Wiley & Sons, 1966.

Hunt, C. C., and Ottoson, D.: Initial burst of primary endings of isolated mammalina muscle spindles. J. Neurophysiol. 39:324–330, 1976.

Iggo, A. (ed.): Handbook of Sensory Physiology. Vol. 2, Somato-Sensory System. New York: Springer-Verlag, 1973.

Jansen, J. K. S.: Spasticity—functional aspects. Acta Neurol. Scand. 1962.

Jasper, H. (ed.): Reticular Formation of the Brain. Boston: Little, Brown, & Co., 1958.

Jones, B.: The importance of memory traces of motor efferent discharge for learning skilled movements. Dev. Med. Child. Neurol. 16:620–628, 1974.

Kenshalo, D. R. (ed.): The Skin Senses. Springfield IL: Charles C Thomas, 1968.

Kimble, D. P. (ed.): The Anatomy of Memory, Learning, Remembering and Forgetting. Palo Alto: Science & Behavior Books, 1965.

Kimura, D.: The asymmetry of the human brain. Scientif. Amer. 228:70–78, 1973.

Knighton, R. S., and Dumke, P. R. (eds.): Pain. Henry Ford Hospital International Symposium. Boston: Little, Brown, & Co., 1966.

Kots, Y. M., and Zhukov, V. I.: Supraspinal control over segmental centers of antagonistic muscles in man. III. Tuning of spinal reciprocal inhibition system during organization preceding voluntary movement. Neuroscience Behav. Physiol. 6:9–15, 1973.

Luria, A. R.: Human Brain and Psychological Process. New York: Harper & Row, translated 1966.

Magni, F., and Willix, W. D.: Cortical control of brain stem reticular neurons. Arch. Ital. Biol. 102:418–433, 1964.

Magni, F.: Afferent connections to reticulo-spinal neurons. Prog. Brain Res. Elsevier 12:246–258, 1964.

Magni, F.: Subcortical and peripheral control of brainstem reticular neurons. Arch. Ital. Biol. 102:434–438, 1964.

Magoun, H. W.: The Waking Brain, ed. 2. Springfield IL, Charles C Thomas, 1963.

Moore, J. C.: Concepts from The Neurobehavioral Sciences. Dubuque: Kendall-Hunt, 1973.

Moore, J. C.: Neuroanatomy Simplified. Dubuque: Kendall-Hunt, 1969.

Morin, C., et al.: Role of the muscular afferents in the inhibition of the antagonist motor nucleus during a voluntary contraction in man. Brain Res. 103:373–376, 1976.

Neff, W. D. (ed.): Contributions to Sensory Physiology, ed. 2. New York: Academic Press, 1967.

Payton, O. D., Hirt, S., and Newton, R. A.: Scientific Bases for Neurophysiologic Approaches to Therapeutic Exercise. Philadelphia: F. A. Davis, 1977.

Piercey, M. F., and Goldfarb, J.: Discharge patterns of Renshaw cells evoked by volleys in ipsilateral cutaneous and high threshold muscle afferents and their relationship to reflexes recorded in ventral roots. J. Neurophysiol. 37:294–302, 1974.

Rispal-Padel, L., et al.: Relations between the ventrolateral thalamic nucleus and motor cortex and their possible role in the central organization of motor control. Brain Res. 60:1–20, 1973.

Ruch, T. C., et al.: Neurophysiology, ed. 2. Philadelphia: W. B. Saunders, 1966.

Rushworth, G.: Some aspects of the pathophysiology of spasticity and rigidity. Clin. Pharmacol. Ther. 1964.

Schultz, D. P.: Sensory Restriction—Effects on Behavior. New York: Academic Press, 1965.

Sherrington, C.: The Integrative Action of The Nervous System. New Haven CN: Yale University Press, 1961.

Speyer, K. M., Ghelarducci, B., and Pompeiano, O.: Gravity responses in main reticular formation. J. Neurophysiol. 37:705–721, 1974.

Tokizane, T., and Shimaza, H.: Functional Differentiation of Human Skeletal Muscle. Tokyo: Tokyo University Press, 1964.

Wagman, I. H., Pierce, D. S., and Burger, R. E.: Proprioceptive influence in volitional control of individual motor units. Nature (Lond) 7:957–958, 1965.

Weeks, Z. R.: Effects of the vestibular system on human development. Part 1. Overview of functions and effects of stimulation. Am. J. Occup. Ther. 33:376–381, 1979.

Wolstencroft, J. H.: Effects of afferent stimuli on reticulospinal neurons. J. Physiol. 1961.

Woodburne, L. S.: The Neural Basis of Behavior. Columbus: Charles E. Merrill Publishing Co., 1967.

Yahr, M. D., and Purpura, D. D.: Neurophysiological Basis of Normal and Abnormal Motor Activities. New York: Raven Press, 1967.

Acknowledgment

My appreciation to Josephine C. Moore, Ph.D., O.T.R., for her continuing efforts to assist all of us in the understanding of the neuroanatomical and neurophysiological aspects of human function.

Section 2

Overview of Sensorimotor Approaches *A. Joy Huss*

This section provides an historical overview of the various sensorimotor approaches, their current status, a statement regarding the application of these principles to occupational therapy, and a bibliography of greater depth for those interested. It is not an exposition in depth but rather an additional tool for the beginner or the uninitiated.

Overview

Fay-Doman-Delacato: Neuromuscular Reflex Therapy

Temple Fay, neurosurgeon, was the forerunner of sensorimotor approaches, beginning in the early 1940s. For nearly two decades he observed, discussed, demonstrated, and wrote about neuromuscular reflex therapy, which he defined as the "utiliza-tion of reflex levels of response to the highest level possible."[1] Much of his work was done prior to the present knowledge and understanding regarding the central nervous system, and it was based on the work of Sherrington. His basic premise was that ontogeny recapitulates phylogeny. Therefore, an individual's neurological development parallels the evolution from fish to amphibian, to reptile, to anthropoid. Since human movement is based on patterns of muscle activity, not on individual muscle response, he believed that if reflex patterns were elicited and utilized properly, functional movement could be established. As a result, his treatment program involved the following six concepts[2]:

1. After careful observation of the patient's level of functioning, including existing reflexes and automatic responses, treatment began with simple patterns of movement utilizing these reflexes.
2. Since in normal development each stage lays the foundation for the next stage, so in treatment it is

essential that lower levels of mobility be developed before expecting higher levels.

3. Reflexes in and of themselves are not abnormal but may indicate pathology if they interfere with refined coordinated movement. Therefore, reflexes can be utilized to develop muscle tone, inhibit antagonists, and lead to higher levels of coordinated movement.

4. Passive exercise patterns which involve the total extremity, not isolated joints, can enhance the sensory feedback mechanisms important for movement.

5. Active or passive patterns done repeatedly will in time lead to the spontaneous development of higher level patterns.

6. The patterns utilized are prone patterns of forward propulsion that can be observed in normal human infants as well as in amphibian and reptilian life forms.

The three basic patterns used are homologous (bunny hop), homolateral (camel walk), and crossed-diagonal (reciprocal).

Homologous is a bilateral-symmetrical pattern. With the head in midline with extension of the neck, the upper extremities are flexed at the shoulder while the lower extremities are extended at the hip. The extremities are then reversed rhythmically with neck flexion. In prone this is not too effective for propulsion, but in the all-fours position it is commonly called the bunny hop.

Homolateral is an ipsilateral pattern with the head, thorax, and pelvis turned toward the flexing upper and lower extremities with extension of the contralateral extremities. The pattern is then reversed leading with the head. In the all-fours this provides a gait similar to that of a camel.

Crossed-diagonal is a more highly integrated pattern with flexion of the upper extremity and extension of the lower extremity on the face side with extension of the lower extremity on the face side with extension of the upper limb with flexion of the lower limb on the opposite side. In the all-fours this provides the typical reciprocal gait pattern seen in higher mammals and human infants.

Following the prone position are the all-fours (hands and knees), plantigrade (hands and feet), and erect postures. All three patterns are utilized in the first three positions. Homolateral and crossed-diagonal are utilized in the erect position. Depending on the level of development, patterns are done passively, active-assistively, or actively. The key elements in determining the program planned for a patient are intellectual and functional motor development levels. Chronological age is less important.

Fay's work has provided the basic foundation for the approach now advocated by Carl Delacato, Ed.D., Robert Doman, M.D., and Glenn Doman, physical therapist. The same patterns of movement are utilized. In addition the program includes selective use of sensory stimulation procedures such as heat, cold, brushing, and pinching to establish hand dominance and a breathing exercise routine to increase the vital capacity.

The program for any given patient is administered at least four times per day for 5 minutes, 7 days a week. Each treatment requires at least three adults, because each extremity must be manipulated smoothly and rhythmically in the proper pattern.

Bobath: Neurodevelopmental Treatment Approach

The neurodevelopmental treatment approach has been developed in England by Berta Bobath, physical therapist, and Karel Bobath, neuropsychiatrist. Their work was begun in the 1940s with the cerebral palsied and adult-acquired hemiplegics. The treatment, however, is appropriate to a wide variety of other dysfunctions of the central nervous system. Treatment foundations are based on the experimental works of Magnus, Sherrington, deKleijn, Rademaker, Schaltenbrand, Walshe, and Weisz.

The concept of neurodevelopment treatment is based on two fundamental principles about the nature of the central nervous system dysfunction: (1) the arrest, or retardation, of normal movement is caused by the interference with normal brain maturation resulting from brain lesion, and (2) the resultant release of abnormal, or immature, postural reflex activity causes the observed abnormal patterns of posture and movement. On the basis of these concepts, treatment techniques have been developed by the Bobaths and others and are continually being added to and refined. Kong, Quilan, Finnie, Mueller, Reye, and Morris are names often associated with neurodevelopmental treatment.

The primary aim of treatment handling is the inhibition of abnormal movement patterns with the simultaneous facilitation of normal righting and equilibrium reactions and other appropriate normal movement patterns. The patient is so handled that the abnormal patterns are blocked and higher level reactions are elicited to give the patient more normal sensory experience. The therapist takes the patient through a series of graded sensory and motor experiences which set the stage for learning new, less stereotyped movement patterns. Through "preparation" activities the therapist normalizes the muscle tone (increasing it in the individuals or body parts where tone is too low and decreasing it in the individuals or body parts where it is too high), moves the patient passively to provide sensory experience to unfamiliar movement patterns, encourages active movement from the patient while still providing guidance control and, eventually, encourages the patient to move actively without control. This sequence may all take place in one treatment session or may involve weeks or months of therapy.

Movement is a physiological necessity. It allows us to maintain normal muscle tone and yet to be prepared to instantaneously change that tone in response to environmental demand. Movement is the primary modality of treatment in neurodevelopmental treatment. Normal movement inhibits abnormal movement, thus normal movement becomes both the process and the goal of therapy. Key points of control are used to influence the movement and balance of tone in the rest of the body. Key points of control are body parts, usually proximal; for example, the trunk and shoulders may be used to prepare the arms for weight bearing and the rest of the body for side-sitting. In addition to facilitation of movement, techniques of tapping, placing, and holding, and compression may be used to change the muscle tone when appropriate.[3]

The primary success of neurodevelopmental treatment is contingent on the therapist's ability to make changes in the muscle tone. Prolonged bracing, extensive surgery, and static positioning are usually incompatible with this treatment, because they do not allow for changes in muscle tone.

As in all good systems of therapy, a thorough initial assessment and frequent reassessment are necessary. The evaluation includes the following: type, strength, and distribution of muscle tone in all positions; abnormal patterns of posture and movement; basic automatic (normal) reactions; general stage of development with awareness of important gaps; contractures and deformities; and other associated handicaps. Readers not familiar with the basic reflex and developmental information are referred to Bobath, Fiorentino, Gesell, and Peiper. On the basis of the initial assessment, a plan of therapy is individualized appropriate to the present level of development and needs of the patient.

Teamwork among occupational therapist, physical therapist, speech therapist, physicians, classroom teacher, and parents is considered an essential aspect of treatment. Therapy is a 24 hour a day process when the whole patient and his/her perceptual systems, learning capabilities, personality, and motor system are influenced by the damage to the central nervous system. Close communication and cooperation in the whole treatment plan are essential to prevent disagreement in approach and confusion for the patient and his/her family.

Rood: Neurophysiological Approach

Margaret S. Rood, occupational therapist and physical therapist, frustrated by the slow improvement of patients with cerebral palsy, began to study the neurophysiological and developmental literature in the late 1930s. Based on the works of Sherrington, Gesell, Denny-Brown. Eldred, Hooker, Magoun, Cooper, Boyd, and others, a method of treatment has evolved since the 1940s. The basic principles utilized are as follows[4]:

1. Motor output is dependent upon sensory input. Thus sensory stimuli are utilized to activate and/or inhibit motor responses.
2. Activation of motor responses follows a normal developmental sequence. All muscles progress through the following stages of development:
   a. Full range of shortening and lengthening with the antagonist. Phasic movement—reciprocal innervation.
   b. A pattern of co-contraction in which antagonistic muscles of one or more joints work together for a holding action. Stability-tonic postural set.
   c. A pattern of heavy work movement superimposed on the co-contraction. Movement in weight-bearing position.
   d. Skill or coordinate movement. Movement in nonweight-bearing position with stabilization at the proximal joints.
3. Since there is interaction within the nervous system between somatic, psychic, and autonomic functions, stimuli can be used to influence one or more directly or indirectly.

This treatment approach can thus be defined as "the activation, facilitation, and inhibition of muscle action, voluntary and involuntary, through the reflex arc."[5]

This treatment approach assumes that an exercise per se is not treatment unless the pattern of response is correct and results in feedback which enhances learning of that response. Treatment or therapy is not in the form of a motor act alone, but rather is the application of stimuli to activate a response, followed by sensory input from a correct response with additional stimuli given to facilitate or inhibit elements in the pattern. The use of stimuli is an integral part of treatment, since sensory factors are essential for the achievement and maintenance of normal motor functions.[6]

Developmental sequences are outlined in Tables 7-2 and 7-3. These patterns are used to evaluate the patient's level of development that determines the level of treatment.

Table 7-2 *Skeletal development sequences.*

Reciprocal Innervation	Stability or Co-innervation	Movement Superimposed on Stability	Skill
1. Withdrawal: total flexion in supine	4. Co-contraction of neck with vertebral extension		
2. Roll over: flexion top side, extension bottom side	5. Prone on elbows static holding with co-contraction neck and shoulder	6. Push back	
		7. Pull forward	8. Belly crawling
3. Pivot prone: total extension in prone except for elbows, which are flexed with arms adducted	9. All-fours: static holding	10. Shifting weight backward-forward, side-to-side, alternate arm-leg	11. Creeping: homologous, homolateral, reciprocal
	12. Standing: static	13. Shifting weight backward-forward, side-to-side	14. Walking: must analyze stance, push off, pick up, and heel strike

Sensory stimulation is provided first for the proprioceptors, utilizing vibration, rubbing pressure into the muscle bellies, joint compression, quick stretch of the muscle to be facilitated, and appropriate vestibular input. If necessary, this is followed by exteroceptive input of light touch and/or rapid brushing. Ice, if used at all, is applied with great caution and only to the extremities. If exteroceptive input is used, there should be a careful follow-up of the patient by the therapist for several hours. Since cutaneous stimuli have a profound effect on the reticular system, there may be adverse rebound effects if exteroceptive stimulation is not used appropriately.

Inhibitory procedures used by Rood include slow stroking, neutral warmth, and slow rolling for overall relaxation and pressure to the muscle insertion for specific relaxation. Slow stroking is an alternate stroking of the posterior primary rami with a firm but light pressure. One hand starts at the cervical area and progresses to the lower lumbar region. As the first hand finishes, the second hand starts. Thus, there is always contact with the patient. This is done for no more than 3 minutes. If the hair growth pattern is irregular, this may be irritating to the patient. Neutral warmth is the wrapping of part or all of the patient in a cotton towel or blanket until the appropriate amount of relaxation is observed. Slow rolling from supine to side and return is also generally inhibitory. The rolling continues until relaxation is seen.

Depending on the type of muscle tone and developmental level of the patient, a treatment program may be all-inhibitory, inhibitory and facilitory, or all-facilitory.

Cortical demand for voluntary effort on the part of the patient is directed through activities that utilize the patterns that have been stimulated. The patient's attention is thus directed to the activity and not to specific movement or stabilizing patterns.

Kabat-Knott-Voss: Proprioceptive Neuromuscular Facilitation

Around 1946, Herman Kabat, physiatrist and neurophysiologist, began the development of a therapy system based on neurophysiological principles outlined by Sherrington, Coghill, McGraw, Gesell, Hellebrandt, and Pavlov. The major emphasis is stimulation of the proprioceptors with active participation by the patient. These principles were ex-

Table 7-3 *Vital function developmental sequences.*

Reciprocal Innervation	Stability or Co-innervation	Movement Superimposed on Stability	Skill
1. Inspiration			
2. Expiration	3. Sucking	4. Swallowing fluids	5. Phonation
		6. Chewing	
		7. Swallowing solids	8. Speech

panded and utilized in treatment by Margaret Knott and Dorothy Voss, both physical therapists. "Proprioceptive neuromuscular facilitation enlists the less involved parts, to promote a balanced antagonism of reflex activity, of muscle groups and of components of motion."[7]

As stated by Knott and Voss in the second edition of *Proprioceptive Neuromuscular Facilitation*, the philosophy of treatment is

> . . . based upon the ideas that all human beings respond in accordance with demand; that existing potentials may be developed more fully; that movements must be specific and directed toward a goal; that activity is necessary to the best development of coordination, strength, and endurance; and that the stronger body parts strengthening weaker parts through cooperation lead toward a goal of optimum function.[8]

The technique is therefore defined as "methods of promoting or hastening the response of the neuromuscular mechanism through stimulation of the proprioceptors."[9]

There has been a gradual evolution of the technique since the 1940s. Initially greatest emphasis was placed on the use of maximal resistance throughout the range of motion. Patterns of movement were utilized that allowed action at two or more joints and that required two component actions of a given muscle. Other factors considered important were stretch for proprioceptive stimulation, positioning to enhance contraction, motion beginning in the strongest part of the range progressing to the weaker part, incorporation of reflexes, and reinforcement through resistance.

In 1949, based on Sherrington's law of successive induction, rhythmic stabilization and slow reversal procedures were added to enhance facilitation of the weaker muscles. In 1951 the patterns of movement were analyzed more thoroughly. In order to apply stretch to maximally elongated muscles, it was found that patterns that were spiral and diagonal were most effective and that they also corresponded more nearly to normal functional patterns of movement.

Since that time the above principles have been incorporated into mat, gait, and self-care activities to assist in motor learning and the development of strength and balance.

Current techniques being used are maximal, but not overpowering resistance; quick stretch; postural and righting reflexes; mass movement patterns with spiral and diagonal components; reversal of antagonists (rhythmic stabilization and slow reversal); and ice (generally used for inhibition and occasionally for facilitation).

The patient is evaluated developmentally, and treatment begun appropriately. In all cases, beginning treatment utilizes the strongest groups of muscles and the most coordinated movements the patient has for reciprocal innervation, irradiation, and summation. Movement patterns are reinforced through simple verbal commands which utilize the patient's voluntary control.

Brunnstrom

Around 1951, Signe Brunnstrom, physical therapist, became concerned with the lack of rehabilitation of the upper extremity in acquired hemiplegia. She studied the research on reflex responses in decerebrate cats and hemiplegia in man. From the research efforts of Riddoch and Buzzard, Magnus and de-Kleijn, and Simons, Brunnstrom selected the effects of associated reactions initiated either by voluntary effort on the noninvolved side or by reflex stimulation, postural reactions resulting from tonic neck and tonic labyrinthine reflexes, and the flexion and extension synergies. After careful observation of over 100 hemiplegic patients, she delineated the stages of recovery and techniques to facilitate the patient's progression from one stage to the next. Thus, treatment consists of developing the potential for "coordinate movement with reflexlike mechanisms, sensory cues, volitional effort and gradation of demand through the stages of recovery."[10]

The stages of recovery follow a definite sequence, and the patient never skips a stage. However, he or she may plateau at any one of the following six stages:

1. Immediately following the vascular insult there appears to be flaccidity with no voluntary movement in the affected extremities.
2. Spasticity begins to develop. The flexion and extension synergies can be stimulated reflexively. They first appear with co-contraction but gradually become more distinct with the flexion synergy dominating the upper extremity and the extension synergy dominating the lower extremity.
3. Spasticity becomes quite severe. However, the synergies can now be voluntarily initiated with some range of motion. Any attempt to use the extremity voluntarily results in a synergy pattern.
4. Spasticity begins to decrease. Simple uncoordinated movements that differ from the basic synergies can be performed slowly and deliberately. Also, reciprocal movements within the synergies are beginning to develop.
5. Spasticity continues to decrease to the point that the patient can perform some functional activities although still slowly and deliberately without eliciting synergies. Some independence of the synergy patterns is achieved, and isolated individual joint movement is possible.

6. Spasticity has almost disappeared. Individual joint motion is freer and has controlled speed and direction. With rapid, reciprocal movement some incoordination may still be present.

Because of the degree of cortical control necessary for hand control, recovery of function in the hand is more difficult and less predictable. Mass grasp does precede mass extension, and thumb motion precedes finger motion.

After evaluation of the patient's stage of recovery and sensory status, treatment aimed at reflex training follows. The steps of treatment are listed:

1. Motion synergies are elicited on a reflex level. Reflexes used include:
   a. tonic neck reflex
   b. tonic labyrinthine reflex
   c. tonic lumbar reflex
   d. resistance to voluntary contraction of noninvolved limb*
   e. sensory stimulation, which includes quick stretch, passive movement, tapping over a muscle belly, surface stroking, positioning, and pressure on muscle belly or tendon.
2. Motion synergies are captured, that is, an effort is made to establish voluntary control of the synergies. This is accomplished by utilization of the following stages:
   a. repetition using facilitation
   b. repetition without using facilitation
   c. working from proximal to distal, concentrating on various components of the synergy with and without the use of facilitation. Reciprocal motion between the two synergies is started with a goal of diminishing the time lag between contraction and relaxation of antagonistic muscles.
3. Motion synergies are conditioned by combining elements of antagonistic synergies starting with the stronger components. At this point, time is also spent on muscles that do not participate in the synergies, such as the serratus anterior and the peroneal muscles. As progress occurs, more complex motions with rapid reciprocation are initiated.
4. The most difficult step is the elicitation of voluntary hand and finger function. Maneuvers such as Souque's phenomenon and imitation synkinesis are helpful.[11]

---

*It is important to note that in the upper extremities resistance to flexion of the noninvolved extremity facilitates flexion in the involved extremity and vice versa. In the lower extremities resistance to flexion in the noninvolved extremity facilitates extension of the involved extremity and vice versa.

Postures and positions used during treatment include supine, sitting, and standing. Visual and verbal cues are used throughout. Volitional effort and functional activities are initiated early, and they are considered necessary if there is to be carry-over by the patient.

Ayres: Sensory Integration Approach to Learning Disorders

A. Jean Ayres, Ph.D., O.T.R., began her studies of children with learning disabilities in the 1950s. She and others observed that the cognitive approach to treatment of such children had led to dissatisfaction of skill training as an end in and of itself, because too many children were still unable to generalize and respond adaptively to their environment. Study of the approaches of Knott, Bobath, Fay, and especially Rood for the physically handicapped, which placed an emphasis on integration of the nervous system at subcortical levels, seemed to have some application to those with learning problems.

Ayres' intensive and extensive research studies of these latter problems, along with intense study of the integrative functions of the nervous system, led to her present and still evolving theoretical framework from which treatment procedures are devised. This is discussed further in the next section of this chapter.

Fuchs: Orthokinetics

Julius Fuchs, orthopedic surgeon, dissatisfied with the static approach of braces, casts, and splints, created devices that provided immediate mobilization as well as support. His work was done in the 1920s, and it was published in German in 1927; however, a description in English was not published until 1955. The principles originally were applied to fractures, scoliosis, and other orthopedic problems. The application to neurological and arthritic dyskinesias was made in the 1950s by Manfred Blashy, physiatrist, and Elsbeth Harrison and Ernest Fuchs, both occupational therapists.

The basic idea in orthokinetics is the use of a segment or cuff composed of elastic and inelastic parts. Several of these put together form the orthokinetic tube. The inelastic or inactive fields cover those parts where support and muscle inactivity are desired. The elastic or active fields cover those parts where muscle activity is desired. The inactive field, thus, becomes the inhibitory field, and the active field the facilitory field.

Originally these cuffs were made of leather and molded directly to the patient. Currently they are made of Ace bandages or sewing elastic 1 to 6 in.

wide, depending on the size of the area of application. The device is usually two or three layers thick for the active field and three to four layers thick in the inactive field. The layers are stitched firmly together to provide the inactive field and left free for the active field. The cuff can be fastened with Velcro.

Among the results claimed by Fuchs and others are (1) rapid relief of pain, (2) increase of muscle strength, (3) increase of range of motion, (4) muscle re-education, and (5) improvement of coordination. I have also noted an increase in girth as muscle bulk fills in.

The cuffs are worn repeatedly to increase the effects. They can be worn all day while the individual is active. This provides continuous sensory input. The greater the imbalance initially between agonist and antagonist muscle groups, the quicker the effects will be noticed.

This is an effective, inexpensive procedure that supplies continuous input when the patient is not "in therapy." It should be further investigated by occupational and physical therapists as to its value as an adjunct to treatment.

Summary

In looking at the various sensorimotor treatment approaches, it is helpful to place them in a continuum of control needed by the patient.

The Fay-Doman-Delacato approach is initially one of passive movement superimposed upon the patient; only later does this call for active participation on the part of the patient.

Rood uses a strong mixture of exteroceptive and proprioceptive input in developmental patterns followed by activity utilizing the stability and mobility components of the patterns. The individual's attention is directed to the activity and not to the patterns per se.

Orthokinetics provides a continuous exteroceptive input followed by proprioceptive feedback as muscles are facilitated and inhibited. The individual is able to use the resultant muscle function in activities of daily living.

Bobath inhibits primitive patterns and then facilitates righting and equilibrium reactions, controlling at key points, so that the nervous system receives feedback only from more normal movement. Whenever possible, cortical control of movement is demanded.

Brunnstrom uses the initial synergy patterns seen in recovery from cerebral vascular insult on both a reflexive level and with conscious control by the patient. Using exteroceptive and proprioceptive input as well as cortical control, these patterns are then broken up and lead to functional movement.

Kabat-Knott-Voss place primary emphasis on proprioceptive input reinforced by visual and verbal cues that demand cortical control by the client. Exteroceptive stimulation is considered primarily in the placement of the therapist's hands.

Thus, when the client is at a level in which cortical control hinders movement, approaches such as Rood, Fuchs, Bobath, and Fay can be utilized. Once cortical control begins to develop and strengthening is needed, Brunnstrom and Kabat-Knott-Voss approaches become appropriate.

Many of the techniques of the various approaches are quite similar. Often it is feasible to employ techniques from various approaches at any given time with any individual. The therapist must know and understand normal human development, neurophysiology, and techniques of evaluation in order to effectively use these treatment approaches.

At the present time there is controversy whether these approaches to the treatment of CNS dysfunction should be used by occupational therapists or whether they are strictly a physical therapy approach. Personally, I hold certification in both professions, and I firmly believe that occupational therapists should know and utilize the underlying principles and techniques of the sensorimotor approaches. It takes appropriate input to organize the CNS for output, and the motor output must be purposeful, goal-directed activity in order for it to be retained and built upon by the CNS. Occupational therapists are in a unique position to utilize purposeful, goal-directed activity on a subcortical level. These approaches will not be effective unless the client is allowed to actively respond to the input in a meaningful way.

References

1. A. J. Phys. Med. NUSTEP, p. 816, 1967.
2. Ibid., p. 817.
3. Manning, J.: Facilitation of movement—the Bobath approach. Physiotherapy (Eng.) 58:403–408, 1972.
4. NUSTEP, p. 900–954.
5. Rood, M. S.: Unpublished class notes, 1958, 1959, 1970, and 1975.
6. NUSTEP, p. 903.
7. Knott, M., and Voss, D. E.: Proprioceptive Neuromuscular Facilitation: Patterns and Techniques, ed. 2. New York: Harper & Row, 1968, p. 14.
8. Ibid., p. 3.
9. Ibid., p. 4.
10. NUSTEP, p. 794.
11. Ibid.

Bibliography

Ayres, A. J.: Occupational therapy for motor disorders resulting from impairment of the central nervous system. Rehab. Lit. 21:10, 1960.

Ayres, A. J.: Perceptual-Motor Dysfunction in Children. Monograph from Greater Cincinnati District, Ohio Occupational Therapy Association Conference, 1964.

Ayres, A. J.: Sensory Integration and Learning Disorders. Los Angeles: Western Psychological Services, 1972.

Bailey, D. M.: The effects of vestibular stimulation on verbalization in chronic schizophrenics. Am. J. Occup. Ther. 32:445–450, 1978.

Banus, B. S., Kent, C. A., Norton, Y., et al.: The Developmental Therapist, ed. 2. Thorofare NJ: Charles B Slack, 1979.

Barnes, M. R., Crutchfield, C. A., and Heriza, C. B.: The Neurophysiological Basis of Patient Treatment. Vol 2, Reflexes in Motor Development. Morgantown, WV: Stokesville Publishing Co., 1978.

Bishop, B.: Vibratory stimulation. Part I—Neurophysiology of motor responses. J.A.P.T.A. 54:1273–1281, 1974.

Bishop, B.: Vibratory stimulation. Part II—Vibratory stimulation as an evaluation tool. J.A.P.T.A. 55:28–34, 1975.

Bishop, B.: Vibratory stimulation. Part III—Possible applications of vibration in treatment of motor dysfunction. J.A.P.T.A. 55:139–143, 1975.

Blashy, M.: Manipulation of the neuromuscular unit in the periphery of the central nervous system. J. So. Med. Assoc. 54:873–879, 1961.

Blashy, M., and Fuchs, R.: Orthokinetics: A new receptor facilitation method. Am. J. Occup. Ther. 13:226–234, 1959.

Blashy, M., Harrison, H. E., and Fuchs, E. M.: Orthokinetics—a preliminary report on recent experiences with a little known rehabilitation therapy. V. A. Bull., 1955.

Bobath, B.: Abnormal Postural Reflex Activity Caused by Brain Lesions. London: Wm. Heinemann Medical Books, 1965.

Bobath, B.: Motor development, its effect on general development, and application to the treatment of cerebral palsy. Physiotherapy (Eng.) 57:526–32, 1971.

Bobath, B.: Adult Hemiplegia: Evaluation and Treatment, ed. 2. London: Wm. Heinemann Medical Books, 1978

Bobath, K.: The motor deficit in patients with cerebral palsy. Clin. Develop. Med. 23:1966.

Bobath, K.: A Neurophysiological Basis for the Treatment of Cerebral Palsy. Philadelphia: J. B. Lippincott, 1980.

Bobath, K., and Bobath, B.: The facilitation of normal postural reactions and movements in the treatment of cerebral palsy. Physiotherapy (Eng.) 50:246–262, 1964.

Bobath, K., and Bobath, B.: The importance of memory traces of motor efferent discharges for learning skilled movements. Dev. Med. Child. Neurol. 16:837–838, 1974.

Brunnstrom, S.: Movement Therapy in Hemiplegia: A Neurophysiological Approach. New York: Harper & Row, 1970.

Child With Central Nervous System Deficit—Report of Two Symposiums. Washington DC: U.S. Dept. of Health, Educ. & Welfare, 1965.

Coryell, J., and Henderson, A.: Role of the asymmetrical tonic neck reflex in hand visualization in normal infants. Am. J. Occup. Ther. 33:255–260, 1979.

Dayhoff, N.: Rethinking stroke: Soft or hard devices to position hands. Am. J. Nurs. 7:1142–1144, 1975.

Doman, G., and Delacato, C.: Children with severe brain injuries. J.A.M.A. 174:257–267, 1960.

Eviatar, L., Eviatar, A., and Naray, I.: Maturation of neurovestibular responses in infants. Dev. Med. Child. Neurol. 16:435–446, 1974.

Farber, S.: Neurorehabilitation: A Multi-Sensory Approach. Philadelphia: W. B. Saunders Co., 1982.

Fay, T.: Basic considerations regarding neuromuscular and reflex therapy. Spastics Quart. 3, 1954.

Fay, T.: Neuromuscular reflex therapy for spastic disorders. J. Florida Med. Assoc. 44, 1958.

Finnie, N.: Handling the Young Cerebral Palsied Child at Home. London: Wm. Heinemann Medical Books, 1968.

Fiorentino, M.: Reflex Testing Methods For Evaluating C.N.S. Development, ed. 2. Springfield IL: Charles C Thomas, 1976.

Fiorentino, M. R.: A Basis for Sensorimotor Development—Normal and Abnormal: The Influence of Primitive, Postural Reflexes on the Development and Distribution of Tone. Springfield IL: Charles C Thomas, 1981.

Fox, J. V. D.: Improving tactile discrimination of the blind: A neurophysiological approach. Am. J. Occup. Ther. 19:5–7, 1965.

Fox, J. V. D.: The olfactory system: Implications for the occupational therapist. Am. J. Occup. Ther. 20:173–177, 1966.

Freeman, J., Gould, V., Merkley, F., and Smith, M.: Project A.D.A.P.T.: A Developmental Curriculum for Infants Exhibiting Developmental Delay. Ventura CA: Ventura County Association for the Retarded, 1975.

Friedlander, B. Z., Sterritt, G. M., Kirk, G. E. (eds): Exceptional Infant: Assessment and Intervention, Vol 3. New York: Brunner/Mazel, 1975.

Gesell, A.: The First Five Years of Life. New York: Harper & Row, 1940.

Gilfoyle, E. M., Grady, A. P., and Moore, J. C.: Children Adapt. Thorofare NJ: Charles B. Slack, 1981.

Goff, B.: The application of recent advances in neurophysiology to Miss M. Rood's concept of neuromuscular facilitation. Physiotherapy (Eng) 58:409–415, 1972.

Griffin, J. W.: Use of proprioceptive stimuli in therapeutic exercise. J.A.P.T.A. 54:1072–1079, 1974.

Griffin, J., and Reddin, G.: Shoulder pain in patients with hemiplegia: A literature review. Phys. Ther. 61:1041–1045, 1981.

Harris, F. A.: In defense of facilitation techniques. Arch. Phys. Med. Rehab. 51:438–441, 1970.

Harris, F. A.: Multiple-loop modulation of motor outflow: A physiological basis for facilitation techniques. J.A.P.T.A. 51:391–396, 1971.

Harris, F. A.: Facilitation techniques in therapeutic exercise. In Basmajian, J. W. (ed.): Therapeutic Exercise, Student Edition. Baltimore: Williams and Wilkins Co., 1980.

Heiniger, M. C., and Randolph, S. L.: Neurophysiological Concepts in Human Behavior: The Tree of Learning. St. Louis: C. V. Mosby, 1981.

Holle, B.: Motor Development in Children, Normal and Retarded. London: Blackwell Scientific Publications, 1976.

Huss, A. J.: Application of Rood technique to treatment of the physical handicapped child. In West, W. (ed.): Occupational Therapy for the Multiply Handicapped Child. Chicago: University of Chicago, 1965.

Huss, A. J.: Clinical application of sensorimotor treatment techniques in physical dysfunction, and, Controversy and confusion in physical dysfunction treatment techniques—clinical aspects. In Zamir, L. (ed.): Expanding Dimensions in Rehabilitation. Springfield IL: Charles C Thomas, 1969.

Johnston, R. M., Bishop, B., and Coffey, G. H.: Mechanical vibration of skeletal muscles. J.A.P.T.A. 50:499–505, 1970.

Kabat, H.: Central facilitation; the basis of treatment for paralysis. Permanente Fnd. Med. Bull. 10, August 1962.

Keshner, E. A.: Reevaluating the theoretical model underlying the neurodevelopmental theory: A literature review. Phys. Ther. 61:1035–1040, 1981.

King, L. J.: Toward a science of adaptive responses. Am. J. Occup. Ther. 32:429–437, 1978.

Knott, M.: Bulbar involvement with good recovery. J.A.P.T.A. 42:38–39, 1962.

Knott, M.: Neuromuscular facilitation in the child with central nervous system deficit. J.A.P.T.A. 46:721–724, 1966.

Knott, M.: Neuromuscular facilitation in the treatment of rheumatoid arthritis. J.A.P.T.A. 44:737–739, 1964.

Knott, M., and Voss, D. E.: Proprioceptive Neuromuscular Facilitation, ed. 2. New York: Harper & Row, 1968.

Koczwara, H.: Use of a vibrator to facilitate motor and kinesthetic behavior in children. J.A.P.T.A. 55:510, 1975.

Kottke, F. J.: Neurophysiologic therapy for stroke. In Licht, S. (ed.): Stroke and Its Rehabilitation. New Haven: Elizabeth Licht Publishers, 1975.

Leiper, C. I., Miller, A., Lang, J., and Herman, R.: Sensory feedback for head control in cerebral palsy. Phys. Ther. 61:512–518, 1981.

Lindblom, U.: On the treatment of spastic paresis. J. Swed. Assoc. Reg. Phys. Ther. 27, Reprint, 1969.

Loomis, J.: Facilitation techniques in hemiplegia—treatment of the arm. J Can. Physiother. Assoc. 25:283–285, 1973.

Mazzo, M. J., and Baez, M. B.: Therapeutic Positioning Equipment for the Multiply Handicapped Child: A Neurodevelopmental Approach to its Design and Development. New York State Occupational Therapy Association.

McCracken, A.: Drool control and tongue thrust therapy for the mentally retarded. Am. J. Occup. Ther. 32:79–85, 1978.

McPherson, J. J.: Objective evaluation of a splint designed to reduce hypertonicity. Am. J. Occup. Ther. 35:189–194, 1981.

Montgomery, P., and Richter, E.: Sensorimotor Integration for Developmentally Disabled Children: A Handbook. Los Angeles: Western Psychological Services, 1977.

Morrison, D., Pothier, P., and Horr, K.: Sensory-Motor Dysfunction and Therapy in Infancy and Early Childhood. Springfield IL: Charles C Thomas, 1978.

Neeman, R.: Techniques of preparing effective orthokinetic cuff. A.O.T.A. Bull. 6:1, 1971.

Neuhaus, B. E., Ascher, E. R., Coullon, B. A., et al.: A survey of rationales for and against hand splinting in hemiplegia. Am. J. Occup. Ther. 35:83–90, 1981.

Norton, Y.: Neurodevelopmental and sensory integration. Am. J. Occup. Ther. 29:93–100, 1975.

Ohwaki, S., et al.: Preference for vibratory and visual stimulation in mentally retarded children. Am. J. Ment. Def. 77:733–736, 1973.

Okoye, R.: Functional Evaluation of the Adult with CNS Dysfunction. Long Island District New York State Occupational Therapy Association, 1976.

Oster, C.: The neurophysiologic treatment of hemiplegia. J. Am. Osteopath. Assoc. 74:124–130, 1974.

Parent, L. H.: Effects of a low-stimulus environment on behavior. Am. J. Occup. Ther. 32:19–25, 1978.

Pearson, P. H., and Williams, C. E. (eds.): Physical Therapy Services in the Developmental Disabilities. Springfield IL: Charles C Thomas, 1972.

Peiper, A.: Cerebral Function in Infancy and Childhood. New York: Consultants Bureau, 1963.

Piercy, J. M.: The place of facilitation in non-neurological problems. Physiotherapy (Eng): 59:2–6, 1973.

Pink, M.: Contralateral effects of upper extremity proprioceptive neuromuscular facilitation patterns. Phys. Ther. 61:1158–1161, 1981.

Price, A.: Neurotherapy and specialization. Am. J. Occup. Ther. 34:809–815, 1980.

Resman, M. H.: Effect of sensory stimulation on eye contact in a profoundly retarded adult. Am. J. Occup. Ther. 35:31–35, 1981.

Reuck, A. V. S., and de Knight, J. (ed.): Myotatic, Kinesthetic and Vestibular Mechanisms. London: Churchill, 1967.

Rood, M. S.: Proprioceptive neuromuscular facilitation and demonstration physiotherapy and occupational therapy. South Africa Cerebral Palsy J. 13:3, 1969.

Rood, M. S.: Use of Reflexes as an Aid in Occupational Therapy. Speech delivered at World Fed. of O.T., Copenhagen, Denmark, August, 1958.

Sattely, C. (ed.): Approaches to the Treatment of Patients with Neuromuscular Dysfunction. Dubuque IA: William C. Brown, 1962.

Schwartzman, R. J., and Bogdonoff, M. D.: Behavioral and anatomical analysis of vibration sensibility. Exp. Neurol. 20:43–51, 1968.

Semans, S.: Physical therapy for motor disorders resulting from brain damage. Rehab. Lit. April, 1959.

Shepherd, R. B.: Physiotherapy in Pediatrics. London: Wm. Heinemann Medical Books, 1974.

Silverman, E. H., and Elfant, I. L.: Dysphagia: An evaluation and treatment program for the adult. Am. J. Occup. Ther. 33:382–392, 1979.

Smith, K. U.: Delayed Sensory Feedback and Behavior. Philadelphia: W. B. Saunders Co., 1962.

Smith, K. U., and Smith, W. M.: Perception and Motion. Philadelphia: W. B. Saunders Co., 1962.

Snook, J. H.: Spasticity reduction splint. Am. J. Occup. Ther. 33:648–651, 1979.

Troyer, B.: Sensorimotor integration: A basis for planning occupational therapy. Am. J. Occup. Ther. 15:51–54, 1961.

Voss, D. E.: Proprioceptive neuromuscular facilitation: Application of patterns and technics in occupational therapy. Am. J. Occup. Ther. 13:191–194, 1959.

Voss, D. E., and Slatinsky, J. P.: Textured cane handle. J.A.P.T.A. 53:1295, 1973.

Weeks, Z. R.: Effects of the vestibular system on human development, Part 2. Effects of vestibular stimulation on mentally retarded, emotionally disturbed, and learning-disabled individuals. Am. J. Occup. Ther. 33:450–457, 1979.

West, W. (ed.): Occupational Therapy for the Multiply Handicapped Child. Chicago: University of Chicago Press, 1965.

Whelan, J. K.: Effects of orthokinetics on upper extremity function of the adult hemiplegic patient. Am. J. Occup. Ther. 18:141–143, 1964.

Yamanaka, T.: Effects of High Frequency Vibration on Muscle Spindles In The Human Body. Zhiba Igakkai Zasshi 40, 1964.

Zamir, L. J. (ed.): Expanding Dimensions in Rehabilitation. Springfield IL: Charles C Thomas, 1969.

Section **3**
Sensory Integrative Theory *Mary Silberzahn*

This summary of literature on the theory of sensory integration as it has been constructed and published by A. Jean Ayres is intended to introduce the reader to selected basic concepts of the theory. The therapeutic application of this body of knowledge requires in-depth study of the theory as cited in the original works of the author. Omitted from this summary is the extensive research underlying the theoretical construction.

The Sensory Integration Process

A theoretical model of the process of sensory integration has been constructed by Ayres. The theory, built on both brain and behavioral research, was developed as a guide to improve neurological dysfunction and to promote learning ability. The research underlying the theory focuses on the development of sensory integrative mechanisms and identification of irregularities in the learning disabled child. "The theory is not considered final: rather, it is seen as a continually evolving formulation of ideas to incorporate information from neurobiological research."[1]

Sensory integration is the neurological process of organizing and processing, or perceiving, sensations for use. The organization of events between the sensation and the response is dependent upon the brain's ability to filter, sort, and integrate a mass of sensory information. The manner in which these events can be influenced is a major concern of the theory.

The objective of the sensory integrative approach to the treatment of learning disabilities is to enhance the brain's ability to develop the capacity to perceive, remember, and motor plan in order to provide a basis for mastery of all academic and other tasks rather than a focus on specific content. The therapeutic approach is directed towards controlling sensory input in order to activate brain mechanisms. Therapy in some, but not all, learning disabled children results in a reduction of the severity of the difficulty and allows specific skills to be learned more rapidly. Thus it "is considered a supplement, not a substitute to formal classroom instruction or tutoring."[2]

Neurophysiological Constructs

The understanding of certain basic principles of brain function on which sensory integrative theory is constructed is essential to the implementation of a therapeutic approach to learning disabilities.

Intermodality Association

The convergence of sensory input on a common neuron or larger structure is one method by which the brain associates sensory input from various sensory modalities. Implications for the therapeutic process lie in the premise that some neurons require convergence of many impulses for discharge. Thus, the summation of stimuli from various sensory modalities, when directed toward a specific response, may be more effective than input from one modality alone.

Sensory Feedback

Awareness from action or feedback from the somatosensory and vestibular systems is essential to organizing and using sensory input for motor performance. For example, appropriate adaptive responses are impossible if the child does not know if he is falling and in which direction he will fall. "The problem is not one of loss of sensation but of inadequate discrimination of the temporal and spatial qualities which, presumably, results in 'hazy' or vague feedback."[3] The therapist should utilize procedures and activities that emphasize the processing of accurate discriminative information. Selection of activities that have simple motor demands and require integrative responses are preferable to more complex motor activities requiring a great many responses that cannot be adequately integrated.

Centrifugal Influence

The ability to suppress part of the sensory flow and to prevent sensory overload is an important regulatory function of the central nervous system. The influences operate in a direction away from the cerebral cortex and toward the periphery to regulate the sensory flow. "Some of the disinhibited behavior, hypersensitivity to sensation, deficient perception and clumsiness can be linked, in one way or another to inadequate centrifugal influences from cortical or subcortical levels."[4] Therapy should be directed toward providing sensory input which is designed to enhance influences operating in a direction away from the cerebral cortex and toward the periphery.

Movement

"One of the most powerful organizers of sensory input is movement which is adaptive to the organism."[5] The theory proposes that the brain will tend to organize itself in response to functional environmental demands resulting in integrative responses. The therapeutic procedure should be concerned with the selection of activities that require organization of a more complex response than previously made.

Developmental Sequence

The importance of the developmental sequence to sensory integration is viewed in terms of phlogeny, ontogeny, and neurodevelopment and developmental stages. "In children, intersensory integration follows a developmental sequence with the most rapid maturation of the function occurring before eight years of age."[6]

The progress of evolution of the brain is, at least in part, a result of the organizing of successful or adaptive responses to environmental demands. "The therapeutic situation attempts to modify both the child's capacity and the environmental demands to make it possible for the child to succeed in organizing a response and thus to proceed with the developmental sequences that eventually result in the capacity for academic learning."[7]

Levels of Brain Function

The concept of levels of function, derived mainly from brain evolution, is that lower structures of the brain are phyletically less complex, and they develop before the higher and more complex structures.

The importance of the brainstem is particularly critical to sensory integrative theory, because it evolved earlier, is an important area for convergence of sensory input, and has widespread influence over the rest of the brain. It is concerned primarily with total massive patterning involving overt responses of the entire body, determined by a relatively simple integration. It contributes to visual perception, especially to the development of an environment scheme or map to which the body relates. The cerebral hemispheres evolved later, enabling more discrete, individualistic motor patterns based on more precise interpretation of sensory information. A general principle of brain function is that higher levels do not function optimally without adequate lower function. Similarly, higher structures never quite lose their dependence on lower structures. "The course of therapy follows a progression similar to that of the developmental course of brain function. Enhancing maturation at the lower, less complex levels of environmental-response function enables a child to become more competent at the higher, more complex levels."[8] Thus, a great deal of the therapeutic emphasis is placed on organization of sensory-integrative mechanisms at the brainstem level.

Sensory Modalities

Knowledge of sensory modalities in terms of neural pathways, intersensory influences, developmental sequence, and contribution to sensory integration is basic to evaluation and treatment of sensory integrative dysfunction. The theory proposes hypotheses of neural functioning as suggestions for exploring therapeutic procedures or as providing tentative explanations for their apparent effectiveness. Because vestibular, tactile, and proprioceptive sensory systems mature earliest, they have received the greatest emphasis in theory development. These modalities have pervasive influence on brain function, mature early, and are important to survival. They provide input from the body for unconscious neural control of sensorimotor activity and to convergent neurons for intersensory association. They contribute to perceptual-motor development including body scheme, motor planning, motor and academic skill development, and psychosocial development. The therapeutic use of motor activity is important to sensory integrative development because of the input to the tactile, vestibular, and other proprioceptive systems. Visual and auditory functions mature later, and they are seen as end products of sensory integration.

Evaluation

Evaluation of sensory integrative dysfunction is both objective and subjective; standardized tests are used to strengthen and increase clinical impressions.

The Southern California Sensory Integration Tests and the Southern California Postrotary Nystagmus Test, a battery of 18 tests, were constructed by Ayres "to detect and to determine the nature of sensory integrative dysfunction."[9] The tests measure parameters statistically identified as related to learning disabilities, which include tactile, kinesthetic, vestibular, and visual senses and aspects of motor planning and motor coordination. The total test battery should be administered to obtain adequate reliability. Dysfunction can be detected by comparing standard scores of a child's performance with the expected performance derived from the normative sample. The nature of sensory integrative dysfunction can be identified by comparing one area of performance that comprises a meaningful cluster (*e.g.,* visual) with other areas of performance (*e.g.,* tactile). The appropriate use of these tests "is dependent upon wide background knowledge of neurobiology, especially that related to sensory integration and processing, and extensive experience with children who have sensory integrative problems."[10] (The reader is referred to the *Southern California Sensory Integration Tests Manual,* the *Southern California Postrotary Nystagmus Test Manual,* and the *Southern California Sensory Integration Interpretation Manual* for extensive coverage of evaluation procedures.)

Subjective assessment relies heavily on the understanding of postural mechanisms and sensory systems in relation to sensory integrative development and function.

Postural Mechanisms

Postural responses, elicited by gravity and movement, influence the sensory integrative process at the brainstem level, and they contribute to neural integration required for academic learning. Principles and functions underlying the therapeutic approach to enhancing postural mechanisms include the antigravity nature of these responses, the brainstem level of organization, the developmental sequence, the rela-

tionship to muscles and muscle receptors, and to extraocular muscle control.

The ability to assume and maintain a prone extension and a supine flexion position is considered to be an indicator of one aspect of sensory integrative development. The tonic labyrinthine reflex (TLR), activated by change of position of the head in space, biases postural changes in the neonate in the direction of gravity. As the more mature antigravity responses develop, the child can assume and maintain the basic motor patterns of flexion when supine and extension when prone. The child who demonstrates an inadequate response will need to be provided with opportunities for a more mature level of response. The prone extension pattern may be reflexively facilitated by riding a scooterboard down an incline in a prone extension position. If this position has previously been difficult, the nervous system may need to be prepared to make an appropriate response. Therapeutic procedures such as brushing, quick stretch, and vibration may be employed previous to the scooter ride.

The tonic neck reflex (TNR), which originates from receptors in the joints and ligaments of the first three cervical vertebrae, reflexively orients the limbs in relation to the head-body angle. The ability of the head to move freely on its axis indicates integration of the primitive TNR and, as such, is another indicator of sensory-motor development. A proposed remedial procedure is for the child to assume and maintain an anti-tonic neck position, a reverse position of the head and forearms in relation to the head.

The integration of primitive reflexes is mainly dependent upon adequate vestibular and proprioceptive functions; the righting reactions involve receptors from several sensory modalities—visual, tactile, proprioceptive, and vestibular.

The righting reactions, including the neck-righting reflex, triggered by sensory input to neck receptors for automatic body turning, represent a more mature response, integrating the TNR and eliciting rotation on the longitudinal axis. Activation of the neck-righting reflex is best promoted by rolling activities replicating the early rolling patterns of the developing infant.

Activities designed to elicit equilibrium reactions in prone, quadruped, and sitting and the protective extension responses are introduced as part of the developmental sequence. These activities should involve trunk and extremities in an attempt to attain and maintain balance. The development of kneel and squat patterns should be encouraged. It is recommended that standing balance not be emphasized in the therapeutic process until the earlier developmental steps have been achieved.

Therapeutic procedures for developing postural

mechanisms are described in *Sensory Integration and Learning Disorders* by Ayres.

Sensory Systems

Integration of the tactile, proprioceptive, and vestibular systems are considered of primary importance because of their contribution to generalized neurological integration and to enhanced perception in other sensory systems. The planning and controlling of sensory input for facilitation of neural development in as near normal a sequence as possible is an important therapeutic consideration.

Tactile System

It is hypothesized that the tactile system has a pervasive, primal, and preparatory influence on generalized neurological integration. It is a primal source of input to the reticular formation by way of both ascending and descending fibers. It has a generalized effect on the neuromuscular system as well as a specific facilitory effect on a given muscle. It is quite probable that tactile input may be facilitory to the cortex. Early maturation of this system is further evidence of its importance to the sensory integrative process.

Because of the prolonged effect and primacy of the tactile system, it is suggested that treatment sessions be initiated with tactile stimulation. It is estimated that a barrage of tactile stimuli will exert a major influence on the nervous system for approximately half an hour. The quality and quantity of the stimuli administered is guided by the child's response. Positive responses are generally considered to be integrating. If overstimulation results in undesired arousal and negatively affects sleep patterns and attention, this response is interpreted as an inability to organize this stimuli adequately, rather than a lack of need of this type of input. It may be advisable to use alternate procedures for a while. The general level of reticular excitation may be inhibited by touch pressure and by slow vestibular stimulation. Light touch, especially when applied directly over the muscle belly, may elicit phasic contraction. The neuromuscular system may be counterbalanced by vestibular stimulation to elicit a tonic response in the muscles.

Vestibular System

The early normalization of vestibular functions provides a background for skill development. Vestibular input is important to the integration of many postural responses and to other types of sensory integrative processes, and it should be introduced early in the treatment program.

The child may be involved passively for generalized stimulation or actively to elicit adaptive responses that tend to have an organizing influence.

Vestibular stimulation may be excitatory or inhibitory to the central nervous system. Excitatory, such as that which occurs from rapid spinning without an adaptive response, may be disorganizing. The child should be carefully observed. Inhibitory influence may be elicited by slow, rhythmical movements. This type of stimulation may inhibit the brainstem centers governing vital functions such as respiration. An activity that demands an adaptive response tends to normalize the sensory input. If the child demonstrates a hypo-responsiveness to vestibular stimulation, the therapeutic approach may be to bombard the system through the many different vestibular receptors. If the child shows anxiety and a hyperresponsive reaction to vestibular stimulation, the therapist may need to employ a slow, safe, nonthreatening approach to the introduction of vestibular stimulation.

Different receptors are stimulated by different planes of movement and different head positions. The horizontal position is considered optimal for horizontal semicircular canal input and more effective for activating the otoliths than the upright position.

Other Proprioceptive Stimuli

Proprioceptive input from joints, bones, and muscles may contribute to sensory integration through organization of locomotion and visual input at the brainstem level. Proprioception is enhanced through muscle contraction, especially against resistance. The therapeutic procedure should include activities such as riding a scooter prone which requires maintained or static contraction. The sensory input is tonic, influencing secondary afferents from the muscle spindle rather than phasic action that affects the primary afferents. Input to the proprioceptors through joint compression or approximation and traction may increase kinesthesia or the conscious sense of joint movement or position. Methods of increasing sensory feedback to proprioceptors may include use of weights for traction or rapid alternating resistance to antagonistic muscles for contraction. Vibration may be used to excite muscles under contraction or to inhibit and lower the central excitatory state over muscles not contracting.

Adaptive Response

Activities that require purposeful, goal-directed actions, or adaptive responses add functional meaning to motion and enhance the sensory integrative process. The therapeutic value of the motor response is dependent upon the accuracy of the somatosensory and vestibular feedback. When combined with emotional involvement and effort, a motor response that requires a level of response more complex than previously demonstrated is considered an adaptive response and integrating to the central nervous system.

Precautions

The therapist must be constantly alert to the potential dangers in providing therapy. Consideration must be given to general safety precautions as well as those incurred in the therapeutic procedure such as tone increase in irregular and hypertonic muscles, sensory overload, over-inhibition, and seizure precipitation. Vestibular stimulation is a particularly powerful therapeutic tool. Its influence on the autonomic nervous system may be recognized by flushing, blanching, perspiring, nausea, or yawning. These signs are indicators that, at least temporarily, the amount of stimulation should be reduced.

Syndromes of Dysfunction

Test data were subjected to factor analysis as a method of investigating, identifying, and clarifying the nature of different types of sensory integrative dysfunction. The relationships of test parameters yielded through repeated studies led to hypothesizing syndromes, or constellations of symptoms, characteristic of dysfunction. Types of neural system disorders are not clear cut, nor consistently defined, but are sufficiently independent to contribute to theory construction from which therapeutic procedures were derived.

A brief description of two types of sensory integrative dysfunction—deficit in hemispheral function and developmental apraxia—is presented. A third type, a deficit in form and space perception, has not been included because, in this theoretical model, it is considered to be an end product of the integration of vestibular, kinesthetic, and tactile stimuli. Treatment procedures are therefore based on concepts of treatment for vestibular, kinesthetic, and tactile dysfunction.

Deficit in Interhemispheral Function

The theory proposes that hemispheric specialization of function is important for greater adaptiveness and specificity of cortical function. The neural basis for learning is considered optimal when language functions are lateralized in the left hemisphere and visuo-spatial functions are in the right hemispheres (in right-handed people).

Central to the theory and treatment of this syndrome is the postulate that the brain stem interhemispheral integrating mechanism is functionally associated with the brain stem postural reflexes and reactions and, furthermore, that inadequate maturation of the brain stem mediated postural reactions interferes with maturation of the interhemispheral integrative mechanism at that level. The resultant dysfunction interferes with the development of specialization of function in the cerebral cortex.[11]

Lack of integration of function of two sides of the body is the most characteristic symptom of a deficit in interhemispheral function. It is hypothesized that the neural mechanisms involved in bilateral integration are directly related to learning problems, especially reading problems. A disorder in the neural system subserving interhemispheral integration includes "disorder in postural and ocular mechanisms, and usually, but not invariably, auditory-language problems, poor right-left discrimination, and deficits in visual form and space perception."[12]

Clinical findings include poorly integrated TLR and TNR, immature righting and equilibrium reactions, and poor eye pursuits. Hypotonic musculature and diminished co-contraction and inadequate postural adjustments such as protective extension, poor weight shift, and poor trunk rotation are frequently observed. There is a tendency toward ipsilateral hand usage and avoidance of midline crossing, difficulty using two hands together in a coordinated manner, and frequently, poorly established hand dominance. The child may appear to be clumsy and may lack flexibility of movement.

Treatment procedures are designed to normalize postural reactions and to develop the capacity to motor plan. It is proposed that function of the two sides of the body will automatically begin to integrate functions. Treatment steps should follow the developmental sequence as much as possible. The treatment program should accomplish the following:
1. normalize the tactile and vestibular systems through activities that provide general stimulation of these sensory systems.
2. utilize neurophysiological procedures and activities to elicit a more mature level of response that encourages integration of primitive reflexes; develop supine flexion and prone extension patterns.
3. provide activities that elicit a postural response such as protective extension and postural background movements.
4. assimilate TNR and activate neck-righting reflex.
5. develop more mature postural reactions through

activities that elicit equilibrium reactions in prone, quadruped, and sitting postures.
6. develop eye and neck musculature.
7. enhance bilateral coordination.
8. develop visuo-spatial perception.

Specific procedures are cited in the original publications.

Developmental Apraxia

Developmental apraxia is defined as "a disorder of sensory integration interfering with the ability to plan and execute skilled or non-habitual motor tasks."[13] The dysfunction is characterized by a clumsiness in motor activity, a lack of knowing how to go about executing an unusual motor task, reduced quality of oral motor proficiency, and inadequate extraocular control. Although skill development usually is slower than age expectation, the child can and does learn splinter skills. Dressing, constructive manipulation, drawing, cutting, pasting, assembling, and learning to write are frequently difficult for an apraxic child.

The somatosensory input that contributes to development of body scheme is inadequate. As a result, the child has difficulty in associating the different anatomical elements of the body and how they work together. He has not developed a sensorimotor awareness of body parts and their potential motions, especially in relation to each other as a basis for motor planning.

Sensory integrative therapy for the apraxic child focuses on "specificity versus non-specificity of sensory process and excitation versus inhibition of sensation."[14] The treatment principles that guide the therapeutic procedure are:
1. enhance sensory integration at the brainstem level; provide generalized tactile, vestibular, and other proprioceptive input.
2. activate joint receptors for enhancement of kinesthesia.
3. develop postural mechanisms.
4. develop the basic motor repertoire: basic gross motor patterns of flexion in supine and extension in prone, portions of the basic flexion and extension synergies, gross diagonal patterns.
5. provide an opportunity for a variety of activities to promote growth of sensory integration in general and to develop a generalized ability to motor plan.
6. require an adaptive motor response to promote organization of the sensory input.

Summary

The theory of sensory integration extends the body of knowledge that focused primarily on motor function to a body of knowledge that considers the interaction between sensory and motor. Procedures such as therapeutic exercise and neuromuscular facilitation may contribute to sensory integrative therapy when they enhance neural integration. Sensory integration cannot, therefore, be considered in isolation. This theoretical model will extend and expand as knowledge increases.

References

1. Ayres, A. J.: Sensorimotor foundations of academic ability. In Cruickshank, W., and Hallahan, D. (eds.): Perceptual and Learning Disabilities in Children, Vol. 2. Syracuse University Press, 1975, p. 36.
2. Ayres, A. J.: Sensory Integration and Learning Disorders. Los Angeles: Western Psychological Services, 1972, p. 2.
3. Ibid., p. 33.
4. Ibid., p. 32.
5. Ibid., p. 36.
6. Ibid., p. 28.
7. Ibid., p. 11.
8. Ibid., p. 12.
9. Ayres, A. J.: Southern California Sensory Integration Tests Manual. Los Angeles: Western Psychological Services, 1972, p. 1.
10. Ayres, A. J.: Southern California Sensory Integration Interpretation Manual. Los Angeles: Western Psychological Services, 1977, p. 1.
11. Ayres: Sensorimotor foundations. In Cruickshank and Hallahan (eds.): Perceptual Learning Disabilities, p. 342.
12. Ibid., p. 336.
13. Ayres: Sensory Integration, p. 165.
14. Ibid., p. 176.

CHAPTER 8

Occupational Behavior Approach *Janice S. Matsutsuyu*

Background

The early proponents of occupational therapy used activities of daily living as a therapeutic focus in alleviating the day to day problems encountered by the chronically disabled. They firmly believed that patients have the capacities, however limited, to be active participants in their own daily lives. They viewed patients as capable of learning and becoming productively engaged in activities that ranged from simple to complex. Programs were carefully designed so that patients would have opportunities to acquire skills and habits. The goals of the early occupational therapy programs included helping patients to recognize a balance between work, rest, play, and sleep, and to gain some measure of self-worth and self-respect.[1-4]

The modalities of arts and crafts, of work and play were regarded as fundamental to occupational therapy programs and provided standards of craftsmanship and sportsmanship. These standards for performance were considered an inherent attribute of normal living. The accepted philosophy was based on moral treatment, "wholesome" living, and the actual practice of daily activities to achieve a balanced rhythm in work, rest, play, and sleep.[1,4]

These early objectives for promoting the health and well-being of chronically disabled patients were revitalized by Mary Reilly in her Eleanor Clarke Slagle Lecture of 1960. She succinctly hypothesized that "Man, through the use of his hands as energized by mind and will, can influence the state of his health."[5] This hypothesis suggests that human beings have a need to master the environment, to alter it, and to improve it. It respects the patient as having capacities to think, to feel, and to learn and assume responsibilities necessary for productive and creative living.[5] Reilly's Slagle lecture renewed occupational therapists' appreciation and understanding of the fundamental basis for clinical practice and challenged clinicians and educators to modernize the early paradigm that legitimized occupational therapy.

Subsequently at the 50th Annual Conference of the American Occupational Therapy Association in 1970, Reilly proposed a number of modernization projects for occupational therapy.[6] One was that "occupational therapy develop an ideology, a sharp demanding theoretical frame of reference to support the quality of the adaptation of patients."[6] She set forth three critical essentials for pursuing this proposal: concern for the accumulated experiences of practice and review of occupational therapy's basic values and beliefs; evaluation of the relevance of new technology and its integration into occupational therapy; and the development of strategies to maximize the utilization of limited resources. Reilly also reminded occupational therapy of the substantial contributions of Slagle, Louis Haas, William Bryan, and L. Cody Marsh, and she highlighted the need to learn more about moral treatment, a humanistic concept which formed the basis for occupational therapy's original values and beliefs.[6]

Occupational behavior proposes a modernization of the original paradigm from an interdisciplinary knowledge base. It focuses on the importance of activities of daily living for chronically disabled and incapacitated patients throughout the life stages. Occupational behavior relies on a studied approach of the constructs associated with day to day behaviors and commonplace occurrences of daily life.

An interdisciplinary study on human behavior provides a useful conceptual framework for the integration of past knowledge with new technology and can be guided by an understanding of human behavior and by the methods of studying it. There is an important shift away from single-focus research (as in the physical sciences) to study that involves a broader interdisciplinary knowledge base. The challenge is to acquire a means of processing such knowledge in a systematic way. General Systems Theory (GST) provides one such means. GST recognizes that universal phenomena are interdependent, while a single phenomenon is studied for its own merits with specific methodology for it.[7–11] The constructs of living open systems and rules of hierarchy in GST can facilitate the rigorous, scholarly development of a paradigm that focuses on activities of daily living.

While medical science guides occupational therapy in the treatment of medical conditions, an interdisciplinary knowledge base for understanding human behavior enriches occupational therapy services. People not only have problems which makes them patients but also resources that may be promoted for healthful daily living.

The goal of enhancing patients' health through the use of activities of daily living to reduce incapacities and to promote capacities, is a complex task. This goal requires occupational therapists to take into account not only medical knowledge and technology but also the qualities of human behaviors that find satisfaction in productive achievement in daily living. Concepts defining disability, incapacity, and intervention are readily found in medicine with its system of diagnosis and subsequent treatment. Less common are concepts for promoting the capacities of the chronically disabled.

The development of such concepts, and research of the applicability of occupational behavior drew on both academic and clinical resources. Mary Reilly at the time of the early studies, held a faculty appointment in the Department of Occupational Therapy, University of Southern California, and she was administrative head of the Rehabilitation Services at the Neuropsychiatric Institute, University of California at Los Angeles.

She first specified her ideas for clinical programming in a 1966 article, "A Psychiatric Occupational Therapy Program as a Teaching Model."[12] This model reflects the conviction that "occupational therapy is, first, a milieu, or a culture, which must be built and functioning (1) before the various kinds of behaviors we call rehabilitative can occur in patients; (2) before the relationship and learning potential of occupational therapy as a treatment can be realized."[12] The model was based on existing concepts in occupational therapy literature. The principles of the specifications served as mandates for developing the clinical occupational therapy program at the Neuropsychiatric Institute, UCLA.

A framework for academic study by graduate occupational therapy students was explained in Reilly's 1969 article, "The Educational Process."[13] The first focus, *patient achievement,* was identified as a direct responsibility of occupational therapy's clinical practice. Reilly believes that the achievement phenomenon is developmental in nature, and that interests, abilities, skills, and habits of competition and cooperation are components in the process of growth of the achievement drive. Robert White,[14] M. Brewster Smith,[15] and David McClelland[16] provide substantive interdisciplinary support for clinicians' need for a deeper understanding of the struggle for competence and achievement by incapacitated patients.

Play and work, the next focus, are the contexts in which competence and achievement are strengthened. The exploration, acquisition, and adaptation of skills are facilitated throughout the developmental stages found in *play and work.* The levels of organization, from simple to complex skills, become the patterns of behavior needed for life roles.

The third focus of the occupational behavior framework is the concept of *role.* Role theory forms a view of a patient who possesses life roles as well as a medical diagnosis. It can be useful in organizing and prioritizing occupational therapy services. Based on social psychology, role theory suggests divisions based on masculine-feminine identification, group membership, and occupational roles. Roe defines occupational role as the activity that takes up the major portion of an individual's day.[17] Occupational role has attributes defining a person's position in society as well as the tasks he or she must do. Therefore, for the purpose of studies in occupational behavior, occupational roles include that of preschooler, student, worker, homemaker, and retiree.[13,18]

The combined parameters of *patient achievement, play and work,* and *roles* offer fruitful and refreshing approaches for clinical programming and graduate studies. By examining the patterns of the behaviors of patients in play, work, and school with their family and peers, further knowledge is gained about reducing incapacities and promoting competence.

Studies in Occupational Behavior

Since the late 1960s there have been over 90 graduate studies related to occupational behavior framework completed at the University of Southern California, Department of Occupational Therapy. Careful attention to the resources to be found in the history of occupational therapy predominates. Clinicians and students have found that clear statements of purpose, the use of crafts, and the concept of activities of daily living (as a view of time at work, play, rest, and sleep) can normalize the social adaptation of disabled persons.

Studies were directed towards (1) gaining knowledge about phenomenological attributes, mainly on work and play; (2) developing clinical instruments to assess patient's functional assets for achievement; and (3) pursuing explanations of role behavior for daily living.

The following section only briefly touches on the three aspects of *patient achievement, work and play,* and *role.* The student is urged to read the original writings of the authors cited in order to pursue a studied approach to occupational behavior.

Patient Achievement

Concepts of competence and efficacy, of individuals as active agents in socialization, and of levels of aspirations for achievement gave direction for the development of clinical instruments and for model building.[14–16,19,20] The first clinical assessment tools were aimed at determining the presence of capacities for competence and achievement. Westphals' Decision Making Inventory is for problem solving through observation of decision making in a task.[21] The presence of interests and ability to discriminate choices is an objective of the Interest Checklist by Matsutsuyu.[22] A Time Inventory for assessing the perception of the value of time and its organization for use was designed by Larrington.[23] A common objective was to describe the patterns of these variables.

Intrinsic motivation as the dynamics of occupational therapy is delineated by Florey,[24] and Rosessler[25] proposes a model for the acquisition of achievement motivation in patients. Kielhofner's conceptual model of temporal adaptation as the un-

derlying basis for the use of time calls attention to continuing study of a rewarding area.[26] Further study on motivation from an occupational therapy clinical view has been done by Burke,[27] and Robinson has written on the competence behavior through the acquisition of rules.[28] These highlight the efforts for further explanations of knowledge base for patient achievement.

Work and Play

Parallel to the study for patient achievement were those studies on work and play. Since there is abundant literature ranging from economics to philosophy, the challenge is that of learning about the socialization of the skills, habits, abilities, attitudes, and interests that become productive behaviors in work and play.

The study of occupational behavior based on the constructs of a living open system and hierarchy acknowledges change brought about by growth and its interruption by illness. Since previous life experiences (*i.e.,* acquired skills, competencies, and achievements) give data that help in understanding a patient's current pattern of daily living, history taking has become necessary for clues for planning for the future.[13,18,29] History of the past socialization experiences of clients is a requisite for assessing the strengths and deficits of competence and achievement for activities of daily living, play, and work behaviors. Occupational History by Moorhead[18,30] and the Play History by Takata[29] were designed to gain a picture of the patient's previous accomplishments and the environmental conditions that promote learning and give satisfaction. Other published work on the dimension of play and work have addressed the complexity of the various interdependent factors which need to be considered.[31–34] The extent of the complexity may be studied in *Play as Exploratory Learning.*[9] Reilly offers scholarly explanations of dimensions of play that form the prerequisites for maturation of work behaviors. The chapters by the contributing authors Takata, Michelman, Knox, Hurff, and Shannon reflect application to patient care.[9]

Role

The concept of roles serves to organize patient data and to make the studies on patient achievement, play, and work relevant to activities of daily living. Study of occupational role development gives beginning explanations of the maturation of role behaviors, role function, and/or dysfunction. The dual lens of viewing a patient with a medical diagnosis and an occupational role integrates the existing occupational therapy technology. Occupational therapy has demonstrated expertise in the treatment of disability incurred by illness, birth defects, or trauma. The added benefit of viewing a patient with life roles maximizes the available capacities for activities of daily living by giving role-relevant purpose to treatment objectives.

Key points were identified in the study of role and role development. One is that the occupational choice process provides a bridge for the transformation of skills and habits, competence, and achievement acquired in childhood play and socialization to the decision making of a career choice.[35-37] A clinical finding concluded that this process, usually associated with adolescence, may reoccur when a change is needed because of disability or because of retirement. Also, the chronically disabled and patients who are dissatisfied with work often have not experienced the process of occupational choice. Therefore, history taking, observation of current function, and guidance through the occupational choice process are useful treatment strategies for most patients.

Since individuals occupy several roles in the course of their lives, skills and habits are interdependent and available for the transition from one role to another. Once skills and habits are acquired, practiced, and routinized, role fulfillment gives valuable feedback of the competencies gained. This fulfillment frees the individual to go on to new skills, and to combine skills for more complex tasks and demanding roles.[35-37] This element of simple to complex for competence and achievement calls attention to the standards of craftsmanship and sportsmanship through graded activities that early occupational therapists used to normalize the social adaptation for daily living.

Further Directions in Occupational Behavior

We have learned, and continue to learn, about the universality of the characteristics and behavior that are activities of daily living (ADL) behavior, and that they are more than what is commonly listed in a ADL Checklist. Work, play, rest, and sleep are patterns of daily behaviors that, throughout civilization, human beings have learned and adapted as their environment has changed. Reilly[9,38] and Montgomery[10] explain from their interdisciplinary study that daily living behavior is a biosocial phenomena, and they propose that learning of adaptive skills for daily living has biological and social basis and attributes.

Their proposal is based on universal formulations of the structure and function of human behavior. For instance, the genetic structure of human beings distinguishes them from other animals, and the capacities to derive rules, to form complex images, to de-

velop and to integrate values, and to form language are distinct human qualities. A human being has a biological basis for gathering and organizing information, in short, for learning. Crucial to this process are autonomous spontaneous activity, the drive to change the environment, central nervous system arousals, as well as curiosity and exploratory behavior. Complex learning takes place as the central nervous system matures. There is an ontogeny of skills in the way specific acts, parts of a skill, and particular features are mastered. Acts are perfected through repetition and then turned into routinized forms; these "subroutines" are combined with others to form a higher order, longer range, skilled sequence.[9,10,38,39]

When skills become habits through repetition, routine tasks can be performed automatically. This permits the individual to attain higher levels of decision making, to direct attention toward new environmental demands, and to acquire additional skills. Information is organized by gaining meaning from the sensory data gathered through information seeking and gathering. The ability to detect differences, and the symbolic capacity for generating images and rules, guide action.[9,10,38,40] Reilly's and Montgomery's findings give further explanations toward discovering the basis of the behaviors and environments involved in activities of daily living.

Summary

The process of adaptation in daily living takes place throughout the life span as a biosocial phenomenon; it is phylogenetically based and ontogenetically observed. Whereas what is biologically inherited prepares the individual for learning, the environment provides opportunities for adaptive learning to occur.

From the clinical viewpoint, the concept of roles and of history taking become the frame for organizing the complex biosocial aspects of daily living behaviors. Role identification and history taking also guide in setting priorities among the many problems encountered by patients needing attention in occupational therapy. Occupational behavior is broad enough to include the age and developmentally related life stages of the patients treated, and it is specific enough to set the parameters for human behaviors relevant to activities of daily living. The development of the original mandate of occupational therapy as the "caretaker" of the behaviors and tasks of daily living is emphasized.

Again, the student is urged to pursue study of the literature for a more comprehensive understanding of the extent of synthesis required for the occupational behavior knowledge and for its clinical application.

References

1. Slagle, E. C.: To organize an occupational therapy department. Occu. Ther. and Rehab. 3:125–130, 1927.
2. Slagle, E. C.: Training aids for mental patients. Occup. Ther. and Rehab. 1:11–14, 1922.
3. Haas, L. J.: Practical Occupational Therapy. Milwaukee: Ruce Pub. Co., 1944.
4. Meyers, A.: The philosophy of occupation therapy. Arch. Occup. Ther. 1:1–10, 1922. (Reprinted in AJOT 31:639–642, 1977.)
5. Reilly, M.: Occupational therapy can be one of the great ideas of the 20th century medicine. Am. J. Occup. Ther. 16:300–308, 1962.
6. Reilly, M.: The modernization of occupational therapy. Am. J. Occup. Ther. 25:243–246, 1971.
7. Bertalanffy, L. von.: General system theory—a critical review. General Systems 7:1–20, 1962. (Reprinted in Buckley, W. (ed.): Modern System Research for Behavioral Scientists. Chicago: Aldine Pub. Co., 1968.
8. Boulding, K. E.: General systems theory—the skeleton of science. Manage. Science 3:197–208, 1956. (Reprinted in Buckley, W. (ed.): Research for the Behavioral Scientists. Chicago: Aldine Pub. Co., 1968.
9. Reilly, M. (ed.): Play as Exploratory Learning, pp. 15–149. Beverly Hills CA: Sage Publications, 1974.
10. Montgomery, M.: An exploratory study of the resources of adaptation for daily living. Unpublished master's thesis, Department of Occupational Therapy, University of Southern California, Los Angeles, CA, 1979.
11. Kielhofner, G.: General systems theory: Implications for theory and action in occupational therapy. Am. J. Occup. Ther. 32:637–645, 1978.
12. Reilly, M.: A psychiatric occupational therapy program as a teaching model. Am. J. Occup. Ther. 20:61–67, 1966.
13. Reilly, M.: The educational process. Am. J. Occup. Ther. 23:299–307, 1969.
14. White, R. B.: Motivation reconsidered: The concept of competence. Psychol. Rev. 66:297, 1959.
15. Smith, M. W.: Competence and socialization. In Clausen, J. (ed.): Socialization and Society, pp. 271–320. Boston: Little, Brown & Co., 1968.
16. McClelland, D.: The Achieving Society, pp. 36–62. New Jersey: D. Van Norstand Co., 1961.
17. Roe, A.: Psychology of Occupations, pp. 3–40. New York: John Wiley & Sons, 1956.
18. Moorhead, L.: The occupational history. Am. J. Occup. Ther. 23:329–334, 1969.
19. White, R. B.: The urge towards competence. Am. J. Occup. Ther. 25:271–274, 1971.
20. Smith, M. B.: Competence and adaptation: A perspective on therapeutic ends and means. Am. J. Occup. Ther. 28:11–15, 1974.
21. Westphal, M.: A study in decision making. Unpublished master's thesis, Department of Occupational Therapy, University of Southern California, Los Angeles, CA, 1967.
22. Matsutsuyu, J.: The interest checklist. Am. J. Occup. Ther. 23:323–328, 1969.
23. Larrington, G.: Exploratory study of the temporal aspect of adaptation functioning. Unpublished masters thesis, Department of Occupational Therapy, University of Southern California, Los Angeles, CA, 1970.
24. Florey, L.: Intrinsic motivation; the dynamics of occupational therapy theory. Am. J. Occup. Ther. 23:319–322, 1969.
25. Rosessler, K.: A model for achievement motive acquisition. Unpublished master's thesis, Department of Occupational Therapy, University of Southern California, Los Angeles, CA, 1969.
26. Kielhofner, G.: Temporal adaptation: A conceptual framework for occupational behavior. Am. J. Occup. Ther. 31:235–242, 1977.
27. Burke, J.: A clinical perspective in motivation: Pawn versus origin. Am. J. Occup. Ther. 31:254–258, 1977.
28. Robinson, A.: Play, the arena for acquisition of rules for competent behavior. Am. J. Occup. Ther. 31:249–253, 1977.
29. Takata, N.: The play history. Am. J. Occup. Ther. 23:314–318, 1969.
30. Florey, L., and Michelman, S.: Occupational Role History: A Screening Tool for Psychiatric Occupational Therapy. Am. J. Occup. Ther. 36:301–308, 1982.
31. Shannon, P.: Work-play theory as the occupational therapy process. Am. J. Occup. Ther. 26:169, 1972.
32. Klavins, R.: Work-play behavior: Cultural influences. Am. J. Occup. Ther. 26:176–179, 1972.
33. Florey, L.: Studies of play: Implication for growth, development, and for clinical practice. Am. J. Occup. Ther. 35:519–523, 1981.
34. Matsutsuyu, J.: Occupational behavior—a perspective on work and play. Am. J. Occup. Ther. 25:391–394, 1971.
35. Pezzuti, L.: An exploration of adolescent feminine and occupational behavior development. Am. J. Occup. Ther. 33:84–91, 1979.
36. Black, M.: The occupational career. Am. J. Occup. Ther. 30:225–228, 1976.
37. Heard, C.: Occupational role acquisition: A perspective on the chronically disabled. Am. J. Occup. Ther. 31:243–247, 1977.
38. Reilly, M.: Lecture at the Occupational Behavior Institute, Boston, MA, 1977.
39. Short, J.: Occupational therapy intervention in role dysfunction. Unpublished master's thesis, Department of Occupational Therapy, University of Southern California, Los Angeles, CA, 1977.
40. Boulding, K. E.: The Image—Knowledge in Life and Society, pp. 3–175. Ann Arbor, MI: University of Michigan Press, 1956.

Bibliography

Black, M.: Adolescent role assessment. Am. J. Occup. Ther. 30:73, 1976.
Bateson, G.: A theory of play and fantasy. Bobbs-Merrill Reprint Series in Social Science, 1955.
Berlyne, D. E.: Curiosity and exploration. Science 52:25–33, 1966.

Bertalanffy, L. von.: General systems theory and psychiatry. In Arieti, S. (ed.): Handbook of American Psychiatry. New York: Basic Books, 1966.

Bockoven, J. S.: Moral Treatment in American Psychiatry. New York: Springer Publishing Co. Inc., 1963.

Bockoven, J. S.: Legacy of moral treatment—1800's to 1910. Am. J. Occup. Ther. 25:223–225, 1971.

Bruner, J.: On coping and defending. In Coleman, J. (ed.): Psychology and Effective Behavior. Glenview, IL: Scott Foresman & Co., 1969.

Bruner, J.: Nature and uses of immaturity. Am. Psychol. 27:687–708, 1972.

Boulding, K. E.: Toward a general theory of growth. General Systems 1:66–75, 1956.

Borys, S.: Implications of interest theory of occupational therapy. Am. J. Occup. Ther 28:35, 1974.

Dunning, H.: Environmental occupational therapy. Am. J. Occup. Ther. 26:292–298, 1972.

Feibleman, J. K.: Theory of integrative levels. Br. J. Philosophy Science 5:59–66, 1955. Reprinted in Coleman, J.: Psychology and Effective Behavior. Glenview, IL: Scott Foresman & Co., 1969.

Florey, L.: An approach to play and play development. Am. J. Occup. Ther. 25:275–280, 1971.

Kielhofner, G., and Burke, J. P.: Occupational therapy after 60 years: An account of changing identity and knowledge. Am. J. Occup. Ther. 30:675–689, 1977.

Kielhofner, G., and Gillette, N.: The impact of specialization on the professionalization and survival of occupational therapy. Am. J. Occup. Ther. 33:20–28, 1979.

Hurff, J.: A play skills inventory; a competency monitoring tool for the 10 year old. Am. J. Occup. Ther. 34:651–656, 1980.

Kuhn, T. S.: The structure of scientific revolutions, 2nd ed. Chicago: University of Chicago Press, 1970.

Koestler, A.: Beyond atomism and holism—the concept of the holon. In Koestler, A., and Smythies, J. R. (eds.): Beyond Reductionism. New York: Macmillan, 1969.

Laszlo, E.: The Systems View of the World. New York: George Braziller, 1972.

Lazare, A.: Hidden conceptual models in clinical psychiatry. N. Engl. J. Med. 288:245–350, 1973.

Michelman, S.: The importance of creative play. Am. J. Occup. Ther. 25:285–290, 1971.

Sarbin, T. R.: Role theory. In Lindzey, G. (ed.): Handbook of Social Psychology. Reading, MA: Addison-Wesley Publishing Co., 1954.

Shannon, P.: The derailment of occupational therapy. Am. J. Occup. Ther. 31:229–234, 1977.

Takata, N.: The play milieu—a preliminary appraisal. Am. J. Occup. Ther. 25:281, 1971.

Turner, R.: Role; sociological aspects. In Sill, D. (ed.): International Encyclopedia of Social Sciences. New York: Macmillan and the Free Press, 1968.

CHAPTER 9

Rehabilitation
Helen L. Hopkins,
Helen D. Smith, and
Elizabeth G. Tiffany

Rehabilitation and Habilitation

The term *rehabilitation* in its broadest sense means restoration of or return to ability. In 1947 the National Council on Rehabilitation defined rehabilitation as "the restoration of the handicapped to the fullest physical, mental, social, vocational and economic usefulness of which they are capable."[1] Procedures were developed to accomplish this purpose.

Medical care is not considered to be complete until each individual with a residual disability has been trained to live and work with his or her remaining capabilities. A vital factor in rehabilitation is motivation or "the will to get well" and to return to society and the community.

Children born with or acquiring disability shortly after birth have not had the opportunity to develop ability to function. The term *rehabilitation* is not appropriate in their cases. Therefore a different term, *habilitation*, is used to indicate development of the ability to function regardless of the disability and the process of learning to live and work with one's capabilities.

Philosophy of Rehabilitation/Habilitation

The philosophy of rehabilitation/habilitation requires that the total capabilities of each individual must be considered. This includes physical, emotional, cognitive, social, cultural, vocational, and economic factors. In 1953 Whitehouse stated that rehabilitation is a social problem whose roots are in the life of a community. He said the rehabilitation center exists for the client and centers around the client's needs. Thus, rehabilitation must be dynamic and must keep step with both scientific advances and changes in society. Rehabilitation includes the concept of prevention or of the exacerbation of dysfunction in all aspects of human activity, thus requiring an on-going process of assessment with follow-up being a necessity.[2]

Rehabilitation is concerned with the intrinsic worth and dignity of the individual. It is, therefore, committed to the restoration of the disabled to a life that is purposeful and satisfying, one that allows each individual the opportunity to function adequately as a family member and as a member of society with the capabilities to meet the responsibilities of that society.[3]

Government Involvement in Rehabilitation/Habilitation

The United States has had state and federal programs of vocational rehabilitation since 1920. Early programs were limited to guidance, vocational training, and placement of the physically handicapped. Training was focused on working around the disability with no concern being given to alleviating or reducing the effect of the disability on the physical and mental capabilities of the individual.

It was not until 1943 when Public Law 113 (Barden-LaFollette Act) was passed that federal and state laws were amended to allow for the provision of medical rehabilitation services. It was recognized at that time that medicine as a whole, using the skills of all those specialized in patient care, must be applied through a team approach to assure restoration of both the physically and the mentally disabled to their highest potential in all aspects of function. To assure the alleviation or reduction of the effect of disability as well as to reach for the highest potential for each individual, rehabilitation became the concern of the physician with the nurse, occupational therapist, physical therapist, speech therapist, psychologist, vocational counselor, and prosthetist/orthotist as members of the rehabilitation team.[4] The client had to be involved in the decision-making processes, and thus he/she was also a member of the rehabilitation team. The client's participation helped promote the development of maximum commitment and optimum function.

In 1954, through Public Law 565, federal laws were expanded to include payment for the training of rehabilitation personnel, expansion of rehabilitation facilities, and support of research.[5] This law helped to alleviate the shortage of qualified personnel, and it caused the development and expansion of rehabilitation centers throughout the country to meet the growing demands for rehabilitation services.

In 1965 a federal law established a National Commission on Architectural Barriers under the Rehabilitation Services Agencies; in 1968 a federal law was passed to eliminate architectural barriers from all governmentally funded buildings. These laws brought to public consciousness the architectural requirements of the physically disabled. As a result, many public places are accessible to handicapped individuals today. Much still needs to be done to make total communities accessible.

In 1973 a law was passed giving the handicapped equal access to schools and jobs. In April 1977, because of nonenforcement of the 1973 law, there were numerous demonstrations by the handicapped who claimed infringement on their civil rights. Thus, Health, Education, and Welfare Secretary, Joseph Califano, Jr., signed regulations for elimination of discrimination in health insurance and government contracts to assure the handicapped equal access to schools and jobs.[6]

Rehabilitation of the Physically Handicapped

World War II precipitated many advances in medicine that preserved the life of many severely disabled individuals. Changes in industrial technology also made it possible for the employment of many of these persons. Manpower shortages gave these individuals the opportunity to demonstrate their productivity and value to the economy.[7] In order to meet the needs and demands of the physically disabled, the dynamic process of rehabilitation was developed. This process viewed each individual as a total person, and it was not concerned with illness or disability alone but with restoration of the person's total capabilities as well. This approach allowed the individual to participate in his or her own rehabilitation, to communicate with others, and to adapt his/her physical environment to meet his/her physical and energy requirements. In this way the person was able to resume his/her self-care, work, and leisure activities by utilizing maximum physical, intellectual, social, and vocational potential.[8]

Rehabilitation centers for the physically disabled were developed immediately after World War II. The first outpatient rehabilitation center was the Institute for the Crippled and Disabled in New York City, which opened under the direction of George G. Deaver, M.D., in 1946. The five objectives for treatment at this center[9] were for the client to

1. gain maximum independence in bed and wheelchair activities,
2. gain maximum use of hands,
3. be able to ambulate and elevate,
4. achieve maximum ability in communication (hear and speak),
5. function in as nearly normal manner as possible.

To achieve these goals, underlying pathology had to be assessed along with the chances of overcoming disability. Deaver said, "Rehabilitation is the medical management of physical disability." He described rehabilitation medicine as active rather than reactive, for it focused on the patient and the patient's function and relationship with others, especially family and community members, rather than solely on treatment of the disease.[10]

The first inpatient rehabilitation center was established at New York City's Bellevue Hospital in 1946 under the direction of Howard A. Rusk, M.D.[11] Subsequently, rehabilitation centers were established throughout the United States, many independent and many affiliated with hospitals with both inpatient and outpatient facilities. In the 1960s many general hospitals throughout the United States established Rehabilitation Centers or Physical Medicine and Rehabilitation departments within their facilities, for it was recognized that to ignore a disability was far more costly than to start rehabilitation early in an individual's hospital stay.[12] It is now the practice in many general hospitals, whether or not they have rehabilitation centers, to begin rehabilitation of physically disabled individuals as soon as the acute phase of the disease or injury is past. Insurance carriers, federal and state rehabilitation agencies, parents, and patients added impetus to the development of this practice.

Occupational Therapy in Rehabilitation of Physically Disabled

Rehabilitation/habilitation as a treatment approach in occupational therapy means a dual approach to problems: (1) helping clients increase the functioning of disabled extremities and overcome disturbances in the ability to function, and (2) helping clients utilize remaining capabilities to reach their highest potential in meeting the demands of daily living. This treatment approach attempts to overcome dysfunction resulting from disease or injury and to enhance the ability to function and better utilize remaining capabilities. This approach uses constructive activity, which is guided by the therapist to achieve the desired physical and psychological results.[13]

Occupational therapy must begin with assessment of capabilities to determine a baseline of function. A treatment plan is established in conjunction with the rehabilitation team and client, keeping in mind the client's goals. The treatment program is then planned so as to eliminate or diminish disability through the use of activity while focusing on the individual's capabilities in all aspects of function. Activities utilized include exercise that can be translated into useful activity, self-care activities (ADL—activities of daily living), expressive or creative activities, intellectual or educational activities, play or leisure activities, prevocational activities, and simulated or actual vocational activities including

homemaking and other work tasks. Energy conservation, joint protection, and work simplification techniques should be included in the rehabilitation program. Reassessment of capabilities and progress must be continued on a regular basis to determine gains made and to prevent problems from developing. Preventive measures such as splinting and positioning must be utilized to eliminate contractures, deformity, skin breakdown, or other secondary problems.

The client's family should be involved in the total process of rehabilitation if there is to be a smooth transition from living in the rehabilitation center to successful integration into the home and community. There must be an increase of independence on the part of the client and less dependence on rehabilitation personnel.

The family must be counseled regarding the role it must play in helping the disabled individual attain maximum capability and independence. Visits to the client's home before discharge, when possible, may assist families in eliminating architectural barriers and in making the transition from rehabilitation facility to home easier. Follow-up through reevaluation within the rehabilitation facility, through home visits, and through utilization of services of community agencies is required for the total success of the rehabilitation process.

Rapid change in society and health care now requires that rehabilitation services be provided at the convenience of the consumer. Rehabilitation services once housed only within a rehabilitation center are now becoming a part of and are available within the community.[14] Many professionals are providing services in such institutions as schools and community centers as well as in the client's home.

Psychiatric Occupational Therapy and Rehabilitation

In the years since the advent of the use of drugs to control the symptoms of mental illness, there has been a marked increase in the kinds of occupational therapy programs that may be defined as rehabilitative. There have been both subtle and dramatic changes in attitudes about mental illness both in society at large and on the part of the providers of services. As mental illness came to be viewed as reversible, the mentally ill person came to be considered as a possible participant in a rehabilitation program. A shift in the emphasis and context of treatment came with the community mental health movement of the 1960s. The patient who previously had been regarded as having potential for only marginal adjustment to the sheltered life of the institution now began to be viewed as potentially able to return to life and productivity "on the outside." Efforts began to be directed toward minimizing the length of the institutional stay of acutely ill people and toward the development of outpatient treatment facilities.

Rehabilitation in psychiatry refers to the development of skills that will enable the individual to return to function successfully in the world outside the institution. This includes being competent in caring for one's daily living needs and adapting to the demands of work and social life. Rehabilitation becomes the focus after the major treatment effort has taken place. Rehabilitation is differentiated from treatment in that its concern is no longer the interruption of or direct intervention in the pathological process of the illness but the improvement and organization of existing strengths and skills of the client and on the development of competence in handling the demands of everyday living. Much of modern psychiatric occupational therapy is directed toward rehabilitation. The differentiation between treatment and rehabilitation in psychiatry itself, however, tends to lack clarity. Perhaps one of the characteristics of work with the mentally ill is that treatment and rehabilitation may need to be, in some cases, continuous and reciprocal.[15]

The psychiatric occupational therapist, working within a rehabilitation context, must first be able to identify clearly the client's existing assets and liabilities and the internal and external areas that may be developed, improved, or changed through the occupational therapy process. Second, the occupational therapist must know the kinds of skills that will be required for the client to function in his/her social and work community. The occupational therapy process, then, is geared to providing experiences and opportunities that are oriented realistically and directly to improving those skills. An important

goal of rehabilitation underlying all other goals is for the client to achieve the ability to know his or her own strengths, limitations, and needs and to have a sense of ways to use the strengths, minimize limitations, and seek to satisfy real needs. In this process, the participation of the occupational therapy staff decreases as the client's ability to assume autonomy increases in the following areas: (1) self-assessment; (2) management of life activities so that a healthy balance of work, play, rest, and sleep is achieved; (3) management of the time requirements of life-schedules, appointments, and pacing oneself through being able to predict how long a given activity may take; and (4) handling of the problem-solving and decision-making demands that present themselves.

A sequence of steps that may be followed in psychiatric rehabilitation in occupational therapy is suggested in Figure 9-1.

Summary

Rehabilitation has been a concept used in the care of the disabled since 1920, but it was limited to vocational rehabilitation at that time. World War II provided the impetus for the concept of rehabilitation to be expanded to include medical rehabilitation services. This concept views each individual as a total person with concern for both restoration of disability and enhancement of capabilities. It utilized a team approach for treatment, and it requires involvement of the patient or client in the evaluation and treatment process.

Since World War II this concept has been used in occupational therapy intervention with both physical and psychosocial dysfunction. It is, however, a concept that may pervade the developmental, occupational behavior or other approaches as well. In order

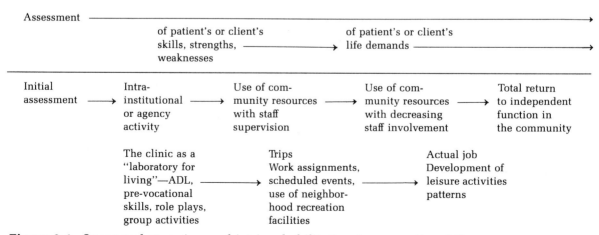

Figure 9-1. Suggested steps in psychiatric rehabilitation in occupational therapy.

to fulfill the expectations of the philosophy of occupational therapy, any approach to treatment must view the individual as a total being and must be concerned for both restoration of a disability and enhancement of capabilities and thereby utilize the rehabilitation concept. It may be possible in the future, therefore, to include the rehabilitation concept as part of other approaches, rather than identifying it as a separate approach to occupational therapy intervention.

References

1. Reggio, A. W.: Rehabilitation—what is it? Am. J. Occup. Ther. 1:149–151, 1947.
2. Whitehouse, F. A.: The rehabilitation center—some aspects of a philosophy. Am. J. Occup. Ther. 7:241, 1953.
3. Licht, S.: Rehabilitation and Medicine. Baltimore: Waverly Press, 1968, pp. 1–13.
4. Rusk, H. A.: Rehabilitation Medicine, ed. 3. St. Louis: C. V. Mosby, 1971, pp. 1–8, and ed. 4, 1977, pp. 1–2.
5. Ibid.
6. Boston Globe, April 29, 1977.
7. Licht: Rehabilitation and Medicine, pp. 1–13.
8. Ibid.
9. Ibid.
10. Ibid.
11. Rusk: Rehabilitation Medicine, pp. 1–8.
12. Licht: Rehabilitation and Medicine, pp. 1–13.
13. Spackman, C. S.: A history of the practice of occupational therapy for restoration of physical function: 1917–1967. Am. J. Occup. Ther. 22:67, 1968.
14. Hightower, M. D.: Rehabilitation—a part of the community or apart from the community. Am. J. Occup. Ther. 28:296–298, 1974.
15. Fidler, G. S., and Fidler, J. W.: Occupational Therapy: A Communication Process in Psychiatry. New York: Macmillan, 1963, p. 27.

PART 4

Evaluation Process
and Procedures

CHAPTER 10

Assessment and Evaluation—An Overview*

Helen D. Smith and Elizabeth G. Tiffany

In 1971 Gillette referred to evaluation as a professional responsibility. She defined the functions of the evaluation process[1] as (1) determining the baseline for objectives and providing the foundation for a treatment program, (2) identifying which problems can and cannot be mediated by occupational therapy, (3) giving some indication of the potential for change, (4) enlisting the cooperation of the client in beginning to assess his or her capabilities and dreams, and (5) helping the client begin a course of action designed to master some of the difficulties he or she has previously tried to master alone.

Evaluation also serves the purpose of keeping the therapist's work current, for it is a spiral, building process. Each treatment session should be assessed, and each target area should be reviewed in order to determine the effectiveness of the activity process and to revise the objectives as they are mastered or found to be

unreachable. Treatment should not persist in a straight line. It is the system of evaluation that is built into the treatment process that ultimately determines the effectiveness of treatment.[2]

In occupational therapy, evaluation is a process of collecting and organizing the relevant information about a client so that the therapist will be able to plan and implement a meaningful, effective program of treatment. Several steps are involved:

1. *The collection of data.* This includes the selection and use of tools and methods by which information is obtained. The frame of reference for treatment will determine the kinds of data that will be sought. The participation of the client in this process is critical to the success of the program.

2. *The organization of the data* into a meaningful, dynamic description of the client's strengths and weaknesses with a focus on those areas in which occupational therapy can be of help. The client, the therapist, and others should be able to understand this description readily.

3. *The setting of treatment objectives.* This involves the use of clinical judgment and predictive assumptions on the part of the therapist. Objectives must be based on the accumulated data, including

---

* The terms *evaluation* and *assessment* have both been used with regard to procedures used in fact-finding preparatory to and during treatment. In general, the term *assessment* refers to the sum of the results of the *evaluation* procedures used. Assessment yields a composite picture of the patient's functioning. Evaluation refers to the data gathered from specific procedures.

the client's goals, the therapist's knowledge about the clinical pathology, and the treatment frame of reference.

4. *Commitment to continuing evaluation* as the occupational therapy plan is carried out. The original objectives and treatment plan need constant reassessment. Changes in the occupational therapy plan are dependent upon the results of ongoing re-evaluation.

The evaluation process thus represents an organized and systematic way of determining a client's needs. It is essential to objective setting, treatment planning, and assessing the effectiveness of the implementation of the treatment plan. Careful evaluation and re-evaluation in occupational therapy also adds significant information to the total treatment program of the team as an aid in setting overall goals and in monitoring the effectiveness of interventions such as medication or treatment in physical therapy.

It is important to recognize that any fair and valid assessment of a client must be based on several sources, yielding a multidimensional picture of the client's status. It should focus on those data that are pertinent to the occupational therapy process. Any assessment procedure, moreover, includes a clear analysis of the context for treatment, the therapist's skills and resources, and activities that could be used in treatment.

Types of Evaluation

Evaluation procedures take many forms. There are specific tests for specific functions (*e.g.*, manual muscle testing). There are more complex or comprehensive assessments that are comprised of data from several tests or procedures. Successful evaluation is dependent upon the ability of the therapist to gain the trust of the client so that a cooperative effort can take place. The therapist must observe and record data accurately, and must make use of a wide range of appropriate information sources that are pertinent to the treatment process.

Medical Records

The medical record provides valuable information about the client, and it gives indications for precautions that must be considered when planning and carrying out treatment. Data gleaned from the medical record add to the baseline information necessary for effective treatment planning.

The past and present medical history, written by the physician, gives the therapist information on the client's health status, former medical problems, present medical or physical findings, diagnoses, precau-

tions, and prognosis. Daily notes by physicians and nurses list medications and treatments being given as well as the patient's responses. Reports and/or evaluations from other specialties (x-ray, dietary, social service, psychiatry, psychology, physical or speech therapy, vocational and/or rehabilitation counselling) are also included. With information from medical records as background, the therapist is ready to move on to the next step in the evaluation process.

Observation

A key to successful evaluation lies in the therapist's skills in observation. The ability to see and to listen well must be accompanied by the ability to sort through the mass of perceptual and conceptual data that may be presented, and to focus on what is relevant to the process.

Human beings communicate information about themselves in a great many ways. There is verbal communication—the choice of words and sentences, their meanings, and the quality of tone and inflection with which the words are said. There are the paralinguistic and nonverbal behaviors that accompany verbal communication—facial expression, gestures, posture, and body movements. Attention to nonverbal communication is especially important to the occupational therapist inasmuch as a large part of the occupational therapy process is doing, not talking. Nonverbal expressions in human beings are established earlier in life than verbal ones, and they rely upon older neurophysiological structures.[3] A third mode of communication is the written form. It can be assumed that the written work has been, in some ways, more carefully considered and censored, and it is less spontaneous than the spoken, although this is not necessarily true. What an individual writes about him or herself may be useful as a representation of a desired or ideal self. The organization and form of the handwriting and placement on the page have been considered as clues to personality, feelings, and cognitive functioning at the time of the writing. Closely related to writing are other forms of psychomotor projection through which communication takes place—the behaviors connected with the use of media and the choice of clothing, colors, and objects an individual has made. Over a longer period of time, an individual communicates much information by the total effect of behavior, especially small, unconscious, and automatic behaviors in a variety of circumstances.

The communication process between the client and the therapist lays a foundation for rapport and trust. The client needs to feel that communications have been heard and understood by someone who has not only some empathy but also some knowledge and skill. The therapists's confidence in his or her abilities and in the profession may be crucial in setting the tone for all future transactions with the client. Four filters affect interactions between people, and they are significant in their potential for distortion of the observation process[4]:

Perceptual—how sensory stimuli such as color of clothing or perfume affect the way the other person is perceived.
Conceptual—the knowledge base that is brought to the interaction.
Role—the way each person perceives the role to be played in the interaction.
Self-esteem—the way each person feels about himself or herself.

It is useful for the therapist to consider these filters and the ways in which they might affect objectivity in observation.

The occupational therapist is in a position to observe the patient or client in a variety of structured and unstructured situations. The interview, formal testing procedures, and planned activities represent structured opportunities for observation. These usually involve some elements of prediction or expectation on the part of the therapist, and they will be discussed in the next sections.

The therapist's opportunities to see and interact with clients in situations that are less planned will vary depending upon the setting. If it is possible for the therapist to interact informally and spontaneously with patients in situations where role differentiation may be less clear, information may be available that otherwise might be difficult to obtain. Different perspectives on values, interests, and functional levels, for example, may be gained by seeing the patient in the local snack shop, in the elevator, or at recreational activities. It is desirable to build some opportunities for informal contact into the evaluation process whenever possible.

Interview

There are occasions when a health professional may wish to interview a client formally or informally. Probably the most important occasion is the initial interview, undertaken as part of the process of evaluation. The initial interview serves several vital purposes. It provides for (1) collection of information about the client to help develop objectives and a plan for treatment, and (2) establishment of understanding on the part of the client about the role of the therapist and purposes of the occupational therapy process, as well as (3) an opportunity for the client to discuss his or her situation and to think about plans for change.

In the *The Helping Interview*[5] Benjamin refers to both external and internal factors that are important and that need careful consideration in preparing for an interview. The external factors are such things as the room in which the interview is to take place and the extent to which the place will be private, free of interruptions and other distractions. Internal factors are the attitudes, knowledge, and feelings that the interviewer brings to the interview. It is important for the therapist to be clear about the purpose of the interview, to know the kinds of information specifically desired, to be self-trusting, and to be honest.

Allen, in a paper presented at the American Occupational Therapy Association Annual Conference in October 1976,[6] points out there are two essential requirements for the therapist to be able to conduct a successful interview with a patient: a solid knowledge base and skills in active listening. These requirements are not simple. They necessitate study, preparation, and practice. The solid knowledge base must underly the therapist's selection of questions or areas to be covered in the interview. It is important that the interview reflect what the therapist knows and that the interview cover areas that will be relevant to occupational therapy. Active listening means that the interviewer plays a vital, deeply involved role that demonstrates genuine respect for the patient or client.

Benjamin[7] delineates three parts to an interview: initiation, development, and closing. In the initiation phase the interviewer explains the purpose of the interview and his or her role in relation to the person interviewed, and begins to establish some level of mutual trust and understanding. It is during the initiation phase that the interviewer should define the parameters of the interview—the amount of time it should take, the kind of material to be discussed, and the uses to be made of the information.

During the development phase the interviewer seeks information and explores issues with the person interviewed. The occupational therapist doing an initial interview as an evaluation procedure should bring some form of outline or a list of planned questions to the interview to be certain that information vital to the future process of setting objectives and treatment planning will be covered. The kinds of questions the occupational therapist may ask should allow the patient to respond with more than a simple "yes" or "no" answer. The occupational therapist needs to have skill in asking one question at a time, tolerating silence, listening carefully, observing both verbal and nonverbal responses, restating or clarifying questions when needed, and encouraging the client to continue or to stay on the track.

Clues marking the end of the interview are either the end of the time defined at the beginning of the interview or the end of the list of questions or issues to be explored. It is important for both the therapist and the client to know that the interview is coming to a close. No new material should be brought up at this point. It is best to plan another time and place to discuss new material. Summarizing the material that has been discussed may be a useful way to terminate the interview as well as to double-check on the accuracy of information gained.

The therapist will need to make notes unless he or she has an unusual memory and time to record the interview later. The purpose of writing notes (or using a tape recorder) should be explained to the client at the beginning of the interview. The client should also be told that he or she may read the notes or listen to the tape and that their sole purpose is to provide valid guidelines for the occupational therapy process.

Sometimes it is useful to have clients answer a simple questionnaire before coming to the interview. The use of the questionnaire has some advantages. It may save time in situations where setting aside 30 to 45 minutes for personal interviewing of each client initially is not feasible. It can provide information about the client's ability to read and to respond in an organized fashion in writing. The disadvantage is that some of the richness of detail and interaction will be lost. A written questionnaire can never completely replace a face-to-face interview.

The kinds of information that are best gained through an interview may vary somewhat according to the client population and the general context for treatment. In general the occupational therapist may learn about education; work experience; leisure interests and pursuits; the way patients' balance their work, sleep, and play and manage time; the quality and extent of their care for their own personal needs (grooming, nutrition, laundry, housekeeping, hygiene); their families or significant people in households; friends or other family members who are supportive; the communities in which they live; their values and familiar objects; their own assessment of their current situations and problems; their own personal goals; and current housing situations including potential architectural barriers.

Knowledge about whether the patient's level of skill has been high enough to accomplish tasks and to fulfill expected social roles successfully provides important clues to the kinds of experiences that should be provided in occupational therapy. The importance of collecting information about this history has been outlined by Moorehead:

> In gathering the occupational history, the investigator is concerned with discovering how and under what conditions the individual patient has learned to approach tasks and role expectations as he does; and

whether he was ever more competent than he now appears. Can the therapist expect that the patient will be able to improve his role skills, and if so, how much? In other words, the investigator asks what a patient's particular life style is in terms of occupational function, so that therapy can be structured for him to build upon his experiences for improved function.[8]

A terminal interview, undertaken just before the client leaves treatment, serves other important functions. It gives the client and therapist an opportunity to look together at what has taken place and to identify some of the things that have been learned in the process. Often the occupational therapy experience may be significant in helping the patient plan how to balance activities at home. For example, the client has learned which activities provide exercise or energy conservation and which are integrative and provide energy release. A final interview helps to reinforce this learning.

Inventories and Check Lists

An adjunct to the interview is the check list, in which the client is asked to respond on paper to questions regarding interests, hobbies, and desires. Janice Matsutsuyu developed the Interest Check List.[9] This list has served as a prototype for many others that have been adapted and used. Another inventory that is useful is the Activities Configuration[10] developed by Sandra Watanabe and used to identify the qualitative aspects of how a person uses time to meet his or her needs in life.

Object History

One useful way of learning about a client's values and the cultural system to which he or she belongs is the object history. It is a flexible evaluation tool, and it may be incorporated into the formal interview or learned about in informal conversation. Written object histories may also be solicited. It may be done individually or in a group. The object history often helps in establishing rapport between the people participating by permitting them to explore their respective backgrounds and experiences. It may also provide some important clues about the beginnings of the patient's pathology. The object history simply asks the client to try to remember something that was important or that he or she valued at earlier periods of life and to explain why it was important or valued. For example, a young man recalled a bush in front of his house where he went to hide as a child whenever he was scolded. In this statement one can learn that the world of nature may represent refuge to him. Another person recalled an erector set with which he felt he could build anything mechanical in the whole world. Thus one can learn that mechanical things represent pleasure in accomplishment for him. A young woman recalled a stereo set to which she used to dance. In this one can learn that social dancing once was important to her. Through the exploration of important nonhuman objects the therapist may learn both the kinds of things that might be integrative to the client and the ability that the client has had in the past to use the nonhuman world to meet emotional needs.

Summary

Over the years, occupational therapists have tended to develop tests and batteries of tests, check lists, and rating scales as the need arose. These tests helped them to evaluate the needs of their own clients within their own contexts. In recent years, a need for reliable, standardized tools has become evident. Occupational therapists have found that they need to identify and employ their tools that are in general use as part of the arduous process of establishing their legitimacy. At the same time, when occupational therapists use tools for which there are standard protocols, and which require additional training or certification (*e.g.,* Southern California Sensori-Integrative tests), it is essential for them to make sure that they are fully qualified to use them.

Evaluation of the client's physical or psychological condition is indicated when a suspected or obvious problem exists. Therapeutic procedures chosen depend upon the patient's diagnosis, medical reports, lifestyle, interests, and needs. Observations made by the therapist, checklists previously prepared by the client, and information gained in interviews also suggest the best directions that treatment planning might take. Evaluation of special areas such as perceptual-motor function, activities of daily living, or prevocational evaluation, and others may also be indicated. The remainder of this section deals with specific evaluation procedures utilized by occupational therapists in problem identification.

References

1. Gillette, N.: Occupational therapy and mental health. In Willard, H. S., and Spackman, C. S. (eds.): Occupational Therapy, ed. 4. Philadelphia: J. B. Lippincott Co., 1971, p. 79.
2. Ibid.
3. Freedman, A., Kaplan, H., and Saddock, B.: Modern Synopsis of Comprehensive Textbook of Psychiatry/II. Baltimore: Williams & Wilkins Co., 1976, p. 146.
4. Fidler, G. S.: Talk given at Medical College of Georgia. Augusta, Georgia, 1976.
5. Benjamin, A.: The Helping Interview. Boston: Houghton Mifflin Co., 1974.
6. Allen, C.: The Performance Status Examination. Paper presented at the American Occupational Therapy Association Annual Conference, San Francisco, October 1976.
7. Benjamin: Helping Interview.
8. Moorehead, L.: The occupational history. Am. J. Occup. Ther. 23:331, 1969.
9. Matsutsuyu, J.: The interest checklist. Am. J. Occup. Ther. 23:323–328, 1969.
10. Watanabe, S.: Activities Configuration. 1968 Regional Institute on the Evaluation Process, Final Report RSA-123-T-68. New York: American Occupational Therapy Association, 1968.

Bibliography

American Psychological Association: Standards for Educational and Psychological Tests and Manuals. Washington, D.C., 1966.

Garrett, A.: Interviewing: Its Principles and Methods. New York: Family Service Association of America, 1972.

Hemphill, B. J. (ed.): The Evaluative Process in Psychiatric Occupational Therapy. Thorofare NJ: Charles B. Slack, 1982.

Hurff, J.: A play skills inventory. In Reilly, M. (ed.): Play as Exploratory Learning. Beverly Hills, Sage Publications, 1974.

Knox, S.: A play scale. In Reilly, M. (ed.): Play as Exploratory Learning. Beverly Hills, Sage Publications, 1974.

Llorens, L.: Projective techniques in occupational therapy. Am. J. Occup. Ther. 21:266, 1967.

Takata, N.: The play history. Am. J. Occup. Ther. 23:314–318, 1969.

CHAPTER 11

Assessment and Evaluation—Specific Evaluation Procedures *Helen D. Smith*

Manual Muscle Testing

Manual muscle testing (M.M.T.) is a procedure that determines the strength of a muscle through manual evaluation (Fig. 11-1). Rating is done by having the patient or client move the part through its full range against gravity and then against gravity and resistance. When the patient or client cannot perform the motion against gravity, the part is positioned to eliminate gravity, and then the muscle power is reevaluated. Manual muscle testing should not be used when spasticity is present, because the increased tone invalidates the results.

Procedure

1. Check the client's passive range of motion (R.O.M.) before beginning M.M.T.
2. Position patient or client so that the muscle will be tested against gravity.
3. Stabilize the joint above the one being tested to prevent substitution of incorrect muscles.
4. Have client perform the motion and observe the performance.
5. Palpate muscle performing the motion to be sure it is contracting.
6. Apply resistance into the opposite motion of the one being performed. (Resistance should be applied before the extreme end of the R.O.M.)
7. Grade the muscle strength.
8. In order to maintain reliability and accuracy, the same therapist should repeat this test on the client at the same time of day.
9. Enter the results of each test, sign and date.

Grading Scale

N Normal—complete R.O.M. against gravity with full resistance.
G Good —complete R.O.M. against gravity with some resistance.
F Fair —complete R.O.M. against gravity.
P Poor —complete R.O.M. with gravity eliminated.
T Trace —evidence of contractility on palpation. No joint motion.
0 Zero —no evidence of contractility.

CLINICAL RECORD—MANUAL MUSCLE EVALUATION

Name _____

Age _____

Diagnosis_____

LEFT   RIGHT

					Examiner's Initials							
					Date							
				ACTION	PRIME MOVERS	INNERVATION	SP. C. LEVEL					
			N E C K					N E C K				
				Flexion	STERNOCLEIDOMASTOID	Spinal Accessory,	C 2-3					
				Extension	EXTENSOR GROUP	Spinal Accessory,	C 1-8					
			T R U N K	Flexion	RECTUS ABDOMINUS		T 5-12	T R U N K				
				Rotation	EXTERNAL OBLIQUE		T 5-12					
					INTERNAL OBLIQUE		T 5-12					
				Extension	Thoracic	Post. Rami Spinal Nerves						
					Lumbar							
				Pelvic Elevation	QUADRATUS LUMBORUM		T 12 L 1-3					
			H I P	Flexion	ILIOPSOAS	Femoral	L 2-4	H I P				
					SARTORIUS	Femoral	L 2-4					
				Extension	GLUTEUS MAXIMUS	Inf. Gluteal	L 5 S 1-2					
				Abduction	GLUTEUS MEDIUS	Superior Gluteal	L 4-5 S 1					
					TENSOR FASCIA LATAE	Superior Gluteal	L 4-5 S 1					
				Adduction		Obturator	L 2-4					
				External Rotation			L 3 S 3					
				Internal Rotation			L 4 S 1					
			K N E E	Flexion	BICEPS FEMORIS	Sciatic	L 5 S 1-2	K N E E				
					SEMITENDINOSUS SEMIMEMBRANOSUS	Tibial	L 5 S 1-3					
				Extension	QUADRICEPS	Femoral	L 2-4					
			A N K L E	Inversion	ANTERIOR TIBIALIS	Deep Peroneal	L 5 S 1-2	A N K L E				
					POSTERIOR TIBIALIS	Tibial	L 4-5 S 1-2					
				Eversion	PERONEUS LONGUS	Sup. Peroneal	L 4-5 S 1					
					PERONEUS BREVIS	Sup. Peroneal	L 4-5 S 1					
				Plantar Flexion	GASTROCNEMIUS	Tibial	S 1-2					
					SOLEUS	Tibial	S 1-2					
			T O E S	Flexion	DIGITORUM LONGUS	Tibial	L 5 S 1-2	T O E S				
					DIGITORUM BREVIS	Tibial	L 5 S 1-2					
				Extension	DIGITORUM LONGUS & BREVIS	Deep Peroneal	L 4-5 S 1					
			H A L L U X	Flexion	HALLUCIS LONGUS	Tibial	L 5 S 1-2	H A L L U X				
					HALLUCIS BREVIS	Tibial	L 5 S 1-2					
				Extension	HALLUCIS LONGUS	Deep Peroneal	L 4-5 S 1-2					

KEY:
- 5 N NORMAL Complete range of motion against gravity with full resistance
- 4 G GOOD Complete range of motion against gravity with some resistance
- 3 F FAIR Complete range of motion against gravity
- 2 P POOR Complete range of motion with gravity eliminated
- 1 T TRACE Evidence of slight contractility. No joint motion
- 0 0 ZERO No evidence of contractility

Figure 11-1. Manual muscle evaluation form. Printed with permission of Moss Rehabilitation Hospital, Department of Physical Therapy, Philadelphia PA.

CLINICAL RECORD—MANUAL MUSCLE EVALUATION (Cont.)

Name _____ Age _____ Diagnosis_____

								SP. C. LEVEL				
LEFT									RIGHT			
			Examiner's Initials									
			Date									
			ACTION	PRIME MOVERS	INNERVATION							
			S C A P U L A	Elevation	UPPER TRAPEZIUS	Spinal Accessory		C_{3-4}	S C A P U L A			
				Adduction	MID TRAPEZIUS	Spinal Accessory		C_{3-4}				
					RHOMBOIDS	Dorsal Scapular		C_{4-5}				
				Abduction	SERRATUS ANTERIOR	Long Thoracic		C_{5-7}				
				Depression	LOWER TRAPEZIUS	Spinal Accessory		C_{3-4}				
			S H O U L D E R	Flexion	ANTERIOR DELTOID	Axillary		C_{5-6}	S H O U L D E R			
				Abduction	MIDDLE DELTOID	Axillary		C_{5-6}				
				Horizontal Adduction	PECTORALIS MAJOR Clavicular	Ant. Thoracic		C_{5-8}				
					Sternal			C_5 T_1				
				Extension	LATISSIMUS DORSI	Thoracodorsal		C_{5-8}				
				Horizontal Abduction	POST. DELTOID	Axillary		C_{5-6}				
				External Rotation				C_{5-6}				
				Internal Rotation				C_{5-8}				
			E L B O W	Flexion	BICEPS	Musculocutaneous		C_{5-6}	E L B O W			
					BRACHIALIS	Musculocutaneous		C_{5-6}				
					BRACHIORADIALIS	Radial		C_6				
				Extension	TRICEPS	Radial		C_{5-8}				
			FORE ARM	Supination	SUPINATOR	Radial		C_6	FORE ARM			
				Pronation	PRONATOR TERES	Median		C_6				
			W R I S T	Flexion	CARPI RADIALIS	Median		C_6	W R I S T			
					CARPI ULNARIS	Ulnar		C_8				
				Extension	CARPI RADIALIS L. & BREV.	Radial		C_{6-7}				
					CARPI ULNARIS	Radial		C_7				
			F I N G E R S	Flexion MP joint	LUMBRICALES 1,2	Median		C_{7-8}	F I N G E R S			
					3,4	Ulnar		C_8				
				Prox. IP joint	DIG. SUBLIMUS	Median		C_7 T_1				
				Dist. IP joint	DIG. PROFUNDUS 1,2	Median		C_8 T_1				
					3,4	Ulnar		C_8 T_1				
				Extension	DIG. EXT. COMMUNIS	Radial		C_6				
				Adduction	INTEROSSEI	Ulnar		C_8 T_1				
				Abduction	INTEROSSEI	Ulnar		C_8 T_1				
				Abduction, digit 4	DIGITI QUINTI	Ulnar		C_8				
				Opposition, digit 4	OPPONENS DIGITI QUINTI	Ulnar		C_8				
			T H U M B	Flexion MP joint	POLL. BREV.	Median		C_{6-8}	T H U M B			
				IP joint	POLL. L.	Median		C_8 T_1				
				Extension MP joint	POLL. BREV.	Radial		C_7				
				IP joint	POLL. L.	Radial		C_7				
				Adduction	ADDUCTOR POLLICIS	Ulnar		C_8				
				Abduction	POLL. L.	Radial		C_7				
					POLL. BREV.	Median		C_{6-7}				
				Opposition	OPPONENS POLLICIS	Median		C_{6-8} T_1				

See Figure 11-1 on page 150 for sample form for manual muscle testing.

Joint Range of Motion—Goniometry

In discussing joint movement it is necessary to understand the basic terminology used to describe joint motions.

Basic Terminology

Anatomical position—the body in an upright, standing position, face forward, upper extremities at the side, forearms supinated, and palms facing forward.

Flexion—a decrease in the angle of a joint as it is being moved.

Extension—a return from flexion.

Hyperextension—a movement beyond extension and past anatomical position.

Abduction—a movement away from the midline of the body.

Adduction—a movement toward the midline of the body and a return from abduction.

Internal rotation—a rotation toward the midline.

External rotation—a rotation away from the midline.

Supination—with elbow positioned at 90 degrees, the palm is turned up.

Pronation—with elbow positioned at 90 degrees, the palm is turned down.

Ulnar deviation—in anatomical position, a movement at the wrist toward the midline.

Radial deviation—in anatomical position, a movement at the wrist away from the midline.

Circumduction—a combination of movements: flexion, abduction, hyperextension, adduction, and extension.

Inversion—turning the sole of the foot toward the midline.

Eversion—turning the sole of the foot away from the midline.

Joint range of motion (R.O.M.) is measured in both upper and lower extremities to determine existing freedom of motion at a joint. This is either done passively (part moved by an outside force) or actively (part moved by muscle contraction, *i.e.*, muscle power.) Causes of decreased R.O.M. can be spasticity, weakness, pain, or a bone block. When a difference is noted between active and passive R.O.M. in the same joint, it is usually an indication of muscle weakness.

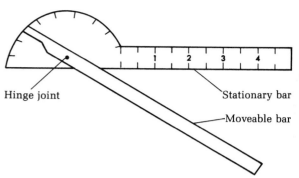

Figure 11-2. Goniometer.

Types of Motion

Passive Motion is movement performed by an outside force. No muscle contraction can be seen or palpated. *Active Motion* is movement performed independently by the individual.

Measurement Tool

The goniometer (Fig. 11-2) is the most frequently used tool for measurement of joint motion. Other methods used either alone or in conjunction with the goniometer are a ruler to measure distance (used especially in hand evaluation); photographs of the client performing the motion(s); outline drawings, for example, tracing the fingers while in abduction; and hand prints made by inking hands on a stamp pad and pressing on paper.

Procedure—180° Scale

1. To maintain reliability and accuracy each time, the same therapist should measure the client using the same method at the same time of day.
2. When measuring the upper extremity, use anatomical position as a starting position when possible. The starting position is recorded at zero degrees. Some exceptions to starting in anatomical position are shoulder internal and external rotation and forearm supination and pronation.
3. Prevent substitution by positioning and stabilizing the joint proximal to the joint being measured.
4. Check both passive and active R.O.M. when indicated.
5. The axis of the goniometer should be aligned with the joint axis.
6. Align the stationary bar parallel to the long axis of the stationary bone.
7. Align the movable bar parallel to the long axis of the movable bone.

8. Measure both the starting position and the maximum range. This indicates the arc through which the part moves, thus giving the freedom of motion at the joint.
9. Compare with opposite extremity or, if amputee, compare with a chart giving average joint R.O.M.
10. Indicate whether active or passive motion is being measured.
11. Record degrees of motion on a R.O.M. form (see Figs. 11-3 and 11-4).
12. When a patient or client is unable to reach zero degrees starting position (the normal position for that joint), indicate by stating number of degrees of motion from zero (example: −10 degrees of elbow extension).
13. Indicate if any pain, swelling, or spasticity is present.
14. Enter the results of each test, sign and date.

Sensory Testing

Sensory testing is performed when the therapist suspects that a sensory problem might exist. A patient or client with neurological disease or damage should always be tested for sensory loss. The following areas are usually examined: tactile sense, temperature, proprioception (position sense), and stereognosis.

General Procedure

1. Explain the test procedure to the client. Ask for feedback to be sure instructions are understood.
2. Occlude vision of the client with a shield such as a folder or cut-out box.
3. Test distally to proximally.
4. Enter the test results, date and sign.

Specific Procedure

1. *Tactile sense:* Test for recognition and localization of sharp and dull stimuli using a cotton ball, pencil, or a safety pin. Test two point discrimination using a compass. Texture discrimination is tested using smooth and rough objects.
2. *Temperature:* Test for the recognition of hot and cold using test tubes filled with hot and cold water.
3. *Proprioception* (position sense): Move body part up or down. Have the client indicate up or down or duplicate the motion with the opposite extremity.
4. *Stereognosis* (ability to recognize the shape of familiar objects by touch): Familiar objects of various size, shape, and weight are placed individually into the palm of the client who is to indicate

what object was placed in the hand. If the object cannot be manipulated, the therapist manipulates the object making sure contact is made with the fingers and thumb. If the client cannot communicate verbally, an alternative is to have him/her point to the duplicate object. Familiar objects such as a coin, key, pencil, or safety pin are examples of objects that are frequently used.

Sample Rating Scale

Intact—A quick, correct response.
Impaired—An incorrect or delayed response.
Absent—No response.

Coordination

Coordination is the working together of muscles or groups of muscles in order to perform a task. Both gross and fine coordination should be evaluated by the therapist. The tests listed in Table 11-1 (pp. 158–167) under the heading Manual Dexterity and Motor Function Tests are recommended. All are standardized and most have reliability and validity information. When these tests are not available, a task such as tossing and catching a bean bag or ball or playing a board game will assist the therapist in judging the patient's coordination ability.

Cognition

Cognition is the mental process by which knowledge is acquired; it is the ability to think and reason. Following disease or injury in which impairment of cognitive functioning is suspected, the following should be evaluated:

1. Ability to follow simple or complex instructions.
2. Ability to carry over learned skills from one day to the next.
3. Ability to attend to a task (attention span).
4. Ability to follow numerous steps in a process.
5. Ability to understand cause and effect.
6. Ability to problem solve.
7. Ability to concentrate.
8. Ability to perform in a logical sequence.
9. Ability to organize parts into a meaningful whole.
10. Ability to interpret signs and symbols.
11. Ability to read.
12. Ability to compute.

Hand and Pinch Strength Testing

Hand strength is measured by the patient's or client's gripping a dynamometer. The dial is calibrated

(Text continues on page 168)

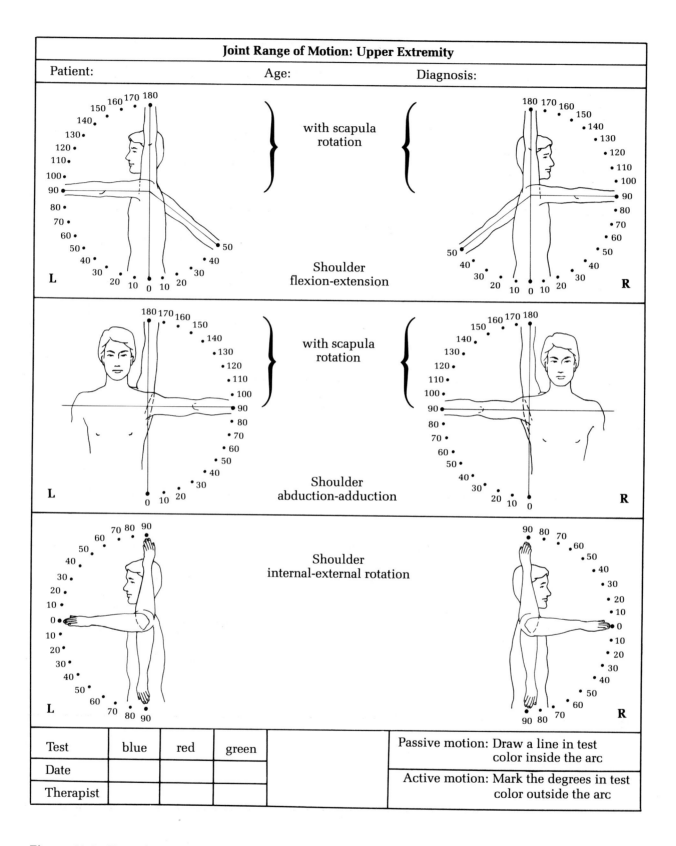

Figure 11-3. Form for measurement of joint range of motion, upper extremity. Redrawn and printed with the permission of Moss Rehabilitation Hospital, Department of Physical Therapy, Philadelphia PA.

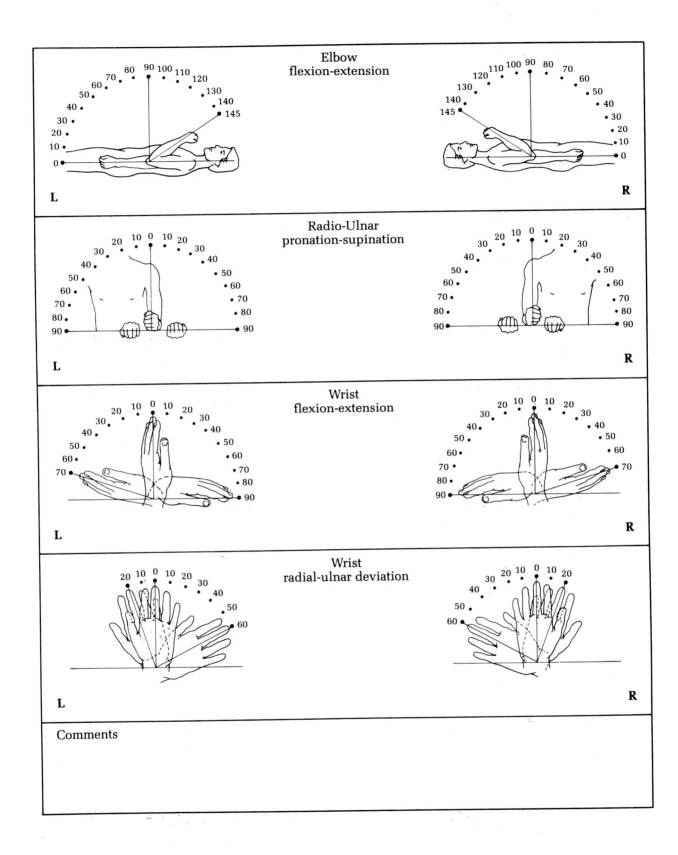

Elbow
flexion-extension

L   R

Radio-Ulnar
pronation-supination

L   R

Wrist
flexion-extension

L   R

Wrist
radial-ulnar deviation

L   R

Comments

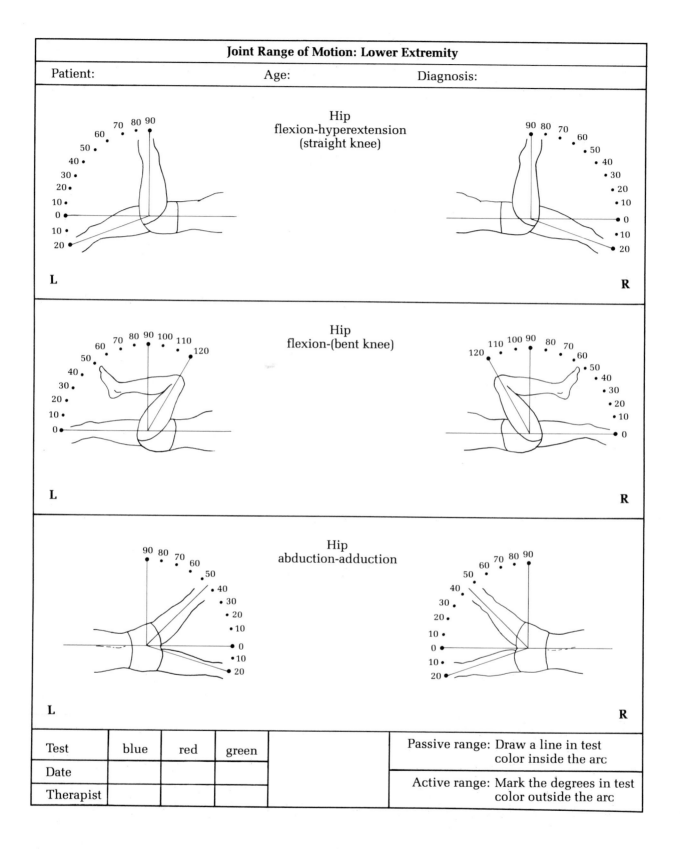

Figure 11-4. Form for measurement of joint range of motion, lower extremity. Redrawn and printed with the permission of Moss Rehabilitation Hospital, Department of Physical Therapy, Philadelphia PA.

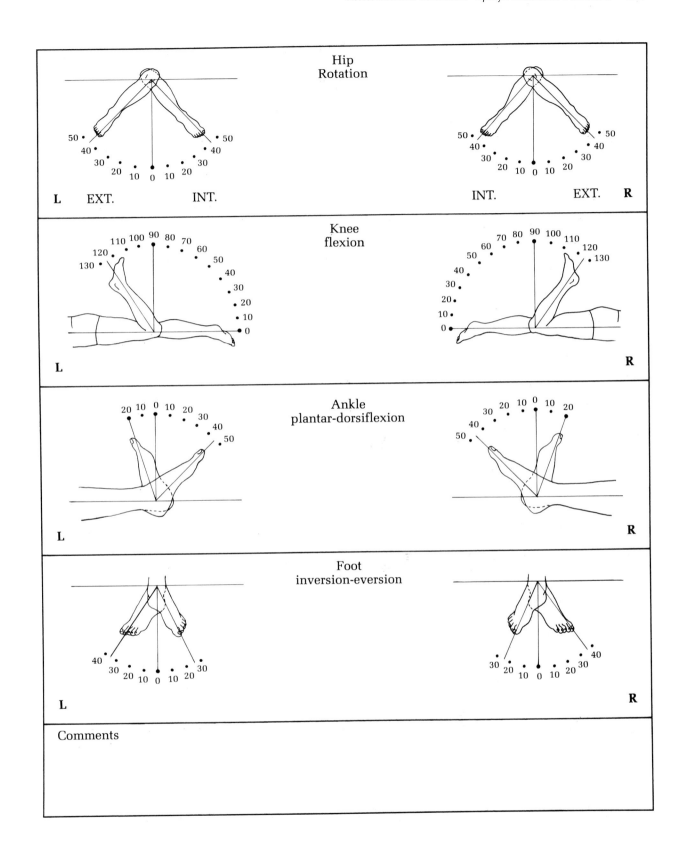

Table 11-1 *Sampling of tests used in evaluation.*

Name	Type	Description	Features	Source
Manual Dexterity and Motor Function Tests				
Jebsen-Taylor Hand Function Test[7]	Individual test to evaluate functional capabilities.	Seven subtests measure major aspects of hand function often used in activities of daily living. Equipment needed: stopwatch	Standardized tasks, objective measurements taken with stopwatch. Norms (360 normal subjects) included. Easy to administer. Test equipment and material-are either made or easily available. Subtests are writing, card turning, picking up small objects, simulated feeding, stacking checkers, picking up large tight objects, picking up large heavy objects. Time: 12–15 min. Age: child–adult	Jebsen, R. et al.: Arch. Phys. Med. Rehab. 50:311, 1969. Sand, P.: Am. J. Occup. Ther. 28:87, 1974.
Purdue Pegboard	Individual test to aid selection of employees for industrial jobs requiring manipulative dexterity.	Measures both gross movements of arms, hands, and fingers and fingertip dexterity. Equipment: stop watch	Two operations: rapid placing of pins in pegboard, assembly of pins, washers, and collars. Norms for male industrial applicants, veterans, college students, female college students, and industrial applicants Time: 12–15 min. Has face validity, low acceptable reliability	Science Research Associates, Inc., 259 East Erie St., Chicago IL, 60611
Minnesota Rate of Manipulation Test	Individual test of manual dexterity.	Designed to measure dexterity of individuals grade 7 to adult.	Five operations resulting in five scores: placing, turning, displacing, 1-hand turning and placing, and 2-hand turning and placing. Form board used—wells and round dics. Time: 30–50 min.	American Guidance Service, Inc., Publishers Bldg., Circle Pines MN, 55014.
(Oseretsky Tests of Motor Proficiency) Revised: The Lincoln-Oseretsky Motor Development Scale	Scale of motor development. Individual test for hand and arm movements measuring speed, dexterity, coordination, and rhythm.	First published in Russian, 1923. Portuguese adaptation, 1943. English translation, 1946. Sloan adaptation, 1948. Items sample variety of motor performances.	Items arranged in order of difficulty. Instructions concise, scoring is specific. Correlations of each item score with age and tentative percentile norms. Separately and combined scores given for sexes. Validated in relation to changes with age.	C. H. Stoelting Co., 424 N. Hohman Ave., Chicago IL, 60624

Table developed from Buros, O. K. (ed.): The Third–Eighth Mental Measurement Yearbooks. Highland Park, NJ: Gryphon Press, 1949–1978.

Manual Dexterity and Function Tests

Test	Description	Details	Publisher
Pennsylvania Bi-Manual Work Sample	Individual test of bi-manual dexterity: finger dexterity of both hands, gross movements of both arms, eye-hand coordination, and indication of use of of both hands.	First part—assembly of 100 nuts and bolts. Second part—dissasembly of nuts and bolts. Two scores—one for each operation. Time: 10 min. assembly and 5 min. disassembly. Reliable. Validity not indicated.	Educational Test Bureau, American Guidance Service, Inc., Publishers Bldg., Circle Pines MN, 55014
Crawford Small Parts Dexterity Test	Individual measure of fine eye-hand coordination and manipulation of small hand tools.	10-inch square board. Round wells for parts to be manipulated, (*i.e.*, pins, collars, and screws): a metal plate containing 42 unthreaded and 42 threaded holes; two metal trays beneath the plate to receive the pins and screws. Tools: a tweezer and a small screwdriver. *Part I*—Examinee picks up pin with tweezer, inserts in small hole in metal plate and places collar over it using preferred hand. *Part II*—Examinee picks up screw, starts it in threaded hole with the fingers, then screws through metal plate with screwdriver, using both hands in operation. Six practice trials. Scored by time required. Time: *Part I*—5 min. *Part II*—10 min. High reliability Face validity	Psychological Corporation, 304 East 45th St., New York NY, 10017

Developmental Tests

Test	Description	Details	Publisher
Bayley Scales of Infant Development	Individual scales of infant development.	A three-part evaluation of a child's development in relation to other children of the same age. Scales include mental, motor, and behavior ratings. Well standardized. No data on validity of motor scale or predictive validity of mental scale. Reliability is satisfactory. Testing Time: 45–90 min. Age: 2–30 mo.	Psychological Corporation, 304 East 45th St., New York NY, 10017
Brazelton Behavioral Assessment Scale	Individual score of infant interactive behavior.	Evaluates the neonate's reaction to stimuli and responses to the environment. Best performance is scored. Photographs of testing procedures are included. Testing time: 20–30 min. Research in progress on test reliability and validity.	J. B. Lippincott Co., East Washington Square, Philadelphia PA, 19105 4 training films: Educational Development Corp., 8 Mifflin Place, Cambridge MA, 02138

Table 11-1 *(continued)*

Name	Type	Description	Features	Source
Brigance Screen	Individual and group screening test for kindergarten and first grade.	Adapted from and cross-referenced to readiness section of the Brigance Inventory of Basic Skills and Inventory of Early Development. Identifies children needing referrals to special services and those needing further assessment and for program planning.	Small group screening, individual screening added 2 or 3 minutes to the time. Cost for manual $19.95. Pads of 30 forms .25 cents per child. Scoring—one scale, 100 points. Rank words to score. No special materials needed. Time: 10–12 min.	Curriculum Associates, Inc., 5 Esquire Rd., N. Billerica MA, 01862
Callier-Azusa Scale (1975)	Individual developmental scale for assessment of deaf, blind, and multi-handicapped children.	Designed to be used in a classroom, this scale is divided into five subscales: motor development, perceptual development, daily living skills, language development, and socialization. Subscales are made up of sequential steps describing developmental milestones.	Examples of behavior are provided for many items. (Behaviors were observed on deaf-blind children.) Lists criteria. Observation period to extend over a 2-week period. Reliability information available from author.	Robert Stillman, PhD, Callier Center for Communication Disorders, University of Texas/Dallas, 1966 Inwood Rd., Dallas TX, 75235
Denver Developmental Screening Test	Individual formalized observations of normal developmental behavior of infants and children.	A screening tool for detecting infants and children with developmental delays. Areas evaluated: gross motor, fine motor, language, and personal-social development.	Standardized on children age 2 wk–6.4 yr. in Denver. High percentage came from professional families. Inexpensive, quick, easy to use. Uses common items. Manual and scoring guide are clear. Reliability and validity vary with age groups.	Ladoca Project and Publishing Foundation, Inc., East 51st Ave. & Lincoln St., Denver CO, 80216
Developmental Screening 0–5 Years	Individual screening inventory of abnormal development.	History and observation ratings in five areas: adaptive, gross motor, fine motor, language, and personal-social. (Selected items were used from the Gesell Developmental Schedules)	Age: 1 yr.–18 mo. No reliability data available. Testing time: 5–30 min.	Knobloch, H., et al.: A developmental screening inventory for infants. Pediatrics 38:1095, 1966.
The Gesell Developmental Tests	Individual scale of developmental levels.	Scale of behavioral observations by age level (5–10) of the mental growth of the child in determining school readiness.	Qualitative measure of motor development, adaptive behavior, and personal-social behavior. Present functional level is evaluated. Time: 20–30 min.	Programs for Education, Box 85, Lumberville PA, 18933

Sensory Integration Tests

Test	Purpose	Description	Details	Source
Developmental Test of Visual-Motor Integration (Berry, K.)	Test to detect children with problems in visual-motor integration.	Subject is presented with 24 geometric forms arranged in order of increasing difficulty which are then copied into a test booklet.	Standardized test that can be group administered. Emphasis is on preschool group. Directions are clear. Separate age norms for each sex. Two Forms: ages 2–15 (long form), ages 2–8 (short form). Reliability and validity information does not appear complete. Time: 10 min.	Follett Educational Corporation, 1010 W. Washington Blvd., Chicago IL, 60607
Marianne Frostig Developmental Test of Visual Perception	Individual and group test measuring visual perception.	Five subtests of visual perception: eye-motor coordination, figure-ground, constancy of shape, position in space, and spatial relations.	Five areas relate to preschool and early elementary academic performance. Group administration possible. Norms for ages 3–8 yr. Reliability appears adequate. Validity information does not appear to be complete. Testing Time: Individual, 30–45 min.; Group, 40–60 min.	Consulting Psychologists Press, Inc., 577 College Ave., Palo Alto CA, 94306
The Imitation of Gestures: A Technique for Studying the Body Schema and Praxis of Children 3 to 6 Years of Age.	Individual test of perceptual motor function.	Berges, J., and Lezine, I.: Clin. Develop. Med., No. 18. Spastic Society Medical Education and Information Unit. London: W. Heinemann Medical Books Ltd., 1965.		Medical Market Research Inc., 227 South 6th St., Philadelphia PA, 19105
Perceptual Forms Test	Individual and group testing for perceptual and readiness evaluation and training.	Two Parts: perceptual forms test and incomplete forms in which subject is required to complete partial drawings. Visual-motor coordination is required. Test used to identify children who might have problems in school achievement.	Geometric forms are copied. Templates are used. Formal scoring on the perceptual form test but not on the incomplete forms. Age: 5–8 yr. Reliability and validity information not complete.	Winter Haven Lions Research Foundation, Inc., P.O. Box 111, Winter Haven FL, 33880
The Purdue Perceptual Motor Survey	Individual test of perceptual motor abilities.	Identifies children with perceptual motor problems that could interfere with learning of academic skills. Eleven subtests: rhythmic writing; walking board; jumping; identification of body parts; imitation of movements; obstacle course; chalkboard; Kraus-Weber; angels-in-the-snow; ocular pursuits; developmental drawing.	Test based on theory. Easy to administer, and instructions and scoring keys are adequate. Reliability and validity information are said to be good. Age: 6–10 yr. Time: 20 min.	Charles E. Merill Publishing Co., 1300 Alum Creek Drive, Columbus OH, 43216

Table 11-1 (continued)

Sensory Integration Tests

Name	Type	Description	Features	Source
Southern California Sensory Integration Tests	Individual tests of perceptual motor development. A series of separate tests.	See individual test listings.		Western Psychological Services, 12031 Wilshire Blvd., Los Angeles CA, 90025
Southern California Figure-Ground Visual Perception Test	Individual test of figure-ground.	Assessment of visual perception of a foreground figure superimposed on a background.	Instructions are well done, scoring is simple. Norms available for children 4–10 yr. Test has face validity. Reliability information is questionable. Time: 5–20 min.	
Southern California Kinesthesia and Tactile Perception Tests	Individual evaluation of dysfunction in somesthetic perception.	Six subtests: kinesthesia; manual form perception; finger identification; graphesthesia; localization of tactile stimuli; double tactile stimuli perception.	Verbal responses are not required. Studies have shown girls tend to score higher than boys. Norms available for 6-mon. intervals from age 4-0 to 8-6. Reliability and validity are said to be moderate. Time: 15–20 min.	
Southern California Motor Accuracy Test	Individual test of motor accuracy.	Assesses the degree of sensori-motor involvement of the CNS in a motor planning task. Involves eye-hand coordination using sensory information from eyes, touch, and proprioceptors.	Requires child to cross midline of body. Both upper extremities are tested and scores are recorded for most accurate and least accurate hand. Norms available for ages 4-0 to 7-11. Reliability and validity are said to be high. Time: 10 min.	
Southern California Perceptual-Motor Tests	Individual evaluation of perceptual motor function.	Six subtests: imitation of posture; crossing midline of body; bilateral motor coordination; standing balance with eyes opened and closed.	Verbal responses not requires except for two items in right-left discrimination. Manual and protocol sheet can easily be followed. Test administration is not difficult. Norms for ages 4–8 yr. No validity data at this time. Time: 20 min.	
Southern California Postrotary Nystagmus test	Individual test of the duration of nystagmus or reflexive eye response to rotary movement.	Passive rotation of S sitting in cross-legged position with head in 30° of flexion on freely turning board 10 times in 20 sec. to the left, stop abruptly, and time duration of involuntary eye movement to the nearest sec.; observe excursion of eye movements. Repeat procedure to the right.	Standardized test. Time: 20 sec. to left / 10 sec. between / 20 sec. to right / 50 sec. total. Reliability: 0.834. Standard error: Boys—3 sec. Girls—2.6 sec. Reliability coefficient: 0.485	

Ayres Space Test	Individual measure of space relations.	Measures speed of perception of stimuli: position in space or directionality and space visualization.	Test consists of 60 items. Form and two blocks presented each time. Difficulty increases throughout test. Norms available from age 3–11 yr. Validity and reliability information appears incomplete. Time: 20–30 min.	University of Illinois Press, Urbana IL, 61801
Illinois Test of Psycholinguistic Abilities (I.T.P.A.)	Individual test of cognitive functioning.	A test of language perception and short-term memory abilities to assist in diagnosing learning problems.	Visual and auditory channels are used for input. Vocal and motor channels are used for output. Norms on children from slightly above average homes, age 2–10 yr. Reliability is said to be moderate. Time: 45–50 min.	Crippled Children and Adults of Rhode Island, Inc., Meeting Street School, 333 Grotto Ave., Providence RI, 02906
Meeting Street School Screening Test	Individual test to determine children with learning difficulties.	Short battery for children, kindergarten to first grade. Four scores: motor patterning; visual-perceptual motor; language; total score.	No reading required. Reliability and validity data do not appear to be complete. Time: 15–20 min.	

Intelligence Tests

Goodenough-Harris Drawing Test	Individual or group test of conceptual and intellectual maturity.	Tests accuracy of observation and development of conceptual thinking. The subject draws a picture of a man, woman, and a self-portrait.	A simple nonverbal test. Norms were established on children 5–15 yr. from four major geographical areas representative of various occupations. Reliability and validity information are said to be adequate. Time: 10–15 min. Age: 3–15 yr.	Harcourt Brace Jovanovich, Inc., 757 3rd Ave., New York NY, 10017
Peabody Picture Vocabulary	Individual test of verbal intelligence.	Untimed test that estimates verbal intelligence by measuring hearing vocabulary. Subject chooses one of four pictures after hearing a word.	No reading required. Standardized age range 2.5–18 yr. Content and item validity are good, and reliability is said to be adequate.	American Guidance Service, Inc., Publishers Bldg., Circle Pines MN, 55014

Psychological Tests

Adaptive Behavior Scales	Individual scale assessing adaptive behavior of the mentally retarded and emotionally maladjusted individual.	Evaluation of subject's effectiveness to cope with environmental demands. Twenty-four areas of social and personal behavior are covered.	Easy to administer but hand-scoring is complex. Norms based on institutionalized retardates beginning at age 3. Has face validity but no data on reliability. Time: Children, 20–25 min.; Adults, 25–30 min.	American Association on Metal Deficiency, 5201 Connecticut Ave. N.W., Washington DC, 20015

Table 11-1 *(continued)*

Name	Type	Description	Features	Source
Psychological Tests				
Vineland Social Maturity Scale	Individual performance scale of social maturity.	Behavioral observations of self-help, self-direction, locomotion, occupation, communication, and social relations. Provides an evaluation of subject's social competency.	Useful tool for evaluating mentally retarded individual. Includes 117 items. Age: birth to maturity. Time: 20–30 min.	Educational Test Bureau, American Guidance Service, Publishers Bldg., Circle Pines MN, 55014
Bender-Gestalt Test	Individual or group projective evaluation of personality dynamics.	Measure nonverbal gestalt functioning in perceptual motor area. The subject copies designs.	Evaluates perceptual motor functioning, neurological impairment, and maladjustment. Scoring system quantified and objective. Most validity research done on scoring system. No data on reliability. Time: 10 min. Age: 4 and over.	American Orthopsychiatric Association, Inc., 1790 Broadway, New York NY, 10019
H-T-P, House-Tree-Person Projective Techniques	Individual and group projective test of personality appraisal.	Freehand drawing by subject of a house, tree, and person. Notes are made by tester of behavior of subject.	Quantitative and qualitative scoring. Achromatic and chromatic drawings. Eight assorted color crayons are used. Ages: 5 and over. No norms for ages 5–14. Time: 60–90 min.	Western Psychological Services, 12031 Wilshire Blvd., Los Angeles CA, 90025
Minnesota Multiphasic Personality Inventory (MMPI)	Individual and group nonprojective test measuring psychopathology.	Assesses the type and degree of emotional dysfunction in adults.	Spanish edition is available. Normative and reliability data has not been changed since 1951. Time: Individual, 30–90 min.; Group, 40–90 min. for complete form and 40–75 min. for short version.	The Psychological Corporation, 304 East 45th St., New York NY, 10017
Nurses' Observation Scale for Inpatient Evaluation (NOSIE)	Nonprojective individual rating scale measuring behavioral status and change.	Highly sensitive ward behavior rating scale that assesses subject's status and change over time.	Seven scores: competence, social interest, personal neatness, irritability, manifest psychosis, and retardation. Easy to use. Norms based on adult male schizophrenics age 55–69. Validity and reliability appear to be adequate. Time: 3–5 min.	Behavioral Arts Center, 90 Calla Ave., Floral Park, New York NY, 11001

Activity Configuration	Pencil and paper schedule with clear legend.	Client lists hourly activities for a typical week with personal assessments of the nature of the activity (recreation, social, work, etc.), autonomy, pleasure, and adequacy. Especially useful with clients who are depressed.	Administration should be accompanied by discussion. Promotes consideration of personal priorities, time management.	Watanabe, S. AOTA 1968 Regional Institute on the Eval. Process. Final Report RSA 123-T-68 NY, 1968, pp. 46–47.
Adolescent Role Assessment	Interview—individual or group admin.	Semi-structured dialogue with specific rating criteria to assess quality of childhood play, family interactions, chores, school skills, work attitudes, and fantasy.	Specific questions to be explored with specific rating criteria so that role expectations may be consistent with values and skills.	Black, M. AJOT 30:73, 1976.
Allen Cognitive Level (ACL)	Individual Cognitive Performance.	Measures cognitive level through performance of prescribed tasks.	Clearly delineated administration. Provides base line for establishment of task expectations and ongoing monitoring of treatment effectiveness.	Allen, Claudia Univ. S. Cal. Med. Ctr. Los Angeles.
Azima Battery	Projective battery.	Assesses mood organization, organization of drives, ego organization, object relations through client's performance in drawing, finger painting, use of clay and plastic media.	Classic psychoanalytically-based assessment, first presented in 1961. Valuable in T_x planning, as change detection, prognosis, effects of drug administration. Heuristic considerations with regard to research, use in family therapy (comparative batteries).	Azima, F. J. Diseases of the Nervous System, Monograph Suppl. 22, 1961, and in Hemphill, B. J. (ed.). The Eval. Process in Psychiatric O.T.
Bay Area Functional Performance Eval. (BAFPE)	Evaluation Battery.	Assesses functional performance in ADL with psychiatric clients. Two subtests—Task Oriented Assessment (TOA) and Social Interaction Scale (SIS). Use of interview, structured and projective tasks, observation.	Clear directions for assessment of ADL, motor skills, sensory motor function, sensation, endurance, cognition, appearance. Rating scale and directions—Research implications—Video Tape available.	Consulting Psychologists Press, Inc. 577 College Ave., Palo Alto CA, 94306

Table 11-1 *(continued)*

Name	Type	Description	Features	Source
Comprehensive Assessment Process	Projective Assessment process, includes structured interviews and group activities.	Administration of initial interview and follow-up interviews, ADL questionnaire, group activity sessions, to yield observations of grooming, levels of awareness, orientation, affect, motor level, self-esteem, attendance, self-direction, task investment, independence, concentration, following instructions, problem solving, decision-making, frustration, tolerance, work tolerance, planning, workmanship, leadership, etc.	Designed to evaluate overall client behaviors—as basis for individualized plans in short-term, acute-care psychiatric treatment facilities. Indications for further research.	Ehrenberg, F. in Hemphill, B. J. (ed.).
Comprehensive Occupational Therapy Evaluation (COTE)	Evaluation Scale	Assesses 25 identified behaviors in three areas: (1) general, (2) interpersonal, and (3) task. Provides guide to observation, interview, tasks, and recording methods.	For use in adult acute psychiatric T_x setting—to enhance observation and reduce subjectivity in reporting, facilitate team communication—enables therapist to report a large volume of comprehensive and pertinent information quickly, in consistent format with defined terminology. Grid with space for daily recording for 16 days.	Brayman, S. F. and Kirby, T. in Hemphill, B. J. (ed.)
Goodman Battery	Projective battery.	Evaluates cognitive and affective ego assets and deficits affecting function. Tasks presented represent decreasing structure—copying to freehand drawing to clay task.	Very specific instructions retest environment, timing, etc. Rating scales. Further research implications.	Evaskus, M. G. in Hemphill, B. J. (ed.)
Interest Check List	Interview with pencil and paper. Check list.	Eighty activities listed with space for client to check interest level (casual, strong, no). Gives indications of client's experience and interests.	Administration should be accompanied by discussion— Classic check list, much adapted and widely used.	Matsutsuyu, J. AJOT 3:327, 1969.

Name	Type	Assesses	Notes	Source
Kohlman Evaluation of Living Skills (KELS)	Structured interview with tasks.	Assesses psychiatric clients' skills in self-care, safety and health, money management, transportation and telephone, work and leisure.	Clear directions for observation, recording, and implications for community living and/or further T_x. Protocol. Videotape available.	Health Sciences Learning Resources Center T 281 SB-56. Univ. of Washington, Seattle WA, 98195 (206)545-1186
Lifestyle Performance Profile	Individual interview.	Assesses performance skills and skill levels as determined by age, culture, and biology in the areas of self-care and maintenance; self needs—extrinsic gratification; service to others.	Data gathered yields information to aid description of skill deficits and strengths, social-cultural expectations for performance, lifestyle performance balance, nature of family, social cultural, economic, and environmental resources or barriers; sensorimotor, cognitive, psychological, and social skill deficits/strengths, individual characteristics, and interests that shape response.	Fidler, G. S. in Hemphill, B. J. (ed.): The Eval. Process in Psychiatric O.T.
Schroeder Block S-I Eval.	Comprehensive Assessment Tools.	Assesses S-I in adult psychiatric clients using specific testing procedures and observation.	Definite procedures, observations, scoring, work sheets, summary sheets required. Research implications.	Schroeder, C. V., Block, M. P., Campbell, E. T., Stowell, M. Adult Psychiatric S-I Eval. San Diego V.A. SBC Research Assoc. La Jolla CA, 1979
Shoemeyen Battery	Projective Battery (one to four clients).	Uses four activities: mosaic tile, clay figure, fingerpainting, sculpture—media and interview-discussion to gain information about attitudes, mood, cognitive and social skills, dexterity, attention, suggestibility, independence, and creativity.	Information gained to aid in team T_x planning—to promote relatively natural therapist-client relationship and collaborative planning and implementation of T_x.	Shoemeyen, C. O.T. orientation and evaluation: A study of procedure and media. AJOT 24:276–279, 1970 and in Hemphill, B. J. (ed.) Shards Teaching Hospital U. of Florida, Gainesville FL

Other

Name	Type	Assesses	Notes	Source
Parachek Geriatric Rating Scale	Geriatric rating scale.	Designed to help in planning treatment programs for the geriatric patient. Areas rated: physical capabilities; self-care skills; social-interaction skills.	Items arranged and rated in developmental sequence. A treatment manual is attached. Time: 3–5 min. once a month.	Greenroom Publishing Co., 8512 East Virginia, Scottsdale AZ, 85257

in either pounds or kilograms, and the indicator will stay at the highest reading until reset manually. An added feature in some dynamometers is an adjustable hand grip.

Pinch strength is measured on a pinch gauge. The dial is calibrated in pounds, and it measures finger prehension force. A quick reading of the dial must be made if the indicator on the dial does not stay at the highest reading point. Both the dynamometer and the pinch gauge can be purchased through suppliers of physical medicine and rehabilitation equipment.

Endurance Testing

The patient or client is often tested for the ability to reach or maintain the necessary energy output required to perform an activity. This is especially important in activities of daily living, homemaker retraining, and work-related activities. The amount of work and the time required to do the work are carefully noted, and work output and time are carefully increased according to the tolerance of the client until either the desired level is reached or the client reaches his or her maximum.

The Physical Capacities Evaluation*

In writing a summary of a client's physical capacities, one should summarize the client's ability, endurance, speed, safety, and strength in all activities tested. The activities that the client was unable to perform should be listed, and it can be stated why he or she was unable to perform each activity. The length of time the test took, the frequency of rest periods, appliances used, the amount of pain or discomfort, and the client's overall work endurance should also be stated. The client's emotional reactions, including his or her emotional tolerance, ability to follow directions, appearance, and cooperativeness are also important. An example of a Physical Capacities Evaluation follows.

* This evaluation procedure is based upon the physical capacities requirements of the *Dictionary of Occupational Titles* (D.O.T.), U.S. Department of Labor. Developed and reprinted with permission of Susan L. Smith, Professional Occupational Therapy Services, Inc., Metairie, Louisiana.

PHYSICAL CAPACITIES EVALUATION

Administrator's Guide for Physical Capacities Evaluation

Performance Rating:
    Within Normal Range (W.N.R.)
    Fair
    Poor
    Unable
    Not appropriate (N.A.)

"Comment" space to be used only for:
    Reason unable to perform
    Other significant performance

Use of exercise mats:
    "Kneeling" and/or "Crawling" if client's knees are tender
    "Reclining" if floor too hard

Standard of comparison:
    "Walking": Army Regulation—66 seconds per 100 yards
    "Climbing" (stairs): Average time between 3 and 5 seconds each way

---

Walking:
    Request:
        1. To walk as ordinarily 100 yd. on rubber tiled flooring.
            A. Performance:
                a. Type of gait:
                b. Appliances used:
                c. Endurance:
                d. Safety:
        2. The client's estimate of distance and length of time he is able to walk.
            A. Estimate:
                a. Distance inside:
                b. Distance outside:
                c. Time inside:
                d. Time outside:

Comment: _____

_____

PHYSICAL CAPACITIES EVALUATION (*continued*)

Running
Request:
1. To run 30 yds on rubber tiled flooring.
    A. Performance:
        a. Endurance:
        b. Type of gait:
        c. Safety:

Comment: _____

_____

Jumping:
Request:
1. To jump from a 19 in. & 30 in. high platform onto rubber tiled flooring landing on both feet.
    A. Performance:
        a. Balance: 19″: _____ 30″: _____
        b. Ability: 19″: _____ 30″: _____
        c. Safety: 19″: _____ 30″: _____

Comment: _____

_____

Climbing
Request:
1. Ramp (8′ × 12° textured brick tile surface): To walk up and down five consecutive times.
    A. Performance:
        a. Gait:
        b. Endurance:
        c. Use of handrail:
        d. Use of appliance:

2. Stairs: (10 steps, 7 in. rise, steel and stone tread) to walk up and down once.
    A. Performance:
        a. Safety:
        b. Endurance:
        c. Speed:
        d. Use of handrail:
        e. Use of appliances:
        f. Foot-over-foot: Foot-by-foot:

3. Curbs: (9 in. and 14 in. high) To climb and descend curbs once.
    A. Performance in reference to public transportation:

        a. Ability: 8″ _____ 14″ _____
        b. Use of appliances:
        c. Safety:

4. Straight ladder (8 rungs, 10 ft. high): to climb up and down five consecutive times.
    A. Performance:
        a. Foot-over-foot: Foot by foot:
        b. Hand-over-hand: Hand on rail:
            Hand-by-hand:
        c. Balance:
        d. Safety:

5. Step Ladder. (6 ft. 10 in. rise): To climb up and down once carrying a 10 lb. paint pail in one hand.
    A. Performance:
        a. Foot-over-foot: Foot-by-foot:
        b. Balance:
        c. Safety:

Comments: _____

_____

PHYSICAL CAPACITIES EVALUATION (*continued*)

Crouching:
Request:
1. To work in a squatting position for 3 minutes placing 1½ lb. cans (4″ × 8″) from the floor to a 19″ high shelf.
   A. Performance:
      a. Ability to carry out task:
      b. Ability to assume position:
      c. Ability to regain standing:
      d. Balance:
      e. Endurance:

Comments: _____

_____

Lifting:
Request:
1. Left Hand—To lift maximum weight from floor to a waist-high surface five consecutive times.
   A. Performance:
      a. Number of lb.;
      b. Ability:
      c. Balance:
      d. Endurance:

2. Right Hand—Same as left
   A. Performance:
      a. Number of lb.:
      b. Ability:
      c. Endurance:
      d. Balance:

3. Both hands—To lift maximum in weighted box from floor to a waist high surface five consecutive times.
   A. Performance:
      a. Ability:
      b. Balance:
      c. Endurance:
      d. Number of lbs.:

Comments: _____

_____

Carrying:
Request:
1. To bilaterally carry maximum weight in weighted boxes 25 yd. while walking on rubber tiled flooring.
   A. Performance:
      a. Number of lb.:
      b. Ability:
      c. Endurance:
      d. Balance:

Comments: _____

_____

Handling:
Administrator's estimate of the maximum weight the testee is able to handle comfortably.
1. Estimate:

Comments: _____

_____

Pushing: Push—Pull
Request:
1. To push a wheelbarrow (heavy duty with inflated rubber tire) for 25 yd. on rubber tiled flooring with maximum load.
   A. Performance:
      a. Ability:
      b. Endurance:
      c. Balance on turning:

PHYSICAL CAPACITIES EVALUATION (*continued*)

   2. To alternately push and pull bilaterally to arm's length the maximum in a weighted box on a waist high rough wooden surface, ten times, both from standing and sitting positions.
      A. Performance:
          a. Number of lb. ＿＿＿＿＿＿   Standing: Sitting:
          b. Ability:

Comments: ＿＿＿＿＿＿＿＿＿＿＿＿＿＿＿＿＿＿＿＿＿＿＿＿＿＿＿＿＿＿＿＿＿＿＿

＿＿＿＿＿＿＿＿＿＿＿＿＿＿＿＿＿＿＿＿＿＿＿＿＿＿＿＿＿＿＿＿＿＿＿＿＿＿＿

Pulling:
  Request:
    1. To pull in a hand-over-hand fashion the maximum weight on a single pulley (¾ in. cotton rope) ten consecutive times.
      A. Performance:
          a. Number of lb.:
          b. Ability:
          c. Endurance:
          d. Balance:

Comments: ＿＿＿＿＿＿＿＿＿＿＿＿＿＿＿＿＿＿＿＿＿＿＿＿＿＿＿＿＿＿＿＿＿＿＿

＿＿＿＿＿＿＿＿＿＿＿＿＿＿＿＿＿＿＿＿＿＿＿＿＿＿＿＿＿＿＿＿＿＿＿＿＿＿＿

Stooping:
  Request:
    1. To perform in 3 min. standing and stooping repeatedly while placing 5 lb. cans (4 in. × 8 in.) from the floor to a 48 in. high shelf.
      A. Performance:
          a. Ability:
          b. Endurance:
          c. Ability to grasp—   Right hand: Left hand:

Comments: ＿＿＿＿＿＿＿＿＿＿＿＿＿＿＿＿＿＿＿＿＿＿＿＿＿＿＿＿＿＿＿＿＿＿＿

＿＿＿＿＿＿＿＿＿＿＿＿＿＿＿＿＿＿＿＿＿＿＿＿＿＿＿＿＿＿＿＿＿＿＿＿＿＿＿

Reaching:
  Request:
    1. Overhead—from a standing position to bimanually reach a 10 lb. box from an overhead shelf; return it to position. To reach with separate hands small objects from the same shelf.
      A. Performance:
          a. Ability: 10 lb.:   Right: Left:
          b. Range of motion
          c. Balance:
          d. Coordination: Grasp:
    2. Forward: Standing—To reach forward and pick up a 10 lb. box from a table with both hands.
      A. Performance:
          a. Balance: Both: Right: Left:
          b. Coordination: Both:
          c. Grasp: Right: Left:
          d. Range of motion: Both: Right: Left:
    3. Forward: Sitting—To reach forward for a small object on the table with separate hands, both directly and across the body.
      A. Performance:
          a. Balance: Both: Right: Left:
          b. Coordination: Both:
          c. Grasp: Right: Left:
          d. Range of motion: Both: Right: Left:
    4. Low: Standing—To pick up small objects on floor from front position with both hands. To pick up same object on right and left sides with separate hands both directly and across body.
      A. Performance:
          a. Balance: Both: Right: Left:
          b. Coordination: Both:
          c. Grasp: Right: Left:
          d. Range of motion: Both: Right: Left:

PHYSICAL CAPACITIES EVALUATION (*continued*)

    5.   Sitting—To reach directly for small object on floor with separate hands at the right, left, and front positions.
        A.   Performance:
           a.   Balance: Right: F. Right: F. Left:
           B.   Range of motion:
           c.   Grasp: Right: Left: F. Right: F. Left:

Comments: _____

_____

Kneeling:
   Request:
      1.   To assume a kneeling position on a rubber tiled floor and maintain it for a 1 min. period.
         A.   Performance:
            a.   Ability to assume position:
            b.   Ability to regain standing:
            c.   Balance:
            d.   Endurance:

Comments: _____

_____

Crawling:
   Request:
      1.   To crawl on rubber tiled flooring 8 ft. forward and then backward with head and shoulders down.
         A.   Performance:
            a.   Type crawl: 4-point: 3-point: Other:
            b.   Speed:
            c.   Agility:

Comments: _____

_____

Reclining:
   Request:
      1.   To assume a backlying position on rubber tiled flooring. When in position.
         A.   Performance:
            a.   Ability to assume position:
            b.   Ability to regain standing:
            c.   Ability to turn: Right: Left: Face:
            d.   Comfort on: Right: Left: Face: Back:

Comments: _____

_____

Turning:
   Request:
      1.   To lift maximum weight in box from the floor, to turn trunk only and place it to the right at waist level and back to floor. Repeat for left side.
         A.   Performance:
            a.   Ability to: Right: Left:
            b.   Balance: Right: Left:
            c.   Endurance:

Comments: _____

_____

Balancing:
   Request:
      1.   To one-leg stand on individual legs for 30 sec. each.
         A.   Performance:
            a.   Ability: Right: _____   Left: _____
            b.   Endurance: Right: _____   Left: _____
            c.   Leg dominance: Right: _____   Left: _____

Comment: _____

_____

PHYSICAL CAPACITIES EVALUATION (*continued*)

Sitting:

With what ability is the client able to get in and out of a straight-backed chair? For an estimated period how long could he sit comfortably and with what type posture?

1. Ability to sit:
2. Ability to rise:
3. Estimated time:
4. Type of posture:

Comment: _____

_____

Standing:

What type of posture and stance does the client exhibit? Client's estimate of time he can stand.

1. Posture:
2. Stance:
3. Estimate of time:

Comment: _____

_____

Hand Grasp:

As measured with a dynamometer, the strength of the client's hand grasp.

1. Broad grasp: Right: _____   Left: _____
2. Tight grasp: Right: _____   Left: _____
3. Hand dominance: Right: _____   Left: _____

Comment: _____

_____

Standardized Tests

Standardized tests of hand function, motor ability, intelligence, learning disability, development, sensorimotor ability, and personality have been incorporated into Table 11-1 (pp. 158–167). Most information was obtained from Buros in *Mental Measurement Yearbooks*[1-6] with additional material from sources indicated in the table. The tests mentioned in the table are referred to in various chapters of this book. This table is not intended to be a complete listing of all tests used by occupational therapists.

References

1. Buros, O. K. (ed.): The Eighth Mental Measurement Yearbook. Highland Park NJ: Gryphon Press, 1978.
2. Buros, O. K. (ed.): The Seventh Mental Measurement Yearbook. Highland Park NJ: Gryphon Press, 1972.
3. Buros, O. K. (ed.): The Sixth Mental Measurement Yearbook. Highland Park NJ: Gryphon Press, 1965.
4. Buros, O. K. (ed.): The Fifth Mental Measurement Yearbook. Highland Park NJ: Gryphon Press, 1959.
5. Buros, O. K. (ed.): The Fourth Mental Measurement Yearbook. Highland Park NJ: Gryphon Press, 1953.
6. Buros, O. K. (ed.): The Third Mental Measurement Yearbook. Highland Park NJ: Gryphon Press, 1949.
7. Jebsen, R., et al.: An objective and standardized test of hand function. Arch. Phys. Med. Rehabil. 50:311, 1969.

Bibliography

Specific Procedures

Abreu, B. C. (ed.): Physical Disabilities Manual. New York: Raven Press, 1981.

Daniels, L., Williams, M., and Worthingham, C.: Muscle Testing Techniques of Manual Examination. Philadelphia: W. B. Saunders, 1980.

Joint Motion: Method of Measuring and Recording. Chicago: American Academy of Orthopaedic Surgeons, 1965.

Kellor, M., et al.: Hand strength and dexterity. Norms for clinical use, age and sex comparisons. Am. J. Occup. Ther. 25:77–83, 1971.

Moberg, E.: Emergency Surgery of the Hand. London: E. S. Livingston Ltd., 1967.

Fedretti, L. W.: Occupational Therapy, Practice Skills for Physical Dysfunction. St. Louis: C. V. Mosby, 1981.

Trombly, C. A., and Scott, A. D.: Occupational Therapy for Physical Dysfunction. Baltimore: Williams & Wilkins, 1977.

Weiss, M. W., and Flatt, A. E.: A pilot study of 198 normal children: Pinch strength and hand size in the growing hand. Am. J. Occup. Ther. 25:10–12, 1971.

Werner, J. L., and Omer, G. E.: A procedure-evaluating cutaneous pressure sensation of the hand. Am. J. Occup. Ther. 24:347–356, 1970.

Willard, H. S., and Spackman, C. S. (eds.): Occupational Therapy, ed. 4. Philadelphia: J. B. Lippincott, 1971.

General

Ayres, A. J.: Interrelationships among perceptual-motor functions in children. Am. J. Occup. Ther. 20:68–71, 1966.

Bell, E., et al.: Hand skill measurement, a gauge for treatment. Am. J. Occup. Ther. 30:80, 1976.

Brayman, S.: Measuring device for joint motion of the hand. Am. J. Occup. Ther. 25:173, 1971.

Brazelton, T. B.: Neonatal Behavioral Assessment Scale. Philadelphia: J. B. Lippincott Co., 1973.

Brown, M., Diller, L., Fordyce, W., et al.: Rehabilitation indicators: Their nature and uses for assessment. In Bolton, B., and Cook, D. (eds.): Rehabilitation Client Assessment. Baltimore: University Park Press, 1980.

Denhoff, E., et al.: Developmental and predictive characteristics of items from the Meeting Street School Screening Test. Develop. Med. Child Neurol. 10:220, 1969.

DeVore, G. L., and Hamilton, G.: Volume measuring of the severely injured hand. Am. J. Occup. Ther. 22:16, 1968.

Erhardt, R. P., Beatty, P. A., and Hertsgaard, D. M.: A Developmental Prehension Assessment for Handicapped Children. Am. J. Occup. Ther. 35:237, 1981.

Fiorentino, M.: Reflex Testing Methods for Evaluating C.N.S. Development, ed. 2. Springfield IL: Charles C Thomas, 1965.

Hasselkus, B. R., and Safrit, M. J.: Measurement in occupational therapy. Am. J. Occup. Ther. 30:429, 1976.

Hurt, S. P.: Considerations in muscle function and their application to disability evaluation and treatment—joint measurement. Am. J. Occup. Ther. (Part 1—1:209, 1947; Part 2—1:281, 1947; Part 3—2:13, 1948.)

Kendall, H. O., Kendall, F. P., and Wadsworth, G. E.: Muscles, Testing and Function. Baltimore: Williams & Wilkins, 1971.

Llorens, L.: An evaluation procedure for children 6–10 years of age. Am. J. Occup. Ther. 21:64, 1967.

MacBain, K., and Hill, R.: A functional assessment for juvenile rheumatoid arthritics. Am. J. Occup. Ther. 26:326, 1973.

McNary, H.: Keynote address—A look at occupational therapy. Am. J. Occup. Ther. 12:203, 1958.

Milani-Comparetti, A., and Gidoni, E.: Routine developmental examination in normal and retarded children. Develop. Med. Child Neurol. 9:631, 1967.

Sand, P., et al.: Hand function in children with myelomeningocele. Am. J. Occup. Ther. 28:87, 1974.

Sand, P., et al.: Hand function measurement with educable mental retardates. Am. J. Occup. Ther. 27:138, 1973.

Skerik, S. K., et al.: Functional evaluation of congenital hand anomalies, Part 1. Am. J. Occup. Ther. 25:98, 1971.

Smith, H. B.: Smith hand function evaluation. Am. J. Occup. Ther. 27:244, 1973.

Stratton, M.: Behavioral Assessment Scale of Oral Functions in Feeding. Am. J. Occup. Ther. 35:719, 1981.

Turner, A. (ed.): The Practice of Occupational Therapy. London: Churchill Livingstone, 1981.

Von Prince, K., and Butler, B.: Measuring sensory functions of the hand in peripheral nerve injuries. Am. J. Occup. Ther. 21:385, 1967.

Weiss, M. W., and Flatt, A. E.: Functional evaluation of the congenitally anomalous hand, Part 2. Am. J. Occup. Ther. 25:139, 1971.

Zimmerman, M.: The functional motion test as an evaluation tool for patients with lower motor neuron disturbances. Am. J. Occup. Ther. 23:49, 1969.

CHAPTER 12

Selected Developmental Reflexes and Reactions— A Literature Search *Gail Tower*

There are many reflex charts and references available to the interested clinical occupational therapist. The very fact that there is not yet one universally acknowledged authority indicates that the definitive word regarding reflexes has not yet been spoken. Until such time, existing reflex charts will be revised, and new ones will appear as studies are conducted and as new knowledge and insight are accumulated. This chart is a compilation of many sources representing the information felt by the author to be most helpful to beginning and practicing clinical therapists. Wherever possible and appropriate, the source of each statement is cited. When no reference is indicated, the author assumes responsibility for the accuracy and applicability of the statements.

Although some authors and clinicians differentiate among the words reflex, reaction, and elicited response, this author has made no attempt to do so; the terms are used interchangeably throughout this section.

Importance of Reflexes to the Therapist

An extensive knowledge of reflexes is important for the clinical therapist. This knowledge (1) can aid in the diagnosis of deviant or abnormal motor behavior in an infant, child, or adult; (2) will help the therapist's understanding of current treatment techniques; (3) will increase the therapist's understanding of normal movement; (4) can aid in determining chronological age in the premature infant and approximate developmental age in the older infant; and (5) may allow prognostication of future motor function in infants and children with problems.

Diagnosis of Abnormal Motor Behavior

Some normal reflexes are normally consistently symmetrical in nature and fairly easy to elicit in the infant of proper age. Examples include the Moro and the upper extremity forward protective extension reflexes. Consistent asymmetrical responses in those reflexes could indicate an orthopedic problem such as a fracture, peripheral nerve injury (such as an Erb's palsy), or a central nervous system lesion (such as hemiplegia).

Abnormality may also be expressed by failure of a given reflex or set of reflexes to develop or occur at the age when they are normally easy to obtain upon testing. This could include any of the primary reflexes which D'Argassies states are perfectly developed in a normal, full-term neonate or those that develop later like righting and equilibrium reactions.[1]

Finally, and of tremendous importance, if the simplest of all reflexes, the stretch reflex, is abnormal, other reflexes will be abnormal. If the stretch reflex is abnormal throughout the body, all reflexes will be abnormal; if the stretch reflex is only abnormal in part of the body, the related reflexes will be abnormal. (The stretch reflex contributes to muscle tone or the background state of muscle readiness which supports all movement. See the section on normal movement for further explanation of the role of the stretch reflex.) The reflexes most commonly associated with an abnormal stretch reflex are the tonic reflexes: the asymmetrical tonic neck reflex, the symmetrical tonic neck reflex, the positive support reaction, and the tonic labyrinthine reflex.* These are the reflexes that help to control and distribute muscle tone throughout the body as it is needed on a prolonged basis. It stands to reason that if the muscle tone is abnormal, then what will be seen is a distribution of abnormal tone in the particular pattern of each reflex. In nearly every case of abnormal tonic reflexes, the distribution pattern of the tone remains the same as it is when muscle tone is normal. What becomes abnormal about these reflexes, in the presence of the abnormal stretch reflex, is the extent to which they "lock" an infant into their own pattern, preventing free and easy movement out of the pattern.

However, the phasic reflexes also distribute muscle tone, in a manner of speaking, via a movement pattern. Since execution of any movement pattern is dependent upon normal background muscle tone, the phasic reflexes will also be executed abnormally, if at all, in the presence of an abnormal stretch reflex.

Reflexes and Normal Movement

Most current treatment techniques for motor disorders, such as those developed and taught by the Bobaths and Ayres, stress the importance of normal reflex activity, including normal muscle tone, for normal movement.[3-6]

One of the ultimate goals of therapy for a client diagnosed as having abnormal movement, is normal movement. Thus therapists must have an intimate knowledge of movement's ingredients and requirements if it is to be the therapeutic goal.

While current literature still refers to *voluntary* versus *reflexive* movement, Evarts has recently stressed that we must no longer look at normal movement as divided into voluntary and reflexive components.[7] This implies two quite different and distinct types of movements, and he points out that for the past decade neuroscientists have been stressing that the only voluntary aspect of movement is the intention to move.

> Reflexes and voluntary improvements are not opposites. This was recognized by Hughlings Jackson a century ago when he wrote that volitional movements are subject to the laws of reflex action. Nevertheless, if voluntary movements cannot be defined by exclusion, that is, as something that does not involve a reflex, how can it (sic) be defined? The most succinct statement I know is one put forward by the Swedish neurophsiologist Ragnar Granit in his recent book *The Purposive Brain: What Is Volitional in Voluntary Movement Is Its Purpose.*[7]

The Bobaths and Martin have contributed much to the clinical therapist's understanding of the roles of reflexes in normal movement, or what they call the normal postural reflex mechanism.[3,8] Of initial importance is the stretch reflex and the background muscle (or postural) tone to which the stretch reflex contributes. This tone must be high enough to support the human in a functional, upright, antigravity position but low enough to allow movement to occur while the individual is upright. Reflexes that help to govern the distribution of muscle (postural) tone throughout the body are referred to as the tonic reflexes, and they include the asymmetrical tonic neck reflex, the symmetrical tonic neck reflex, the positive support reflex, and the tonic labyrinthine reflex. While these reflexes are most potent and, thus, most obvious at specific ages during infancy, they remain with us throughout life, and they are most evident at times of stress or fatigue.[9-12] They are often also seen to dominate tone distribution in the brain damaged.[3,13-17]

The righting reactions are next in importance in developing the normal postural reflex mechanism and in laying the foundation for movement patterns. These allow the human to move from the horizontal, gravity, dependent position at birth to the controlled, upright position of the adult. They help align the head vertically against gravity (labyrinthine and optical righting acting on the head.). This becomes the human's usual point of reference for body movements for the duration of life. Righting reactions produce control of the body in midline positions, which must be present before controlled movement across the midline and away from the midline can occur.

---

* The tonic labyrinthine reflex is not included on the chart as there are very few sources discussing its role in human development. Animal studies indicate that in the abnormal, brain-damaged state the labyrinths distribute increased extensor tone in the supine animal and decreased extensor tone in the prone animal. In the side-lying animal, extension is increased in the underneath extremities, while flexion is increased in those extremities uppermost.[2] Bobath says the same elements are present in the child with cerebral palsy.[3]

Finally, equilibrium reactions (ERs) develop after the infant has practiced all possible movement combinations using the righting reactions. ERs include muscle tone and movement changes throughout the entire body in response to shifts in the body's center of gravity or ". . . to compensate for changes in the direction of the force of gravity."[18] Without ERs, the human being would behave like a statue in the upright position; when tipped to one side or another he or she would simply topple. The clinical therapist must always keep in mind that total body movements usually involve a shift in the center of gravity that entails an equilibrium response. Since human beings are capable of shifting their center of gravity in a variety of directions, nearly all somatic musculature must be prepared to respond when needed in an equilibrium reaction. Equilibrium reactions are both tonic and phasic in nature, and both must be present for normal movement to occur. In fact, ERs might be thought of as the very matrix of mature human movement.

Determining Age

The primary reflexes that are present at birth begin developing *in utero* and follow a definitive maturation schedule. While it is possible to use reflexes to determine the chronological age of a premature infant, Dubowitz and Dubowitz have pointed out that more accurate assessment of gestational age results from combining the evaluation of neurological signs with external physical characteristics.[19] It is beyond the scope and intent of this paper to educate the reader sufficiently for safe and accurate handling of data regarding the fragile premature infant. The reader is referred to the clinical manual by Dubowitz and Dubowitz for an excellent introduction.[19]

In determining the developmental age of an older infant through reflex testing, the therapist is urged to exercise extreme caution. The most consistent rule in child development seems to be that there is no rule governing normal development that has not been broken by dozens of normal infants. One glance at the accompanying reflex chart reveals the tremendous variation in *normal* times given by the world's experts on reflexes, most of whom have an intimate and extensive knowledge of human infants.

Prognostication

Parents of children diagnosed as abnormal are anxious to know how far their child will progress in the developmental sequence including movement potential. Bleck[20] and Capute, *et al.*,[14] have published separate studies of the relationship between reflex findings and future ambulation in children with abnormal movement. In both studies the authors reported that they were able to predict whether a child would ambulate functionally based upon the outcome of reflex testing. (Bleck reported that the prognosis was 94.5% accurate in the 73 children he studied.)

Capute, *et al.*, included four tonic reflexes in the group of seven primitive reflexes assessed. The authors pointed out that these four (the asymmetrical tonic neck reflex, the symmetrical tonic neck reflex, the tonic labyrinthine reflex, and the positive support reaction) were the only ones of the seven tested that were statistically associated with walking outcome. (The other three reflexes were derotational righting, the Moro reflex, and the Galant reflex.) It is interesting to note that all of the reflexes associated prognostically with ambulation were reflexes responsible for distributing muscle tone within the body.

Extreme care must be taken in utilizing the information just reported. All of the children studied were "older"—10 months to 21.5 years. When younger infants are followed and regularly assessed the findings may be different as Campbell's preliminary data are showing.[21] In her longitudinal study of infants at risk for central nervous system (CNS) deficit the infants are assessed initially during the neonatal period and then regularly thereafter. Five of the first seven infants studied exhibited positive tonic reflex activity at six months of age, a time thought by most to indicate CNS abnormality. Testing of the same infants at one year revealed that only one of the five could be definitely diagnosed as abnormal in movement.

It is clear that more research and age related data are needed before definitive statements can be made about the use of reflexes for prognosticating motor outcome.

Organization and Utilization of the Chart

Design of the Chart

The design is similar to that used by Milani-Comparetti and Gidoni,[22] Hoskins and Squires,[23] and Wilson,[24] all of which have been used clinically by many therapists. This chart, however, incorporates some additional parameters believed essential to accurate reflex testing and which should also help the clinical therapist design a treatment program.

Muscle Tone

Muscle tone should be assessed by the therapist before asking for movement. Neither excessively low nor excessively high tone will support movement throughout normal ranges and patterns at normal speeds.[3] Unfortunately muscle tone remains as difficult to assess objectively in a clinic as it is to define.* Passive range of motion and deep tendon reflexes are the classical and current methods of assessing muscle tone. Since normal tone encompasses a broad range, experience plays a major part in any therapist's accuracy of tone assessment.

At birth and for the first 1 to 2 months of life, the infant's extremities are normally dominated by flexor tone (physiological flexion), while the neck and trunk are generally low tone throughout. This produces a different range of motion than is seen at one year.[27] As antigravity control develops in a cephalocaudal direction, the extension component is often ahead of the flexion component (at least in the upper body) by as much as 2 months in some children. By 6 months the infant has developed good flexor and extensor control in the trunk, while the background tone in the arms is much lower than at birth and allows full active motion to occur. The legs at 6 months are able to extend against gravity in standing, giving the infant good support.[28]

Resting Postures

Resting postures are basically a reflection of the background muscle tone present in the infant at rest. When an infant is sleeping or in deep relaxation, muscle tone falls so low as to approach flaccidity. An experienced therapist can assess much from simply looking at an infant's postures. In the normal infant, no single position dominates or obligates the infant. For example, although the 2-month-old lies primarily with the head to one side or other and the arms and legs abducted away from the body, unable to function in midline, frequent head turnings and arm and leg motions (regardless of head position) demonstrate that the infant is not "trapped" in one single body alignment or posture. By 4 months the infant has achieved enough flexor control to lie with the head in the midline and to bring the hands to the midline to play with them. The legs are abducted at the hips, flexed at the knees, and the plantar surfaces of the feet frequently touch. The infant also, of course, moves in and out of this posture.

Active Movement Patterns

Active movement patterns are generally characterized as normally primitive, normally mature, or

---

* While muscle tone is classically defined as the resistance encountered when passively moving a limb[25] the reader is referred to R. Granit's recent comments concerning tone.[26]

abnormal. A typical primitive pattern is seen in the externally rotated, scissored legs of the neonate during primary walking. A typical abnormal movement pattern is seen in the internally rotated, scissored legs of the ambulatory child with spastic diplegia. A normal mature movement pattern is seen during the execution of equilibrium reactions. A detailed study of normal infants from birth until the acquisition of mature running skills is necessary to assess accurately and to categorize the gross movement patterns seen in children in the clinic.

Primary Reflexes

Primary reflexes are so characteristically perfect in the normal neonate according to S. Saint-Anne D'Argassies that they may be used to aid in diagnosing abnormality.[1] These reflexes fall into all four of the categories used to classify reflexes according to their functional purpose. The initial role of reflex activity is to support survival of the helpless being at birth (*e.g.,* rooting and sucking). Another purpose, lifelong in nature, is protection of the organism (*e.g.,* Galant, crossed extension, equilibrium reactions, and protective extension of the arms). A third group of reflexes are precursors to or necessary prerequisites of more complex movement patterns (*e.g.,* primary standing and walking, positive support, the righting reactions, the tonic reflexes, and the equilibrium reactions). A fourth purpose of reflex activity is to serve as a precursor to learning and the development of intelligence.[29] Obviously these categories are not mutually exclusive.

As can be seen from the chart, most of the primary reflexes are rapidly incorporated into more mature movement patterns, and most can no longer be easily elicited beyond the first 3 months of life.

Tone Distributing Reflexes

Tone distributing reflexes may dominate resting postures for only brief spans of time in the normal infant[30] but never do so again in the normal individual. That is not to say that they stop distributing tone, however. Roberts says that, in quadripeds at least, their role becomes more complex with development, as they begin interacting to provide trunk support in equilibrium reactions in the more mature individual.[31]

Prehensile Reactions

Prehensile reactions are obviously involved with the development of hand function. While the exact relationship between the primary grasp reflex and the mature instinctual grasp has yet to be elaborated,

Touwen feels that the diminution of the former is unnecessary for development of the latter so long as the background muscle tone is normal.[32]

Righting and Equilibrium Reactions

The righting reactions and equilibrium/protective extension reactions are the last movement oriented reflexes to emerge in the developing infant. They are critical, however, to normal, mature movement. Without ERs ambulation will be abnormal or absent. Without ERs the infant will be unable to free his arms from their initial role of supporting the trunk (in prone or sitting) thus blocking the development of fine hand control. Without practicing all possible movement patterns through the righting reactions the infant cannot develop the ERs. It is through the righting and equilibrium reactions that the infant is able to shift weight and free the extremities from weight bearing allowing controlled stepping and grasp to occur, the ultimate in the human beings ability to translate the body in space.

Of all the reflexes mentioned, the symmetrical tonic neck reflex and the tonic labyrinthine reflex are the least tested and talked about in the normal infant. Both are more frequently discussed as present in central nervous system dysfunction.[2,3,5,13-15]

An outlined description of each reflex given in Table 12-1 follows. The reflexes in parentheses following the reflex being described refer to those tested in the same way as the one presented or to a response so similar that, in the author's opinion, it tests the same area of integrity.

Tremendous variation was found in the literature regarding reflex development. Average ages, regarding the time of initial appearance (emergence) and the time when a particular response is fading out of the infant's consistent behavioral repertoire (integration), are available from most of the authorities cited in this literature search. However, the normal age suggested by one authority may vary by as much as 6 months (in the extreme case, 3 years) from the age given by another authority. The shaded areas of the profile represent the normal time cited most frequently in the literature during which the response was most consistently active. The solid arrows pointing right encompass the youngest age given when a reflex begins to fade (tail of arrow) and the oldest age for normal integration (point of arrow.) The wavy arrows pointing left include the youngest age at which a reaction begins to appear (point) and the oldest age for normal appearance (tail).

The references were selected on the basis of clinical relevance and research integrity and as occupying the time-tested position of national or international authority. It is not, however, an exhaustive list.

Grading

Grading of the chart is similar to the method employed by others.[22-24] Reflex responses should be elicited several times before passing judgment upon a grade. It is important to note that a positive reflex response at any given time is dependent upon the central state of the nervous system. In other words, the preoccupation or activity of motor neurons at the moment of testing will influence the response seen. This is vividly illustrated in neonatal testing where there are at least three factors having direct bearing upon the testing:

1. The physiological state of the infant may directly influence whether or not a response is obtained.[27,33]
2. The amount and type of analgesic or anesthetic, especially central nervous system depressants, used upon the mother during the labor-delivery process may affect the reflex response of the infant.[33,34]
3. The reflexes present in the newborn actually emerge at various times during the gestational period. Results of reflex testing will be a result of both the health and the age of the nervous system in the neonate, along with the above two factors.[19,35,36]

The grading symbols are easy to remember and record: NP refers to *normally present*, AP to *abnormally present*, (−) to *absent*, and D to *doubtful*. By recording directly upon the chart one can see at a glance whether an absent reflex is normally or abnormally absent. Further elaboration of the grades may be done at the bottom of the chart under comments.

Directions

Record the name, age of the infant (adjusted for prematurity),* and the date. Record the appropriate grade directly upon the chart using a different color pencil for each testing session. Record appropriate clarifying comments on the bottom of the chart. Generally it will be beneficial to begin observations and testing at the top of the chart and work down. Whether one tests reflexes appropriate to infants older or younger than the one currently being tested depends upon the developmental age and the abilities of the infant. If an infant is being formally tested, there is usually a problem or suspected prob-

---

* Determine the infant's chronological age by subtracting his birthdate from the date of testing, converting years to months and months to weeks as needed. Next subtract the exact number of days and weeks premature from his chronological age. This will be the infant's "actual" postconceptual age.

Table 12-1 *A Literature Search for a Profile of Selected Developmental Reflexes and Reactions*

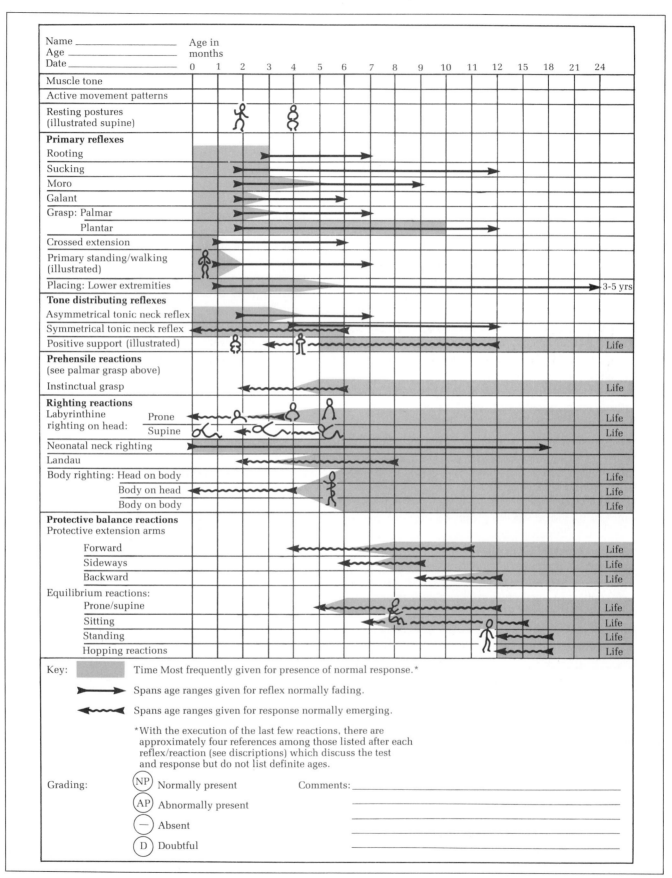

lem about which the parents are seeking information. The beginning therapist will probably want to test the entire list of reflexes (at least up to and including those listed that are age appropriate) rather than risk omitting possibly significant findings by inappropriately skipping some reflexes. The experienced therapist will know where to begin and which reflexes are important to evaluate.

Descriptions

Rooting Reflex

(Reaction of the four cardinal points)[1,17,24,33,35-45]

Procedure: Place infant supine with head in midline and hands secured against chest. Examiner uses a finger to lightly stroke the perioral skin at the corners of the mouth and the middle of the upper and lower lips.

Response: "After stimulation of the corners of the mouth, there is directed head turning towards the stimulated side. With stimulation of the upper lip there is opening of the mouth and retroflexion of the head. Following stimulation of the lower lip, the mouth opens and the jaw drops. In all instances the infant tries to suck the stimulating finger."[24]

Comments:
1. The tongue generally seeks the stimulus also.
2. This response may be difficult to elicit in satiated or occupied (crying, defecating, etc.) infants who may turn away from the stimulus.

Sucking Reflex[17,24,27,33,35,37,40,42,43,45]

Procedure: With the infant supine and head in midline, the examiner inserts a fingertip or nipple into the infant's mouth.

Response: The infant will suck vigorously and rhythmically.

Comments:
1. The soft palate is probably the most sensitive area for eliciting sucking followed by the inside of the mouth and the lips.[33]
2. Sucking may be depressed in infants whose mothers received CNS depressants during the labor-delivery process.[34]
3. Only five of the references[4,5,15,24,45] include an age of integration, and they vary from 2 months to 1 year.

Moro Reflex[1,13,15,17,20,22-24,27,32,35-40,42,43,45-51,54]

Procedure: The examiner holds the infant in a semiseated position, supporting the head in midline with one hand and the back with the other. The infant's

hands should be free, and the neck muscles should be relaxed. Let the head suddenly drop a few centimeters before stopping it or abruptly lower the whole body a few centimeters.

Response: Initially the arms abduct at the shoulders and extend at the elbows and fingers, and the back may arch. This is followed by an adduction-flexion movement back toward the midline. Response in the legs is varied depending upon their initial starting position.

Comments:
1. The Moro reflex is considered one of the most consistently seen and one of the easiest responses to elicit in a normal neonate.
2. A normal response is very sudden in nature so the test should be carried out more than once to observe all response components.
3. An absent or asymmetrical response is generally considered to be indicative of some abnormality, for example, fractured clavicle, cerebral hemorrhage.
4. A Moro reflex may be seen in response to several different stimuli. Another commonly used stimulus is to slap the table on either side of the supine lying infant's head so as to jar the head.
5. Integration occurs as control of neck flexion develops.
6. This reflex may also stimulate crying.

Galant Reflex (incurvation reflex)[1,17,24,27,37,39,42,43,45,54]

Procedure: The infant is placed in prone and the examiner runs a fingernail from shoulder to buttocks about 3 cm. lateral from the vertebral column on either side in turn.

Response: The trunk briskly curves away from the stimulus producing folds in the skin.

Comments:
1. This reflex is considered one of the most constant in the neonatal state.
2. Stimulation of the lateral portion of the trunk produces a greater response than close to the midline.

Palmar Grasp (hand grasp, tonic finger flexion, tonic grasp)[1,15,17,22,24,27,32,35-43,45,47,49,50,52]

Procedure: With the infant supine, head in midline, the examiner inserts his index fingers into the infant's hands from the ulnar side and presses against the palmar surface.

Response: The infant's fingers will strongly flex around the examiner's fingers.

Comments:
1. Sucking facilitates the response.
2. Light contact on the dorsum of the hand inhibits the response and facilitates opening of the hand: the avoidance reaction.
3. Some authorities feel this reflex must be inhibited before voluntary grasp may be developed,[39,42,45] while others feel there is no definitive relationship between the disappearance of the palmar grasp and the appearance of the voluntary grasp.[2,32]

Plantar Grasp (tonic reaction of the toe flexors, tonic plantar grasp, foot grasp)[1,16,22–24,27,37,39,40,42,43,45,50,52]

Procedure: With the infant supine the examiner presses the shaft of one finger along the metatarsophalangeal groove of the soles of the feet.

Response: There is a strong flexion of the toes as if to grasp the finger.

Comment: The response is strongest with the foot in dorsiflexion.

Flexor Withdrawal (withdrawal reflex, defense reflex)*[23,24,27,35,37,39,40,42,43,45,48,55]

Procedure: Place the infant supine with head in the midline and legs relaxed, that is, semiflexed. The examiner applies a noxious stimulus, for example, pinprick, to the sole of each foot in turn.

Response: There is abrupt flexion of the hip and knee and dorsiflexion of the foot on the stimulated side resulting in withdrawal of the leg.

Comments:
1. The response may be diminished in a normal neonate born breech with extended legs.
2. Only five of the references[23,24,37,45,48] include an age of integration.

Crossed Extension*[1,15,16,23,24,27,35,37,39,40,42,45,48,55]

Procedure: With the infant relaxed in supine, head in the midline, the examiner extends one leg, holds it down, and pricks the sole of the extended leg with a pin.

Response: There is a slow flexion of the unstimulated free leg followed by extension and finally adduction.

---

* Although ages of integration are given for these reflexes, all nociceptive and protective responses are present for life.

Primary Standing (primary righting, neonatal positive support neonatal righting)[13,15–17,22–24,35,37–40,43–45,50,54,55]

Procedure: The examiner suspends the infant vertically by supporting the trunk under the axilla. The soles of the infant's feet are then brought into firm contact with the table top.

Response: There is a general mobilization of extensor tone in the legs and trunk for partial, flat-footed weight bearing. The neonate does not, however, extend hips and knees or trunk fully as later in the positive support reaction.

Comment: An infant may continue to bear weight on his legs in this position throughout the course of development until the positive support for normal standing is fully developed. However, an infant may pass through a period referred to as astasia abasia, refusing to take any weight on the legs (astasia) or step (abasia) until the positive support emerges for standing.

Primary Walking (stepping response, spontaneous stepping, automatic walking, reflex stepping, walking reflex)[1,13,15–17,23,24,27,35,37–40,42–45,49]

Procedure: The examiner supports the infant under the arms and holds the infant in a standing, weight-bearing position on the table. Tip the trunk slightly forward and gently move the infant forward.

Response: The infant will rhythmically step, alternating legs, in a heel-toe gait. The hips and knees remain in some flexion during this walking.

Comments:
1. It is not true walking because there is little participation of the trunk and only partial weight bearing.
2. The legs may adduct or even cross in the normal neonate, but not internally rotate.
3. This may be absent in infants born of breech delivery.

Placing (proprioceptive placing, limb placement reflex, tactile placing)[1,11,13,15,17,20,23,27,35,37,39,42,43,55]

Procedure: The examiner suspends the infant vertically by supporting the trunk under the axilla. The infant is then moved so the dorsum of the foot makes contact with the under edge of a table.

Response: The infant will flex hip and knee, lifting the foot above the table, and then extend the leg, placing the foot firmly on the table top.

Comments:

1. This response is usually tested one foot at a time. If both feet are simultaneously touched, the normal infant will often place one leg before the other.
2. Vision is not required for this response. Visual placing of the limbs occurs at a later date.
3. The times reported in the literature for integration of this reflex vary from 1 month to 5 years.
4. The same reflex is present in the hands.[15,24,37,38,45,48]

Neonatal Neck Righting[15,23,37,42,43,48,49]

Procedure: Place the infant supine with head and trunk symmetrical. The examiner passively rotates the infant's head fully to one side.

Response: The trunk rotates as a whole in the direction of the head.

Comment: Some references do not distinguish between the trunk rolling as a whole seen in the neonate and young infant and the segmental rolling seen later in response to the same procedure.[37,43] Many more references are available regarding the latter response. (See Body Righting Reactions.)

Asymmetrical Tonic Neck Reflex (A.T.N.R.)[13,15,20,22−24,27,30,37,39,40,42,43,45,47,48,50,53,54,56,57]

Procedure: Place the infant supine with the head in midline, shoulders horizontal. The examiner passively laterally rotates the head to one side and holds the head in that position while observing the response. Repeat to the other side.

Response: Rotation of the head produces extension of the "face" arm and leg and flexion of the "skull" arm and leg. The legs often participate less vigorously than the arms.

Comments:

1. Infants may assume this position by actively turning their heads.
2. This response is never consistently obligatory in a normal infant.
3. There may be a response delay of many seconds in infants with CNS pathology.
4. The response may be manifested only through distribution of muscle tone which the examiner must then feel by passively moving the extremities.
5. Coryell & Cardinali[30] recently reported the greatest effect of the ATNR on the legs was during the first week of life, and the greatest effect on the arms occurred about the sixth week of life.

6. Head position affected limb mobility in that the "face" arm moved significantly more than the "skull" arm.[30]
7. This reflex is associated with the development of antigravity extension control in the neck and trunk.

Symmetrical Tonic Neck Reflex (S.T.N.R.)[15,20,22−24,37,42,45,48,54]

Procedure: Place the infant on hands and knees or prone over examiner's knees if unable to assume the quadriped position. Passively extend and flex the head.

Response: Extension of the infant's head results in extension of the arms and flexion of the legs. Flexion of the head results in flexion of the arms and extension of the legs.

Comments:

1. As with the A.T.N.R., the response may be manifested more by tone changes in the extremities than by actual movement.
2. There is a paucity of information in the literature regarding this reflex in the human. In addition, there is *considerable* variance regarding time of appearance and of integration.

Labyrinthine Righting (otolith righting, head righting)[15,17,22−24,36−40,42−45,47,48,56]

Procedure: Suspend the infant vertically, supporting under the axilla. Tilt the body anteriorly, posteriorly, and laterally to each side.

Response: The infant will right the head to vertical from all of the positions.

Comments:

1. Vision is not required so the infant may be blindfolded to eliminate its effects.
2. It is generally felt that the response is first manifested in the prone position at birth or shortly after, then in the upright by 2 to 4 months and finally in supine by about 5 to 6 months, yielding normal head control. Several of the references do not differentiate the position of the infant but generally state that the reaction begins at a given time and persists throughout life.

Landau Reflex (horizontal or prone suspension in space)[1,15,17,22−24,37,39,40,42,43,45,48,50,55,58]

Procedure: The examiner supports the infant prone in space so the trunk is resting on the examiner's hands (arms) with the infant's head and hips free of support.

Response: The head extends to above the horizontal, extensor tone in the back increases, and the back arches and the hips extend.

Comments:

1. There is great variance in the literature regarding the length of time that this response persists (past 6 to 8 months) in the normal infant.
2. The Landau reflex demonstrates the development of antigravity extension in the prone position, and it is dependent upon head righting for initiation.
3. Lack of response may be insignificant, dependent upon other test results.

Body Righting Reactions (rotative neck righting, derotative righting segmental rolling, body righting on head, body righting on body)[8,13,15,16,22,37,40,42,43,48–50,55,59]

Procedure: (a) Place the infant supine with head and body symmetrical. The examiner passively flexes the infant's leg and then adducts it across the infant's body, thereby rotating the pelvis or (b) the examiner passively rotates the infant's head to one side.

Response: Depending upon the body part passively rotated, the infant will actively, segmentally rotate the rest of the trunk, for example, in (a) above, the infant's shoulders will rotate followed by the head and in (b) above, the infant's shoulders will rotate after the head followed by the hips.

Comment: There is more reference in the literature to the righting reactions in animals than in humans[9,59] where the body righting reactions are separated into neck righting (see Neonatal Neck Righting), body righting on the body, and body righting on the head.

Positive Support[1,13,15–17,22,24,37,39,40,43,45,47,49,50,55–57]

Procedure: The examiner supports the infant under the axilla, suspends the infant vertically in space, and lowers the infant so the soles of the feet firmly contact the floor.

Response: The infant will bear full body weight with knees, hips, and trunk extended.

Comment: An infant who is pulling himself or herself to standing or is walking exhibits a positive support reaction.

Instinctual Grasp (voluntary grasp)[17,37–40,42,47,50,52,60,61,62]

Procedure: With the infant in any position in which the arms and hands are free, the examiner lightly strokes any portion of the infant's hand.

Response: The infant will grope after the stimulus and grasp it.

Comments:

1. Vision does not play a role in this response.[37,52,61] Some authorities describe visually directed grasp, which is not generally considered to be reflexive in nature.[57,62] Other authorities simply speak of the development of voluntary grasp without specifically referring to vision.[17,38–40,42,47,50,60] These references were included because there appeared to be general agreement regarding age of emergence with the references to instinctual grasp.[37,52,61]
2. As the instinctual grasp is emerging, a response can only be obtained by contacting the radial portion of the hand which results in supination.
3. Be aware of the avoiding response which is withdrawal (and opening) of the hand from a lighter contactual stimulus than the instinctual grasp requires and is part of the normal reflex repertoire of an infant. It is most easily elicited between 3 and 8 weeks of age.[61]

Protective Extension—Forward (parachute, supporting response)[1,13,15–17,20,22,23,37–40,43,46,48,50,55]

Procedure: The examiner suspends the infant horizontally in space by supporting under the axilla. The infant is lowered head first at moderate speed toward a flat surface.

Response: As the infant approaches the surface, the upper extremities are extended in front of him/her as if to break the fall. The wrists extend and fingers extend and abduct when the reflex is fully developed.

Comments:

1. Vision is not required for a positive response.
2. The functional interpretation of this reaction is that it is needed for the infant to be able to support himself in sitting. Only one authority, however, differentiated a forward response in sitting from that described above. The child is tipped forward to elicit the response rather than the downward plunge.[22]

Protective Extension—Side (lateral propping)[1,15,22,24,37,39,45]

Procedure: Place the infant on a flat surface in a symmetrical sitting position with the legs out in front and hands and arms free. Push the child on either shoulder in turn with enough force to cause the infant to lose his or her balance to either side. Guard the infant against falling in the event that the response is not developed.

Response: The infant will stop the fall by rapid abduction of the arm and extension of elbow, wrist, and fingers resulting in a weight-bearing (support) reaction against the flat surface.

Comments:

1. Many authors do not test separately from the protective extension—forward reflex for this response although five of the references state that this reaction develops later than the protective extension forward.
2. The range of the five authors was 6 to 9 months for time of emergence, so this range is used as the average time on the chart.

Protective Extension—Back (posterior propping) [15,22,24,37,39,45]

Procedure: Place the infant on a flat surface in a symmetrical sitting posture with his legs out in front and his hands and arms free. Push the infant backward with enough force to cause a loss of balance. Guard the infant against falling in the event that the response is not developed.

Response: The infant will stop the fall by rapidly extending both arms behind him, resulting in a weight-bearing (support) reaction against the flat surface.

Comment: "The full reaction is backward extension of both arms, but more frequently an element of trunk rotation comes in and the reaction is seen in one arm only."[22]

Equilibrium Reaction—Prone/Supine (balance reaction, tilting reaction) [15,16,22–24,37,45,48,63]

Procedure: Place the infant prone on a tiltboard or on a firm pillow on your lap so that he or she may be tipped from side to side. Tip the infant slowly to one side and then the other, guarding against his or her falling off.

Response: The infant's trunk will curve, concavity of the spine toward the elevated side of the lap or board, the upper arm and leg abduct and the lower arm and leg increase in support tone (extension).

Comments:

1. While this reaction is emerging, the infant may only be able to respond to a slow tilt, but when fully developed the infant should respond to a faster tilt.
2. The same reaction emerges 1 to 2 months later if the infant is tested in supine. [15,16,22–24,37,45,48,63]

Equilibrium Reaction—Sitting (balance reaction, tilting reaction) [1,15,22,24,37,45,48,63]

Procedure: Place the infant sitting symmetrically on a tiltboard. Slowly tilt the board to either side of the infant and then in an anteroposterior direction or with the infant sitting on the edge of a table or stool slip your hand under one buttock and tip his weight onto the other. Repeat to opposite side.

Response: "To lateral tilt, the body remains upright, and is flexed against the tilt with the concavity of the spine upward, the neck is flexed laterally and the head slightly rotated with the face toward the upper side. The arm and leg on the upper side are abducted while those on the lower side are adducted and extended. To anterior tilt, the body remains upright, the spine extends, and the limbs are retracted. To posterior tilt the body remains upright with the spine flexing and the arms are extended at the shoulders, elbow extended."[24]

Comments:

1. While this reaction is emerging, the infant may only be able to respond to a slow tilt, but when fully developed the infant should respond to a faster tilt.
2. A diagonal tilt backward onto either hip results in a compensatory diagonal flexion of the trunk forward.
3. The most important and initial element of response is in the trunk and head.

Equilibrium Reaction—Standing (balance reaction, tilting reaction) [15,22,24,37,45,63]

Procedure: Place the infant standing in the center of the tilt board. Tip the infant to either side and then anteroposteriorly, or with the infant standing on a firm surface place your hands on his hips and shift his weight over onto the lateral border of one foot and then repeat on other leg.

Response: To a lateral tilt the body is flexed against the tilt with the concavity of the spine upward. The upper leg is flexed and the upper arm is abducted. The lower leg is extended and strongly braced. To an anterior tilt the infant leans back, the legs extend, and the arms extend and retract. To a posterior tilt the child leans forward, legs extend, and the arms are flexed at the shoulders and extended at the elbows.[5]

Comment: While this reaction is emerging, the infant may only be able to respond to a slow tilt, but when fully developed the infant should respond to a faster tilt.

Hopping Reaction (stagger reactions, shifting reaction, see-saw reaction, balance reactions)[8,15,24,37,45,48,56,63]

Procedure: While the child stands on the floor, the examiner pushes the child forward, to the sides, and backward.

Response: The child protects himself against falling by making the appropriate correcting movements of flexion, extension, abduction, or adduction of the legs to restore his or her center of gravity.

Comment: These reactions in the legs are in a sense the lower extremity equivalent of protective extension of the arms, for example, when the center of gravity has been displaced too far and too rapidly for the trunk to bring it back over the base of support, then the base of support (legs) is rapidly moved under the center of gravity to prevent falling.

References

1. Saint-Anne D'Argassies, S.: Neurodevelopmental symptoms during the first year of life. Develop. Med. Child Neurol. 14:235–246, 1972.
2. Twitchell, T. E.: Attitudinal reflexes. In The Child with Central Nervous System Deficit, Report of Two Symposiums. Washington DC: U.S. Dept. of Health, Education, and Welfare, 1965.
3. Bobath, K.: A Neurophysiological Basis for the Treatment of Cerebral Palsy. Philadelphia: J. B. Lippincott, 1980.
4. Bobath, B.: Adult Hemiplegia: Evaluation and Treatment. 2nd ed. London: William Heinemann Medical Books Limited, 1978.
5. Bobath, K., and Bobath, B.: Cerebral Palsy in Physical Therapy Services. In Pearson, P. H., and Williams, C. E. (eds.): The Developmental Disabilities. Springfield IL: Charles C Thomas, 1972.
6. Henderson A., Llorens, L., Gilfoyle, E. et al.: The Development of Sensory Integrative Theory and Practice: A Collection of the Works of A. Jean Ayres. Dubuque, IA: Kendall/Hunt Publishing Company, 1974.
7. Evarts, E. V.: Brain Mechanisms of Movement. Sci. Am. 241:3:164–179, 1979.
8. Martin, J. P.: The Basal Ganglia and Posture. London: Pitman Publishing Co., 1967.
9. Hellebrandt, F. A., Schade, M. S., and Carns, M. L.: Methods of Evoking the Tonic Neck Reflexes in Normal Human Subjects. Am. J. Phys. Med. 41:90–139, 1962.
10. Hirt, S.: The Tonic Neck Reflex Mechanism in the Normal Human Adult. Am. J. Phys. Med. 46:362–369, 1967.
11. Ikai, M.: Tonic Neck Reflex in Normal Persons. Jap. J. Physiol. 1:118–124, 1950.
12. Waterland, J.: The Supportive Framework for Willed Movement. Am. J. Phys. Med. 46:266–279, 1967.
13. Paine, R. S., et al.: Evolution of postural reflexes in normal infants and in the presence of chronic brain syndromes. In Kopp, C. (ed.): Readings in Early Development for Occupational and Physical Therapy Students. Springfield IL: Charles C Thomas, 1971.
14. Capute, A. J., Accardo, I. F., Vining, P. G. et al.: Primitive Reflex Profile: A Pilot Study. Phys. Ther. 58:1061–1065, 1978.
15. Bobath, B.: Abnormal Postural Reflex Activity Caused by Brain Lesions. New York: Wm. Heinman Medical Books, 1975.
16. Bobath, B., and Bobath, K.: Motor Development in the Different Types of Cerebral Palsy. New York: Wm. Heinman Medical Books, 1975.
17. Fiorentino, M. R.: Normal and Abnormal Development, The Influence of Primitive Reflexes on Motor Development. Springfield IL: Charles C Thomas, 1972.
18. Baloh, R. W., and Honrubia, V.: Clinical Neurophysiology of the Vestibular System. Philadelphia: F. A. Davis, 1979.
19. Dubowitz, L. M. S., Dubowitz, V.: Gestational Age of the Newborn. Reading MA: Addison-Wesley Publishing Co., 1977.
20. Bleck, E. E.: Locomotor prognosis in cerebral palsy. Develop. Med. Child Neurol. 17:18–25, 1975.
21. Campbell, S. R.: Developmental Sequences in Infants at High Risk For Central Nervous System Dysfunction: The Recovery Process in the First Year of Life. Presented by the first author at the 3rd Annual Conference of the Michigan Association For Infant Mental Health, University of Michigan, Ann Arbor, Michigan, April 1979.
22. Milani-Comparetti, A., and Gidoni, E. A.: Routine developmental examination in normal and retarded children. Develop. Med. Child Neruol. 9:631–638, 1965.
23. Hoskins, T., and Squires, J.: Developmental assessment: A test for gross motor and reflex development Phys. Ther. 53:117–126, 1973.
24. Wilson, J.: A developmental reflex test. In Vulpe, S.: The Vulpe Assessment Battery. Downview, Toronto, Canada: National Institute for Mental Retardation, 1979.
25. Mathews, P. B. C.: Mammalian Muscle Receptors and Their Central Connections. Baltimore: Williams & Wilkins, 1972.
26. Granit, R.: Some comments on "Tone." In Granit, R., and Pompeiano, O. (eds.): Reflex Control of Posture and Movement. New York: Elsevier/North-Holland Biomedical Press, 1979.
27. Prechtl, H., and Beintema, D.: The Neurological Examination of the Full Term Newborn Infant. Spastics International Medical Publications. New York: Wm. Heinman Medical Books, 1964.
28. Bly, L.: Normal Motor Development Lecture given at the Northeastern Regional NDTA Conference, Boston, November 7, 1980.
29. Ginsburg, H., and Opper, S.: Piaget's Theory of Intellectual Development, 2nd ed. Englewood Cliffs NJ: Prentice-Hall Inc., 1979.

30. Coryell, J., Cardinali, N.: The asymmetrical tonic neck reflex in normal full-term infants. Phys. Ther. 59:747–753, 1979.

31. Roberts, T. D. M.: Reflex Balance. Nature 244:156–158, 1973.

32. Touwen, B. C. L.: A study on the development of some motor phenomena in infancy. Develop. Med. Child Neurol. 13:435–446, 1971.

33. Brazelton, T. B.: Infants and Mothers, Differences in Development. New York: Dell Publishing Co., 1969.

34. Kron, R., Stein, M., and Goddard, K.: Newborn sucking behavior affected by obstetric sedations. In Stone, L. J., Smith, H., and Murphy, L. B. (eds.): The Competent Infant, Research and Commentary. New York: Basic Books, 1973.

35. Saint-Anne D'Argassies, S.: Neurological maturation of the premature infant of 28–41 weeks gestational age. In Falkner, F. (ed.): Human Development. Philadelphia: W. B. Saunders, 1966.

36. Schulte, F. J.: Neurophysiological Aspects of Development. In Mead Johnson Symposium on Perinatal and Developmental Medicine No. 6: Biologic and Clinical Aspects of Brain Development, 1975.

37. Heriza, C., and Wilson, J.: Reflex Developmental Evaluation Research Form. Presentation, American Physical Therapy Association National Convention, New Orleans, 1976.

38. Andre, T., and Autgaerden, S.: Locomotion from pre- to post-natal life. Clin. Develop. Med., No. 24, Spastic Society Educational and Informational Unit. New York: Wm. Heinman, 1966.

39. André-Thomas, Chesni, Y., and Saint-Anne D'Argassies, S.: The Neurological Examination of the Infant. Clin. Develop. Med., No. 1. Spastics International Medical Publications. New York: Wm. Heinman, 1966.

40. Dekaban, A.: Neurology of Early Childhood. Baltimore: Williams & Wilkins, 1970.

41. Humphrey, T.: Some correlations between the appearance of human fetal reflexes and the development of the nervous system. In Progress in Brain Research 4. New York: Elsevier Publishing Co., 1964.

42. Illingsworth, R. S.: The Development of the Infant and Young Child. New York: Churchill Livingstone, 1974.

43. Peiper, A.: Cerebral Function in Infancy and Childhood. New York: Consultants Bureau, 1963.

44. Twitchell, T. E.: Normal motor development. In The Child with Central Nervous System Deficit, Report of Two Symposiums. Washington DC: U.S. Dept. of Health, Education, and Welfare, 1965.

45. Barnes, M. R., Crutchfield, A. C. A., and Heriza, C. B.: The Neurophysiological Basis of Patient Treatment Vol II: Reflexes in Motor Development. Morgantown WV: Stokesville Publishing Company, 1978.

46. Bench, J., et al.: A comparison between the neonatal sound-evoked startle response and the head drop (Moro) reflex. Develop. Med. Child Neurol. 17:18–25, 1975.

47. Caplan, F.: The First Twelve Months of Life. New York: Grossett & Dunlap, 1973.

48. Fiorentino, M. R.: Reflex Testing Methods for Evaluating CNS Development. Springfield IL: Charles C Thomas, 1965.

49. McGraw, M. B.: The Neuromuscular Maturation of the Human Infant. New York: Hafner Press, 1963.

50. Paine, R. S., and Oppe, T. S. E.: Neurological Examination of Children. Philadelphia: J. B. Lippincott, 1966.

51. Parmalee, A. H.: A critical evaluation of the Moro reflex. Pediatr. 33:773–788, 1964.

52. Seyffarth, H., and Denny-Brown, D.: The grasp reflex and the instinctive grasp reaction. Brain 71:9–183, 1948.

53. Parr, C., et al.: A developmental study of the asymmetrical tonic neck reflex. Develop. Med. Child Neurol. 16:329–339, 1974.

54. Capute, et al. Primitive Reflex Profile.

55. Rushworth, G.: On postural and righting reflexes. In Kopp, C. (ed.): Readings in Early Development for Occupational and Physical Therapy Students. Springfield IL: Charles C Thomas, 1971.

56. Twitchell, T. E.: Variation and abnormalities of motor development. In The Child with Central Nervous System Deficit, Report of Two Symposiums. Washington DC: U.S. Dept. of Health, Education, and Welfare, 1965.

57. Gesell, A., and Amatruda, C. S.: Developmental Diagnosis. New York: Harper & Row, 1974.

58. Cupps, C., Plescia, M., and Houser, C.: The Landau reaction: A clinical and electromyographic analysis. Develop. Med. Child Neurol. 18:41–53, 1976.

59. Roberts, T.: Neurophysiology of Postural Mechanisms. London: Butterworths, 1967.

60. Humphrey, T.: Postnatal repetition of human prenatal activity sequences with some suggestions of their neuroanatomical basis. In Robinson, R. J. (ed.): Brain and Early Behavior. New York: Academic Press, 1969.

61. Twitchell, T. E.: Reflex mechanisms and the development of prehension. In Connolly, K. (ed.): Mechanisms of Motor Skill Development. New York: Academic Press, 1970.

62. White, B., Castle, P., and Held, R.: Observations on the development of visually directed reaching. In Kopp, C. (ed.): Readings in Early Development for Occupational and Physical Therapy Students. Springfield IL: Charles C Thomas, 1971.

63. Weisz, S.: Studies in equilibrium reaction. J. Nerv. Mental Dis. 18:150–162, 1938.

CHAPTER 13

Assessment and Evaluation—Life Work Tasks

Maude H. Malick
and
Bonnie Sherry Almasy

Activities of Daily Living

The concept of Activities of Daily Living (ADL) has always encompassed feeding, dressing, and personal hygiene activities that are basic to an individual's independence. The loss of independence in these basic activities has a traumatic effect on body image, and they may also affect those persons associated with the patient. However, careful assessment, goal setting, planning, and training programs can be geared for accomplishment of short- and long-term goals that aim at self-sufficiency for a patient who is either temporarily or permanently disabled. Dependency in self-care is often the first sign of depression or the major cause of depression. Therefore, early recognition of patient needs and ADL training are essential, especially in acute care settings. Conversely, a chronically disabled person who can be independent in self-care activities requires far less custodial care and, thus, they can be cared for in a more independent unit in a community setting.

The traditional program of ADL has been an integral part of all occupational therapy programs no matter what the setting, disability, or age group. Assessment and training can take place in the home,

school, acute care hospital, rehabilitation center, special school, institution, long-term care agency, or nursing home. Many tests are available for self-care assessment with simple grading forms providing ready reference to the nursing and health team. Cognition and judgment should enter into the assessment process. Merely accomplishing a task does not constitute competency. In many cases simple self-help devices are useful, but they should not be used unless essential. Devices such as built up handles, attachments to faucet handles, reachers, overhead rings, and mats to anchor plates and tableware are very simple aids that can make a great difference in independence. Simple energy saving techniques and planning can also change dependence to independence. In all cases, safety should be a prime concern.

ADL in its broadest sense encompasses independence in the home, at work, and in the community. In this sense the individual should be assessed regarding ability to make judgments, function in a community setting, communicate with others, carry out acceptable social behavior, and manage his or her own lifestyle financially, socially, vocationally, and avocationally.

A grant to develop "Rehabilitation Indicators: A

Method for Enhancing Accountability" was awarded New York University Medical Center, Institute of Rehabilitation Medicine, in 1976, with Doctors Diller, Fordyce, and Jacobs as codirectors. An ADL Task Force chaired by Carl Granger, M.D., developed and explored levels of ADL performance indicating the scope of skills assessed under activities of daily living. As a result of this task force meeting and others throughout the country, rehabilitation indicators (RI), which describe a client's behavior and environment, were developed. Four types of RIs have been developed: status, activity pattern, skill, and environment. Phrases have been written to describe what clients actually do, what clients demonstrate they can do, and what clients plan to do. The field testing of this project has not yet been completed; thus a full report or description is premature.*

A health/disability scale, used to delineate the aspects of ADL function, is given in Table 13-1. In many cases substitution using strengths in one area to compensate for deficits in another area can be effective. For example, speech and communication skills can supplement writing skills.

R. M. Klein and B. J. Bell have developed an ADL scale using behavioral measurements to evaluate patient self-care skills. This scale is an objective and valid measure of ADL, and it has been shown to have a high degree of inter-rater reliability. Based on an activity analysis of self-care skills, the scale mirrors the typical breakdown of self-care activities that would be used in an occupational therapy evaluation and treatment. Each activity is broken down into separate behavioral segments, and each is rated separately. (See Fig. 13-1). The choice for rating is a simple yes or no. The clients receive either full score for

---

* Further information can be obtained from Margaret Brown, Project Coordinator, New York University Medical Center, Institute of Rehabilitation Medicine, 400 East 34th Street, New York NY 10016.

performance without human assistance, or they receive no points for any amount of dependence, excluding the independent use of adaptive equipment. This relieves the rater from having to make subjective judgments as to the amount of assistance required. The problem areas can be quickly identified. A treatment plan can easily be developed from the items that are negatively scored. The positive items then constitute an accumulation of skills that is reaching towards total independence. The client receives a score in each of six areas of self-care: dressing, bathing/hygiene, elimination, mobility, eating, and emergency telephone communication (see Fig. 13-2). All of the self-care items rated in the scale are applicable to all persons, able bodied or disabled. It is also applicable to children, although not yet standardized to age levels. Having many steps that are components of one overall behavior allows relatively slow but steady progress to be identified and plotted. This gives the client, occupational therapist, and team members a sense of accomplishment.

The statistical reliability of this test was determined using independent ratings by pairs of experienced occupational therapists and rehabilitation nurses. Each pair independently rated patients at the same point in time, and their scores were compared. There was a 92% agreement between pairs of raters for all items on all patients. This high reliability is due largely to the dichotomous (independent or dependent) rating and the careful analysis and breakdown of each activity.

Validity measurements reflect the functional abilities actually existing with each client. To measure validity, clients were contacted following discharge from a rehabilitation center. By means of a structured interview, a determination was made of the number of hours attendant care was received per week. The correlation coefficient between the Klein-Bell score at discharge and hours per week of attendant care is $-.86$ ($p < .01$). This is a consistent relationship that indicates that the lower the score on the

Table 13-1 *Health/disability scale determining illness and dependency or health and independence.*

	Internal Limitations (Basic Survival)	*External Obstacles/adaptations (Role Identification)*
Bodily functions	Self-care	Household tasks
Mobility in space	Mobility	Use of transportation
Communication	Speech, hearing, vision	Aids, equipment, devices, etc.
Social	Appropriateness and self-presentation	Social competence in confronting and using support systems
Cognitive	Orientation, problem solving, etc.	Management of personal affairs
Emotional	Tolerance of psychological stress, orientation to goals, phobias, anxiety, depression	Acting out behaviors, motivation

Shorts/Pants

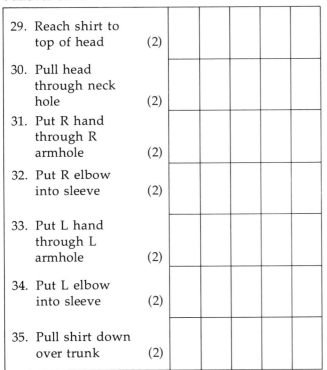

Pullover Shirt

Figure 13-1. Sample items from Klein-Bell ADL scale.

Klein-Bell ADL Scale, the greater amount of assistance is required.

This scale gives the user a reliable and valid measure of patient performance that assists in meeting many clinical, administrative, research, and educational needs. Other assessment and training techniques described by Lawton in 1963[1] are as valid today as when they were written.

Homemaker Rehabilitation

Homemakers constitute the largest group among the disabled. With current figures exceeding 10 million, it is essential both socially and economically that the rehabilitation process be utilized in helping the individual re-establish his or her place in family, home, and community. Physical rehabilitation services encompass those techniques that are instrumental in developing physical residual capabilities, whether it be by training or re-education, with emphasis on modifications of performance or task completion. The home economist introduces to rehabilitation a set of tools that can be utilized in the development of a comprehensive homemaker rehabilitation program.

The recent metamorphosis of "homemaking" into "homemaker rehabilitation" has necessitated a broadening of the definition to be in tune with the emerging holistic concerns of rehabilitation. It is essential in any program to incorporate methods for coping with the individual's physical, personal, and social needs while putting emphasis on promoting self-integration as well as integration into family and society.

The rehabilitation process must include provisions for the personal and social needs, goals, and resources of each potential homemaker. According to Switzer[2]:

> Homemaking activities—whether carried out by men, women or children—contribute to the welfare and stability of the family and to its economic productiveness and well-being. Homemaking itself is a composite of physical tasks, managerial functions, spirit, emotional climate that holds the family or personality together and fosters development. Damage to this process at any point weakens its total capacity to function. Where possible, the damage must be repaired; where this is not possible, other measures must be taken. Perhaps the environment can be changed so that the function can continue; perhaps the other areas of the complex must be brought to greater prominence and use; perhaps the very depths of personality must be touched and a new role learned.

The Rehabilitation Act of 1973 and the Social Services Act of 1974 emphasize the pertinence and urgency of developing comprehensive programs for enabling the homebound individual to realize his or her potential. Homemaking is now a viable occupation and should be considered as such when funding is necessary for implementing the rehabilitation process. Schwab[3] says disabled homemakers with a recent rehabilitation experience exhibit positive changes in self-perception in relation to household

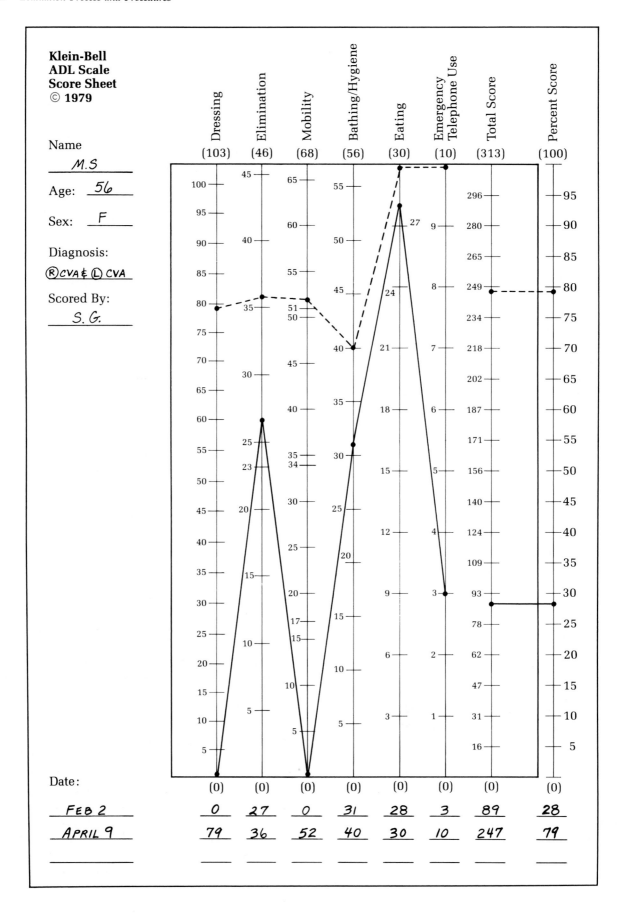

**Klein-Bell
ADL Scale
Score Sheet
© 1979**

Name

M.S

Age: 56

Sex: F

Diagnosis:

Ⓡ CVA & Ⓛ CVA

Scored By:

S. G.

Date:	Dressing (103) (0)	Elimination (46) (0)	Mobility (68) (0)	Bathing/Hygiene (56) (0)	Eating (30) (0)	Emergency Telephone Use (10) (0)	Total Score (313) (0)	Percent Score (100) (0)
FEB 2	0	27	0	31	28	3	89	28
APRIL 9	79	36	52	40	30	10	247	79

tasks. The self-respect and self-confidence derived from this experience can transfer to other activities, which may make the individual more productive, even in terms of competitive employment.

The 1978 amendments to the Rehabilitation Act of 1973 established Title VII "Comprehensive Services for Independent Living." The Independent Living (IL) Center programming is administered by the state vocational rehabilitation agencies. They provide the following:
1. a grant program for IL centers;
2. an IL program for older blind persons;
3. a protection and advocacy program to guard the rights of severely disabled persons.

The goal of Centers for Independent Living is to assure the provision of services to severely handicapped persons so they may live more independently in family and community and/or so they may secure and maintain appropriate employment with the maximum possible degree of self-direction.

Homemaking programs traditionally have encompassed the teaching and assessment of basic work skills. These programs include the utilization of work simplification techniques to promote time and energy conservation concurrently providing therapeutic exercise, teaching the use of prostheses or orthotic equipment, promoting psychological gains through satisfactory performance, and assisting constructive planning for home adjustment. However, a homemaker by definition is "one who manages his or her own household." Thus the inclusion of the management factor in the process of homemaker training is essential. Educational programs that aid the homemaker in developing managerial expertise

◄ **Figure 13-2.** A section of the Klein-Bell ADL Scale. The graph depicts Klein-Bell ADL Scale scores for a client who sustained bilateral CVAs.

M.S. is a 56-year-old female who sustained a right internal capsule CVA with resulting left hemiparesis. Two weeks after this event she underwent her initial ADL evaluation. Nine days after that evaluation she sustained a second CVA, this time the left hemisphere with resulting right hemiparesis and dysarthria. The scores presented represent only her initial and final evaluations. Her ADL score decreased after the second CVA, however, she steadily improved and was discharged to her home with a companion/attendant.

An instructional video-tape with scales and manual for scoring is available from: Distribution, Health Sciences Learning Resources Center, T-245 Health Science Building, SB-56, University of Washington WA 98195.

strengthen the entire rehabilitation process. Although the actual managerial processes remain unchanged, disability may alter the individual's goals or resources and the demands on those resources.

Management is the means by which an individual uses available assets to accomplish a goal. The concept is easy for the disabled homemaker to comprehend as well as implement. As an essential part of the rehabilitation team, the homemaker is responsible for assisting in the development of her own program and, primarily, for setting her own goals.

Management means not only the performance of tasks but also control. It is essential that the homemaker does not feel out of control.

Physical or mental disability necessitates many changes. Because of accident or illness the homemaker may have to cope with changes that are out of his or her realm of control, and he or she may be unable to set realistic goals freely. It is the therapist's role to assist the homemaker in using management skills to bring about the change in an orderly way. This involves the homemaker's adapting to alternatives and finding outside resources in the family. Although functioning may be limited in one area, resources can be channeled in new directions. Tasks do not need to be limited to one member of the family. All family resources must be considered when faced with decision making.

Sometimes the disabled homemaker is so distraught by the changes in herself/himself that he/she may bypass an essential step in the decision-making process and therefore must be given guidance. The process involved in decision making is relatively simple. It is as follows:
1. State the problem.
2. Seek and explore alternatives.
3. Discuss possible solutions.
4. Choose one alternative.
5. Accept the responsibility for the decision made.

The working through of this process provides the family with a better communication system, which in turn leads to greater satisfaction with the ultimate decision.[4]

The managerial aspects of the homemaker training program necessarily affect all other areas of concentration. Possessing rehabilitative skills, the homemaker needs to explore all areas in which he or she will be involved, either as a participant or as a manager. The rehabilitation home economist is trained specifically in these areas, which so frequently elude the therapist. With a strong background of knowledge in family relationships, foods and nutrition, clothing and textiles, child development, equipment, family economics, home management and housing, the home economist proves to be an essential member of the rehabilitation team and one who can be instrumental in the development of a truly comprehensive homemaker rehabilitation program.

Today's homemaker rehabilitation programs have grown and expanded in many new and exciting directions, all aimed towards the goal of producing home managers who are functioning to their capacity in all areas. Among the most important areas of concentration is the fulfillment of nutritional needs. This includes basic food preparation skills with emphasis on planning, purchasing, and serving nutritious meals that meet all dietary needs. Assistance with financial management, and information on budgeting, spending, and saving can be incorporated in the basic program. Selection, care, and adaptation of clothing is yet another facet of the program that can make the handicapped homemaker a more effective and efficient home manager. Child care can consume a good portion of the homemaker's day. With instruction on purchasing functional equipment and clothing as well as techniques regarding actual feeding, dressing, and bathing of children, the handicapped homemaker can resume many tasks that previously were allocated to other family members or to hired help.

Today's homemaker training programs are the keystone in the structure of rehabilitation that enables the disabled person to build a new life with an emphasis on ability and not disability.

Recording and Scoring of Function in ADL and Homemaking

Because the entire rehabilitation process is directed towards change in the total patient profile—change in attitude, ability, activity, awareness, and aptitude for the program—it is necessary to record changes and use these records in the upgrading of the client's program. It is essential to establish a scale of performance and a code for noting the levels of performance before an evaluation begins. There are potentially as many scales and codes as there are therapists. Experimentation may be necessary to find one that is flexible and functional for use in various treatment settings. However, all therapists in a department should use the same recording system, or patients functioning at the same level may receive differing reports from various therapists. This can be confusing, especially when reporting to other treatment departments. Several ADL and homemaking charts

with codes are included as examples (Figs. 13-3 to 13-6).

In order to note a change, a baseline, that is, a point of reference or the initial evaluation, is needed. It is from this that the program develops. The information gleaned from the initial evaluation should be used in setting the goal towards which the therapist and patient will be working. The general levels of functioning, tolerance, and attitude are to be determined. Once a program is established, it is of paramount importance to note daily changes and periodic differences in levels of improvement. These are easily coded and marked on the scales. A progress chart frequently provides some motivation for the patient as a visual and concrete indication that he or she is improving.

Daily reports often take the form of short notes that include activity performed; level of success; tolerance; attitude; pertinent observations including physical limitations such as perceptual, visual, and hearing deficits; use of adapted or standard equipment; ability to solve problems, read, and follow directions; mental reliability (*e.g.*, disorientation or hallucination); and general method of approaching the activity (*e.g.*, precise or careless). Positive or negative changes noted on the chart are indicators of a need for program adaptation. Retraining may be indicated or, possibly, the program may need to be accelerated. It often is helpful for the family to see the coded scales when the therapist explains alterations in the program. Carry-over on home visits generally is greater when the family is aware of the exact level of functioning that can and should be expected.

Not all information relating to progress or condition can be included on a checklist based on observations or testing. Many factors not able to be coded and scaled will influence the patient's performance. These should not be neglected. Each chart should include space for impressions and subjective observations. Records should be accurate and concise, but they should contain all pertinent information. The treatment goals should be noted. In most cases the physician will make referrals indicating general treatment procedures.

The final report, usually a discharge summary, should include the results of the initial evaluation, the treatment procedures, the results of the final evaluation, the final level of functioning, the achievement of goals, prognosis, and recommendations for maximal carry-over upon discharge. This final report often goes to the sponsoring agency and to agencies that may be working with the patient on an out-patient or home program.

(*Text continues on page 202*)

ACTIVITIES OF DAILY LIVING EVALUATION

NAME: _____ AGE: _____ CASE #: _____

DIAGNOSIS: _____ PRECAUTIONS: _____

CODE

PERFORMANCE SCALE

I   *Independent*—Patient can accomplish activity consistently without assistance or supervision.

A   *Assistance*—Patient can accomplish activity with some level of physical assistance.
A-1   Assistance Minimum
A-2   Assistance Moderate
A-3   Assistance Maximum

S   *Supervision*—Patient requires supervision of another person due to either physical or mental limitations.
S-V   Verbal Cueing
S-G   Gestural Cueing
S-P   Physical Cueing

D   *Dependent*—Patient unable to help in activity.

PLACE OF ACTIVITY

C   Regular Chair
W   Wheelchair
B-1   Bed—Sitting on edge
B-2   Bed—Sitting up
B-3   Bed—Supine

TIME

N   Within normal limits
X   Excessive

THERAPIST:

DATES	Perf.	Place	Time	Perf.	Place	Time	Perf.	Place	Time	COMMENTS (EQUIP.)
UPPER TRUNK & ARMS										
SHIRT/BLOUSE—ON/OFF										
BRA/UNDERSHIRT—ON/OFF										
SWEATER/COAT—ON/OFF										
SPLINT/PROSTHESIS—ON/OFF										
LOWER TRUNK, LEGS & FEET										
TROUSERS/SLACKS—ON/OFF										
SHORTS/PANTIES—ON/OFF										
SOCKS/HOSE—ON/OFF										
SHOES—ON/OFF										
PROSTHESIS/ORTHOSIS—ON/OFF										
SHOE LACES										
MISC. ARTICLES										
FEEDING										
PERSONAL HYGIENE										

Figure 13-3. From the Harmarville Rehabilitation Center, Pittsburgh PA. Reprinted with permission.

(Illustration on facing page.)

Figure 13-4. Code used when stating goals for homemaker evaluation. Goals are established after the patient has been interviewed and is seen working in the area. At the time of discharge from the area, it is determined whether or not he has reached the set goal.

A Independent Homemaker—Patient appears capable of performing all homemaking activities without assistance or supervision.

B Independent Light Homemaker—Patient appears capable of performing all light homemaking activities without assistance or supervision.

C Good Partial Homemaker—Patient appears capable of performing most light homemaking activities independently. May require assistance with some heavier or very complex tasks.

D Partial Homemaker—Patient appears capable of performing some light homemaking activities independently or with minimal assistance with heavy or complex activities. May be limited in performing certain activities by physical inadequacy.

E Partial Homemaker with Assistance—Patient appears capable of performing many light homemaking activities but requires assistance in at least one aspect of most of these activities. May be limited by tolerance or mental ability.

F Partial Homemaker with Supervision—Patient appears to require general supervision while performing most homemaking activities but physically performs well.

G Simple Partial Homemaker—Patient appears capable of performing simple, repetitive homemaking activities without supervision or assistance. May need to be set up at an activity but able to follow through.

H Simple Partial Homemaker with Supervision—Patient appears to require supervision to perform even simple repetitive tasks.

I Not Feasible—Patient did not appear capable of working on a homemaking evaluation at the time as a result of either physical or mental insufficiency.

J Incomplete—Homemaking evaluation had been initiated but not completed because of medical problems, early discharge, or referral to another program.

K Refused—Patient was referred to the Homemaking area for an evaluation but refused to attend the program.

From the Harmarville Rehabilitation Center, Pittsburgh PA. Reprinted with permission.

HOMEMAKING EVALUATION AND TREATMENT

Name: Age: Date Referred:

Address: Visual Difficulty:

Disability:

Mobility Status:_____independent_____W/C_____cane_____crutches_____walker

Dominant Hand: R   L   Limitations:

Goal: Special Diet:

Discharge Plans:

Household members and ages:
1.
2.
3.
4.
5.

Available help within or outside of family:

Description of home or apartment: _____floors _____stairs _____rooms

Are bath facilities functional? _____kitchen facilities functional? _____
(X) Patient formerly responsible for:

( ) Patient wants to return to doing:

( ) ( ) Food preparation
( ) ( ) Serving and cleaning
( ) ( ) Washing dishes
( ) ( ) Grocery shopping
( ) ( ) Meal planning
( ) ( ) Budgeting
( ) ( ) Child care
( ) ( ) Bed making   SKETCH PROBLEM AREA
( ) ( ) Laundry—facilities in home _____
( ) ( ) Ironing
( ) ( ) Cleaning
( ) ( ) Sewing

Special problems:

Special interests:

Patient's attitude toward homemaking:

Family's attitude toward patient's role as homemaker and toward family help:

Figure 13-4. (Legend on facing page)

HOUSEHOLD ACTIVITIES PERFORMANCE EVALUATION

MEAL PREPARATION ACTIVITIES	Perf.	Place	Time	Perf.	Place	Time	Perf.	Place	Time	Perf.	Place	Time	Perf.	Place	Time	COMMENTS Equip. & Devices
DATE																
1. Turn on water																
2. Turn on stove																
3. Pour hot liquid																
4. Open package																
5. Open jars																
6. Use can openers																
7. Use refrigerator																
8. Bend to low cupboards																
9. Reach high cupboards																
10. Peel vegetables																
11. Use sharp tools																
12. Measures																
13. Use oven																
14. Use range																
15. Stir against resistance																
16. Use electric mixer																
17. Cut with shears																
18. Read directions																
19. Follow directions																
MEAL SERVICE																
1. Set and clear table																
2. Carry items to table																
3. Wash dishes																
4. Dry dishes																
5. Clean area																
6. Wring out dishcloth																
CLEANING ACTIVITIES																
1. Retrieve objects from floor																
2. Wipe up spills																
3. Make bed																
4. Use dust mop																
5. Vacuum																
6. Use dust pan																
7. Clean bathtub																
8. Sweep with broom																
9. Dust high surfaces																
10. Dust low surfaces																
11. Clean refrigerator																

HOUSEHOLD ACTIVITIES PERFORMANCE EVALUATION (*continued*)

LAUNDRY ACTIVITIES	Perf.	Place	Time	Perf.	Place	Time	Perf.	Place	Time	Perf.	Place	Time	Perf.	Place	Time
1. Sort clothes															
2. Wash lingerie															
3. Iron															
4. Fold clothes															
5. Set up board															
6. Use washing machine															
SEWING ACTIVITIES															
1. Thread needle															
2. Make a knot															
3. Sew buttons															
4. Use machine															
5. Diversional activity															
MARKETING ACTIVITIES															
1. Make out list															
2. Put groceries away															
CHILD CARE ACTIVITIES															
1. Bathe															
2. Dress															
3. Feed															

CODES

Performance
X—unnecessary
A—independent
B—with assistance
C—impossible
D—training needed

Place
W—wheelchair
O—ambulatory
Θ—ambulatory with
  assistive devices

Time
N—within normal limits
X—excessive

Figure 13-5. From Harmarville Rehabilitation Center, Pittsburgh PA. Reprinted with permission.

HOMEMAKING FOLLOW-UP QUESTIONNAIRE

Please complete and return this form in the enclosed, stamped, self-addressed envelope.

1. What are your present living arrangements? (where and with whom)

2. Have you made any changes to your home since you left the Rehabilitation Center? (grab bars, ramp, moved)

3. Did you make any changes before leaving the Center?

4. Are there any changes that need to be made in your home that we can assist you with?

5. Do you do most of your work from the wheelchair, with a walker, crutches, quad cane, conventional cane, or walking independently?

   What were you using when you left the Rehabilitation Center? _____

   _____

		ALWAYS	SOMETIMES	NEVER
6.	Do you prepare your own meals?	_____	_____	_____
7.	Do you do your own dishes?	_____	_____	_____
8.	Do you do your own dusting?	_____	_____	_____
9.	Do you do your own vacuuming?	_____	_____	_____
10.	Do you do your own mopping?	_____	_____	_____
11.	Do you do your own laundry?	_____	_____	_____
12.	Do you fold the laundry?	_____	_____	_____
13.	Do you do your own bedmaking?	_____	_____	_____

14. List any other homemaking activities that you do. _____

   _____

15. Do you use any special homemaking equipment, such as spike board, rubber placemat, etc? _____

16. Could you benefit from the use of any equipment you had used in the Homemaking area at the Rehabilitation Center? _____ Which ones? _____

17. Do you receive help with any of your homemaking activities?
    Which jobs? _____
    How often? _____
    By whom? _____

18. What is the most difficult homemaking activity that you try to do?

19. Do you receive help for any of your personal care?

    What type? (Grooming, dressing, bathing, toilet, eating, etc.)

    How often? _____
    By whom? _____

HOMEMAKING FOLLOW-UP QUESTIONNAIRE (continued)

20. Are you presently receiving services from a community agency? _____
If yes, which one: (VNA, Home Health Care, Outpatient Treatment)

21. Are you on a special diet? _____
If so, what kind? _____
Have you lost weight? _____ If so, how much? _____
Have you gained weight? _____ If so, how much? _____

22. What activities are you involved with outside your home: (such as shopping, visiting, driving, church or other)

23. Are you satisfied with the progress you have made since leaving the Center? Comments.

24. Would a home visit from one of our Rehabilitation Home Economists be of help to you now? _____
For what purpose?

25. Do you have any questions, comments, or special problems?

Name:
Address:
Phone:

Figure 13-6. From Harmarville Rehabilitation Center, Pittsburgh PA. Reprinted with permission.

Case Study

Susan A. is a spry, spunky, 82-year-old widow. She had been living alone in a high rise for the elderly not far from the business district of a small milltown in Pennsylvania. Although she has had two strokes, the most recent 1½ years ago, and has a history of heart trouble, she has returned to independent living following a 6-week stay at a comprehensive rehabilitation center.

Susan tells her story:

"I was always a busy lady, active with my family and at church. My husband was hurt badly in a mill accident just after we were married. We had to live some way, so I turned our house into a guest home. My whole life was spent making people comfortable and happy. It wasn't easy. I've had heart trouble for about 30 years now and then I got a stroke on my left side about 18 years ago. My daughter died of rheumatic heart disease. She left a wonderful husband and two sons. The boys still see me often and send money if I need it.

"After my husband died, about 10 years back, I sold the house and moved into this apartment near my sisters. The place is really nice—we have elevators, a laundry room, even grab bars in the bathroom for us old folks.

"Just over a year ago, I fell down getting out of bed. By crawling across the floor, I finally got to the phone for help. An ambulance took me to the hospital. It was another stroke, on the left side again. I could shrug my shoulder but couldn't move my hand at all. Two people had to hold me to let me walk. For the first time I was really afraid. There was no one who could take care of me and I surely couldn't do much for myself. Although I could feed myself a little I couldn't fix my hair or put on my bra, panties, or slacks. Couldn't tie my shoes either. Housework was unthinkable with one hand. I thought they'd make me go to some home for old people. Just to get better and go back to my apartment was all I wanted.

"My doctor thought I could make some progress at a rehabilitation center. I'm sure glad I went. They had special groups for discussion about strokes. I got to talk to a lot of people who were in the same shape as I was. They gave me therapy on my arm and showed me how to walk with a cane. A lady from ADL worked with me and showed me how to dress and feed myself. I got my hair cut on beauty shop day so I could take care of it myself.

"One of my other classes was homemaking. I told them I didn't need any cooking lessons, but they showed me how to cook my favorite meals with one hand, even how to peel potatoes. I was supposed to be on a 2 gram sodium diet, but I had never followed it because I didn't know what it was. At homemaking they showed me how to eat what I like and still stay on my diet. I learned lots of tricks too, so I wouldn't get so tired doing my work. I used to think it was lazy to sit to work but it's just plain smart!

"I never had much money. I was a regular tightwad. The rehabilitation home economist showed me how to save money in many ways. Now I have a little left over to save for my old age. We went grocery shopping too. My sisters thought it was too hard for me to walk and push a cart too, but I did it.

"The therapists got me in pretty good shape at the rehabilitation center but I was still a little leery about going home to stay by myself. Oh, I wanted to but, with my stroke, wasn't sure I could. My sisters wanted me to move in with them, but at my age it's better to live by yourself.

"The rehabilitation center had an apartment right in the building. I didn't want to stay there; my doctor had other ideas. I think he thought I couldn't do it—I showed him. I stayed there just like I was at home by myself. I washed and dressed myself, took my pills, made the bed, cooked my meals, did laundry, and dusted around the apartment. I did my exercises and had my social worker in for tea. I thought I could do it, but it sure gave me confidence to know for sure. It gave me a real big lift—I was ready to go home.

"My sisters insisted that I get meals-on-wheels. I did for a few weeks, but the food wasn't so hot. I started cooking on my own again. The spikeboard I made in occupational therapy was a big help.

"After I was home for a few weeks the homemaking therapist came to see me. She brought the long-handled sponge and long shoehorn I had asked for. She showed me how to arrange things in the kitchen to make it easier for me to reach. I showed her how I fixed my calendar so I don't get mixed up about when to take my pills. I learned how to get in the tub at the center so I bought those stick-on flowers so I don't slip. I think the therapist was surprised at how well I was doing. Guess I surprised myself too."

Six months later Susan was evaluated on an out-patient visit. Because of her persistence in doing the prescribed exercises and wearing her cock-up splint, she was gaining function in her left hand. Ambulation status was independent. She reported actively participating in apartment activities and utilizing Adult Services for transportation to visit and shop. Figure 13-7 shows Susan's chart.

OCCUPATIONAL THERAPY DEPT.—ADL PROGRAM

NAME _S. A._ Independent _✕_ blue

Admitted _1-8-82_ Some Help _////_ yellow

Discharged _2-10-82_ All Help _XXXX_ red

	1-8-82	1-15-82	1-23-82	2-1-82		
Comb Hair	////	✕	✕	✕	✕	
Brush Teeth	✕	✕	✕	✕	✕	
Shave						
Dress Self						
Undershirt—bra	XXX	////	////	✕	✕	
Shirt	////	✕	✕	✕	✕	
Shorts—Pants	////	////	////		✕	
Trousers	////	////	////	////	✕	
Dress	////	✕	✕	✕	✕	
Socks—Stockings	////	////	✕	✕	✕	
Shoes	////		✕	✕	✕	
Ties Laces	XXX	////	////	////	✕	
Braces						
Feed Self	////	////	✕	✕	✕	
Cut Meat	XXX	XXX	////	✕	✕	

Figure 13-7. Sample form for case study.

Discharge Summary

Mrs. Susan A was referred to the Occupational Therapy Department for a homemaking evaluation by Dr. Jones. She was initially seen in the area in her wheelchair and progressed to ambulation with a one-point cane. Balance appeared good. Tolerance was within normal limits. She appeared alert and oriented to time, person, and place. She was pleasant, cooperative, and very well-motivated to work in the area and to resume independent living.

GOAL: Good partial homemaker. This goal was achieved.

Mrs. A's program included:

1. Vegetable preparation—used spikeboard safely and appropriately.
2. Food preparation—successfully read and followed directions, opened packages, used range, oven, and refrigerator while ambulating.
3. Dishwashing—worked with no apparent difficulty from standing position.
4. Bedmaking—balance and tolerance appeared good. Works neatly and efficiently.
5. Vacuuming—difficulty was noted when patient attempted to move furniture.
6. Laundry—effectively used coin operated facilities.
7. Received instruction in work simplification techniques and management principles. Comprehension appeared good.
8. Received instruction on 2 gm. Na diet and meal planning.
9. Completed 48 hour apartment living experience with excellent results.

Mrs. A was discharged from the program on 2/10/82. At this time she appeared capable of living independently in her apartment in a high rise for the elderly. She will receive homemaker services once every 2 weeks to assist with heavy homemaking tasks. She appeared determined to utilize skills developed in program. A home visit is planned for 2 weeks post-discharge. She will be seen for outpatient evaluation at 3-month intervals.

Jane Doe
Rehabilitation Home Economist

INITIAL INTERVIEW: 1/17/82
DATE DISCONTINUED: 2/10/82
THERAPY SESSIONS: 20
EQUIPMENT: Long sponge, rubber mat, spikeboard □

References

1. Lawton, E. B.: Activities of Daily Living for Physical Rehabilitation. New York: McGraw-Hill, 1963.
2. Switzer, M. W.: Foreword. In Rehabilitation of Physically Handicapped in Homemaking Activities. Proceedings of a Workshop, Highland Park IL, 1963. U.S. Department of Health, Education and Welfare.
3. Schwab, L. O.: Self Perception of Physically Disabled Homemakers. Ed.D. Thesis, University of Nebraska, 1966.
4. Gross, I., and Crandall, E. W.: Management for Modern Families. New York: Appleton-Century-Crofts, 1963.

Bibliography

Abreu, B. C.: Physical Disabilities Manual. New York, Raven, 1981.

After A Stroke: Patient and Family Guide. Pittsburgh: Harmarville Rehabilitation Center, Inc., 1981.

Barrier-Free Site Design. HUD Publication, 1976. Available from Superintendent of Documents, U.S. Government Printing Office, Washington DC.

Barton, D. H.: Self-help clothing. Harvest Years, March 19–23, 1973.

Beppler, M. C., and Knoll, M. M.: The disabled homemaker: Organizational activities, family participation, and rehabilitation success. Rehab. Lit. 35:200–206, 1974.

Bertelsen, J.: Small Group Homes for the Handicapped and Disabled: An Annotated Bibliography. U.S. Department of Housing and Urban Development, 1977.

Bowe, F.: Rehabilitating America: Toward Independence for Disabled and Elderly People. Harper & Row, 1980.

Bryce, T. E.: A home economist on the rehabilitation team. Am. J. Occup. Ther. 23:258–262, 1969.

Clothes for the Physically Handicapped Homemaker. Washington DC: Agricultural Research Service, U.S. Department of Agriculture, Home Economic Research Report #12, June 1971.

Clothing for Wheelchair Users, 1971. Disabled Living Foundation, 346 Kensington High Street, London W14.

Clothing for the Incontinent Older Child, 1972. Disabled Living Foundation, 346 Kensington High Street, London W14.

Cole, J. A., et al.: New Options. Houston: TIRR, 1979.

Cole, J. A., et al.: New Options Training Manual. Houston: TIRR, 1979.

Davis, W. M.: Aids to Make You Able, ed. 2. Fred Sammons, 1979.

Diffrient, N., Tilley, A. R., and Bardagiy, J. C.: Humanscale 1/2/3. Designer: Henry Dreyfuss Associates. Cambridge MA: M.I.T. Press, 1974.

El-Ghatit, Z., Melvin, J. L., and Poole, M. A.: Training apartment in community for spinal cord injured patients: A model. Arch. Phys. Med. & Rehab. 61:90–92, 1980.

Frieden, L.: Independent Living Models. Rehab. Lit. July–August:169–173, 1980.

Frieden, L., Richards, L., Cole, J., and Bailey, D.: A glossary for independent living. ILRU Sourcebook: A Technical Assistance Manual on Independent Living. Houston: TIRR (Institute for Rehabilitation and Research), 1979. Vol. 41, July–August, 1980.

Friend, S. D., Saccagnine, J., and Sullivan, M.: Meeting the clothing needs of handicapped children. J. Home Economics, May, 1973.

Frith, G. H.: The use of professionals in achieving independent living for severely handicapped persons. Rehab. Lit. 42:18–20, 1981.

Garee, B.: Ideas for Making Your Home Accessible. Bloomington IL: Accent Special Publishers, 1979.

Goldsmith, S.: Designing for the Disabled, ed. 2. New York: McGraw-Hill, 1967.

Harkness, S. P., and Groom, J. N., Jr.: Building Without Barriers for the Disabled. The Architect Collaborative Inc., Whitney Library of Design, Cambridge MA, 1976.

Harmarville Rehabilitation Center, Inc. Handicapped Homemaker Follow-Up Study. P.O. Box 11460, Guys Run Road, Pittsburgh PA 15238, 1972.

Hirschber, G., Lewis, L., and Vaugham, P.: Rehabilitation: A Manual for the Care of the Disabled and Elderly, ed. 2. Philadelphia: J. B. Lippincott, 1976.

I.C.T.A. Information Center, Bromma, Sweden.

Jay, P.: Help Yourselves; A Handbook for Hemiplegics and Their Families, ed. 3. Jan. Henry Pubs., 1979.

Klein, R. M., Bell, B. J.: Self Care Skills: Behavioral Measurement with the Klein-Bell ADL Scale. Arch. Phys. Med. Rehab. In press.

Kliment, S. A.: Into the Mainstream: A Syllabus for a Barrier-Free Environment. Prepared under a grant to the American Institute of Architects by the Rehabilitation Services Administration of the Department of

Health, Education, and Welfare, Washington DC, 1975.

Klinger, J. L.: Self Help Manual for Arthritic Patients. New York: The Arthritis Foundation, 1974.

Klinger, J. L., Friedman, F. H., and Sullivan, R. A.: Mealtime Manual for the Aged and Handicapped. New York: Simon and Schuster, 1970.

Knoll, C. S., and Schwab, L. O.: The outlook for homemaking in rehabilitation. J. Home Economics, Jan:39–41, 1974.

Krusen, F. H.: Handbook of Physical Medicine and Rehabilitation. Philadelphia: W. B. Saunders, 1971.

Lifehez, R., and Winslow, B.: Design for Independent Living: The Environment and Physically Disabled People. Watson-Guptill Publishers, 1980.

Lowman, E. W., and Klinger, J. L.: Aids to Independent Living: Self Help for the Handicapped. New York: McGraw-Hill, 1970.

Making Facilities Accessible to the Physically Handicapped. Albany: New York State University Construction Fund, 1974.

Malick, M.: Manual on Dynamic Hand Splinting. Pittsburgh PA: Harmarville Rehabilitation Center, 1978.

Malick, M.: Manual on Static Hand Splinting. Pittsburgh PA: Harmarville Rehabilitation Center, 1979.

May, E. E., Waggoner, N. R., and Hotte, E. B.: Independent Living for the Handicapped and the Elderly. Boston: Houghton, Mifflin Co., 1974.

McHugh, H. F.: The 1977 Family as Consumers. J. Home Economics, January, 1977.

Mondale, W. F.: Government policy, stress and the family. J. Home Economics, November, 1976.

Morgan, M.: Beyond disability: A broader definition of architectural barriers. A/A Journal 65:50–54, 1976.

National Center for Health Statistics. Use of Special Aids, United States, 1977. Hyattsville, Maryland: U.S. Dept. of Health and Human Services, 1980.

Nau, L.: Why not family rehabilitation? J. Rehabil. 39:14–17, 1973.

Newton, A.: Clothing: A rehabilitation tool for the handicapped. J. Home Economics, April:2, 1973.

Nichols, P., and Hamilton, E. A.: Rehabilitation Medicine: The Management of Physical Disabilities, London: Butterworth, 1976.

Olson, S. C., and Meredith, D. K.: Wheelchair Interiors. National Easter Seal Society for Crippled Children and Adults, Chicago, 1973.

Palmer, M. L., and Toms, J. E.: Manual for Functional Training. Philadelphia, F. A. Davis, 1980.

Pan, E., Backer, T. E., and Vash, C. L. (eds.): Annual review of rehabilitation, vol. 1. New York: Springer, 1980.

Parmenter, T. R.: Vocational Training for Independent Living. New York, World Rehabilitation Fund, 1980.

Pflueger, S. S.: Independent Living. Washington Institute for Research Utilization, 1977.

Power, P. W., and Dell Orto, A. E.: Role of the Family in the Rehabilitation of the Physically Disabled. Baltimore: University Park Press, 1980.

Rednick, S. S.: The Physically Handicapped Student in the Regular Classroom. A Guide for Teaching Housing and Home Care. Danville IL: Interstate Printers and Publishers, 1976.

Reference List on Self Help Devices for the Handicapped. Chicago: National Easter Seal Society for Crippled Children and Adults, 1972.

Rusk, H. A.: Manual for Training the Disabled Homemaker. New York: Rehabilitation Monograph VII, Institute of Rehabilitation Medicine, 1970.

Rusk, H. A.: Rehabilitation Medicine, ed. 4. St. Louis: C. V. Mosby, 1977.

Sargent, Jean Vieth: An Easier Way—Handbook for the Elderly and Handicapped, The Iowa State University Press, Ames, Iowa, 1981.

Schwab, L. O.: Rehabilitation of physically disabled women in a family oriented program. Rehabil. Lit. 36:34–47, 1975.

Schwab, L. O., and Fadul, R.: Are we prepared for the new rehabilitation legislation? J. Home Economics, March:33–34, 1975.

Simkins, J.: The Value of Independent Living. New York: World Rehabilitation Fund, 1979.

Slater, S. B., Sussman, M. B., and Straud, M. W.: Participation in household activities as a prognostic factor in rehabilitation. Arch. Phys. Med. Rehabil. 51:1970.

Smith, B. C., and Fry, R.: Instructional Materials in Independent Living. Menomonie WI: Stout Vocational Rehabilitation Institute, 1978.

Technical Handbook for Facilities Engineering and Construction Manual. Section 4.12: Design of Barrier-Free Facilities. Washington DC: U.S. Department of Health, Education, and Welfare, 1974.

Walker, J. M.: A Guide to Organizations, Agencies and Federal Programs for Handicapped Americans. Washington DC: Handicapped American Reports, 1979.

Watkins, S. M.: Designing functional clothing. J. Home Economics, November:33–38, 1974.

Wedin, C. S., and Nygren, L. G. (eds.): Housing Perspectives, Individuals and Families. Minneapolis: Burgess Publishing Co., 1976.

Wheeler, V. H.: Planning Kitchens for Handicapped Homemakers. Rehabilitation Monograph 27. New York: Institute of Rehabilitation Medicine, 1966.

Wilshere, E. R.: Equipment for the disabled: Hoists, walking aids. Oxford, England: Oxford Regional Health Authority, 1980.

Yost, A. C.: The rehabilitation home economist. J. Home Economics, 72:50–53, 1980.

Zimmerman, M. E.: Occupational therapy in the A.D.L. program. In Willard, H. S., and Spackman, C. S. (eds.): Occupational Therapy ed. 4. Philadelphia: J. B. Lippincott, 1971, pp. 217–256.

CHAPTER 14

Prevocational and Vocational Assessment *Dorothy L. Kester*

Prevocational Evaluation. Vocational Evaluation. Work Evaluation. What are they? What is their purpose? Who is involved? Are these terms synonymous? Do some people use one term to mean different things, or do some people use different terms to mean one thing?

The use of the work potential evaluation has become a logical and necessary step in the rehabilitation process of many disabled persons. These persons need to define and refine their knowledge of their abilities, disabilities, potentials, behaviors, interests, and job requirements. Such knowledge is also needed by vocational rehabilitation counselors, job trainers, and employers who are working with clients toward vocational success. Evaluation of work potential was developed in order to help clients obtain this knowledge. Different types of evaluations vary as to breadth and depth of investigation.

The *prevocational evaluation* focuses on areas determined by the occupational therapists providing the service. Major factors evaluated include activities of daily living (ADL), educational abilities, and physical capacities and deficits. *Work evaluation* assesses vocational strengths and weaknesses through the utilization of real or simulated work. *Vocational eval-uation* involves the assessment of pertinent medical, psychological, educational, social, environmental, cultural, and vocational factors. In other words, all factors that could affect successful employment are evaluated. This is an interdisciplinary assessment coordinated by the vocational counselor.

The vocational counselor needs definitive information about the client. The scope of the necessary information is far-ranging because of individual client problems and needs. The counselor wants assistance in differentiating the client who will benefit from remediation before evaluation, the one who requires only evaluation to determine feasibility of placement on, or return to, a specific job, the one who is ready for a full vocational evaluation to determine vocational potentials, and the one who does not have vocational potential.

The counselor needs to receive precise information about the client's strengths and weaknesses in areas such as dexterity, discrimination, work speed, quality of work, short- and long-term memory, ability to understand written and verbal instructions, and job skills. This information, however, can be of no benefit or can be misleading to the counselor if other factors affecting employment are not also reported. These factors include interpersonal relationships with coworkers and supervisors, work behavior, motivation, interests in addition to those enumerated in interest tests, work readiness, health, self-care, transportation problems, or family concerns such as need for day care for children or unwillingness to leave the children or a disabled spouse.

No matter how well informed the counselor becomes, there are times when counseling and planning with clients can fail if the clients do not have sufficient self-knowledge or an awareness of their potentials and the world of work. If the evaluation system provides experiences that the client can easily relate to real jobs (vocational exploration) and the client is provided with input regarding performance, then the client and the counselor can choose a placement more accurately. This increases the probability of successful employment. This is especially true if the client must develop completely new skills, whether because of a catastrophic disability, long-term illness, institutionalization, or lack of work experience. Clients need to "see for themselves" that they can do the job.

To be most effective the evaluation must provide information to the counselor in as many areas as possible and must increase the client's knowledge in areas of personal and vocational exploration. Such an evaluation speeds the client's return to employment, ensures client and employer satisfaction, and eliminates trial-and-error methods that are costly in time, money, and self-confidence for both the client and the counselor.

History

No special methods were utilized in determining vocational placement for the handicapped throughout most of recorded history. Handicapped individuals were on their own, as was anyone else seeking employment. People tried their parents' occupation or what appeared to be something they could do. If failures occurred, other jobs were chosen by trial-and-error until the individual succeeded or became too frustrated to do anything.

It was not until the 20th century, especially during World War I, that any attempt at systematic placement assistance was made. The first method was trial in several trade training classes in order to select the course in which the person was interested and had shown potential. The first objective method involved analyzing and charting the specific demands of jobs such as physical, visual, auditory, verbal, and environmental factors. Clients were evaluated for their capacity to fulfill the same list of demands. By comparing the client's checklist to those of a variety of jobs, some job might be found that the individual

was capable of performing well. Consideration was given to skill factors in this method, but consideration of interest was minimal.

World War I appears to have been the impetus for the broadening of psychometric testing, which increased consideration of interests, skills, and potentials. Job performance tests, which developed during World War II, further broadened the scope of these evaluations.

In 1936 the Institute for Crippled and Disabled (I.C.D.) recognized that traditional psychometric and employment batteries utilized for able-bodied job applicants were not suitable for the majority of persons with physical disabilities. Although these batteries provided some of the necessary information, more in-depth information, closely related to actual work, was needed by both the counselors and the clients. However, it was not until 1953 that the move to develop actual tasks finally gained widespread acceptance and broadened to include both physical and psychological disabilities. Since then techniques for evaluation have undergone many changes and will continue to do so.

In 1954 new laws were written stating that the minimum vocational requirement could be met only if a prevocational evaluation unit with sufficient space, equipment, and personnel was available as part of the vocational rehabilitation process.

In the late 1950s the majority of evaluators were occupational therapists, but now evaluators from other disciplines are in the majority. Several universities have developed departments for the education and training of vocational evaluators.

The Occupational Therapist in Work Evaluation

For many occupational therapists, the evaluator's role, which helps finalize the client's rehabilitation, is rewarding. The goals of occupational therapy programs, by their very nature, should always be aimed towards furthering vocational goals. Work evaluation is a specialty directly related to occupational therapy, with its primary emphasis geared to discovering appropriate vocational goals. Skills already acquired by occupational therapists must be enhanced and some new skills learned in order to do work evaluations. The personal and professional knowledges relevant to occupational therapy are already pertinent to work evaluation.

The occupational therapist is interested in working with people. The therapist must develop an ability to observe and perceive, learn how to analyze what was seen and heard, and relate this knowledge to a patient's problems and goals. When this is combined with an ability to learn the techniques and tool-handling skills of a wide variety of tasks, the therapist has achieved a versatility essential to a work evaluator.

Other factors that give the occupational therapist the capability of performing work evaluations include knowledge of disabling conditions and the problems involved, focus on minimizing the problems and maximizing the assets, knowledge of methods for achieving a therapeutic relationship, and skill in techniques for motivating and teaching "problem" patients.

The need to relate *with* patients and clients and to educate them is present in both occupational therapy and vocational evaluation. Behavioral techniques must be developed and the job market in the community must be investigated in depth. Reality must be emphasized when working with a client and in reporting. Although Tender Loving Care (TLC), motivational techniques, and so forth play an important role with many clients, it is essential that the client knows the "cold facts" of reality before the end of the evaluation.

Vocational Evaluation— An Overview

The comprehensive Vocational Evaluation includes a complete spectrum of factors that might affect the client's vocational placement and success, and it involves persons who are not always housed in the same facility. The Work Evaluations vary in nature, and they may be performed in a variety of situations. The type of evaluation used varies with the comprehensiveness of the centers, the clients served, the informational needs of the counselors, and the backgrounds of the evaluators.

Timing for providing these evaluations varies to some extent but, to be most effective, the client should be at or near his maximal potential prior to evaluation. Information from other disciplines, prior contacts, counseling, testing, and rehabilitation should be utilized. Examples are counselor intake interview, contacts, and counseling; medical evaluation and pertinent treatment; psychological testing; physical or psychiatric rehabilitation; and work and personal adjustment reports.

Reports of the evaluation should not repeat information previously known to the counselor, but they should confirm or refute continuation of previously noted problems and assets.

An effective aid in job placement is the *Dictionary of Occupational Titles* (D.O.T.), 4th edition. This publication indexes, cross indexes, and describes tasks of, and trait requirements of, all jobs. Two recent

aids are the *Guide for Occupational Exploration* (GOE), which clusters jobs by interest areas, worker groups, and subgroups; and *Selected Characteristics of Occupations Defined in the D.O.T.*, which provides data about physical demands, environmental conditions, and training time. These are supplemental resources to the D.O.T.; all three are available from the Department of Labor.

Another aid is the *Classification of Jobs According to Worker Trait Factors* (an addendum to the 1977 edition of the D.O.T.), arranged and edited by Timothy F. Field and Janet E. Field. This volume is used by combining assessments of previous work history and academic achievement with present functioning to determine transferable skills to related jobs; it is available from VDARE Service Bureau, Inc., P. O. Box 55, Roswell, Georgia 30077 (404/992-0700).

Work Sample Evaluations

These evaluations consist of samples of actual job tasks or a simulation of actual tasks used to determine job skills or isolated traits such as finger dexterity. They are used in settings such as rehabilitation centers, vocational rehabilitation centers, special schools, hospitals, and other institutions.

Comprehensive Expedited Vocational Evaluation

This fairly new concept in vocational evaluation was designed to decrease the time lag which has always existed between the time a potential vocational rehabilitation client first seeks services and the completion of the diagnostic studies necessary to determine eligibility for services as a vocationally handicapped individual.

In the past there has often been several months wait for the first examination; a second examination was recommended requiring another long wait for an appointment and report. This is no longer true; with the expedited procedure, the counselor usually has all reports in hand within a month.

The state Division of Vocational Rehabilitation may contract with one agency to provide, or to arrange for, these evaluations expeditiously. The core battery consisting of a general medical examination, social service evaluation, psychological testing, and work evaluation are performed within a 3-day period, and reports are sent to the counselor within 7 working days. Physical/functional and/or sensorimotor evaluations can be provided as part of the core group or upon indication that the information is pertinent to determining eligibility or planning goals.

Contractual arrangements are made with specialists for any pertinent evaluation that cannot be performed within the physical plant.

Any services recommended as a result of the evaluations are cleared with the counselor before proceeding. This type of evaluation can also be offered to insurance companies or other service-providing agencies.

Situational or Simulated Job Tryout

In this evaluation the client is placed in actual work situations in a sheltered workshop, institution, or other appropriate place.

Job Tryout

In this vocational evaluation the client is placed on an actual job in industry. Prior evaluation has not always taken place.

Commercial Systems of Evaluation*

The number of commercially available evaluation systems is increasing. Some of the main systems are included here.

Hester Evaluation System

This system was originally developed by Goodwill Industries of Chicago to assess the physically and mentally handicapped, but it is now described as appropriate to all populations.

This battery is not really a work sample system, but a battery of psychological tests and ratings correlated with the D.O.T. Twenty-six performance and paper and pencil tests provide 28 ability scores in seven major categories: unilateral and bilateral motor ability, perceptual accuracy and perceptual motor coordination, intelligence, achievement, and physical strengths. Each test or apparatus is packaged and used independently, and only two tests use expendable materials.

No preliminary screening or specific order of administration is required, there is little client involvement during actual testing, and the atmosphere is formal. The entire battery requires approximately 5 hours.

Instructions are read aloud to the client, and many are also demonstrated; the client should fully understand instructions prior to starting each test, because

no assistance is given during administration. The emphasis in scoring is on time to completion or number of responses. No quality scores are reported, no behavioral observations are made, and vocational exploration is minimal. Results must be sent out for computer scoring; specific job title recommendations are included in the print-out. This system is probably most effective if used for screening at the start of the evaluation process.

Staff and clients were used for norming, but the norm group is not fully described, and no norms are given. Test-retest reliability is high; validity is based on several factor analyses, but very little information is provided. The system is available from:

Evaluations Systems, Inc.
640 North LaSalle Street
Suite 698
Chicago IL 60610

McCarron–Dial Work Evaluation System

This system was developed by Lawrence T. McCarron and Jack G. Dial for use with the mentally retarded and chronically mentally ill. It can also be used with persons who are neurologically impaired, or those with visual or hearing impairment or specific learning disabilities. It involves eight widely accepted instruments based on five neuropsychological factors: verbal-cognitive, sensory, fine and gross motor activities, emotional, and integration-coping. The first three factors involve instruments that are primarily psychometric in nature, that require a formal testing site, and that can be performed in 1 day. The last two factors involve specific instruments and systematic observation in a work situation such as a sheltered workshop, and 2 weeks of testing is recommended.

Five separate systems (including the psychometric battery) are aimed at specific target groups, packaged separately, and each has its own manual. The only expendable items are the answer sheets, and the scoring and reporting forms.

Many tasks are timed; the emphasis in scoring is on quality of performance. The combined scores for each task area are converted to percentile, and they are plotted on a profile sheet. Work performance as well as work and personal behaviors are included in the scoring, utilizing five-point scales. The final report format includes a profile, narrative summaries for each of the five factors, and recommendations.

Several groups of disabled clients were used to acquire norms; reliability is in the high .80s to low .90s, and a considerable amount of validity data is included in the manuals. Some detailed, well-designed studies have been conducted using this tool.

---

* Information has been adapted from *A Comparison of Commercial Vocational Evaluation Systems* by K. F. Botterbusch and A. B. Sax.

This system attempts to combine useful psychometric testing with performance and behavior observation in one prediction tool. No clear guidelines are given for cut-off points. It is available from:

McCarron-Dial Systems
P. O. Box 45628
Dallas TX 75245

Philadelphia Jewish Employment and Vocational System

This system was originally designed for the disadvantaged, and it is now being used for the special needs population. The 28 work samples are based on the Worker Trait Group Organization of the D.O.T., and they are arranged in ten worker trait groups. Each work sample is packaged individually. The manual provides detailed administration and scoring instructions as well as illustrations of proper set-up and common errors. The work samples are administered in order of difficulty; time and quality are given equal weight. Client-evaluator contact is minimized, and feedback on performance and behavior follows the evaluation process.

The final report utilizes standardized forms for work sample recording, daily observational summaries, and a feedback report. This includes a ranking of work sample performance, recommended worker trait groups with rationale, and space for extensive written comments on performance and behavior. Because of the correlations with the D.O.T., many kinds of jobs are covered in the recommendations, which could be broadened further by the counselor familiar with the D.O.T.

Norming information is inadequate. No data are available regarding reliability, and results of studies done by the U.S. Department of Labor on validity have not been released to the public.

This is a well-integrated highly-standardized system, which emphasizes accurate observation and recording of pertinent information. A major problem is the abstract nature of many of the work samples, which affects the client's ability to relate them to real jobs. This system is available from:

Vocational Research Institute
Jewish Employment and Vocational Service
1700 Sansom Street, Ninth Floor
Philadelphia PA 19103

Talent Assessment Programs

This battery is applicable to disadvantaged, handicapped, and emotionally disturbed people. It is based on occupational clusters of related jobs. The ten tests are geared to assess perceptions and dexterities. Each work sample is independent and packaged individually. Two of the samples must be given at specified times, the others are interchangeable. Information in the manual is general; it includes minimal instructions, no specifications for materials needed, and only outlines of set-ups and administration instructions. The instructions are given orally and no reading is required, but because of the nature of the tests, there is little client-evaluator contact. The battery can be administered in about 2½ hours. Scoring for errors is not completely defined in the manual; the emphasis is on time that is converted to a percentile. Behaviors do not appear to be rated. The final report includes a profile sheet, a form for recording job possibility clusters, and space for a narrative report and recommendations.

This system does not provide any direct vocational information to the client. It was normed against seven groups, primarily young people. Reliability is stated, but no data is available on validity.

Although this system is accepted for specific factors, it is not a system that provides a true vocational evaluation. The developers suggest that other assessment devices be used as well. Information may be obtained from:

Talent Assessment, Inc.
P. O. Box 5087
Jacksonville FL 32207

Tower System

The tower system is an outgrowth of a system developed by the Institute for Crippled and Disabled (I.C.D.) in 1936. It contains 93 work samples arranged into 14 job training areas. The samples are grouped by area, and they are not individually packaged; each facility must construct its own hardware and equipment.

Administration of the complete battery takes 3 weeks. It is progressive within each area, but choice of areas is at the discretion of the evaluator. A realistic work setting and atmosphere is stressed. Instructions are written, but they should be supplemented as needed before the client proceeds. Client-evaluator contact is not specified, but it is taken for granted. The client is exposed to many training areas, and he/she can be given additional specific occupational information.

In scoring this system, time and work quality are given equal weight, criteria are carefully defined, and scoring aids are extensive. Scoring is on a five-point scale. Work factors and work behaviors are mentioned minimally, and they are not specifically defined.

Standardized forms are utilized for recording and

reporting each work sample and job area; others are available for including in the final report. A narrative summary utilizes both a standardized outline and a section giving global ratings directly related to the work samples.

Client, but not industrial, norms are available; reliability data is not available, and validity data is open to question.

This system, based on job analysis, is very useful in evaluating clients, but it applies only to a narrow group of jobs unless the counselor utilizes the D.O.T. to broaden the scope. Lack of precise definitions of performance, behaviors, and adequate norms are the major weaknesses of the system. Information is available through:

I. C. D. Rehabilitation and Research Center
340 East 24th Street
New York NY 10010

Also available from the same source, but addressed to Micro TOWER, is Micro TOWER, which was aimed at the general rehabilitation population, but it can be used with special education students, the disadvantaged, and adult offenders. It is basically a group aptitude test using work sample methodology to measure seven aptitudes.

Thirteen work samples, measuring eight specific aptitudes plus general learning ability, are organized into five major groups. The tests need not be given in any specific order, client involvement is emphasized, and formal feedback is given. Several well-written and detailed manuals are provided; few expendable materials are required, and cassette administration tapes are available.

Total testing time is approximately 15 hours, plus 4 to 5 hours if group discussions are included. Emphasis is on quality of work produced in a set time period; forms are used for recording, and reporting combines forms and a narrative report.

Norms are available on 19 groups, reliability is high, and construct validity is reported.

Valpar Component Work Sample Series

Developed by Valpar Corporation for industrially injured workers, the Valpar component work sample series involves a worker trait and work factor approach based on task analysis. There are presently 16 work samples that are used individually rather than as a group. Each sample is self-contained, mostly in lockable cases; minimal expendable materials are required.

The order of administration is at the discretion of the evaluator, as is feedback on performance. The time required is not given, but it is estimated at an hour or less per work sample. Instructions are given orally and by demonstration; reading is not required unless inherent to the task, and client involvement is minimal. The manuals are clear and detailed; all work samples recycle themselves, so little preparation is required.

Scoring emphasizes time and quality, then scores are converted to percentiles and are combined to provide total performance scores; 17 work behaviors are rated. The samples are each rated on standard forms, but no combined final report form is used.

Reliability estimates are fairly high, but they cannot be accurately assessed; data is available for validity.

This series is well designed, appealing to clients, easy to administer, and combines well with another system, but many aspects of an integrated system are lacking. As a consequence of the abstract nature of the samples, vocational exploration is limited. Since this series was not developed as an evaluation system, the manuals indicate areas for further evaluation. Contact may be made with:

Valpar Corporation
3801 East 34th Street
Tucson AZ 85713

Vocational Evaluation System

Developed by Singer Education Division, this system has an unspecified target group and basis. There are 25 work stations, each located in a separate carrel, the order of administration being left to the discretion of the evaluator. The possibility of client-evaluator contact is close as a result of frequent checkpoints. A system is included for self-ratings of interest and performance. Audiovisual instruction, with a controllable rate of advancement, is utilized for all the work samples; written material occasionally supplements the program. The client is able to gain a fairly high degree of vocational exploration because of the format of the work samples. From 2 to 2½ hours should be allowed for each work station.

Scoring focuses on timing intervals, work behaviors, work performance, error, and quality, with the emphasis on time and quality. Five-point scales are used, and forms are provided. It is recommended that the final report include the forms and a narrative report. Adequate, descriptive norming information is provided, reliability is moderately good, and three validity studies have been done.

The 25 work stations of this system include mostly skilled trades. The built-in career exploration and occupational information are strong points of this system, but this information is often gained at the expense of increased knowledge of the client's potential. Many of the procedures are not clarified in the manual. Information is available from:

Singer Educational Division
Career Systems
80 Commerce Drive
Rochester NY 14623

Wide Range Employment Sample Test

This test, developed by Guidance Associates of Delaware, Inc., does not have a designated target group. The ten samples, developed for a sheltered workshop dealing with mentally retarded and physically handicapped, are fairly low level. Each sample is independent in nature, but the samples are not individually packaged. They are usually administered in numerical order, and it is assumed that there should be client-evaluator involvement. Administration time is about 1 and 1½ hours for one client and 2 hours for small groups. Instructions are oral with demonstration; no reading is required.

The samples are timed by stopwatch, and times are rated on a nineteen-point scale. Errors are checked against clearly defined criteria, totaled for all ten tasks, and compared to a norms table. There is no indication that work performance and behaviors are observed. The final report combines a summary of results form with narrative commentary.

Norming was done on three major groups and is well defined; reliability is high, and the reported validity is encouraging.

This system appears to be most appropriate for determining assignments for clients new to a sheltered workshop, and an emphasis on retesting should determine the client's ability to improve with practice. The major problems include lack of behavioral observations and failure to relate results to the competitive job market. The samples are not appropriate for adding to the client's job awareness. Tests may be obtained from:

Guidance Associates of Delaware, Inc.
1526 Gilpin Avenue
Wilmington DE 19806

Physical and Functional Evaluation

This evaluation requires a maximum of 1 day, and it is designed primarily for two purposes: it helps eliminate the client who really cannot be helped because of severe physical limitations and who cannot perform any of the more sedentary tasks because of educational and/or mental deficits, and it is geared to discovering the client who has employment potential despite limitations.

A standardized test battery is utilized to analyze the ability to perform and to tolerate physical activities such as sitting, standing, walking, lifting, and handling. Tasks are used to provide basic information about potential skill levels. For example, math, reading, and mechanical skills can be tested concurrently with sitting tolerance. This knowledge can be utilized for planning during further testing if employment potential is indicated.

A sample form is shown (see Physical Capacities Evaluation). Norms have not been filled in since they vary depending on the tasks in the individual center's test battery. The norms are recorded for comparison with the client's actual tolerances and strengths that are entered in the limits column. A narrative section includes observations, a summary, and recommendations. The report should define the limitations created by the disability and the capacities remaining despite the disability.

Case Study

Mr. L. D. was 60 years old and mildly retarded with minimal schooling. He had a lumbar disk problem and ulcers for 35 years, osteoarthritis, parkinsonism, emphysema, hypertension, history of alcoholism, loss of memory, and personality disorder. His work history included farming, labor force, and truck driving. He is now unable even to help around the house.

Because of legal technicalities, further evaluation was required to prove lack of work potential.

Mr. D. tolerated sitting for 5-minute periods of time and standing for 1 minute. He required 45 seconds to walk 80 feet with rests, and he was breathing heavily before he had reached 40 feet. He braced his hand on the table during the standing, and on the second attempt hand tremor was so great that the table shook. Strength of grip was only 10 pounds, unless he stabilized his arm against his side. Scores for all capacities were in the zero column. □

Work Tolerance Evaluation

This evaluation includes a physical and functional evaluation with special emphasis on tolerances for those actions and capacities required for a specific job or type of job. For the client who has been unemployed for some time as a result of illness or injury, it also includes an evaluation of ability to perform a full day's work. The length of the evaluation varies with the length of lay-off and severity of the problem, but

PHYSICAL CAPACITIES EVALUATION

Name: _____   Date: _____

	NORMS	N	G	F	P	O	LIMITS	COMMENTS
1. Sitting								
Standing								
Walking								
Stooping								
Kneeling								
Crouching								
Crawling								
2. Climbing								
Balancing								
3. Lifting (Unilateral)								
Lifting (Bilateral)								
Carrying								
Pushing								
Pulling								
4. Reaching								
Handling								
Fingering								
Feeling								
Placing								
5. Talking								
Hearing								
6. Seeing								
a. Acuity								
b. Depth perception								
c. Field of vision								
d. Accommodation								
e. Color vision								

FUNCTIONAL TOLERANCES

1. Standing								
2. Sitting								
3. General mobility								
4. Fine work								
5. Rapid work								
6. Repetitive work								
7. Sequential work								
a. Short cycle								
b. Long cycle								
8. Stamina								

Norms are based on D.O.T. Standards

KEY: O—Unable to perform, or impractical
P—Performed with assistance, improvement needed
F—Performed without assistance, but improvement needed to be adequate
G—Adequate for practical performance even though affected by disability
N—Performance not affected by disability

Sample form for a physical functional evaluation. From Delaware Curative Workshop, Wilmington. Reprinted with permission.

it should always be longer than 1 day, because the client can frequently tolerate much more for 1 day than he can on a sustained basis.

The battery used varies with the goals for the individual client, but the closer the activities relate to the job the more effective the evaluation. In many cases, if the requirements of the activities are graded for stress, tolerance increases as the evaluation proceeds.

Case Study

On Mr. F. J.'s stock clerk job a bicycle was used on level ground for delivering some of the materials; activity was intermittent. Items were stored at all heights, but none weighed more than 25 pounds. After recovery from a posterior myocardial infarction, he required nitroglycerine infrequently. His physician and his counselor were positive that he could safely return to his job, but the employer was reluctant.

Mr. F. J. was admitted for an evaluation of his tolerance for activity, and he was seen for 2 successive days.

On the first day, periods of active tasks were alternated with more sedentary ones. The active tasks included:

Bicycling—15 min.—no resistance, no pulse change, some shortness of breath.
Lifting—41 lb. from floor to waist height one time
    37 lb. from chair to head height one time
    37 lb. from floor to head height 11
    times—some shortness of breath noted.
Stair climbing—seven round trips on eight steps
    with a pulse increase from 72 to 104.

The other tasks on the check sheet were performed as a group without a rest period.

On the second day, two sedentary tasks were performed, and the active tasks were performed without rest periods. Printing was done on a hand press on which the handle must be raised in an arc (up and away from the body) from waist height to head height; graded springs were used to resist raising the handle. The schedule was as follows:

Printing—15 min.—30 lb. handle on the right
    15 min.—25 lb., no symptoms
Bicycling—15 min.—28 lb. resistance, no symptoms
Lifting—3 min.—61 lb. one time from 12 in. to waist
    height
    53 lb. six times—pulse increased
    from 72 to 80 (Normal increase can
    be up to 30 units.)
Sedentary task—7 min.

Lifting—6 min.—41 lb.—ten times from 12 in. to
    waist height—pulse increased to 92
Sedentary task—15 min.
Bicycling—15 min.—40 lb.
Printing—15 min.—50 lb. resistance

Mr. F. J. was able to perform resistive tasks for a 2-hour period with minimal rest and minimal symptomatology. Shortness of breath or pulse rise was noted only with repetitive stairclimbing and repetitive lifting of more than 30 pounds to head height or more than 50 pounds to waist height.

This was adequate tolerance for the intermittently active type of job described. The actual report provided sufficient evidence so that the employer allowed him to return to work. □

Specific Vocational Evaluation

This evaluation is designed to determine ability to perform a specific new job or type of work, to analyze ability to return to a prior employer in a previous or new job, to substantiate or repudiate prior information, or to help the client realize his potential (or lack of potential) for that specific work.

The process involves appropriate commercial work samples, if available, augmented by increasingly definitive tasks. A physical and functional evaluation, and at least pertinent aspects of a tolerance evaluation, should be included. This evaluation varies in length from 1 to several days.

Case Study

Mr. M. C. was 41 years old. His physical condition following an accident at work had deteriorated. When admitted, he required two canes and he had a body posture that placed stress on his hands and arms to the extent that his sense of touch was being affected. His hands were large and heavy.

His only vocational interest was to be a locksmith, which all previous testing ruled out as a possibility. He was admitted for a Specific Work Evaluation to determine his aptitude for this. Emphasis was placed on testing general physical tolerance, manual dexterity, and mechanical comprehension. His overall endurance and lower extremity and trunk strength were poor. He leaned heavily on his canes when ambulating, and he had considerable difficulty moving from a sitting to a standing position.

His manual dexterity proved to be higher on functional tasks than on tests, varying from below average to well above the norm. For example, his scores on the Crawford Small Parts Dexterity Test ranged from the 8th to the 43rd percentiles. When given actual job-related tasks, such as simple lock or cigarette lighter repair, he performed at a higher level of manual skill, handling small parts, springs, and so forth in the usual manner or finding a method that counteracted the large size of his fingers.

Scores on the Bennett Mechanical Comprehension Tests, added to give a complete picture of his potential, were in the 80th percentile when compared to industrial applicants. Actual work samples were satisfactorily completed well within required standards.

This job-relevant information provided his counselor with specific information, and a correspondence course was purchased for him. Before he had finished the course, Mr. C was semiemployed by a locksmith near his home and, after completion, he opened his own shop. □

Sensorimotor Evaluation

The sensorimotor evaluation, either partial or complete, is given to persons of all ages on the same basis that it is used for children. For example, those who have had difficulty learning, cannot function to expected capacities, appear to have visual or coordination problems, poor visual or physical tolerance not from obvious causes, and/or have hyper or hypoactive behavior can undergo this evaluation. In other words, it is given to those who should benefit from training or further education but who seem unable to do so.

The purposes are to diagnose any sensorimotor dysfunction, whether primary or secondary in nature, and to assist with planning by analyzing the effect of any dysfunction on vocational potentials.

The battery consists of a standardized sensorimotor battery, which includes all levels of sensorimotor development plus age-appropriate vocationally-oriented tests that provide perceptual information. This evaluation has been utilized during the process of other evaluations or as a separate entity for clients who are having unexpected difficulties in training programs.

Since sensorimotor battery scoring is available only for children, and it has no real meaning to the counselors, it has been necessary to develop age/goal appropriate forms and scores. The scoring system being developed converts raw scores for both time and accuracy into percentile scores; these are recorded on a chart-type form (see Sensorimotor Evaluation), which breaks results down into the basic Sheltered Workshop and industrially pertinent performance levels. This form becomes part of the final report, in combination with a narrative section designed to educate counselors and supervisors, to relate both the limitations and the abilities to behavioral and vocational limitations and potentials, to provide management suggestions and to recommend remediation and/or the need for other evaluations, as well as job areas to avoid or consider in determining vocational goals.

Two case summaries are presented: one adolescent, one adult.

Case Studies

O. B. was a husky 16-year-old who looked older. His speech development was slow, and he had received therapy. He participated in sports, apparently doing well, but he had problems with his peers. He had a long history of school-related problems. These problems were increasing, as were family tensions and pressures. Testing placed his grade levels at 5 for reading, 3.5 for spelling, and 7 for math. He avoided fine tasks, was heavy handed, and his family perceived him as careless, lazy, unwilling to stick to a task, and poorly motivated.

Test results and observations made during the evaluation indicated that sensorimotor dysfunction played a major role in many of his problems. The asymmetrical tonic neck reflex and tonic labyrinthine response were incompletely integrated, crossing of the midline was avoided, vision was used minimally to assist balance, and laterality was not completely automatic.

Reception and interpretation of tactile stimuli were more highly developed on the left, and symptoms of tactile sensitivity and poor tolerance became increasingly pronounced as testing progressed. In order to provide auditory reinforcement, his handling of the pieces on the Minnesota Rate of Manipulation Test and The Minnesota Spatial Relations Test became increasingly heavy as his tactile tolerance was reached. He also became more "careless", barely raising the pieces if they could be slid into place. The effects of the preceding problems were most pronounced on tasks requiring combined gross and fine motor functions and/or bilateral use of the hands.

Much manipulation of body and materials was noted during visual-motor tasks; minimal shoulder motion was used on the right, and midline crossing was avoided, especially by the left hand. When copying designs he demonstrated difficulty with closure, directionality, and crossing of any previously drawn lines.

The major factors affecting visual ability were poor visual memory, visual tolerance, and figure

Sensorimotor Evaluation

Name _____   Date_____

Equilibrium/Gross Motor Functions

	↓ Scale	0–30%	31–50%	51–70%	71–100%	↑ Scale
Oculomotor functioning—Tracking						
Convergence						
Equilibrium—Static, eyes Open						
eyes Closed						
Active, eyes Open						
eyes Closed						
Crossing own midline						
Right-left discrimination—Self						
Space						
Mirror						
Minnesota rate of manipulation test						
Unilateral placement						
Bilateral placement						
Bilateral with manipulation						
Horizontal motion-hand transfer						

Tactile Perceptions and Functions

	↓ Scale	0–30%	31–50%	51–70%	71–100%	↑ Scale
Tactile form perception						
Finger identification						
Kester's kinesthesia test—Lines						
Numbers						
O'Connor test of finger dexterity						
Grooved pegboard						
Kester's washer test						
Kester's collation						

Visual Perceptions and Functions

	↓ Scale	0–30%	31–50%	51–70%	71–100%	↑ Scale
Position in space—Adjacent pictures						
Adjacent pages						
Memory						
Figure-ground—Concrete Section						
Symbolic section						
Color vision						
Color collation—Pale colors						
Intense colors						

Visual Motor Functioning

	↓ Scale	0–30%	31–50%	51–70%	71–100%	↑ Scale
Purdue pegboard—Placement						
Assembly						
Kester's line marking						
Kester's mazes						
Design copying test—Dotted Grid						
Beery copying test—Frame						
Minnesota spatial relations test						

ground perception. Convergence was poor, and near focus was inadequate. Perseveration was noted on visual and visual-motor tasks.

Auditory discrimination, selective attention, sequential memory, translation from sounds to symbols, and processing were deficient.

(Although nowhere near an ideal solution, in some cases evaluation alone can produce results. Confirmation that there is a basis for many of the problems can ease the pressures, producing a more relaxed attitude which in itself allows the person to function at a higher level.)

With this client much more was attained even though he could not attend the remediation program. He was provided with a home program that he did follow with the help of his family.

His mother observed the evaluation; her observations and discussions with the evaluator provided an understanding of the depth of his problems. She was able to relate what she saw and heard to problems seen at home and in school. Notes she took during this time enabled her to communicate her new knowledge and understanding to the rest of the family and to relate remediative suggestions on the home program list to activities done by him at home.

Communication from the mother was fairly frequent until the family moved out of state. Each telephone call provided further evidence of increase in O. B.'s ego strength and family togetherness in solving this problem. □

M. C. is an intelligent young woman whose mild physical and facial mannerisms distracted slightly from her attractiveness. Pronounced lack of self-confidence about abilities and intelligence was evident. M. C. was divorced and was caring for her 12-year-old daughter who had recently been diagnosed and treated for sensorimotor dysfunction.

All previous employment had been as a secretary; the most recent position was terminated when she was admitted to a psychiatric hospital. Evaluation indicated that she had excellent potential for a variety of occupations and that her previous vocational choice in all probability contributed to her present problems. Findings included mild oculomotor and right-left discrimination deficiencies, poor tactile reception, slow visual processing speed, poor visual tolerance, difficulty with symbolic representations, obvious stress when doing paper and pencil tasks, distractibility for auditory stimuli, and deficient assimilation of auditory stimuli. Interestingly, her findings were very similar to those of her adopted daughter, so she started joining in the daughter's home program even before starting remediation.

M. C. received remediation for a short period of time, learned to use a template to eliminate undesired visual stimuli, started to learn relaxation techniques and then continued in an aerobic dance program, and with the use of a tape recorder to eliminate note-taking (purchased by her Vocational Rehabilitation counselor) started courses in criminal justice in hopes of becoming a probation officer.

Improved self-confidence had been noted, and receiving an "A" in her first course in no way interfered with this progress. □

Summary

As a summary to this chapter, the best way to demonstrate the value and use of work evaluations is to present a case study in which all levels of evaluation and some aspects of adjustment were required.

Case Study

Mrs. H. H. was seen over a period of 3 months. Her major disability was a psychoneurotic disorder with depressive reaction, but hypertensive vascular disease, alcoholism, and a long medical history contributed. Discomfort from a previously fractured coccyx limited sitting tolerance. Educational level was high average except for math that tested at the seventh grade; intellectual potential was superior. She had checked hats in a hotel for 10 years.

Mrs. H. H. was admitted for a work evaluation. She was given a commercial work sample battery, a partial perceptual battery, and a physical and functional evaluation. Extra time was taken for this because of her depression and poor self-esteem.

She complained of arthritis, primarily in her right hand and buttocks, and she had high blood pressure. The only vocationally limiting physical factor was poor tolerance for continuous standing or sitting. She was a perfectionist who did not believe she had any saleable abilities. Reaction to even minor failures was exaggerated and resulted in temporary increase in her depression. She had the additional pressure of her son's return home with all of the problems of the younger generation, including drug addiction.

On admission, she worked slowly, neatly, methodically, and carefully. On most tasks quality was average to superior, but speed was inferior. She found unexpected abilities as the evaluation progressed. Her confidence and speed increased while her depression decreased and her blood pressure lowered. Originally she required a fairly high amount of T.L.C. and a great deal of flexibility in length of time given for a specific task. Some flexibility in stated time standards for tasks during the first week also added to her self-confidence.

Perceptions were average or above, stereognosis was within normal limits although sensation was slightly diminished in the right hand, and motor planning was above average.

Mrs. H. H. did well on all types of tasks involving precision such as drafting, lettering, copying, paper cutting, printing on a hand press, and electronics other than cable tying. Clerical work was average or above except for mathematics, spelling was superior, and use of English was above average. She had some difficulty learning to use new tools, but once she learned the basic techniques she was able to amplify them.

At first she had difficulty concentrating in noisy surroundings, but later she was able to work both alone or among others. She was able to teach other clients jobs with which she was familiar (this was done, at first, to "help the evaluator" who pretended to be too busy to provide needed assistance).

She discovered an interest and ability in artistic work, especially copying. Her work was precise, her sense of color good, and the work was calming to her. She also demonstrated an interest and ability in food preparation, but her tolerance for continuous standing was too limited for many jobs in this area.

Considering the overall picture, it was felt that work in an art, printing, or layout department would be the best vocational choice. It was also felt that Mrs. H. H. would have difficulty learning in a formal setting, but she would be able to function, at this stage, in a more sheltered training situation. Some degree of T.L.C. was still required.

A conference was held including the evaluator, the vocational rehabilitation counselor, and two people from the sheltered workshop who could provide layout training. As a result of this, a specific work evaluation and tolerance (emotional, in this case) evaluation were begun at the center. A second purpose for this method of evaluation was to acquaint her with her future supervisor while still in a familiar setting. A second report was written concerning a conference with the workshop personnel so as to put into the records her need for financial assistance for medical purposes. Actual work was brought and demonstrated to her, and results were discussed with her.

The transition was made to the sheltered workshop; she was hired after a period of on-the-job training and, before long, she was capable of teaching other trainees new work as she learned it herself.

Mrs. H. H. was made aware of her capabilities through the evaluation. This, and the adjustment techniques that were used, provided her with the confidence needed for success. □

Bibliography

Brewer, E., Miller, J., and Ray, J.: The effect of vocational evaluation and work adjustment on clients' attitude toward work. Voc. Eval. Work Adjustment Bull. 8:18–25, 1975.

Bottersbusch, K. F., and Sax, A. B.: A Comparison of Commercial Vocational Evaluation Systems. Menomonie WI: 1980. Materials Development Center, Stout Rehabilitation Institute, University of Wisconsin, 1980.

Dinneen, T.: Work evaluation as a technique for improving self-concept. Voc. Eval. Work Adjustment Bull. 8:28–34, 1975.

Granofsky, J.: A Manual for Occupational Therapists on Prevocational Exploration. Dubuque IA: W. C. Brown Book Co., 1959.

Hoffman, P. R.: Work evaluation, an overview. Work Evaluation in Rehabilitation, Reprint Series RS-70-2, 3-18, 1969.

Olshansky, S.: Reply to Kipstein and Lores. Rehabil. Lit. 36:142, 1975.

Raymond, E.: Measuring the interpersonal aspects of work behavior. Voc. Eval. Work Adjustment Bull. 8:19–23, 1975.

Roberts, C. L.: Definitions, objectives and goals in work evaluation. Work Evaluation in Rehabilitation, Reprint Series RS-70-2, 19-30, 1969.

Persons interested in more definitive information on adjustment techniques, will find articles in journals such as:

Journal of Rehabilitation, published by the National Rehabilitation Association.

Vocational Evaluation and Work Adjustment Bulletin, published quarterly by the Vocational Evaluation and Work Adjustment Association, a division of the National Rehabilitation Association.

The American Journal of Occupational Therapy.

Many of the available articles are indexed in Psychological Abstracts and Rehabilitation Literature. The University of Wisconsin-Stout, Menomonie WI, 54751, maintains a Materials Development Center for such materials, which can be borrowed or purchased.

PART 5

General Treatment Process and Procedures

CHAPTER 15

Therapeutic Application of Activity

Helen L. Hopkins,
Helen D. Smith, and
Elizabeth G. Tiffany

The things human beings do and the objects human beings make provide a bridge between their inner reality and their external world. In their activities they show their concern with how to survive, be comfortable, have pleasure, solve problems, express themselves, and be related with others and the wider world of society. They experience themselves and come to know their strengths and weaknesses or limits through the things they do. The roles they assume have inherent functions, skills, and behaviors that are necessary to support them. There are, for example, characteristic activities that are necessary for the student, parent, store manager, beach bum, and so forth. It is probably for these reasons, more than for any others, that occupational therapy, with its emphasis on the use of activity to promote function, came into being.

Characteristics of Occupational Therapy Activity

The term *occupation* in occupational therapy "is in the context of man's goal-directed use of time, energy, interest and attention."[1] Thus occupation is used in the context of being occupied productively in activities that "are primary agents for learning and development and an essential source of satisfaction."[2] (See Chapter 3). Activities as used in occupational therapy should have at least eight characteristics:

1. *Be goal directed.* Activities should have some purpose or reason for their use to be considered occupational therapy activity. "Busy work," in its keeping hands occupied, may be of some value to the client, but generally it is not chosen with a specific goal in mind.

2. *Have significance at some level to the client.* Activities should have value and usefulness to the client, even though the value may be one that will be realized only at some future date. This indicates that the activity may seem to have no immediate value in reaching a specified goal, but will make it possible to reach that goal in a week, a month, or sometime later. The activity should have some relationship to the roles the individual plays in society.

3. *Require client involvement at some level* (either mental or physical). Activities require "doing" or participation on the part of the client. The individual engaged in the activity should be involved

in the process of determining the activity as well as in the performance of it and thus receives self-gratification from the results. He or she is not a recipient but rather a participant. Participation may be active or passive.

4. *Be geared to prevention of malfunction and/or maintenance or improvement of function and quality of life.* The choice and type of activity is dependent upon the client level of function and ability to participate; however, the goal is clear.

5. *Reflect client involvement in life task situations* (ADL, play, work). Activities are used to acquire or redevelop those skills essential for fulfillment of life roles. Activities provide for development of competence in the performance of those tasks essential to the life roles of each individual.

6. *Relate to the interests of the client.* Involvement in the choice of activity is vital. Commitment to the tasks will be attained only if client goals and interests are considered and are met.

7. *Be adaptable and gradable.* Activity must be age appropriate, be able to be increased or decreased in complexity, and be graded in time and strength required.

8. *Be determined through occupational therapist's professional judgment based on knowledge.* Knowledge of human development, medical pathology, interpersonal relationships, and value of activity to the person are required to make the match between client problems and the activities that will be most meaningful and serviceable in reaching the therapeutic goals of the occupational therapy process.

Factors to Be Considered in Selection of Appropriate Activities

Therapeutic application of activity to meet the specific needs of each client requires that the choice of activity be made on the basis of those activity properties that seem to have an impact on the previously identified problems. Consideration must be given to all factors that may have an impact on the individual's ability to function, including physical, psychosocial, cultural, and economic factors. The activity may need to be adapted in order to provide the desired amount of complexity, the correct exercise, or the desired amount of social interaction. Successful completion of the activity chosen promotes development of competence. Client interest and involvement may be enhanced by providing feedback on progress. Some activities, utilized in the treatment of physical dysfunction, allow the use of biofeedback as a means of providing an indication of correct use of

muscles and adequate performance. Interaction between the therapist and the client, which provides reassurance and encouragement as well as accurate perception of function, is vital to the therapeutic process.

In conditions involving physical dysfunction, the activities are selected for their physical restorative powers as well as for their psychological and psychosocial properties. They must be constructive as well as provide the desired exercise. This enables the client to translate the motion, strength, and coordination gained to normal activity, thus providing the additional psychological value of success in achievement. Activities used for treatment of physical disabilities must be adaptable so they can provide specific exercise for affected joints or muscles. Activities used should be in accord with the following criteria to meet physical restoration requirements[3]:

1. *Provide action rather than position.* Activity should provide for alternate contraction and relaxation of muscles. Activities should be analyzed from a kinesiological point of view to determine components of the activity, motions required to perform the activity, muscle power required, and the range of motion and strengthening the activity can provide.

2. *Require repetition of the motion.* Activity should permit repetition of the desired motion for an indefinite but controllable number of times.

3. *Permit gradation in range of motion, resistance, and coordination.* Activity should allow a greater range of motion than is permitted by the limitation found in the joint so the activity can allow for increase of *joint range*. *Resistance* is required in order to strengthen a muscle. Thus the activity should be gradable in the amount of resistance it provides so that resistance can be increased as power returns. When *coordination* is affected, the activity should be graded so that it provides exercise requiring gross coordination and working toward fine coordination. The activity may also be varied or adapted through positioning or by changing the way the task is performed.

The psychosocial aspects of activities need to be considered in the treatment of clients with all kinds of disabilities, but certain psychodynamic properties are of primary consideration in psychiatric occupational therapy. These include the following[4]:

1. Property of materials—resistive, pliable, controlled, or messy, as well as the sensory input they provide (tactile, auditory, olfactory, visual, proprioceptive).

2. Complexity of the activity—number of steps in the activity, repetition required.

3. Preparation required—prearrangement of supplies, adaptation of environment.

4. Amount and type of directions—verbal or written directions, diagrams, demonstration.
5. Structure and controls (rules) inherent in the activity.
6. Predictability of results.
7. Type of learning required—old learning, adapted old learning, or new learning.
8. Decision making required on part of patient.
9. Attention span—minutes or hours.
10. Interaction—solitary, parallel, interaction with peers, small group, large group, cooperation.
11. Communication—nonverbal, little, oral directions, reading, writing.
12. Motivation—creative, gratifying, intellectually challenging, affect on others, relevance to life space and roles.
13. Time—completion of activity in one session or sessions, quick success, delayed gratification.

In working in the field of pediatrics, a combination of psychosocial, psychodynamic, physical, and developmental factors must be considered. The activities may be required to provide specific aspects relating to normal growth and development, must be age appropriate in complexity and dexterity required, yet may need to provide some aspects that promote physical function and that promote psychological well-being.

Prevocational activities are selected on the basis of their ability to contribute to work-related skills. (See Chap. 17.) They must be selected for their relationship to the components of the actual work requirements. These include such aspects as physical performance, coordination required, concentration needed, speed and accuracy involved, endurance needed, routinization and boredom factors, initiative and decision making required.

For individuals with sensory-integration problems (cognitive-perceptual-motor dysfunction), sensory stimuli presented by the activity must be analyzed along with the "intersensory-integrative mechanisms involved and the motor response required."[5] Thus tactile, kinesthetic, visual, auditory, and olfactory sensory modalities must be analyzed for each activity along with the type of response required including motor, visual, and verbal. Activity analysis in this area requires the analysis of the neurological integration of input from the senses and the muscular response to this stimulation and ingration, and it is therefore called the neurobehavioral approach to activity analysis. Activities must be analyzed with all the components in mind in order to choose the most appropriate one to meet all therapeutic requirements.[6]

In selecting an activity to be used in the therapeutic process, the therapist must answer five basic questions:

1. *How* do you do the activity? The therapist must know the basic components of the activity, the process involved, the tools, equipment, and supplies needed, and he or she must know how to do it well enough to be able to teach it successfully.
2. *What* activity is most appropriate to meet the requirements of the situation? The therapist must assess the problems involved, the needs, interests, and preferences of the patient/client, and, with the individual, must determine the activity that best meets the requirements for therapeutic intervention.
3. *Why* was a specific activity chosen? The therapist must be able to determine the reason for the choice of activity on the basis of a rationale for this choice that is consistent with the overall treatment rationale.
4. *Where* will the activity be performed? The therapist may be constrained in the choice of an activity because of the location or situation within which the activity will be carried out. For example, if the activity is to be done by an individual in bed, it cannot be too messy or require large tools or equipment.
5. *When* will the activity be carried out? The time of day or season of the year may influence the type of activity that is relevant. For example, self-care activities are most logically carried out at the time of day when they are usually done, for example, bathing and dressing before breakfast. Activities that are relevant may be dictated by the time of year, for example, making decorations or presents at Christmas.

Activity Analysis

The therapist's skill in activity analysis is critical in determining the validity of his or her use of activities. There are many approaches used in occupational therapy to analyze activities. The nature of activity analysis used will be influenced by the therapist's frame of reference for treatment. Some occupational therapists have undertaken the task of analyzing the major activities that are used and of keeping these analyses on file for reference when doing treatment planning. In some instances, activity analyses have been adapted to record evaluative data acquired in the use of specific activities as evaluation.

The accompanying sample form (see Activity Analysis Form) is one form of activity analysis, focusing on the skills requirements of the activity and built on the concept of the developmental wheel described in Chapter 4 (see Fig. 4-1). This analysis may easily be adapted to record evaluative data.

ACTIVITY ANALYSIS FORM

Activity analyzed:
Average time required for completion:
Average number of sessions required to complete:
Brief description: (include criteria for determining success)

Activity Characteristics   *Explanations*

Activity Characteristics	Skill required ✓	Degree Low Medium High	Is activity gradable? How?

A. MOTOR
    1. Position:
        a. activity
        b. patient/client
    2. Motion(s) components
        a. joints involved
        b. motion(s) involved
    3. Muscles utilized
    4. Direction of resistance			

5. Action rather than position
6. Repetition of motion(s)
7. Rhythm developed
8. Maintained contraction (static)
9. Manual dexterity
10. Gross motor
11. Fine motor
12. Bilateral
13. Unilateral
14. Endurance
15. Rate of performance
16. Grading adaptability
    a. R.O.M.
    b. resistance
    c. coordination
    d. substitution			

B. SENSORY
    1. Visual
    2. Auditory (impact on)
    3. Gustatory
    4. Olfactory
    5. Tactile
        a. temperature of material
        b. texture of material
        c. heavy to light touch			

C. COGNITIVE
    1. Organizational ability
    2. Problem solving ability
        a. planning
        b. trial and error
    3. Logical thinking
    4. Concentration
    5. Attention span
    6. Written/oral/demonstration directions
        a. complex
        b. simple
    7. Reading
    8. Seriation
    9. Interpret signs & symbols
    10. Multiple processing/steps involved
    11. Creativity
    12. Use of imagination
    13. Establish goal & carry out means to attain it
    14. Causal relationships involved (perceive cause & effect)
    15. Centering			

Activity Characteristics	Skill required √	Degree Low Medium High	Is activity gradable? How?
16. Perceive viewpoint of others			
17. Test reality			
D. PERCEPTUAL			
1. Sensory integration required			
2. Differentiation			
a. Figure-ground			
b. Space relationships			
c. Object constancy			
d. Kinesthesia			
e. Proprioception			
f. Stereognosis			
g. Form constancy			
h. Color perception			
i. Auditory perception			
3. Tactile integration			
4. Motor planning			
5. Bilateral integration			
6. Body scheme			
7. Vestibular			
E. EMOTIONAL			
1. Passive or aggressive motion			
2. Destructive			
3. Gratification			
a. immediate			
b. delayed			
4. Structured			
5. Unstructured			
6. Allows control			
7. Success/failure possibility			
8. Independence			
9. Dependence			
10. Symbolism involved			
11. Reality testing			
12. Handle feelings			
13. Impulse control			
F. SOCIAL			
1. Interaction required			
2. Isolating activity			
3. Group activity			
4. Competition			
5. Responsibility involved			
6. Communication necessary			
7. Work in small groups			
8. Work in large groups			
9. Work with one other person			
10. Test reality			
11. Control—lead			
12. Follow—cooperate			

G. CULTURAL
   1. Relevancy to personal
      a. Value system
      b. Life situations

H. COMMON TO ALL
   1. Age appropriateness
   2. Safety precautions & hazards
   3. Sexual identification
   4. Space required
   5. Equipment needed
   6. Vocational application
   7. Cost
   8. Adaptability

Methods of Instruction

In order to use activity as therapeutic intervention, each occupational therapist must become adept in giving individuals or groups instructions in the processes involved. Therapists must also learn to make astute observations regarding how the activity is approached, the way it is carried out, and the work habits exhibited in the performance of the activity. These nonverbal cues can assist the therapist in determining the actual functional level of the individual.

Occupational therapists must know how to teach the processes involved in an activity so that the client understands clearly what is to be done, yet requires a minimum amount of correction and supervision. The better the instruction, the more chance of successful accomplishment. The more successful the experiences, the more competency gained. It is therefore vital that the therapist determine the complexity of the activity so that it is within the ability of the individual to assure successful accomplishment.

Preparation for Instruction

Successful instruction is dependent upon preparation done by the therapist before instruction begins. The therapist should analyze the processes and the steps involved in the procedure along with the key points involved in the performance of the activity. This is called the *breakdown of the activity*. The *important steps* are the component parts of the total activity, while the *key points* are the specific steps involved in performance of the activity (Table 15-1).

The therapist should have the proper tools, necessary materials, and equipment ready for use before beginning instruction. The work area should be arranged properly with a minimum amount of clutter so that work can be conducted with safety and without strain. Before beginning, consideration must be given to how much of the total activity may be accomplished in one session. A simple activity with few steps or component parts may be taught in a half-hour session, while a more complex activity with many steps may require several sessions to accomplish. The activity of typing, for example, with three steps, may be accomplished in one session with many individuals and might be considered to be one unit of learning. However, becoming adept in typing could not be completed in one session, and it will require additional learning units to acquire skill. Activities such as dressing may have several units of learning such as (1) put on shirt and button, (2) put on slacks and fasten, (3) put on socks, and (4) put on shoes and tie. Each unit may need to be taught in one or more sessions with repetition required for competence.

Steps in Instruction[7]

After the therapist has made all preparations, instruction may begin using a combination of verbal directions and demonstration. There are four basic steps used in instruction: (1) preparation of the patient/client, (2) presentation of the activity, (3) try out performance, and (4) follow-up.

Step 1. Preparation of the Patient/Client
1. Establish rapport between the therapist and indi-

Table 15-1 *Example of breakdown of an activity.*

Activity: Typewriting on Standard Typewriter Important steps	Key points
1. Insert paper in typewriter	1. Pick up paper
	2. Insert paper at back of platen
	3. Pull paper release lever forward
	4. Slide paper to typing level and adjust
	5. Snap paper release into place
2. Type	1. Place fingers on "home" keys
	2. Type to end of line
	3. Push carriage return lever to return carriage that moves paper to next line
3. Take paper out of typewriter	1. Pull paper release forward
	2. Remove paper
	3. Snap paper release into place

vidual to be instructed in order to allay fear and encourage participation.

2. Find out how much the individual knows about the activity so that instruction may be geared accordingly.
3. Involve the individual in the activity in order to assure interest in it. Be sure the individual understands the purpose and value of performance of the activity.
4. Place the individual in comfortable and correct position for performance of the activity. When demonstrating, work at the side of the individual so that the process may easily be seen. Do *not* work opposite or a reverse mental image may be developed. (When teaching an individual with hand dominance different from that of the therapist, it may be appropriate to instruct while sitting opposite the individual.)

Step 2. Presentation of the Activity

1. Give verbal directions as well as demonstration of the process. Written directions and diagrams may be helpful, depending on the complexity of the activity and the learning ability and preferences of the individual.
2. Present instruction slowly and patiently.
3. Teach process step by step, stressing key points.
4. Teach no more than can be mastered at one time.

Step 3. Try out Performance

1. The individual should perform the activity either step by step with the therapist or immediately after being shown.
2. Correct errors as they occur. If possible they should be anticipated so they can be avoided.
3. Have individual explain process.
4. Have individual repeat activity several times to be sure individual knows it and can perform it correctly.

Step 4. Follow-Up

1. Put the individual on his or her own. Allow individual to work independently.
2. Designate the person who can help if difficulties arise.
3. Check progress frequently to correct errors and to assure success in performance. Less frequent checks are sufficient as competence increases.

Adaptation in Instruction

Adaptation in the method of instruction and preparation for instruction may be required for persons having special problems. The visually handicapped, for example, must have the work area precisely and consistently arranged, with every tool or piece of equipment in the same place for each session. Since use of sensation is vital to learning with the visually handicapped, opportunity must be provided and emphasized for tactile input in every step of the process. Verbal instructions must be more specific and very clearly stated.

Individuals with cognitive problems, or those having difficulty following directions, require modification in the instructions in order to be able to perform. The activity must be simplified as much as possible so that only one or two step operations are required. Directions must be given one step at a time and must be clear, concise, consistent, and concrete.

Special adaptations must be made for those individuals having any specific physical dysfunction. For example, an individual who can use only one hand should be instructed by the therapist who demonstrates using only one hand. This requires that the therapist must learn to do the activity successfully with one hand in order to demonstrate adequately.

References

1. Occupational therapy—its definition and functions. Am. J. Occup. Ther. 20:204–205, 1976.
2. Ibid.
3. Willard, H. S., and Spackman, C. S. (eds.): Occupational Therapy, ed. 4. Philadelphia: J. B. Lippincott, 1971, pp. 171–182.
4. Activity analysis. Occupational Therapy Dept., Norristown State Hospital, Norristown PA, 1977.
5. Llorens, L.: Activity analysis for cognitive-perceptual-motor dysfunction. Am. J. Occup. Ther. 27:453–456, 1973.
6. Ibid.
7. Willard H. S., and Spackman, C. S.: Occupational Therapy, ed. 4, Philadelphia PA: J. B. Lippincott, 1971, pp. 44–45.

CHAPTER 16

Activities of Daily Living and Homemaking

Maude H. Malick and Bonnie Sherry Almasy

Activities of Daily Living (ADL)

Numerous techniques for training in activities of daily living (ADL) have been explored and devised, but the primary component for success always is the patient's motivation. The patient must understand what his or her needs and deficits are, and he/she must understand the purpose and goal of the training. The patient will then be more cooperative and more willing to follow through with personal care. The therapist and patient must assess abilities and determine together which accomplishments are best done in bed, in a chair, in a wheelchair, or standing.

Often simple assistive devices such as grab bars, an overhead ring, or sliding board can aid in gross positioning. These devices (easily constructed) are not orthotic devices, but they can make the difference between independence and dependence. An overhead ring or a braided rope attached to the foot of the bed can permit a patient to pull himself up to a sitting position and comfortably transfer with or without a sliding board to a wheelchair or glide-about chair. Once trunk balance can be maintained, a patient may proceed with self-care activities in a chair.

In any disability group it is important that the patient reach maximum physical strength, balance, and skill through a structured exercise and activity program. The occupational therapist should work closely with the physical therapist in developing maximum muscle and joint function so that the patient can be trained to use the maximum of his/her abilities and to substitute for any deficits. In the case of the spinal cord injured patient, the development of muscle strength in the upper extremities is vitally important in order to do useful transfers and self-care activities.[1] At the same time energy conservation and fatigue must be considered, especially when scheduling a patient for training.

ADL is of primary concern when priorities must be set. Muriel Zimmerman states there is a direct corollary in planning physical therapy and occupational therapy activities. "Mat exercises, for instance, precede and coincide with sitting up in bed and transferring from the bed to the wheelchair. However, the needs and interest of the individual patients should always be considered. Independent eating may be started as soon as a patient can sit comfortably in bed or in a wheelchair, and in some instances it may be started while the patient is being tilted on tilt-bed or tilt-board."[2] "After the initial test, the patient is scheduled for training sessions in activities in which he is deficient and which are deemed suitable. He may merely need a few practice periods, with or without special guidance or equipment, or he may need carefully planned and supervised methods of procedure, such as sequence of performance, and the placement of the body or the hands, with repeated practice."[3]

In all self-care and dressing procedures there are some basic considerations that should be employed.

1. The bed, chair, or wheelchair should be positioned properly. All pieces of clothing and self-care items should be placed within easy reach of the patient and stored in a convenient location.
2. Patients should be encouraged to do tasks independently as much as possible. The patient's own ingenuity is an important factor.
3. Little or no adaptive equipment should be used unless it is absolutely necessary and then primarily for safety or to reduce energy and time consumption.
4. All safety precautions should be observed, especially when the patient's stability is in question. The wheelchair should be locked while transferring and during dressing procedures. For example, the patient himself may need to be stabilized by hooking his arm over the wheelchair back if necessary.

Physical disability may be increased when edema and loss of sensation exist. The therapist must instruct the patient to prevent injury from burns or trauma to the affected extremity through use of vision and by placing the extremity in a comfortable, anatomically-sound position. When training a patient, the treatment plan must include precautions if there is a loss of depth perception or if there is hemianopsia or stereognosis.

Independence without assistive devices is most desirable, but many patients cannot manage without some special equipment or even start without an aid. Assistive devices, when wisely selected and designed, can provide independence and often increase safety, speed, and group acceptance. ADL training can be started with an assistive device and later, as physical gains are made, the device can be discarded. Perhaps one of the simplest devices is a built-up handle for an eating utensil or a simple spoon holder with the spoon fitting into a pocket of a simple elastic band (Fig. 16-1). When insufficient wrist stability exists, a simple ADL splint can be made either volarly or, as in Figure 16-1, dorsally. These are most frequently used with the quadriplegic, multiple sclerosis, or muscular dystrophy patient. A clamp or plate guard and a dycem place mat are frequently used to give better food and plate control (Fig. 16-2).

Many ADL techniques for the physically hand-

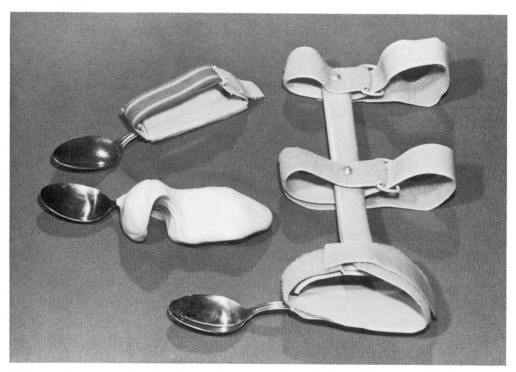

Figure 16-1. Assistive devices to aid in holding eating utensils.

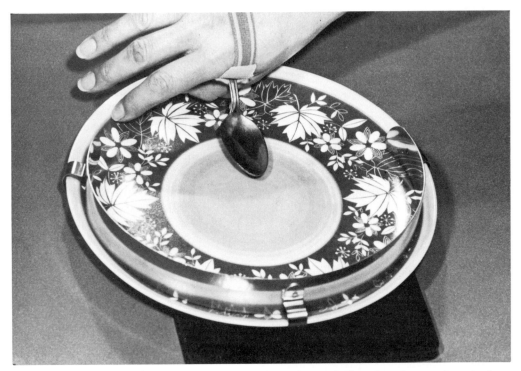

Figure 16-2. A dycem pad and plate guard used to stabilize the plate and control food spillage.

icapped have been developed. We recommend the techniques that follow. Many of these, additionally, are outlined and illustrated in *Physical Management for the Quadriplegic Patient*.[4]

ADL for the Hemiplegic Patient

Feeding

A rocker knife allows the individual to cut food with one hand.

Dressing Techniques

I. Shirts, pajama jackets, robes, and dresses opening completely down the front.
  Recommended Style:
  a. Action-back blouses.
  b. Polyester-cotton, nylon, or seersucker.
  c. Full skirts on dresses so they slip easily over the hips.
  d. Loosely fitting sleeves.
  e. Garments should be loose fitting.
  f. Clothes fastening in the front.
  Procedure:
  Method A:
  1. Put garment on affected arm first, working sleeve on completely.

2. Pull material over affected shoulder and throw it around to the back. "Walk" unaffected hand around collar and slip shirt over unaffected side.
3. Put the unaffected arm in the armhole and adjust (arm should be directed downward rather than over the head).
4. Button.
5. Remove from unaffected arm first, then from shoulder, and last from affected arm.
Method B:
1. Position shirt on lap with inside of shirt up and collar closest to the patient.
2. Put garment on affected arm first, working sleeve up over the elbow.
3. Put unaffected arm into sleeve, then raise the unaffected arm and let the garment slip over head and down the back. (With a shirt, gathering the garment up the middle of the back from hemline to collar or holding onto tail may make it easier to guide over the head.)
4. To remove the garment—make sure garment is free in back, with unaffected arm gather the garment up in back of neck (or take hold of collar), put over the head, and remove first from the unaffected arm and then from the affected arm.

Comments:
1. Sleeve on unaffected side should be buttoned before garment is put on. Button can be secured with elastic thread if cuff is too tight.
2. Button hook may be helpful.

II. Men's trousers and shorts, women's underwear and slacks.
Recommended Style:
a. Boxer style may be easier to manage than zipper. A loop may be attached to zipper to help pull up.
b. Trousers should be loose fitting.
Procedure:
Method A (Sitting Position):
1. Sit on side of bed or in straight arm chair or wheelchair.
2. Cross hemiplegic leg over good leg. Balance is best maintained if the good leg is brought to a point directly in front of the midline of the body.
3. Slip trouser onto hemiplegic leg, uncross the leg.
4. Slip on opposite trouser leg and work trousers up to the hips.
5. Wiggle from side to side, pulling the pants over the hips, or
6. Place affected arm in the pocket to prevent garment from dropping to the floor while the patient stands up to pull trousers over the hips. Suspenders, if fastened before the patient stands, will prevent trousers from dropping, while the patient gets his balance. (Alternative method is to slip the finger into the belt loop.)
7. Sit down to fasten the front or side opening.
Method B (Lying Position):
1. Put clothing on affected leg first and remove from unaffected leg last.
2. Bend affected leg at the knee and hip using unaffected hand. Slip on the pant leg, then put unaffected leg into the other pant leg.
3. Work over the hips either by rolling from side to side or hiking the hips with the uninvolved knee and hip bent.

III. Slips and dresses for women and undershirts and pullover shirts for men.
Recommended Style: Garments should be loose fitting. Dacron and nylon jersey are preferable.
Procedure:
Method A:
1. Position clothing on lap with neck of garment at the knees and back of garment on top.
2. Put affected arm through strap or sleeve.
3. Put unaffected arm through strap or sleeve.
4. Slip garment over the head.

Method B:
1. Gather clothing in unaffected arm and slip over affected arm.
2. Slip over head.
3. Put unaffected arm through strap or sleeve.
Method C:
1. Drop slip over head to the waist.
2. Pull strap over the affected arm and then over the unaffected arm.

IV. Stockings.
Recommended Style:
a. Stockings with tight elastic bands are to be avoided.
b. Stretch stockings are recommended. (They are more difficult to apply but eliminate wrinkles.)
c. Avoid sheer stockings, which are easily snagged.
Procedure:
1. Sit on edge of bed or in a straight chair with arms.
2. Cross affected leg over good leg or prop on a stool.
3. Open top of stocking by inserting the thumb and first two fingers near the cuff and spreading the fingers apart.
4. Put the great toe in first and work over the rest of the foot, alleviating all wrinkles.
Comments: Stockings must be kept free from wrinkles, which may cause pressure areas.

V. Brassieres.
Recommended Style: Front opening style may be easiest to apply.
Procedure:
Method A (Conventional Style):
1. Anchor bra strap with thumb of affected hand, pull around to front.
2. Hook bra in front at the waist and slip around to the back.
3. Place affected arm through the shoulder strap and then place the unaffected arm through the other strap.
Comments: Elastic may be added to the straps for ease in applying.

VI. Shoes and short leg braces.
Procedure:
1. Apply the brace while in bed if balance is poor.
2. Sit on the edge of the bed or in a chair if balance is good.
3. Cross hemiplegic leg over unaffected leg. Balance is best maintained if the unaffected leg is brought to a point directly in front of the midline of the body.
4. Slip the toes into the shoe while holding the

short leg brace in the unaffected hand by the metal bar. Insert toes sideways first, then slip the shoe around to the correct position to avoid catching the toes on the outer edge of the shoe.

5. Place the shoehorn, long-handled if necessary, into the shoe from the side to the back.
6. Frequently the back of the shoe will buckle and the broad part of the shoehorn will be under the heel. Place affected leg on floor or a stool, place pressure on the knee with the unaffected hand, and put weight on the affected foot. The shoehorn is now in a position where the patient's heel is pressing on it.
7. Bring the shoehorn up slowly, flat against the heel and inside the back of the shoe, but do not pull out.
8. Continue to press on knee and put weight on the foot, intermittently moving the shoehorn until the foot slips into shoe and the back of the shoe is straight.
9. Remove the shoehorn and lace the shoe. Elastic shoe laces can be used if the patient has difficulty tying a bow using the one-handed shoe tie method.
10. Press the Velcro closure together or fasten the buckle to stabilize the brace to the leg calf.

Hygiene and Grooming

Recommended Equipment:
a. Electric razor for safety. (Norelco is suggested.)
b. Long-handled bath sponges with a place in the sponge for soap permits the patient to reach nearly all parts of the body.
c. Use bath tub stools or chair inside tub for safe transfers and use hand held shower hose for bathing.
d. Suction cups attached to handbrushes are recommended to enable patient to scrub nails and hand on unaffected side. These brushes are also used for washing dentures (place a wash rag in the sink basin for safety).
e. Bath mitt with soap pocket.
f. Mirror fastening around neck or on knee.
g. Nail file secured to table with masking tape or adhesive.
h. Long lipsticks may be easier to manage.
i. Rubber spool or Velcro hook curlers can be applied with one hand.
j. Toilet articles packaged under pressure or in plastic bottles, such as spray deodorant, are easier and safer to use than those in screwtop glass jars.
k. Combs with long or built-up handles may be of value.

ADL for the Paraplegic Patient

Dressing

I. Shirts, pajama jackets, robes, and dresses opening completely down the front.
Recommended Style:
a. Material should be wrinkle-resistant, smooth, and durable.
b. Action-back blouses, roomy sleeves, full skirts that slip easily over the hips.
Procedure:
1. Balance body by putting palms of hands on mattress on either side of body.
2. Seek assistance or elevate bed backrest if balance is poor. With backrest elevated, both hands are available.
3. Method of putting clothing on does not usually create a problem; however, if difficulty is encountered, the following method is suggested: with garment open on the lap, collar toward patient's chest, put arms into sleeves and pull up over elbows. Then, holding on to the shirt tail or back of dress, pull over head, adjust, and button.

II. Men's trousers and shorts, women's underwear or slacks.
Recommended Style:
a. Slacks are easier to fasten if they have a front zipper closure. However, in some instances, zippers in the side seams are easier to apply over braces.
b. Wear loose fitting clothes for ease in getting over braces.
c. If the patient is incontinent, pants should close with snap opening in front.
Procedure:
1. Sit on bed and pull knees into a flexed position.
2. Hold the top of the trousers and flip the pants down to the feet.
3. Work pant legs over the feet and pull up to the hips.
4. Roll from hip to hip in a semi-reclining position and pull up the garment.

III. Slips and skirts.
Recommended Style:
a. Loose fitting half slips.
b. Full skirts for ease in pulling over hips and for better appearance over braces.
Procedure:
1. Sit on bed, slip garment over head, and let it drop to waist.
2. Roll from hip to hip in a semi-reclining position and pull the garment down over the hips and thighs.

IV. Shoes.
  Recommended Style: Shoes should be of oxford type if braces are to be attached.
  Procedure:
  Method A:
  1. Pull one knee at a time into flexed position with hands while in sitting position on bed and, supporting leg with upper arms, slip on shoe.
  Method B:
  1. Sit on edge of bed or in wheelchair for back support.
  2. Bend one knee to a flexed position, supporting leg with upper arm, and slip shoe on.
  Method C:
  1. Patient sits on edge of bed or in wheelchair for back support.
  2. Patient crosses one leg over the other and slips shoe on.
 V. Stockings.
  Recommended Style:
  a. Socks with tight elastic bands should be avoided.
  b. Service-weight nylons are recommended for women.
  c. Stockings should fit smoothly since any wrinkles may cause pressure areas.

Hygiene and Grooming

1. A spray hose is helpful in bathing. The patient should keep a finger over the spray to determine sudden temperature change in water.
2. Long-handled bath brushes with soap insert are helpful for ease in reaching all parts of the body.
3. Soap bars attached to a cord around the neck may be helpful.

ADL for the Quadriplegic Patient

Dressing Activities

These suggestions depend on the level of lesion of the patient.
1. Zippers and Velcro fastenings facilitate dressing.
2. Blouses should be cut with extra length.
3. Garments should be loose fitting.

Feeding

It may be helpful to have:
1. Leather or plastic cuff with a pocket to hold fork or spoon.
2. Combination spoon-fork (spork).
3. Plate guard to aid in getting food on spoon.

4. Double suction cup or dycem plastic mat to stabilize plate.
5. Long plastic straw.

Grooming

1. ADL splint attachments help in using razor, toothbrush, and comb. When an Engen reciprocal wrist orthosis or wrist-driven flexor-hinge hand splint is used, few assistive devices are needed.
2. A cigarette holder or a robot smoker for safety and a mouth stick for turning pages, painting, typing, writing, and dialing the telephone can be made if needed.
3. Bath tub bench or chair for safe bath tub transfers and hand held shower for bathing can be used.
4. Sliding board for transfer to wheelchair, bath tub or car is helpful.

In the case of a C_4-level quadriplegic, sophisticated environmental control systems can be made using electronic techniques and utilizing external power sources (Fig. 16-3). Battery power sources have been far more successful than carbon dioxide power. Powered wheelchairs and mobile carts have been perfected, and they are easily available. They should be prescribed carefully, because many options are available. The telephone companies have many options in communication aids available for the handicapped, such as push button dialing, voice controls, and amplifiers. These may vary depending on the region or country in which the patient lives.

ADL for Patients with Limited Range of Motion

Generally there are no standard procedures for activities of daily living for patients with limited range of motion (ROM). However the following adaptations may prove helpful.

Dressing Activities

1. Larger size clothing, made of materials which may have some stretch.
2. Adapted styles of clothing.
3. Larger buttons or zippers with a loop on the pull tab.
4. Long shoehorn.
5. Reaching tongs of all types.
6. Elastic shoe laces.
7. Stocking aids: garter attached to string, garters sewn on wooden hoop at end of straps, commercial aids.
8. Tabs sewed on clothing to facilitate use of hook on a long handle.

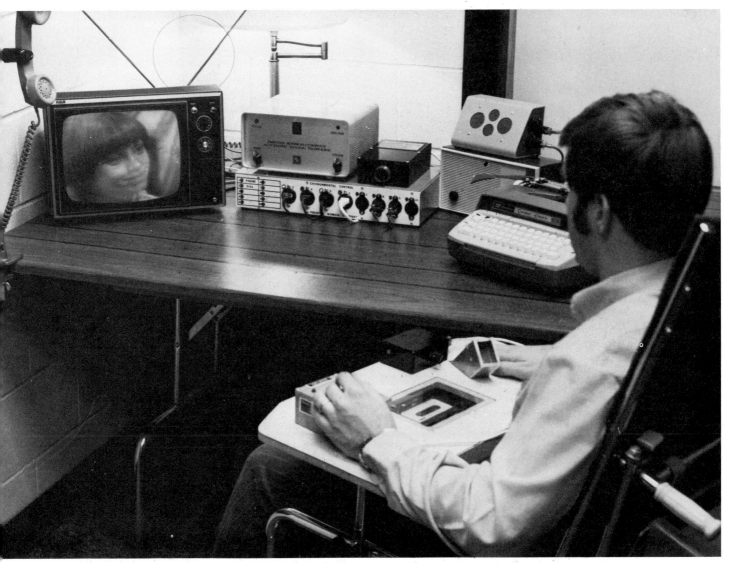

Figure 16-3. Environment control for the severely disabled. The subject can operate household appliances (telephone, lamp, intercom, radio) through environmental control packages. He controls powered wheelchair, onboard tape recorder, lights, horn, power recline, and remote control table top appliances through DU-IT wheelchair control system. (Prentke Romich Co. and Romich, Berry and Bayer, Inc.)

Feeding

1. Built-up handles on utensils.
2. Elongated handles.
3. Plastic straw if ROM is limited in shoulder and when it is difficult to pick up a glass or cup.

Hygiene and Grooming

1. Hand-held shower for bathing or shampooing hair.
2. Reachers to hold washcloth, powder puff, and so forth.
3. Long-handled combs, toothbrush.
4. Long lipstick.
5. Long-handled bath brush with soap container.
6. Extended handle for safety on electric razor.
7. Spray type deodorant.
8. Extended or built-up handles on water faucets.

Homemaking
Energy Saving Techniques

The current definition of homemaker rehabilitation reflects the blending of the traditional treatment procedures with contemporary managerial techniques and philosophies. Without losing sight of the holistic approach to homemaker rehabilitation, it is necessary to consider the actual treatment methods involved in each area. The introduction of basic energy saving techniques is of prime importance regardless of disability.

The homemaker must be made aware of new demands or limitations placed on his or her energy. Use of a wheelchair or walking device requires an extra expenditure of energy. Cardiac problems or arthritis may necessitate stopping or altering some activities. One of the most difficult areas of homemaker rehabilitation is that of helping the patient feel comfortable with and accepting the new rate and method of work. Many individuals become frustrated with initial attempts at activity. Frustration, fear, and mental stress can drain energy faster than the actual performance of some tasks. Efforts should be made to provide an atmosphere for training and evaluation that is pleasant, conducive to learning, and allows for exhibition of maximum performance.

Decision making is an integral part of work simplification. The decisions made may indicate role reversal, hiring help, compromise of priority, or modifications in the home. Many homemakers see work simplification techniques as the lazy way to work, and they are uncomfortable with accepting new methods, products, or equipment. If the attitude cannot be changed, these feelings should be respected and, if at all feasible, alternate methods that are acceptable to the homemaker in meeting her standards should be instituted. Efficiency may suffer but the degree of carry-over at home will be increased. Making the homemaker aware of results of time and motion studies and demonstrating analysis of activity may build a discriminating attitude toward expenditures of energy.

The homemaker should first question the reason for doing each task. Is it necessary? Many tasks or at least portions of tasks can be eliminated. Is the homemaker best suited to do this task? Many family members may be capable of assuming the responsibility. The homemaker may, in turn, assume activities more in tune with present abilities. It is important to consider when a task must be completed in relation to other planned activities. It may be necessary to alternate the tasks of a passive nature with more active tasks. Discussion of how a task should be completed will provide an opportunity to introduce convenience foods and appropriate small appliances or assistive devices. Many individuals are concerned with excessive cost but, in terms of the cost of time and energy saved, the homemaker cannot afford to limit herself to old methods or equipment. *Rehabilitation Monograph VIII*[5] offers assistance in developing an improved method in work simplification techniques and principles:

1. Use both hands to work, in opposite and symmetrical motions if possible, smooth flowing path motions in a curve with no angles such as dusting and washing windows.
2. Lay out work areas within normal reach. Work where the areas of both hands overlap and arrange supplies in a semicircle within normal reach.
3. Slide—do not lift and carry. Slide pots from sink to range. Use a wheeled table where work surfaces are broken.
4. Fixed work stations. Have a special place to do each job so that supplies and equipment may always be kept there ready for immediate use.
5. Select equipment that may be used for more than one job; eliminate unnecessary motions. Use recipes that emphasize the "one bowl method" and quick mixing.
6. Avoid holding—use utensils with a flat base, suction cups, rubber mats, or electric mixers to free both hands.
7. Let gravity work—a laundry chute, a pan below the level of the cutting board.
8. Pre-position tools. Store small tools in such a way that they are in the right position to grasp and start work immediately. Hand utensils separately within sight.

9. Locate machine control and switches within easy reach. Select household appliances with control located within easy reach for standing or sitting, depending on which position will be used. Change the location of switches if possible or insert switches in electric cord for easier use.
10. Sit to work whenever possible. Sit to iron, work at the sink, prepare vegetables, mix foods. Find a comfortable chair and adjust the workplace height to it or, if this cannot be changed, fit the chair to the workplace.
11. Select work place height appropriate for the worker and for the job. The jobs requiring hand activity will need a higher work surface than those requiring arm motion or pressure. There are no "standard heights," as body proportions differ.
12. Working conditions. If the surrounding conditions are good, the job will be pleasanter and less tiring. Good light, directed toward the work, good ventilation, comfortable clothing, pleasing colors, and order set the stage for work without strain.*

Incoordination

Incoordination can be caused by a variety of diseases or conditions such as Parkinson's disease, multiple sclerosis, and cerebral palsy. Regardless of the specific cause, it is necessary to attempt to use the affected extremity to develop coordination. Homemaking tasks may provide a productive form of exercise.

Before introducing specific techniques, it is especially important to allay any of the patient's fears that could aggravate the coordination problem or hinder safe functioning. Fatigue, also, can influence the degree of spasticity or incoordination. In order to promote working in a relaxed, rested manner at home the patient should be made aware of factors that could influence performance.

Energy saving techniques are an essential part of any program, and management of time and energy should be practiced with all activities. Convenience foods that eliminate the need for extensive cutting, chopping, or mixing should be recommended. Easy open packages and containers are helpful. Substitution of a technique such as sliding instead of lifting or the use of equipment such as a wheelchair lap tray or wheeled cart will promote safer functioning. Weighted utensils and items with double handles that can be gripped easily will partially counteract the

* Courtesy—Rehabilitation Monograph VIII, A Manual for Training the Disabled Homemaker, Institute of Rehabilitation Medicine, New York University Medical Center, New York, New York 1967.

affects of the incoordination. Stabilization can be achieved by utilizing a spikeboard, rubber mats, or sponges. Blenders, crockpots, and electric skillets are often essential kitchen aids when placed at appropriate heights on stationary work surfaces. A coffee urn can be utilized as a constant source of hot water for instant soups, cereals, and beverages; it negates the need for using the range. Oversized bowls can contain food that would normally be spilled by extraneous movements. Long mitts promote oven safety. Meals that meet nutritional needs yet simplify the food preparation process can be planned.

One-Handed Techniques

It is important for the one-handed individual to plan a work schedule that allows for periods of rest and for alternating heavy and light tasks. The patient should organize all equipment and supplies, adjust the work height, and use the utility cart, sliding technique, or wheelchair tray to assist in transporting items. Consider convenience foods and the use of small equipment to assist in any activity. If difficulty is noted in reading or following directions, it may be necessary to enlarge print or simplify instructions. If hemianopsia is a problem, compensation as well as general awareness of the affected extremity should be taught for safety's sake. Lack of sensation in the affected extremity can be extremely dangerous, particularly when the task involves use of a knife, hot liquids, or appliances. If poor balance is noted, suggest sitting to work, especially when attempting to use oven or refrigerator. The use of long tongs and proper storage techniques can eliminate some problems caused by inadequate balance. Organizational ability can be easily assessed in such simple activities as setting the table or separating utensils in a silverware drawer. Many homemakers may acquire good return of affected extremities but still experience difficulty in using good judgment or in problem solving. This can create more difficulties than the physical dysfunction.

Emphasis should be placed on activities that the patient can complete easily and safely. Families should be made aware of all limitations as well as abilities. Self-help catalogs have many gadgets for the individual with the use of one hand. While some equipment may be necessary for independent functioning, it should be stressed that most homemaking activities can be completed with nothing more than the proper technique.

A spikeboard, two aluminum or stainless steel nails on a board, becomes a second hand to stabilize everything from potatoes to cupcakes to meat. A rubber mat can be used to hold bowls, pans, or plates. Packages or jars can be stabilized for easy opening by using the knees or a partially opened drawer. Teeth or scissors are helpful in opening many types of packaging. Jar openers and electric can openers are also useful aids that promote independence. Each person should be allowed to experiment with various techniques and pieces of equipment to encourage the problem-solving method at home.

The Arthritic Patient

The arthritic homemaker may find it crucial to conserve energy and protect his/her joints from undue stress. Some homemaking tasks provide good exercise, and they actually may be beneficial. All activities must be monitored with regard to joint stress produced, amount of time required in one position, and contribution to general fatigue. It is important to emphasize the following:

1. Sit when possible but not for prolonged periods of time.
2. Use fingers in extension whenever possible, for example, in dishwashing and dusting.
3. Stress should not be put on the thumb or fingers. Utilize palms or wrist and attempt to distribute the weight of an object evenly. Use both hands when possible.
4. Utilize proper work height. Avoid tasks that put undue stress on joints such as scrubbing, wringing, or opening jars.
5. Slide equipment and supplies when possible rather than carrying them. Use the utility cart.
6. Prevent lifting of heavy items, bending, and reaching by careful storage. Use of light weight bowls, utensils, and appliances is recommended.
7. Avoid prolonged holding of a book, needlework, pencil, or telephone.

The arthritic homemaker, attempting to function at home, will be well aware of his/her limitations. Adapted equipment may be required in addition to demonstration and training in proper techniques. A few well-chosen items early in the treatment program may eliminate the need for restriction of activity or increase in the number of devices necessary as the disease progresses. The homemaker must fully understand the reasoning behind the instructions being given, or he/she may perform activities in a manner which could be detrimental. *The Self-Help Manual for Arthritic Patients* from the Arthritis Foundation[6] answers many questions on equipment needs and specific task techniques.

Because of the general nature of the progression of arthritis, the homemaker may have psychological problems of varying degrees. The therapist may be instrumental in easing psychological problems as well as easing pain and increasing function in the affected joints.

The Quadriplegic Patient

A quadriplegic individual functioning effectively in the home provides a study in management principles.

Brain power, not manpower, must be emphasized. The quadriplegic patient must be equiped with knowledge and skills to organize and manage effectively. Introduced in the early stages of rehabilitation, basic management skills can help allay the feelings of total helplessness. Financial management, childrearing theories, diet instructions, and meal planning are mental tasks that can be accomplished to provide positive reinforcement and increase motivation. With use of telephone and typing skills, manually or by mouth, it is possible to assume tasks such as ordering groceries, paying bills, and being the family's social secretary. It is important that families be involved, especially when role reversals or modifications are indicated.

The subject of home modification can be approached when both the patient and family exhibit signs of acceptance of the disability and an understanding of the permanence of the situation. Although the rehabilitation process for quadriplegic patients generally is lengthy, the extent of home modification may necessitate early initiation. Weekend visits will be more pleasurable and better indicators of postdischarge success if the home is adequately modified. The degree of modification indicated is dependent on the functional level of the patient. Possibly the home would best be designed for the ease of the attendant or the family caring for the patient. *Building Without Barriers for the Disabled*[7] is one of many possible sources of information relat-

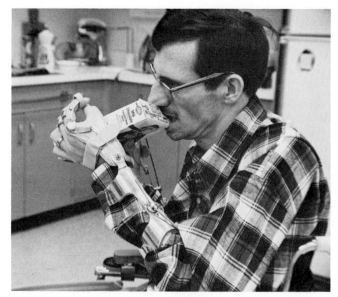

Figure 16-4. Teeth and tenodesis splints work together effectively to open packages.

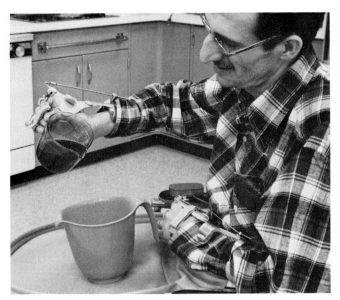

Figure 16-5. A light-weight measuring cup, bowl with a handle, and vinyl lap tray promote independence for the quadriplegic patient with natural or mechanical tenodesis functioning.

ing to home modification. Home-planning consultants and rehabilitation home economists are being utilized by innovative rehabilitation facilities to work with the patient and families in the planning process.

For those quadriplegics (generally C_5 and below) who will be assuming some or most homemaking tasks, special attention should be given to equipment selection and utilization of work simplification techniques (Figs. 16-4 and 16-5). The use of such small appliances as electric skillet, can opener, coffee urn, toaster-oven, or slow cooker can provide a great degree of independence (Fig. 16-6). Convenience foods

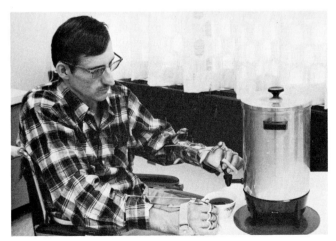

Figure 16-6. An urn, stabilized with a rubber mat, provides a source of hot water for instant cereals, soups, and beverages.

provide a simple but adequate source of nutritional needs. *Mealtime Manual for the Aged and Handicapped*[8] offers specific suggestions for use and selection of adapted equipment and appliances. Because of the patient's loss of sensation, safety should be a prime consideration, especially with use of heat or sharp objects.

Clothing

A large portion of the activities of daily living program is directed towards gaining independence in dressing. It is obvious that certain types of clothing may be more comfortable, safer, easier to care for, or provide for a greater degree of independence. Many sources illustrate styles of clothing particularly suitable for different disabilities. One such source is *Independent Living for the Handicapped and the Elderly*.[9] Clothing does more than merely cover the body. It can provide a method of self-expression and promote confidence and acceptance in society. Personal preferences vary. This must be considered when making recommendations. General considerations include that clothing:
1. be strong enough to take abrasion caused by orthotic devices or sliding transfer techniques to a wheelchair;
2. have openings that are easily accessible and fasteners that are operable by individuals with limited arm movement or poor hand coordination;
3. provide for ease of movement in a wheelchair or with assistive devices for ambulation;
4. be attractive as well as functional.

The homemaker may have actual experience in adapting clothing to make it more functional or to conceal a deformity or device. Basic safety precautions should be taken with persons having decreased reaction time, incoordination, or assistive devices. Discourage the wearing of loose-sleeved garments over open flame or near equipment. Keep slacks and skirts of appropriate length and width to allow ambulation with assistive devices or safe use of a wheelchair. Fireproof garments are recommended.

Emphasis should be placed on the type of fabric selected. Consideration should include allergy or irritations, washability (especially where incontinence is a problem), required ironing, wrinkling, absorption of or resistance to perspiration, and color-fastness. Laundering techniques that are proper for varying types of garments and fabrics include type of detergent, water temperature, use of softener and prewash soaks. These may reduce amount of time and energy expended by the homemaker. Proper technique for laundering slings or support garments will lengthen the life of these costly items.

Care should be taken, especially in selection of undergarments. They must be functional for the wearer, and they must permit independence in dressing and toileting. Fit should not interfere with circulation nor cause skin breakdown by binding or rubbing. A fabric that absorbs perspiration is generally most comfortable. Certain garments may be adapted or eliminated entirely for comfort or ease in dressing—quadriplegic males frequently find undershorts restrictive and nonfunctional for them. The Fashion Able Company offers a wide selection of adapted undergarments and swimwear.

Child Care Techniques

Many disabled persons find themselves responsible not only for their own care but also for that of small children. Modern technology has lightened the task with the advent of disposable diapers and bottles and with premixed formulas. However, the greatest problem is the fear and uncertainty surrounding the resumption of this responsible role. Children also are capable of sensing the confidence, or lack of it, and they will respond accordingly.

The introduction of the parents or grandparent to child care techniques is an integral part of the program that can make the transition to home easier and more comfortable for the entire family. A weighted doll can be utilized in developing basic skills of dressing, feeding, and bathing. The homemaker should be made aware of products on the market that make child care easier. Even if some items are costly, it may be more economical monetarily and psychologically than hiring an assistant. Use of these products save time and energy, and they allow the parent to spend time with the child. A severely disabled person can offer much to the development of a child by offering love and by teaching, playing, and helping the child develop self-confidence and skills. It may be necessary to introduce some basic considerations for selection and use of equipment.[10]

1. Is the equipment manageable within physical limitations?
2. Can height be adjusted easily?
3. Can equipment be moved easily?
4. Are controls easily used?
5. Can it be cared for and cleaned easily?
6. Is it sufficiently sturdy and durable?
7. Is it multipurpose and able to be used over a long period of time?
8. Is it adapted to growth of the child?
9. Is it safe for the child as well as the parent?
10. Will it promote early independence in children?

Children can learn at an early age to assist with dressing and feeding. With well-selected self-help clothing, supervision, and encouragement, they soon become independent. Usually around 4 years of age children express interest in helping, and they should be given the opportunity to be contributing members of the household. The homemaker's management principles may come into use here, with the utilization of family resources.

The disabled parent should be forewarned that discipline of small children may be a problem. However, children generally respond best when they have responsibility in accord with their age and have rules and standards for behavior. A parent's tone of voice or look can be a sufficient indicator of displeasure. Children are by nature flexible beings who can adapt to almost any situation if given proper guidance and stimulation. Guiding a child's development can be a rewarding experience for any homemaker.

Dietary Considerations

The incorporation of nutrition principles is an essential part of any homemaker rehabilitation program. Nutritional needs are established and prescribed by the physician or dietitian, but the homemaker rehabilitation area provides a natural area for testing, training, and explaining dietary plans. The American Dietetic Association offers many audiovisual aids, posters, and pamphlets that are helpful in teaching nutrition.

New demands are being placed on the homemaker's body; the patient must realize this. Depending upon one's level of activity, wheelchair use may indicate an increase or decrease in caloric needs for the day. Age is another determining factor. Many patients experience weight gains during long periods of inactivity during hospitalization. The homemaker can better comprehend the need for a change in diet if he/she understands the reasons for these changes.

Excess weight is a factor that severely limits a handicapped homemaker in reaching his or her potential. Transfers are more difficult and dressing problems are increased. More energy is required to ambulate or perform other physical activity. General tolerance is reduced. Prostheses, if used, often do not fit correctly. Weight control is especially crucial for the cardiac patient or the patient with pulmonary problems. Diabetic diets are prevalent among the amputee population. Many are so frightened by diabetes that they no longer enjoy food. Practice in planning and preparing meals can alleviate the fear, and it offers a better chance for effective carry-over.

Introduction of new food preparation methods may be helpful. For example, teach broiling instead of frying foods, or introduce new products such as sugar substitutes. Take a diet history, if possible, including premorbid eating patterns. Using this as a

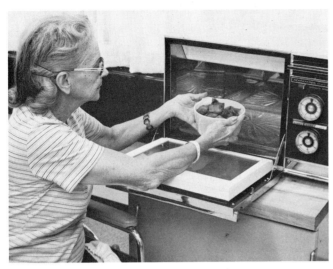

Figure 16-7. Fast, no mess cooking in a microwave oven can encourage those who live alone or are on modified diets to prepare meals that meet their nutritional needs.

guide, assist the homemaker in planning nutritious meals. In explaining a diet it often is necessary to go beyond the general exchange list given by the doctor or dietitian. Cultural, religious, and family customs must be taken into consideration as well as cost and nutritional needs. Emphasis should be placed on planning foods that are not only relatively easy to prepare but also are nutritious (Fig. 16-7).

Basic nutrition principles are essential not only for the homemaker but also for the family. Often it is necessary to emphasize the manner in which the patient's dietary restrictions can be coordinated with family food planning. A trip to the grocery store, in addition to enabling the therapist to determine tolerance, the patient's use of money, and social interactions, also gives the homemaker a practical experience of reading food labels and seeing products on the market that are permitted by the diet. Many special diet foods are expensive and not necessarily indicated. Effective substitutes should be noted for those people on limited budgets. The use of food stamps or other government-sponsored assistance programs should be explained, and the homemaker may be referred to the appropriate agency if indicated. Successful carry-over is predictable if the patient is made aware of the extent of assistance available.

Financial Management

Frequently, because of circumstances surrounding an accident or illness, a family discovers that its previous financial plan is no longer adequate. In planning for disposition of the patient, the therapist and family may find it helpful to go over the new demands on financial resources. Arrangements may have to be made for home modifications, special equipment, nursing care, household help, a new vehicle or means of transportation, tutors for children, or medical expenses and supplies.

For a budget to be flexible and functional it is necessary to involve the entire family. Budgeting is not easy but, when seriously undertaken, should result in a realistic plan for utilization of family financial and other related resources. Five basic steps are needed:
1. Record items and services required by the family for the allotted portion of time.
2. Estimate the cost involved and total each category.
3. Estimate anticipated income.
4. Bring anticipated income and anticipated expenditures into balance.
5. Evaluate plans for realistic chance of success.

Gross and Crandel's *Management for Modern Families* [11] can serve as a guide for budget preparation. A budget cannot be made *for* a family; the therapist can only *guide* the family in devising a plan that is suitable for its own needs and flexible enough to change with its needs. Once the budget is established, the homemaker, though limited physically, may be responsible for keeping the family's records, paying bills, and determining need for future expenditures or changes in the budget.

Training Apartment

In addition to the basic homemaker training and evaluation center, a training apartment provides an essential setting for an important portion of the evaluation process (Figs. 16-8 and 16-9). According to the Procedures and Policies established for the use of the Harmarville Rehabilitation Center apartment,[12] the purposes of a trial stay in the training apartment are as follows:
1. To evaluate patient and family capabilities in a homelike situation. Apartment use must be indicated therapeutically.
2. To evaluate physical and/or emotional needs of a patient and/or family.
3. To reinforce and follow through on patient care procedures in preparation for home visit or discharge. To document level of performance of patient and/or family in a protected but independent area.

The staff, including all appropriate treatment departments and therapy services, and the family should meet after an apartment stay to discuss the experience, make possible changes in program or

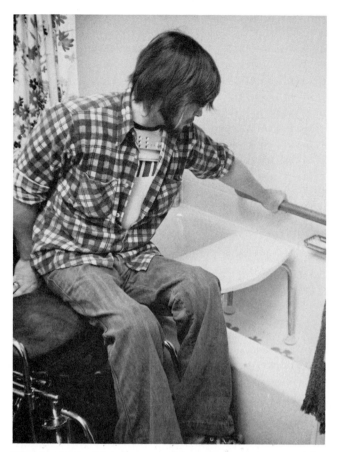

Figure 16-8. The homemaking apartment provides an opportunity for the patient to care for himself independently, thus preparing for independent living.

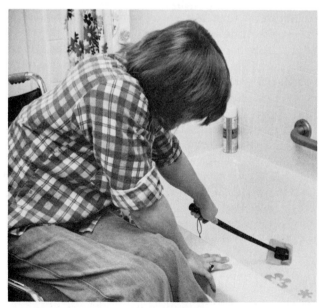

Figure 16-9. The homemaking apartment provides an opportunity for the patient to test his knowledge and skills in the care of his own home.

treatment plan, provide for extended family education, and plan for appropriate disposition for the patient. In addition to being an educational tool, an apartment stay can provide a means for boosting the morale and confidence of the patient and family. On a daily basis the apartment lends itself to use as a training area for activities of daily living and for the evaluation of large scale homemaking tasks such as bedmaking and vacuuming.

Home Visits

It is necessary to know the patient's home situation when establishing a treatment plan. Therefore the therapist must first evaluate the living situation so that the initial teaching of skills and information will be pertinent and appropriate. Often the patient or family can provide adequate information, but if problems are indicated in any area, a home visit may be necessary. It may be advantageous to include the patient when making the home visit. Questions can be answered and fears quelled.

The occupational therapist and rehabilitation home economist or other members of the rehabilitation team, such as the physical therapist, may participate in the evaluation. The following questions should be considered:

1. Is at least one entrance accessible to the patient? Are railings or ramps indicated?
2. Are doorways wide enough for wheelchair traffic?
3. Do doorsills, rugs, or floor coverings hinder safe ambulation?
4. Is furniture placed to provide for a good traffic pattern? Is it sturdy enough for safe transfers?
5. Are the telephone, light switches, television, and radio accessible? Is bathroom adequate for safe transfers? Are grab bars, elevated seats, mats, bathstools, or plumbing modifications indicated?
6. Is the bedroom large enough for independent transfer? Are needed items placed conveniently? Is a commode chair indicated? Are closet spaces enough to accommodate needs? Are storage areas accessible?
7. Is the kitchen of adequate size for safe functioning? Are range, sink, refrigerator, and cupboards accessible for safe use?
8. Are laundry facilities accessible?
9. Is the children's play area available for supervision?

Post-discharge home visits provide a good form of follow-up. The visitor can assess the adjustment to the home situation and the degree of carry-over, make recommendations concerning the problems that might have come to light since discharge, evaluate the effectiveness of the home program and the need for additional services or equipment, and make any necessary referrals to appropriate agencies. Results of the postdischarge evaluation should be shared with all involved departments.

A follow-up questionnaire can be used as an indicator of the necessity of a home visit, or it can serve as an indicator of the effectiveness of the homemaker rehabilitation program.

Architectural Design Considerations and Selection

In the Home

It is necessary to evaluate the home circumstances when planning a rehabilitation program, and often it is necessary to suggest modifications for making the home environment functional. This initial preparation maximizes the affects of the rehabilitation process.

Timing is important in initiating the subject of home modifications with the patient and family. The patient who has not yet accepted the disability may reject any plans because they seem to be an indication that the disability is indeed permanent. The family also must be ready to accept, cooperate, and be supportive. Both the family and patient must see the need for change, and they must be willing to work with the therapist in assessing the modifications necessary in light of the patient's physical ability. Sometimes it is helpful to have the patient sketch a floor plan and list, if possible, inaccessible areas. A home visit may be necessary to obtain measurements or to assess a difficult situation. The family can help by supplying photographs or measurements of the home.

Much has been written concerning home modifications with special emphasis on the kitchen and bathroom. Special requirements have been established for wheelchair functioning, proper work heights, and storage areas (Fig. 16-10). The basic mixing, sink, and range centers have been developed with specifications for equipment and storage techniques. Each of the three types of kitchens—U, L, and aisle—has advantages and disadvantages; these depend on the homemaker, the disability, and the family situation.

Most people are unable to remodel extensively and some, especially apartment dwellers, find it impossible to make any structural changes. Ingenuity and perseverance are needed, and they can make even the most unlikely places livable. The therapist can merely make recommendations for modifications based on the following guidelines:

1. The dwelling must provide adequate space for entrance and exit. Doorways should be 36 in. wide and ramps 30 to 40 in. wide. Inclines should be of approximately 6 degrees or 1 in. to 1 ft. and should be equipped with railings.
2. Doorsills should be eliminated where possible. The dwelling should enable free movement throughout. Throw rugs should be removed and thick carpets avoided. Nonskid floors are preferred. Furniture should be arranged appropriately to allow a free flowing traffic pattern. Doors may be eliminated or changed to sliding or folding doors or curtains. Bathing and toileting facilities should be provided with grab bars and nonskid flooring. Wall switches should be within easy reach, 36 in. from the floor, and outlets should be 24 in. from the floor. The communication system should be within reach and of a type usable by the patient.
3. The kitchen should be functional and meet needs as determined by the homemaking evaluation.
4. Heating and air conditioning systems may be essential for some disabilities.

Figure 16-11 is a sample of a sketch of bathroom facilities.

In Society

The rehabilitation process cannot be considered totally successful until all disabled individuals are freed from manmade environmental restrictions. Making the home accessible is an important first step, but the individual must not be shut out or shut in by barriers outside the home. In addition to physical barriers there are attitudinal barriers. These are broken each time a disabled individual takes his or her place in society.

Architectural and transportation barriers, however, are not so easily eliminated. Stairs, curbs, heavy doors, inaccessible restrooms and telephones, and public transportation restrict independence of those individuals with mobility limitations. This group includes not only the wheelchair bound but also the blind, deaf, those with assistive walking devices, and those with curtailed mobility as a result of the aging process, arthritis, or other limiting conditions. A barrier-free environment would provide freer access for all.

Federal and state governments and public and nonprofit groups are becoming involved in breaking through the barriers that are keeping the disabled from using public buildings, housing, theaters, stores, recreational facilities, restaurants, and public transportation. In the early 1960s the President's Committee on Employment for the Handicapped,

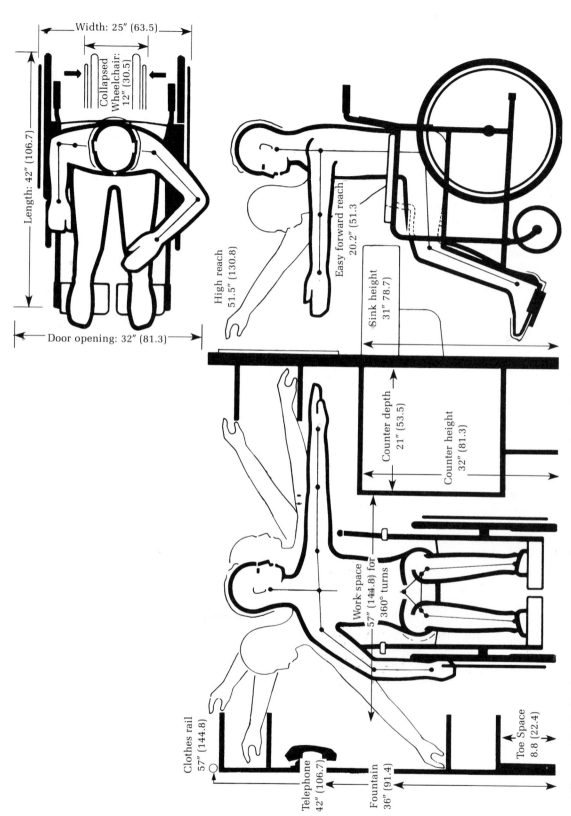

Width: 25" (63.5)

Collapsed Wheelchair: 12" (30.5)

Length: 42" (106.7)

Door opening: 32" (81.3)

High reach 51.5" (130.8)

Easy forward reach 20.2" (51.3)

Sink height 31" 78.7)

Counter depth 21" (53.5)

Counter height 32" (81.3)

Work space 57" (144.8) for 360° turns

Clothes rail 57" (144.8)

Telephone 42" (106.7)

Fountain 36" (91.4)

Toe Space 8.8 (22.4)

Figure 16-10. Basic measurements and proportions can be utilized when planning home modifications. (Measurements are given in inches and centimeters.) (Adapted from Diffrient, N., Tilley, A. R., and Bardagey, J.: Humanscale 1/2/3. (Designer: Henry Dreyfuss Associates.) Cambridge MA: MIT Press, 1974.)

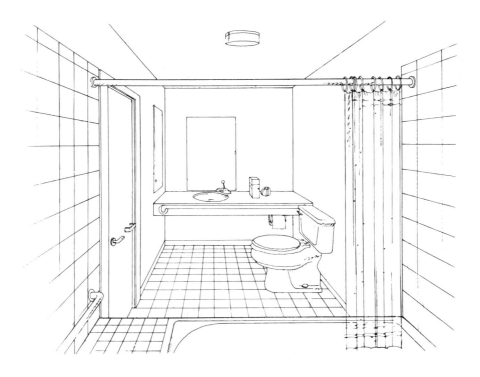

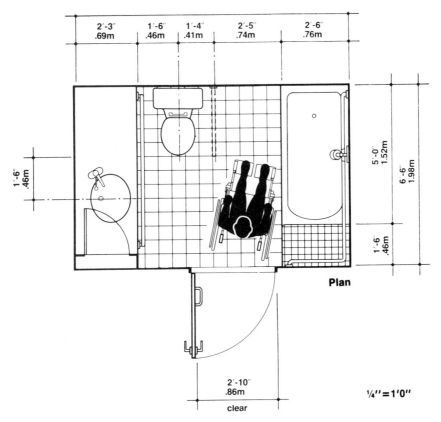

Figure 16-11. Two views of a bathroom suitable for the use of most disabled persons. (Courtesy of Harkness, S. P., and Groom, J. N., Jr.: Building Without Barriers for the Disabled. The Architect Collaborative Inc., Whitney Library of Design, Cambridge MA, 1976.)

with the Easter Seal Society for Crippled Children and Adults, led a campaign that made the public aware of this discrimination. Enactment of the Architectural Barriers Act of 1968 ensured that certain federally funded buildings and facilities would be designed so as to be accessible and usable by the physically handicapped. Federal legislation has established standards, which were revised in 1976, for providing accessibility as prescribed by the American National Standards Institute (ANSI). The Architectural and Transportation Barriers Compoiance Board was created by the Rehabilitation Act of 1973. By 1974 every state and the District of Columbia had required the elimination of architectural barriers in public buildings either through legislation, building codes, or executive directives.[13]

The International Symbol of Access (Fig. 16-12), officially in use since 1969, has been of assistance to millions throughout the world in the location, identification, and use of facilities designed for the disabled. The symbol signifies barrier free facilities: ramped entry ways, restrooms with wide stalls and grab bars, 30 in. wide doorways, ground level entry, telephones, drinking fountains, elevator controls within reach, and/or reserved and enlarged parking spaces near accessible entries. The display of this symbol also serves as a means of educating the public to the problems of accessibility faced by the disabled person. The symbol has increased general awareness, and it acts as a catalyst for the elimination of environmental barriers.

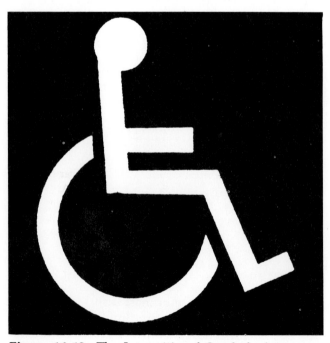

Figure 16-12. The International Symbol of Access.

References

1. Ford, J., and Duckworth, B.: Physical Management for the Quadriplegic Patient. Philadelphia: F. A. Davis, 1974.
2. Zimmerman, M. E.: Homemaking training units for rehabilitation centers. Am. J. Occup. Ther. 20:226, 1966.
3. Zimmerman, M. E.: Activities of daily living. In Willard, H. S., and Spackman, C. S. (eds.): Occupational Therapy, ed. 4. Philadelphia: J. B. Lippincott Co., 1971, pp. 217–256.
4. Ford and Duckworth: Physical Management for Quadriplegic Patient.
5. Rusk, H. A.: A Manual for Training the Disabled Homemaker. Rehabilitation Monograph VIII, pp. 49–50. New York: Institute of Rehabilitation Medicine, 1970.
6. Klinger, J. L.: Self-Help Manual for Arthritic Patients. New York: Arthritis Foundation, 1974.
7. Harkness, S. P., and Groom, J. N., Jr.: Building Without Barriers for the Disabled. The Architect Collaborative Inc., Whitney Library of Design, Cambridge MA, 1976.
8. Klinger, J. L., Friedman, F. H., and Sullivan, R. A.: Mealtime Manual for the Aged and Handicapped. New York: Simon & Schuster, 1970.
9. May, E. E., Waggoner, N. R., and Hotte, E. B.: Independent Living for the Handicapped and the Elderly. Boston: Houghton Mifflin Co., 1974.
10. Waggoner, N. R., and Reedy, G. N.: Child Care Equipment for Physically Handicapped Mothers, Suggestions for Selection and Adaptation. School of Home Economics, University of Connecticut, Storrs CN, 1961.
11. Gross, J. H., and Crandall, E. W.: Management for Modern Families. New York: Appleton-Century-Crofts, 1963.
12. Handicapped Homemaker Follow-up Study. Harmarville Rehabilitation Center, Pittsburgh PA, 1972.
13. Further Action Needed to Make All Public Buildings Accessible to the Physically Handicapped. Report to Congress by Comptroller General of the United States, July 1975.

Bibliography

Accent on Living Buyer's Guide: Your Number One Source of Information on Products for the Disabled. Bloomington IL: Cheever Publisher, 1979.

Access in the 80's: Problems and Solutions. Worchester MA: The Society, [1980]. Massachusetts Easter Seal Society, 27 Harvard St., Worchester, MA 01608.

American Automobile Association: The Handicapped Driver's Mobility Guide. Falls Church VA: The Association, 1981.

American National Standard Specifications for Making Buildings and Facilities Accessible to and Usable by Physically Handicapped People. New York: American National Standards Institute, 1980.

Anderson, H.: The Disabled Homemaker. Springfield IL: Charles C. Thomas, 1981.

Architectural Barriers Removal: Resource Guide. Office for Handicapped Individuals and Architectural and Transportation Barriers Compliance Board, 1979.

Architectural and Transportation Barrier Compliance Board. Resource Guide to Literature on Barrier-free Environments, with selected annotations. ed. 2. Washington DC: The Board, 1980.

Barrier-Free Site Design. HUD Publication. 1974. (Available from Superintendent of Documents, U.S. Government Printing Office, Washington DC.)

Hammerman, S., and Duncan, B. (eds.): Barrier-Free Design: Report of U.N. Expert Group Mtg. on Barrier-Free Design. New York: Rehab. Intern., 1975.

Barton, D. H.: Self-help clothing. Harvest Years, pp. 19–23, March:19–23, 1973.

Beppler, M. D., and Knoll, M. M.: The disabled homemaker: Organizational activities, family participation, and rehabilitation success. Rehab. Lit. 35:200–206, 1974.

Bryce, T. E.: A home economist on the rehabilitation team. Am. J. Occup. Ther. 23:258–262, 1969.

Cary, J. R.: How to create interiors for the disabled; a guidebook for family and friend. New York: Pan Theon, 1978.

Carver, V., and Rodda, M.: Disability and the Environment. New York: Schocken, 1978.

Chasin, J., and Saltman, J.: Wheelchair in the kitchen: A guide to easier living for the handicapped homemaker. Paralized Veterans of America, 1978.

Chollet, D.: A cost-benefit analysis of accessibility. Washington DC: U.S. Department of Housing and Urban Development, 1979.

Clothes for the Physically Handicapped Homemaker. Washington DC: Agricultural Research Service, U.S. Department of Agriculture, Home Economic Research Report #12, June 1971.

Clothing for disabled people. Rehab. Brief published by Rehab. Research Inst., College of Health Related Professions, Univ. of Florida, Gainsville FL, 1981.

Clothing for the incontinent older child. London: Disabled Living Foundation, March 1972.

Clothing for Wheelchair Users. London: Disabled Living Foundation, September 1971.

Friend, S. D., Zaccagnine, J., and Sullivan, M.: Meeting the clothing needs of handicapped children. J. Home Ec. 65:25–27, 1973.

Gallender, C. N., and Gallender, D.: Dietary Problems and Diets for the Handicapped. Springfield IL. Charles C. Thomas, 1979.

Gallender, D.: Eating Handicaps. Illustrated Techniques for Feeding Disorders. Springfield IL. Charles C. Thomas, 1979.

Goldsmith, S.: Designing for the Disabled, ed. 2. New York: McGraw-Hill, 1967.

Guthrie, J. L., Crist, K., Dienicki, D., and Walls, R.: Homemaker Rehabilitation in the Age of Accountability. Rehab. Lit. 42:90–93, 1981.

Hale, G.: The Source Book for the Disabled: An Illustrated Guide for Easier and More Independent Living for Physically Disabled People, Their Families, and Friends. New York: Paddington Press (95 Madison Ave., New York, NY 10016), 1977.

Hoffman, A.: Clothing for the Handicapped, The Aged, and Other People with Special Needs. Springfield IL: Charles C. Thomas, 1979.

I Can Do It! Cookbook for People with very Special Needs. Newport Beach CA: K&H Publishing Co., 1979.

Jay, P. E.: Help Yourselves—A Handbook for Hemiplegics and Their Families, ed. 3, London: Butterworths, 1979.

Jones, M.: Accessibility Standards. Springfield IL: Capital Development Board, 1978.

Kernaleguen, A.: Clothing Designs for the Handicapped. Edmonton, Alberta: University of Alberta, 1978.

Kliment, S. A.: Into the Mainstream: A Syllabus for a Barrier-Free Environment. Prepared under a grant to the American Institute of Architects by the Rehabilitation Services Administration of the Department of Health, Education, and Welfare, June 1975.

Klinger, J. L.: Mealtime Manual for People with Disabilities and the Aging. Campbell Soup Co. and Institute of Rehab. Med., 1978.

Knoll, C. S., and Schwab, L. O.: The outlook for homemaking in rehabilitation. J. Home Ec. January:39–41, 1974.

Krusen, F. H.: Handbook of Physical Medicine and Rehabilitation. Philadelphia: W. B. Saunders Co., 1971.

Laurie, G.: Housing and home services for the disabled. Hagerstown MD: Harper & Row, 1977.

Learning to Live with Disability: A Guidebook for Families. Falls Church VA: Natl. Rehab. Information Center (4407 8th St., N.E., Washington DC 20017), 1980.

Levitan-Rheingold, N., Boettke Holte, E., and Mandel, D.: Learning to dress: A fundamental skill toward independence for the disabled. Rehab. Lit. 41:72–75, 1980.

Lowman, E. W., and Klinger, J. L.: Aids to Independent Living: Self Help for the Handicapped. New York: McGraw-Hill, 1970.

Making Facilities Accessible to the Physically Handicapped. Albany NY: New York State University Construction Fund, 1974.

Malick, M.: Manual on Dynamic Hand Splinting. Pittsburgh PA: Harmarville Rehabilitation Center, 1979.

Malick, M.: Manual on Static Hand Splinting. Pittsburgh PA: Harmarville Rehabilitation Center, 1978.

McHugh, H. F.: The 1977 family as consumers. J. Home Ec. 69:6–8, 1977.

Mealtimes for Severely and Profoundly Handicapped Persons: New Concepts and Attitudes. Baltimore: University Park Press, 1980.

Mondale, K.: Standardization and the handicapped. Bromma, Sweden: Int. Com. on Technical Aids, Housing and Transport (Information Center, Box 303, S-161 26, Bromma, Sweden), 1980.

Mondale, W. F.: Government policy, stress and the family. J. Home Ec. 68:11–15, 1976.

Morgan, M.: Beyond disability: A broader definition of architectural barriers. Am. Inst. Architects J. 65:50–54, 1976.

Nau, L.: Why not family rehabilitation. J. Rehabil. 39:14–17, 1973.

Nessley, E., and King, R. R.: Textile Fabric and Clothing Needs of Paraplegic and Quadriplegic Persons Confined to Wheelchairs. J. Rehab. 46:63–67, 1980.

Newton, A.: Clothing: A rehabilitation tool for the handicapped J. Home Ec. 65:29–30, 1973.

Olson, S. C., and Meredith, D. K.: Wheelchair Interiors. Chicago: National Easter Seal Society for Crippled Children and Adults, 1973.

Patient/Family Rehab. Handbook for the Spinal Cord Injured. Pittsburgh PA: Harmarville Rehabilitation Center, 1981.

Rednick, S. S.: The physically handicapped student in the regular classroom. In A Guide for Teaching Housing and Home Care. Danville IL: Interstate Printers and Publishers, 1976.

Reference List on Self-Help Devices for the Handicapped. Chicago: National Easter Seal Society for Crippled Children and Adults, 1972.

Resource Manual of Canadian Information Services for the Physically Disabled, ed. 2. Toronto: Canadian Rehab. Council for the Disabled, 1980.

Roessler, R. T.: Training Independent Living Specialists. J. Rehab. 47:36–39, 1981.

Rusk, H. A.: Rehabilitation Medicine, ed. 4. St. Louis: C. V. Mosby, 1977.

Schwab, L. O.: Rehabilitation of physically disabled women in a family oriented program. Rehab. Lit. 36:34–47, 1975.

Schwab, L. O. and Fadul, R.: Are we prepared for the new rehabilitation legislation? J. Home Ec. 67:33–34, 1975.

Shannon, E., Reich, N.: Clothing and Related Needs of Physically Handicapped Persons. Rehab. Lit. 40:2–6, 1979.

Slater, S. B., Sussman, M. B., and Straud, M. W.: Participation in household activities as a prognostic factor in rehabilitation. Arch. Phys. Med. Rehab. 51:605–610, 1970.

Sorensen, R. J.: Design for Accessibility. New York: McGraw-Hill, 1979.

Steinfeld, E.: et al. Access to the Built Environment: A Review of the Literature. Washington DC: U.S. Dept. of Housing and Urban Development, 1979.

Step-by-Step Pictorial Cookbook. St. Louis: Ralston Purina Co., 1979.

Strebel, M. B.: Adaptations and techniques for the disabled homemaker, ed. 5. Minneapolis: Sister Kenny Inst., 1978.

Svensson, E.: Rebuilding: A Few Examples of how Accessibility Can Be Improved in Public Buildings. Bromma, Sweden: ICTS Information Center, 1980.

Technical Handbook for Facilities Engineering and Construction Manual. Section 4.12: Design of Barrier-Free Facilities. Washington DC: U.S. Dept. of Health, Education, and Welfare, 1974.

Uncommon Cookbook. Easter Seal Rehab. Center of S.W. Conn., 1978.

Van Vechten, D., Pless, I. B.: Housing and transportation: Twin barriers in independence. Rehab. Lit. 37:202–221, 1976.

Watkins, S. M.: Designing functional clothing. J. Home Ec. 66:33–38, 1974.

Wedin, C. S., and Nygren, L. G. (eds.): Housing Perspectives, Individuals and Families. Minneapolis MN: Burgess Publishing Co., 1976.

Wheeler, V. H.: Planning Kitchens for Handicapped Homemakers. Rehabilitation Monograph 27. New York Institute of Rehabilitation Medicine, New York University Medical Center, 1966.

Wilshere, E. R.: Equipment for the Disabled: Housing and Furniture. Brighton, England: Oxford Reg. Health Authority (2 Foredown Dr., Portsdale, Brighton BN4 2BB, England), 1979.

Wittmeyer, M. B., and Stolov, W. C.: Educating wheelchair patients on home architectural barriers. Am. J. Occup. Ther. 32:557–564, 1978.

Wittmeyer, M., and Barrett, V.: Housing Accessibility Checklist. Seattle: University of Washington, 1980.

Yost, Schroeder, Rainey: Home Economics Rehabilitation, A Selected, Annotated Bibliography. Columbia MO: University of Missouri-Columbia (206 Whitten Hall, Columbia MO 65201), 1977.

Special Issue Independent Living

Arch. Phys. Med. Rehab. Vol. 60, October, 1979.

Berrol, S.: Independent living programs: The role of the able-bodied professional. Pp. 456–457.

Bowe, F. G.: Transportation: A key to independent living. Pp. 483–486.

Cole, J. A.: What's new about independent living? Pp. 458–462.

DeJong, G.: Independent living: From social movement to analytic paradigm. Pp. 435–476.

Lifchez, R.: The environment as a support system for independent living. Pp. 467–476.

Tate, D. G., Jarvis, R. L., and Juhr, G. D.: International efforts in independent living. Pp. 462–467.

Verville, R. E.: Federal legislative history of independent living programs. Pp. 447–451.

Addresses

American Home Economics Association
2010 Massachusetts Avenue
Washington DC 20036

American Dietetics Association
Publication Department
430 N. Michigan Avenue
Chicago IL 60611

ICTA Information Center
(International Center on Technical Aids)
IACK S-161 03
Bromma 3, Sweden

National Center for a Barrier-free Environment
Suite 1006
1140 Connecticut Avenue, NW
Washington, DC 20036

Schools Offering Homemaker Rehabilitation Programs: University of Missouri-Columbia, University of Nebraska-Lincoln, and University of West Virginia.

CHAPTER 17

Prevocational Training *Dorothy L. Kester*

For many handicapped persons the need to fulfill the self-actualizing feeling of "I can do it too" has priority in the choice of employment. This need is true in direct proportion to the degree of the disability. Just as the reasons for working and for choice of work vary with individuals, so do the reasons and magnitude of the problems that bar people from successful employment.

Problems

Physical or Medical

It is possible for an apparently minor physical problem to create a complete barrier to returning to work. Consider the house painter trying to paint a ceiling if neck motion were limited, moving the ladder if shoulder motion were limited, or climbing the ladder if hip, knee, or ankle movement were painful. Performance of the same occupation would be hindered by limited tolerance for general physical activity following a cardiovascular accident or respiratory ailment, even if ability to perform the specific activities were not affected. Consider the typist with cervical pain, a fractured finger or coccyx, tenosynovitis, or limited visual tolerance.

Some conditions are temporary and do not prevent return to previous employment, even before remediation is complete. Other disabilities that are more permanent in nature might not preclude return to work if adaptive devices or environmental changes could compensate for the personal limitation. A third category involves the permanent medical or physical disability that is severe enough to prevent return to previous employment. In this case, or in the case of a person who has never worked, vocational evaluation is available to determine potentials, but adjustment programs are also frequently required because of mental, emotional, and social problems or other personal problems.

Mental, Emotional and Social

In the areas of mental, emotional, and social dysfunction there are problems that may appear to be minor in the home or in many social situations but which are actually major deterrents to employment.

Limited cognitive abilities automatically limit vocational choices but do not preclude employment. Limited concentration, distractibility, or psychological pressures that limit tolerance for specific activities might preclude employment even though job skills are present. Job skills are meaningless if interpersonal relationships or problem behaviors create friction or reduce productivity.

Life Survival Skills

Deficiencies in life survival skills are other problem areas that can render job skills meaningless. Grooming, hygiene, and safety skills are as important to the employer and co-workers as they are to the employee. Poor time and money concepts, as well as poor social relationships, affect employment success, and lack of transportation skills can nullify any possibility of employment.

Job Survival Skills

Factors included under job survival skills overlap some of the other problem areas as well as adding different dimensions. Although it may seem redundant to include life survival skills and interpersonal relationships here, there are differences between the requirements of social and vocational situations. In social situations, for instance, it is possible to choose one's associates, but the personalities of one's co-workers are usually more diverse, since associates are determined at least in part by the job and the situation.

Sensorimotor Dysfunction

Sensorimotor dysfunction does not disappear as the person grows older. The poor motor, tactile, visual, auditory, or cognitive skills and tolerances remain; emotional and behavioral problems intensify, and ego strength and ability to tolerate stress continue to decrease. Vocational choice is limited or, in many cases, is absent.

Those who do have the ability to perform higher-level occupations frequently yield to the stresses and end up in lower-level jobs. Another group of individuals might have abilities commensurate with employment, but these are negated by emotional or behavioral problems severe enough to prevent success.

Cognitive Dysfunction

Deficiencies in math, reading, reading comprehension, and spatial and temporal concepts and relationships, and limited ability to deal with abstractions and mental manipulations are problems that may stem from a variety of causes such as retardation, sensorimotor dysfunction, or emotional disturbance. Whatever the cause, these problems, in themselves, limit vocational choice and, if combined with other problems, decrease vocational potential even further.

Remediation Programs

All of the previously mentioned problems may be evaluated and diminished or solved by the occupational therapist, and he or she may design appropriate remediation programs. However, some of the occupational therapy skills must be refined or taken into new dimensions, and other skills must be learned.

All of the adjustment programs involve changing some form of behavior—physical, emotional, social, vocational, and so forth. A variety of techniques should be used to produce these changes, but the evaluative techniques are basic to all of the remediation programs. In many ways these programs could be considered "continuing evaluation," because without a continual evaluation of status there is no foundation on which to determine at any given time what has changed, what needs to be changed, what techniques might work, or when the client reaches the point of having made maximum gains from the program.

Work Tolerance

Work tolerance programs are designed to improve physical abilities, to compensate for disabilities, and/or to improve poor physical tolerances that interfere with successful employment potential for a specific job or for work in general. Work tolerance programs start with physical and functional evaluations, measurement of joint range of motion, and other pertinent objective measurement techniques. For example, the Minnesota Rate of Manipulation Test is used to measure speed of performance. Frequency of re-testing varies with the length of the program, but must be done on or near the day of completion in order to provide meaningful information about the client's accomplishments. The programs are most effective when traditional occupational therapy techniques are combined with job-related tasks that are graded to increase the degree of function and/or tolerance required.

Individual programs vary considerably depending on the cause and degree of the disability, duration of inactivity, specific difficulties noted the first day, speed of change, and attitude of the client, especially fear of activity. The occupational therapist's knowledge of symptoms and precautions is especially helpful in the early stages of the program for determining whether the client is performing appropriately, underdoing, or possibly pushing too hard. Many clients need help in achieving a more realistic awareness of their capacities through activity combined with counseling. They will not be convinced by purely verbal techniques that they are capable of more activity, but must experience it. This experiencing is most meaningful if the tasks are related to the client's work.

These programs follow many of the rules of traditional occupational therapy programs, such as

1. The activities must be within the client's capability but should offer a challenge.
2. The activities must be graded to increase the patient's capability.
3. In order to create change, the effort required and/or the time spent on a given type of activity must increase.

In reporting to the counselor, whether verbally or in writing, information about present status, expected gains, and potentials must be factual. Motivation, attitudes, behaviors, and emotional status are as important as the physical findings and should, therefore, be included. Check lists or other forms are a concise method for recording these facts, but usually cannot provide adequate information. Examples of task performance are more meaningful in many cases, but are also inadequate without qualifying narrative or interpretive additions. The narrative section should include specific, objective personal and work behavior observations, present status, work readiness, summary, and recommendations. The recommendations are the most important part of a report; all of the other facts merely provide background information leading to those conclusions.

Case Summary

Mr. B. V. was referred for a five-day work tolerance program to determine whether he could return to kitchen installation work following his heart attack.

He was a sturdy-appearing young man whose ability to perform the tests for physical activities was unaffected, except for his ability to lift and carry. He was able, after five days, to lift or carry only slightly above half of the average load for a man of his age and build. He found, however, that this amount created no problems and was confident that with further work at home he would be able to lift the required weights by the time he returned to work.

Activity on the first day consisted of alternating sedentary and active work, with the amount and level of the active work increasing each day. By the fifth day he was working primarily on active tasks, such as large wood projects.

He worked accurately and neatly on all assigned tasks, had no difficulty with tasks involving spatial relationships or cognitive functions, and performed well on the basic skill requirements for machine shop work.

Mr. B. V. gained an understanding of the degree to which he could safely push himself in order to regain further strength and tolerance. He was able to return to kitchen installation work shortly after discharge from the program. □

Adjustment Training

There are two major types of adjustment training: personal adjustment training and work adjustment training. Although they differ in their overall objectives, they share some similarities and actually overlap in terms of individual goals. Methods used for both training programs are similar in that they use work as the therapeutic medium. Differences in techniques result primarily from the type and philosophy of the facility and the type and severity of the client's disability. The techniques vary from learning by experience to well-organized behavioral techniques.

Work itself is used as a major catalyst, but many other techniques are also required. Personal, social, and vocational counseling with individuals and groups, role playing, behavior modification, skill training, audiovisuals, guest experts, and field trips are some of the tools that can be helpful with all clients. These tools are usually necessary with those clients who have either a severe dysfunction or a combination of dysfunctions.

Concurrently with the above techniques, the work and working space can be manipulated to accelerate the rehabilitation process. Depending on the facility, use of either simulated or actual jobs provide a flexible, yet controlled, realistic work environment for the client. At the same time the client is gaining work experience, social, emotional, and vocational behaviors and skills are being evaluated. Long-range goals and short-range objectives for rehabilitation are determined and procedures planned.

The work assigned might be graded from sedentary to active or the reverse, from gross motor to fine motor, from minimal to high requirements for speed and/or accuracy, from working alone to cooperating with others, or from a task on which speed and attention are externally controlled, as on an assembly line, to one that is self-controlled.

The client might be placed on a specific job primarily for the example peers will set or for the feedback peers will contribute. This peer feedback is often much more effective than that provided by the supervisors or counselors. Charting or graphing of behaviors, work rhythm, accuracy, and productivity is also an effective means of providing immediate feedback as well as demonstrating progress or regression. Other effective feedback techniques include use of video tape, self-evaluations, tokens, or remuneration.

Group sessions, even when geared for specific learning experiences such as job survival skills, are an economical means of providing other necessary knowledge and skills. These skills include such factors as peer interaction, self-esteem, emotional awareness, attentiveness, and amount and appropriateness of verbal and nonverbal responses.

Generalization and oversimplification are necessary when discussing different personalities. There is no specific rule for determining the sequence of the learning hierarchy. Each client has an optimal time to learn a specific skill. Each client differs also as to how much he or she will learn and by which method or combination of methods he or she learns best. The occupational therapist must develop the ability to determine those times, places, and methods for each client.

Personal Adjustment Training

One of the types of adjustment training is personal adjustment training (P.A.T.). The major goals of P.A.T. are the following:
1. Decrease behaviors adversely affecting vocational potential.
2. Improve interpersonal relationships.
3. Normalize work-related behaviors.
4. Maximize life survival skills.
5. Improve use of leisure time.
6. Maximize acceptance of the disability.

An important part of this program might involve social as well as personal adjustment. Basic math, basic reading or survival vocabulary, personal hygiene, health, grooming, dress, manners, appropriate behavioral reaction patterns, social relations, use of leisure time, table manners, relations with peer groups and authority figures, recreation, and dating are areas given attention in personal adjustment training. Persons who need help with these skills usually require assistance with money-handling, concepts and awareness of time, transportation, appropriate self-expression, human sexuality, desirable character and behavior traits, making friends, and building ego strength and self-confidence combined with accepting limitations. In many cases it is also important to assist the family in accepting the client's disability in order to help develop realistic goals for the client.

Work Adjustment Training

The second type of adjustment training is work adjustment. The three major goals of work adjustment training (W.A.T.) are the following:

1. Maximize vocational potential.
2. Maximize potential for independent living.
3. Maximize potential for emotional and vocational self-support.

A "pure" work adjustment training program involves knowledge of, and skill in, meeting the requirements of work. It includes such factors as punctuality, attendance, independence and self-support, understanding the relationship of work to daily living, relationships with co-workers, and acceptance of supervision and authority. However, frequently there is no such thing as pure work adjustment. Poor vocational knowledge or skills usually go hand-in-hand with, or result from, poor personal adjustment. To ignore the developmental hierarchy of these factors can create the additional behavioral and emotional problems of crises, frustrations on the part of the client and work adjustment counselor, and even failure. If the client has not learned what a job is, why people work, or why responsibility, dependability, independence, willingness to accept help, handling of frustrations, personal relationships, health, and hygiene are important, the client has not learned how to keep a job. It is unrealistic, therefore, to teach him how to find a job, fill out applications, or handle a job interview.

New dimensions are added to the value of work itself at this level. In the W.A.T. program the emphasis of the work itself shifts to improving interpersonal relationships, effective use of abilities and acceptance of disabilities, adjustment to work pressures, derivation of work satisfaction, and development of a realistic self-concept as a worker. Many of the skills dealt with in a P.A.T. program are also included in W.A.T. in order to develop the skills to a more mature level.

Once the personal aspects have been developed, the client is ready to continue with the work skills. Learning how to look for and apply for work, how to fill out an application, what is involved in an interview, and what to expect on a new job requires a variety of methods and much practice. Guest speakers and field trips should be added at this time, if they have not been used before, to provide more realistic experiences directly related to the world of work.

Vocational-Educational Program

The vocational-educational program is a newer, more complex type of program that was developed for adolescents and young adults with sensorimotor dysfunction. The goals of this program include the following:
1. All P.A.T. goals
2. All W.A.T. goals

3. Maximize sensorimotor integration
4. Maximize educational skills

Sensorimotor dysfunction, in itself, affects vocational potential in many ways: gross motor, fine motor, and tactile problems affect physical skills; apraxia affects visual-motor skills; and visual dysfunction affects visual and visual-motor skills. Each aspect of dysfunction interacts with and compounds the problems created by the others. For instance, tactile dysfunction and poor spatial and temporal skills affect potential for all types of employment. The person's speed of learning, ability to deal with abstractions, emotional, social, and behavioral maturation, as well as self-concepts and ego strength, are also directly affected by the sensorimotor dysfunction.

Sensorimotor dysfunction also compounds the difficulties of the rehabilitation process. The following is an example of this situation.

Previous testing may have indicated potential for a specific type of work, such as janitorial, in which the client is interested. In the training program, however, unexpected difficulties arise when the job is broken down into specific tasks. For example, the client stops working after doing only part of the task, ignores obviously dirty areas when cleaning and says he or she can't see anything wrong when told to redo the area, stops to stare into space or have a conversation with a co-worker, can't schedule his or her own work, or doesn't start the second task when the first is completed.

When corrected or told to redo a task, the client insists it was done correctly and becomes irate or otherwise behaves inappropriately. The supervisor considers him or her lazy, sloppy, inattentive, and explosive. The supervisor may not realize that the client's time concepts are poor, that the client is unable to conceive of the sequence from task to task or within a task, that poor visual perceptions prevent the client from seeing that the job is not done correctly, and that the client's low self-esteem and poor emotional maturity cause him or her to take the correction as an accusation and one more example of failure.

As a result of behavior problems in combination with unacceptable job performance, the client is discontinued from the training program. The counselor finds another, supposedly easier type of training and the same problems arise; eventually, the case is closed and the client is on his or her own. The person has become increasingly frustrated and, as the frustration increases, self-esteem and willingness to try decrease even further.

A special program is needed for this type of client. Since most multi-faceted problems are best remediated through a multi-faceted attack, the most effective program for this type of client is one that in-

cludes all aspects of the P.A.T. and the W.A.T. programs, with additional emphasis placed on educational remediation, adding sensorimotor remediation, and an understanding by the staff of the ramifications of sensorimotor dysfunction. Adolescents and young adults do accept sensorimotor remediation and become increasingly motivated as change is realized. Self-esteem, willingness to try new things, speed of learning, accuracy of work, and behavior all improve as sensorimotor functioning improves and ego strengths increase. Because of the complexity of these problems and the length of time they have existed, the rehabilitation process is also a lengthy one.

The results that can be attained by the preceding programs are demonstrated by the following case summary.

Case Summary

F. W. is a 19-year-old male who has received special services from a minimum of 10 special facilities. Minor surgery was performed at 18 months of age, following which he stopped making any attempts to speak. His family was counseled by a crippled children's service; his condition was diagnosed as aphasia, and he received speech therapy. Upon reaching school age, he was placed in special education, spent two years at an institute of logopedics, then returned to the public school system for a work experience program. During this time he and his parents were also seen by child guidance services. Many psychological assessments were attempted, each resulting in minimal objective information. However, clinical judgments indicated that F. W. had much more potential than testing could indicate, considering his lack of communication and response, shyness, retiring nature, and extremely immature behaviors.

At age 16, at the request of the school program director, he became a vocational rehabilitation client and was admitted to the recently developed vocational-education program at the center.

For months after admission, F. W. insisted on keeping his lunch with him, refused to remove his coat, pulled the coat over his head, and turned his back or actually hid if asked to do anything when other persons were in the area. He hid if any new person appeared and, if talked to firmly, hid for the rest of the day. Communication consisted of grunts and gestures, primarily to indicate that something hurt. Educational skills consisted of counting to three and recognizing most letters of the alphabet. Balance, equilibrium reaction, and sensorimotor development were poor. Despite these behaviors, it became apparent that he learned physical tasks easily and liked challenges when he worked alone.

He required several months to feel comfortable with persons he saw every day, and six months to be willing to do anything in a group situation except woodwork. Once comfortable, he was willing to attempt new things if he thought he was helping. Following conferences with the staff, his family allowed him to help with increasingly difficult tasks at home.

As self-confidence increased, he began to communicate verbally. A speech evaluation was performed when his speech consisted primarily of nouns strung together with an occasional uninflected verb and a few adjectives. Auditory comprehension for language was at a 6-year level, but auditory memory, fine discrimination, and usage were lower. Therapy was recommended and instituted.

Behaviors, skills, and motivation improved slowly. He no longer blushed when new people or groups appeared, and he worked with new staff members with little hesitation. He did not yet fully understand the productivity aspects of employment, but willingly accepted new challenges. Work quality was very good when he understood what was wanted.

Sensorimotor development improved considerably in all areas. He was functioning at approximately the first-grade level in reading and math, major gains were made in his sight knowledge of words, and he was beginning to use phonics to sound out words. He functioned semi-independently in simple addition and possessed some skills in money handling and telling time. Dramatic gains were noted in the amount and variety of verbal output and the use of simple grammatical structures. Speech was not clear, but he willingly repeated whatever was not understood. Quantity of speech was close to normal with his peers, and he talked on the telephone nightly with one co-worker.

At a conference his parents requested our assistance with a familial decision. Was F. W. now ready for an out-of-state move they had been planning for several years but had delayed because of his progress? They would investigate possibilities for continuing speech, educational, social, and vocational programs. We concurred with this decision, recommending that social and vocational factors be the primary considerations.

The family decided not to move because several of the other children were in senior high school. F. W. was admitted to a work activities program in a sheltered workshop, and performed adequately to well on a variety of increasingly difficult jobs. He contacts the director of the vocational education program periodically to inform her about his work, his experiences at the Special Olympics, his "girls," and the dances he attends. □

Adult Sensorimotor Remediation

The Adult Sensorimotor Remediation program is proving to be effective and requires an average of 24 remediation sessions. Remediation is provided either individually or in compatible small groups, and emphasis is placed on decreasing or developing techniques to compensate for the specific functional deficiencies of each client. Some activities used are either the same as, or adapted from, activities used with younger persons; but most of the activities are appropriate to age and vocation or vocational goal.

Dysfunction may not be eliminated or even substantially reduced, and results depend upon level of motivation. However, most clients improve in their self-concepts and ability to function, learn to live with their problems, and develop an awareness of previously unsuspected abilities. Many clients continue to carry on recommended remediation programs after discharge, and some are able to adapt or generalize what they have learned to other situations.

Case Summary

P. E. is an obese man with a multitude of medical, physical, and personal problems, including vertigo. He has a master's degree in counseling, and had been employed as a counselor but had not succeeded. He is presently employed as a college admissions clerk but had been having major difficulty filling in the forms, finding course numbers in the catalogs, remembering and/or writing the numbers correctly and entering the numbers in the proper place, and making other related errors. He has also been having difficulty coping with the pressure of telephone call interruptions and the realization that students were waiting for assistance.

Some of the functional problems delineated by evaluation were defective oculomotor functioning with nausea or dizziness created by eye motion, deficient equilibrium, gross motor and tactile functioning, deficient visual memory and spatial discrimination, extremely poor visual speed and tolerance, and deficient auditory figure-ground and memory. Visual figure-ground was accurate, but speed was significantly below scale. Direct remediation resulted in considerable improvement in functioning and awareness, with some improvement in self-concepts, but perhaps more important, his ability to organize, analyze, or problem solve has improved, and the dizziness, which was created by visual activity and job-related problems, has decreased. Analysis of the work environment revealed that the forms the client used were poor copies, with many blurred or spotted areas, and two forms that required similar information were reversed, right to left. The environment was noisy, interruptions were frequent, and the work pace was hectic.

As a result of the analysis of the work environment the forms were redone for clarity and consistency. He was taught to use a template to eliminate unnecessary stimuli and help him focus on the desired stimuli. Although these changes helped job performance, it was noted that the work continued to involve his areas of greatest deficits and to increase his negative feelings about himself. The recommendation was made that he should explore other opportunities in the counseling field and continue with personal counseling for support during the job change.

Follow-up revealed that Mr. E. is working in a small, quiet office, but is still feeling pressure from interruptions and waiting students. Realizing his glasses need changing, he has made an appointment with a developmental optometrist, who will evaluate function as well as acuity, and provide an exercise program if feasible. Job opportunities are scarce in his state; he is being asked to return to a previous school system position in another state, but has refused because his family is reluctant to move. □

Bibliography

Botterbusch, K. F., and Sax, A. B.: A Comparison of Commercial Vocational Evaluation Systems. Menomonie, WI: Materials Development Center, Stout Rehabilitation Institute, University of Wisconsin, 1980.

Brewer, E., Miller, J., and Ray, J.: The effect of vocational evaluation and work adjustment on clients' attitude toward work. Vocational Evaluation and Work Adjustment Bulletin. 8:18–25, 1975.

Dinneen, T.: Work evaluation as a technique for improving self-concept. Vocational Evaluation and Work Adjustment Bulletin. 8:28–34, 1975.

Granofsky, J.: A Manual for Occupational Therapists on Prevocational Exploration. Dubuque, IA: W. C. Brown Book Co., 1959.

Hoffman, P. R.: Work evaluation, an overview. Work Evaluation in Rehabilitation, Reprint Series RS-70-2, 3–18, 1969.

Olshansky, S.: Reply to Kipstein and Lores. Rehabil. Lit. 36:142, 1975.

Raymond, E.: Measuring the interpersonal aspects of work behavior. Vocational Evaluation and Work Adjustment Bulletin. 8:19–23, 1975

Roberts, C. L.: Definitions, objectives and goals in work evaluation. Work Evaluation in Rehabilitation, Reprint Series RS-70-2, 19–30, 1969.

Recommended Periodicals and Journals

National Rehabilitation Association: *Journal of Rehabilitation* Vocational Evaluation and Work Adjustment Association, a division of the National Rehabilitation Association: *Vocational Evaluation and Work Adjustment Bulletin.*

The American Journal of Occupational Therapy.

Many of the available articles are indexed in Psychological Abstracts and Rehabilitation Literature. The University of Wisconsin-Stout, Menomonie, WI, 54751, maintains a Materials Development Center for such materials, which can be borrowed or purchased.

CHAPTER 18

Biofeedback *Abby Abildness*

Biofeedback Revolution in Medicine

In its present state, biofeedback employs simple devices to detect signs of inner physiological activity. These tools have been used for acquiring evaluative information in medical and biological research for many years. Now biofeedback is used not only to diagnose disease, but also to provide feedback to the patient about his or her own state, and to enable the patient to improve by using cortical control.

The use of biofeedback for self-control has developed in the behavioral sciences over the past twenty years. This has excited and challenged a wide variety of health-care professionals. Through awareness of the patient's internal psychophysiological status, patients and therapists can learn together to manipulate the patient's internal homeostasis to promote changes in maladaptive behavioral responses. The exciting implication is that the therapist–patient relationship changes from the professional's imposing treatment on the patient to the therapist's facilitating the patient's ability to change internal psychophysiology. This can reduce the need for medications, which can have harmful side effects, decrease the need for adaptive equipment, and reduce environmental stress as the patient gains self-control.

Overall, feedback has an impact not only on preventive and restorative comprehensive health-care alternatives, but, through its emphasis on self-control, on medicine's philosophical and psychophysiological concept of human beings.

Electronic feedback of internal physiological events is given to patients in the form of visual or auditory signals. Biofeedback machines have transducers that detect heart rate, blood pressure, muscle tension, peripheral blood flow, skin temperature, sweat gland activity, and brain wave rhythms. Machines detect much more subtle changes than can be perceived otherwise, and thus give feedback on minute biological changes. The feedback process consists of five operations, as schematically diagramed in Figure 18-1:

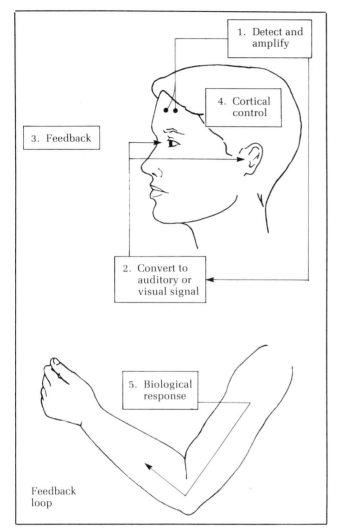

Figure 18-1 Five operations in the biofeedback process.

1. Detection and amplification of bioelectric potentials that are otherwise subliminal and undetected
2. Conversion of bioelectric signals to auditory and visual signals that are understandable to the individual
3. Instantaneous feedback of the status of, and changes in, biological state
4. Triggered cortical awareness of biological status enabling an individual to learn volitional control of biological state
5. Biological response with continuous feedback as an operant reinforcer to enable skilled execution of the biological response, as for instance, a motor response

It is critical for accurate learning that the feedback be continuous, instantaneous, and directly proportional to the biological change. The instrument's feedback becomes the reinforcer stimulating learning that is "shaped" by the therapist to obtain the desired behavioral outcome.

Biofeedback is not intended as a treatment in itself, but as an adjunct to traditional occupational therapy procedures. It enhances possibilities for restoring health by providing information needed by the patient in order to gain control of internal biological events previously thought to be uncontrollable.

The Feedback Concept in Occupational Therapy

The effectiveness of biofeedback is determined by its integration into a therapist's total treatment framework. Individuals can readily use biofeedback sensory aids to learn to change physiological or psychological arousal, but unless the learned skill is applied to functional daily life, it is useless. Biofeedback should be one of a variety of means used to achieve goals.

Biofeedback offers crucial advantages in the early stages of treatment, because it focuses on cortical remediation of psychophysiological ills. Its unique asset is its capacity to register the psychological and physiological aspects of disordered functioning simultaneously. Biofeedback demonstrates to patients their ability to control physiology. It also provides direct information about the symptom to be changed. Finally, it monitors physiological changes during treatment.

Overall treatment advantages documented by multiple sources include the following:
1. Reduced training time: Patients achieve desired goals more rapidly when biofeedback is used.
2. Cost effectiveness: Therapist time and hospitalizations are shortened.
3. Enhanced initiation of motion or emotion that could not otherwise be elicited
4. Objective evaluative data for documenting treatment progress or effectiveness
5. Improved client self-image by increasing responsibility to self-manage treatment
6. Longer-lasting effects owing to development of cortical awareness and control.

Biofeedback in Continuous Activity Analysis

Biofeedback technology offers invaluable adjunctive, objective, evaluative information for analysis of activities and their therapeutic effects. Continuous monitoring of specific biological parameters during prescribed functional activities will demonstrate the degree of appropriateness of each. Some examples of monitoring include the following:

1. *Electromyography* (EMG) monitoring of triceps during reaching, grasp, and release activities in different planes to determine strength, endurance, and appropriate relaxation of contraction
2. *Galvanic skin response* (GSR) or sweat response monitoring of psychiatric clients involved in individual or group activities to determine stress or relaxation effects
3. *Heart Rate* monitoring during exercise for cardiac patients to determine actual limits of physical demand provided by the activity

Biofeedback alerts patients to the strength of their psychophysiological behavior, but not to the nature of the reaction. Therapists should use other clinical skills to explore the meaning and clinical significance of the behavioral response.

Major Biofeedback Applications to Physical Dysfunction

Biofeedback in Neuromuscular Re-education

Traditional neurodevelopmental rehabilitation procedures are aimed at providing appropriate proprioceptive input for the patient. EMG biofeedback can detect latent motor unit potentials existing in seemingly paralyzed muscles. This information is relayed to the patient by using intact auditory and visual systems rather than neurologically impaired proprioceptors. Biofeedback enhances the neurodevelopmental treatment process by providing information about actual motor responses too slight to be sensed by the patient or therapist otherwise.

When injury occurs to the upper or lower motor neuron, electrical impulses from the brain to the muscle are interrupted, and the muscle may become paralyzed. Marinacci has determined that a few active motor units may remain in the muscle even if it appears to be totally paralyzed.[1] But the patient and therapist may have no means of detecting the potential for recruiting other motor units and regaining some functional control. The EMG biofeedback machine detects and amplifies these electrical potentials either to enable patients to learn to elicit a motor act or as feedback for accurate execution.

Normal learned motor responses occur through proprioceptive feedback of muscle tension and position, indicating how movement was performed.

Biofeedback technology can provide information of exact tension changes, but coordinated motor control requires position feedback, which must come from the client's and therapist's observation of the limb performing a functional task.

Spasticity or hypertonicity may also develop owing to diminished proprioceptive information concerning muscular tension, causing a loss of the inhibiting or modulating influences of the brain on the lower motor neurons. In the case of excessive tension, biofeedback provides information regarding exact tension levels, enabling the patient to learn to relax the tension internally.

The ability to substitute for absent, impaired, or faulty kinesthetic feedback is the most important advantage of EMG biofeedback as an adjunct treatment tool in neuromuscular re-education. At first, patients rely heavily on feedback display representations of actual motor activity. But as the ability to initiate and terminate contraction develops, they become less dependent on electronic cues and more reliant on associated internal sensory cues and visual observation of limb changes.

Examples of Clinical Applications

Cerebrovascular Accident

Most neuromuscular biofeedback research has been done with stroke patients two to five years after injury to ensure no possibility of spontaneous recovery. After standard rehabilitation attempts had maximized motion, biofeedback greatly increased strength and volitional control, even in muscles previously thought to be paralyzed. A representative study compared biofeedback to standard physical therapy, and showed biofeedback to excell in strengthening the anterior tibialis muscle and in reducing the need for short leg braces in most cases.[2]

Spinal Cord Injury

Biofeedback training facilitates development of full motor potential at, or sometimes below, the identified cord lesion. It is believed that spinal shock impairs the brain's ability to detect minimal proprioceptive signals. Biofeedback externally and artificially provides the necessary feedback to facilitate motor activity otherwise undetected, and may functionally lower the cord lesion.

Cerebral Palsy

Biofeedback efforts in cerebral palsy are aimed at regaining motor control in characteristic disorders of posture, gait, and involuntary athetoid movements. Harris and his associates identify athetoid movements as faulty kinesthetic monitoring.[3] Accurate simultaneous biofeedback of opposing muscles encourages coordinated motor control. Special head control caps have also been devised to enhance postural control. Tape recorder feedback is heard when the patient sits erect, and diminishes in proportion to the degree of slouch.

Peripheral Nerve Injury

Feedback from isolated muscles can be used to prevent substitution problems and to encourage peripheral nerve regeneration following disease or crushing.

Rehabilitation Engineering Feedback Tools for Activity Analysis and Training

Biofeedback instrumentation adaptations may be among the most important contributions of occupational therapists to the field of biofeedback. Electrokinesiological devices have already been developed at Emory University and at Boston University.[4,5] These include electrogoniometers for elbow, wrist and finger joints, and pressure feedback devices for grasp and prehension strengthening. Each of these devices has calibrated threshold settings that allow for setting multiple strength or range-of-motion goals during prescribed activities. They are useful for evaluating range and strength changes, as well as the therapeutic value of functional tasks. A bioconverter has been reported by Brown and Basmajian to provide more motivating feedback to children.[6] It can send EMG signals through any household appliance or electrical toy, thus increasing the child's attention span and perseverance in performing accurate motor tasks in order to see electrical toys move.

Other occupational therapy evaluative and treatment tools could lend themselves to feedback adaptations. It simply requires a creative therapist who understands the feedback concept and its therapeutic use. The therapist can present the type of feedback required to a biomedical engineer or electronic technician, who can devise simple adaptations at minimal costs.

Heart Rate

Heart rate biofeedback is one of the most widely researched areas. Because heart rate responses are such sensitive indicators of stress and anxiety, and because nervous regulation of heart beat is relatively simple, heart rate has been easy to control through conditioning procedures. Cardiac arrhythmias are the predominant category for clinical treatment. The direct relationship between nerve stimulation and heart rate lends itself to modification by higher cerebral control. It is chiefly limited by the integrity of nerve connections. The strength of biofeedback applicability to certain pathological conditions of heart beat conduction by way of neural involvement can positively relieve any emotional overlay aggravating the conditions.

Blood Pressure

Because of the psychogenic nature of blood pressure variability, biofeedback treatment is part of a program dealing with underlying stresses. Biofeedback can help patients recognize the role of emotion in the precipitation of their illness; it can also help them to identify harmful emotion-arousing situations or conditions. It facilitates control over overt activities associated with emotional arousal and autonomic responses.

Temperature Self-Regulation (With Raynaud's Disease)

Initial temperature clinical applications were applied to Raynaud's disease, in which paroxysms of cutaneous vasospasm occur, causing reduced blood flow. Peripheral constriction causes pain, skin discoloration, and ulcers, and can lead to gangrene of the digits. Skin temperature, being a measure of peripheral vascular activity, can be internally raised to cause vasodilation and relax sympathetic activity.

Control is recognized when the treatment is effective during the coldest months of the year and is maintained over seasonal variation. Maintenance and generalization of the learned behavior change (temperature control) must be programmed by continued logging of vasospastic attacks. Learned control must be practiced frequently for short periods to prevent or terminate episodic symptoms.

Temperature training is being expanded to encompass inflammatory arthritis, wound healing, tumorous growth reduction, diabetic peripheral neuropathies, and renal blood flow problems. Trained vasodilation and vasoconstriction alter blood flow to specific regions.

Respiration (with Bronchial Asthma)

Biofeedback relaxation training can increase peak respiratory flow rates in asthmatic children.[7] A counterconditioning desensitization approach reduces frequency, duration, and severity of attacks, as patients learn to develop bronchodilation as an antagonistic approach to bronchoconstriction. Children develop a sense of self-confidence in controlling mild attacks, which lessens fear and apprehension believed to induce natural asthmatic attacks.

Biofeedback with Psychosomatic and Psychopathological Disorders

Biofeedback counterconditioning strategies are designed to bring mastery of psychobiologic stress by developing awareness of certain stress indices (muscle tension, increased blood pressure, increased sweating) and learning to inhibit them. Awareness of ability to change or control stress reactions internally, rather than be controlled by them, increases the patients' potential to be healed. For example, the bronchial asthmatic who senses the beginning signs of an attack can intervene and stop or minimize the attack, rather than fear its onset and heighten its effects.

Many epidemiological studies initially investigating psychoses and psychosomatic symptoms have shown that conditions producing psychological stress greatly increase the risk of adverse consequences, such as psychiatric hospitalizations, stomach lesions, diabetes, hypertension, and many other medical complaints.[8] Stress is usually accompanied by a generalized arousal of the neuromuscular, autonomic, and central nervous systems. Once stimulated, people with psychosomatic or psychiatric symptoms will experience maladaptive, heightened arousal more frequently and for longer periods of time, and have difficulty returning to pre-stress levels. Specific physiological patterns of arousal to stress may vary. One person may show greater cardiovascular changes, while another may have gastrointestinal or neuromuscular alterations. Therefore, a stress profile must be taken using various biofeedback machines, as part of a complete medical and behavioral analysis. This will provide information about the physiological systems that should be altered in order to promote healthful responses to stress.

Feedback dermography is used to measure generalized arousal mechanisms. It monitors ongoing skin conductance characteristics by detecting the direct current potential between two electrodes on the skin's surface. Physiologically, current is primarily mediated by sweat gland activity and activated by smpathetic nervous system stimulation. During evaluation or treatment the dermograph feedback magnitude will reflect the intensity and nature of anxiety-provoking topics discussed or events experienced.

Patients having stress-related disorders typically demonstrate multiple symptoms and initially need a generalized relaxation training approach. Lowering physiological arousal to provide relief of psychiatric symptoms is based on Jacobson's premise that anxiety is incompatible with relaxation and that controlled relaxation is sufficient to provide relief from physical or emotional stress.[9]

By first using feedback machines reflecting generalized emotional responses and progressing to those measuring specific functions, such as heart rate or isolated muscle tension, patients are taught control over generalized arousal and then isolated physiological functions applied to real life stressors. Patients actively perform self-monitoring, and document for themselves symptom changes. Instrument feedback facilitates awareness of tension levels, and how to monitor and inhibit them cortically. This enhances simple relaxation strategies by enabling patients to realize their progress with relaxation techniques, and to decide which techniques are most effective.

Psychotherapeutic Applications

Neurosis

Neurosis, in physiological terms, is a form of neuromuscular hypertension complicated by pathological habit formation. Excessive tension begins to control the individual as he or she loses an internal locus of control. As an adjunct to insight therapy, biofeedback promotes self-awareness as patients learn their physiological response to stress, and learn to produce more appropriate responses. As they learn to relax, mental tension is relieved. Reasoning becomes clearer and verbalizations more coherent. Confidence gained in the ability to control oneself increases independence, which decreases reliance on external substances such as medications.

Phobia

Electrodermal feedback has been used as a physiological measure of the autonomic components of phobic responses to identify the specific fear. This enhances accuracy in development of a stress hierarchy, or graded stress situations, for patients not in touch with their emotions. Feedback alerts patients when relaxation is achieved in each progressive stress situation and helps them to determine when they may move to the next level.

Drug Addiction (Substance Abuse)

Biofeedback is used to offer an alternative to anxiety-relieving addictive substances. Many addicts cannot withstand withdrawal from the substance without some type of alternative. They feel unable to overcome powerful drives to use substances that fill an emotional void. Biofeedback and relaxation alternatives help addicts to gain control of their psychophysiological arousal, thus decreasing the need for the substance. Biofeedback can be preferable for anxiety reduction since it has functional specificity and does not need to subdue the entire central nervous system.

Pain

Biofeedback deals directly with muscle or vascular tension levels resulting in pain. Biofeedback provides a means of developing awareness of tension levels, as well as their triggering stimuli, thereby enabling patients to recognize early pain and abate it before it becomes incapacitating. Pain applications most frequently discussed include migraine headaches, bruxism, low back syndrome, cancer, and spasticity pain associated with neurological disorders.

The Occupational Therapist's Role in Biofeedback Training

The therapist should plan and monitor treatment with biofeedback, viewing it as one tool for accomplishing total treatment goals. The therapist acts as coach and educator, and teaches the patient to interact and derive meaning from the biofeedback. Changes are observed in physiological activity as the patient develops ability to alter feedback displays, and verbal cues are provided to encourage the development of cortical awareness of physiological change. The therapist must be aware of other aspects of the patient's homeostasis being affected by changes in the monitored system.

Since biofeedback strategies do not specifically address a person's maladaptive appraisals and behaviors in the natural environment, the therapist must guide the patient to translate learned internal control skills into real-life behavioral adaptations. If environmental modifications have already been made, they may no longer be necessary once internal control is achieved. Observing internal control on biofeedback displays is a reinforcer in itself, yet a greater motivational challenge is to be able to achieve more gratifying personal activity goals.

Note

Therapists should take care to apply the biofeedback tools within the behavioral context for which they were intended. They should be cognizant of the medical risks of using electrical equipment improperly. Material in this chapter is intended to inform therapists about the potential of biofeedback; it is not a training manual in the use of biofeedback machines. Other educational resources should be studied to develop expertise in the use of biofeedback technology.

References

1. Marinacci, A., and Horande, M.: Electromyogram in neuromuscular re-education. Bull. Los Angeles Neurol. Soc. 25:57–71, 1960.
2. Basmajian, J. V., Kukulka, C. G., Narayan, M. G., and Takebe, K.: Biofeedback treatment of foot drop after stroke compared with standard rehabilitation technique: Effects on voluntary control and strength. Arch. Phys. Med. Rehabil. 56:231–236, 1975.
3. Harris, F. A., Spelman, F. A., and Hyner, J. W.: Electronic sensory aids as treatment for cerebral-palsied children, inaproprioception: Part II. Phys. Ther. 54:354–365, 1974.
4. Trombly, C. A., and Cole, J. M.: Electromyographic study of four hand muscles during selected activities. Am. J. Occup. Ther. 33:440–449, 1979.
5. Brown, D. M., Dibaucher, G. A., and Basmajian, J. V.: Feedback goniometers for hand rehabilitation. Am. J. Occup. Ther. 33:458–463, 1979.
6. Brown, D. M., and Basmajian, J. V.: Bioconverter for upper extremity rehabilitation. Am. J. Phys. Med. 57:233–238, 1978.
7. Kotses, H., Glaus, K. O., Crawford, P. L., Edwards, J. E., and Sherr, M. S.: Operant reduction of frontalis EMG activity in the treatment of asthma in children. J. Psychosom. Res. 20:453–459, 1976.
8. Miller, N. E.: Biofeedback and visceral learning. Ann. Rev. Psychol. 29:373–404, 1978.
9. Jacobson, E.: Progressive Relaxation. Chicago: University of Chicago Press, 1942.

PART 6

Implementation of Occupational Therapy

CHAPTER 19

Psychiatry and Mental Health *Elizabeth G. Tiffany*

The term *mental health* covers a broad spectrum of concerns that have been of primary interest to occupational therapists since occupational therapy had its beginnings. In all parts of life, the mental health of the individual is a vital component of adaptation. What then of "mental illness," or of the shades of emotional, cognitive, and psychomotor problems in adaptation which become the focus of psychiatric intervention?

If we look for definitions, perhaps the most effective one today is a functional one. People who, through the centuries, have been called mentally ill, psychiatrically disabled, or maladjusted have been those who have lacked the ability to organize their thoughts, feelings, attitudes, and actions in a way that would permit them to function within society for either a brief or extended period of time. Such a broad definition seems necessary. The phrase "ability to organize" allows for a wide range of etiologies, which include physiological, toxic, psychological, social, and others. Such a definition allows for some consideration of the severe psychological pathologies that sometimes accompany physical illness or trauma and require very special attention if the process of

rehabilitation is to be effective. It does not exclude the possibility that the mentally retarded or the neurologically impaired may also have components of psychiatric disability. The phrase "within society" allows for the possibility that the environments and social systems in which people live are varied and that what constitutes healthy behavior in one may be seen as highly undesirable, perverted, or ill in another. We find that, at the outer edges of our definition, the distinctions between "mental" and "physical," "individual" and "societal," tend to become blurred.

Occupational therapy, like medicine, is concerned with the restoration or maintenance of function in people who are ill or otherwise disabled. Like medicine, occupational therapy must always reflect and act upon the base of knowledge of the time. What is known and understood about people and their functioning dictates what is perceived as possible. Like medicine, occupational therapy will always be bound to some degree by the values of the time and the place in which it provides service. Occupational therapy, like medicine, is practiced by people, individuals who bring to their profession their own personal strengths and weaknesses, value systems, needs, and unique ways of perceiving, thinking, feeling, and acting. These factors explain some of the differences one finds in occupational therapy practice, especially in psychiatric settings. They also give urgency to the need to define clearly and in depth the underlying premises of psychiatric occupational therapy practice.

The purpose of this chapter is to examine the principles and practices of occupational therapy as applied to the treatment of mental illness.

SECTION 1
Historical Roots

On close perusal of the history of psychiatric occupational therapy, it is evident that there are threads of thought which are woven into the fabric of the profession as a whole. These constant strands of thought are what have given the profession its consistent uniqueness throughout the years.

Competence, mastery, self-image, motivation, total function, adaptation, integration, satisfaction—these are some of the key words that appear throughout the literature of occupational therapy. A thoughtful look at their meanings reveals a fundamental belief which has prevailed throughout the history of occupational therapy: the belief that human beings are whole, that mind and body are intricately linked, and that anything that impinges upon or influences one must affect the other. Dunton, one of the founders of occupational therapy, said in 1922, "The primary objects to be obtained by occupational therapy may be divided into two groups, mental and physical, although it is impossible to divorce these functions."[1] To work toward the restoration of function in their physically disabled clients, occupational therapists have relied upon psychological involvement in the *meanings* attached to the *doing* process. To work toward restoration of function in their mentally ill clients, occupational therapists have used movement, doing, touching, sensing, that is, physical factors. In working with all kinds of clients, occupational therapists must be concerned with factors such as stress, anxiety, tension, and learning, all of which have long been demonstrated to have both emotional and physical components.

Moral Treatment—Work and Productivity Equate with Dignity

It is generally thought that the principles of "moral treatment" formed the base for modern psychiatric practice and for the specific concern with the uses of activity for treatment as we know it in occupational therapy. What are the tenets of moral treatment which, in the late eighteenth century, were so great a departure from the existing beliefs and practices with regard to the mentally ill? Moral treatment was based on the belief that mental illness occurred as the result of physical and psychological, not mystical, factors. Environmental stresses were recognized as major causes. Therefore, attention to a patient's environment or milieu was a primary concern, and institutions for the mentally ill gave attention to providing pleasant surroundings, kind and consistent treatment, and opportunities for patients to be productive. There was a belief that, no matter how ill or bizarre the patient appeared, there were still healthy parts to his or her personality; therefore treatment should include ways for the patient to develop self-esteem.

The institution to which the mentally ill were sent became their community. At a time when cultural and social systems were homogeneous and communication and transportation methods were limited, the establishment of a fairly uniform institutional community was quite possible. Patients were committed to institutional care for long periods of time, and in some instances for life. Moral treatment sought to develop in the institutional community a sense of family living. The milieu was one of daily routines, with chores and responsibilities shared by staff and patients for the good of all. Staff members provided role models for the patients. When staff members and patients both came from the same kinds of cultural and ethnic backgrounds, as they often did during this period, such a milieu could be quite successful.

Because the work ethic was dominant in society, work prevailed as a major means for the individual to experience satisfaction and purpose in life. "The patient is now one of our best workers, and in other respects improves much . . . I had the most rational conversation with him that I had ever had . . . It was truly pleasing to discover such rationality."[2] So wrote Isaac Bonsall, who, in 1817, became the first superintendent of the Friends Asylum in Frankford, located in Philadelphia. Bonsall was describing the effect of occupation on a severely disturbed patient.

The Beginning of the Profession of Occupational Therapy

Occupational therapy developed into an identified profession during the years after World War I (see Chap. 1). At that time Doctor Adolf Meyer and Eleanor Clarke Slagle developed the use of carefully planned goals and methods for promoting health through the use of activities. It was in the 1920s that Meyer restated the principles of moral treatment and gave a context and philosophy for the development of the profession of occupational therapy.[3] At the same time Slagle began training occupational "therapeutists." She divided their rehabilitation efforts into three distinct groups: those directed toward patients who in all likelihood would continue their lives within the institution, those directed toward return to the community, and those directed toward prevention through the use of a pre-hospital work clinic. The approaches of Meyer and Slagle to the use of activities and relationships, examined in the light of today's knowledge and practice, were remarkably modern—they emphasized developmental needs and had a sense of the importance of preparing the individual patient for functioning within society.[4]

In the 1920s, behaviorism dominated psychology while psychoanalytical theory dominated psychiatry. The pioneers in occupational therapy, however, focused on the patient's outer reality and functional behavior. In the institutional setting, the patient was involved in work assignments. These assignments seemed effective in promoting adjustment.

William Rush Dunton, Jr., the psychiatrist whose commitment and belief in the principles of occupational therapy were at the cornerstone of the profession, wrote several books and articles on the subject. In *Prescribing Occupational Therapy*, published in 1928, he systematically categorized activities and kinds of patients. He thoughtfully delineated principles for matching activities with the needs of patients in a way that could be therapeutic. He classified activities in terms of their demands for attention, repetition, physical or intellectual effort, social factors, and criteria for rest, surprise, or creativity. He simplified the categories of mental disorders and suggested the kinds of activities that could be most desirable and most therapeutic with each category. He also described the importance of the therapist's approach and attitude for each:

For the manic—steady, quieting activity to reduce motor restlessness and train concentration; sedative activity, rhythmic and repetitive, with little variety

For the depressed—stimulating activity, although initially the therapist may need to give a preliminary course of stereotyped activity. The activity should have the potential for replacing the patient's preoccupations with depressive ideation. The therapist must use tact and be sensitive.

For the demented (dementia praecox or schizophrenia)—reeducation activities to train better habits of thought and action. Social activities which would place the individual into simple, structured work with others—activities which demand constant attention to overcome daydreaming, and activities to emphasize reality contact

For the paranoid—activities which would create or stimulate interest in concrete things—such as caring for goldfish or canaries, working in hospital industries

For the psychoneurotic—activities to reduce egocentricity and to allow for the sublimation of repressed conflicts[5]

In Dunton's work we see a major attempt to analyze activities, to categorize patient needs, and to suggest therapist approaches. He considered the core of the occupational therapy process to be making the correct matches among these elements.

Other proponents of the clear, deliberate application of activities to meet specific patient needs were Louis J. Haas and L. Cody Marsh. Haas' publications, *Practical Occupational Therapy* and *Occupational Therapy for the Mentally and Nervously Ill*, contain interesting, detailed descriptions of crafts projects, in addition to theoretical formulations about the use of crafts.[6,7] Haas stated emphatically that "being busy is not necessarily therapeutic."

Marsh, in a speech at the Sixteenth Annual Conference of the American Occupational Therapy Association, defined the uses of carefully matched work assignments as therapy.[8]

Occupational Therapists as Aides to the Psychiatrist

In the 1930s and 1940s psychiatric occupational therapists clearly identified themselves as aides to the psychiatrist in providing treatment for the mentally ill. The occupational therapist's activities included music, psychodrama, bibliotherapy, recreation, work, and arts and crafts. In effect, occupational therapy was concerned with the whole person and his or her total life of work and play within the institutional setting.

At the same time that occupational therapy developed as a profession there began a search for theoretical concepts that would provide frames of reference for treatment. Therapists began to be dissatisfied with basing their practice purely on intuitive and empirical success. Occupational therapists saw their roles as closely aligned with the psychiatrist responsible for patients. The situation in which they worked involved a written prescription from the psychiatrist or physician before the occupational therapist could initiate treatment. The prescription gave basic information about the patient, including special precautions, and requested that the occupational therapist provide specified services. The occupational therapist's areas of service to the psychiatrist included the following: (1) diagnostic aid (through the observation of the patient's behavior and performance in occupational therapy), (2) facilitating the patient's adjustment to the hospital environment, (3) supplementing shock therapy, (4) supplementing psychoanalytical therapy, and (5) habit training.[9]

Psychoanalytical Bases and Some Research

The theoretical base for occupational therapy as a true intervention and treatment modality within a psychoanalytical frame of reference was specified by William C. Menninger. His six categories of the functions of activities as treatment are as follows: (1) as an outlet for aggression and hostility, (2) to provide opportunities for advantageous identifications, (3) as atonement for guilt, (4) as a means of obtaining love, (5) to provide opportunities to act out fantasies, and (6) to allow for an experience of creative work.[10] The occupational therapist working within this context needed to have basic knowledge of the principles of psychoanalytical psychiatry and especially of defense mechanisms, as well as a sensitivity to the potentials of given activities for fulfilling the functions described above.

Although intuition, common sense, and empirical success provided the only guidelines in the selection of activities, it is evident from the literature of the time that there were tendencies to seek a more scientific base and to define occupational therapy professionally.

Electric and insulin shock therapies were being employed. These presented special challenges to the occupational therapist. The psychiatric casualties of World War II provided impetus for the development of programs under the Veterans Administration. One is struck by the number of articles written by physicians in collaboration with occupational therapists during this period.

Training Programs for Aides

Obviously, for the number of patients hospitalized, there were never enough trained therapists, especially as training programs grew longer and more academic. The professional occupational therapist, in many instances, became a program planner and a supervisor of aides, particularly in the large hospitals. It became a major concern of professional therapists to find ways to transmit theoretical knowledge to untrained staff members and to facilitate the communication of treatment goals and methods. In the large hospitals, psychiatrically trained physicians were also in short supply. Although the psychiatrist's written prescription could serve an important purpose, effective communication of this kind often was more an ideal than a reality.

On the Threshold of Radical Changes

At the beginning of the 1950s, in addition to shock therapies, psychosurgery in the form of the prefrontal lobotomy was added to the list of medical attempts to cure the mentally ill, or at least to provide symptomatic relief. Occupational therapists had to find ways to work effectively with the lobotomized patient. It was often discouraging. Psychosurgery, although initially considered promising, was to be a short-lived form of treatment.

Psychodynamic principles for treatment and activity analysis were explored in greater depth in the 1950s. The occupational therapist began to look at the patient's behavior and symptoms in terms of "externalized or internalized aggression, projection, withdrawal and regression."[11] Gail Fidler, in an article in the *American Journal of Occupational Therapy* in 1948, presented an outline of activity analysis through which the materials, tools, actions, and interpersonal relationship potentials of activities could be explored.[12] Professional occupational therapists attempted to match activities with patient needs based on this kind of thinking.

TIME: 1949

PLACE: An Occupational Therapy Shop in a private psychiatric hospital.

The occupational therapist enters her office, a screened off area in the back of the bright, pleasantly decorated large room known as the "O.T. Shop." (A sign, carefully painted in old English script, hangs outside the door to designate this fact.) She stops for a moment to smooth her starched white uniform and notes that she will soon have to have her hair cut or fasten it up. On her desk lies a copy of *Discovering Ourselves* by Strecker and Appel,[13] an old book, but one which she finds stimulating and helpful not only in understanding her patients but also in understanding herself.

Her patients have just left and the day is about over. There were ten in this last group, men from the locked ward. An attendant brought them down to her shop and stayed with them for the hour they were there. She thinks, with satisfaction, how much better it is in this bright new area, compared with the dingy basement shop next to the boiler room. It was more than the change that felt good—it was the idea that the hospital superintendent really seemed to appreciate and support occupational therapy. Until the shop was moved two months before she had needed to take supplies to the men on the ward. It seems so much better to get them out of that atmosphere. Here, she could give them so many more things. There are floor looms, where patients can beat out their hostility on rugs. And there is a bicycle jigsaw and a workbench. Good masculine activities. And, of course, the radio, so they could have music. The only drawback is that the men can come only when they're on good behavior. That's a problem she's been thinking a lot about. She was planning to get together with the ward personnel to see if there would be some way to put a punching bag up, or something, right on the ward, for the men to use whenever they began to feel upset.

Now, however, her mind was focused on one patient. He was new in the hospital and she had already received a written prescription for occupational therapy from his doctor. She thumbed through a pile of cards on her desk until she found his prescription. The card read:

| NAME: John Jones   AGE: 31 |
| DIAGNOSIS: Schizophrenia, paranoid type |
| O.T. PRESCRIPTION: Activities to divert attention from hallucinations, improve reality testing and attention span, increase socialization |
| PRECAUTIONS: Patient has auditory hallucinations. May become assaultive. Currently being treated with insulin coma therapy. Observe for insulin reactions. |
| PHYSICIAN: *M. Brown, M.D.* |
| WARD: 5B |

John Jones had come to O.T. that day. He seemed mild-mannered and polite but a little vague in his thinking, probably because he'd had an insulin treatment earlier. That was the problem with the patients who were getting insulin or electric shock therapy. They sometimes seemed to forget everything or be really out of touch. John Jones had picked copper tooling to do. This had seemed a good choice to the occupational therapist because it would require some planning and attention; its actions involved hard pressure but also controlling, and it was masculine. He already was planning to use it as a gift. He had chosen a picture of two sheep, with a little lamb standing between them. When he started to work on it, he seemed able to follow the directions all right. He said that the little lamb reminded him of himself, in between his mother and his wife. The occupational therapist jots down a little note to mention that to his doctor. She also decides to set aside time to read John Jones' chart before he comes to the shop tomorrow.

The occupational therapist then opens a cabinet and takes down rolls of brightly colored crepe paper, some construction paper, paste, and a box of blunt-pointed scissors. She places these items on a cart, ready to take to the women's locked ward first thing in the morning. They would need an early start to make the decorations for the party that evening.

One more thing, before she could call it a day. She picks up the telephone and calls the lady in charge of the hospital auxiliary. She needs to check out a few more details about the O.T. sale next week.

"Sometimes," she thinks, "I really do feel like a jack-of-all-trades but I like what I'm doing and I feel sure that the activities I give my patients help them. They know I'm interested in them and accept them as human beings." She remembers, in a flash, having seen the movie *The Snake Pit* the week before. "Thank goodness it doesn't have to be like that anymore," she thinks as she locks up the cabinets and desk, puts on her coat, and leaves. □

Psychopharmacology— New Possibilities

The mid-1950s saw a major revolution take place in mental hospitals. The introduction of psychopharmacology, the use of tranquilizers and psychic energizers, opened a new world of possibilities. The medicines seemed to reduce most of the gross pathological symptoms and acting out behaviors that previously had interfered with treatment. Social psychiatry and anthropology explored new vistas for handling the problem of mental illness. Maxwell Jones' "therapeutic community" in England received attention.[14] The therapeutic milieu, opendoor policies, halfway house, family treatment, aftercare services, and volunteer involvement all became possibilities.

The American Psychiatric Association, in 1952, published the first edition of *Diagnostic and Statistical Manual of Mental Disorders,* the first official manual to give descriptions of diagnostic categories of mental problems. These descriptions reflected the view of Adolf Meyer that mental disorders were reactions of the personality to psychological, social, and biological factors.

Occupational therapists at this time began to look in greater depth than previously at the social adaptation of their patients and to focus on the meaning and use of activities and their interpersonal components in the treatment process. Two major events took place in psychiatric occupational therapy. One was a book. The other was a study that culminated in a book. In 1954, *Introduction to Psychiatric Occupational Therapy* was written and published by Gail S. Fidler, OTR and Jay W. Fidler, M.D. This book represented professional occupational therapy as the use of productive activities as treatment in a collaborative effort between the occupational therapist and the psychotherapist. It suggested the concept of the occupational therapy area as a laboratory in which the patient could experiment with new ways of handling emotions and developing living skills. It presented a much refined, psychoanalytically flavored activity analysis process, suggested ways in which groups could be used to facilitate treatment, and encouraged the study of projective techniques. While acknowledging that many occupational therapists were working without psychiatric supervision to the extent described, it encouraged occupational therapists to formulate treatment goals and programs in the most meaningful way on their own and to work toward effective communications with all involved staff. The Fidlers candidly stated, "These views cannot be presented without the realization that occupational therapy is a young field and that there are great potentialities for future development. This is especially emphasized by the fact that the entire field of psychiatry is still in its youth and therefore any of the subsidiary techniques must also be as elementary if not more so."[15]

In 1956, following a two-year study funded by a grant to the American Occupational Therapy Association by the National Institute of Mental Health, a conference of leaders in the field of psychiatric occupational therapy was held at Boiling Springs, Pennsylvania. Under the leadership of Elizabeth P. Ridgway and Gail S. Fidler, the participants explored and questioned many emerging issues of psychiatric occupational therapy practice. These were identified as *use of self, use of group and group techniques, use of activities, creation of the therapeutic milieu, development of special treatment goals as a supplement to psychotherapy,* contributions to psychodynamic formulations through the *use of personality, social, and skills evaluations* and, finally, *bridging the gap between community living and the hospital.*[16] In her introduction to the published proceedings of the conference, Wilma West said, "Several developments and changes in the treatment of psychiatric patients during recent years made this project a timely one. These include an awareness of the reversibility of the process of mental illness, the growth of the team approach and resulting collaboration of all concerned, utilization of group interaction and an increasing emphasis on the total individual and the milieu in which he functions."[17] This is a fair assessment of the state of psychiatric occupational therapy at that time.

TIME: 1957

PLACE: O.T. Shop in a large, progressive state institution

Barbara and Jack, registered occupational therapists, are seated at the end of a long table near a window in the large, somewhat cluttered O.T. room. They've just come back from lunch and are working together warping a table loom. Two copies of the *American Journal of Occupational Therapy* lie on the windowsill.

Barbara comments to Jack, "Did you see the article in the September Journal about the study they made—the one that proved that if the occupational therapist is able to work on developing relationships with the patients, the patients become more active?"[18]

Jack replies, "Nope. But it makes sense, doesn't it? I know that sometimes it looks as if I'm goofing off when I just sit and talk with the guys from Ward B but they really do seem to want to come to O.T. and I think I get further with them . . . you know . . . it's like they trust me more."

"Yes," Barbara says, and adds, "By the way, has Dr. Brown started having team meetings for Ward B? He said he wanted to because soon they want to make it an open ward. He wants to start having ward meetings for all the patients too. He really wants to make sure that everybody's involved in the changes."

Jack recalls, "They're supposed to start next week, at eight o'clock Wednesday morning. That's the time when most of the nurses and attendants are around. I wonder how it will work. Incidentally, since you mentioned the Journal, I did look at that article about changes in O.T. due to tranquilizing drugs.[19] Did you see it? I guess because I'm a recently graduated O.T. I'm not so aware of the differences the new drugs are making. I know the things they told us about in school, the kinds of crazy actions we heard about. Well, I just haven't seen them, at least not many of them. What worries me, though, is that half the time I feel as if I'm working with zombies. The article says that a lot of your time and energy used to go into finding ways to channel excess drives, controlling hyperactivity, and so forth. Is that true? I almost think that would make O.T. more interesting!"

Replying to Jack's comments, Barbara says, "Oh, I don't know about that. It got pretty wild sometimes. Now, in some ways it seems easier, but in other ways it seems harder—like working through a mask. And we've got a whole new set of things to watch for, and report. By the way, has Dick complained to you about his eyesight? He was trying to draw the squares on that chessboard he's making and he was having an awful time. Said everything was going blurry on him. Better check it out. Uh-oh, it's one o'clock and the crowd is about to arrive."

They fasten down the pieces of warp with tape, open the supply cabinets, and unlock the O.T. room doors. Jack says, "See you," and retreats through a back door which leads to the men's shop.

A group of twenty women, in hospital dresses, presses through the door. Two nursing aides accompany the group. As if preprogrammed, they go to the supply cabinets, take out boxes neatly labeled with their names, and seat themselves around the table. Some begin to work on embroidery and some on knitting; one goes to an upright loom on which a braided rug has been started. Two of the women, apparently new, stand still until the aides talk them into taking seats at the table. Barbara sits down near them and suggests to them that they draw some pictures. She gives them crayons and construction paper. Barbara is uncomfortable. She has been reading, for the second time, the book, *Introduction to Psychiatric Occupational Therapy*.[20] The scene before her seems so very far removed from the exciting ideas about what O.T. could be. She begins to think about things they could do, especially if the hospital really goes into teams.

She moves about the group of patients, offering help to some, encouraging others, stopping to listen while one complains about a problem in the dining room, occasionally chatting with the whole group

about some current event and trying to interest the group in planning an afternoon party to which they would invite their doctors, visitors, or any special friends. The atmosphere is quiet and subdued. It is hard to feel enthusiasm. On another level, Barbara's mind is racing ahead. She's devising a form—one which would list the kinds of information we get about patients when they do activities—the way they use the materials and the way they relate to the O.T. and to each other. And she's planning a new method for reporting to the doctors and nurses. And, remembering that the hospital has just hired a volunteer director, she's thinking about ways volunteers can help them in new kinds of activities. She'll have to talk to Jack about all this. □

Government Action Spurs Community Mental Health

The Mental Health Study Act was passed in 1955, establishing the Joint Commission on Mental Illness and Health. The charge of the Commission was to establish priorities and viable methods of services for the mentally ill. *Action for Mental Health*, the report of the commission, was published in 1961.[21] This report proposed a concerted attack on mental illness in the following ways: (1) better distribution and community-oriented philosophical reorientation of psychiatrists; (2) increasing participation of lay people at various levels in programs of prevention, treatment, and rehabilitation; (3) shift of emphasis from institutional to community services; (4) plans for shared federal, state, and local funding of community mental health centers. Thus was launched the community mental health movement.

In 1963, the Community Mental Health Act was passed, mandating the National Institute of Mental Health to establish and fund community mental health centers in local "catchment" areas with populations from 75,000 to 200,000. This gave impetus to the development of new approaches to treatment. Transactional analysis, gestalt therapy, and milieu therapy came to the fore. Family therapy became a treatment of choice for some individuals, with the interesting premise that the mentally ill person in a family may simply be expressing the symptoms for a whole family's pathology.[22] Behavioral approaches to treatment such as desensitization and operant conditioning techniques, developed by Joseph Wolpe and others, grew rapidly.[23] "Token economies" or behaviorally-oriented milieus were developed and seemed promising, particularly in treating the long-term chronically disabled and institutionalized mentally ill, the mentally retarded, and some kinds of childhood psychoses.

Research efforts were intensified in the areas of biochemistry, neurophysiology, as well as metabolic, enzyme, and genetic abnormalities. Psychosomatic illnesses were explored in greater depth. The wholeness of human function and the connections between mind, body, and emotions were proven repeatedly. Each new research finding, it seemed, pointed to new questions and new areas for exploration. Research efforts and techniques were aided by the enormous capabilities introduced by the growth of computer technology.

There was a shift away from emphasis on the long-term, deep methods of treatment by psychoanalysis, and a concerted effort was turned to explore ways in which individuals could be returned to function as rapidly as possible. Partial hospitalization programs opened so that patients could continue to live their lives in the community and attend treatment programs during the day or evening. Mental health professionals, including occupational therapists, began to visit the homes of their patients, and to look into important aspects of work and recreation in the community. Patients, in some settings, began to be called clients, residents, or members. The atmosphere of psychiatry had taken on a new and optimistic perspective.

Creative Chaos

The worlds in which psychiatric occupational therapists worked were greatly expanded by these changes. The spirit of experimentation, of questioning, and of unrest which characterized society as a whole during the 1960s permeated occupational therapy as well. Knowledge grew and new techniques were developed for the management of the mentally ill.

The second *Diagnostic and Statistical Manual of Mental Disorders* (DSM-II), of the American Psychiatric Association, was published in 1968 and represented an effort to base the classification of mental disorders on the comparable section of the eighth revision of the *International Classification of Diseases* (ICD-8) that was published at the same time. This edition of the *Diagnostic and Statistical Manual*, like the *International Classification of Diseases* did not attempt to define the diagnostic categories in terms of a theoretical framework, as the previous one had done, but simply gave descriptions of the classifications.

The Fidlers published a second book in 1963, *Occupational Therapy: A Communication Process in Psychiatry*.[24] They emphasized the enormous potential of the occupational therapy process as another vital language for communication, especially in view of its use of the nonverbal and its work regarding object relationships. They identified three major emphases for occupational therapy in psychiatry: (1) *treatment*, directly applied intervention in a pathological process to effect change in the patient, with subcategories defined as *psychoanalytic, supportive,* and *directive* (repressive); (2) the *mental health process,* by enhancing the milieu and supporting the healthy parts of the individual; and (3) *rehabilitation*, helping the patient to learn to use existing strengths more effectively. This book provided carefully analyzed and synthesized material, especially regarding the meaning of activities and interpersonal transactions in the activity process. Though strongest in its psychoanalytical orientation, it acknowledged as well the changes which were taking place both in psychiatry as a whole and in psychiatric occupational therapy.

The early 1960s were also influenced by the development of instruments for evaluation or assessment of the client. This was a period when there was significant interest in the use of the *Azima Battery*.[25] Gail Fidler also developed a battery, similar to the Azima Battery, through which information about a client's psychodynamics could be obtained.[26] These two batteries, and a number of local modifications of them, used art media and clay. The client's behavior and his or her projections were interpreted to provide meaningful data to aid in treatment planning.

Cognitive-Perceptual-Motor Research

Another very significant development was taking place during the 1960s. A. Jean Ayres was beginning to publish her observations of perceptual motor development and dysfunction in children.[27] Her research, which is still going on, was based on neurophysiology, and seemed to point to some areas of major concern to the occupational therapist working in psychiatry. Lorna Jean King, in Arizona, began a daring experiment with chronic schizophrenics and exhaustive research in the literature on perception, neurophysiology, and mental illness. She adapted and applied the theoretical base and some of the techniques developed by Ayres. The results of her work with severely regressed, institutionalized, chronically ill schizophrenic patients were most encouraging. By the end of the 1960s, it appeared that continued research and application of *sensory motor integrative* techniques for certain groups of patients was indeed indicated and contained heuristic value in terms of other, related psychiatric concerns.

Developmental Theory

In psychological and educational circles during this time there was a growth of interest in the work of Piaget. Developmental theory and especially theories of cognitive development were being explored generally. Psychiatric occupational therapists began to explore the significance of Piaget's work as it might relate to the occupational therapy process in psychiatry.

Activities Therapists

It should be noted that, with the increased attention to direct services for the mentally ill, there were not enough trained occupational therapists to fill the critically needed positions in both institutions and community. New activity specialties grew up: therapeutic recreation, art, music, dance, drama, and horticulture. These specialties grew from at least two roots: (1) independently and in a parallel stream of thought with occupational therapy, based on existing knowledge in education and psychology; and (2) as an outgrowth of the training of workers in occupational therapy in the two decades preceding. Each new discipline using activities has sought to develop its own professional identity, its own special areas of practice, and its own research base. Taking as its foundation the same base as occupational therapy, that activity can be used for evaluation and for treatment, the new activity specialties presented a challenge to occupational therapy to refine its own theory and practice and to work toward developing viable ways of communicating and cooperating with them.

American Occupational Therapy Association Funded for Consultant

Under the Social Rehabilitation Services Grant (#123), the American Occupational Therapy Association was funded in 1964 to have a full-time consultant in psychiatric rehabilitation in the National Office. Through the efforts of this consultant, and with the backing of the American Occupational Therapy Association, a number of regional and national institutes were held across the United States. The main foci of these workshops, which were held between 1964 and 1968, were supervision, group process, object relations, and education. In addition to the effects of deepening the knowledge base and strengthening the skills of practicing therapists, there was a concomitant development of a sense of community among them, as they shared together in the search for greater professional effectiveness.

The project director for this particular grant was June Mazer. Actually, the project RSA#123 had been started in 1958 as a consultancy program in physical dysfunction; at that time Irene Hollis was director. Mary Alice Coombs joined the project in 1961, and it became a joint physical-psychiatric consultancy. In December, 1962, the physical dysfunction phase was concluded. The psychiatric phase continued until 1968. Fourteen regional institutes were held on group process, administration, object relations, and evaluation, and twenty-one national institutes were held on education and advanced object relations.

Search for a Comprehensive Theory

The Psychiatric Special Interest Group of the Council on Practice of the American Occupational Therapy Association became especially active on a nationwide basis during the 1960s. There was a surge of interest in exploring ways to incorporate the expanding approaches and the ever-widening knowledge base into occupational therapy practice. Local special interest groups flourished in many areas. These groups became forums in which practicing therapists studied together, shared their questions and their ideas, and supported each other as they faced the critical issues which were emerging in psychiatry as a whole. The Psychiatric Special Interest Group, on a national level, participated in a number of special projects.

In 1968 the *American Journal of Occupational Therapy* invited occupational therapists practicing in psychiatry to submit papers describing the application of concepts to practice. The resulting issue of the *American Journal of Occupational Therapy* might be considered a landmark as the authors attempted to define theoretical frames of reference and to describe viable approaches to their use. The words of the introduction to the special section describe the situation of occupational therapy in psychiatry at that time: "It is evident that many therapists are involved in the struggle to formulate and/or apply various theories in their practices, even though none of the submitted papers proposed a truly comprehensive theory of occupational therapy. Each article is accompanied by critical discussions and an author's response. We hope that these will stimulate further critical thinking and discussion. Our dream is that this special section may herald the beginning of a period rich in clinical exploration and research."[28] The four articles and the conference report included in this issue focused attention on the difficulties of developing such a comprehensive theory. The authors identified the work still to be done by describing both their thought and their practice.[29,30,31,32,33]

Following the institutes on object relations in 1967, a small group of therapists met in Albion, Michigan, to attempt to relate "a large number of divergent theories and thoughts to a specific framework that would include all aspects of the organism."[34] The object relations institutes and their culminating seminar attempted to explore in some depth the existing knowledge bases in anthropology, sociology, psychology, neurophysiology, and philosophy, as well as in psychiatry. There seemed to be little doubt that all of these could be significant in contributing to the knowledge base of occupational therapy. This was a most ambitious task and the problem seemed to be one of providing bridges between all the possibilities. The charge was stated, "A necessary step toward building a body of knowledge specifically related to the kind of experience occupational therapy is able to provide is a frame of reference which utilizes a truly holistic developmental approach."[35]

The climate of optimism, enthusiasm, and investigation characterizing psychiatric occupational therapy at this time was reflected in a number of articles which were published during 1969 and 1970. Mary Reilly and her colleagues and students at the University of Southern California began to make their contributions to the field through the study of the work-play continuum, the patient's real world, and concepts of competence as the keys to the theoretical base of psychiatric occupational therapy.

The "occupational behavior" frame of reference for occupational therapy in psychiatry, as explored and proposed by Reilly, has taken the earliest principles and approaches of occupational therapy, as practiced in "moral treatment" and expressed in 1922 by Adolf Meyer, and examined them in depth and in the light of current psychological and sociological literature. This group proposed that occupational therapy shift its "initial perspective of patients from diagnostic labels to those of occupational roles of worker, student, housewife, retiree, preschooler and even career patient. . . ."[36] Occupational therapists were urged to look into the influences of the experiences found in childhood play.

In 1970 a symposium, "The Skill Continuum from Play through Work," was conducted in Boston under the sponsorship of the United States Department of Health, Education and Welfare (HEW), Maternal and Child Health Service. The papers presented at this symposium were published in the *American Journal of Occupational Therapy* in September 1971.[37,38,39,40,41,42,43,44] The important message of this orientation was expressed by Matsutsuyu: "It was found that the perspective based on pathology held few guidelines for working knowledge of healthy function. It is not enough to accept the definition of

health as the absence of disease."[45] The framework for this thinking had been expressed earlier by Reilly when she said: "Play, in a chronological or longitudinal sense, we believe, is the antecedent preparation area for work. In a cross-sectional sense, we have found it clinically useful to see an adult social-recreation pattern of behavior as a sublatent support to a work pattern. The entire developmental continuum of play and work we designate as occupational behavior."[46]

TIME: 1969

PLACE: The O.T. office in a day program in a mental hospital of medium size

Alice W., the occupational therapist, sits at her desk, writing a note. She has just finished working with a group that is planning an issue of the program's newspaper. The clients in the group are Don, a middle-aged man who is just recovering from a depression; Marie, an obese young woman whose obsessive-compulsive tendencies have interfered with her ability to work at her job; and Jim, a 19-year-old man who is suffering from an anxiety neurosis.

"How can I express what seemed to be happening when Jim and Don and Marie were starting to plan the next issue of the newspaper?" she thinks, her pen poised above the paper. "It was as if Don and Marie were Jim's mother and father, and he was their little child. And Jim seemed to fit right into that role. Maybe it's because Don and Marie really have had a lot more experience with the paper. On the other hand, we have seen so much of Jim's dependency in just about every aspect of his life. We've seen it in our evaluations too. This is probably just another expression of that. Putting the paper out could be a good way to help him grow, because he certainly has the basic skills. I'll talk with Don and Marie about letting Jim do the typing first . . . then maybe they'll show him how to do the paste-up, if he's interested."

At this point, there's a knock on the door, and a pleasant-faced woman, the unit's social worker, pokes her head in and says, "They're going to run the videotape of the activity group again, so the group can watch. Maybe you'd better be there for the feedback session."

Alice gets up and goes to the door saying, "You bet. I want to have another look at the way Jim handled the situation. I have a feeling he may want to talk about it. By the way did you want to borrow my Arieti?[47] And sometime could you let me look at your *Freedom to Learn?*"[48] □

Accountability

In American society the early 1970s were a time of some disenchantment. Out of the chaotic and creative flux of the late 1960s there emerged a public tiredness. The Vietnam War dragged on, draining off money and manpower that more and more Americans began to feel could be better used. Government spending priorities moved further away from the social and health concerns of the 1960s. The economy seemed doomed to increasing inflation as a worldwide problem. Watergate set off widespread questions about trust and accountability, which had ramifications beyond the political arena, touching business, education, and health care delivery systems.

The focus of the consumer movement on greater personal involvement, concern for human rights, and issues of responsibility and accountability led to some important changes in the way mental illness and its treatment were viewed. There was a general increase of public interest in abnormal psychology, nurtured by the use of psychological themes in the media and popular literature, and by the development of opportunities to study about it at all educational levels. This interest and knowledge, coupled with a growing concern for clients' rights led to questions and demands with regard to mental health practices. The lay population, no longer altogether naïve, sought to define health care in terms of its costs, benefits, risks and hazards. It became increasingly important for all health professionals to justify their services. This meant clearly defining their goals and methods and the populations to be served. Reporting systems needed refinement to be consistent with professional aims and relevant to patients' needs.

A new chaos and creative flux developed in society as a whole. The Civil Rights Movement begun in the 1950s extended into concerns that profoundly affected health-care professionals. It aroused consciousness of inequities suffered by many segments of the population. The Women's Movement mobilized many people into action to change some of society's most fundamental attitudes and practices. The elderly and the handicapped organized to demand long overdue rights, opportunities, and concern. Homosexuality no longer was considered an illness in itself, and people with varying sexual orientations "came out of the closet." Other taboos were lifted. Death and dying, as part of the continuum of living, became a subject of conversation and study. *Patients' rights* became a major concern. The nation experienced what Alvin Toffler called "future shock."[49] People continued to be increasingly bombarded with facts, new orientations, and the rapid fabrication and just as rapid decline of

materials, ideas, and fads. All of this has had enormous significance to occupational therapy, a profession with a commitment to help others to "do for themselves."

Legal Decisions

The United States legal systems lent support to these developments. In 1971, in a milestone decision, the Alabama Courts (Wyatt vs. Stickney) ruled that an individual who has been involuntarily confined to a mental institution has a right to treatment—as opposed to simply maintenance or incarceration. Minimum standards for institutional staffing and treatment were spelled out.[50] In 1975, a United States Supreme Court decision (O'Connor vs. Donaldson) ruled that "a finding of mental illness alone cannot justify a state's locking a person up against his will and keeping him indefinitely in a simple custodial confinement. . . . In short, a state cannot constitutionally confine without more (than custodial care) a non-dangerous individual who is capable of surviving safely in freedom by himself or with the help of willing and responsible family members or friends."[51]

Across the country, states were compelled to look into their laws, policies, and practices regarding institutional management of the mentally ill. There were a number of local changes in laws which reflected three broad themes: (1) access to mental health care; (2) the rights of mental patients to receive or to refuse treatment; and (3) social acceptance of deviance.

Occupational therapy was forced during the late 1960s and early 1970s to look carefully at its uses of work as therapy. For many years, in some of the large public institutions, patients had been assigned to work in the laundry, maintenance shops, farm, and a variety of other areas. Frequently in these assignments patients were able to experience the success of developing real proficiency at given tasks and the sense of being contributing, productive members of the institutional community. Unfortunately, the very positive personal effects which these work assignments had on some patients, also, within the institutional setting, tended to reinforce their need to stay in the hospital. There was not enough attention given the total milieu of the institution and not enough effort put into helping the patients generalize their skills so they could use them in the world outside the institution. From the standpoint of the public it appeared that patient labor was being seriously exploited.

The question of institutional peonage was brought into the courts. (The case, Nelson Eugene Souder vs. Peter J. Brennan, Civil Action 482-73, resulted in a law in April 1974 requiring that patients be paid the statutory minimum wage for performing work within the institutional setting. The date when vigorous enforcement was to proceed was set as December 1, 1974.) Therefore, the assignment of patients to work without pay in situations that benefited the institution became illegal. The act resulting from the above-mentioned court action required that institutions provide pay for patients' work. Few institutions could afford either this or the necessary staff and paperwork to justify work as therapy. There were some patients, the seriously institutionalized and chronic, who lost in the process their one successful, however rote, activity. And so, a concomitant, and possibly resultant, movement took place to develop more community, business, and industrial contacts so that patients could be given work assignments in the real world with real remuneration. Occupational therapists needed to examine this concept.

New Preventive Models

In 1971 Geraldine Finn presented the Eleanor Clarke Slagle Lecture at the Annual Conference of the American Occupational Therapy Association in Cleveland. Her lecture discussed the societal and technological changes which had taken place during the preceding decades and examined the efforts that had been made at Boston State Hospital to shift occupational therapy services to a prevention model. She identified nine major issues which were part of that process:

1. The function of primary institutions in maintaining the health of the people of a community and the need for occupational therapists to understand the functions, goals and policies of these primary institutions
2. The planning of appropriate programs and services based on man's need to engage in interaction with the objects of his environment in order to maintain his health throughout his life
3. The need to reinterpret the body of knowledge available within the profession of occupational therapy in order to apply it in the service of keeping people healthy rather than in helping people minimize their disabilities
4. The creation of new associations of our available knowledge in order to respond more accurately to the pressing reality needs of today
5. The establishment of an organizational model which will allow translation of abstract plans about activities, human action and the delivery of health services into concrete actions
6. The presence of risk taking and its ramifications on one's ability to function and persevere when faced with an unfamiliar environment

7. The necessity of reexamining communication patterns to ensure real communications among people
8. The need to create a climate of acceptance for a planned program and the development of the skills needed to assist others in seeing the value of these programs
9. The role of supervision in maintaining the performance and professional growth of the staff members[52]*

The kinds of programs described by Finn included early intervention programs for children, consultation services to teachers, inservice programs on developmental screening, and program planning, outreach programs for the elderly, workshops for mothers and preschool children, inservice programs on perceptual-motor development for mental health workers, development of new models of parent education and counseling and the introduction of knowledge about developmental levels of human performance in a community drug program.[53]

In 1977, President Carter appointed a Commission on Mental Health to study and make recommendations regarding the status of mental health and mental health services in this country. Their findings led to the following statement: "Because of the pluralistic nature of the American Society and cultural order, social problems and social deviances, when applied to mental health issues, must be approached from a cultural relativity frame of reference."[54]

Thus, during the 1970s, the psychiatric occupational therapist was plunged into a new and challenging set of perspectives. In many ways the occupational therapist was beginning to accept and identify with a peer professional role along with physicians, social workers, psychologists, and nurses. The search for a unifying theory of occupational therapy had disclosed in sharp relief the unique contributions that could be made by the therapist. The occupational therapist as an "aid to the physician" gave way to the occupational therapist as a co-professional cooperating with a number of other disciplines in the treatment of the mentally ill in at least some of the newer and less traditional settings. The contexts for treatment and the constitution of the treatment teams were considerably extended. By 1970 occupational therapists were working in schools, community programs, and homes in addition to the traditional settings. In some of the more traditional settings, nontraditional staffing patterns and new approaches were being explored.

---

* Reprinted with permission of the *American Journal of Occupational Therapy*.

As popular trends in psychiatry gained momentum and prominence, many occupational therapists working in psychiatry saw the value of learning and gaining skills in their use. Transactional analysis, gestalt therapy, meditation, bioenergetics, assertiveness and effectiveness training, and a variety of humanistic and self-actualization group techniques are just a few of the movements which were beginning to offer new avenues to the development of healthier, more productive and satisfying lives in the general (normal to mildly neurotic) population. Some occupational therapists, as well as psychologists, social workers, and others, saw in these techniques opportunities for enhancing the treatment of their clients. With varying degrees of effectiveness, they incorporated them into existing treatment techniques. This happened most readily and most often in those settings where the occupational therapist's role was blended with the roles of other members of the treatment team.

The work of Anne C. Mosey, Lela Llorens, and others gave further impetus to occupational therapists in several parts of the country to study and articulate the principles of human development as a basic frame of reference for psychiatric occupational therapy. This approach led to further interest in perceptual and cognitive functioning and the concepts of stress and regression.

The 1970s saw the resurgence of interest in, and attention to, the significance of societal attitudes, values, and varying life styles. Community-based programs, partial hospitalization, and home treatment programs have made it essential for occupational therapists to consider the impact of these social changes as well as the impact of their own personal value systems on all aspects of treatment.

In some areas, psychiatric occupational therapists began to experiment and work with behavioral approaches to treatment. Usually working within a team and in a setting where *behavior therapy* was being used, therapists developed methods of treatment based upon schedules of reinforcement, operant conditioning, modeling, shaping, and chaining procedures. For some patients, these techniques proved useful in changing or extinguishing undesirable behavior patterns and in establishing and reinforcing healthy behavior patterns.

At the same time, neurophysiological knowledge and neurophysiological approaches to treatment have been continuing to gain momentum; they promise to make a very significant impact on psychiatric practice. Refinement and development of the work of Ayres and King have continued. There has been increased attention to the effects of the functions of the reticular activating system. In 1975 Josephine Moore, in her Eleanor Clarke Slagle Lecture at the Annual Conference of the American Occupational Therapy Association in Milwaukee, "Behavior, Bias and the Limbic System," spoke eloquently of the need for greater consideration of the influence of basic neurophysiological mechanisms in determining human feelings and actions.[55]

The search for clean conceptual models, clear frames of reference, and a unifying theory of occupational therapy continued to be a preoccupation of the profession as a whole during the 1970s. The work of several prominent occupational therapists during this period and a special consciousness on the part of the American Occupational Therapy Association sought to provide guidelines to practice.

In her book, *Three Frames of Reference for Mental Health,* published in 1970, Mosey discussed three different conceptual approaches to psychiatric occupational therapy: (1) psychoanalytic, (2) acquisitional, and (3) developmental. She suggested that each of these three frames of reference define specific aspects of the occupational therapy process.[56] According to Mosey, each frame of reference has postulates regarding the nature of the individual, the characteristics of health and illness, and viable approaches to evaluation and treatment. Clarity with regard to the frame of reference used in treatment is seen as highly desirable. It permits the therapist to tap into and utilize a specific body of knowledge. It encourages consistency among expectations, goal-setting, and approaches to evaluation and treatment.

Mental Health Task Force Makes Recommendations

In 1975 a special task force comprised of psychiatric occupational therapists was appointed by the American Occupational Therapy Association. Their charge was to identify issues of concern in the practice of occupational therapy in mental health and to recommend solutions to identified problems. They surveyed practice in psychiatric occupational therapy and, based on their assessment of the status of occupational therapy in psychiatry, made their recommendations. The recommendations were published in the American Occupational Therapy Association newspaper in September 1976. The task force reported that "mental health practice lacks standardized clinical techniques and therefore is dependent on a conceptualization of the fundamental value of performance which has never been clearly articulated."[57] The task force went on to make recommendations geared to refining the knowledge base and strengthening the technology of occupational therapy practice. Specific recommendations were made regarding research, graduate education, continuing education, and the definition of occupational therapy practice in psychiatry. Although the work of this task force was addressed to psychiatric occupational therapy practice, it had serious implications for the profession as a whole.

TIME: 1977

PLACE: Kitchen area of a Community Mental Health Center

Bill (a registered occupational therapist with five years of experience in psychiatry) and Rona (an occupational therapy student in the sixth week of her second fieldwork experience) are having a cup of coffee before starting the day. They are in the kitchen, an area partitioned off from a pleasant livingroom, part of the program's small ADL apartment. Bill and Rona have a pile of papers spread out on the table in front of them. They have been discussing the clients.

Rona comments, "I finished checking out Roberta yesterday. It didn't work at all to place her in the group on Monday. She just went into her shell and stayed there. So I decided to work with her on a one-to-one basis for a while. She has a lot of rote skills, old familiar schemes, I guess, at a pretty high level—things like making coffee and setting the table—but when she tries something she never did before, or when there's some special emotional strain, she falls apart unless we give her a lot of structure. She seems able to handle only about two steps at a time, so you have to stay near. I think it's really important to give her that support. Don't you?"

Bill comments, "She certainly needs to succeed. Just watch that she doesn't get too dependent."

Rona replies, "I know. That's tricky, and I may need help to recognize it if it's happening. I was thinking—you know, her husband is going to stop by for lunch today. I thought I'd have her make something like grilled cheese sandwiches—which I'm sure she can handle—but use ready-mades like potato chips and tomatoes, and finish it out with ice cream for dessert. She's coming in at ten o'clock to decide the menu and seems to feel okay about going down the street to buy the food. I just think it's important for her to make the meal, but it can't be too complicated. What do you think?"

Bill says, "Sounds good to me. You're using her integrated skills well and that's probably important, because, while it's neat that her husband is coming, it's bound to be somewhat stressful. You know—he's been doing most of the cooking at their house for a couple of years! Good luck."

Bill leaves Rona and goes down a short hall to his office to check his schedule of activities for the day. A 9:30 meeting with the director to review the budget. The meeting would be sticky. Everybody's looking for ways to cut corners and save money. At 10:30, he would work with a small group of clients, men and women, in the workshop next to the kitchen. They would be doing simple repairs to broken pieces of furniture which they had brought in to the center. Most of the work was gluing and clamping, but there were some minor painting and refinishing jobs. He had found that this activity was good, both as evaluation and as treatment.

In the afternoon he would be taking Rona with him to the home of one of their clients. Mrs. Smith, the client, was 45 years old. An arthritic condition prevented her from getting out of the house. She was depressed and anxious. An occupational therapy program had been started to see if there were ways she could be helped to handle her basic activities of daily living. The situation was difficult because her family were all hard-working, energetic people, who were used to having Mrs. Smith depend on them, but who tended also to resent it silently. And the house was full of architectural barriers.

Somewhere, Bill was going to have to fit in time to read over the AOTA Mental Health Task Force Report again, because there was going to be a local hearing about it that evening. He had read it once and had felt excited about parts, depressed about other parts, and disturbed about some but not all of the recommendations.

"It could matter a lot, how this gets handled!" he thinks. □

In 1977, the Mental Health Specialty Section of the American Occupational Therapy Association expressed concern about the need for valid and reliable evaluation tools. A series of activities designed to survey the field and to encourage the development and standardization of methods and techniques for evaluation of clients in mental health was launched.

In 1978, Lorna Jean King, as the Eleanor Clarke Slagle lecturer, eloquently addressed the need for occupational therapy to have a comprehensive, unifying theory. She suggested that the adaptive process could be considered the unifying principle of occupational therapy. King identified the four unique features of adaptation in the individual human experience as: (1) active participation in adjustment to different conditions or environments; (2) adaptation as called forth by the demands of the environment; (3) adaptation as most efficiently organized subcortically; and (4) the adaptive response as self-reinforcing. She stated that, "I am implying that the essential purpose of occupational therapy is to stimulate and guide the adaptive processes through which an individual may best survive and develop."[58]

A landmark meeting of the American Occupational Therapy Association officers, the Representative Assembly, and academic and clinical leaders took place in Scottsdale, Arizona in the fall of 1978. At this meeting, major issues of education, clinical practice, and research in occupational therapy were discussed, and the status of occupational therapy as a true profession was analyzed. Papers were presented by ten leaders in the field, who thoughtfully and provocatively addressed the history, philosophy, current status, and future of occupational therapy. Resolutions were generated to affirm a philosophical base, to encourage support for research, and to reassess the levels of preparation required for entry into practice. These resolutions and the decisions which ensued had a significant effect on the field of occupational therapy as a whole. The impact was experienced in the field of psychiatry, especially in the momentum that developed around the standardization and dissemination of instruments and methods of evaluation, and in an increase in the publication of books and articles.[59,60]

A New Diagnostic and Statistical Manual

In 1980, the American Psychiatric Association published the *Diagnostic and Statistical Manual of Mental Disorders*, Third Edition, (DSM-III), a task that had been laboriously and conscientiously undertaken over a period of six years by its Task Force on Nomenclature and Statistics. The DSM-III, while compatible with the Ninth Edition of the *International Classification of Diseases* (ICD), is not identical to it. It was prepared to reflect the current state of knowledge in such a way as to be clinically useful and to provide a basis for research and administration. Mental disorder is conceptualized in terms of significant behavior or psychological syndromes or patterns that cause individuals to experience subjective distress or functional disability. An important feature of the DSM-III is its multiaxial system for evaluation. This system recommends consideration of the individual in terms of five different dimensions or *Axes*: (I) clinical syndromes; (II) personality or specific developmental disorders; (III) physical disorders; (IV) severity of psychosocial stressors; and (V) highest level of adaptive functioning during the past year. The developers of the DSM-III state that this revision represents only "one still frame in the ongoing process of attempting to better understand mental disorders."[61]

The major classifications representing the categories within Axis I are as follow: Disorders Usually First Evident in Infancy, Childhood or Adolescence; Organic Mental Disorders; Substance Use Disorders; Schizophrenic Disorders; Paranoid Disorders; Psychotic Disorders Not Elsewhere Classified; Affective Disorders; Anxiety Disorders; Somatoform Disorders; Dissociative Disorders; Psychosexual Disorders; Factitious Disorders; Disorders of Impulse Control Not Elsewhere Classified; and Adjustment Disorders. Unlike DSM-II, DSM-III does not have a separate category for Neurotic Disorders but includes them under Affective, Anxiety, Somatoform, Dissociative and Psychosexual classifications. Personality disorders are categorized for inclusion under Axis II. Psychiatric factors affecting physical condition are categorized for inclusion under Axis III, and codes are given for conditions that are not attributable to a mental disease but are a focus of attention or treatment.

The significance of the DSM-III to occupational therapists lies in its attempt to take a holistic approach to understanding mental disorders. Certainly, adding the considerations of Axes IV and V (Psychosocial Stressors and the Highest Level of Adaptive Functioning) underscores concerns which have special importance to the occupational therapist.

There has always been some controversy over the usefulness of diagnostic labels when one is working with people in a treatment context. The practice raises the issue of depersonalization or of predisposing the professional to perceive a classical picture or fantasy patient, rather than a unique human being with a personal gestalt which is different from that of any other person. On the other hand, a diagnosis represents a compilation of research and experience with large numbers of people over a long period of time, and as such, presents important guidelines for understanding the disease process, methods for treating it, and certain expectations regarding its prognosis. It is a professional responsibility for mental health professionals to recognize both aspects of this issue and to seek to achieve the balance in their use of diagnosis that will serve their clients best.

American Psychiatric Association—American Occupational Therapy Task Force

The Commission on Psychiatric Therapies of the American Psychiatric Association began a study of the existent therapies in practice and asked the American Occupational Therapy Association to join in the effort to prepare a report. A committee of occupational therapists, chaired by Gail Fidler, addressed the background, practice, and issues of psychiatric occupational therapy in its paper entitled "Overview of Occupational Therapy," which was submitted to the American Psychiatric Association in May of 1981.[62] This report emphasized the neurobiological and sociocultural framework for understanding human experience and behavior as underlying the practice of occupational therapy. It stressed the emphasis of occupational therapy on the value of purposeful activity in the development of a person's sense of competence and worth, and underscored the "integrative, adaptive qualities of doing, and the significance of doing in the acquisition of age-specific, culturally relevant performance skills."[63] It outlined the psychiatric contexts within which occupational therapy works and emphasized the need for continuing research into the relationship between purposeful activity and neurophysiological integration.

New Publications

The year 1980 also saw the beginning of a journal, *Occupational Therapy in Mental Health*, providing another medium through which practice and research issues might be shared.[64] The American Occupational Therapy Association also began work on the publication of a journal of research for the field as a whole.[65]

Cognitive Approach

During this period, the study of cognitive function and dysfunction as critical aspects of mental health and mental illness continued under the leadership of Claudia Allen in California. Defining cognitive function as the quality of thought that an individual uses in doing a task, Allen suggested that the occupational therapist is in a unique position. Using the knowledge of task analysis and of human cognitive levels, the occupational therapist can evaluate cognitive function and provide specific remediation where dysfunction exists. This is a far more specific and focused approach to occupational therapy in psychiatry than most, and one which presents new directions and new challenges for refining practice.[66]

There is, in the 1980s, increasingly productive interest and research in the biochemical and biogenetic bases of human emotional and cognitive functioning. Health-care professionals need to be able to understand and use the knowledge gained from this research. The occupational therapist's skills in observation of the task behaviors of patients are important factors in the effective use of medications and other biological treatments.

Societal Influences on Mental Health

The delivery of health care is related to factors that affect the nature of society as a whole. On the one hand, the development of electronic devices, video games, and home computers, as well as the flights of the Columbia space shuttle, have captured the popular imagination, suggesting unlimited potential for "progress." But this optimism is countered by vast economic and political problems—runaway inflation, assassinations, military intervention and military takeovers, unemployment, economic dislocations, terrorism by small hit-squads and established governments, cut backs in social services. People are bombarded by the news media. Immediate and vivid coverage of devasting events invites mass empathy; but the feeling that they can do nothing to control world-scale occurrences causes people to retreat into despair or numbness. The threat of nuclear destruction, by accident or conscious act of war, is changing the consciousness of human civilization—in one direction or the other. Some choose to deny, for political reasons. Others have no choice but to deny, because the threat is too great to comprehend; but they suffer a growing sense of powerlessness in their denial. Broad segments of the Western European population, as well as many members of the scientific and medical establishments in the United States, claim it is pathological to continue such denial, and have set out to oppose the destruction. All of these factors combine to compromise the mental health of individuals on a broad scale. "Burn-out" and stress management have become clichés, especially among people who work in human services. Self-help and group-help programs designed to aid people in developing and using coping strategies are proliferating.

The community mental health movement in many places has lacked adequate financial support or structural understanding. In most metropolitan areas there are thousands of formerly institutionalized individuals who are barely existing in the community—the fortunate ones in "good" boarding homes or independent living facilities. Too many of them are literally homeless and are known as "bag-ladies" or "vent-people," living on the streets, seeking warmth, shelter, and food wherever they can be found.

All of these factors, the positive and the negative, are powerful influences on thinking and behavior. To mental health professionals, and everyone else, the crisis exists as a danger or an opportunity.

TIME: 1982

PLACE: Community Mental Health Center in a Large City

Marvin Horn, OTR, and Carie Davis, mental health aide, are seated at a table, in a large room. The room is divided into areas, by the placement of furniture. There is a work area with a long table and folding chairs and cupboards along the wall, a socialization area, with a coffee urn, a couch, some soft chairs and a coffee table, and a library area with tables, chairs, and bookshelves half full of paperback books and well-used magazines. Large bright posters are taped to the walls and there are two bulletin boards on which schedules and notices have been posted. One section of the wall has large windows that look out on the busy street below. Potted plants line the window sill. There are several folding chairs placed facing out of the window.

Marvin and Carie have just said good-bye to their group, 20 former state hospital patients who leave on the center's bus each day at 3:30 p.m. to be delivered to their respective boarding homes. About six more travel independently by public transportation to their families' homes.

Carie calls Marvin's attention to the chairs at the window. They both sigh. No matter how often they have tried to find substitute activities to staring out the window, it seems that there are always a few clients who prefer to withdraw in this way. (But is it really withdrawal? Marvin wonders.) The last activity that afternoon had been a current events discussion group. This is a daily activity, in which clients are encouraged as "homework" to bring in news items to discuss with the group. Marvin and Carie talk about some of the clients.

Carie says, "Mary's too good for this group. She is so much smarter and with it in every way. How come they keep her here?"

Marvin replies, "It's a strange thing—she has tried other programs, but she always goes to pieces. I think she's scared and this group makes her feel superior. She's beginning to sound that way in group therapy—that's why we're doing some special individual treatment sessions . . . It's old Joe I'm worried about."

"Yeah—!" says Carie, "Now he's bragging about getting some money from his buddy who plays the casinos—and some slick guy wants to sell him a car! I don't think he even knows how to drive." Marvin grunts and frowns. He had done some evaluations with Joe and it was evident that it would take intensive work to help him to develop even basic living skills like money management and the ability to recognize when he needs to ask for assistance.

Carie gets up to straighten the room and prepare supplies for the next day's activities. Marvin picks up a pen and poises it over a blank paper. There are so many clients and such a limited staff! Staff burn-out has become a real problem and they were trying to find ways to reorganize themselves to deal with it. Marvin was hoping to convince his administrator to add a position for a COTA to replace the mental health aide who just left. He decided to put the request in writing. There was no point in going home because there was a supper meeting of the local community board to discuss plans for getting support for further program development. Marvin knows that the big issue is to decide whether to mount a fund-raising campaign or to cut back further on the existing program. A good movie would be in order after this meeting! □

References

1. Dunton, W. R.: Prescribing Occupational Therapy. Springfield IL: Charles C Thomas, Publishers, 1928, p. 9.
2. Bonsall, I. I: In Van Atta, K.: An Account of the Events Surrounding the Origin of the Friends Hospital. Philadelphia: Williams Brothers Printing Co., 1976, p. 24.
3. Meyer, A.: The philosophy of occupational therapy. Arch. Occup. Ther. 1:5, 1922, pp. 1–10.
4. Slagle, E. C.: Training aides for mental patients. Arch. Occup. Ther. 1:14, 1922.
5. Dunton: Prescribing Occupational Therapy.
6. Haas, L. J.: Practical Occupational Therapy. Milwaukee WI: Bruce Publishing Co., 1944.
7. Haas, L. J.: Occupational Therapy for the Mentally and Nervously Ill. Milwaukee WI: Bruce Publishing Co., 1925.
8. Marsh, L. C.: Shall we apply industrial psychiatry to psychiatry? Occup. Ther. Rehab. 12:1, 1932.
9. Wade, B.: Occupational therapy for patients with mental disease. In Willard, H. S., and Spackman, C. S. (eds.): Principles of Occupational Therapy, ed. 1. Philadelphia: J. B. Lippincott Co., 1947, pp. 99–109.
10. Menninger, W. C.: Psychiatric hospital therapy designed to meet unconscious needs. Amer. J. Psychiat. 93:347, 1936.
11. Wade, B., and Franciscus, M. L.: Occupational therapy for the mentally ill. In Willard, H. S., and Spackman, C. S. (eds.): Occupational Therapy, ed. 2. Philadelphia: J. B. Lippincott Co., 1954, pp. 103–108.
12. Fidler, G. S.: Psychological evaluation of occupational therapy activities. Am. J. Occup. Ther. 2:284, 1948.
13. Strecker, E. A., and Appel, K. E.: Discovering Ourselves, ed. 2. New York: Macmillan Co., 1948.

14. Jones, M.: The Therapeutic Community. New York: Basic Books, 1953.
15. Fidler, G. S., and Fidler, J. W.: Introduction to Psychiatric Occupational Therapy. New York: Harper and Row Publishers, 1954, p. 170.
16. West, W. (ed.): Changing Concepts and Practices in Psychiatric Occupational Therapy. New York: American Occupational Therapy Association, 1959.
17. Ibid, p. xi.
18. Niswander, G. D., Haslerud, G. M., and Dixey, E.: The effect of the professional activity of the occupational therapist on the behavior of acute mental patients. Am. J. Occup. Ther. 11:273, 1957.
19. Elkins, H. K., and Van Vlack, N. M.: Changes in occupational therapy due to the tranquilizing drugs. Am. J. Occup. Ther. 11:269–271, 1957.
20. Fidler and Fidler: Introduction to Psychiatric Occupational Therapy.
21. Action for Mental Health. Joint Commission on Mental Illness and Mental Health. New York: John Wiley & Sons, 1961.
22. Nagy, I., and Framo, J.: Intensive Family Therapy. New York: Harper and Row Publishers, 1965.
23. Wolpe, J.: Psychotherapy by Reciprocal Inhibition. Palo Alto: Stanford University Press, 1958.
24. Fidler, G. S., and Fidler, J. W.: Occupational Therapy: A Communication Process in Psychiatry. New York: Macmillan Co., 1963.
25. Azima, F. J.: The Azima Battery. In Mazer, I. (ed.): Materials from the 1968 Regional Institutes sponsored by the American Occupational Therapy Association on the Evaluation Process. Final Report R.S.A.-123-T-68. New York: American Occupational Therapy Association, 1968.
26. Fidler, G. S.: Diagnostic battery, scoring and summary. In Mazer, J. (ed.): Materials from the 1968 Regional Institutes sponsored by the American Occupational Therapy Association on the Evaluation Process. Final Report R.S.-123-T-68. New York: American Occupational Therapy Association, 1968.
27. Ayres, A. J.: The development of body scheme in children. Am. J. Occup. Ther. 15:3, 1961.
28. Mazer, J., and Mosey, A. C.: Introduction to Special Section: Theories of psychiatric occupational therapy. Am. J. Occup. Ther. 22:398–399, 1968.
29. Diasio, K.: Psychiatric occupational therapy: Search for a conceptual framework in the light of psychoanalytic ego psychology and learning theory. Am. J. Occup. Ther. 22:400–414, 1968.
30. Tempone, V., and Smith, A.: Psychiatric occupational therapy within a learning theory context. Am. J. Occup. Ther. 22:415–425, 1968.
31. Mosey, A. C.: Recapitulation of ontogenesis. Am. J. Occup. Ther. 22: 426–438, 1968.
32. Watanabe, S.: Four concepts basic to the occupational therapy process. Am. J. Occup. Ther. 22: 439–450, 1968.
33. Mazer, J.: Toward an integrated theory of occupational therapy. Am. J. Occup. Ther. 22: 451–456, 1968.
34. Mazer, J.: Ibid.
35. Ibid., p. 456.
36. Matsutsuyu, J.: Occupational behavior: A perspective on work and play. Am. J. Occup. Ther. 25:292, 1971.
37. White, R. W.: The urge towards competence. Am. J. Occup. Ther. 25:271–274, 1971.
38. Florey, L.: An approach to play and play development. Am. J. Occup. Ther. 25: 275–280, 1971.
39. Takata, N.: The play milieu. Am. J. Occup. Ther. 25:281–284, 1971.
40. Michelman, S.: The importance of creative play. Am. J. Occup. Ther. 25:285–290, 1971.
41. Maurer, P.: Antecedents of work behavior. Am. J. Occup. Ther. 25:294–297, 1971.
42. Bailey, D.: Vocational theories and work habits related to childhood development. Am. J. Occup. Ther. 25:298–302, 1971.
43. Johnson, J.: Considerations of work as therapy in the rehabilitation process. Am. J. Occup. Ther. 25:303–307, 1971.
44. Matsutsuyu, J.: Occupational behavior: A perspective on work and play. Am. J. Occup. Ther. 25:291–294, 1971.
45. Ibid, p. 291.
46. Reilly, M.: The educational process. Am. J. Occup. Ther. 23:302, 1969.
47. Arieti, S.: The Intrapsychic Self. New York: Basic Books, 1967.
48. Rogers, C.: Freedom to Learn. Columbus OH: Charles E. Merrill Co., 1969.
49. Toffler, A.: Future Shock. New York: Random House, 1970.
50. Goldstein, M. J., Baker, B. L., and Jamison, K. R.: Abnormal Psychology: Experiences, Origins and Interventions. Boston: Little Brown and Co., 1980, pp. 616–622.
51. Ibid.
52. Finn, G.: The occupational therapist in prevention programs. Am. J. Occup. Ther. 26:65, 1972.
53. Ibid.
54. President's Commission on Mental Health: Task Panel Reports. Vol. III Appendix. Washington, D.C.: U.S. Government Printing Office, 1978.
55. Moore, J.: Behavior, bias and the limbic system. Am. J. Occup. Ther. 30: 11–19, 1976.
56. Mosey, A. C.: Three Frames of Reference for Mental Health. Thorofare, NJ: Charles B. Slack, 1970.
57. A Report of the American Occupational Therapy Association Mental Health Task Force: Occup. Ther. Newspaper 30, 1976.
58. King, L. J.: Toward a science of adaptive responses. Am. J. Occup. Ther. 32:429–444, 1978.
59. American Occupational Therapy Association: Occupational Therapy 2001 A.D. Rockville, MD: American Occupational Therapy Association, Inc., 1979.
60. American Occupational Therapy Association Representative Assembly Proceedings. Am. J. Occup. Ther. 33:785, 1979.
61. American Psychiatric Association: Diagnostic and Statistical Manual of Mental Disorders, Edition III (DSM-III). Washington, D.C.: American Psychiatric Association, 1980.

62. Fidler, G. S. (chair), Shapiro, D., Falk-Kessler, J., Ellsworth, P., Gillette, N., and Parkin, J.: Overview of Occupational Therapy. Report submitted to American Psychiatric Association Commission on Psychiatric Therapies, 1981.
63. Ibid.
64. Occupational Therapy in Mental Health: A Journal of Psychosocial Practice and Research. New York: Haworth Press.
65. American Occupational Therapy Foundation. Journal of Research. Rockville, MD: American Occupational Therapy Foundation, 1981.
66. Allen, C.: Workshop on Assessment in Mental Health. Friends Hospital, Philadelphia, April, 1981.

SECTION 2
Models for Practice: Approaches to the Psychiatric Occupational Therapy Process

Conceptual models for psychiatry at the present time are drawn from the knowledge bases of the biological and social sciences. There has been a continuous expansion of knowledge in response to new research findings and to the changes in society as a whole. Through the years at least six schools of thought in psychiatry have evolved, and these have provided conceptual bases from which the prevailing frames of reference for psychiatric occupational therapy have been derived. These schools of thought may be identified as (1) biophysical, (2) intrapsychic, (3) behavioral, (4) sociocultural, (5) phenomenological, and (6) integrative.[1] Table 19-1 summarizes some of the major streams of thought in psychiatry.

In the *biophysical* school of thought, research and theoretical formulations focus on problems in the basic anatomical, physiological, and neurophysiological structures of the individual. These include biochemical and metabolic imbalance as well as abnormality or dysfunction as a result of trauma, disease, genetic, and congenital aberrations. In occupational therapy, the *sensory integrative* frame of reference relies heavily upon the conceptual bases and theoretical formulations of the biophysical school of thought.

In the *intrapsychic* school of thought, the concern is with unconscious processes, conflicts based on repressed material, and the health of conflict resolution in each of the successive stages of psychosexual development. The *psychoanalytic* frame of reference takes its conceptual basis and theoretical formulations from the intrapsychic school of thought.

The *behavioral* school of thought is based upon hypotheses and scientifically controlled laboratory research into the ways in which learning is acquired. It is concerned with the specific observable behaviors of individuals and does not acknowledge or attempt to work with unconscious material or thought processes. The *behavior therapy* frame of reference is clearly based on this school of thought.

The *sociocultural* school of thought places major emphasis on the effects of community, cultural, and social forces on the individual. These are seen frequently as defining what constitutes psychiatric illness as well as directly contributing to an individual's ability to function adaptively. The concepts and theories of this school of thought comprise the background for many of the occupational therapy approaches, but are especially influential in the *developmental* and *occupational behavior* frames of reference.

In the *phenomenological* school of thought, major interest is in the individual's perception of self and others, as well as in the effects of societal values on this type of perception. The phenomenological school of thought incorporates knowledge and perspectives from the intrapsychic and sociocultural schools; its concern is highly individualized. The school of thought has lent itself well to preventive and self-actualization approaches. Some of its theoretical premises and conceptual bases may be incorporated into *psychoanalytic, developmental,* and *occupational behavior* frames of reference in occupational therapy.

Another term for the *integrative* school of thought is *biopsychosocial.* This is a comprehensive approach which considers that psychological processes and human behavior are determined by dynamic and complex interrelationships of physical, emotional, social, and cultural processes. The *developmental* and *occupational behavior* frames of reference in occupational therapy rely upon the broad spectrum of knowledge that characterizes this school of thought.[2,3]

It is obvious that these approaches are not totally equal or parallel in their spheres of concern. There are

Table 19-1 *Major Streams of Thought in Psychiatry*

School of thought	Basic Ideas	Major Proponents	Treatment Modes
Biophysical	Biophysical defects; deficits in anatomy, physiology, biochemistry, genetics, and metabolism.	Emil Kraepelin Eugen Bleuler Franz Kallman William Sheldon Ernst Kretschmer Kurt Goldstein	Psychopharmacology, insulin and electric shock, psychosurgery Nutritional and special dietetic concerns Emphasis on present
Psychoanalytic intrapsychic	Unconscious processes and conflicts (repressed material) in early years of life. Defense mechanisms maybe maladaptive or inadequate. Concepts of id vs. superego Disruptions or trauma in sequence of development lead to pathology. There are many variations on this original theme.	Sigmund Freud Anna Freud Carl Jung Karen Horney Harry Stack Sullivan Otto Rank Alfred Adler Erich Fromm Franz Alexander Frieda Fromm-Reichmann Sandor Ferencz Paul Schilder Sandor Rado Theodor Reik Melanie Klein Wilhelm Reich	Psychoanalytic therapy Psychotherapy Use of free association, dreams, and projective techniques to uncover unconscious material Support for ego functions Reconstruction through catharsis, insight, use of transference phenomena Exploration of the past
Behavioral	All behavior is learned. Reinforcements shape behavior. Differences explained in terms of reinforcement patterns.	B. F. Skinner John Dollard Neal Miller H. J. Eysenck Joseph Wolpe	Behavior therapies: operant conditioning; reciprocal inhibition; desensitization Biofeedback techniques
Phenomenological	Individual's perception of the world is warped, distorted. Experience leads to self-concept. Loss of personal potentials, feelings and values (self-ness) in assuming others externally imposed. Social isolation in "mass" society.	Rollo May Carl Rogers Viktor Frankl R. D. Laing Albert Ellis Frederick Perls Eric Berne William Glasser Aaron Beck	Existential analysis Rational therapy Gestalt therapy Transactional analysis Reality therapy Some exploration of past but emphasis on present Humanistic psychiatry Cognitive therapy
Sociocultural	Community, culture, social forces of primary importance.	Thomas Scheff Erving Goffman Maxwell Jones	Milieu therapy Prevention programs Community psychiatry Emphasis on present
Integrative biopsychosocial	Biological and psychological unity. Psychological processes are multidetermined, multidimensional, include social, and cultural processes and development.	Adolf Meyer Roy Grinker Paul Meehl	Focus on coping strategies, competence A great variety of treatment modes and development of understanding about all factors Emphasis on present

Adapted from Millon, T.: Theories of Psychopathology and Personality. Philadelphia: W. B. Saunders Co., 1973 and Freedman, A. M., Kaplan, H. I., and Sadock, B. J.: Modern Synopsis of Comprehensive Textbook of Psychiatry/II. Baltimore: Williams and Wilkins Co., 1976.

overlapping areas, and it is possible to refine or limit further the perspective from which the client and treatment planning are understood, as in Allen's cognitive approach.[4] Briggs, Duncombe, Howe, and Schwartzberg suggest a *humanistic model* for occupational therapy.[5] The occupational behavior approach is far broader in its view of human functioning than are the behavioral or sensory integrative approaches. Both the sensory integrative and psychoanalytic approaches contain critical developmental aspects. The consideration of adaptation from a developmental perspective is an important component of the occupational behavior and humanistic approaches.

Sensory Integrative Perspectives

The mentally ill frequently are found to have perceptual difficulties, some of which may be due to the primary disease process and some of which may be due to more transitory factors such as stress or medication. The perceptual process is the core of an individual's ability to organize, integrate, and interpret internal and external or environmental stimuli. Perceptual ability is developed; the earliest experiences of infancy and childhood are critical to the process. Beginning with early tactile and kinesthetic percepts, children develop concepts of their bodies. If this process is interrupted, or if the neurological system is in some way dysfunctional, the resultant perceptual distortions may prevent normal interactions between the individual and the environment and make reality testing and the establishment of healthy, functional cognitive and motor abilities difficult. The resultant distortions in object relationships, both human and nonhuman, may lead to further emotional distress, which may ultimately result in serious forms of maladaptation or mental illness.

The functions of the brain in integrating and screening the sensory stimuli with which human beings are continuously bombarded are of monumental importance in determining human behavior. King, building on the research of Ayres into sensory integration in learning disorders, has developed an exceedingly well documented body of knowledge about sensory integrative dysfunction in patients diagnosed as having schizophrenia. Observation of large numbers of institutionalized chronic schizophrenics yielded a common picture: S-shaped posture; shuffling gait; inability to raise arms over head; immobility of the head and shoulder girdle; tendency to hold arms and legs in a flexed, adducted, and internally rotated position; lack of normal hand function; weakness of grip; and lack of motivation. Her hypothesis, based on observation and a search of the literature, is as follows: "Some individuals have defective proprioceptive feedback mechanisms, the ves-

tibular component in particular being first underreactive, and second, underactive in its role in the sensorimotor integration process. This defect, whether genetic, developmental, or the result of trauma, constitutes an important etiological or prodromal factor in process and reactive schizophrenia."[6]

King also indicates that the paranoid schizophrenic syndrome is distinctly different from that of process and reactive schizophrenia. One of the most universal problems of the process and reactive schizophrenic seems to be in the area of perceptual constancy. It is not difficult to understand how this problem would seriously hamper the development of healthy concepts of self, other people, and objects and would interfere with the process of reality testing.

Some of the basic principles underlying the sensory integrative approach to treatment are the following:

1. Early life (probably including prenatal) experiences of vestibular, proprioceptive, and tactile stimulation are important in personality development.
2. Neurological immaturity has a related emotional overlay, which may take the form of full-blown illness.
3. The tactile sense is critical for an individual to learn about the environment and about himself or herself as a differentiated entity.
4. Perceptual constancy is necessary to provide a predictable basis on which to build learning. Lack of visual or auditory perceptual constancy seriously distorts an individual's ability to adapt to both the human and nonhuman environment.
5. When a client's perceptual deficits are identified and understood, a multidimensional remedial approach may be used to help him or her. Movement and sensory activities, carefully selected, have the potential of facilitating or acting as true remediation.

King has experimented and worked with neurophysiological approaches to remediation of sensorimotor integrative dysfunction and has experienced empirical success with these methods. In general, the activities of sensory integration are gross motor ones, selected with two important requirements: (1) that the conscious attention of the patient *must not be centered on the motor process, but on the outcome or object,* and (2) that the *activity must be pleasurable.* The subcorticalization of the experience is most important. It has been Lorna King's observation that when patients make gains in sensory integration, the gains tend to be permanent, and the

	Alerting, Stimulating		Inhibiting, Calming
Vestibular	Fast, sudden, jerky, intense		Slow, rhythmic, even
Tactile	Light touch	Pressure touch	Pressure touch, rhythmic
Temperature	Cool		Warm—neutral
Position	Head up, chest out		Head down

Figure 19-1. Effects of activities in terms of neurophysiological mechanisms. Adapted from King, L. J.: Psychiatric Occupational Therapy Workshop, Temple University, Philadelphia, 1977.

success of the process usually motivates patients to continue.[7]

The specific kinds of activities are ones which involve vestibular stimulation, heavy work, proprioceptive feedback, sensory input, and awareness of space and form. Both recreational and task-oriented activities may incorporate these elements. Attention may also be directed to the potential of activities in terms of their alerting or stimulating effects and inhibiting or slowing effects. Figure 19-1 gives these general characteristics.

King's work is making a significant impact on the treatment of a heretofore difficult population. She has broken ground for continuing important research.[7]

Behavior Therapy Perspectives

From the behavior therapy perspective, there are four systems that determine the way learning takes place: positive reinforcement, negative reinforcement, punishment, and extinction. *Positive reinforcement* is a pleasing or need-fulfilling event; *negative reinforcement* is the withdrawal of an unpleasant or aversive stimulus when a change of behavior has taken place; *punishment* refers to the presentation of an unpleasant stimulus; *extinction* is the withdrawal of a pleasing stimulus or the bombardment with the original reinforcer with a resultant decrease in the behavior.

For example, a parent's smiles and praise when the child brings home a good report card are a form of positive reinforcement. The child learns that good grades please his or her parents; if that is important, the child has learned to work for good grades. When a child works very hard to get good grades in order to avoid being nagged and scolded, the child has learned to do so through negative reinforcement. Punishment is the presentation of an unpleasant or

aversive stimulus or the withdrawal of a pleasant stimulus following the occurrence of some undesirable behavior. The child might be punished for receiving poor grades by being spanked or scolded or by not being allowed to go out to play. If parents stop praising the child for receiving good grades, the child may stop trying to please them in that way, or, if the parents give too much praise too continuously, the effect will be one of *satiation* and the child will stop trying. These are two examples of extinction.

The behavior therapy perspective is based on scientific laboratory research, originally done with laboratory animals. In terms of treatment procedures, it may permit highly controlled procedures for helping people change their behaviors. Patterns of behavior, even very complex ones, may be altered or reversed, and new ones may be established, if one is able to identify and use effective schedules of reinforcement. The behavioral approaches are concerned with the existing behavior-environment relationships of the individual. The behaviorally oriented therapist, then, would look at the things which an individual *said* or *did* reflecting problems in the areas of self-concept, reality testing, object relationships, coping with feelings, and organizing thinking. The large problems would be seen in terms of the component specific behaviors. Words like "self-concept," "reality testing," and "object relationships" would not be used. One would state instead, for example, something like "the client will initiate a conversation with another client." Certainly, this is a piece of several larger areas of concern, but it is a small, observable, and measurable behavior. Behaviors are identified clearly and specifically and are treated directly. Concern is for the individual's unique and individual patterns of response to feedback.

Sieg[8] has defined behavior therapy in the following way: "the emphasis is on designing conditions which will change the behavior and thus alleviate the problem, rather than delving into psychic or mental reasons for the problem." She describes the process of designing a program to include the following considerations:[9] (1) Identifying the terminal behavior, which means clearly and specifically what behavior needs to be increased, decreased, or shaped. This behavior should be observable and measurable. (2) Counting the behavior, which must be done initially, before treatment, to establish the baseline of data upon which treatment will build. Counting or measuring then is done continuously as treatment proceeds. The measured data are recorded, charted, and provided to the client as feedback. (3) Selecting a reinforcer, which involves identifying what supports the behavior, and individualizing the reinforcement so that it will be successful and fair for a given client. (4) Selecting a schedule for reinforcement on the basis of learning theory; the therapist must determine the schedule of reinforcement for the particular client and behavior. (5) If new behavior is to be established, techniques of behavior modification are used. The first is *shaping* in which reinforcement is given for each successive approximation to the desired behavior. The second is *chaining,* in which reinforcement is given for behaviors related to a specific behavior which has been established. (The occurrence of the established behavior is treated as the stimulus for another response which is related. Very complex behavior patterns may be developed through the step by step shaping and chaining of series of responses.) Finally, the therapist (or another person) may *model* the desired behavior and receive reinforcement in the presence of the client. The client may then be reinforced for successful imitation of the behavior.[10]

Behavioral techniques are often unconsciously or automatically applied in life and in many therapeutic circumstances. Behavioral therapy makes the process specifiable and controllable and may be useful to help some clients meet certain desired therapeutic goals.

A useful tool in treatment using behavioral learning theory is biofeedback. Through the use of biofeedback equipment and techniques, individuals can learn to identify the early physical signs of stress, before these are experienced on a conscious or cognitive level. Strategies, such as relaxation, for controlling or coping with anxiety early can similarly be learned. Coupling the two processes of stress identification and coping strategies has been found to be an extremely effective method for averting less healthy attempts at coping, such as excessive drinking, drug use, or outbursts of rage. Once control has been accomplished and the fear of loss of control and its consequences is diminished, the individual is likely to be in a state in which it will be possible to work on the resolution of more basic conflicts and the development of healthy patterns of adaptation. Biofeedback techniques are being used successfully in the treatment of hand injuries and other physical problems. Their effectiveness in psychiatric practice has only begun to be explored.

Psychoanalytic Perspectives

Psychoanalytic theory has been extensively studied, and many new perspectives based on psychoanalytic theory have developed over the years. The literature is rich in materials that amplify and modify the basic Freudian formulations.

From the psychoanalytic perspective, the client is understood in terms of the powerful interplay between the id or primary drives, the superego or the demands of society, and the ego functions that have developed to mediate their conflict. It is a major function of the ego to maintain contact with reality, and it is the ego that develops ways to help the individual defend against the demands of the id and the superego. Ego functions are clearly and directly related to self-concept, reality testing, object relationships, coping with feelings, and the capacity to organize one's thinking and actions.

The client may also be understood in terms of stages of psychosexual development. Character traits and modes of achieving pleasure or need-satisfaction may be traced to the oral, anal, genital, latency, and phallic stages of development.

In approaching the evaluation and treatment of a client within a psychoanalytic frame of reference, one is concerned with behavior as the overt manifestation of unconscious processes mediated by the ego. All communication and other forms of behavior have both real and symbolic meanings. In therapy, there is a primary concern for the health of the functions of the ego in reality testing, providing effective defense mechanisms and satisfactory interpersonal relationships, and synthesizing all of human experience into logical and adaptive modes of thinking, feeling, and acting. The relationship that develops between the client and therapist is a dynamic one through which the client may be helped to explore, relive, develop insight, and change. The nonhuman objects—the materials, tools, and actions—used in occupational therapy are facilitators to these processes. The ego strength of the therapist is an important factor in the relationship that develops.

It is possible to add the dimension of a psychoanalytic perspective to the basic understanding one has of the client and to focus on providing opportunities for developing and supporting the functions of the ego which will be adaptive. To provide treatment which is purely psychoanalytically based, however, requires that the therapist have thorough self-knowledge as well as a strong theoretical base in psychoanalytic principles.

Developmental Perspectives

Considered developmentally, the client may be seen to be functioning at any given time at levels which are comparable to those which are experienced in the process of growth and development. The basic principles which relate to the developmental perspective in psychiatry include the following:
1. The individual grows, matures, and learns in a sequential way. Each gain in structure or function provides the base upon which each new gain is built.
2. The physical, sensory, perceptual, emotional, cognitive, and social aspects of human growth and development are intricately interwoven, and

issues, stresses, or gains that take place in any one area will bring about changes in the others.

3. There are special issues and opportunities that present themselves at each period of human development. Through the process of adaptation, the individual explores these issues and opportunities, solves problems, learns, and grows.

4. Under stress of any kind it is a human characteristic to regress to earlier levels of function. Regression may be very brief (seconds or minutes) or may be long-term, depending upon the nature of the stress and the basic health or strength of the individual. Individuals may choose regressive activities deliberately as a method of preserving balance in their lives.

5. In providing experiences to facilitate growth and adaptation, one should consider the developmental issues which present themselves at the client's functional level and the conditions which will make successful achievement possible.

Llorens has been a primary spokesperson for the developmental perspective in occupational therapy. She speaks of occupational therapy as a process of facilitating growth, as well as mastery of self and the environment through a recognition of the needs, abilities, and issues of the growing child.[11] These principles have been translated into a highly successful approach to treatment with adult psychiatric clients.

Mosey, in her "Recapitulation of Ontogenesis," refers to seven adaptive skills on a development continuum and offers suggestions for approaches to treatment to help the client to develop or to regain them.[12]

Between 1971 and 1973, taking Piagetian formulations of cognitive development, Allen and Lewis developed an approach to understanding the client whose ability to organize thoughts and actions has regressed to early levels as a result of the stress of the illness.[13] The levels with which occupational therapy may be concerned are characterized in terms of the infant's process of exploring and learning about the world: (1) focus on one's own bodily movements, (2) interest in the effects of one's actions on the environment, (3) use of familiar schemes to achieve an end result, (4) use of trial and error to solve problems, and (5) use of thoughts and images to solve problems. By a thorough knowledge of the Piagetian concepts about the ways the child understands cause and effect, object permanence, and time, and about the conditions that help the child to learn, it is possible to think in terms of structuring occupational therapy experiences through which the client can experience himself or herself as whole and able. Careful identification and use of existing familiar and well inte-

grated "schemes" in an occupational therapy program is an important part of this approach.

An example of the developmental approach to treatment is described by Levy in her careful analysis of a movement approach to the treatment of severely disorganized psychotic patients. Table 19-2 describes the levels of cognition and the behaviors that may be expected at each level. The therapist involves clients in body movement and exercise patterns planned to help in the building of basic cognitive skills. Levy writes: "A significant manifestation of a schizophrenic break is the regression of thought processes to early developmental levels of functioning. Remission from that break hinges on rebuilding the steps toward integrated cognition in developmental order. Movement is the plane on which primal learning must take place, and it is this cognitive level that must be integrated before higher-level thought processes can evolve."[14]

In the use of the developmental approach, it is important to note that many normal, healthy, mature adult activities do, in fact, require no more skill than some of the activities of infancy and childhood. For example, hiking, jogging, swimming and many other

Table 19-2 *Piaget's Stages and Predictable Behaviors in the Adult Psychotic*

	Cognition	Behaviors
Stage 1	Functional assimilation	Will perform available schemata
	Generalizing assimilation	Will generalize available schemata to new situations
Stage 2	Able to repeat behavior of models if similar to own behaviors (approximately, at first)	Will imitate if his own body movements are modeled for him
	Beginning to be interested in moderately novel events, actively seeks new stimulation	Will respond to introduction of moderately novel movements
Stage 3	Beginning to perceive effect on environment	Gross-motor activities critical
	Is learning to imitate new behaviors	Is learning direct imitation through progressively more accurate imitation
Stage 4	Is able to imitate directly simple new behaviors	Is able to deal with object-oriented activity

From Levy, L.: Movement therapy for psychiatric patients. Reprinted with permission of the American Occupational Therapy Association, Inc. Copyright 1969, Am J Occup Ther 28, No. 6: 354.

basic physical activities are at a movement level. Most simple craft activities and some activities of daily living may be broken down and presented in such a way as to meet early levels of integration.

Occupational Behavior Perspectives

Roles and routines characterize the lives of most human beings. We became psychologically and physically attuned to taking care of our basic needs and to fulfilling the expectations and responsibilities that are part of our lives. In the course of a day and in the course of a lifetime, routines and roles change. Some are normal role changes. The *cashier* in the supermarket may be the *mother* of a school-aged child, the *wife* of an accountant, and the *best bowler* on the church bowling team. Vacation times and weekends permit changes by choice in routines and in roles. But illness and personal crises often cause major disruptions in routines and readjustment of roles.

In the process of development there are factors that enable human beings to establish both the stability and the flexibility needed to support themselves in assuming their roles within society, in carrying out life routines with minimal expenditures of energy, and in coping successfully with changes. Piaget and others have referred to the fact that infants are innately curious and that it is a basic human characteristic to seek stimulation and to value novelty. As children grow and develop they integrate both *knowledge* about the world and the *habits and skills* necessary for living in it. They learn the extent of their abilities to control or to be controlled by other people and events. They learn the "rules" of making things happen. The integrate a sense of time, as it is defined by the culture and society in which they live.

Reilly[15] has described three phases of play through which people learn. The first is a period of *exploration*. When confronted with something new, one is curious and may try to learn about it. New experiences of oneself, new objects, new people, and new procedures bring about a state of arousal. If the novelty is too great, the individual may be afraid and seek to avoid it. If it is too little, there may be no interest evoked. But if the conditions are safe the individual learns rules and develops feelings of hope and trust in the initial exploration of objects and relationships. The second phase is one in which the individual strives to develop *competence*. Through practice and repeated opportunities to experience the effects of one's skills, one develops confidence. The third phase is one in which the individual builds on the trust and self-confidence and works toward *achievement* in terms of externally defined standards

as well as those standards which have developed within.

The occupational behavior frame of reference is concerned with clients from the perspective of the roles and the balance of their lives. Play is seen as significant both in childhood and in adulthood to develop and support the knowledge and skills required for carrying out the life roles of society. A strong knowledge base in sociology and psychology as well as in psychiatry is required in order to understand both illness and health in our society. Building upon this base, then, the major concern of the occupational therapist working within this frame of reference is to prevent and reduce the incapacities which result from illness.

Reilly specified six parts of an occupational therapy program based on the occupational behavior frame of reference:[16]

1. The program should incorporate examination of the client's life roles and identification of the skills to support them.
2. The program should reflect developmental stages which help the individual to acquire life skills.
3. The program should provide "natural and legitimate" decision-making opportunities to the client.
4. The milieu must acknowledge competencies, arouse curiosity, deepen appreciation, and demand appropriate behavior across the full spectrum of human abilities.
5. Occupational therapists must recognize and plan for the balance of work, play, and rest in the patient's total life space.
6. The structure of the program should be tailored to the patient and his or her own opportunities to practice life skills.

Humanistic Approaches

The humanistic model for treatment in occupational therapy, as described by Briggs, Duncombe, Howe, and Schwartzberg,[17] is grounded in existential philosophy. Occupational therapy is attuned to the principle of facilitating the client's own personal search for purpose, meaning, and self-actualization. Within this model, it becomes important for the therapist to "focus on the client's perception of the discrepancies between what he would like to be able to do or be and what he presently feels he can accomplish."[18] It is important for the therapist to achieve a clear understanding of the client's own experience of the environment. This understanding will lead to the selection of activities based on considerations of the potential meanings to the client and the opportunities they present (1) for mastery, (2) for continued self-exploration, (3) for choice, (4) for responsibility, (5) for feedback potential, and (6) for congruence with the client's interests, values and cultural background. The humanistic model is one which is frequently employed in outpatient or primary prevention contexts. Clients need to show "potential for growth and a need for self-enhancement."[19] Verbal ability and fairly high cognitive functioning are important to the success of humanistic treatment techniques. It is clear, however, that the attitude and philosophy underlying this model are compatible with occupational therapy as a whole.

References

1. Millon, T.: Theories of Psychopathology and Personality. Philadelphia: W.B. Saunders Co., 1973.
2. Ibid.
3. Freedman, A. M., Kaplan, H. I., and Sadock, B.J.: Modern Synopsis of Comprehensive Textbook of Psychiatry/II. Baltimore: Williams and Wilkins Co., 1976.
4. Allen, C.: Workshop on Assessment in Mental Health. Friends Hospital, Philadelphia, 1981.
5. Briggs, A. K., Duncombe, L. W., Howe, M., and Schwartzberg, S. L.: Case Simulations in Psychosocial Occupational Therapy. Philadelphia: F. A. Davis, 1979.
6. King, L. J.: A sensory integrative approach to schizophrenia. Am. J. Occup. Ther. 28:529–536, 1974.
7. King, L. J.: Psychiatric Occupational Therapy Workshop, Temple University, Philadelphia, 1977.
8. Sieg, K.: Applying the behavioral model to the O.T. model. Am. J. Occup. Ther. 28:422, 1974.
9. Ibid., pp. 421–428.
10. Norman, C. W.: Behavior modification: A perspective. Am. J. Occup. Ther. 30:491–497, 1976.
11. Llorens, L.: Facilitating growth and development: The promise of occupational therapy. Am. J. Occup. Ther. 24:93–101, 1970.
12. Mosey, A. C.: Recapitulation of ontogenesis. Am. J. Occup. Ther. 22:426–438, 1968.
13. Allen, C., and Lewis, N.: Workshop series notes. Philadelphia and Baltimore, 1972.
14. Levy, L.: Movement therapy for psychiatric patients. Am. J. Occup. Ther. 28:354–357, 1974.
15. Reilly, M. (ed.): Play as Exploratory Learning. Beverly Hills, CA.: Sage Publishing Co., 1974.
16. Reilly, M.: A psychiatric O.T. program as a teaching model. Am. J. Occup. Ther. 20:66–7, 1966.
17. Briggs, A. K., Duncombe, L. W., Howe, M., and Schwartzberg, S. L.: Case Simulations in Psychosocial Occupational Therapy. Philadelphia, F.A. Davis, 1979.
18. Ibid., p. 101.
19. Ibid., p. 102.

SECTION 3
The Four Elements in the Psychiatric Occupational Therapy Process

It is evident, in exploring the history of psychiatric occupational therapy, that, in spite of developments and changes in society as a whole and in the theoretical and conceptual bases of psychiatry, the psychiatric occupational therapy process has been consistent in at least one characteristic. It has consciously and deliberately developed methods for using the interactions among four basic elements to promote and maintain function. The four basic elements considered in occupational therapy are (1) the *client*, or individual who needs help, (2) the *therapist*, or individual who is the helper, (3) the *activity*, and (4) the *context* in which the helping takes place.

The frames of reference that are used in the helping process determine the perspective from which the client's problems are understood, the kind of relationship which is fostered between the therapist and client, the nature of activities used in treatment, and the total context for treatment. Each frame of reference provides its dimensions of understanding about the occupational therapy process; each suggests a way of going about the processes of evaluation, setting objectives, planning and implementing the occupational therapy program.

These factors are the essence of psychiatric occupational therapy. In this part of the chapter, perspectives on these four elements as a foundation for a subsequent consideration of the psychiatric occupational therapy process are explored.

The Client

When an individual seeks psychiatric treatment, the need to do so arises out of problems that are acutely felt. Sometimes it is the client who feels the need and takes the initiative in seeking help, but often, because of the nature of the illness, other people, often family members, friends, work associates, or neighbors, may need to take some responsibility for seeing that the client receives care and treatment. Sometimes, when an individual becomes very ill or severely disturbed, especially if this occurs in a public place, it is the police who are charged with the responsibility for getting the client to a hospital.

What are the problems which make it necessary for an individual to require psychiatric help? They include confusion, disorientation, distortions of perceptions or thoughts, feeling of being bombarded by stimuli, anxiety, depression, despair, impulsive outbursts, inability to organize, inability to handle feelings, inability to communicate or to relate to others, lack of capacity for pleasure, deficits in judgment in the management of personal or work life, lack of balance in routines of waking and sleeping, tactile defensiveness, poor sense of time, and, frequently, lack of ability to recognize or assess the self or problems. All of these are experienced in some degree by most people at times of stress. It would seem that there are several factors that determine whether experiences may be considered symptomatic of mental illness. These factors are (1) the severity of the problem, whether it is experienced so acutely that it threatens to cause harm to the individual or to the people around him or her, (2) the length of time the problem is experienced, and (3) the ability of the individual to recognize and undertake measures to change the condition or simply to "bounce back" spontaneously. It is useful to think of mental conditions as degrees of psychiatric function and dysfunction on a continuum that goes from health to illness. In doing so, it is possible to take into account a number of important considerations, such as environmental stress and cultural perspectives, as well as the stress of disease, trauma, or deficit. It also encourages the consideration of preventive as well as treatment, maintenance, and rehabilitation measures.

Underlying the presenting problems of the client, there are at least five major areas that are important, including the client's concept of self, ability to test reality, object relationships, ability to cope with feelings, and organization of thoughts and actions.

Concept of self refers to the knowledge and feelings a person has about himself or herself. It includes awareness of one's body and bodily functions, a sense of one's ability to control one's actions, and a sense of competence in doing the tasks of everyday living. Self-esteem and the way a person feels that others see him or her are part of self-concept.

Reality testing refers to the process by which individuals can know that what they perceive, think, and feel is real. It is closely related to self-concept in that one must be able to recognize reality to know one's own strengths, assets, weaknesses, and limits. As in self-concept, reality testing takes place both at a con-crete body-experience level and at an abstract social-emotional level. The ability of an individual to process information received from the world is the key to reality testing.

Object relationships refer to the kinds of interactions that take place between an individual and the external world. Objects are both human and nonhuman. Objects meet human needs; through objects we learn about the world; objects are the recipients of our expressions of feelings. The term, object relationships, which springs from psychoanalytic thought, refers to the kinds of perceptions one has of others and the effectiveness with which one gets along with others. It is closely meshed with self-concept and with reality testing.

Coping with feelings refers to the ways in which individuals handle their moods and emotions. All human beings experience some measure of fear, anger, joy, sadness, depression, and elation in the normal course of living. Sometimes strong feelings occur in response to specific events. Sometimes feelings are part of a general mood. They may be felt intensely or mildly. They may debilitate the person who is experiencing them or may be the cause of actions that are destructive to self or others. They may on the other hand energize and enhance one's concept of self and relationships with others. Feelings are powerful motivators to action and bear a direct but complex relationship to thought processes.

Organizing one's thoughts and actions refers to all those cognitive functions which are necessary for an individual to plan a course of action and follow it, to recognize cause-and-effect relationships, to be able to problem solve and to have clear, functional concepts of time and space.

Medication and the Client

The introduction of psychopharmacology produced a revolution in the treatment of psychiatric problems. With the increased knowledge of the biochemical aspects of mental and emotional functioning, it has become possible, with medication, to reduce psychotic symptoms (hallucinations, delusions, bizarre ideation, and so forth), control debilitating depressive or manic states, relieve anxiety, and promote relaxation. Many clients have become more socially acceptable and more accessible to therapeutic intervention because of the effects of medication. While their use has certainly made it possible for clients to function better, it has also produced some new sets of problems. The therapist who works with clients who are receiving medication needs to be aware of the possiblity of side-effects.[1] In addition to the fact that side-effects may be extremely troublesome and upsetting to the client, it is essential that they be monitored closely, so

Table 19-3 *Major Medications Used in Psychiatry and Their Effects*

Major Medication Group (Some common trade names)	Therapeutic Effects	Possible Adverse Reactions
NEUROLEPTIC DRUGS (Examples: Thorazine, Mellaril, Compazine, Prolixin, Stelazine, Haldol, Taractan, Serpasil)	Modify affective states, decrease psychotic ideation, normalize psycho-motor behavior, promote greater responsivity	Parkinson-like syndrome, tardive dyskinesia, restlessness, dystonia, akinesia, dryness in mouth and throat, constipation, appetite and weight gain, nausea, urinary retention, skin erup-tions, edema, contact dermatitis, sexual function changes, amenorrhea, jaundice, photosensitivity
PSYCHOANALEPTIC DRUGS Antidepressants, affective mod-ulators, mood elevators (Examples: Aventyl, Elavil, Norpramin, Vivactil, Sinequan, MAO inhibitors such as Nardil, Parnate)	Lessen depression in severely depressed psychotic patients Promotes brightening of activities in psychomotor, cognitive, affective function	Dry mouth, blurred near vision, consti-pation, urinary retention, tachycardia, heart block, severe headache, dizzi-ness, rapid pulse, orthostatic/postural hypotension, skin rash, photosensi-tivity
ANXIOLYTIC DRUGS Minor tranquilizers, mild tranquilizers, antianxiety drugs, sedatives (Examples: Equanil, Miltown, Librium, Valium, Atarax, Trancopal)	Reduce anxiety, cause muscle relaxation, anticonvulsive	Habituation with withdrawal symptoms, drowsiness, sedation, ataxia, suicide potential (through overdose or in combination with alcohol), dizziness, lessened sex drive
PSYCHOSTIMULANTS Cerebral stimulants (Examples: Benzedrine, Dexedrine, Metrazol, Ritalin, Desoxyn)	Transient increase in psychomotor activity with adults (In treatment of hyperkinetic syndrome in children: sedation)	Restlessness, irritability, tension, insomnia, weight loss, confusion, angina, high blood pressure, head-ache, diarrhea, cramps
ANTIMANIC AGENTS (Example: Lithium carbonate)	Effective treatment of bipolar disorder (manic–depressive psychosis). Reduc-tion in severity of mood swing	Nausea, abdominal cramps, vomiting, diarrhea, thirst, edema
SOMNIFACIENTS Sedatives (Examples: Barbiturates—Amytol, Butisol, Luminal, Nembutal, Seconal; Non-barbiturates—Dalmane, Doriden, Quaalude, Valmid)	Sleeping medication, anti-convulsant	Addiction with serious withdrawal risk (convulsions, death), slow speech, slow respiration, slow thinking, slow physical movement, high suicide potential (in combination with alcohol or other medications)
ANTICHOLINERGIC DRUGS Used in combination with phenothiazines (neuroleptics) to prevent parkinsonian syndrome. (Examples: Artane, Pipanol, Cogentin, Kemadin)	Reverses parkinsonian syndrome	Dry mouth, blurred vision, constipation

The following general forms of drug toxicity are serious and should be watched for in all clients who are taking medication:[1]

Sensitivity Reactions: Dermatologic eruptions, angioneurotic edema, inflammation of the oral cavity and larynx, exfoli-ative dermatitis, asthmatic symptoms

Blood Dyscrasias: Sore throat, fever, glandular swelling, bleeding from mucous membranes, cutaneous lesions, petechiae, purpura

Information summarized from materials by Peter Doukas, Ph.D., School of Pharmacy, Temple University, Philadelphia, PA, and Doris A. Smith, M.Ed., OTR, Department of Occupational Therapy, Western Michigan University, Kalamazoo, MI.

that changes in medication will be made when necessary. Signs of general drug toxicity are very serious and it is imperative for these to receive *immediate* attention, as they may indicate life-threatening reactions to drugs. Table 19-3 lists some common medications and their effects. Because psychopharmacology is in a continual state of developing new drugs and refining their uses, each mental health professional should check on the medications his or her clients are receiving, become aware of possible side-effects, and keeping this knowledge up-to-date.

The Therapist

The therapist is only one of many new people to whom the client is exposed when he or she becomes involved in treatment situations. Because psychiatric problems most frequently manifest themselves in chaotic, confused, or destructive interpersonal relationships, the interactions between the therapist and the client may be critical to the desired processes of growth and change.

Although the therapist's role is usually defined by the context, it may not always be entirely clear to the client. It is therefore vital that the therapist be quite clear about his or her role. In the occupational therapy process, the therapist's "use of self" means bringing together knowledge, skills, caring, and basic personality strengths to help the client overcome difficulties and maximize abilities. A therapist is a helper. The kind of helper may vary. The therapist may help by teaching, giving support, aiding in communication, engineering opportunities for growth, confronting problems, clarifying, reinforcing progress, or promoting plans for the future. In the therapeutic context the therapist may be friendly but never the client's "friend," "buddy," or close confidante. This means that the therapist especially must monitor the influence of personal needs and feelings. If, for example, a therapist has a strong need to prove that occupational therapy will cure a client, the therapist risks feeling angry if the client rejects help offered or may feel disappointed if the client fails to respond. Either reaction would be a distortion and ultimately not helpful to the client. Because the maintenance of objectivity within the relationship is important, it is helpful and often necessary for the therapist to have another professional with whom to discuss feelings and events as they arise.

People with psychiatric problems may have great difficulty in developing healthy and health-promoting relationships with other people. Often the relationships that they have experienced either just before becoming ill or throughout longer periods of their lives have been negative. The precedents for human relationships may be fraught with distortions. There may be unrealistic positive or negative expectations of authority figures. Other human beings may be perceived as lacking constancy or predictability or as being threatening or hurtful. On the other hand, the emotional needs of the client may be so powerful as to cloak the reality of the situation in a cloud of wish-fulfillment. Frank has referred to the problems of avoidance, selective inattention, and self-fulfilling prophecy on the part of the client.[2] Fear of being hurt or of an unknown new mode of behavior may function to prevent the client's correction of a pathological self-image. It is the task of the therapist to break through these problems and to develop with the client a new, different set of transactions, ones that will "confirm healthy expectations and disappoint pathological ones."

Initially it is necessary to gain some measure of the client's trust. Trust is a feeling that is based on the perception of the therapist's ability and caring. Trust potentiates motivation. A client who trusts the therapist will be more easily motivated to participate in the occupational therapy process than one who does not feel trust. The issues of trust and motivation are important throughout the entire time the therapist and client are involved with one another.

How are trust and motivation developed? In the therapeutic context there may be many factors. Apart from the direct interpersonal experiences of the therapist and client, there may be the distant uninvolved appraisal the client may make of the therapist based on observations of the transactions between the therapist and other clients or other staff members. There may be the "halo" effect of the encouragement to be involved in occupational therapy from the client's physician, other staff members, or other clients. The client may have made a simple, uncritical judgment based on wish-fulfillment that, if the therapist is on the staff, the therapist must know how to help.

It is, however, in the direct interpersonal transactions between the therapist and the client that true and effective trust is established and reinforced. It is first necessary for the therapist to communicate empathy for the client's feelings and respect for the client as a human being. Such communication may be very simple, like a nod, or asking the client how he or she wishes to be called rather than automatically using a first name, nickname, or a formal name.[3] Communication must be clear and consistent throughout the total process. This is not always easy. The silent, nonverbal client who may be depressed and despairing, for example, may show a strong wish to avoid involvement. The client who may be acting out feelings with hostile language or behavior may seem to be trying to "put the therapist off." The paranoid person who is suspicious or the schizophrenic client who is prompted by hallucinations to behave strangely may make it difficult for the therapist to communicate empathy and respect. Yet, it is these people who most need to feel they are cared for and valued in spite of the strange or threatening behaviors they show. Unless they feel valued it is not really worth the effort for them to invest in making changes. The therapist too must be able to recognize the pain that underlies their behavior in order to wish to invest in making a change process possible. Sometimes this means sitting silently with a client. Sometimes it means confronting behavior or setting clear limits in a way that indicates an expectation that change is possible. It always means maintaining a clear contact with reality and being willing to communicate that reality to the client who needs to know that the therapist can be counted on to point out what is real.

The therapist's own self-confidence and self-knowledge are critical to the development of a truly therapeutic relationship. It is the therapist's knowledge base, combined with the therapist's personal trust in his or her own skills, that make it possible for the therapist to have the confidence necessary to instill confidence in the client. What the therapist knows about the disease or deficit, about the client, and about the kinds of interventions occupational therapy can make will determine the effectiveness of what is communicated about the program. If the client experiences the program as effective, this will promote trust and motivation.

There are a number of fears which often inhibit a client's willingness to participate in occupational therapy. Many of the ordinary things which are part of normal living, such as sometimes expressing anger, or receiving anger expressed by someone else, or making a mistake, may be perceived by the client as extremely risky. In the therapeutic relationship an important contribution may be made when the therapist who is trusted expresses or receives anger without becoming upset, or makes a mistake and is able to admit it.

There are certain other issues that may emerge in the course of a therapeutic relationship in occupational therapy. Among these are dependency, control, and transference. The ultimate goal of the program is to facilitate the client's ability to function as successfully as possible. This means recognizing the issues when they arise, often naming them with the client, and planning strategies for dealing with them. The frame of reference within which the therapist is working will determine the way in which issues are perceived and the kinds of strategies that may be used. For example, dependent behavior will be identified in terms of specific, dependent actions within a *behavioral* frame of reference, and the therapist's role

will be to try to develop reinforcement schedules to effect a reduction in the specific behavior. Dependent behavior within a *developmental* frame of reference will be seen in terms of the sequence of developmental needs,[4] and the therapist will try to construct strategies for the client to experience success at the existing level of function so that a sense of competence is fostered, promoting the ability to move toward greater independence.

The *occupational behavior* frame of reference would approach the problem similarly, but with some major considerations being given to the role and functions expected of the client in society. Dependency, viewed *psychoanalytically*, would be regarded as a manifestation of deeper, unconscious needs. As such, it might be dealt with on a symbolic reenactment basis, in which the therapist allows the client to use the activities and the relationship of the occupational therapy process to explore and to relive in a more positive way the events that originally fostered pathological growth. The *sensory integrative* approach would focus primarily on promoting the client's basic perceptual and motor abilities in order to foster a better body image and more effective reality testing. This in turn would lead to a greater sense of or desire for independence in functioning.

At all stages in the course of the therapeutic relationship, initiation, implementation, and termination, it is important to remember that the relationship is a dynamic one involving both therapist and client. Their concepts of themselves and others, as well as their values and biases, will affect the quality and extent of their commitment to a program of change. In this way, an authentic, acting, feeling self on the part of the therapist lends strength to the relationship.

The Activity

It has been said that activity is the bridge between one's inner reality and the external world. It is through our activities that we are connected with life and with other human beings. Through the activities in which we engage, we learn about the world, test our knowledge, practice skills, express our feelings, experience pleasure, take care of our needs for survival, develop competence, and achieve mastery over our destinies.

Some element of volition is involved in mental, physical, and social activities. It is this type of volitional activity that is important in the occupational therapy process. The use of activity, which is carefully planned to facilitate change in the client, is a unique characteristic of occupational therapy. The activities used in psychiatric occupational therapy are highly influenced by the total treatment context, but also may be significant in *determining* the nature of that context. Limitations on the kinds of activities which may be used are imposed by the environment, materials, or resources available as well as the extent of the therapist's knowledge, skill, interests, and creativity.

In 1981, Fidler referred to the concept of the purposefulness of activities as fundamental to the occupational therapy process. She suggested that two assumptions are made about the meaning and use of activities.

> One assumption fundamental to the use of purposeful activity may be expressed as: A society's values and norms *weight* certain tasks and activities. Mastery and competence in those activities and tasks that are valued and given priority by one's society or social group have greater meaning in describing and defining one's social efficacy than mastery and competence in activities carrying less social significance. This assumption speaks to the social relevance of an activity.
>
> A second assumption may be framed as: An individual's unique neurobiology and psychology *weight* certain tasks and activities so that mastery and competence in these are more readily achieved and have greater meaning to that individual in terms of intrinsic gratification, personal pleasure, and satisfaction. This assumption relates to matching an activity to the person.[5]

She went on to refer to the idea that every given activity has social, cultural and personal meanings that are "describably real and symbolic."

With these ideas in mind, occupational therapists in psychiatry have used activities in a number of ways. General categories into which occupational therapy activities may fall include body movement and exercise, individual and team sports, games, crafts, personal hygiene and grooming, activities of daily living or life skills, prevocational practice, horticulture, work, and creative activity.

Activities may be used as part of the initial assessment process and have, inherently, a function in the ongoing evaluation process. Observation or measurement of the client's performance, behavior, and end product in the execution of an activity can yield much valuable information to aid in determining the directions of treatment. The realtively objective nature of data obtained in the activity process is valuable to the therapist and to other members of the treatment team. But most importantly, it is valuable to the client.

A difficult problem that is encountered with a large number of psychiatrically ill clients is their inability to understand their personal assets and limitations. Often activities that involve manipulating objects, tools, and materials, and producing something finished at the end, provide concrete evidence which can be used to help the client to test reality about himself or herself.

Activities used within a group context or on a dyadic interaction basis, may provide a focus around which the individuals involved can relate to one another. When working together on a task, individuals have an opportunity to explore and practice dimensions of interpersonal relationships in ways that may be either provocative or "safe."

Freely creative or projective activities have long been employed within the psychoanalytic frame of reference, as a communication link with unconscious processes and, as such, have made useful diagnostic contributions.

Occupational therapy is concerned with promoting the ability of clients to function in their own worlds. Activities can provide the ground for exploration and learning, practicing, and achieving mastery. They permit function from the simplest, developmentally earliest, and nonverbal levels to the most complex, most mature levels. It is the task of the occupational therapist to understand the meaning of activity and to know how to determine the potential of each given activity for promoting performance.

Activity Analysis

Activity analysis is essential in making a match between the needs, interests, and abilities of the client and the activities that will help to bring about growth or change. Activities may be analyzed with respect to a number of important dimensions. The frame of reference may determine which dimensions of the activity are to be emphasized and the depth with which some of the dimensions are to be explored and exploited. At this point in the development of psychiatric occupational therapy there is no universally accepted method of activity analysis. In general, it is useful to think of the several aspects of experience or functional requirements of the activity, then analyze each of these in terms of its gradability. Time requirements and cultural implications of the activity should also be explored.

Activity analysis based upon a *behavioral* frame of reference will be concerned especially with the specification and seriation of the component parts of the activity, their potential as or need for reinforcement contingencies, and the measurability of data. Activity analysis based upon a *psychoanalytic* frame of reference will pay special attention to the symbolic, expressive, and interpersonal aspects of the activity. Based upon a *sensory integrative* frame of reference, it will be focused primarily on the sensory, perceptual, and physical aspects of the activity, especially in terms of the kinds of input which may be experienced. From a *developmental* perspective, it will

Figure 19-2. Activity analysis in a long-term hospital setting. Developed by the Occupational Therapy Staff of Norristown State Hospital, Norristown PA. Printed with permission.

ACTIVITY ANALYSIS

I. General Information
   A. Name of Activity
   B. Specific Purpose of Activity according to treatment goals

   C. Type of Activity—work related, leisure time, culturally determined, economic implications, role identification, sexual connotation.

II. Materials
   A. Specific Materials
   B. Nature of these materials
   Resistive _____
   Pliable _____
   Controlled _____
   Messy _____
   C. Sensory Input
   Tactile _____
   Auditory _____
   Olfactory _____
   Visual _____
   Taste _____
   Kinesthetic (joint movement) _____
   D. Color
   A. Number and names
   B. Variability (light to dark)

III. Parts of Activity
   A. Number of parts _____
   B. Complexity of part—one step repeated _____, two steps repeated _____, more than two steps repeated _____ .

IV. Preparation
   A. Precutting
   B. Provide pattern
   C. Provide sample
   D. Pre-arrangement of supplies (explain)
   E. Re-arrangement of environment (explain)

V. Directions
   A. Demonstration with assistance
   B. Demonstration of each part
   C. Demonstration of whole task
   D. Verbal: part/whole
   E. Written: part/whole

VI. Amount of structure and controls (rules) inherent in activity

VII. Predictability of Results

VIII. Learning Required

	Whole Task	Part One	Part Two	Part Three	Part Four
Old	_____	_____	_____	_____	_____
Adapted Old	_____	_____	_____	_____	_____
New	_____	_____	_____	_____	_____

IX. Decisions required by patient (explain)

X.   Attention span (hours, minutes)

XI.   Interaction: solitary, parallel play, interaction with one other person, interaction in small group, interaction in large group, competition, cooperation, taking turns.

XII.   Communication: little required, nonverbal communication, one word, 10–15 words necessary, common environmental words, reciprocal language, oral directions, reading, writing.

XIII.   Motivation: useful, decorative, prestigious, successful, intellectually challenging, effect on others, creative, gratifying.

XIV.   Additional Comments:

Figure 19-3. Sample of activity analysis form for one specific activity.

ACTIVITY ANALYSIS   *Activity:* digging and planting a garden plot

Time Requirement (average range for successful completion):   one hour.

Average no. of sessions required to complete: one, but may be done in several short sessions, if needed.

Brief Description (including criteria for determining success):

Garden plot 5′ × 5′. Requires digging with spade, raking to remove stones, marking out three rows, planting seeds or small plants.

Success may be determined by the extent to which all the ground is turned over and stone free, and the planting is completed.

Characteristics of Activity	Input	Skills	How can activity be graded?
Physical:			
Gross motor	X	X	The preparation of the 5′ × 5′ plot in advance will determine the amount of physical work required. A new area will require far more effort than a previously dug area.
Fine Motor	X	X	
Strength	X	X	
Rhythm	X	X	
Repetition	X	X	The nature of the seeds or plants will determine how much fine motor skill is required.
Coordination		X	
Passive			
Active		X	
Sensory:			
Tactile	X	X	The kinds of tools provided, the kinds of seeds or plants; their relative size, texture, fragility, fragrance. Use of hose or can to water.
Visual	X	X	
Auditory	X		
Olfactory	X		
Gustatory			
Perceptual:			
Tactile	X	X	The kinds of tools, seeds or plants; the amount of lifting, bending, stooping.
Visual space	X	X	
Visual form	X	X	
Vestibular	X	X	

Figure 19-3 (*continued*)

Proprioceptive	X	X	
Kinesthetic	X	X	
Part—Whole		X	
Auditory—Language	possibly		
Auditory figure—Ground	possibly		
Visual figure—Ground	X	X	
Bilateral integration	X	X	
Body scheme	X	X	
Motor planning	X	X	
Cognitive:			
			Immediate feedback with regard to effects of digging, raking, and changes made in the plot.
Object permanence	X	X	
Causality	X	X	
			Delayed feedback with regard to growth of plants or harvest crop.
Goal establishment		X	
Goal implementation		X	
			Therapist may grade means of instruction from use of immediate imitation to verbal or written directions.
Imitation		X	
Trial-and-error problem solving		X	
Seriation		X	Instructions may involve degrees of seriation.
Organize parts into whole		X	
			Most of the skills involved rely on schemes which are familiar, even if total activity is not.
Interpret signs, symbols		X	
Cognitive:			
Read			
Use imagination, creativity			
Perceive viewpoint of others			
Test reality		X	
Decenter		X	
Logical thinking			
Hypothetical thinking			
Social-Emotional:			
			The activity is highly gradable with regard to leadership, dependence, number of interpersonal interactions involved.
Control, lead		X	
Follow, cooperate		X	
Independence		X	
			The heavy work component may be useful in terms of emotional expression or sublimation.
Dependence		X	
Impulse control		X	
Handle feelings		X	
Work with one other person		X	
Work in a small group		X	
Work in a large group			
Test reality (consensual validation)	X	X	
Play	possibly		

Cultural implications of the activity, with attention to factors which would indicate its relevance to individual life situations:

Activity is familiar to most clients from suburban or rural areas. To city dwellers, the activity may be less relevant, although it tends to be the kind of "new" activity which can be interesting because of its implications for providing a valuable product. The activity is fairly universally understood.

be concerned with the parallels between levels of functioning required or expected and developmental levels. In the *occupational behavior* frame of reference, activity analysis will be concerned with developmental levels and the potential of the activity for providing meaningful opportunities for individuals to develop competence and balance within their life roles in society.

There is little doubt that there is a vital need in occupational therapy for in-depth research into the actual meanings of activity as used in occupational therapy and into certain other aspects, such as the transfer of learning.

Figures 19-2 and 19-3 are examples of activity analyses as they might be used in specific psychiatric settings.

The Context

The settings in which psychiatric occupational therapists currently practice in psychiatry have become varied and complex. Now, in addition to hospitals, one finds therapists working with clients in community centers, satellite clinics, schools, centers for specialized populations, homes, and correctional institutions, to name a few new settings. In terms of space, this means that the occupational therapist does not always work with clients in a well-equipped, well-defined place, such as the Occupational Therapy Shop of a large state hospital. It means that the occupational therapist may often be challenged to plan how to carry out treatment in environments which are not easily controllable but which are close to or part of the realities of the client's life.

The teams with whom occupational therapists work have also become more diversified in the past decade. Instead of, or in addition to, the traditional medical team, occupational therapists in some settings may find themselves working with teachers, business persons, politicians, and members of the clergy as well as the family, friends, and neighbors of the client. Occupational therapists must broaden their knowledge base to include deeper understanding of social, economic, cultural, and political factors and forces. These factors challenge occupational therapists to become more sensitive to the significance of personal biases and value systems as they affect interpersonal transactions within these contexts.

There is a special need for the occupational therapist to be flexible enough to work in a role which often seems very much blended with the roles of others. This may present either a problem or an opportunity, depending upon how confident the occupational therapist is about the principles of occupational therapy practice and its conceptual bases.

References

1. Doukas, P.: A Brief Discussion of General Principles of Drug Action and Certain Agents Affecting the Central Nervous System. Unpublished manuscript. Philadelphia: Temple University, 1981.
2. Frank Jerome: The therapeutic use of self. Am. J. Occup. Ther. 12:215. 1958.
3. Purtilo, R.: Health Professional/Patient Interaction. Philadelphia: W.B. Saunders Co., 1978.
4. Mosey, A. C.: Recapitulation of ontogenesis. Am. J. Occup. Ther. 22:427, 1968.
5. Fidler, G. S.: From crafts to competence. Am. J. Occup. Ther. 35:569, 1981.

SECTION **4**

The Occupational Therapy Process: Treatment, Maintenance, Rehabilitation, and Prevention

The process of bringing together the client, the therapist, the activity, and the context for the purpose of providing treatment, maintenance, rehabilitation, or preventive services is the essence of occupational therapy. The context and the status of the client usually determine whether the process is geared to treatment, maintenance of function, rehabilitation, or prevention, although often the therapist may move from treatment to rehabilitation to prevention as the client is helped to achieve increasing autonomy and competence.

The treatment process is one of intervening directly in the pathology of the client and of effecting changes or interruptions in the illness itself. Behavior therapy techniques and sensory integration techniques in psychiatry are often clearly geared to treatment. So are many of the psychoanalytically based techniques. Maintenance of function refers to the process which must take place when dealing with clients who have chronic debilitating or deteriorating conditions. Occupational therapy then is based on strengths and geared to the promotion of optimum functioning as long as possible. The developmental and occupational behavior frames of reference place greater emphasis on building upon the strengths and healthy parts of the client; they therefore seem to make their major contributions in the areas of rehabilitation, maintenance, and prevention.

There are five sequential parts to the occupational therapy process: initial assessment, development of objectives, development of plan, implementation of the plan, and termination of the program. Evaluation of the client's progress, keeping records, and making reports are ongoing or periodic processes which keep the program current, relevant, and effective. Table 19-4 provides an example of the occupational therapy process as it would take place in an hypothetical treatment situation.

Assessment/Evaluation

It is essential that the occupational therapist gain a baseline of information about the client before initiating or proceeding with the development of objectives, a plan, and a program. Assessment requires the collection of data and the organization of the data into a meaningful description of the client. In addition to providing an understanding of the client's current illness or problems and their effect on his or her life, it should incorporate information about his or her work, social and cultural worlds, value systems, skills, and interests.

The occupational therapist needs to have the knowledge and judgment to determine what information will be relevant and essential to provide a meaningful occupational therapy program within the chosen frame of reference. There must also be a commitment to an attitude of ongoing evaluation, through which the effectiveness of the program will be determined.

The evaluation process is often helpful in eliciting the interest and cooperation of the client. The establishment of motivation on the part of the client to be involved in occupational therapy is often accomplished through early and continuing collaboration in assessing the problem.

Assessment and evaluation techniques and methods have received much attention in recent years. Some newly developed techniques and some of the older techniques have been subjected to tests for their reliability and validity and to standardization procedures. Some of these have been listed in Chapter 11. Table 11-1 lists some of the newer procedures as a quick reference. Some techniques have been described in the literature but have not yet been fully developed or standardized. It is important for the therapist to be aware of the status of procedures being used and to follow their protocols carefully.

The sections which follow will describe some of the standard ways of doing assessment or evaluation in psychiatric occupational therapy, including observation, getting data from other sources, interviewing, projective techniques, activity evaluation, developmental evaluation, ADL evaluation, prevocational evaluation, perceptual-motor evaluation, inventories, and check lists.

Observation

The skill of the therapist in observing well is critical to all kinds of assessment procedures. The therapist must be able to see, listen to, and pay attention to the

Table 19-4 *One Example: Occupational Therapy Process in Psychiatry*

The client, Ms. S., is a 26-year-old unmarried woman. She lives alone in a small apartment in the downtown area of a small city. She works as a clerk in a super-market. She became anxious and depressed following transfer to a new location in her job. She has been unable to work or take care of her meals, laundry, and cleaning. After a brief hospitalization during which she received treatment, she was transferred to the day program of a community mental health center. This chart shows the process of treatment and rehabilitation in occupational therapy.

Initial Assessment	Objectives	Plan	Implementation	Reevaluation	Termination
METHODS USED: Interview, activities configuration, interest inventory, activity battery, records, and team conference	LONG TERM: Ms. S. will be able to set priorities on her time and energy.	Starting with follow-ing a standard schedule of the center, Ms. S. will be encouraged to plan for substitute activities of her own choosing, gradually incorporating activ-ities which are part of her normal life routine.	Ms. S. started working with a task group, attend-ing weekly, joined bowling activity. Followed written schedule of standard activities.	Observation and periodic interviews to review progress	Treatment on a daily basis was weaned gradually.
INFORMATION GAINED: *Family:* out of touch *Friends:* a few good friends	SHORT TERM: Ms. S. will be able to plan a schedule of activities for a typical day and follow it with encouragement from therapist.		Completed indi-vidual project of a datebook and calendar for personal use	Ms. S. was initially reluctant but gained interest after a few minor successes.	Evening program is still providing encouragement and support.
Education: finished high school, started but did not finish beauty culture course	SHORT TERM: Ms. S. will be able to complete one simple task within reason-able time frame.	Support of therapist, other staff and patient group to be gradually lifted as Ms. S. gains feel-ings of competence	Began to incorporate personal marketing weekly and to schedule house-cleaning in her apartment	She spent a long time on the datebook, but afterwards began to be inter-ested in filling in plans of her own.	
Work: present job since high school. Considers work "a drag," but says she was "pretty good at it."			Eventually returned to job—came to center twice a week in the evening for therapy		
Interests: television, bowling, paperback mysteries					
Self-care: used to be "fussy" but in illness unable to cope or care very much					
Self-assessment: feels "all apart"—but not so hopeless as before hospitalization. Wants to get better					
STRENGTHS: able to work cooperatively and can carry out a task with support. Motivated to improve					
PROBLEMS: decision making, meeting time requirements					

intangible feeling tones, which are part of the client's acts and communications, as well as to the more obvious and measurable behaviors. The occupational therapist is in a particularly advantageous position because in the use of carefully planned activities there is a structure for controlled as well as spontaneous observation. Activities provide opportunities for nonverbal and verbal communication to take place.

It is important to think about the know about the kinds of things which may be observed. In a task that involves perceptual motor skill, for example, the therapist must be sensitive to the fact that, if the client consistently changes hands to cross the midline, it may be important; or in a group activity, if a client consistently sits outside of the main circle, it means something. Standardized assessment procedures usually provide guides to observation of relevant behaviors or responses. Before using one of these methods, it is important to review not only the methods to be used but the kinds of general and specific behaviors that might be observed.

Sensitivity to seeing, hearing, and feeling the communications of others is a variable which is subject to a number of factors. Some people are naturally better observers than others. It is possible, however, for one to develop skills in observation. In addition to basic ability, the perceptual and cognitive "sets" of the observer are important. What will be attended to is directly influenced by what the observer knows about the client and the situation or task in which he or she may be involved and by the expectations which this knowledge may have engendered. One's perceptual and cognitive sets are further influenced by personal biases and value systems and by the level of anxiety or other emotional factors which might enter into the situation. It is important to be aware that this is true and, with that awareness, in the clinical setting, to work toward the achievement of as much objectification as possible. Objectification of the process of observation is helped by planning ahead or by seeking consensual validation from others who may also have been in a position to observe the client.

Interview

An interview is a planned conservation, conducted for a specified purpose. For most clients, the initial interview with the occupational therapist launches the occupational therapy process. It is in the initial interview that the first contact may be made to establish understanding about the purposes of further evaluation and the occupational therapy program it-self. It is in the initial interview that the client has an opportunity to share information about his or her problems and situation and to begin to think about making changes.

The therapist needs to plan the interview so that there will be time to explore fully the aspects of the client's history and current status which will be helpful in setting objectives. The types of information gained may depend upon the frame of reference, but there are general areas which provide important information regardless of frame of reference. These might include the client's interests and skills, most recent living situation, existing support systems, what the client thinks about his or her illness, and what the client's hopes for the future are. Other questions that can provide valuable information relate to the client's history. What is the client's educational background? Where, and at what kinds of jobs, did the client work? How did the client feel about school or work? If he or she left school or work, why? It is in such questions that the therapist gains information about the strengths and weaknesses and the assets and liabilities which have characterized the client's life before illness. The questions the therapist asks the client in the course of the interview will communicate the tone and the interest of the occupational therapist and the nature of the occupational therapy program. The therapist needs to be clear and knowledgeable in the choice of questions, so that they will encourage realistic expectations on the part of the client with regard to occupational therapy.

The environment in which the interview takes place is important. It should be comfortable, quiet, and as distraction-free as possible. This is not always easy to achieve, but it can make a big difference in the success of the interview.

The therapist should clearly state at the outset the purpose of the interview and his or her role in relation to the client. This allows for some further explanation of the purpose of occupational therapy. The therapist's attitudes in the initial interview are the keystone for the rapport and continuing relationship that will be developed. It is essential to feel and to communicate respect, interest, and empathy for the client and confidence that the process will be beneficial.

The information that has been gained in the interview should be available to the client. The notes that the therapist makes during the interview should be made openly. It may be useful for the client to review them. When the interview is reaching its conclusion, the therapist should make this clear to the client. A summary or review of the discussion is often a helpful way to conclude the interview. The therapist will want to let the client know what is to happen next and make an appointment for future contacts and assessment procedures.

There may be other occasions to use the interview technique as an ongoing evaluation procedure. At the termination of the occupational therapy program, especially, an interview may be of great value. It provides an opportunity to review and assess the progress which has been made and to reinforce the learning which has taken place.

Data from Other Sources

There is a wealth of information available from assessment efforts when a team of coprofessionals work together. The pooling of data from all team members may yield a coherent and valid picture of the client. It is essential that the occupational therapist be clear about the pieces of information contributed by team members so that unnecessary duplication of effort (and aggravation to the client) will not occur. For example, a social worker may be able to provide much needed information about the client's home and family.

Psychological tests may give information about certain aspects of the client's intelligence or unconscious motivations. Some tests commonly used by psychologists contain information of special value in developing an occupational therapy plan. The psychiatric occupational therapist may especially wish to check out results in such tests as the Wechsler or Stanford-Binet for intelligence, the Rorschach, Thematic Apperception, and Minnesota Multiphasic Personality Inventory for personality orientation and unconscious material, and the Bender-Gestalt or Draw-a-Person for organic disease. The observations of ward personnel, the charted medications, and comments about transactions between the psychiatrist and client are also significant to understanding the gestalt of the client in the treatment setting.

Activity Evaluation

The careful identification of skills required to carry out activities is the key to treatment in occupational therapy as a whole; the continuing observation of a client's performance is the key to the essential process of ongoing evaluation. Certain specified, uniform tasks, which call upon identified skills for their accomplishment, lend themselves well to the processes of initial and periodic evaluation. The success of the use of activities as evaluation tools relies upon the accuracy and detail of activity analysis. The therapist must be quite clear about the kinds of information

that may be gained through the use of a specified task. Almost any task may be used evaluatively, but it is important that the therapist have a clear idea about the skills and time requirements for "normal" performance. It is generally useful to select activities that may be completed in one session, although there may be times when the evaluation of a client's ability to postpone gratification or of a client's frustration tolerance may indicate the use of longer-term projects.

One advantage to the use of activities as evaluation procedures is that the range of traits that can be tested is great and there is wide flexibility in planning. A second advantage is that the use of activities may promote a truly cooperative effort between the client and the therapist in the implementation of treatment. Their heuristic value to the client is in terms of the client's own wishes to feel and to function better. This is easily communicated around activities performance. Establishing the validity and reliability of activity evaluation procedures, however, constitutes one of the major disadvantages of the technique and one of the major challenges to the profession of occupational therapy.

Mosey suggests the use of concepts of present and future levels of functioning as part of the evaluation. "Future" levels of functioning refer to those skills that are related to the client's "anticipated, expected environment."[1] As examples, consider the mother who expects to regain the ability to care for her three children, cook for her family, and keep the house in order; the factory worker who will return to a job requiring attention and manual dexterity, not to mention getting up at five o'clock in the morning; the office manager who will need skills in interpersonal relationships and problem solving. Evaluation of present skills in relation to future demands gives the occupational therapy process a reality and validity which can usually be communicated and mutually understood.

Developmental Assessment

The collection and organization of data in terms of the normal developmental continuum have proven to be useful and empirically successful in the occupational therapy process. Although in psychiatric occupational therapy there has always been some attention to the process of development and to developmental approaches using Freud's concepts of psychosexual development or Erikson's eight crises and the age-specific educational theories, the publication of Mosey's "Recapitulation of Ontogenesis" focused attention on specific ways in which clients could be assessed and treated in terms of adaptive skill development.[2] The organization of adaptive skills may be assessed by a number of different methods and then charted to give a picture of the client. The evaluation of adaptive skills lends itself well to treatment planning.

Another method, developed by Allen and Lewis, focuses on developmental levels of cognitive skills. The identification of cognitive levels in such a plan is based on the ways in which the client uses imitation and perceives causality, object permanence, and time. Levels of functioning are determined in terms of Piagetian concepts of sensorimotor development and the cognitive gains that are made in normal development during this period. Developmental approaches to evaluation presuppose the importance of identifying the client's current level of functioning as the necessary starting point of treatment. People who are mentally ill regress to earlier stages of development and earlier levels of functioning. The therapist needs to identify not only in what areas and to what levels regression has taken place at a given point in time, but also what circumstances or activities tend to make the client function well and experience success or function poorly and further regress. The Piagetian concept of "familiar schemes" is important, and developmental evaluations should include some attention to activities the client knows well and can perform easily.

An example of developmental assessment using one specific activity is the Allen Cognitive Level Test which uses the task of leather-lacing a key case. The processes used in this task are graded and correlated with levels of cognitive functioning.[3] The data yielded in this evaluation provide important information about the client's level of function. This information can be used to determine directions for treatment.

Techniques such as interview, activities configuration, and interest and activities evaluations all lend themselves well to contributing to the data used in developmental assessment. In certain settings and with certain kinds of clients, perceptual testing may also be important.

Perceptual-Motor Evaluation

Testing procedures described elsewhere in this book (Chap. 11) have been adapted by therapists for use with psychiatrically disabled clients. These are especially important in pediatric psychiatric problems and with the chronically institutionalized patient. Because most of the standard procedures have been developed and standardized for pediatric popula-

tions, their use with adult populations can only indicate trends or possible areas of difficulty. Some therapists have incorporated the Bender-Gestalt, Draw-a-Person, and Purdue tests into their standard testing battery. At the present time, the therapist's ability to observe and identify perceptual-motor performance in a variety of sensory motor activities would seem the basic tool. Walking with a shuffling gait, evidence of auditory or tactile defensiveness, visual or auditory constancy problems, inability to cross the midline in the performance of tasks, rocking behavior, awkwardness, and inaccurate motions are some of the clues indicating the possibility of sensory integrative dysfunction.

Projective Techniques

There is a degree of projection in everything we do and in all things that we produce. As Hammer notes, "One's way of walking, whether proudly, boldly, timidly, arrogantly, self-consciously or stridently; one's way of hammering a nail, whether confidently, impatiently, irritatedly, rhythmically or joyfully; even one's way of lacing a shoe, whether one alloplastically places one's foot on a hydrant or fence post thus bringing the shoe up to one's self, or whether one autoplastically brings one's self all the way down to the ground to encounter the shoe lace—all reflect some fact of one's personality."[4]

This element of projection of otherwise often inexpressible parts of the personality in an important part of the total occupational therapy process. Sensitivity to the symbolic as well as the concrete representations in all aspects of doing activities is a primary requirement of good observation. Procedures known as projective tests or techniques are geared specifically to allowing communication of unconscious material in this way.

In settings where the frame of reference for treatment is primarily psychoanalytic, the use of projective techniques may be indicated as a standard form of evaluation. The vast array of unconscious material which a client might present in clay, drawings, or other free-form media has frequently encouraged occupational therapists to work in close collaboration with other therapists, usually psychiatrists. Projective techniques can yield a wide range of diagnostically useful information. The success of the occupational therapist in the use of these techniques is dependent upon a number of factors including (1) the therapist's sophistication about psychodynamics and psychoanalytic theory and practice, (2) the nature of the client population, and (3) the quality and extent of the therapist's own emotional maturity and self-knowledge.

Art, dance, and music therapists rely heavily upon projection as a primary point of entry and ongoing evaluation technique in the therapeutic process. There are a number of projective *testing* procedures, however, which may be used. Standardized tests such as the Thematic Apperception Test and the Rorschach are tools of the clinical psychologist and require specialized training for administering and interpreting. Occupational therapists have developed and adapted some procedures that lend themselves well to the occupational therapy setting.

The prototype of the occupational therapy projective techniques in the Azima Battery.[5] In this, the client is asked to produce something, using first pencil, then fingerpaints, then clay. In this way, the person moves from the simplest two-dimensional, achromatic mode to a more primitive, less controllable, chromatic, two-dimensional mode, and finally to a three-dimensional, regressive mode. In working with the three different materials, the client produces unconscious material. The subtle movement to earlier developmental stages in the sequence is experienced symbolically and often unconsciously through the feeling of the media. This appears to elicit progressively deeper levels of repressed material.

Other projective techniques that have been developed by occupational therapists include the Fidler Diagnostic Battery, the Magazine Picture Collage, and variations of the Draw-a-Person technique.[6,7] These techniques have proven empirically useful; there have been some attempts to standardize them, but there is still much to be done in this area.

Some therapists have sought training and incorporated the use of standardized procedures, such as the House-Tree-Person, or Person-in-the-Rain tests into their evaluation batteries.[8] Group projective techniques, in which the interactional elements of personality are especially communicated, are another interesting variation. Among these would be the production of group drawings, collages, and fingerpaintings.

The sophisticated therapist may learn much about the client's feelings, conflicts, self-image, values, and cognitive processes through the themes and organization created in projective techniques. There are, of course, some important principles that must be understood before undertaking these kinds of evaluation procedures including those that follow:

1. If the frame of reference for treatment is geared to "sealing over" unconscious material, projective techniques are inappropriate.
2. There must be *consensual validation* regarding the nature of the client's productions. This means that the therapist will discuss with the client the pictures or forms which have been produced. The client may or may not wish to explain their meanings. The therapist should allow the client to take the lead in doing this.
3. There should be no interpretation of unconscious materials or symbols with the client. The therapist and client together should discuss only the material as it is presented.
4. Validation of the information gained in a projective technique should be sought in other observation and evaluation methods. The use of projective materials alone is seldom complete enough for the occupational therapist's purposes.
5. It is important to recognize that these procedures may be fatiguing to the client, and the therapist should plan a time after the testing for him or her to rest with some form of activity that is known to be integrating and nonthreatening.
6. Because projective techniques tend to release more material of a personal nature than some other techniques, the need for the therapist to respect confidentiality is especially important.

Activities of Daily Living, Life Skills

The assessment of activities of daily living in psychiatry must be based on the therapist's knowledge of the demands that may be placed upon the client in his or her daily life. Several therapists have developed lists of the kinds of activities of daily living that should be assessed with most clients. Such activities as basic hygiene and grooming, care for clothing and other possessions, cooking, cleaning, shopping, budgeting, using public transportation, reading a map, understanding and following a timetable, and using the telephone are all part of daily living for most people. Attention to the client's ability to do these things is very important. The client should be assessed in terms of his or her current situation and in terms of his or her future expected situation.[9]

One method of assessing activities of daily living or life skills is to use a questionnaire or interview, and then to try out the various skills. For an outpatient, or the client about to be discharged, a visit to the home may be appropriate. The therapist may learn that life skills for his or her farmer client include getting up at daybreak and tending the chickens and cows or that life skills for an urban secretary include being able to make complicated carpooling arrangements to get to work or that life skills for a mother may mean dealing with the neighborhood children who come to play with her own children.

Prevocational Evaluation

Much of the occupational therapist's work with a client may be directed toward developing skills that may be used in the work world of the client. The kinds of problems that many psychiatrically ill clients encounter with regard to work, and that should be assessed and dealt with in occupational therapy, generally fit into categories that apply to other areas of their lives, for instance, the ability to organize, to manage time requirements, to get along with other people, to relate to authority figures, to adapt to changes, and to solve problems. It is vital that these kinds of considerations be assessed along with specific skills evaluation procedures. They are probably best assessed through observation of the client in a variety of activities that are structured to provide opportunities for the client to work with other people.

Skills assessments such as have been described in the other chapters may have an important place in the occupational therapist's repertoire in psychiatry. Usually occupational therapists articulate prevocational assessment programs with those provided by other services or agencies, such as Vocational Adjustment Services or the Bureau of Vocational Rehabilitation, and the extent to which the occupational therapist evaluates for specific skills is determined by the kinds of services provided by the other agencies. It is vital that this very important aspect of the client's life should not be overlooked.

Development of Objectives

The tone of the process of assessment is one which should lead directly to the setting of objectives. Objectives are based on the data gained in the process of assessment and, like assessment, should be subject to review and revision as the occupational therapy process is going on. It takes skill to include the client in setting objectives, but it is essential to try to do so. The depressed client, who is caught in a web of static and despairing images about himself or herself, or the psychotic schizophrenic client, who seems to be functioning at a preverbal level, may be difficult to communicate with, but it is nevertheless vital for the therapist to share the objectives which are developed with the client in some way.

The factors that contribute to objectives include information about the client, objectives and frame of reference of the total treatment team, knowledge about the disease process or deficit and the client's prognosis, knowledge about the client's expected future environment, and the realistic possibilities for implementing a plan to achieve the objectives. As objectives are developed it is important to consider the ways in which it will be possible to measure the degrees of success that have been reached in achieving them.

Overall objectives are usually developed by the team. Occupational therapy long-term objectives are designed to promote progress toward the overall objectives. Short-term objectives are developed to provide a series of sequential small steps to bring about progress toward the long-term objective. In the example of the occupational therapy process in Table 19-4, Ms. S's long-term objective was that she should be able to "set priorities on her time and energy." The first short-term objective in accordance with it was that she would be able to "complete one simple task within a reasonable time frame." A subsequent short-term objective was for her to be able to "plan a schedule of activities for a typical day and follow it with encouragment from the therapist." Short-term objectives should represent small increments in the development of healthy patterns of functioning. If it happens that, after assessment, there are no legitimate reasons for developing objectives, occupational therapy probably is not indicated for the client.

Development of a Plan

Initial assessment data about the patient and the objectives for treatment must be translated into a plan of action. A well-designed plan describes for each of the objectives the kinds of activities that will be used, the nature of the therapist's relationship with the client, and the setting in which treatment is to take place. The treatment plan must describe possibilities that can be implemented realistically, taking into consideration any limitations of time, space, and staffing. The treatment plan should be developed in collaboration with the client, or, at least, shared with him or her so that there can be some degree of mutual understanding about the occupational therapy process. In some settings, it is standard practice to have the client sign the treatment plan as a means to achieving this end.

The kinds of considerations that are important in developing the plan include the following: (1) the meaning of the activities to the client, (2) the suitability of the activities for facilitating progress toward meeting the treatment objectives, (3) the consistency of the plan with the predominant frame of reference for treatment and the methods being used in other services, (4) the accuracy with which the activities are matched to the client's current level of functioning, (5) the gradability of the activities to accommodate increased function or regression, (6) the adaptability of the activities to meet special needs, and (7) the potential for a successful experience in doing the activities.

Just as the treatment objectives represent an action-oriented summary of the assessment of the client, the treatment plan represents a synthesis of the theapist's knowledge of the potential of activities and relationships as facilitators of growth and performance. A treatment plan is stated in reference to each short-term objective and needs to be flexible enough to permit changes if reevaluation suggests that the plan is not working.

The thoroughness of the therapist's kowledge, the sensitivity with which the therapist has evaluated client's needs, assets, and limitations, and the soundness of the therapist's professional judgment are put to the test as the therapist develops a treatment plan. The plan must be realistic and must relate clearly to the treatment objectives that have been developed.

Implementation of the Plan

The purpose of initial assessment, objective setting, and the development of a plan is to make it possible for clients to be involved in therapeutic programs that are designed as carefully as possible to meet their needs. In one sense the occupational therapy program is a test of the validity of those other measures and of the skill of the therapist in carrying out the plan.

Depending upon the setting and the frame of reference, the therapist may be directly involved with the client or may work in cooperative efforts with other team members in carrying out the program. In some settings the therapist may be only consultative to other services, to community agencies, or to the client, since the program may involve the use of resources away from the primary treatment center. In some instances clients are transferred or discharged before the occupational therapy program can be considered complete. It is a professional responsibility for the occupational therapist to consider and carry out ways of ensuring as much as possible that the client will have continuity in the program.

The issue of trust and confidence is critical to the implementation of the program. The therapist has been able to secure the client's interest in the program and motivation to invest in it. It is therefore vital that the therapist build upon this by maintaining his or her own consistent interest and involvement.

There are three parts of the implementation process. In the orientation phase the therapist reviews the objectives and the plan which have been developed and describes the way the program will be carried out. During the development phase the events of the program should be shown to correlate closely with the objectives that have been set. Formal or informal methods of evaluation of the client's progress should be used. If continuing evaluation indicates that the plan is not working or that the client's needs have changed, it is important to review the objectives and plan as may seem to be indicated. When objectives have been met, or if they become irrelevant, it is time either to terminate the program or to think of new plans to meet new objectives. At the termination of the program, it is a good idea to review with the client the progress that has been made and, perhaps, to work with the client on future plans and future objectives.

Choice of Activities in the Program

The development of the occupational therapy program requires translating the objectives into specific activities. The activities must fulfill the requirements of (1) relevance to the objectives and (2) meaning to the client within his or her normal life space. There are a number of factors which enter into these considerations. Is the activity to be designed so that a success experience may be assured? Are objects and finished products important? Or is the process itself the most important factor? Is body movement important? Are the dynamics of working in a group a factor to be considered? Should the activity be one that involves verbal expression and transactions with others? What about the dimension of time? Is immediate feedback or an immediate result important, or should there be moderate or prolonged delays? These questions can be answered first by looking at the initial assessment of the client. On the basis of that information, and with the knowledge and skills in activity analysis, the therapist should be able to match activities, plans, and objectives.

In many settings, occupational therapy takes place within a group, and the dynamics of the group provide one of the important dimensions of the treatment process. Groups can provide an opportunity for clients to experience and practice interpersonal relationship skills. The focus of the individual within a group is one which is often effectively directed, using

Chart 19-1 *DEVELOPMENTAL GROUPS* *

I. *Aggregate of Individuals*—The individual may interact with one other person, usually the therapist. There is no attempt by an individual to promote interaction outside of the one-to-one relationship.

II. *Parallel Group*—An aggregate of persons who work on individual tasks with minimal requirement for interaction. The leader meets the social–emotional needs of each individual.
  A. Goals:
    1. Increase awareness of self, others, and the environment.
    2. Improve ability to tolerate a nonthreatening group.
    3. Develop beginning sharing behaviors.
    4. Increase attention span.
    5. Reclaim old skills.
  B. Behavioral characteristics:
    1. Attention span—variable (5 min. to 1 hr.).
    2. Verbal but not disruptive.
    3. Nonverbal—(1) quiet (2) withdrawn (3) limited interaction.
    4. Difficulty performing tasks independently.
    5. Requires a structured activity for success to occur.
    6. Ability to attend to individual tasks in the presence of others.
  C. Size and time factors:
    1. 6 to 12 participants.
    2. Length of time variable (20 min. to 1 hr.).

III. *Project Level Group*—Group members interact in a short-term task with others for the length of the task.
  A. Goals:
    To facilitate interaction, verbal and nonverbal, in a short-term task with others. The duration of the relationship is determined by the group activity.
  B. Behavioral characteristics:
    1. Exploration and testing of others, i.e., development of trust.
    2. Difficulty in participating in shared tasks.
    3. Inability to seek assistance of a peer in carrying out a task.
    4. Avoids giving assistance to a peer or provides inadequate assistance.
    5. Fear that others may interfere with task completion.
    6. Tendency to work alone, avoiding contact with others.
    7. Lack of understanding that one must help others to receive help from others.
    8. Minimal interaction outside of task place.
    9. Trial-and-error behavior is observed in the group.

C. Size and time factors:
  1. 4 to 10 participants.
  2. Length of time variable (30 min. to 1 hr.).
D. Role of therapist:
  1. Therapist must meet the social and emotional needs of individual group members.
  2. Provides and/or helps the group to select tasks which require interaction of two or more persons for completion.
  3. Therapist usually must provide each group member with specific aspect of the activity to work on and individual instruction when necessary.
  4. All materials and tools and equipment must usually be prepared prior to start of each group session.

IV. *Egocentric–Cooperative*—Group members interact cooperatively and competitively in a long-term task (major emphasis of individuals continues to be self-interest).
  A. Goals:
    1. Group members will be able to select, implement, and execute long-term projects through shared interaction and/or individual response. The therapist provides suggestions and guidelines.
    2. Group members will be able to recognize and respect the rights of others.
    3. Group members will perceive themselves as belonging to the group both during and after sessions.
    4. Group members will be able to engage in cooperative and/or competitive behavior.
    5. Group members will be able to assume various group membership roles.
  B. Behavioral characteristics:
    1. Difficulty engaging in cooperative tasks.
    2. Preoccupied with competition or avoids competition.
    3. Inability to conform to goals or norms of the group.
    4. Disregard for the rights of others.
    5. Disrespect for authority.
    6. Compulsive, indiscriminate conformity to any authority figure.
  C. Size and time factors:
    1. 6 to 8 participants.
    2. Length of time—1 hr.
  D. Role of therapist:
    1. Primarily a resource person.
    2. Therapist provides minimal assistance (i.e., suggestions, encouragement) so that the group selects plans and executes tasks with much independence.
    3. Offers support *and guidance* and continues

to satisfy a considerable portion of the individual's social–emotional needs.
V. **Cooperative Group**—Group members satisfy the social–emotional needs of others while interacting in a task, in a same sex peer group.
   A. Goals:
      1. Increase the individual's ability to express both positive and negative affect in a group.
      2. Be able to perceive the needs of others.
      3. Be able to meet the needs of others.
      4. Become cohesive as a group.
   B. Behavioral characteristics:
      1. Verbal and aware of other members.
      2. Can engage in a shared task.
      3. Difficulty in accurately perceiving the needs of others.
      4. Difficulty in expressing both positive and negative affect in a group.
      5. Difficulty in meeting the needs of others.
      6. Attention span adequate to length of task.
      7. Task is secondary to need fulfillment.
   C. Size and time factors:
      1. 10 to 12 participants.
      2. Minimum time—1½ hr.
   D. Role of therapist:
      1. Does not function as an authority.

2. Assists in finding resources (acts as advisor).
3. Offers some support and some need satisfaction.
VI. *Mature Group*—Group members assume those task and social–emotional roles that promote the general welfare and goal attainment of a heterogeneous group. Leadership is shared.
   A. Goals:
      1. Be able to interact with group members who vary in age, interest, ability, and cultural background.
      2. Be able to assume roles somewhat foreign to the individual's usual pattern of behavior.
      3. Be able to maintain a proper balance between task accomplishment and satisfaction of the social–emotional needs of group members.
      4. Be able to maintain a sense of self-integrity and individuality concomitant with productive participation in a group.
   B. Size and time factors:
      1. 10 to 15 participants.
      2. No time limit.

* Developed by the Occupational Therapy Staff of Norristown State Hospital, Norristown PA. Printed with their permission.
Reference: Mosey, A. C.: Occupational Therapy: Theory and Practice. Medford, MA: Pothier Bros., 1968.

a developmental frame of reference. Chart 19-1 describes developmental group levels.[10]

Figure 19-4 is a schematic representation of the levels on which activities may be experienced and the kinds of activities that promote healthy function at these levels. It is offered as one form of guide to the selection of activities as treatment in occupational therapy.

At the core there is body awareness experience, where movement and sensory input activities are of value. At this level the *process* of the activity is important, and automatic and noncortical performance is the measure of success. The focus of the activity is *individual,* although it may be done in a group. It is *nonverbal* but there may be some value in the use of simple naming of the actions or objects presented.[11] It is *immediate,* involving the integration of experiences as they occur.

The second ring is the body effectiveness experience, where one experiences the capability of the body to perform according to some internalized image or standard (exocept). *Individual* sports ac-

tivities such as swimming, hiking, jogging, climbing or jumping, dancing, and some forms of heavy work may provide for this experience. These activities are primarily *nonverbal* and *process* oriented. They may be accomplished in groups but their focus is *individual.* They involve minimal relationships with external objects apart from the environment in which they take place. They also, like the first experience, involve *immediate* experience.

The third ring refers to the experience of performing actions that have an impact on objects or the environment. One experiences the effects of coordination of thoughts and actions, but on a level which is *individual* and personal, not social. It is here that the wide range of crafts activities are especially useful in promoting the ability to see cause-and-effect relationships, object permanence, and problem solving. Some of the basic activities of daily living, such as grooming, hygiene, and simple cooking, also fit this grouping as do individual hobbies, such as collecting stones, birdwatching, and simple horticulture. These activities *may use but do not depend upon verbal activ-*

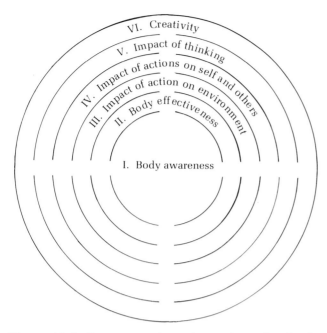

Figure 19-4. Representation of experience levels. See text for explanation of corresponding activities.

ity. They are primarily *nonverbal*. End *products* as well as *processes* are important. The time frame is short, with *minimal delay* between start and completion.

The fourth ring refers to the coordination of thought, body, and other-relatedness. One experiences the impact of actions and behavior on self and others. At this level we begin to think of using *group* activities by choice as a way of furthering treatment objectives. At this level all kinds of group tasks (including crafts), games, social activities, and more advanced forms of life skills, such as using the telephone and public transportation, shopping or caring for pets may be appropriate. This level is both *verbal* and *nonverbal* and *process* and *product* oriented. There may be some *delay* between start and completion.

The fifth ring refers to the experience of the impact of thought. At this level the individual may be involved in purely intellectual pursuits—reading, learning a language, doing mathematics, art, or music appreciation. These activities may be undertaken as an *individual* or in a *group*. They are more *process* than *product* oriented and tend to be highly *verbal*. The time frame is highly flexible and may involve *considerable delay* between start and completion.

The final, outside ring refers to the creative experience, that level at which the individual is able to use his or her experiences from all levels and produce something which is new and different and an expression of the self. At this level art, humor, writing, and some forms of planning are used. It is a level which is indicative of high integration and it is one which is seen only occasionally or briefly. It may be either *verbal* or *nonverbal* and is both *process* and *product* oriented.[12] The time frame is highly *flexible*.

The "normal" individual experiences all or most of these levels in the course of living. At each of the levels it is possible to conceptualize movement from issues of survival to the achievement of mastery. A program that will allow the client to experience levels of mastery as a stimulus to exploration of new levels should be planned.

Other issues that must be addressed in the occupational therapy program include the development of autonomy and balance in the client's life. The achievement and maintenance of health may be measured by the degree of control people have over their life activities and the extent to which they have been able to internalize and act upon a sense of balance uniquely suited to themselves. The hospitalized client has very little autonomy in his or her life; concern for balance in rest, activity, and sleep is reflected in the hospital schedule. Even clients who are not hospitalized but who are seen in outpatient centers seem to have major problems in these two areas. The occupational therapist, in the use of activities as treatment, is in an excellent position to help plan for the development and maintenance of the client's own sense of autonomy and balance.

Finally, a word about the meaning of the activities of the treatment program to the client. In reviewing the data from evaluation procedures, and in targeting the areas for treatment in occupational therapy, one finds important clues as to the level and mode for effective communication. If a client is seen to be functioning at the core area of body awareness, then communication will be nonverbal, and the meaning of the activity will be *in its experience*. King's research has shown that the pleasure derived from activities that effectively meet the client's level of functioning have a remarkable potentiating effect.[13] Effectively meeting the client's level of functioning means that communication has taken place.

Records and Reports

Because the occupational therapist seldom, if ever, works in isolation, it is essential that accurate records be made and kept current, and that adequate systems of reporting to other members of the treatment team be worked out. Although systems for both record-keeping and reporting vary from setting to setting, their functions remain the same: (1) to provide clear, objective data about the client to aid in guiding future directions of treatment; (2) to permit congruent articulation between occupational therapy and other services; (3) to provide the necessary justification for the cost of treatment, especially where fiscal intermediaries, Professional Standards Review Organization (PSRO), or other forms of utilization review may be concerned.

Four kinds of notes may be written: an *initial note*, giving the results of assessment procedures and the objectives and plan for treatment; *ongoing progress* notes, reporting change or progress toward the specified objectives; *special reports* of incidents, accidents, or especially notable progress; and a *final discharge* summary.

The results of the lengthy initial assessment process may be recorded first in some detail and filed for reference in the occupational therapy office, but it is advisable for the occupational therapist to learn to write a *succinct* report that synthesizes the important factors to be considered and which supports the stated treatment objectives and treatment plan. The report, which becomes part of the client's chart, is designed for the purpose of communicating to others; its completeness and clarity are vital.

The written report of the occupational therapy assessment and treatment process has gained greater importance as the public has demanded greater accountability on the part of health care providers. The written note needs to be more than a brief description of what or how treatment has taken place. It should contain a clear statement of the objectives of treatment and of the progress of the client toward achievement of those goals. A note written at the termination of treatment should contain information about the status of the client at discharge compared to his or her status earlier.

The SOAP note, used in some centers, provides a framework for incorporating the important information. SOAP is an acronym for the organization of data as follows: *Subjective:* the client's view of the problem; *Objective:* the clinical findings with regard to the problem; *Assessment:* a listing of important data from the evaluation; *Plan:* a statement of the goals of treatment, the environment and modalities to be used, and the personnel to carry out treatment.

The same principles apply to oral reporting, which is done in team meetings or conferences. The dimension that may be added in the conference situation is that it frequently becomes a forum for pooling of information and for problem solving among all members of the treatment team. In this situation, it is especially important for the occupational therapist to be able to articulate clearly the objectives of the program and the baseline of information and knowledge that serve as their foundation.

References

1. Mosey, A. C.: Activities Therapy. New York: Raven Press, 1973, pp. 90–93.
2. Mosey, A. C.: Recapitulation of ontogenesis. Am. J. Occup. Ther. 22:426–438, 1968.
3. Allen, C., and Moore, D.: The Allen Cognitive Level Test. Los Angeles: University of Southern California, 1981.
4. Hammer, E.: The Clinical Application of Projective Drawings. Springfield, Il.: Charles C Thomas, 1967, p. 5.
5. Azima, F. J.: The Azima Battery. In Mazer, J. (ed.): Materials from the 1968 Regional Institutes sponsored by the American Occupational Therapy Association on the Evaluation Process. Final Report R.S.A.-123-T-68. American Occupational Therapy Association, New York, 1968.
6. Fidler, G. S.: Diagnostic Battery, scoring and summary. In Mazer, J. (ed.): Materials from the 1968 Regional Institutes sponsored by the American Occupational Therapy Association on the Evaluation Process. Final Report R.S.A.-T-68. American Occupational Therapy Association, New York, 1968.
7. Lerner, C., and Ross, G.: The Magazine Picture Collage: Development of an objective scoring system. Am. J. Occup. Ther. 31:156–161, 1977.
8. Hammer, op. cit., p. 5.
9. Mosey, op. cit., pp. 90–93.
10. Mosey, A. C.: Occupational Therapy: Theory and Practice. Medford, MA: Pothier Bros., 1968.
11. Arieti, S.: The Intrapsychic Self. New York: Basic Books, 1967, pp. 100–101.
12. Ibid., pp. 327–413.
13. King, L. J.: A sensory integrative approach to schizophrenia. Am. J. Occup. Ther. 28:529–536, 1974.

SECTION 5
Contexts or Settings for Treatment

There are three levels of mental health services: primary, secondary, and tertiary care. These must be part of any consideration of the contexts within which occupational therapists may function. The first, *primary care or prevention*, is an area that has only recently been formally addressed by mental health professionals. *Secondary care* is defined here as direct intervention in dysfunctional processes or disease. *Tertiary care* has the goal of maintenance of an optimum level of function within the limitations imposed by the disease or the client's environmental circumstances. Secondary and tertiary care have been the traditional concerns of mental health professionals.

Occupational therapists who work in psychiatry are involved in more innovative programs than can be described here—programs such as providing inservice education to law enforcement officers, working in industrial stress management settings, and developing community programs for the prevention of adolescent adjustment problems. The descriptions offered here are presented not as models, but rather as examples of current occupational therapy practice. References and resources are also provided for the reader who wishes to explore them in greater depth.

Primary Prevention

Primary prevention represents an aspect of mental health that is in one sense a "natural" for occupational therapists. Inherent in occupational therapy is a recognition that healthy growth experiences are important, and that the skillful and knowledgable application of activities can promote health. The occupational therapist is increasingly finding a role as both consultant and practitioner in assessing mental health needs and designing mental health programs, in a variety of nonmedical settings. Ellsworth and Rumbaugh and Jaffe are among those who describe their roles as consultants to community projects in which their skills were used on a broad base to develop programs of activities to promote health.[1,2] On a more specific basis, occupational therapists may function either within programs designed to help individuals to identify and reduce stress, or in crisis intervention programs. Ellsworth and Rumbaugh, for example, suggest that occupational therapy can have a direct service role within community programs of primary prevention of drug abuse by participating in volunteer training within the commu-

nity, practical parenting courses and mothers' study groups within the family, developmental screening, and organized youth activities for children. Occupational therapists who work with the severely disabled or the terminally ill have a major concern for the psychosocial adjustment of their clients and often have a clearly identified role in support programs for relatives and friends. It is apparent that occupational therapists can make a contribution in a number of areas in which they have only begun to be involved—child abuse prevention, effective parenting, women in transition, elder citizens' activity groups and social clubs.

Large Public Institutions

Large public institutions include state, county, and federal facilities and institutions run by the Veterans Administration. These hospitals, which evolved during the past 100 years, have provided care for great numbers of people who were unable to function in their homes and communities as a result of emotional problems or actual mental illness. By its nature, because of its being supported by public money, and because there were, until recently, few other kinds of services available, the large public hospital tended to become a catch-all for a wide range of society's problem people, not all of them mentally ill. Many of the large public hospitals were originally built some distance away from population centers. This may have reflected the prevailing attitude of fear that characterized public thinking about mental illness 50 to 100 years ago. The large public hospital usually spread over many acres of ground and incorporated services and functions to make it a fairly self-sufficient community. One may find a farm, stores, post office, laundry, one or more chapels, maintenance services, theater, recreation center, snack bar, medical surgical hospital, and a range of other facilities that make the large institution not unlike a small town.

In a great many of the large institutions, the number of trained professionals has been low. It is not unusual for a physician to have 100 or 200 patients assigned to him or her for care. The use of medications is extensive.

The large public institutions have been changing radically in recent years. Large numbers of patients who have been identified as "chronic" but not dangerous and perhaps capable of existing in the outside community have been discharged. Services within the institution now include components of primary, secondary, and tertiary care.

The stable population found today in the large public institution includes many severely and chronically disabled patients with schizophrenic diagnoses, organic brain syndromes, or senile psychoses. These patients are considered unable to manage to live outside the institution. Many such institutions have, in addition, special units for children, adolescents, drug or alcohol addiction problems, and court-committed cases. The acute care unit or services for newly admitted patients are generally short-term facilities in which screening is done, care is given to individuals during the acute phase of their illnesses, and every effort is made to prevent long-term hospitalization. Whenever possible, clients are referred to partial hospitalization programs or to community facilities or outpatient departments for continued care. All of these may or may not be on the grounds or part of the institution's programs.

Since the advent of psychopharmacology and the proliferation of outpatient and community services to the mentally ill, there has been a major overhauling of the large public institutions. States have approached their mental hospital systems in a variety of ways, but a central theme has been one of working toward decentralization, returning as many of the inpatients as possible to the community. This has meant, for many clients who had been hospitalized for a significant part of their lives, leaving the security of the institution to live in boarding homes or group living situations in the community. It is obvious that some major efforts have been needed to make adjustment possible. The large public hospitals have been leaders in the development of partial hospitalization programs and such projects as quarter-way or half-way houses and satellite clinics.

Treatment frames of reference in the large public institution are highly variable and, in some cases, would best be termed eclectic. Some sections of an institution may be developed around a behavior therapy frame of reference or "token economy"; others may follow a "reality therapy" model and rely heavily upon the development of a therapeutic community; many institutions have sections that are oriented to modified forms of the psychoanalytic frame of reference.

The occupational therapist has had an important role to play in the large public institution, and it has become increasingly important for the occupational therapist to articulate services with other members of a very complex treatment, maintenance, or rehabilitation team, which includes physicians (who may or may not be psychiatrically trained), nurses, psychiatric aides, social workers, psychologists, dietitians, rehabilitation workers, therapeutic recreators, work

adjustment therapists, art, music, dance, and education therapists, and volunteers. Frequently the occupational therapy department is part of a larger "Activities Therapy" or "Adjunctive Therapy" department, which includes the other activities oriented workers and professionals. The occupational therapy department may be quite large and may be staffed with a number of on-the-job trained aides or therapeutic workers. Because of the large number of clients to be treated, they are usually seen in groups, although treatment itself may be individually oriented.

Case Study*

Miss Agatha Simpson is 40 years old and has spent 23 years in the state hospital. She has a diagnosis of "schizophrenia/chronic undifferentiated type." She had a 12th grade education and worked briefly as a waitress and sales clerk prior to her hospitalization. Data collection in preparation for setting treatment goals in occupational therapy showed the following: flat affect, withdrawal from participation in activities, hostility toward other people, poor judgment, short attention span, little verbalization (mumbles), auditory hallucinations. She is right-handed, needs help in using the shower and in grooming but is independent in her dressing. She is oriented to place, person, and the year and month (not the day). She dresses in her own clothing, but is slightly disheveled, with food stains on her clothes. Her sensory integrative assessment showed the following: tactile defensiveness, difficulty in crossing the midline, hesitance in identifying body parts (trouble with touching her elbows), poor performance in motor planning, difficulty in assuming postures requiring crossing the hands across the midline, good visual memory and awareness of body parts. Her person drawing was complete. She did not know her own age (said that she was 56.)

Several of Miss Simpson's difficulties, such as hostility, problems with showering and self-care, may be influenced by the combined problems of tactile defensiveness, bilateral coordination problems, and difficulties with midline crossing.

During the first four treatment sessions, the occupational therapist will observe which types of sensory integrative stimulation will elicit positive responses from Miss Simpson.

* Prepared by Wilma Wiener and Nancy Nonini, Norristown State Hospital, Norristown, PA.

HALEY STATE HOSPITAL*

OCCUPATIONAL THERAPY ASSESSMENT

PATIENT: DOE, John
AGE: 30   *SEX:* Male
DIAGNOSIS: Paranoid Schizophrenic
ASSESSMENT DATE: 2/20/82

Presentation of Self:

John was cooperative when approached a second time for assessment. He presents as a somewhat disheveled, unshaven 30-year-old white male. Affect was slightly depressed and speech remained rambling and loose throughout the 45 minute session. Patient appeared confused and vague regarding his problems, stating reason for hospitalization was that he had "freaked out" because he was not able to find his girlfriend at the hospital. Reality testing is poor—patient denies having tried to hurt father prior to admission. Ability to perceive assets and limitations is poor and unrealistic—problem area was described as getting back together with Joanne (girlfriend). Strength cited was "I'm together." Patient does not appear to be reliable information source at this time.

Cognitive Skills:

John is able to utilize overt trial and error problem-solving. He works at opposite extremes—sometimes impulsively with little attention paid to detail in a careless haphazard manner. On the tile task he barely noticed the design and quickly began to assemble the tiles in a diagonal criss-cross pattern instead of a cross. (It should be noted that he had been given this task by another therapist on a previous admission—that design utilized a criss-cross pattern). However, perceptual inconsistencies cannot be ruled out. He was able to correct his mistakes when the sample was represented and with additional assistance from the therapist. On the second task, more difficult than the first, utilizing organizational skills and judgment, his cognitive difficulties became more apparent. He attempted to use a complicated system to center the square, drawing random dots on the paper. It was obvious from his continual rambling remarks that he was not only having difficulty organizing his thought processes, but decision making and judgment were decreased. His preoccupation with centering the square made it impossible for him to complete the task in the allotted time period, suggesting difficulty in stress situations. Patient is able to follow two-step concrete verbal directions.

Social Skills:

Patient's rambling, tangential speech is vague and loose. John had to be redirected to questioning. Social judgment is decreased—at one point when discussing recreational interests he became verbally hostile in a sexually explicit manner upon describing his exercise program. He appears to have difficulties interacting in a casual one-to-one relationship and is obsessed with finding a girlfriend.

Drive Object Skills:

Patient shows difficulty in setting goals and carrying them out in even simple concrete tasks due to cognitive dysfunction. He is unable to gain adequate need satisfaction from others due to decreased judgment and impaired reality testing. The possibilities of underlying hostility towards females and difficulties with sexual identity exist. Patient appears poorly motivated. He does not want to return to a work situation if he must make adjustments in his work style. (*i.e.,* following directions, working more quickly). His goals are vague and unrealistic for his abilities.

Summary of Functional Level:

Strengths:
1. Cooperative.
2. Oriented x 3.

3. Able to follow two-step concrete verbal directions.
4. Able to utilize overt trial and error problem-solving.
5. Reported recreational interests.
6. Has own apartment.

Weaknesses:
1. Difficulty channeling anger in an appropriate fashion.
2. Unreliable informant.
3. Poor A.D.L. skills.
4. Decreased cognitive functioning, memory, judgment, organizational skills, decision making.
5. Poor insight into problem areas.
6. Difficulty interacting in a casual one-to-one relationship, possible hostility towards females.
7. Decreased motivation; difficulty investing energy outside of self.
8. Difficulty setting goals and carrying them out.

Specific Skills & Interests:

Mostly solitary activities—playing guitar, writing poems, exercising.

Goal: Unspecific—"to use my mind in whatever capacity."

Vocational: Patient claims he held job 10 years ago at General Electric as a welder. No verification seen on chart.

Carole L. Pollack

Carole L. Pollack, B.S., OTR
Occupational Therapy Department

* Prepared by Carole Pollack, Haverford State Hospital.

Goals and Treatment Plan:

Short-term goals, Stage 1:
1. Reduce aversive responses to light touch. Method: use patient-controlled tactile stimulation through rubbing upper extremities with varied textured materials and lotion.
2. Decrease withdrawal as evidenced by increased time engaged in purposeful activities of up to 15 minutes per session. Method: encourage participation in activities of her choosing, activities which provide vestibular stimulation.

Short-term goals, Stage 2:
1. Increase attention span as evidenced by active, uninterrupted participation in simple gross motor tasks. Method: encourage and guide patient's participation in gross motor activities for progressively longer time periods as tolerated.
2. Decrease avoidance of midline crossing and increase bilateral coordination. Method:

encourage participation in vestibular activities which demand and elicit spontaneous adaptive responses.

Short-term goals, Stage 3:
1. Continue to increase attention span and improve midline crossing. Method: patient to engage in a series of graded cognitive, fine motor tasks.
2. Decrease hostility to other people. Method: patient to engage in familiar cognitive, fine motor tasks in a small group.

Long-term goal: Patient will enter the hospital sheltered workshop.
Time Frame: Two years. □

Evaluation and reporting procedures in many large public institutions are specified and standardized in accordance with a government agency. The occupational therapist may, in addition, develop and use a battery of tests and procedures in order to develop viable treatment plans. Any or all of the procedures described earlier in this chapter may be incorporated into the evaluation.

Common problems encountered in the large public hospital include the following: sensory integrative dysfunction; inability to manage self-care, personal hygiene and grooming, time, and activities of daily living; body image distortions; sexual identification problems, and problems with reality testing. One finds in the large public hospital such programs as groups oriented to cooking, grooming, shopping, exercise, gardening, and current events as well as gross motor and sensory integrative activities. Much of the activity of occupational therapy is currently oriented to the preparation of the patient for leaving the institution or for becoming as active as possible if leaving the institution is not feasible. The challenge has been to find ways to develop some degree of autonomy in people who have lived with none for a long time.

Private Hospitals

Private hospitals are generally concerned with treatment or secondary care, although many of them have established community programs geared either to primary prevention or to aftercare or maintenance (tertiary care).

There are different kinds of private hospitals for psychiatric care and treatment. In general there are hospitals that are staffed with psychiatrists and other professionals and geared to provide team-based services coordinated around clearly defined and shared goals of treatment. There are also hospitals that have been developed to provide a safe, pleasant "rest" for patients who are receiving private, individualized treatment from their psychiatrists, who are not, as a rule, part of the regular hospital staff. The role of the occupational therapist in each of these situations is different and these roles will be dealt with separately.

Private hospitals are expensive, so that their patients have tended to be, in general, from a segment of the population that is economically advantaged. Insurance coverage and such programs as Medicaid and Medicare have recently, however, made limited hospitalization in private hospitals possible for all people. Hospitalization periods tend to be short, up to ninety days, as compared with those for the large public hospital. Usually the problems treated are acute. Patients requiring longer hospitalization may be referred to other facilities, such as the large public hospital, or, whenever possible, to partial hospitalization facilities or community mental health centers. In general one sees far less of the long-term chroni-

cally institutionalized client in the private hospital than in the public hospital, but chronic, long-standing problems of adjustment are not uncommon.

The occupational therapist in a team-oriented hospital usually works with at least one psychiatrist, nurses, aides, social workers, psychologist, therapeutic recreation workers, and possibly a number of other activities therapists specializing in art, music, drama, dance, horticulture, and so forth. The size and diversity of the treatment team is dependent upon the size and orientation of the hospital. In smaller hospitals, the occupational therapist working with a staff of aides, therapeutic workers, and volunteers, may be responsible for all activity planning.

In the second type of hospital, if the occupational therapist is on the staff, the department may be charged with carrying out activities in all areas. Occupational therapy is, on one hand, less guided here because there is no treatment team structure. The range of activities and the extent to which occupational therapy is free to develop therapeutic programs is limited primarily by the occupational therapist's own creativity or by administrative policies. Occupational therapy evaluations and reports may or may not be valued, depending upon the orientation of the private psychiatrist. Often, the registered therapist serves as a consultant, not a regular staff member, to such hospitals. The primary goal then is to provide guidance and inservice education.

Fair Meadows Institute*

PATIENT: Doe, Jane

AGE: 30   SEX: Female

MARITAL STATUS: Divorced, 18 months

EDUCATION: 11th grade

ADMITTING DIAGNOSIS Depressive Neurosis
Mixed Personality Disorder
Continuous Alcohol Dependence

Final Diagnosis

Same as above.

This was the patient's first admission. Her length of stay in the hospital was 45 days.

Brief History

This mother of three children (aged 2, 5, and 7) worked until recently as a clerk in a department store. She has had a long history of dealing with feelings of anxiety and depression by

* Prepared by Jack Schweiker and staff, Fairmont Institute, Philadelphia, PA.

self-medicating and the use of alcohol. Her use of alcohol has precipitated problems in her marriage, work life, and family life. A sparse history of her marriage indicated that her husband of 7½ years was a heavy drinker who frequently abused her physically.

Status on Admission

Cooperative and alert, her speech was coherent and goal directed, without any loosening of association. In terms of affective status she had a depressed mood and admitted to thinking about suicide. Her judgment appeared to be fair. There were no evidences of delusions or hallucinations. She was oriented 3X. Her memory was intact and she seemed to be of above average intelligence. She stated that she was having "a bad anxiety attack" and that drinking was her "way out" but she realized that it was too much.

Assessment Information

Affective Problems: anxiety; withdrawal; feelings of guilt, depressed mood; feelings of inferiority; inability to express emotions; lack of confidence
Physical Problems: difficulty sleeping, lack of energy
Cognitive Problems: indecisiveness; inability to maintain attention
Self-Organization: poor judgment; poor self concept; projection of blame; denial
Behavior: passive-dependent; alcohol dependent

Hospital Goals

Short term:
1. Reduction in cognitive, affective, motivational, or somatic aspects of depression
2. Decrease anxiety
3. Reduction in self-defeating behavior

Long term: Reduction in drug and alcohol misuse
Discharge Plans: Participation in Alcoholics Anonymous; follow-up by psychiatrist at Fair Meadows Institute

Course of Treatment in Occupational Therapy

Ms. Doe was seen in occupational therapy sessions four times a week. She was involved in continuous long-term activities and participated in a time/leisure study group. At first she had difficulty talking and was passive and guarded. She had a low energy level and difficulty with any goal-directed behavior. She needed much support from the therapist to invest herself in any activity. She lacked confidence in her ability to succeed at any task, was disorganized, had difficulty making decisions, and was frightened to take even very small risks. She depended upon the therapist for decision-making and problem-solving. At times she seemed

overwhelmed and was easily frustrated when under stress. She showed little understanding of her values and needs and an inability to receive satisfaction from her environment.

Occupational Therapy Goals

Short-term goals: decrease social withdrawal; increase confidence; increase ability to approach tasks; decrease frustration; increase energy level
Long-term goals: increase recognition of needs and values and satisfaction and assertion of self; decrease passive behavior; increase ability to make decisions and take risks

Summary

Upon discharge, Ms. Doe had made substantial changes and showed marked improvement in the direction of the goals of both the hospital and of occupational therapy. Her organization and approach to tasks had improved, and she was able to identify and complete activities independently and successfully. She was able to explore and recognize past behavior patterns and had a better understanding of her values, needs, and of ways of gaining satisfaction from her environment. During the two weeks prior to discharge, her occupational therapy program involved exploring the local YMCA's special program for women on evenings and weekends with baby-sitting and children's activities provided. She began to use family swimming privileges and to attend three of the women's groups: assertiveness training, aerobic dancing, and an elementary course in business management. She also became first a group member, and later an advocate, for a community program developed to aid battered women. □

General Practice/General Hospital

It has been estimated that as many as 70% of patients who go to their physicians have significant emotional complaints.[3] Although only a few of these patients would be given formal psychiatric diagnoses, their emotional problems are important enough to warrant attention.[4] There is evidence to suggest that there are several kinds of associations between psychiatric and physical disorders, personality styles, and characteristic responses to stress.[5]

Occupational therapists may be called upon to treat individuals with combinations of major physical illness or dysfunction and associated psychiatric problems in a variety of contexts, including private practice, as consultants to primary care physicians, in home health agencies, and in the acute care general hospital. The depressions which follow major surgery or the diagnosis of terminal illness, the loss of a sense of reality following any extended period in an intensive care unit, and the adjustment to a long period of convalescence are only a few of the situations in which the knowledge and skills of psychiatric occupational therapy may be applied. The therapist in such situations is involved in both primary and secondary care.

The inpatient ward of a general hospital usually provides emergency or acute care and services to people whose problems have become of such an overwhelming nature that they are unable to continue to function. The patient may be referred from the medical or surgical units of the hospital or by a private physician, often after a precipitous or critical incident such as a suicide attempt. Length of stay in such a facility is usually quite short, often less than two or three weeks.

The inpatient psychiatric ward may be staffed with a dynamic psychiatric team, including psychiatrists, nurses, social workers, psychologist, and occupational therapists. Where this is true the team effort is primarily geared to two major goals: (1) evaluation so that relevant referrals can be made for continued treatment, and (2) provision of a therapeutic climate to provide for optimal rapid reconstitution on the part of the patient.

The kinds of evaluations used by occupational therapy depend upon the treatment frame of reference. Generally, however, occupational therapists use interviews, screening methods to determine organic problems, activity evaluations, and possibly some projective techniques.

Treatment methods are limited to short-term group and individual projects geared to objectives such as increasing reality testing, attention span, and the ability to organize. The understanding and participation of the patient in his or her program is vital, especially if total discharge is imminent.

In such centers, evaluation and reporting techniques used in occupational therapy need to be efficient and accurate as well as rapidly communicated and well coordinated with the efforts of the total staff.

Community Mental Health Centers

Satellite programs, aftercare centers, and community mental health centers have become extensive in terms of the kinds of services offered. Based in "catchment areas" of 75,000 to 200,000 in population, these centers have been developed to care for the mental health and mental retardation needs of the people as close to their homes as possible. The kinds of programs that have been incorporated into community mental

health centers include outpatient therapy, crisis intervention, emergency inpatient care, group homes, geriatric programs, therapeutic services to children and adolescents, addiction programs, and a variety of outreach services within the community. Community mental health centers are usually administered and staffed by both professional and lay mental health workers. They have boards of directors composed of community leaders. The community boards may serve as advisory or as governing bodies, and, in most instances, are very active in determining policies and staffing for the centers. Centers are often funded through federal and state sources.

Part of the client population is made up of formerly hospitalized individuals who have been discharged to live at home, in boarding homes, or in group homes. This group of individuals usually attends the center regularly for activities that have been designed primarily to help in adjustment to life outside the hospital.

The occupational therapist may work in several of the programs of the community mental health center. The teams with which he or she works include a psychiatrist, psychologist, social worker, nurse, other activity workers, and, most important, the members of the community. In a community-based service, the objectives of the occupational therapy programs must be geared to helping clients to function optimally in a non-institutional setting and may use community facilities such as neighborhood recreation centers, shopping areas, swimming pools, and ballparks. One innovative approach in community mental health has been to develop programs that are open to the "normal" population as well as to the designated clients. In this way, occupational therapy may get very much involved in preventive programs and health maintenance programs.

Important issues which may be addressed in such a setting include a client's lack of any sense of autonomy; lack of self-esteem; lack of ability to manage the ordinary demands of daily living including grooming, self-care, sense of time, and organization; lack of assertiveness; need for leisure time interests, habits, and pursuits; need for contact with other people in the community; and fears about jobs and money. See the accompanying example of an evaluation used in a community health center.

The occupational therapist and the community mental health center team are usually involved in preventive services to the public. Often, through counseling and through the use of activities, hospitalization may be avoided. The occupational therapist's concern in the use of activities here may be centered around helping the client to achieve the establishment of healthy patterns and balance in living, especially the ability to both pace himself or herself and to assess the need for help before it is too late.

OCCUPATIONAL THERAPY FUNCTIONAL EVALUATION*

Name _____ BSU # _____

Address _____ Telephone # _____

Initial Evaluation (date) _____ Reevaluation _____

A. Concept of Self

1. Activities of Daily Living:
   a. Care of Clothing
      _____ Is able to fold clothes
      _____ Is able to perform simple mending
      _____ Washes clothes by hand
      _____ Is able to use washer and dryer
   b. Care of Living Area:
      _____ Can dust
      _____ Can sweep with a broom
      _____ Operates a vacuum cleaner
      _____ Mops a floor
      _____ Dries dishes
      _____ Washes dishes
      _____ Can set the table with silverware, glass, and dishes
   c. Food Preparation:
      _____ Serves self food
      _____ Can prepare one dish or part of a meal
      _____ Can plan for and prepare a simple nutritious meal
      _____ Can plan nutritious meals for one week
      _____ Needs supervision when shopping for food
      _____ Can shop for food independently
   d. Standardized Evaluation of Living Skills:

2. Specific Skills and Interests:

3. Affect (specify):

4. Reality Orientation:
   Is oriented to the following items:
   _____ Day of week
   _____ Month
   _____ Date
   _____ Year
   _____ Next holiday
   _____ Client's home address
   _____ Name of Day Treatment Program
   _____ Location of Day Treatment Program
   _____ County of residence
   _____ State of residence
   _____ Name of President of U.S.A.
   _____ One current event

5. Need Satisfaction:
   _____ Feelings of self not being worthy of need satisfaction—unable to respond to therapist
   _____ Relies on therapist to satisfy his/her needs
   _____ Invests energy in another person, but emphasis is on self and what self can get
   _____ Feels satisfied by one-to-one peer give-and-take relationship
   _____ Needs may be met through cooperation in groups

6. Dependency:
   _____ Unable to sustain effort despite continued assistance
   _____ Is able to follow through only with continued encouragement
   _____ Needs some encouragement to follow through
   _____ Persists on own with task until completion

7. Ability to Organize Stimuli:
   _____ Is easily distracted—requires highly structured environment
   _____ Is distracted by external stimuli—can work in a structured environment
   _____ Is sometimes distracted by external stimuli—needs some structure
   _____ Is not easily distracted by external stimuli—needs very little structure

8. Maintains Focus and Attention on Program Activities:
   _____ Hardly ever
   _____ Occasionally
   _____ Approximately half the time
   _____ Frequently
   _____ Nearly always

9. Responsibility:
   _____ Client rejects all responsibility
   _____ Is unpredictable and hesitant
   _____ Therapist perceives needs; asks client to assume responsibility; client follows through with _____ without _____ assistance
   _____ Client perceives needs but has difficulty accepting responsibility
   _____ Client recognizes and accepts responsibility independently; can be depended on

10. Frustration Tolerance and Impulse Control:
    _____ Is apt to lose control, easily becomes angry
    _____ Tends to respond to frustration by withdrawal or anger
    _____ With support, can exercise appropriate control
    _____ Has appropriate emotional control, tolerates frustration without difficulty

11. Assertiveness:
    _____ Hardly ever
    _____ Occasionally
    _____ Approximately half the time
    _____ Frequently
    _____ Nearly always

B. Task Orientation

1. Learning:
   _____ Can imitate several familiar schemes, previously organized into a skill
   _____ Can expand a familiar skill
   _____ Can adapt a familiar skill
   _____ Can imitate new, unfamiliar schemes
   _____ Can imitate new, unfamiliar skills (series of schemes)
   _____ Can expand or adapt new skills

2. Ability to Follow Directions:
   OLD   NEW
   _____   _____ Needs to be physically assisted through motions of activity
   _____   _____ Requires specific step-by-step demonstrations, able to do _____ number of steps at a time
   _____   _____ Follows simple verbal instructions when accompanied by step-by-step demonstration
   _____   _____ Follows simple verbal instructions when accompanied by illustrations
   _____   _____ Follows simple verbal instructions of entire process when accompanied by illustrations
   _____   _____ Follows simple verbal instructions when accompanied by sample
   _____   _____ Follows simple verbal instructions
   _____   _____ Follows complex verbal instructions
   _____   _____ Follows written instructions

3. Decision Making:
   _____ Unable to make decisions
   _____ Relies on others for decisions
   _____ Hesitant—needs to check with others
   _____ Makes some decisions independently
   _____ Makes decisions with ease; capable of independent decision making

4. Validation of Judgments:
   _____ Judgments are unrealistic
   _____ Judgments are usually idiosyncratic and unrealistic—can maintain some control with therapist's guidance
   _____ With tasks that are personally filled with emotion a deterioration of judgment is exhibited
   _____ Seeks help to check judgments on tasks which are difficult
   _____ Can use cultural norms to assess acts realistically and objectively

5. Critical Evaluation:
   _____ Refuses to listen to critical evaluation or to recognize errors
   _____ Tends to avoid situations with error risks
   _____ Has difficulty tolerating error
   _____ Has difficulty tolerating error, degrading the value of the task
   _____ Accepts criticism, but withdraws
   _____ Accepts criticism, profits, but expresses hostility
   _____ Can tolerate making mistakes and profits from critical evaluation

6. Adheres to Rules and Regulations:
   _____ Hardly ever
   _____ Occasionally
   _____ Approximately half the time
   _____ Frequently
   _____ Nearly always

C. Concept of Others

1. Communication Skills:
   _____ Mute
   _____ Cannot communicate in organized, understandable way
   _____ Has great difficulty communicating thoughts, ideas, feelings
   _____ Communication is vague but understandable
   _____ Makes self understood, focusing on essential, appropriate factors

2. Group Skills:
   _____ Isolates self from group
   _____ Works on fringes of group; observes members; only therapist-client interaction
   _____ Does tasks while associates are present; interaction with associates is limited
   _____ Engages in a shared, give and take relationship with peers
   _____ Can work competitively

3. Relationship to the Therapist:
_____ Openly defiant of therapist
_____ Questions therapist
_____ Works with therapist appropri-
ately _____ inappropriately _____

D. Motor Skills

1. Motor Learning:
   Gross   *Fine*
   _____   _____ Has difficulty or cannot learn simple motor skills
   _____   _____ Is able to learn simple motor skills
   _____   _____ Is able to learn average motor skills
   _____   _____ Learns complex motor skills

2. Motor Performance:
   (a) Handedness: Right _____
                  Left _____
   (b) Performs gross motor tasks within *normal limits*:
   _____ Walking
   _____ Climbing stairs
   _____ Catching medium ball
   _____ Running
   _____ Sitting
   _____ Moving to music (rhythms)
   _____ Transfers object from one hand to another
   _____ Needs further evaluation
   (c) Performs fine motor tasks within *normal limits*
   _____ Palmar grasp (holding a pencil)
   _____ Pincer grasp (sewing)

_____ Combination grasp (crocheting)
_____ Finger dexterity (making paper flowers)

3. Physical Limitations:
_____ None
_____ Visual impairment (Specify)

_____ Hearing impairment (Specify)

E. Summary of Functioning:

1. Areas of Strength:

2. Areas of Weakness:

3. Significant Changes:

4. Client's Personal Goals:

5. O.T. Treatment Goals and Recommended Activities:

By _____
Title _____

* Christine Hischmann, Mary Goble, and Mary Rogosky, 1977. Revised 1981 for use in rural after-care program, out-patient.

Addiction Programs*

Centers for the inpatient treatment of those people addicted by drug and alcohol may be located in urban or rural settings, may be private and independent, or may be part of a larger institutional system such as a state hospital or community mental health center. Such centers may be staffed by psychiatrists, psychologists, social workers, nurses, counselors, activities therapists, educational counselors or teachers, and a criminal justice liaison person. An important feature of many addiction programs is that staff posi-

tions at different levels are made available to residents (clients) as they recover from their addiction. The incorporation of recovered addicts into staff positions is a valuable addition to the program and provides therapeutic incentives to the ex-addict.

Most inpatient, drug-free addiction programs are developed around a therapeutic community model that is psychologically oriented, promotes shared responsibilities, and gives a fair amount of freedom to the residents. Most of the therapeutic efforts of these programs are group oriented. Reality therapy, behavior modification, and developmental approaches are commonly used.

Usually the clients or residents in inpatient drug-

_____

* Betty B. Neves, OTR, furnished information on this topic.

free addiction programs are there voluntarily, although they have committed themselves to the program as an alternative to going to jail. Many initially enter the program with the intention of "drying out" so that they may return to their lives on the outside. They represent a wide range of population variables with regard to age, sex, intelligence, family background and socioeconomic status.

The one outstanding personality characteristic that has been observed by people who have worked closely with addicts is that they seem to have an exceedingly low level of self-esteem. Other characteristics include regression to oral (or earlier) levels of emotional need gratification, underlying depression, limited coping strategies, low frustration tolerance, and a need for intensity of experience. They appear to have some deficit in their ability to process information from the environment. This last deficit, coupled with an apparent need for intensity of experience, raises the question of perceptual or sensory integrative dysfunction. In fact, the apparent need of the addict to avoid responsibility and to flee reality, to lack trust, and to show impulsiveness may be symptomatic of some more basic problems. Motivating the client or resident to stay in treatment beyond the "drying out" period is a major concern for all the staff.

The occupational therapist working in an addiction program may use a number of evaluative techniques. Interviews, activities configurations, observation in activities and in other group settings, and consultation with other staff are the commonly used approaches. The use of sensory integrative methods of assessment may also prove useful.

The need for continual, completely honest and clear communication that is both verbal and nonverbal is essential in the therapist's relationship with the client. The therapist needs to be, in this area especially, aware of personal biases and values, honest about them, and willing to risk anger or embarrassment if in doing so a responsible concern for the client can be communicated.

In order to meet objectives for treatment in occupational therapy, activities should be designed to include provisions for success, developing reality testing, gaining social status, and experiencing clear, strong sensory input. The addict usually needs to develop ways to assess his or her own abilities and problems realistically, and also needs to learn ways to incorporate into his or her life style the advances made. Activities, especially crafts, sports, and games, lend themselves especially well to the kinds of deliberate and tangible confrontations with self needed to make this possible.

In the area of drug addiction, efforts are being expended on prevention programs. It has been found that activities are a most viable alternative to the use of drugs. Occupational therapy has an important contribution to make in programs designed to reach the early user or abuser of alcohol or drugs.

There is an overall sequence to team treatment goals for the addicted person, starting with admission into the program.* At each point in the process of rehabilitation, occupational therapy intervention is geared to working toward its specific goal. The initial, or detoxification, process may be a very painful and critical one for the client. Following detoxification, there is the need to restore the client's physical health. Often clients are not only physically worn down or malnourished as a result of their addiction, but they may also have sustained injuries as a result of accidents or fights. When this is the case, occupational therapy services may be called upon to help in the restoration of physical function. The restoration of emotional stability is the next goal for the client. During this period, occupational therapy needs to be geared to the presentation of reality in concrete terms, and to the accomplishment of activities in which success can be experienced. The restoration of physical health and emotional stability must take place before the client can be expected to be motivated to undertake the deeper and more difficult aspects of treatment. As the client becomes interested in rehabilitation, part of the motivation process will involve early planning for future goals, and this must be done so that the painful process of challenging destructive defenses, and developing insight will seem worthwhile. The process of building self-esteem must also begin. As the client approaches discharge from treatment, the occupational therapist, with the team, will need to be involved in facilitating the client's plans for the future.

Partial Hospitalization: Day and Evening Programs

Partial hospitalization programs make it possible for the client to continue to live in the community while receiving treatment on a regular basis. The client who is seen in partial hospitalization programs frequently has been transferred from an inpatient program. The day or evening program may be viewed as a step toward totally independent living. For others, the day or evening program represents an early intervention step, hopefully to prevent more extensive hospitalization.

Many clients who attend partial hospitalization programs are individuals whose adjustment to life

---

* Sequential Goal Model, adapted from program at Eagleville Hospital and Rehabilitation Center, Eagleville, PA.

has been somewhat marginal for some time. The task of a day program staff is one of providing rehabilitation. Most programs are group and milieu oriented. The team, consisting of psychiatrists, psychologists, social workers, nurses, occupational therapists, and therapeutic recreators, usually is closely knit and there may be much blending of roles. The total team, for example, may become trained and responsible for such activities as group therapy and psychodrama.

In settings such as these, the occupational therapist has a special responsibility for providing opportunities for the client to use activities in ways that are relevant to his or her life. Occupational therapy may, for example, develop activity groups built upon problems clients express they have in shopping, using transportation, and balancing their life routines. The occupational therapy model that incorporates the development of skills in managing time or balancing work, rest, play, and sleep in their life space is one which is valuable in the partial hospitalization program especially. Planning for the weekend and practicing skills for making friends may be special issues for these clients, as many of them experience great stress from long empty periods during which they have little sense of how to use the time. Having fun in a social setting may also be an important part of the program.

Evaluation procedures in day or evening programs tend to be informal, unless otherwise specified by the hospital or agency. Interview, observation in group activities, and consultation with other staff members are the most commonly used methods. The interest inventory and activities configuration or an adaptation of these methods have proven to be especially useful. Efforts are frequently made to deemphasize the medical or institutional atmosphere and to develop a sense of community which is normalized in its atmosphere.

Children's Centers

Children who are hospitalized in inpatient facilities usually are psychotic or so seriously hampered by neurotic or behavior disorders that it is impossible for them to function in a normal setting. Children with less severe problems may be seen in school settings or in outpatient facilities such as those connected with the community mental health center.

Children's inpatient facilities frequently are part of a larger institution, but they may be administered and staffed independently. The concept of team is of utmost importance because of the need for sick children to experience consistent treatment. Teams in children's psychiatric facilities consist of psychiatrists, nurses, child care workers, social workers, psychologists, teachers, and a variety of activities

therapists. Ideally there is round-the-clock planning for hospitalized children. Parent counseling and family therapy may be an important part of the total program.

Treatment frames of reference in children's centers are usually well defined; psychoanalytic, developmental, occupational behavior, sensory integration, and behavior modification may be used. The occupational therapist and all other workers in a children's setting, regardless of treatment frame of reference, need to have strong, basic knowledge of human development and the ability to work in close collaboration with other members of the team, especially with the child care workers and the teachers. The occupational therapist may or may not be involved in parent counseling or family treatment, but the addition of occupational therapy for these groups is seen as highly desirable.

Occupational therapy evaluation procedures, especially those related to sensory integration, developmental levels, and play, can be of diagnostic value. For purposes of treatment planning in occupational therapy, evaluation may be accomplished in the use of perceptual tests, activities evaluations, observation, and interview. The play inventory techniques described by Takata are especially useful.[6] Occupational therapy may offer play activities to provide sensory motor experience, interactions with others, and the development of basic cognitive skills.

Adolescent Programs

Special inpatient and outpatient treatment facilities have been developed to provide services to troubled or emotionally disturbed adolescents. Treatment teams in these programs are similar to those of children's facilities, and it is equally important for all staff members to have a strong knowledge base in human development.

The kinds of problems presented by adolescents range widely from full-blown psychotic schizophrenic and depressive reactions through neuroses, personality disorders, and mild to severe but transient situational episodes. The normal adolescent world has its special symbols and important objects, different from those of childhood or adulthood, and even the psychotic adolescent needs to have these symbols and objects. The skill of the therapist may well be in knowing how to incorporate the activities that are common to adolescence into projects that meet emotional and cognitive developmental needs of a much earlier period.

The Adolescent Role Assessment, a semistructured interview developed by Maureen Black, helps the therapist to focus on the developmental strengths and weaknesses of adolescents, as these are man-

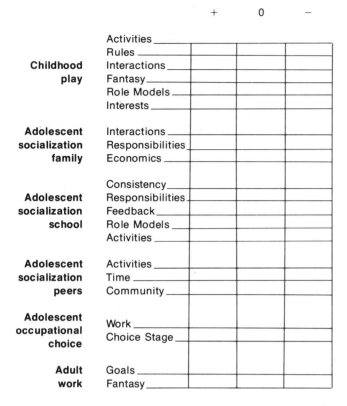

		+	0	−
Childhood play	Activities			
	Rules			
	Interactions			
	Fantasy			
	Role Models			
	Interests			
Adolescent socialization family	Interactions			
	Responsibilities			
	Economics			
Adolescent socialization school	Consistency			
	Responsibilities			
	Feedback			
	Role Models			
	Activities			
Adolescent socialization peers	Activities			
	Time			
	Community			
Adolescent occupational choice	Work			
	Choice Stage			
Adult work	Goals			
	Fantasy			

Figure 19-5. Adolescent role assessment scoring. (Black, M. M.: Adolescent role assessment. Reprinted with the permission of The American Occupational Therapy Association, Inc., Copyright 1976, American Journal of Occupational Therapy, No 2, p. 79)

ifested in the maturation of their growing understanding of role expectations.[7] The interview is one which is conducted in casual dialogue. Its findings provide a guide to therapists in working with clients to identify issues to address in treatment programs.

Figure 19-5 is the summary scoring sheet of the areas covered. The entire interview is listed in the reference.

Geriatric Programs

Many kinds of programs have been designed to meet the needs of the geriatric population. The occupational therapist with special knowledge and skills in geropsychiatry has an important contribution to make in these programs.

There are community based programs, which serve the function of helping the elderly to maintain and improve their abilities to live productively in society. These programs reach clients who have never been hospitalized or treated for psychiatric disorders but who, as they have grown older, have experienced the debilitating effects of decreasing sensory function and other effects of the aging process and have become less able to cope with the demands of everyday

living. The role of the occupational therapist in a community geriatric center is clearly one of providing preventive services. The occupational therapist who works in one of these centers may be involved cooperatively with many different kinds of people. Centers may be part of the outreach program of a church, a settlement house, a special housing project or apartment for the aging, or a school system. The personnel connected with these agencies may be deeply invested in the success of their programs. The range of activities that evolves out of such programs is very wide and may be limited only by financial factors and the ingenuity of the leaders (staff or clients). Musical groups, crafts boutiques, and even small business services are not beyond the possibilities, especially since the major goal is to provide the elderly with opportunities to develop and maintain their fullest sense of productivity and capability.

Inpatient programs for elderly psychotic clients are usually part of a large institution. Many of these clients are people who have been long hospitalized with chronic psychiatric conditions and have grown old living in the institution. Others have developed psychoses as a result of illness, stress, or organic deterioration in the process of aging.

The staffing for such programs usually includes physicians, nurses, social workers, volunteers, and activity workers, including occupational therapists, with psychological services consulting. Where the clients are infirm or physically ill there is a heavy weighting in favor of nursing services.

Occupational therapy can make a vital contribution in several ways to these clients. The reality orientation which is provided through involvement in activities is much needed. Sensory input activities such as working with fragrant or colorful objects, feeling textures, and tasting good food are the elements of some basic activities designed to help the client to maintain contact with the world. Other kinds of activities, dependent upon the client's physical condition and level of contact, might include discussion groups, cooking groups, preparations for special events like a party or community outing, exercise sessions, and folk dancing.

Home Treatment

Occupational therapists are beginning to provide services to clients in the home setting for psychiatric problems. It has, however, been a practice of some occupational therapists working within a hospital or partial hospitalization program to begin to explore with clients the home and community settings from which they come and to which they will return. This has been of great value in helping the occupational therapist know more clearly the demands that may be made upon the clients away from the treatment setting. It thus becomes easier for the occupational therapist to help to plan relevant activities for each client.

Watanabe describes four concepts as being critical to consider in the psychiatric home treatment process: (1) life space, (2) mastery, (3) life tasks, and (4) responsibility.[8] These represent long-term targets around which short-term goals and short-term occupational therapy tasks could be developed in the home treatment setting.

When an occupational therapist goes into the home of the client, the occupational therapist is in the client's territory. The occupational therapist's skills in observation and interviewing the client and other significant people, such as family members, close neighbors, or the local grocer, are critical. There is probably no more directly beneficial way to conduct treatment for some clients than in their own homes where their own objects, rituals, and routines can be observed and worked with, provided these things are not so emotionally charged as to contraindicate treatment in that setting at that particular time.

The home treatment team usually consists of nurses, social workers, and physical therapists in addition to the occupational therapist, with the physician as a referral source and consultant. The occupational therapist must be able to provide clear reports that promote coordination of effort.

Frequently the home treatment occupational therapist who is seeing a case for physical dysfunction encounters significant emotional overlays or full-blown mental illness. The occupational therapist then needs to call upon a psychiatric knowledge base to provide the needed services. Home treatment is discussed in detail in Chapters 36 and 37.

Correctional Institutions

One of society's on-going dilemmas is the extent to which it is possible to plan and carry out programs of rehabilitation for convicted criminals. This is an area of practice which may develop more fully in time. Much depends upon the direction of public attitudes and policies with regard to the prison system, and upon the sophistication of knowledge and techniques for identifying, on an individual basis, the individuals who might show potential for rehabilitation. Occupational therapists who have explored the prison systems have frequently felt that it would be possible to apply occupational therapy evaluation, goal setting, and programs to help inmates to develop living skills that might prevent recidivism. The few programs that have been described have relied heavily upon working with prison officials and staff and have focused on reality-oriented approaches to work, leisure, and self-care.[9,10,11]

References

1. Ellsworth, P. D., and Rumbaugh, J. H.: Community organization and planning consultation. Occupational Therapy in Mental Health: A Journal of Psychosocial Practice and Research 1:33–55, Spring, 1980.
2. Jaffe, E.: The role of the occupational therapist as a community consultant: Primary prevention in mental health programming. Occupational Therapy in Mental Health: A Journal of Psychosocial Practice and Research 1:47–62, Summer, 1980.
3. Daniels, R. S.: Is psychiatry a "primary medical care specialty?" Psychiatric Opinion 13:34–36, 1976.
4. Shepherd, M.: The prevalence and distribution of psychiatric illness in general practice. Journal of the Royal College of General Practice 23:16–19, 1973.
5. Granville-Grossman, K.: The relationship between physical and psychiatric disorder. In Maxwell H. (ed.): Integrated Medicine: The Human Approach. Bristol, England: John Wright and Sons, Ltd., 1976, pp. 78–86.
6. Takata, N.: The play history. Am. J. Occup. Ther. 23:314–318, 1969.
7. Black, M. M.: Adolescent role assessment. Am. J. Occup. Ther. 30:73–79, 1976.
8. Watanabe, S.: Four concepts basic to the occupational therapy process. Am. J. Occup. Ther. 22:439–445, 1968.
9. Davis, J., and Freides, C.: Exploring occupational therapy in Philadelphia prisons. Unpublished manuscript. Philadelphia: Temple University, 1981.
10. Platt, N. P., Martell, D. L., and Clements, P. A.: Level I field placement at a federal correctional institution. Am. J. Occup. Ther. 31:385–387, 1977.
11. Penner, D. A.: Correctional institutions: An overview. Am. J. Occup. Ther. 22:517–524, 1978.

Bibliography
Primary Prevention

Aguilera, D. C., and Messick, J. M.: Crisis Intervention Theory and Methodology. St. Louis: C. V. Mosby Co., 1978.
Ethridge, D. A.: The management view of the future of occupational therapy in mental health. Am. J. Occup. Ther. 30:623–628, 1976.
Finn, G.: The occupational therapist in preventive programs. Am. J. Occup. Ther. 26:59–66, 1972.
Freeman, A. M., Sack, R. L., Berger, P. A.: Psychiatry for the Primary Care Physician. Baltimore: Williams and Wilkins Co., 1979.

Hospital

Allard, I.: A study of the effects of occupational therapy upon perceptual inaccuracies of the schizophrenic. Am. J. Occup. Ther. 23:115, 1969.
Bachrach, L. L.: A conceptual approach to deinstitutionalization. Hospital and Community Psychiatry 29:9, 1978.
Casanova, J. S., and Ferber, J.: Comprehensive evaluation of living skills. Am. J. Occup. Ther. 30:143–147, 1976.

Gray, M.: Effects of hospitalization on work-play behavior. Am. J. Occup. Ther. 26:180–185, 1972.

Heine, D. B.: Daily living group. Am. J. Occup. Ther. 29:628–630, 1975.

King, L. J.: A sensory integrative approach to schizophrenia. Am. J. Occup. Ther. 28:529–536, 1974.

Kolodner, E.: Neighborhood extension of activity therapy. Am. J. Occup. Ther. 27:381–383, 1973.

Levy, L.: Movement therapy for psychiatric patients. Am. J. Occup. Ther. 28:354, 1974.

Mann, W. C.: A quarterway house for adult psychiatric patients. Am. J. Occup. Ther. 30:646–647, 1976.

General Practice/General Hospital

Corry, S., Sebastian, V., and Mosey, A. C.: Acute short-term treatment in psychiatry. Am. J. Occup. Ther. 28:401–406, 1974.

Holmes, C., and Bauer, W.: Establishing an occupational therapy department in a community hospital. Am. J. Occup. Ther. 24:219–226, 1970.

Hyman, M., and Metzker, J. R.: Occupational therapy in an emergency psychiatric setting. Am. J. Occup. Ther. 24:280–283, 1970.

McDonald, S. S.: Looking in on Gates-10. Pa. Gazette 75:32–36, 1977.

Community Mental Health Centers

Auerbach, E.: Community involvement: The Bernal Heights Ladies' Club. Am. J. Occup. Ther. 28:272, 1974.

Baum, C. M.: Independent living: A critical role for occupational therapy. Am. J. Occup. Ther. 34:12, 1980.

Becker, R. E., and Page, M.: Psychotherapeutically oriented rehabilitation in chronic mental illness. Am. J. Occup. Ther. 27:34–38, 1973.

Broekema, M. C., Danz, K. H., and Schloemer, C. U.: Occupational therapy in a community afercare program. Am. J. Occup. Ther. 29:22–27, 1975.

Cromwell, F. S., and Kielhofner, G.: An educational strategy for occupational therapy community service. Am. J. Occup. Ther. 30:629–633, 1976.

Johnson, T. P., Vinnicombe, B. J., Merrill, G. W.: The independent living skills evaluation. Occupational Therapy In Mental Health: A Journal of Psychosocial Practice and Research 1:5–18, Summer, 1980.

Laukaran, V.: Toward a model of occupational therapy for community health. Am. J. Occup. Ther. 31:71–74, 1977.

Webb, L.: The therapeutic social club. Am. J. Occup. Ther. 27:81–84, 1973.

Addiction Programs

De Angelis, G. G.: Theoretical and clinical approaches to the treatment of adolescent drug addiction. Am. J. Occup. Ther. 30:87–93, 1976.

Dohner, V. A.: Alternatives to drugs—a new approach to drug education. J. Drug Ed. 2:3–22, 1972.

Freudenberger, H. J.: The therapeutic community revisited. Am. J. Drug Alcohol Abuse 3:33–50, 1976.

Jones, K. L., Shainberg, L. W., and Byer, C. O.: Drugs and Alcohol. New York: Harper and Row Publishers, 1969.

Reese, C. C.: Forced treatment of the adolescent drug abuser. Am. J. Occup. Ther. 28:540–545, 1974.

Rinella, V.: Rehabilitation or bust: The impact of criminal justice system referrals on the treatment of drug addicts and alcoholics in a therapeutic community. Am. J. Drug Alcohol Abuse 3:181–184, 1976.

Sendy, E., Shorgz, V., and Alkane, H. (eds.): Developments in the Field of Drug Abuse. Proceedings 1974 of the National Association for the Prevention of Addiction in Narcotics, Cambridge, MA: Schenkman Publishing Co., 1975.

Slobetz, F. W.: The role of occupational therapy in heroin detoxification. Am. J. Occup. Ther. 24:340–346, 1970.

Partial Hospitalization

Deacon, S., Dunning, E., and Dease, R.: A job clinic for psychotic clients in remission. Am. J. Occup. Ther. 28:144–147, 1974.

Kuenstler, G.: A planning group for psychiatric outpatients. Am. J. Occup. Ther. 30:634–639, 1976.

Linn, M. W., Caffey, E. M., Klett, C. J., Hogarty, G. S., and Lamb, H. R.: Day treatment and psychotropic drugs in the aftercare of schizophrenic patients. Archives of General Psychiatry 36, 1978.

Schechter, L.: Occupational therapy in a psychiatric day hospital. Am. J. Occup. Ther. 28:151–153, 1974.

Solberg, N. A., and Chueh, W.: Performance in occupational therapy as a predictor of successful prevocational training. Am. J. Occup. Ther. 30:481–486, 1976.

West, O. L., Casarino, J. P., Dibella, G., and Gross, R. A.: Partial hospitalization: Guidelines for standards. Psychiatric Annals 10:3, 1980.

Children's Centers

Ayres, A. J., and Heskett, W.: Sensory integrative dysfunction in a young schizophrenic girl. J. Autism Childhood Schizophrenia 2:174–181, 1972.

Barker, P., and Muir, A. M.: The role of occupational therapy in a children's in-patient psychiatric unit. Am. J. Occup. Ther. 23:431–436, 1969.

DiLeo, J. H.: Children's Drawings as Diagnostic Aids. New York: Brunner Mazel, 1973.

Fahl, M. A.: Emotionally disturbed children: Effects of cooperative and competitive activity on peer interaction. Am. J. Occup. Ther. 24:31–33, 1970.

Florey, L.: An approach to play and play development. Am. J. Occup. Ther. 25:275–284, 1971.

Herman, B. E.: A sensory integrative approach to the psychotic child. Occupational Therapy in Mental Health: A Journal of Psychosocial Practice and Research 1:57–68, Spring, 1980.

Hindmarsh, W. A.: Play diagnosis and play therapy. Am. J. Occup. Ther. 33:11, 1979.

Hurff, J.: Play skills inventory: A competency monitoring tool for the ten-year old. Am. J. Occup. Ther. 34:10, 1980.

Hurff, J.: A play skills inventory. In Reilly, M. (ed.): Play as Exploratory Learning. Beverly Hills: Sage Publications, 1974, pp. 247–266.

Kohler, E. S.: The effect of activity/environment on emotionally disturbed children. Am. J. Occup. Ther. 34:7, 1980.

Knox, S.: A play scale. In Reilly, M. (ed.).: Play as Exploratory Learning. Beverly Hills: Sage Publications, 1974, pp. 247–266.

Llorens, L.: Facilitating growth and development: The promise of occupational therapy. Am. J. Occup. Ther. 24:93–101, 1970.

Llorens, L.: Occupational therapy in community child health. Am. J. Occup. Ther. 25:335–339, 1971.

Llorens, L.: The effects of stress on growth and development. Am. J. Occup. Ther. 28:82–86, 1974.

Llorens, L., et al.: The effects of a CPM training approach on children with behavior maladjustment. Am. J. Occup. Ther. 23:502–512, 1969.

Loveland, C. A., and Little, V. L.: The occupational therapist in the juvenile correctional system. Am. J. Occup. Ther. 28:537–539, 1974.

Masagatani, G.: Hand-gesturing behavior in psychotic children. Am. J. Occup. Ther. 27:24–29, 1973.

Michelman, S.: The importance of creative play. Am. J. Occup. Ther. 25:285–290, 1971.

Shaefer, C. E. (ed.): Therapeutic Uses of Child's Play. New York: Jason Aronson, Inc., 1976.

Takata, N.: Play as prescription. In Reilly, M. (ed.): Play as Exploratory Learning. Beverly Hills: Sage Publishing Co., 1974, pp. 209–246.

Takata, N.: The play milieu. Am. J. Occup. Ther. 25:281–284, 1971.

Adolescent Programs

Caplan, G., and Lebovici, S.: Adolescence: Psychosocial Perspectives. New York: Basic Books, 1969.

Jodrell, R. D., and Sanson-Fisher, R.: An experiment involving disturbed adolescent girls. Am. J. Occup. Ther. 29:620–629, 1975.

Mosey, A. C.: The treatment of pathological distortion of body image. Am. J. Occup. Ther. 23:413–416, 1969.

Pezzuti, L.: An exploration of adolescent feminine and occupational behavior development. Am. J. Occup. Ther. 33:84, 1979.

Shannon, P. D.: Occupational choice: Decision-making play. In Reilly, M. (ed.): Play as Exploratory Learning. Beverly Hills: Sage Publishing Co., 1974, pp. 285–313.

Geriatric Programs

Anderson, E.: A continuity of care plan for long-term patients. Am. J. Public Health 5:2, 1964.

Butler, R., and Lewis, N.: Aging and Mental Health: Positive Psychological Approaches. St. Louis: C. V. Mosby Co., 1975.

Deichman, E., and O'Kane, C.: Working with the Elderly—A Training Manual. Buffalo, NY: D.O.K. Publishing, Inc., 1975.

Hasselkus, B. R.: Aging and the human nervous system. Am. J. Occup. Ther. 28:16–21, 1974.

Hasselkus, B. R., and Kiernat, J. M.: Independent living for the elderly. Am. J. Occup. Ther. 27:181–188, 1973.

Hasselkus, B. R., and Safrit, M. J.: Measurement in occupational therapy. Am. J. Occup. Ther. 30:429–436, 1976.

Kiernat, J. M.: The use of life review activity with confused nursing home residents. Am. J. Occup. Ther. 33:306–310, 1979.

Leslie, D. K., and McLure, J. W.: Exercises for the Elderly. Iowa City: University of Iowa Graphic Series, 1975.

Lewis, S.: A patient-determined approach within a state hospital. Gerontologist 15:146–149, 1973.

Lewis, S., Paire, J., Stravinskas, L., and Kilgour, W.: Occupational therapy in a geropsychiatric unit. Osteopathic Annals 6:56–62, 1978.

Lewis, S.: The Mature Years: A Geriatric Occupational Therapy Text. Thorofare, N.J.: Charles B. Slack, 1979.

Lewis, S.: Occupational therapy and geriatrics: Assuming a leadership position. Am. J. Occup. Ther. 29:459, 1975.

Murphy, E. C.: Organic brain syndrome. Paper prepared for Geriatric Care Symposium, Norristown State Hospital, Norristown, PA, April, 1976.

Nystrom, E.: The elderly. Am. J. Occup. Ther. 28:337–345, 1974.

Parachek, J. F.: Parachek Geriatric Rating Scale. (Written in cooperation with L. J. King.) Scottsdale, AZ: Greenroom Publications, 1976.

Shafer, A. L.: Providing supportive services to the elderly. Am. J. Occup. Ther. 25:423–427, 1971.

Weg, R.: The changing physiology of aging. Am. J. Occup. Ther. 27:213–217, 1973.

Correctional Institutions

Paulson, C. P.: Juvenile delinquency and occupational choice. Am. J. Occup. Ther. 34:517–524, 1978.

Home Treatment

Rozycka, M. F.: The maintenance of community mental health with the family as the unit of treatment. Unpublished manuscript.

SECTION 6
Summary and Challenge for the Future

As theory and practice in psychiatric occupational therapy are traced through the years, a pattern emerges that indicates that the profession has maintained certain consistent awareness and concerns. The therapist has sought to promote in clients a sense of wholeness as well as the ability to adapt and to function as fully as possible. To do this, the therapist has tried to maintain a level of awareness and sophistication that keeps pace with growing knowledge and advancing technology, and with the expanding consciousness that has characterized both health care and society in general.

Allying itself with psychiatry, occupational therapy has been subject to the excitement, dilemmas, and ambiguities that have characterized the development of psychiatric practice. As psychiatry has grown and become more diversified, it has had to become more responsive to and interested in the changes, diversification, and growth that have taken place in the social sciences. Changes in society have been close to revolutionary. These changes have forced psychiatry and all of its related professions and services, including occupational therapy, to develop new alliances and new perspectives.

There has been a need to develop broader concepts of health and illness and to accommodate to greater demands for preventive services, in addition to providing for treatment, maintenance, and rehabilitation. The move has been away from institutional care and toward diverse community programs. Creativity and frustration tolerance have been challenged as fiscal constraints make it difficult to accomplish what needs to be done. Psychiatric practice and occupational therapy seem to be in a period of disequilibrium, out of which the development of new levels of understanding and adaptation could grow.

To date, the psychiatric occupational therapist has had only embryonic conceptual models and frames of reference to address some of the issues that present themselves. Nevertheless, issues have been there to be addressed. What about the great numbers of chronic institutionalized ex-patients who have been discharged to live in the obscurity of boardinghouse rooms, nursing homes, bus stations, and the streets? What about the runaway adolescent who seems unable to find stability in life? What about the segment of an increasingly aged population, which is neither sick nor well, but which might be helped to continue to be productive, contributing members of society? What about the effects of more leisure time? What

about the agony of unemployment and its stress on the individual? What about the increase in computer technology and the devaluation of the work ethic? What about the effects of increasing consciousness of racism, sexism, agism, and the rights of the handicapped? What role do we have in helping our clients to understand sexuality? Should we accommodate to new approaches or fads in popular mental health self-help? How do we work with other activities therapy professionals? How can we maintain our commitment and work within the constraints imposed by some standards that are well meaning but seem to be depersonalizing to the client? How do we deal with increasingly complex concerns for accountability and legality? How can we be involved productively in the important developments in biogenetic and biochemical research? How can we relate what we know about human adaptation and activities to these developments? Are we ready to discard some of our long cherished assumptions if we learn that they are not scientifically accurate?

These are only a few of the issues that call upon us to explore, study, think, adapt, grow and act as a true profession. Some of them are critical and some even painful. Some of them are truly exciting.

If one were to characterize the trends, directions, and, in fact, major goals of psychiatric occupational therapy in recent years, one would find three important themes. First, with the increasing sense of urgency that emanates from newly acquired knowledge, there has been the need to establish strong scientifically based support for the apparent therapeutic effects of our practice. Second, there have been significant efforts to promote an identity and public visibility for occupational therapy as a distinct profession. Third, there has been a continuing need to examine the models which best represent our bases for practice whether they are medical, sociological, or biopsychosocial. These concerns are pervasive and must be considered not only in practice but in the arenas of education and research as well. The future appears to promise opportunities and challenges for the occupational therapist who works in the area of mental health. Perhaps the most demanding of the challenges will be to achieve true professionalism in a way that will most effectively serve our ultimate purpose, to be able to help our clients to achieve the highest possible quality of life and function.

There is no way that a single chapter on occupational therapy practice in psychiatry and mental

Psychiatry and Mental Health **331**

health can begin to provide the depth or the breadth of the knowledge base that is required to function within even one of its frames of reference or one of its contexts. Rather, it is hoped that this chapter, its references and bibliographies, will present a challenge and some resources for working toward refining the knowledge and defining the practice presented here.

General Bibliography

Alexander, F., and Selesnick, S.: The History of Psychiatry. New York: Harper & Row Publishers, 1966.

Allen, C.: The performance status examination. Paper presented at the Annual Conference of the American Occupational Therapy Association, San Francisco, 1976.

Arieti, S.: The Intrapsychic Self. New York: Basic Books, 1967.

Ayres, A. J.: Sensory Integration and Learning Disorders. Los Angeles: Western Psychological Services, 1972.

Ayres, A. J., and Heskett, W.: Sensory integrative dysfunction in a young schizophrenic girl. J. Autism Childhood Schizophrenia 2:174–181, 1972.

Azima, H., and Azima, F. J.: Outline of a dynamic theory of occupational therapy. Am. J. Occup. Ther. 23:215, 1959.

Bachrach, L. L.: A conceptual approach to deinstitutionalization. Hospital and Community Psychiatry 29:9, 1978.

Beck, A.: Cognitive Therapy and The Emotional Disorders. New York: International Universities Press, 1976.

Bendroth, S., and Southam, M.: Objective evaluation of projective material. Am. J. Occup. Ther. 27:78–80, 1973.

Benjamin, A.: The Helping Interview. Boston: Houghton Mifflin Co., 1974.

Bloomer, J.: The consumer of therapy in mental health. Am. J. Occup. Ther. 32:10, 1978.

Brayman, S., Kirby, T. F., Misenheimer, A. M., Short, M. J.: Comprehensive occupational therapy evaluation scale. Am. J. Occup. Ther. 30:137–141, 1976.

Briggs, A. K., Duncombe, L. W., Howe, M. C., and Schwartzberg, S. L.: Case Simulations in Psychosocial Occupational Therapy. Philadelphia: F. A. Davis, 1979.

Bruner, J.: On voluntary action and its hierarchical structure. In Koestler, A., and Smithies, J. R. (eds.): Beyond Reductionism. Boston: Beacon Press, 1969.

Burke, J. P.: A clinical perspective on motivation: Pawn vs. origin. Am. J. Occup. Ther. 31:254–258, 1977.

Carroll, J. F. X.: Staff burnout as a form of ecological dysfunction. Contemporary Drug Problems. Summer, 1979, pp. 207–225.

Casanova, J., and Ferber, J.: Comprehensive Evaluation of Living Skills. Am. J. Occup. Ther. 30:143–147, 1976.

Coleman, J. C.: Life stress and maladaptive behavior. Am. J. Occup. Ther. 27:129–179, 1973.

Conte, J. R., and Conte, W. R.: The use of conceptual models in occupational therapy. Am. J. Occup. Ther. 31:262–264, 1977.

Cousins, N.: Anatomy of an Illness. New York: W. W. Norton Co., 1979.

Cutting, D.: A review of projective techniques. In Mazer, J. (ed.): Materials from the 1968 Regional Institutes sponsored by the American Occupational Therapy Association on the Evaluation Process. Final Report R.S.A.-123-T-68. New York: American Occupational Therapy Association, 1968.

Cynkin, S.: Occupational Therapy: Toward Health Through Activities. Boston: Little, Brown and Co., 1979.

Diasio, K.: Occupational therapy in mental health: a time of challenge. Occupational Therapy in Mental Health 1:1–10, Spring, 1980.

Diasio, K., and Moyer, E.: On psychosocial assessment. Occupational Therapy in Mental Health 1:1–3, Summer, 1980.

Doukas, P. H.: A brief discussion of general principles of drug action and certain agents affecting the central nervous system. Unpublished Manuscript. Philadelphia: Temple University, 1981.

Dubovsky, S. L., Weissberg, M. P.: Clinical Psychiatry in Primary Care. Baltimore: Williams and Wilkins Co., 1978.

DuCette, J., and Wolk, S.: Cognitive and motivational correlates of generalized expectancies for control. J. Personality Social Psychol. 26:420–426, 1973.

Ellsworth, P. D., and Colman, A. D.: The application of operant conditioning principles to work group experience. Am. J. Occup. Ther. 23:495–501, 1969.

Ethridge, D. A.: The management view of the future of occupational therapy in mental health. Am. J. Occup. Ther. 30:623–628, 1976.

Fidler, G. S., and Fidler, J. W.: Doing and becoming: Purposeful action and self-actualization. Am. J. Occup. Ther. 32:305–310, 1978.

Fidler, G. S.: From crafts to competence. Am. J. Occup. Ther. 35:568–673, 1981.

Fidler, G. S.: Professional or nonprofessional. In 2001 A.D. Rockville, Md.: American Occupational Therapy Association, 1979.

Fidler, G. S.: The Task-oriented group as a context for treatment. Am. J. Occup. Ther. 23:1, 1969.

Florey, L.: An approach to play and play development. Am. J. Occup. Ther. 25:275–284, 1969.

Florey, L.: Intrinsic motivation: The dynamics of occupational therapy theory. Am. J. Occup. Ther. 23:319–322, 1969.

Frank, J.: The therapeutic use of self. Am. J. Occup. Ther. 12:4, 1958.

Freedman, A. M., and Kaplan, H. I. (eds.): The Child—His Psychological and Cultural Development, Vol. II, New York: Atheneum, 1972.

Freedman, A. M., Kaplan, H. I., and Sadock, B. J.: Modern Synopsis of Comprehensive Textbook of Psychiatry/II. Baltimore: Williams & Wilkins Co., 1976.

Freud, S.: The Ego and Mechanisms of Defense. New York: International Universities Press, 1946.

Gillette, N.: Occupational therapy and mental health. In Willard, H. S., and Spackman, C. S. (eds.): Occupational Therapy, ed. 4. Philadelphia: J. B. Lippincott Co., 1971.

Glasser, W.: Reality Therapy. New York: Harper and Row Publishers, 1965.

Goldstein, A. P., Gershaw, N. J., and Spafkin, R. P.: Struc-

332 *Implementation of Occupational Therapy*

tured learning therapy: Development and evaluation. Am. J. Occup. Ther. 33:154–158, 1979.

Goldstein, M. J., Baker, B. L., and Jamison, K. R.: Abnormal Psychology: Experiences, Origins and Interventions. Boston: Little, Brown and Co., 1980.

Goodwin, D. W., and Guze, S. B.: Psychiatric Diagnosis. New York: Oxford University Press, 1979.

Gregory, I., and Smeltzer, D. J.: Psychiatry. Boston: Little, Brown and Co., 1977.

Haas, L. J.: Occupational Therapy for the Mentally and Nervously Ill. Milwaukee, WI: Bruce Publishing Co., 1925.

Hall, E. T.: The Hidden Dimension. Garden City: Doubleday and Co., 1966.

Hemphill, B. J.: Mental Health Evaluations Used in Occupational Therapy. Thorofare, N.J.: Charles B. Slack, 1981.

Hightower-Vandamm, M.: Take three giant steps—backwards. Am. J. Occup. Ther. 35:8, 1981.

Kielhofner, G.: Temporal adaptation. Am. J. Occup. Ther. 31:235–242, 1977.

King, L. J.: Creative caring. Am. J. Occup. Ther. 34:522–534, 1980.

King, L. J.: Toward a science of adaptive responses. Am. J. Occup. Ther. 32:429–444, 1978.

Kolodner, E.: Neighborhood extension of activity therapy. Am. J. Occup. Ther. 27:381–383, 1973.

Laukaran, V. H.: Toward a model of occupational therapy for community health. Am. J. Occup. Ther. 31:71–72, 1977.

Lawn, E. C., and O'Kane, C. P.: Psychosocial symbols as communication media. Am. J. Occup. Ther. 27:30–33, 1973.

Levy, L.: Movement therapy for psychiatric patients. Am. J. Occup. Ther. 28:354, 1974.

Line, J.: Case method as a scientific form of clinical thinking. Am. J. Occup. Ther. 23:308, 1969.

Llorens, L.: Projective techniques in occupational therapy. Am. J. Occup. Ther. 21:4, 1967.

Matsutsuyu, J.: The interest check list. Am. J. Occup. Ther. 23:323–328, 1969.

Matsutsuyu, J.: Occupational behavior: A perspective on work and play. Am. J. Occup. Ther. 25:291–294, 1971.

Mazer, J., and Mosey, A. C.: Toward an integrated theory of occupational therapy. Am. J. Occup. Ther. 22:451–456, 1968.

McClelland, D. C., Atkinson, J. W., and Lowell, E. L.: The Achievement Motive. New York: Appleton-Century-Crofts, 1953.

Meyer, A.: The philosophy of occupational therapy. Arch. Occup. Ther. 1:5, 1922.

Millon, T.: Theories of Psychopathology and Personality. Philadelphia: W. B. Saunders Co., 1973.

Moore, J.: Behavior, bias and the limbic system. Am. J. Occup. Ther. 30:11–19, 1976.

Moorhead, L.: The occupational history. Am. J. Occup. Ther. 23:331, 1969.

Mosey, A. C.: An alternative: The biopsychosocial model. Am. J. Occup. Ther. 28:137–143, 1974.

Mosey, A. C.: A model for occupational therapy. Occup. Ther. in Mental Health 1:11–31, Spring, 1980.

Mosey, A. C.: The concept and use of developmental groups. Am. J. Occup. Ther. 24:273–275, 1970.

Neville, A.: Temporal adaptation: Application with short-term psychiatric patients. Am. J. Occup. Ther. 24:193–196, 1980.

Overbaugh, T. E., and Bucher, B.: Use of operant conditioning to improve behavior of a severely deteriorated psychotic. Am. J. Occup. Ther. 24:423–427, 1970.

Piaget, J.: Play, Dreams and Imitation in Children. New York: W. W. Norton & Co., 1962.

Piaget, J.: The Construction of Reality in the Child. New York: Basic Books, 1954.

Piaget, J.: The Origins of Intelligence in Children. New York: International Universities Press, 1952.

Pines, A., and Maslach, C.: Characteristics of staff burnout in mental health settings. Hospital and Community Psychiatry 29:4, 1978.

Purtilo, R.: Health Professional/Patient Interaction. Philadelphia: W. B. Saunders, 1978.

Reilly, M.: A psychiatric occupational therapy program as a teaching model. Am. J. Occup. Ther. 20:66–67, 1966.

Reilly, M.: Occupational therapy can be one of the greatest ideas of twentieth century medicine. Am. J. Occup. Ther. 16:1, 1962.

Reilly, M. (ed.): Play as Exploratory Learning. Beverly Hills: Sage Publishing Co., 1974.

Reilly, M.: The educational process. Am. J. Occup. Ther. 23:299–307, 1969.

Robinson, A. L.: Play, the arena for acquisition of rules for competent behavior. Am. J. Occup. Ther. 31:248–253, 1977.

Rogers, C.: Freedom to Learn. Columbus: Charles E. Merrill, 1969.

Searles, H.: The Nonhuman Environment. New York: International Universities Press, 1960.

Shannon, P. D.: The derailment of occupational therapy. Am. J. Occup. Ther. 31:229–230, 1977.

Sieg, K.: Applying the behavioral model to the occupational therapy model. Am. J. Occup. Ther. 28:421–428, 1974.

Smith, D.: Psychotropic drugs and their effect on the occupational therapy process. Presented at the Mental Health Specialty Section Institute, Wilmington, Delaware, August, 1981.

Smith, M. B.: Competence and adaptation: A perspective on therapeutic ends and means. Am. J. Occup. Ther. 28:11, 1974.

Stein, F.: Three facets of psychiatric occupational therapy models for research. Am. J. Occup. Ther. 23:491–494, 1969.

Van Allen, R., and Loeber, R.: Work assessment of psychiatric patients: A critical review of published scales. Can. J. Behavioral Science 4:101–117, 1972.

Watts, F. N.: Modification of employment handicaps of psychiatric patients by behavioral methods. Am. J. Occup. Ther. 30:487–490, 1976.

Watanabe, S.: Four concepts basic to the occupational therapy process. Am. J. Occup. Ther. 30:487–490, 1968.

Watanabe, S.: The activities configuration. In Mazer, J. (ed.): Materials from the 1968 Regional Institutes sponsored by the American Occupational Therapy Association on the Evaluation process. Final Report, New York: American Occupational Therapy Association, 1968.

Wheelis, A.: How People Change. New York: Harper and Row, 1979.

White, R. W.: Competence and the growth of personality. In Masserman, J. (ed.): The Ego. New York: Grune and Stratton, 1967.

White, R. W.: Motivation reconsidered: The concept of competence. Psycholog. Rev. 66:297–333, 1959.

Wolk, S. and DuCette, J.: The moderating effect of locus of control on achievement motivation. J. Personality 41:59–70, 1973.

Acknowledgments

Appreciation is expressed to all the patients, colleagues, and students who, over the years, have contributed to my learning. Special thanks to Christine Hischmann of the Tunkhannock Counseling Service, Doris Kaplan, Wilma Wiener, Nancy Nonini, and the O.T. staff of the Norristown State Hospital, Carol Tengdin, Carole Pollack, and the O.T. staff of the Haverford State Hospital, and Jack Schweiker and the O.T. staff of Fairmount Institute, for providing illustrative materials; to Claudia Allen, Gail Fidler, and Lorna J. King for the challenge, stimulation, and encouragement they have given over the years, and to Jennifer S. Tiffany, for her continuing moral support and editorial help.

CHAPTER 20

Mental Retardation   *Reba M. Sebelist*

Sam is a 17-year-old male who demonstrates symptoms of mental retardation,[1] His parents were told by social service agencies staff members, physicians, and well-meaning friends to care for his physical needs but not to expect much mental progress. Not being really sure what the term "mentally retarded" meant, Sam's parents decided to keep him at home rather than to institutionalize him as recommended. Siblings were expected to help care for him and to give in to all his whims—a truly one-sided arrangement.

The lack of guidance, assistance, and respite care have produced a family filled with confusion and guilt because of both their lack of ability to meet Sam's obvious needs and their concern for his future care.

Being nonverbal and incontinent, Sam evidences his frustrations by kicking out and biting himself when thwarted in both physical and mental actions, refusing to attempt new or unfamiliar activities, and meeting his ego needs through voluntarily eating only a few favored foods. Lack of educational opportunities has limited his world a great deal, with most of his learning coming from general television viewing. Contacts with persons other than his family are rare because of his unpredictable behavior. This results in a small confined world for Sam and a restriction of human contact and opportunity for the whole family. □

This is a composite case history with mostly negative connotations, yet one which would probably be matched in reality anywhere in the country. Although this is a nation of skills and opportunities, that promises rights for all, this is not true for all citizens. The physically and mentally handicapped have been the recipients of much physical and verbal abuse. Mentally retarded individuals have been locked in bedrooms by families who were confused about what to do, full of guilt regarding "why did this happen to us," upset by their inability to cope, and ashamed. They feared that relatives, neighbors, or friends might discover their supposed disgrace.

As demeaning as this physical abuse might be to the mentally retarded, verbal abuse is much more destructive of human worth. Terms such as "dummy," "moron," "low-grade," and "kids" have a much more dehumanizing effect. After hearing these designations over the years, individuals begin to refer to themselves and their peers in the same

335

manner—a self-perpetuating process of breaking down their sense of worth.

Well-meaning groups have attempted to change labels from early ones like "idiot" or "imbecile" to "trainable" or "educable." These new, supposedly complimentary terms are now being fought by organizations such as the National Association for Retarded Citizens (NARC), which changed its name from the National Association for Retarded Children. Throughout this chapter, the retarded are referred to as individuals who have feelings, rights, obligations, and ego needs.

Changing of designation is a long and slow but positive experience. Society is being forced to observe the change evidenced by retarded individuals when positive acceptance is given to them upon completion of success experiences. Accomplishing this goal is not a matter of simply "watering down" everyday procedures but rather constructing ones that are at the correct levels of development and skill for the individuals concerned. Nothing succeeds like success, as the cliché states—the retarded are people who respond to success experiences.

Definition

What is mental retardation? The *Random House Dictionary of the English Language* refers one to the term "mental deficiency," which it defines as "lack of some mental power or powers associated with normal intellectual development resulting in an inability of the individual to function fully or adequately in everyday life."[2] This definition does not differ significantly from the one developed in 1973 by the American Association on Mental Deficiency (AAMD): "Mental retardation refers to significantly subaverage general intellectual functioning existing concurrently with deficits in adaptive behavior and manifested during the developmental period."[3]

It is apparent from the definitions that the mentally retarded do not demonstrate only one area of difficulty but do, indeed, manifest an interaction of multiple factors among which are sociocultural, psychological, and physical influences. A more extensive discussion of the AAMD definition with emphasis on the effect of the various factors is available in *Occupational Therapy for Mentally Retarded Children*.[4]

Therapy for Mentally Retarded Children—Mental Retardation versus Mental Illness

Frequently the public does not comprehend the difference between mental retardation and mental ill-

Table 20-1 *Differences Between Mental Retardation and Mental Illness*

Mental retardation	Mental illness
Primary defect in intellect	Intellect relatively unimpaired
Usually oriented in time and place	Difficulty with time and place orientation
Not curable, long term	Often significant cure possible
May not differ in aptitude, interests, and feelings	Cluster of behaviors differing from normal

ness. Some very basic differences are indicated in Table 20-1.

Incidence

The people known as mentally retarded comprise approximately 3% of any given population. The greatest number of these individuals demonstrate symptoms at birth or shortly thereafter. The remaining, acquired retardates, are mentally retarded as a result of problems occurring after the neonatal period.

Within this 3% there is a further percentage breakdown based on the individual functioning level. Those considered to be profoundly retarded comprise $1^5/_{10}$%, severely retarded $3^5/_{10}$%, moderately retarded 6%, and mildly retarded 89%.[5]

Using 3% of a *given* population as a point of reference it would be simple to deny need for individualized special programming. However, when placed into perspective as 3% of the *total* population, a very large number of individuals emerge who require aid in meeting particular needs.

Historical Perspective

An historical review provides an understanding of the specialty area of mental retardation as well as the motivating forces of those currently involved with planning and demanding accountability.

History tells us that in early times the mentally retarded were ignored, received little or no care, or were placed in the woods to fend for themselves or die. Life for the average person was short and living arduous; hence it was extremely difficult to support those who were different and required extra care. Another reason for the desertion and persecution of these individuals is that they were thought to be possessed by demons.

During the Middle Ages the role of the court jester was usually filled by a retarded individual. Observation of art of the time shows individuals now diagnosed as having Down's syndrome filling the role. Frequently, when these individuals lived with their families, they filled the role of "village idiot." Those who fill the role today run errands, carry messages, and so forth for a small tip but, more importantly, in order to gain social acceptance and a sense of self-worth.

Various religious orders became so distressed with the lack of physical care, the ridicule, and the abuse given the retarded that they built sheltered communities. Unfortunately, along with the kindly intended isolation, a sense of hopelessness grew. No change was envisioned. Good care and shelter were provided, but there was little mental stimulation; this in turn caused more regression and deterioration.

In the 1800s, Jean Itard, a physician who worked with the deaf, became involved with a boy about 12 years of age who had been captured in the forest of Aveyron, France.[6] The lad had been diagnosed as severely retarded by Pinel, an associate of Itard. Feeling that intellectual performance and potential could be affected by environmental stimulation and opportunity, Itard began working with sensorimotor techniques to achieve this goal. Initially he began working with Victor (his name for the young man) through the sense of hearing. After occluding visual stimuli he bombarded Victor with auditory stimuli and required from him an acceptable response. Next he required discrimination of types of noises, proceeding afterwards to verbal clues. As soon as possible, the blindfold was removed, but Victor would frequently request its use to rule out extraneous visual distractions. Itard concluded this probably was an attempt by Victor to reduce visual stimuli from his most frequently used, and highly sophisticated sense. When Victor was able to respond to emotions such as anger, sadness, and happiness in vocalizations, Itard proceeded to the sense of touch. Following a similar procedure he then proceeded to the senses of smell and taste. This was a very promising sequence of training but one which was soon to be discarded only to be resumed in the latter part of the 1900s. Itard worked with Victor for five years, and although gains were made by this previously animalistic "Wild Boy of Aveyron," they were not sufficient for him to fit into the "dandified" Paris society; Itard felt he had failed. He did indeed fail if we use the goal of fitting into that society as a criterion; nonetheless, his greatest contribution was to effect attitudinal change regarding the mentally retarded.

Seguin, a student of Itard, elaborated upon Itard's work and developed what he called the "physiological method" of training. After coming to the United States, Seguin became a prime mover in the opening of residential facilities such as Fernald in Massachusetts and Germantown (now Elwyn) in Pennsylvania. His involvement led to the establishment of an organization, now the American Association on Mental Deficiency (AAMD).

As with most specialty areas, unqualified persons promised cures that they could not effect, since mental retardation is not a curable illness but a condition. Many felt that if the condition could not be cured, time, money, and energy expended were wasted. As a result, these unqualified persons caused a reversal in feelings regarding the potential of the mentally retarded and negated the work of Itard and Seguin, with a resultant return to the sense of hopelessness.

This attitude of futility continued with the development of larger residential facilities mostly in isolated areas. Society was convincing itself that it was meeting the needs of the mentally retarded by assuring them care for their basic physical needs, while at the same time showing little concern for psychosocial and mental needs.

This sheltering and "protective" care continued for many years. By the end of World War II emphasis shifted, and programming was demanded by the NARC to meet the needs of all retarded individuals regardless of age, thereby permitting the recognition of the adult population. Organizations such as AAMD had functioned to assist the professionals serving the mentally retarded but did not hold themselves responsible for defining and justifying the service provided. Now, however, for the first time, professionals were being held accountable for both resultant behavioral change in clients and the utilization of funds.

Following lengthy litigation between the Commonwealth of Pennsylvania and parents, regarding the availability of educational opportunities for the mentally retarded, a Right to Education Consent Agreement was implemented in 1973.[7] This guarantees educational opportunities for all mentally and physically handicapped to an age of 21 years. This was indeed a major accomplishment for the parents, who were supported in the action by the Pennsylvania Association for Retarded Citizens (PARC), an affiliate of NARC. Many other states utilized this Agreement as a model in legal actions for defining and providing educational and theapeutic programs.

Public Law 94-142, The Education For All Handicapped Children Act, was passed by the federal government in 1975. The major effect of this act on occupational therapy has been that all special education programs were to have physical or occupational therapists available, either on their staffs or as consultants, by September 1977.

A positive change has now been seen in the role of training centers. Funds had not always been available to provide personnel to effect change. Society had been content to have the retarded isolated or institutionalized to recieve mostly custodial care. Professionals had not assumed responsibility for preparation to work with the mentally retarded. Pressure from organizations such as NARC, along with federal and state regulations, have forced accountability by staff. They, in turn, have demanded and are receiving more efficient and appropriate training from colleges, universities, and professional schools, which are producing staff members less hesitant to assume responsibility for education and training.

Etiology

The AAMD definition of mental retardation refers to causation as occurring during the developmental periods of the life cycle. Most frequently this is associated with an interruption in the sequence of one of three time frames, prenatal, perinatal(neonatal), or postnatal. Each stage may have its own particular etiological component but may also include a causation crossing all three periods, thus demonstrating the multiplicity of factors involved with mental retardation (see Table 20-2). Only a sampling of causation is identified here; more comprehensive information may be investigated in *Birth Defects Compendium, Atlas of Mental Retardation,* and *Mental Retardation.*[8,9,10]

Methods of Classification

Intelligence Quotient

For many years the only method used to designate the functioning level of the retarded was the measurement of intellectual skills. The evaluator would utilize instruments and issue an IQ score. These scores have both positive and negative aspects. The skilled evaluator is a valued program team member. Conversely, an inexperienced evaluator can do irreparable damage.

The IQ score with a descriptive statement frequently would influence the amount of effort expended on an individual. It would then remain on the record permanently. Staff members with large case loads would have to set priorities. An individual who scored 40 to 45 would most often be chosen for participation in a program before one who scored 20 to 25. Little thought was given to motivation, previous program exposure, or plateauing. The individual with the low score might be motivated and ready for change. It is not only unfair but also unrealistic and

Table 20-2 *Causation of Mental Retardation and Developmental Period of Occurrence*

Causation	Prenatal	Perinatal	Postnatal
Infection	X	X	X
Trauma	X	X	X
Genetic Disorders	X		
Drugs or Intoxication	X	X	X
Prematurity		X	
Low Birth Weight		X	
Anoxia	X	X	X
Parental Age and Health	X		
Sensory Deprivation		X	X
Cultural Deprivation		X	X

weak programming to base decisions on IQ evaluations only.

A skilled evaluator, who looks at the total person, the physical abilities and limitations, verbal or nonverbal communicative state, and so forth, and then chooses an evaluation instrument that is appropriate, can do invaluable work. This type of evaluator elicits responses that produce a higher functioning level and aids the treatment team in developmentally designed programming.

Many states require that a numerical IQ score be given. This information is useful for record keeping, statistics, and research but is not in itself meaningful for the goal-directed team.

Medical Diagnosis or Causation

The World Health Organization (WHO) has been concerned with obtaining uniform information for international sharing. WHO feels this process would clarify communication in addition to encouraging sharing for improvement of international health concerns.

In the United States, to implement the request of WHO, the International Classification of Diseases has been utilized by the medical team in an attempt to classify mental retardation according to etiology or causation.

Initially a number from 310 to 315, based on intellectual functioning according to the Revised Stanford-Binet Tests of Intelligence Forms L and M, is assigned: 310 for borderline, 311 for mild, 312 for moderate, 313 for severe, and 314 for profound retardation. The 315 designation is for those who have not been assigned a specific functioning level but who demonstrate behaviors associated with retardation.

Following this number is a fourth digit signifying a clinical subcategory based on etiology: .0 following infection and intoxication, .1 following trauma or physical agent, .2 with disorders of metabolism, growth, or nutrition, .3 associated with gross brain disease (postnatal), .4 associated with diseases and conditions resulting from unknown prenatal influence, .5 with chromosomal abnormality, .6 associated with prematurity, .7 following major psychiatric disorder, .8 with psychosocial (environmental) deprivation, .9 with other (and unspecified) conditions. There may come to be a fifth and sixth digit listed as a means of further pinpointing causation.

Hence, for example, the numerical designation 314.5 indicates that an individual is profoundly retarded as a result of chromosomal abnormality. The greatest value of this type of classification is the ease of comprehension and research usage. This system does, however, remove the human element while social agencies and families are attempting through legal maneuverings to give human dignity to the mentally retarded.

Information including numerical designations desired by the mental retardation section of the Inernational Classification of Diseases is available in the *Diagnostic and Statistical Manual of Mental Disorders* (DSM-II).[11]

It is desirable to know the etiological factors, but this information is not essential for program planning. Combining the two classifications provides information regarding the IQ and the etiological factors but does not indicate what the individual is capable of doing, and thus should not be used in isolation as a determinant for training.

Education

A frequently-used classification method is one that was designed for use by educators. Terms such as life support, dependent, trainable, and educable are assigned. These terms are meaningful to those who use them daily but are relatively useless to the general population.

The use of case histories for providing relevant information has been frustrating because the focus in the past has been one of describing what has been done and includes neither past nor present performance levels of the individual. The use of the educational terms also reinforces in most instances the same lack of information.

Adaptive Behavior Level

The AAMD definition refers to impairment in adaptive behavior as being demonstrable in the mentally retarded. As early as 1955, Sloan and Birch began defining these behaviors.[12] A Monograph Supplement to the *American Journal of Mental Deficiency* pre-

pared by Heber gives four levels of behavior with the following three appropriate age groupings.[13] Descriptive paragraphs are given for Levels 1, 2, 3, and 4, with Level 4 referring to maximal ability and vocational adequacy. Useful as this information was, it still was not an adequate system of classification. Thus, it was updated in 1973 with age level delineation of skills in areas such as activities of daily living, communication, physical, social, self-motivation, and occupation.[14] This method now offers quick reference, with information indicating at what level on the developmental continuum the individual is functioning. It also provides a possible recommendation for setting achievable goals.

In 1974, the AAMD issued a revision of the Adaptive Behavior Scale.[15] This revision has a more comprehensive method of evaluating adaptive behavior and will be discussed more fully in the Assessment segment.

Composite Classification

Finally, a compilation of information that is meaningful is evolving. From the generic term of mental retardation it is possible to progress through the use of demonstrable IQ score, etiological factors with indications of possible progressive deteriorating conditions, educators' designation, and conclude with adaptive behavioral levels. A combination of all these factors is not only desirable but essential for designing a program to meet the needs of the individual.

Assessment

As with all aspects of programming for the mentally retarded, assessment must be a combined effort. Some well-staffed centers are implementing a decentralized system of management, which can be an asset for evaluating abilities and limitations. A group of experienced professionals is charged with the responsibility of devising composite evaluative measures affecting the full range of activities existing at the center. This composite evaluation device is administered by either the professional services staff or by other qualified evaluators working in the unit. The results of the testing are shared with the combined staff working with the involved individual.

Not only is the more structured and formal assessment utilized, but also the professional services staff meets with the direct care staff to learn the individual's level of response in the residential unit, and, with representatives of other program staff, to ascertain behaviors, gains, regressions, or plateauing.

In addition, the professional service staff observes each individual in a variety of program experiences for on-site evaluation and completion of an all-inclusive assessment.

This sophisticated level of assessment will not be possible in all centers because of size of staff and assigned multiple responsibilities. However, a complete goal-oriented training program cannot exist without evaluative measurements, for, if no initial or reevaluative information is available, change cannot be measured. However there continue to be programs in which change is recorded only through periodic subjective progress notes without an initial assessment having been performed.

Regardless of the sophistication of the assessment team or the materials used, the most important factor is the relevance of the instruments used for measuring the desired results. As the use of a standardized test written in English is unfair to a Spanish-speaking person so, also, is one for the mentally retarded that is not level appropriate. After defining the purpose of a specific assessment and the goals to be achieved, the instrument with the greatest potential for determining the functional level of the individual is chosen and administered.

There is a controversy regarding where assessments should be done. Valid arguments can be presented to substantiate various points of view. Concerns include questions of where the activity is usually done, the discomfort of the individual being evaluated in a strange setting, the distractibility of the individual, and so on. Just as it is true that most people function better in a familiar environment, it also follows that the distractions of that same area might affect performance. The professional doing the assessment must make the decision regarding the location, time of day, and family members present when choosing the optimal setting.

A representative listing of some instruments having demonstrated their potential usefulness with the mentally retarded follows. Although the list is incomplete, it is presented to illustrate the scope of available formal instruments. With most mentally retarded individuals, the number of areas to be assessed is such that one or more program areas may be involved in doing the evaluations that are peculiar to the contribution of their disciplines. A more comprehensive description of each of these instruments and their validity and reliability can be found in *The Eighth Mental Measurement Yearbook*, edited by Buros.[16] With all screening devices it is essential to remember that they are only as useful as the skill of the evaluator in comprehending the behaviors of the mentally retarded.

Many occupational therapy departments devise evaluation forms to meet the requirements of their service. The tool can be as simple or as complex as desired but should elicit such information as physical status, mental functioning level, and adaptive behavioral level. Other information contained is dependent on the age level served, the type of program, and the relationship of the department to other program services. It is suggested that an instrument based on the type described by Currie is most useful.[17] This type of instrument evaluates neuromuscular status, perceptual-motor abilities, activities of daily living, and performance abilities.

Many therapists use evaluative instruments from the following listing.

Intelligence and Developmental Scales

BAYLEY SCALES OF INFANT DEVELOPMENT. Devised for use with infants from 2 to 30 months of age, this instrument has a mental scale, motor scale, and an infant behavior record. It does not predict potential abilities but does establish an infant's current status in relation to others of the same age. The instrument aids in recognition and diagnosis of sensory and neurological defects as well as emotional distress or disturbance. It is standardized and has good reliability.

DENVER DEVELOPMENTAL SCREENING TEST. This is a screening device for children from 2 weeks to 6 years of age. Four sections evaluate gross motor, fine motor-adaptive, communication, and personal-social development. The score sheet with its key gives the average age by which each skill should be attained. In addition, the score sheet provides columns for reevaluation, thus producing a quick composite reference. This is a practical, efficient evaluative tool.

PEABODY PICTURE VOCABULARY TEST. This instrument was devised for use with persons aged 2½ to 18 years. The individual responds to verbal clues by indicating the correct picture from a choice of four. Negative features of this instrument are that directions are given in English, thus making it invalid for persons who speak other languages. It does not take colloquialisms into account. A very useful instrument for nonverbal individuals, it only requires pointing to the correct picture. The motorically involved can also be evaluated as the test pictures are of a good size and are well-separated on the page. The positive aspects of this test outweigh its negative features.

STANFORD-BINET INTELLIGENCE SCALE (IQ). This very old instrument was devised for use with individuals aged 2 years or older. The current third revision was published in 1960 and combines items from Forms L and M to become the Revised Version Form L-M. This utilization of the better items is felt to produce a more valid instrument. The instrument relies heavily on verbal ability. It requires the use of six different items from a possible seven for each age level. Although this tool has good validity, it does not adequately evaluate older severely-retarded individuals.

WECHSLER INTELLIGENCE SCALE FOR CHILDREN. A stable general purpose scale, this instrument was devised for use with individuals from 5 to 15 years of age. From the composite of twelve subtests, information is accumulated for verbal, performance, and full scale scores. The division of items in this scale is based on content rather than level of difficulty. Some evaluators consider this the reason why the scale is easy to administer as well as successful in gaining responses from children. Individually administered, this instrument is valid in measuring immediate mental functioning.

ILLINOIS TEST OF PSYCHOLINGUISTIC ABILITIES. The recommended age range for use of this instrument is 2 to 10 years. In the development of this tool, the original purpose was to produce a device to be used as a diagnostic tool for analyzing intellectual deficits in the learning disabled and mentally retarded. Nine subtests evaluate communication performance in decoding, association, and encoding; levels of language organization; and channels of input and output of language. Although there are areas needing some revision, this instrument has served the purpose of diagnosing learning difficulties. A practical, valid test, it can be a valuable tool.

GOODENOUGH-HARRIS DRAWING TEST. The age range of this test is 3 to 15 years. This updating of the Draw-a-Man test presents an opportunity to use a quick, nonthreatening instrument that frequently evokes useful verbal comments while the individual is completing the task. Of vital importance in the use of this instrument is the *purpose* for the use. As a result of motoric difficulties and impaired mental functioning the retarded individual responds not only as a definite individual but also as one who has obvious aberrance. Recognizing these limitations, the evaluator must know how to administer the test and be skilled in the use of the information it evokes.

Adaptive Behavior Scales

VINELAND SOCIAL MATURITY SCALE. This instrument has been widely used although no true standardization has been done. Results are based on the experience of the developer. An important feature of this instrument is that the information comes from a general population sample. Because of the subjective

nature of this test, the relationship between the evaluator and the individual being tested may have either a "halo" or negative effect on scoring. It provides a useful broad evaluation of adaptive behaviors.

ADAPTIVE BEHAVIOR SCALE. This instrument was published by the American Association on Mental Deficiency in 1969 and is composed of two scales, one for ages 3 to 12 and the other for ages 13 and older. The tool was developed for use with the mentally retarded and emotionally maladjusted.

The scale devised for adults, 13 years and older, measures behaviors in the areas of independent functioning, physical development, economic activity, language development, number and time concept, occupation-domestic, occupation-general, self-direction, responsibilities, and socialization in Part One. Part Two evaluates factors such as violent and destructive behavior, antisocial behavior, rebellious behavior, untrustworthy behavior, withdrawal, stereotyped behavior, and odd mannerisms, inappropriate interpersonal manners, unacceptable vocal habits, self-abusive behavior, hyperactive tendencies, sexually aberrant behavior, and psychological disturbances. Since many of the behaviors listed have more than one item to be evaluated, the final score totals the assigned point values from each item.

This is a broad scale and when utilized presents a global view of the individual. The scale is a well-constructed and easily administered tool that has much to offer in assessment of easily discernible areas for habilitation training.

An updated revision of this scale was published by the AAMD in 1974. This edition tends to be more refined and, with increased data collection, should evidence greater validity and reliability. The Profile Summary makes it possible to study a composite survey of the individual's behavioral changes. Careful use of different colors in plotting scores would produce a meaningful and valuable record of the individual over a period of time.

Perceptual Motor Instruments

MARIANNE FROSTIG DEVELOPMENTAL TEST OF VISUAL PERCEPTION, THIRD EDITION. The age range recommended for this test is 3 to 8 years. Measuring visual perceptual skills in five areas, the instrument contributes valuable data to the clinical team. The global scores have reasonable reliability.

Although this tool is a good instrument, the value of its use with the mentally retarded is limited to individuals with higher levels of functioning. Low scores are not necessarily an indication to start perceptual training but might rather indicate that the instrument was not the most appropriate one for testing the individual.

THE PURDUE PERCEPTUAL MOTOR SURVEY. This tool was designed for use with children 6 to 10 years of age and aids in identification of children lacking in perceptual motor abilities necessary for acquiring academic skills. As such, it has potential for use with the so-called borderline and mildly retarded but is not useful with the severely or profoundly retarded. It is an action or performance survey. Thus, it is easily administered to the individual who cannot read.

Habilitation Training

The training of a mentally retarded individual requires the cooperation of many persons filling a variety of roles. The mentally retarded individual, dependent upon his or her functioning level and comprehension, must be a team member. Lack of desire and motivation or a high degree of resistance could interfere with the success of a well-planned developmentally-appropriate training sequence.

The family must be involved in a positive manner and must be given much encouragement and reinforcement in an attempt to allay unwarranted guilt feelings. The family members must be aided in adjusting to the fact that progress will be slow, gains small and in some cases minimal, and yet they must be demanding and supportive of the retarded individual so that the greatest level of achievement possible is obtained.

The individual may require drugs to aid in control of seizures or aberrant behavior or may use dietary supplements. For example, an individual having causative phenylketonuria (PKU) requires a dietary supplement for maintenance or prevention of further changes. Although physicians and nurses are busy, most will respond to questioning about the individual's medication record. In turn, the medical representatives have the responsibility of informing other team members of changes in the medicinal regimen, especially if consequences or side effects, which could influence the program, are anticipated. Physicians are becoming more aware of the type of contribution the occupational therapist may make relative to observation of drug reactions, but it is the responsibility of the occupational therapists to make their skills and contributions clear.

The psychologist and social case worker are vital team members. They frequently can elicit from the individual or the family information that is important to program development. The skill of these people can be helpful in the evaluation and compilation of program goals and can forge another link in the development of a total program team.

The staff members considered to be giving direct service vary with almost every center; they are the persons who have daily contact with the individual. They are known by a variety of names: mental retardation aides, child care workers, resident living aides, and so forth. This group provides a vital source of information because they see retarded individuals for extended periods of time; they can report on specific needs, the carry-over of learning from therapies, the reaction of the individual to peers and activity, the individual's tolerance of frustrations and response to daily living situations.

The interaction of physical therapists, occupational therapist, speech therapists, teachers, recreation therapists, and other concerned persons should occur not only at unit staff meetings but whenever a concern arises. The staff should feel free to discuss problems without having to follow a rigid bureaucratic process; however, the staff does have the responsibility to share information with supervisors so they can be aware and able to contribute to the program.

Each and every staff member must have a concern for the retarded individual. The dietary staff will cooperate if time is taken to explain why a special food or preparation is needed. The carpenter might help by making large pieces of equipment, such as relaxation chairs, standing tables, and prone boards. These support staff members can be involved in the program; they are able to give much worthwhile help.

The occupational therapist is not working in an isolated area but must offer aid and solicit the same from the total staff. Specifically, occupational therapists are working with a team to develop level appropriate training to aid each individual. The team must set realistic goals, be able to accept slow progress in achieving them, be content to accept temporary plateauing when it occurs, and be prepared to increase training emphasis when the individual evidences readiness for progression in the program.

Roles of Occupational Therapy

Occupational therapy assists in improving the individual's ability to meet the demands of his or her culture with satisfaction and in a manner that is acceptable to and compatible with that environment. It is essential that the occupational therapist have a knowledge not only of normal growth and development but also of the cultural and social requirements the particular individual must fulfill. Those from a ghetto in a large urban area have different demands to meet than do those from the farming heartlands. In addition, there must be an awareness of the differences resulting from their social, cultural, and value systems, since these too affect program implementation and cooperation of both the individual and the family.

The diversity of skills possessed by occupational therapists makes it possible for them to fill a variety of roles both in administration and in providing direct service. In a small understaffed center, the occupational therapist may be expected to be the one providing recreational activities in addition to occupational therapy. In other settings the implementation of an approved work training program may be the occupational therapist's responsibility. As staff is acquired in other disciplines, the occupational therapist is able to relinquish some of these extra duties.

Larger, more completely staffed centers for the mentally retarded present different types of roles. Here, the occupational therapist is delegated responsibilities traditionally assigned to him or her. The therapist is, in addition, able to have frequent contact with members of other disciplines. Each discipline can be an extension of the others. The occupational therapist might prepare an individual for physical therapy treatment and yet accomplish an occupational therapy goal—that of teaching self-dressing. The teacher reinforces physical and occupational therapy by using adapted equipment or proper positioning. The era in which each discipline was viewed as an isolated entity is past, and the occupational therapist must become a working member of the team.

Occasionally the occupational therapist is placed in an administrative role. One difficulty here might be keeping occupational therapy in its proper perspective as a part of the team. Members of all disciplines must become contributing members of the team coordinated by an administrator, whose major responsibility is to utilize the skills of each as required by the mentally retarded individual at a given time.

In centers for habilitation training of the mentally retarded, occupational therapy methods have followed the traditional use of arts and crafts with increased use of appropriate neurodevelopmental activities to aid each individual's sequential development. Both of these approaches are valid. The major decision is which form of treatment should be used to meet the needs of the individual being served.

Traditional

Initially there were few available trained staff who understood the needs of the retarded for participation in gainful activity. Little activity was available beyond occasional entertainment. This lack of activity produced fertile ground for regression (even in those with a higher functioning level), self-abuse, public masturbation, fights, broken windows, destroyed furniture, and torn clothing. These negative behaviors reinforced society's attitude that the retarded person could not be taught or benefit from positive experiences.

A few determined staff members would not accept this attitude and began implementing arts and crafts activities based on the premise that busy work is better than idle hands. This was a positive step for some individuals, as was evidenced by improved ego strength. Much fine work was produced, but usually little thought was given to the individual's symptoms, interests, or desired goals. A negative feature of the arts and crafts programs was that most were self-funded: individuals had to produce in order to buy supplies, making production the primary function of the activity.

The low institutional housekeeping budgets produced another type of traditional programming—that of the individual's doing much of the work around the institution that was not done by paid help. Properly assigned and supervised work within the institution is a useful therapeutic tool. However, the mentally retarded person was often put to work in areas of need (laundry, grounds, kitchen) for long hours with little or no compensation beyond a pinch of tobacco, a cigar, or a cup of coffee. Days off were unheard of, with the retarded individual frequently doing more physically demanding labor than the paid staff.

This type of abuse led to involvement by labor unions. After much discussion, numerous law suits, and negotiations, the pendulum has swung to the other extreme. Individuals may work only if they agree, sign a voluntary consent form, and receive the minimum wage or prevailing wage, whichever is higher, pro rated to the level of performance. This federal regulation affects the use of therapeutic work as a part of habilitation since many refuse to participate in it voluntarily. Also, most live-in centers have not been given increased funds either to hire the retarded individual or to employ additional staff.[18]

Both types of activities described had much to offer but were abused. Occupational therapists involved in both types of programs were distressed by what was happening, and joined other team members in designing program goals indicating availability and quality of program which would produce the potential for change in individuals served.

Current

As an example of current practice, the system developed in one state is described. In Pennsylvania, the directors of occupational therapy departments serving the Commonwealth Department of Public Welfare Office of Mental Retardation institutions for the mentally retarded defined major program areas in which occupational therapy has a valid contribution to make toward eliciting behavioral change. The list is not to be considered a complete, all-inclusive one but one that is subject to revision and updating. Each of the areas is discussed more fully later in the chapter but is recorded here for a global view of their thinking. Some areas are evaluation, maintenance, research, resource, and consultancy. The areas listed cannot be considered as separate entities as there are many situations in which their functions overlap. They were difficult to define and are impossible to separate; therefore staff must be prepared to see needs in one or more program areas, set priorities, and plan the program accordingly.

There also appears to be a variety of function and program types to meet specific needs. The group of directors of occupational therapy had difficulty in separating the role responsibilities but have listed them for more clarity of comprehension.

Although these program areas were defined for institutional training, they are also relevant to community centers that provide day care, special education, preschool, and infant stimulation programs.

The Occupational Therapy Program

Assessment/Evaluation

The intent of evaluation is to appraise and assess functioning levels of the individual. This may be done for program placement within the occupational therapy service or upon the request of a member of another discipline. A physician, psychologist, or community agency may ask that evaluation be done in order to determine the readiness of the individual for program or to determine the individual's current functioning level.

Instruments for screening aid in determining the need for further evaluation in specific areas. However, if it has been determined previously that the individual presents symptoms of physical or mental retardation, then further screening is repetitious and unnecessary. Assessment should then be used to determine the level of function of the individual.

Most therapists use a selected battery of instruments. One caution is that the chosen battery must be appropriate and produce meaningful results. A department may assemble a collection of standardized tests with good reliability and validity that produces results to meet their needs. Others may devise a composite battery of their own, combining appropri-

ate materials for their needs. No one instrument or battery will fill all needs. How extensive the battery should be is dependent upon the function of the center, the age of individuals served, and the basic goals of the service. It would be meaningless for a preschool program to compile a prevocational interest and skill battery, or for an infant stimulation program to develop a battery on cognitive tasks or refinements of self-care. The type of battery promulgated by Currie[19] is broad enough in scope to cover many age and involvement levels but can be limited to meet specific needs.

Evaluation is not a one-time experience. It is an ongoing process to provide current and updated information on level of ability. Within the training process one must be careful, however, not to teach items used in the test. It is easy to elicit good scores on evaluation yet have poor results in performance if an individual has become test-wise. Evaluation is necessary but must be utilized with care and skill.

A major responsibility of the occupational therapist is the preparation of clear, concise, and comprehensive reports. If occupational therapists are to function usefully as evaluators they must produce reports that are understandable, meaningful, and useful. Long reports are meaningless because they may not be read thoroughly.

Neurodevelopmental Sequence

All individuals follow an essentially similar sequential pattern of development. Some, the gifted, progress more rapidly; some, the retarded, progress more slowly. But for each there is a sequential pattern to be followed. The mentally retarded persons have had their sequence interrupted in some manner—physical, mental, emotional, or as a result of multiple factors. They will therefore require special training in order to progress along the developmental sequence.

For years, well-meaning and skilled therapists were using adaptive support devices such as braces and splints in order to get individuals into the upright position and ambulating. When the individuals did not progress it was determined that they were too handicapped, too retarded, or too uncooperative. Little thought was given to developmental sequence.

Frustration on the part of the staff and lack of progress on the part of the individual caused a review of programs of different types and goals. Staff began to question whether the goals were appropriate for the skill level of the individual. Finally various techniques aimed at developmentally-realistic goals evolved, with therapists providing sensory stimuli to the individual in order to aid the integration process and permit performance of a motor act. Of vital importance is the awareness of normal growth patterns, the proper level, and type of sensory input needed to achieve the desired result. A person, for example, must have head control before sitting and be able to knee-stand before standing in the upright position.

As in many other areas of dysfunction there is no one technique to meet all the needs. The occupational therapist must evaluate and, after determining the technique most appropriate, proceed with program implementation. There must be constant contact with specialists from other disciplines to utilize their skills and achieve the greatest potential function for the individual in this highly specialized treatment process.

Multiply Handicapped

Many individuals who are designated as mentally retarded are also multiply handicapped. Some are blind, deaf, nonverbal, cerebral palsied, or have missing or incomplete body parts. Many of these involvements alone would demand much adjustment in life style and learning process. When coupled with mental retardation, these problems are severely compounded. A sensory disturbance may be the only manifestation, but more often it is accompanied by a motor disturbance, which indeed produces a complex training need.

There is much overlapping in this program area. The primary need may be in the neurodevelopmental level or in the area of activities of daily living. The role of the occupational therapist must be to determine the need, set the priority for the service, and proceed to implement the indicated program.

Emotionally Disturbed

This program area encompasses a wide scope of problems ranging from the difficulties of mildly and moderately involved individuals to the persons who demonstrate autistic-like behaviors.

The multiple problems faced by the mildly and moderately retarded do not preclude emotional disturbances. Frequently they are alert enough to recognize their difference, feel society's rejection acutely, and yet strongly want to be a part of that society. Many internalize their feelings and develop physical malfunctions such as ulcers and colitis. Occupational therapy can aid these individuals by providing an outlet for, and encouraging the release of, feelings. The release felt while using the beater on a floor loom or wedging clay is immeasurable, and it also is a positive, acceptable behavior. The results derived from the use of various activities are shared with the program team for use by all those working with the individual.

Programming for those who demonstrate autistic-like behavior must first determine whether the individual is profoundly retarded or is demonstrating

such symptoms as a result of extreme emotional distress. The assistance of the total program team is vital in making this decision before goals can be set and programming instituted.

This is an expensive type of programming initially because it requires a one-to-one relationship, but the results are gratifying to the total team. The occupational therapist may be the original worker in the process or may be called upon as a consultant or resource person.

Activities of Daily Living

The majority of mentally retarded individuals appear unable to meet daily self-care needs because of their functioning level. For years, the staff and families of the mentally retarded, in the interest of saving time, have met these needs. On rare occasions inability to learn is the main cause for the individual's not performing self-care activities. More frequently the mentally retarded person has not been required or permitted to undertake his or her own self-care. The behaviors demonstrated by the retarded in this area are often related to the demands made upon them.

It is unfair if the individual is given an unpressed buttonless shirt or blouse and then criticized for sloppy appearance. Likewise, if open zippers are permitted, the therapist is negligent in training for community living. Similarly there should not be one dress code for the retarded persons and another for the staff. There must be consistency in what is expected or accepted.

Use of cosmetics and hair styling should be realistic and meet reasonable current standards. Proper use of cosmetics is a useful tool in teaching body scheme and image.

Self-feeding for some individuals is a slow process and often staff have done the feeding. Frequently, small, inexpensive, dishwasher-safe adapted utensils can be made and utilized for more independent self-feeding.[20] More involved adaptations may require greater on-site assistance from the occupational therapist and demand the training of other staff members in their use and purpose. Adapted equipment should be kept as simple as possible in construction in order to encourage use by all staff.

Self-care in personal hygiene is a topic frequently avoided by most disciplines. The use of the toilet and toilet tissue and handwashing must be encouraged. Teaching of self-care for menstrual needs is increasing. Unfortunately, little is being done to instruct individuals about or to discuss these bodily functions.

Sex education must be faced realistically, and the occupational therapist must be prepared to explain or answer questions in a manner comprehensible to the individual. The use of proper names for body parts is encouraged. One should not expect that a lesson explained once is learned. As with all individuals, the retarded have normal urges and are concerned about them. The therapist should answer questions factually and truly in a manner that can be understood.[21]

A successful method of teaching self-care in feeding, dressing, and personal hygiene is the process known as *chaining*. *Forward chaining* means building upon a series of simple steps, to develop a more complex series, and finally to complete the task. For example, the donning of slacks would progress from having the individual insert his feet into the leg openings, to pulling up the trousers, and finally to fastening them. For some individuals, *backward chaining* is an easier learning process. This involves having the individual first complete the task—buttoning, fastening the clamp, pulling up the zipper—and then expanding to include the pulling up process, and finally the insertion of feet into the leg openings. Each procedure ends with the same result, but the manner used is dependent upon the individual's perceptions and physical status. Chaining can be utilized for teaching most activities of self-care through individualized occupational therapy training as well as through sharing the process with the direct care staff for reinforcement and implementation.

Vocational Exploration

The extent of the role of occupational therapy in this area varies according to the roles taken by members of the other disciplines. It may be that, in one setting, a registered occupational therapist has the responsibility for evaluating potential, planning, and implementing the total program. In a larger, more completely staffed center, the occupational therapist's role could be that of evaluation through offering work experiences for exploration and determination of readiness for progression to workshop assignment.

It is imperative that the therapist be aware of the individual's feelings toward work and those of his or her culture. To many, the ability to work is a sign of health and usefulness. Unfortunately many mentally retarded persons feel they do not have any responsibility in this area. The occupational therapist can be of value to the team by attempting to motivate the individual to become involved in a work training experience.

Maintenance

For the want of a better term, the descriptive word "maintenance" is used to designate programming for those who have reached what is probably their maximum level of functioning. The goal is to prevent regression.

The individual with a progressive disorder needs assistance in retaining ability in range of motion, activities of daily living, and cognition for as long as possible. The aid that the therapist can give the individual and the family is important. There are few progressive disorders causing mental deterioration among those diagnosed as mentally retarded. However, those that do exist require additional skill and effort from the program team.

The normal aging process and the acquisition of additional physical or neurological involvements compound the care and responsibility of the program teams. A senile 80-year-old mentally retarded individual may demonstrate behaviors similar to those seen throughout his or her lifetime but will probably demonstrate less skill than other eighty-year-old senile individuals. This individual requires an evaluation and adjustment of goals by the program team to assist in functioning at his or her highest level.

Although the term maintenance can be interpreted negatively, in this aspect of programming it is given a positive connotation and is meant to be an area in which therapy is not only desired but strongly indicated.

Research

Unfortunately few occupational therapists have been involved in the area of research, and those working with the mentally retarded have been just as remiss. A wise man once said something to the effect that, "It is not the so-called retarded who are retarded. It is those who work with them who are lacking in skill to provide aid." Occupational therapists are involved in providing facilitation of change and are attempting to meet current needs, but understaffing, heavy case loads, and required paperwork have frequently been used as excuses for avoiding involvement in research.

Many times a therapist may say a patient has reached his or her maximum level of function, when this may be an evasive statement for not knowing what to do next. The frustration felt by an individual who apparently cannot control drooling is an excellent example of an aspect of training where joining with the speech therapist in research might produce results for improvement in chewing, swallowing, cosmetic appearance, and ego strength for the involved individual.

Research does demand time, but the occupational therapist has the responsiblity to become more involved in sharing findings with others. Research projects also improve level of skill.

Resource and Consultancy

The increase in numbers of small facilities providing interim care, extended care, and community living arrangements, and the requirement that such centers have a registered occupational therapist as a consultant in order to meet government regulations for funding, provides another potential role for the therapist working with the mentally retarded.

Agencies such as AAMD and NARC have encouraged the return to community centers of those who can profit from living in such settings. Being closer to the family has been desired by many but the level of functioning requires more care than the family can provide. In addition, many mentally retarded persons with no families can be placed in a center where they might go to a workshop and return to minimal supervision at nighttime. Others who require more skilled care may be placed closer to their families so family members may visit them more easily.

The role of occupational therapy can be that of assisting the staff in providing needed adaptations for self-care, in developing an activity program that is therapeutic, and in aiding the staff to meet the particular needs of the mentally retarded individuals so that they may adjust more easily to a new and different life style.

Composite Treatment

The mentally retarded develop acute or chronic physical or emotionally disabling conditions, as does the non-retarded population. Special intervention techniques must be implemented to remediate the secondary condition. The overall concern, however, remains the elicitation of behavioral change in regard to the level of mental retardation.

Following is a sampling of the types of programming occupational therapists may emphasize during five broad age periods of the individual.

During the *pre-school period* it would be essential to first assess and then remediate through early intervention and neurodevelopmental techniques. Second, would include encouraging the development of self motivation, a skill useful throughout the individual's life. Third is the use of play. *Biology of Play*[22] is a most valuable resource during this period to assist in bridging the next developmental stage.

Early school age would probably include continuation of neurodevelopmental training with appropriate reevaluation. The child should be placed in a school environment compatible with his or her functioning level. The occupational therapist can assist with adaptive and seating devices to alleviate physical dysfunction. Modalities are also used to aid in cognitive development. Motor behavior evaluation and remediation techniques as described by Beter and colleagues would be a valuable tool for use with the early school child.[23] The expansion of living skills is most important at this age level.

Adolescent years would evidence, if needed, continued utilization of previously employed modalities and techniques for evaluation and assessment. In addition, the occupational therapist may be involved in prevocational exploration. Activities of daily living would be expanded and include basic sex education.

For the *adult years* there would be increased emphasis on community living, including work responsibilities and behaviors, and basic finances and budgeting. Dating, sex education, marriage, and homemaking skills may be included in further expansion of daily living skills.

During the *aging years* it is essential that the occupational therapist be able to differentiate between the mental retardation component and that of the normal aging process. One must continually reassess skills in order to maintain the individual's maximum functional level. With improved medical care the mentally retarded are living longer, thus extending the demands upon the therapeutic team.

For an occupational therapist to provide an adequate and meaningful program for all ages of mentally retarded individuals it is essential to have a broad base in understanding normal growth and development. However, just as important is the assistance to the individual when an aberration does occur.

Case Study

Carol, at the time of admission to occupational therapy, was a 12-year old diagnosed as profoundly mentally retarded with autistic-like behavior.

An illegitimate daughter of a borderline intelligent mother, Carol was rejected at birth. The infant was placed in a foster home but was transferred many times because she was unable to adjust. She was a difficult feeder and poor sleeper, essentially a silent child and apparently fearful of human contact. Rimland, in his work *Infantile Autism*, advances the theory that this type of behavior may evolve as a result of maternal rejection in utero.[24] If one agrees with this theory then the behavior can be explained. However, for occupational therapists in a training center, the main concern was how to evoke behavioral change in Carol.

Admission behavior was that of a nonverbal, incontinent, pretty, fairly-well-nourished adolescent who spent her waking time pacing or moving in a whirling pattern. Sleep habits were poor. Carol had difficulty relating to humans but did have an attachment to a rolled bib which she used to slap herself. The palm of her right hand was used to slap her face with enough intensity to cause bleeding on occasions.

In an attempt to restrict self-abusive behavior, Carol was dressed in a jumpsuit with hand pockets which was laced up the back. This protective procedure was deemed necessary by medical service but further compounded Carol's withdrawal by limiting her sporadic positive hand movements.

It was impossible to utilize formal evaluative procedures, so goals were determined as a result of extended observation of Carol in her residential area. The goals determined after discussion with the program team involved the following: (1) obtain eye contact and pleasurable human contact, (2) negate self-abusive behavior, and (3) develop self-feeding, since this was her one area of voluntary human contact.

It was decided that liquids were an acceptable primary reward so they were given with secondary verbal praise and physical contact when possible.

Much time was spent in aiding Carol to react to her human environment: walking with her, waiting for her to walk by (when she stopped she was given a drink), and reaching to touch her. Finally the big day came when she voluntarily reached to touch the therapist. Concurrently, reduction in self-abusive behavior occurred, permitting removal of the jumpsuit and the use of dresses and other normal attire.

The decision was made to progress to self-feeding, because food is an oral reinforcer and fulfills a very basic survival need. First, Carol was fed while standing in her living unit. Next, the therapist sat making it necessary for Carol to come to the spoon, while being encouraged to sit beside the worker. Finally she was able to sit at a table while being fed. The next step was to aid her in grasping, filling, and inserting the spoon into her mouth. Physical assistance was reduced to pressure on the ulnar border of her hand, then discontinued. Other residents who also were beginning self-feeders were added to the table with Carol who was able at the end of about 18 months to self-feed with acceptable behaviors for her developmental stage.

The improved contact with her environment and demonstrated reactions aided in determining the next goal—that of toilet training and self-care in this area.

As the residential life staff had 24-hour contact with Carol it was determined to use this staff for toilet training and resultant self-care. It was shown that the utilization of the residential life staff encouraged carry over of program goals and reinforced the transdisciplinary team concept.

Small but meaningful gains were made, giving Carol an increased sense of self-worth through actions that meet physical and psychosocial requirements. □

Advancements and Future Prospects

Accountability

One outstanding advancement is the demand for accountability. Families, community agencies, funding sources, and professional organizations are demanding proof of the results of time, energy, and funds expended. Staff no longer can report impressive-looking statistics for attendance at mass activities, numbers of pounds of food served, tons of laundry washed, or gallons of water used. They are expected to produce behavioral change in individuals, with some exhibiting extreme change which will permit independent living, apart from the family unit. In others, seemingly minimal change in self-care is seen; these changes permit more active participation within an institutional community. These extremes on the continuum are dependent on degrees of change that are obtainable based on the individual's skill level. If an individual can sit in a chair rather than lie down, self-feed rather than be fed, or be continent rather than wear diapers, the time and energy spent in training are justified.

Family Contribution

Publications like *Mothers Can Help*[25] will be of assistance for family involvement and carry over of the treatment goals. The treatment techniques will need to be demonstrated and explained so that appropriate use by families is insured and treatment is reinforced.

Involvement of families must continue to increase. Initially families were encouraged to institutionalize and forget a retarded family member. For those who conformed to this counsel, there was development of increased guilt and shame. This was compounded, on the rare occasions that they were permitted to visit, by the lack of recognition on the part of the mentally retarded individual and in some instances by lack of interest on the part of the staff. For those who kept the family member at home, stress was placed on the total family by a society that did not understand, gaped, and commented on aberrant behaviors. Fortunately these types of abuse have lessened, and families are being involved as a total unit in a variety of community treatment activities.

The increased involvement of the family unit is only one product of family counseling. The family is being given help in adjusting to the needs of any member who is mentally retarded; it is aided in deciding where and when to go for assistance and in comprehending how to obtain and ask the maximum level of function of the retarded individual. The family is helped in planning for the care of the individual when the primary family can no longer meet his or her needs.

Medical Advances

Advances have been made medically that will make the prevention of mental retardation caused by some factors a reality. Genetic counseling will be of immeasurable importance. Individuals who have potential for conceiving an involved child will be so informed and counseled.

Those known as high-risk mothers because of age, exposure to infection, and possible genetic complications have access to the amniocentesis procedure. This involves the removal of amniotic fluid, which contains fetal cells. The fluid is analyzed relative to a number of metabolic disorders and chromosomal content, with the recommended remediation being given by the physician.

Much progress has been made with an even greater prospect for the future as a result of prenatal care. Early care during pregnancy will aid in improving the nutrition of both the mother and the baby. Various medical and dietary supplements providing a well-balanced diet will aid in the reduction of premature births as well as in the prevention of disorders, such as hypothyroidism, that result from endocrine imbalances.

Some geographical areas are now developing a high-risk registry. Individuals considered to be potential candidates for extended care are listed in the registry and observed closely with therapeutic intervention occurring as early as possible.

Increased use of tests at birth, such as those for phenylketonuria, will determine if there will be a need for dietary supplements for the baby. The use of the supplement may not totally eliminate the effect of these causative factors but will surely reduce the potentially severe level of retardation.

Legal Rights and Obligations

Much has been written about the legal rights of the mentally retarded. Relevant federal legislation has been enacted since 1827. An historical overview has been compiled by Chinn and his colleagues that will enable the reader to follow actions leading to the enactment of Public Law 94-142, Education for All Handicapped Children Act on November 28, 1975.[10]

The right to an education to the extent of the individual's potential is mandated in Public Law 94-142. Expansion of programs such as infant stimulation may decrease the numbers of those considered retarded as a result of insufficient stimulation during the early and formative years.

In addition, the process of mainstreaming is required in states receiving special federal funds. Mainstreaming is defined as educational programming in the least restrictive environment along a continuum of seven levels—from those who can function in a regular classroom to those homebound or in institutional settings. Education is defined broadly so that the individual receives service compatible with his or her functioning level.

Other legal issues include voting, securing and maintaining employment, appropriate housing, marriage, and parenthood. With each of these rights come obligations and responsibilities, such as total housing rental and upkeep, taxes, and involvement with the community and family.

Combined with legal rights and responsibilities is an awareness of ethical and societal concerns. With expanded freedom and legal rights the mentally retarded should be afforded societal opportunities but must be expected to conform to the mores of their culture.

Future Prospects

What does the future hold in store for the mentally retarded? When a study is made of all potential causative factors of mental retardation, it is apparent that the current advances will not eliminate retardation. Many causes, such as unknown prenatal influences or trauma, are not yet preventable, but the gains made recently do present a positive indication for future reduction of the incidence of mental retardation and for more efficient care for those affected.

References

1. Smith, D. W., and Marshall, R. E. (eds.): Introduction to Clinical Pediatrics. Philadelphia: W. B. Saunders Co., 1972, p. 181.
2. Stein, J. (ed.): The Random House Dictionary of the English Language. New York: Random House, 1967.
3. Grossman, H. J. (ed.): Manual on Terminology and Classification in Mental Retardation. Baltimore: Garamond/Pridemark, 1973.
4. Copeland, M., Ford, L., and Solon, S.: Occupational Therapy for Mentally Retarded Children. Baltimore: University Park Press, 1976, p. 27.
5. Ibid.
6. Itard, J.: The Wild Boy of Aveyron. Century Psychology Series. Englewood Cliffs NJ: Prentice-Hall, 1962.
7. Goldberg, I., and Lippman, L.: Right to Education. New York: Teachers College, Columbia University, 1973.
8. Bergsma, D. (ed.): Birth Defects Compendium, ed. 2. National Foundation—March of Dimes New York: Alan R. Liss, Inc., 1979.
9. Gellis, S. and Feingold, M.: Atlas of Mental Retarda-

tion Syndromes. Washington, DC. U.S. Government Printing Office, 1968.
10. Chinn, P., Drew, C., Logan, D.: Mental Retardation. St. Louis, MO: C.V. Mosby, 1979.
11. Diagnostic and Statistical Manual of Mental Disorders (DSM—II), ed. 2 American Psychiatric Association, Washington DC, 1968.
12. Heber, R. (ed.): A Manual on Terminology and Classification in Mental Retardation. Monograph Supplement to Am. J. Mental Deficiency, ed. 2. American Association on Mental Deficiency, Springfield IL, 1961, p. 64.
13. Ibid., p. 63.
14. Grossman: Manual on Terminology and Classification, p. 23.
15. Nihira, K., Foster, R., Shellhaas, M., and Leland, H.: AAMD Adaptive Behavior Scale for Children and Adults, 1974 Revision. The American Association on Mental Deficiency, Washington, DC, 1974.
16. Buros, O. K. (ed.): The Eighth Mental Measurement Yearbook. Highland, Park IL: Gryphon Press, 1978.
17. Currie, C.: Evaluating function of mentally retarded children through use of toys and play activities. Am. J. Occup. Ther. 23:1, 1969.
18. Employment of Patient Workers in Hospitals and Institutions at Subminimum Wages, U.S. Department of Labor, Washington DC. U.S. Government Printing Office, 1975.
19. Currie: Evaluating function of mentally retarded children.
20. Nathan, C.: Please Help Us Help Ourselves. Occupational Therapy Department, Indiana University Medical Center, Indianapolis, 1970.
21. De la Cruz, F. F., and LaVeck, G. D.: Human Sexuality and the Mentally Retarded. New York: Brunner-Mazel, 1973.
22. Tizard, B., and Harvey, D. (eds.): Biology of Play. Philadelphia: J.B. Lippincott, 1977.
23. Beter, T., Cragin, W., and Drury, F.: The Mentally Retarded Child and His Motor Behavior. Springfield, IL: Charles C Thomas, 1972.
24. Rimland, B.: Infantile Autism. New York: Appleton-Century-Crofts, 1964.
25. Cliff, S., Gray, J., and Nymann, C.: Mothers Can Help. El Paso TX: Guynes Printing, 1974.

Bibliography

Diagnostic and Statistical Manual of Mental Disorders ed. 3, American Psychiatric Association, Washington, D.C., 1980.
Anderson, F.: Fay's First Fifty: Activities for the Young and the Severely Handicapped. Augusta GA: Strothers Printing, 1974.
Arnold, L. E. (ed.): Helping Parents Help Their Children. New York: Brunner/Mazel, 1978.
Banus, B. S.: The Developmental Therapist. Thorofare NJ: Charles Slack, 1971.
Banus, B. S. et al: The Developmental Therapist ed. 2. Thorofare NJ: Charles B. Slack, 1979.

Batshaw, M. L. and Perret, Y. M.: Children with Handicaps: A Medical Primer. Baltimore: Paul H. Brookes, 1981.
Baumeister, A. A.: Mental Retardation. Chicago: Aldine Publishing Co., 1967.
Bergsma, D. (ed.): Birth Defects Compendium, ed. 2. National Foundation-March of Dimes, New York: Alan R. Liss, Inc., 1979.
Beter, T. R. and Cragin, W. E.: The Mentally Retarded Child and His Motor Behavior. Springfield IL: Charles C Thomas, 1972.
Breines, E.: Perception: Its Development and Recapitulation. Leban NJ: Geri-Rehab, Inc., 1981.
Brolin, D. E.: Vocational Preparation of Retarded Citizens. Columbus OH: Charles E. Merrill, 1976.
Buros, O. K. (ed.): Tests in Print II. Highland Park IL: The Gryphon Press, 1974.
Capute, A. J. et al: Primitive Reflex Profile. Baltimore: University Park Press, 1978.
Carter, C. H.: Handbook of Mental Retardation Syndromes, ed. 3. Springfield IL: Charles C. Thomas, 1975.
Carter, C. H.: Medical Aspects of Mental Retardation. Springfield IL: Charles C. Thomas, 1978.
Cohen, D. and Stern, V.: Observing and Recording the Behavior of Young Children (2nd Ed.). New York: Teachers College, Columbia University, 1978.
Cole, M. et al: The Cultural Context of Learning and Thinking. New York: Basic Books, 1971.
Cratty, B. J.: Motor Activity and the Education of Retardates. Philadelphia: Lea and Febiger, 1969.
Ellis, N.: Handbook and of Mental Deficiency. New York: McGraw-Hill Book Co., 1963.
Erickson, M. L.: Assessment and Management of Developmental Changes in Children. St. Louis, MO: C. V. Mosby, 1976.
Fairchild, T. N. and Parks, A. L.: Mainstreaming the Mentally Retarded Child. Austin TE: Learning Concepts, 1977.
Fiorentino, M. R.: Normal and Abnormal Development. Springfield IL: Charles C. Thomas, 1976.
Fiorentino, M. R.: Reflex Testing Methods For Evaluating CNS Development. Springfield IL: Charles C Thomas, 1972.
Flavell, J. H.: The Developmental Psychology of Jean Piaget. New York: Van Nostrand Reinhold, 1963.
Gellis, S. S. and Feingold, M.: Atlas of Mental Retardation Syndromes. Washington DC: U.S. Government Printing Office, 1968.
Gordon, T.: Parent Effectiveness Training. New York: Peter H. Wyden, Inc., 1970.
Hamilton, J. C., and Segal, R. M. (eds.): Proceedings of a Consultation Conference on the Gerontological Aspects of Mental Retardation. Ann Arbor MI: University of Michigan, 1975.
Haynes, U.: A Developmental Approach to Case Finding. Washington DC: U.S. Government Printing Office, 1967.
Houts, P., Scott, R., and Leaser, J.: Goal Planning with the Mentally Retarded. Milton S. Hershey Medical Center of the Pennsylvania State University, Hershey, 1973.

Kindred, M. et al. (ed.): The Mentally Retarded Citizen and the Law. New York: The Free Press, 1976.

Koch, R., and Dobson, J. (eds.): The Mentally Retarded Child and His Family. New York: Brunner-Mazel, 1971.

Koestler, F. A. (ed.): Reference Handbook for Continuing Education in Occupational Therapy. Dubuque: Kendall/Hunt, 1970.

Krajicek, M. J., and Tearney, A. I. (eds.): Detection of Developmental Problems in Children. Baltimore: University Park Press, 1977.

Magrab, P. R. (ed.): Psychological Management of Pediatric Problems Vol I: Early Life Conditions and Chronic Diseases. Baltimore: University Park Press, 1978.

Magrab, P. R. (ed.): Psychological Management of Pediatric Problems Vol II: Sensorineural Conditions and Social Concerns. Baltimore: University Park Press, 1978.

Meier, J.: Screening and Assessment of Young Children at Developmental Risk. Report of the President's Committee on Mental Retardation, Washington DC: U.S. Government Printing Office, 1973.

Moore, J. C.: Neuroanatomy Simplified. Dubuque: Kendall/Hunt, 1969.

Mysak, E. D.: Principles of a Reflex Therapy Approach to Cerebral Palsy. New York: Teachers College Columbia University, 1963.

Price, A., Gilfoyle, E., and Myers, C. (eds.): Research in Sensory Integrative Development. American Occupational Therapy Association, Rockville MD, 1976.

Robinson, N. M., and Robinson, H. B.: The Mentally Retarded Child: A Psychological Approach ed. 2. New York: McGraw-Hill, 1976.

Rothstein, J.: Mental Retardation. New York: Holt, Rinehart & Winston, 1961.

Schiefelbusch, R. L. (ed.): Language of the Mentally Retarded. Baltimore: University Park Press, 1972.

Seguin, E.: Idiocy and Its Treatment. (reprinted) New York: Teachers College Columbia University, 1907.

Smith, D. W. (ed.): Introduction to Clinical Pediatrics, ed. 2. Philadelphia: W.B. Saunders, 1977.

Smith, D. W.: Recognizable Patterns of Human Malformation. Philadelphia: W. B. Saunders, 1970.

The Child with Central Nervous System Deficit. Children's Bureau Publication Number 432-1965, Washington DC: U.S. Government Printing Office, 1965.

Turnbull, H. R. III (ed.): Consent Handbook, American Association on Mental Deficiency, Washington D.C., 1977.

West, W. (ed.): Occupational Therapy for the Mentally Handicapped Child. Chicago: University of Illinois, 1965.

Wolfensberger, W.: Normalization. National Institute on Mental Retardation, Toronto, 1972.

Recommended Periodicals and Journals

American Association on Mental Deficiency:
AMERICAN JOURNAL OF MENTAL DEFICIENCY
MENTAL RETARDATION
American Occupational Therapy Association:
AMERICAN JOURNAL OF OCCUPATIONAL THERAPY
American Orthopsychiatric Association:
AMERICAN JOURNAL OF ORTHOPSYCHIATRY
American Physical Therapy Association:
PHYSICAL THERAPY
American Speech-Language-Hearing Association:
ASHA
JOURNAL OF SPEECH AND HEARING DISORDERS
Council for Exceptional Children:
EXCEPTIONAL CHILDREN
Haworth Press:
SOCIAL WORK IN HEALTH CARE
Insight Publishing Company, Inc.:
PEDIATRIC ANNALS
Macmillan Journals Ltd.:
NURSING TIMES
National Association for Retarded Citizens:
ACTION TOGETHER/INFORMATION EXCHANGE
National Rehabilitation Association:
JOURNAL OF REHABILITATION
Perceptual and Motor Skills:
PERCEPTUAL AND MOTOR SKILLS
Professional Press, Inc.:
JOURNAL OF LEARNING DISABILITIES
Society for the Experimental Analysis of Behavior
JOURNAL OF APPLIED BEHAVIOR ANALYSIS

CHAPTER 21

Functional Restoration— Theory, Principles, and Techniques *Elinor Anne Spencer*

so much
depends upon

a red wheel
barrow

glazed with rain
water

beside the white
chickens

William Carlos Williams*

The outward simplicity and inherent complexity of Williams' poem is analogous to the occurrence of debilitating disease or injury to an individual and the resulting impact on the individual's life. While the poem conveys a simple, colorful, pastoral image, there is an underlying current of symbolism which adds meaning and dimension to the purely visual. So too, functional restoration embodies the totality of human potential.

---

* Williams, William Carlos. In Richards, Mary Caroline: Centering. Middletown, CT: Weslyan University Press, 1964, pp. 79–80.

Whether precipitated by known factors or caused by a sudden accident, the effects of disability are demonstrated in both psychological and physical responses. They may reach to some degree into all areas of an individual's life and contacts, necessitating adjustments in life patterns and directions. The extent of these adjustments depends on three major factors related to the individual: premorbid situation, prognosis, and goals. These factors will be explored and referred to frequently throughout the chapter.

In preparation for practice, the student occupational therapist learns the structure and behavior of the human body both within the context of the normal range of development and as related to deviations from the norm. Academic and clinical experience include the complete developmental continuum from birth through death. In this chapter and the one that follows, two major areas are given attention: (1) theory, principles, and techniques related to evaluating and treating the individual with physical dysfunction, and (2) identification and description of major disability areas with recommendations for specific evaluation and treatment approaches. The therapist is advised to augment the approaches included here with additional information from other chapters in this book as well as from the publications and resources listed at the end of these chapters.

Specific techniques mentioned may be applicable for use with a variety of diseases or disabilities. Since people have different needs, it is important to use the appropriate approach with each patient, and it is often impractical to use the same approach with all patients. Many theorists and clinicians have published their approaches; these should be explored by the therapist in order to choose appropriate techniques for each patient treated. Preliminary relevant, accurate, and complete evaluation procedures are necessary to determine the use of techniques.

Although there is reference to expensive commercial equipment used in large hospital or rehabilitation center treatment programs, the occupational therapist can use ingenuity and creativity in adapting whatever resources are available to the treatment program at hand. As the occupational therapist's goal is related to functional restoration of performance abilities, virtually any setting is adaptable to therapeutic use if it is one in which the client must perform.

Although the focus of this chapter is on physical dysfunction, it is essential to acknowledge the psychological impact of physical dysfunction on the individual and its resultant effect on potential functional restoration. In the recuperation process the mind and the body may work together or against each other. Effective functional restoration depends on the development of self-awareness, motivation, and effort with regard to the acceptance of insurmountable limitations and the achievement of realistic goals.

Basic Principles

The following principles are basic to functional restoration through occupational therapy:

1. *Correlation of the occupational therapy program* with the medical condition of the patient, assessment information, motivation and goals of the patient, the family and home situation, other treatment methods and services being received by the patient, medical and functional prognosis, and discharge planning

2. *Correlation of physical treatment procedures* with (a) the patient's level of receptivity, and (b) the patient's behavior

3. *Use of therapeutic positioning of the body* for rest and for therapy, using equipment appropriate to the individual's need and level of function and using principles of body mechanics

4. *Use of therapeutic relationships* during evaluation and treatment sessions between: (a) patient and therapist, (b) patient and patient, and (c) patient and group

5. *Use of purposeful activity* during evaluation and treatment procedures

6. *Use of a variety of evaluation techniques* including: (a) observation, (b) interview, (c) standardized tests, and (d) performance tests

7. *Use of the environment* to aid in adjustment and adaptation by the patient for functional living, including: (a) adjusting the setting for appropriate and effective evaluation of the patient's functional level, (b) adapting the level of stimuli for tolerance and interaction, (c) adjusting for successful and satisfying daily living activity, and (d) insuring self-worth through productive and social activity

8. *Use of activity analysis* in: (a) choice of activity for evaluation and treatment, and (b) choice of treatment method as related to the therapeutic value of the selected activity

9. *Use of activities of daily living* in evaluation and treatment to provide: (a) body awareness and acceptance, (b) daily exercise, and (c) indication of independent skill level and assistance needed

10. *Use of adaptive devices and equipment* to: (a) obtain maximum involvement in functional physical activity, (b) provide independence in daily self-care activities, and (c) provide self-esteem and self-worth in task completion

11. *Use of work simplification and energy conservation techniques* for: (a) motivation, accomplishment, and productivity, (b) maximum achievable independent living functions, and (c) successful task accomplishment

12. *Use of community resources* for: (a) successful community re-entry, (b) continued level of independence post-discharge, (c) social stimulation and benefit, and (d) independence in continuing rehabilitation goals

The development of occupational therapy practice has been influenced by medical concepts and practice with regard to life support systems, diagnostic accuracy, awareness of and referral to allied medical or therapeutic services, effect of medicines on patients' behaviors and functions, and technical development with regard to equipment and devices.

Occupational therapists have participated in the growth of therapeutic services by joining team efforts with associated physicians and professionals and by developing specific techniques. A multitude of treatment techniques is available for use with a patient. Characteristic of an eclectic approach has been the adaptation of some techniques used successfully with children to the treatment of adults. Further, sensory integration, useful in the psychiatric setting to encourage both physical and mental health, is now adapted for use in the physical rehabilitation setting to serve the patient suffering such disability as cerebrovascular accident (CVA) or head trauma.

Therapy has progressed from localized treatment of the injured part to work with the whole patient. This has been formalized into what is called "holistic therapy." Occupational therapists have long been taught to see and to treat the whole person. Indeed, it is on this basis that the occupational therapist determines the present and potential functional ability of the patient and then designs the treatment plan.

The material in this chapter is directed toward gaining an understanding of how to detect dysfunction and how to effect restoration of function as it relates to performance.

Impact of Disability

The impact of disease or injury causing physical and mental disability can be devastating to a person's present and future life. Although the long-term implications of the condition may not be recognized by the individual in the early stages of disability, they can affect the person and his family in a variety of ways over a period of time.

Characteristics of Onset

Sudden onset of manifestations and symptom complexes from external trauma is characteristic of spinal cord injury, brain injury, fractures, peripheral nerve injury, and amputation. These injuries are often caused by accidents involving cars, sports, industrial machinery, falls, or weapons, and usually affect the young or middle adult population. Although the manifestations may result in permanent limitations, the injuries are generally non-progressive in their symptoms. In older adults, lower extremity amputations also may be a result of poor circulation, and lower extremity fractures are commonly caused by falls.

Some neurological conditions are characterized by sudden onset resulting from internal trauma such as cerebrovascular accident (CVA, stroke). Pathology in the nervous system (polio, Guillain-Barré) also may have a sudden onset.

Insidious and progressive diseases such as multiple sclerosis, Parkinson's disease, and arthritis may show intermittent exacerbations and remissions in the disease process and may vary in duration. Myasthenia gravis and amyotropic lateral sclerosis are also progressive neurological diseases.

Impact

Sudden disability forces many sorts of adjustments when the disability impinges on the person's daily lifestyle and habits. The disease or disability takes on a unique meaning for each individual, related to age, family status, lifestyle, educational or vocational status, self-concept, general responsibilities, and interests. When daily living patterns are suddenly changed, the individual experiences an effect on motivation, emotional and social reactions, and general abilities.

The immediate or resultant difference between what was and what is may result in confusion, fear, questions, insecurity, feelings of inadequacy, or disequilibrium. A previous level of understanding may be replaced by unknown and unfamiliar or unacceptable conditions or situations. In order to establish a relationship which will help the individual to regain self-acceptance, the occupational therapist must begin by finding out the social significance of his or her medical condition to the patient, or what its impact will be on his or her lifestyle.

The patient with a sudden, imposed disability maintains the self-concept, self-awareness, and responses of an able-bodied person. If the patient has suddenly and possibly unknowingly made the transition from the ability context to the disability context, he or she must make the transition back. This is the rehabilitation process.

The therapist learns as much as possible about the family, environment, lifestyle, experience, achievements, and goals the individual had before becoming disabled. The process of rebuilding or rehabilitating begins with guidelines already set by the person before the intervention of disease or trauma.

Figure 21-1 illustrates the ability/disability/ability pattern with types of changes characteristic of the premorbid, trauma or disease, and post-trauma or disease periods. In the premorbid lifestyle the patient has begun to form a pattern of individuality. As a result of trauma or disease, a person experiences sud-

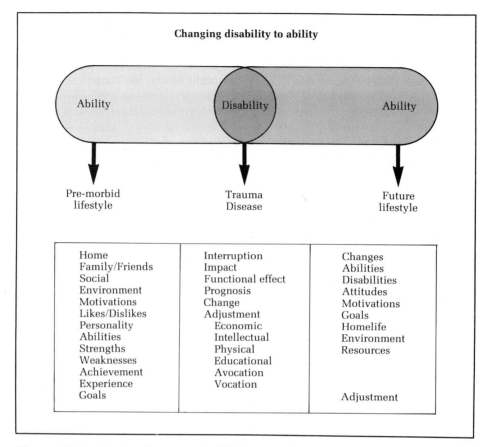

Figure 21-1. Areas of premorbid life experiences and achievement, areas affected by trauma and/or disease, and aspects of planning lifestyle for the future.

den change in anticipated security, expectations, and challenges. Once the immediate and early trauma period is past, having experienced temporary or permanent disability, each individual will look ahead to a new group of adjustment areas. In the post-trauma period, the individual regains or adjusts to the premorbid lifestyle. In the effort to change disability to ability, the patient deals with the areas listed in Figure 21-1.

The Role of Therapy

The rebuilding of a lifestyle demands a creative, realistic, and practical day-to-day adaptive approach to daily living skills, activities, and tolerance. The patient knows the *meaning of ability* in functioning, but must learn the *meaning of disability*. The therapist is able to challenge the patient to become an independently functioning individual, both mentally and physically, and to aid him or her in maintaining a balance in all abilities, no matter how well or how poorly developed.

The therapist sets the stage for attitudes regarding the physical setting, the techniques used, the indi-

vidual, the staff members, and the other patients. By constructing an environment conducive to optimum functional performance, the therapist conveys personal attitudes with regard to characteristics of diagnosis, disability, and behaviors demonstrated by the patients. The therapist provides respect, dignity, and reality to the patient during the initial period of fear, stress, confusion, or denial so that the patient can achieve self-awareness and self-respect as well as understanding of the situation, a sense of support from others, and acceptance of the therapist and the rehabilitation program. The therapist helps the patient to achieve integration reconciliation between predisability life and the life imposed by disability, between the known self and the unknown or new self. In programming for success, the therapist assumes a positive attitude. If the therapist's behavior does not convince the patient that occupational therapy is important, the patient will not respond well.

The following are some specific areas where the impact of disability will be experienced by functional restoration patients. What each patient experiences in these areas will affect the rehabilitation process.

Premorbid Personal Development

The premorbid level of personal development in all areas of function provides the person suffering from dysfunction with ways in which to deal with the effects on his present life, which has suddenly come to be made up of unfamiliar events and patterns. The prognosis for the future is determined by the premorbid characteristics the person has to invest in the process of rehabilitation.

As shown in Figure 21-2, disease or trauma occurs to persons at various stages of development or maturity. Preceding experiences, abilities, and problems affect the rehabilitation process and either enhance or hinder the accomplishment of goals. Good physical and mental development may aid in adjusting to future challenges.

A child born with a congenital disability experiences early life development *with* the disability, and it becomes part of the body image. The disability is a part of him or her as he or she grows. In this way, the congenitally disabled adult shows a high level of developmental integration because he lacks experiential guidelines to "normal" functioning. In contrast, the adolescent, young or older adult who has experienced a period of life as an able-bodied person knows the implications of loss of function in reference to previous life experience. It appears that the higher the physical, mental or social achievement the person has reached premorbidly, the greater the challenge in accepting loss and developing positive alternative goals for the future in accordance with the balance of permanent functional deficits and assets. The stage of development and the age of the person can be both advantageous and disadvantageous to necessary adjustments.

Social

Social interaction is essential for healthy human development, whether a person is gregarious or shy. At some point a person has need of others. When tragedy occurs, friends and family rally, but the duration of their commitment to the needs of the traumatized person will depend on the nature of the disability, the demands on people, the ability to give and personality of the individual, and the duration of need. The sequelae of disability (disfigurement, assistive devices, pathological motor patterns, presence of tremors, drooling, peculiar voice patterns, or deviations in normal behavioral or intellectual patterns) present a challenge to continuing social contact on a long-term basis.

In the social milieu the disabled person is faced with a new arena of behavior, one in which gains in self-awareness are challenged by a complex environment. Strong self-concepts and awareness are essential for expanding perceptions and reactions to include others and to become able to function effectively within a group. Here, as well as in the nonhuman (object) environment, gains in the ability to function will depend on the type and level of opportunities available. In order to interact with a group, the patient must be able to perform at the level expected by the group; otherwise, the patient will not be included as a significant member in the group.

Educational

The impact of disability can have a variety of effects on the educational development of the person. A child injured by a stray gunshot bullet during hunting season, resulting in permanent paraplegia, may be compelled to use a wheelchair as his or her principal means of locomotion. The child is dependent on ramps, curb cuts, and wide doorways for access to school, classrooms, and bathrooms. Although public schools in rural and urban environments are required to be accessible to wheelchair users, many are not.

The person suffering a head injury from an automobile accident may suffer damage to perceptual or intellectual centers in the brain, thus hindering the visualization and retention of information necessary for the learning process, preventing continuation of academic studies. The spinal cord injured person may not have the interest in or premorbid ability to pursue high academic goals which could be outlets to compensate for the loss of normal physical function.

Financial

Economic implications of disability can be devastating for both an individual and the individual's family. Financial assistance is available according to age, level of financial assets, type of illness or disability, duration, vocational or educational prognosis, governmental benefits, private insurance coverage, and liability coverage. Without the benefit of financial aid, rehabilitation costs can result in a drain of individual or family resources. Possible expenses include outlays for surgery, special treatment, assistive devices, wheelchairs, special home equipment, home modifications, adapted transportation aids, home health care, personal care attendant, outpatient treatment, follow-up, and adaptation to the employment site.

Premorbid lifestyle and psychological attitudes can assist the individual in coping with the struggle to regain continuity in life and to set new goals to achieve physical and emotional satisfaction. The occupational therapist must learn when and how each patient can work through each concern most beneficially.

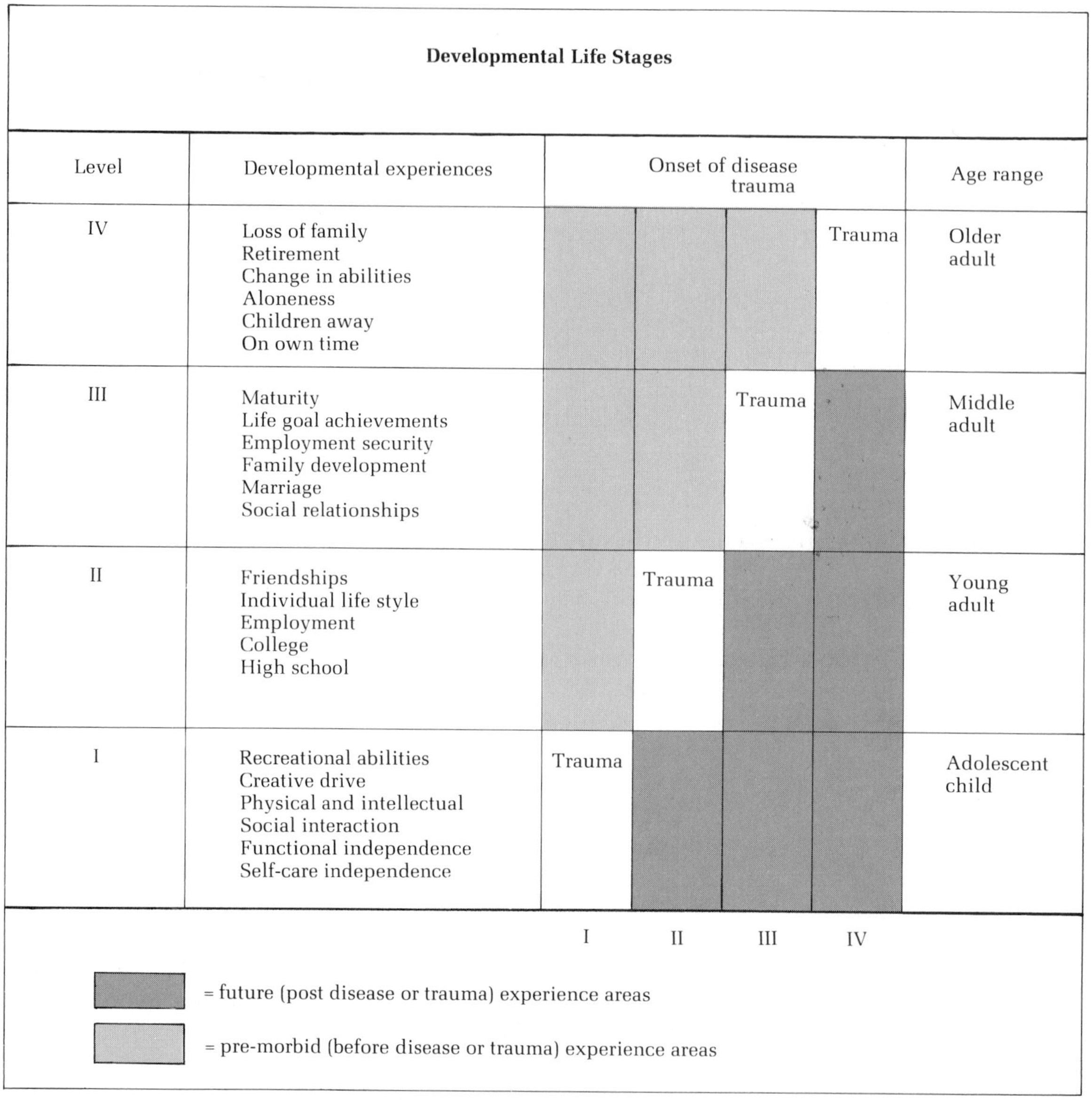

Developmental Life Stages

Level	Developmental experiences	Onset of disease trauma				Age range
IV	Loss of family Retirement Change in abilities Aloneness Children away On own time				Trauma	Older adult
III	Maturity Life goal achievements Employment security Family development Marriage Social relationships			Trauma		Middle adult
II	Friendships Individual life style Employment College High school		Trauma			Young adult
I	Recreational abilities Creative drive Physical and intellectual Social interaction Functional independence Self-care independence	Trauma				Adolescent child
		I	II	III	IV	

■ = future (post disease or trauma) experience areas

■ = pre-morbid (before disease or trauma) experience areas

Figure 21-2. The determination of age and developmental levels, life goal setting, and achievement extant at the time of the occurrence of disease or trauma are crucial to the planning of an appropriate treatment program.

The graph shows that the person is engaged in a certain level of development of life tasks at the occurrence of trauma or disease. Physical and psychological development resulting from the medical condition will be hindered or enhanced by what the person has gained.

A young child, disabled early in life, will approach and adjust to new life experience growing as a disabled person. An adult, disabled in midlife, has more life experience with which to adjust to his disability. Thus, premorbid development, experience, and attitudes have a crucial effect on the life adjustment of a disabled person.

Personal Attitudes That Inhibit Rehabilitation

1. Denial or rejection of the reality of long-term disability
2. Acceptance of societal attitudes that disabled persons are not "normal" or are socially and intellectually inferior
3. Fear of the unknown
4. Dislike of self due to inability or deformity
5. Rejection of therapy as unnecessary in adapting to disability and achieving ability
6. Development of dependency resulting from decreased self-value
7. Rejection of association with disabled people

Personal Associations Affecting Rehabilitation*

Recreation:	fun, skill, talent, game, leisure, physical, win, group
Therapy:	discipline, shame, parent-child, pain, discomfort, fear, anger, helpful
Paralysis:	dumb, inferior, cripple, stupid, useless, unknown, frightening, confining
Disabled:	bad, unpleasant, dumb, inconvenient, impatient, unattractive, someone else, childlike
Man:	able-bodied, masculine, strong, controlling, manipulating, smart, social
Woman:	attractive, weak, subordinate, mother, kind, supporting, loving
Dependent:	children, old people, women, undesirable, lazy, reversible, weak, sick, poor
Work:	remunerative, masculine, hard, strong, difficult
Leisure:	nonremunerative, fun, frivolous, social, relaxing
Well:	normal, walking, talking, doing, working, desirable, non-dependent, able-bodied, independent, capable
Ill:	dependent, lazy, non-desirable, controllable, non-controllable, unmasculine, unproductive

* Personal attitudes, concepts, associations, taboos, and experiences can hinder or enhance a person's positive role in the rehabilitation effort.

Theoretical Basis for Therapy

Occupational therapy is based on the belief that people are capable of relating to the human and nonhuman environments in a manner which is self-directed, purposeful, meaningful, and satisfying. Throughout the developmental continuum from birth to death, human beings experience growth by adapting to the challenges and stresses confronted in daily living. Adaptation is enhanced, thwarted, encouraged, or delayed by the individual's singular or composite abilities to progress through the myriad of learning experiences toward integration of sensorimotor and cognitive awareness and function necessary to accomplish meaningful tasks.

The occupational therapist's greatest challenge is to motivate a person toward self-direction and achievement for personal satisfaction. To this end the occupational therapist organizes the patient's immediate environment to provide opportunities for successful achievement of independent and productive functions.

The following criteria are suggested to ensure adequate and appropriate provision of occupational therapy services:
1. That the recipient of services can benefit from them
2. That occupational therapy services provide the opportunity for the recipient to improve and to gain functional abilities related to daily living requirements and desires
3. That the occupational therapist assist the recipient in learning about his or her medical condition and its resultant ability/disability pattern as related to the goal of the patient's assuming responsibility for the rehabilitation program
4. That the relationship between the occupational therapist and the patient be one in which the therapist lends support, guidance, and opportunity to the patient to achieve independent functions at his or her own speed, ability, and tolerance—not at that of the therapist
5. That the occupational therapist regard function qualitatively to enhance the patient's regard for and ability to function within the limits and range of individual goals and potentials.

Environment

In order to reach independence at any level, the disabled person must achieve enough control over the natural and the man-made environments to be able to achieve his or her goals with self-respect and satisfaction. Although there may be limitations which render the individual "handicapped" in specific situations, the extent to which the person with temporary or permanent disability can accomplish his or her goals is dependent on this control. The following are steps helpful in gaining self-confidence and strength to cope with the challenges of the natural and the man-made environments:

1. Ability to determine what one can do independently
2. Ability to determine what one can do with some assistance
3. Ability to determine what one cannot do without assistance
4. Ability to ask for assistance and get it
5. Ability to know whom to ask for assistance
6. Ability to instruct the person giving assistance
7. Ability to adjust to changes imposed by disability (appearance, special equipment, changes in abilities)
8. Development of knowledge of available resources (people, services, equipment, construction)
9. Development of knowledge of rights
10. Development of knowledge and acceptance of physical and mental tolerance

(See section on Environmental Factors, pp. 364–366 for more details.)

Performance

For the disabled individual, reaching previous physical activity levels or potential may seem inconceivable or unachievable; this feeling may result in decreased motivation to achieve at any level. This patient may be described as "unmotivated" because his or her goals may differ from the rehabilitation goals. The therapist must be sensitive to the patient's physical and mental levels, reactions, and apprehensions with regard to acceptance and tolerance of limitations and changes in ability imposed by the medical condition. The therapist is challenged to assist the patient in developing a "path of achievement" in accordance with medical and personal goals, the current medical condition, and the medical prognosis. Generally, patients need and benefit from assistance in channeling and controlling their energies into appropriate outlets designed to result in realistic, positive feedback regarding their current abilities.

One of the basic practices of occupational therapy is the use of performance as feedback to assist the patient in becoming involved in self-initiated, *purposeful activity* (see Fig. 21-3). Adaptive techniques to assist in the achievement of independent functions (self-care, social interactions, planning and initiating tasks) are often employed.

To perform is: to do
to carry out
to fulfill
to carry to completion
to accomplish

In occupational therapy, observation and evaluation of a person in the act of performing a task provide the therapist with a picture of the abilities and the limitations the person has in the accomplishment of a given task.

As a treatment facilitator, performance provides the experience of *doing,* from which the patient can gain an indication of whether or not he or she is able to accomplish the task and how well he or she can do it. Thus the patient gains feedback for self-awareness. Performance of a specific movement (repetitive reaching, supination, or any other specific drill) may increase function for use in task completion. To effect a feeling of self-worth, what a person does must be meaningful to him. Since people value the opinions of others, the patient will also derive self-worth when significant persons recognize accomplishments.

Successful performance appropriate to a person's level of functioning facilitates a sense of personal ability. Increasing the demand challenges increased ability which, when gained, provides additional feedback for self-worth. Levels of performance also serve as an indicator of *in*ability and are important for the person's awareness of reality in adjusting to living with permanent disability. Patients develop self-awareness in the performance of tasks and develop realistic self-concepts and goals through the experience of learning their own levels of accomplishment.

From the very beginnings of development, the human being progresses through life experiences and growth in a delicate balance of physical and psychological impressions, reactions, effects, and behaviors. They are interdependent and interchanging and stand in a cause-and-effect relationship to function. The mind and the body work together in providing feedback from function to effect change, adaptation, and improvement in the ability to relate to people, things, and tasks.

As the person is motivated to act, the mind designs the task for the body to perform. The nature of performance determines the sensory feedback which serves to motivate for continuation or for change in

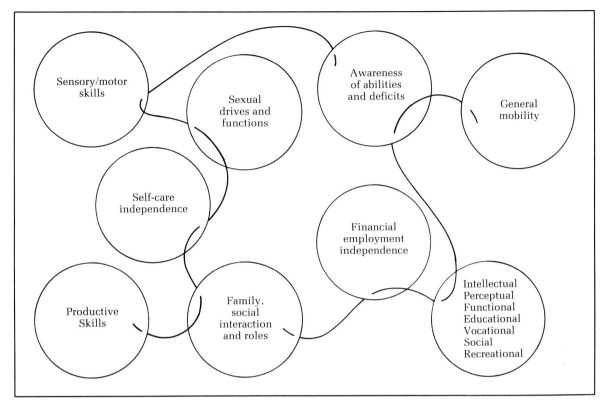

Figure 21-3. For the patient, the experience of and feedback from performance in one area of function can facilitate motivation and accomplishment in another. The timely interrelationship of tasks is connected by the thread of achievement.

the performance. The performer gains an awareness of social and personal acceptance dependent on the quality and appropriateness of the performance.

Therapeutic Relationship

The therapist must attempt to recognize the impact of evaluation and treatment methods on the patient's level of awareness and acceptance of disability. At the same time, the professional must be aware of his or her own limitations and must not feel *personally* rejected if the patient balks at the treatment program.

In her distinction between the *Sick Role* and the *Disabled Role,* Daniels states that choice of role affects the type and value of health care given to and received by the patient.[1] She describes the patient in the Sick Role as receiving care focused on noncontinuing or acute illness, with the medical treatment directed by a physician. In this role the person "acts sick" and responds to the authority of the physician, lacking the knowledge and experience to care for her or himself.

During the initial acute care phase of disability, a person may respond to this Sick Role due to the overwhelming nature of the onset of symptoms and

hospitalization. The patient avoids anxiety and uncomfortable feelings of confusion and helplessness by reaching out for protective denial of the implications to use as a crutch or as a retreat from reality. The unwanted reality may be severe damage to body parts and bodily functions implying undesirable long-term personal and social implications. Vargo states that, in this denial stage, "the individual is not emotionally prepared to accept the reality and the implications of the disability and consequently will deny that such a disability exists."[2]

During this period the patient attempts to regain old abilities, interests, and habits (if only in fantasy) in a desperate attempt to deny the temporary or permanent loss of them. The admission of these fantasies may be repressed in euphoric and cooperative behavior to minimize the anxiety which surfaces in anger or hostility when the patient is challenged to dig into true feelings. As there may be many unfamiliar new medical procedures during this time, the patient may slide into the beginning of a habit of dependency, encouraged by the necessity to fit into an unfamiliar, authoritative, medical system. With the prime focus on the person being medical, the disabled person becomes hypersensitive to his or her own thoughts. The patient may try to ward off the fearful recognition that his or her body represents a nonintegrated group of parts and no longer functions totally within control. Fear and confusion may lead to feelings of shame and rejection of his or her body. This effectively blocks the patient's investment in rehabilitative measures and places the full responsibility for motivation to get well on the shoulders of those serving him or her.

Daniels states that the Sick Role should not be applied to a disabled person, for this can result in undertreatment (not enough information being provided to the patient regarding the medical condition and treatment), overtreatment (too much or inappropriate care is given), or mistreatment (decisions regarding the medical condition and treatment are made without consulting the patient).

To avoid these errors, the health care providers should use the Disabled Role, according to Daniels. She describes this as a continuous process in which the treatment is centered around the patient and the patient's goals, coordinating care with lifestyle, and working through cooperation. In this role the patient seeks rehabilitation, accepts disability as a personal characteristic, and through growing knowledge of the disability, takes an authoritative role in his or her own care.

The Disabled Role is often difficult to follow in a general hospital setting, where care is directed toward acute medical intervention. However, a disabled person hospitalized for acute distress should be allowed to carry out as much self-care as possible as being treated for the long-term disability rather than for the acute illness constitutes "overtreatment"; "interrupted established routines can injure the self-sufficiency of the disabled person."[3] This, of course, refers to the patient who has already been through the process of rehabilitation and has been living in the community as a disabled person.

The hospitalization of the newly disabled patient may terminate during the denial stage, with the patient unreconciled to future implications of disability and unprepared to leave the sterile protection of the medically-oriented environment. In acknowledging the patient's difficulty in accepting alternatives to prior decisions and actions, Granger states that the occupational therapist "introduces unfamiliar devices and techniques that substitute for actions that have become difficult or impossible due to functional loss" which may be "direct non-verbal confrontation with existing deficits" necessitating "recognition of the permanence of the impairment."[4]

After the period of autocratic denial of disability and unsuccessful attempts to regain the reality of the past, the affected person reaches a stage of beginning to recognize the facts regarding the condition and passes into a period of bitter mourning where the fantasy of denial can no longer be maintained. Medical changes begin to plateau, and the patient sees that his or her new life does not fit into old patterns. During this depression the patient may consider suicide or wish for death, become uncooperative toward care, and hurt both family members and those most able to aid him or her in improving the condition.

Heijn states that "a patient must be able to mourn his losses to see the options in a restricted life."[5] A patient puts limited effort into learning new methods if she or he insists on holding onto past and out-of-reach methods. In adjusting to a new body image, the patient must accept a new or adapted lifestyle and indeed may wish to change it. The strength for these life changes is won by developing a new sense of self-worth by participating in experiences that allow abilities to grow and to be accepted. Although the patient benefits from the support of loved ones, the patient will be the best teacher of how they can accept and adapt to him or her.

Self-worth is developed through trial and result, whether successful or unsuccessful. One's concept of ability is proven through the successful accomplishment of tasks and recognition by oneself and others. When the opportunity to repeat the same successful performance is removed by the inability to perform a part or all of the task, one may doubt one's future ability and the gradual destruction of self-confidence and motivation may begin. Then self-worth must be regained by the acceptance of one's actual ability.

Although the patient may not be aware of what has happened to disrupt normal function or of the implications and potentials of progressive functional restoration, the patient is acutely aware of a *selfness* inside. Although physical abilities may be lacking, the patient focuses on personal signs of achievement. The patient may even hold on to destructive concepts of over-judging and anticipating gains. The therapist must remember that the patient's views are as important as those of the treatment team. Only if the patient's views are known and respected is the therapist able to assist the patient in developing positive ideas about himself or herself.

Value of Activity

The theory expressed by Mary Reilly, Ed.D., OTR, "that man, through the use of his hands as they are energized by mind and will can influence the state of his own health," has long guided the occupational therapist in the use of manual activity for therapeutic purposes.[6] The therapeutic value of the activity provided is dependent on its meaning to the person performing it.

Activity provides the patient with information

about what he or she is capable of doing. When presented with a situation in which to perform, the patient can deny neither ability nor inability related to a specific task. Although the patient may object to the nature of the activity and reject its importance and significance to rehabilitation, performing it does provide the patient with important gauges for measuring his or her own abilities and attitudes.

A. Jean Ayres suggests that doing the activity is a more meaningful way to improve human functioning than is thinking or talking about the activity. She further suggests that the brain needs information from gravity, movement receptors, muscles, joints, and the skin of the entire body for effective integration:

> The interaction of the sensory and motor systems through all their countless interconnections is what gives meaning to sensation and purposefulness to movement.[7]

Ayers describes purposeful activities as things which begin, continue, and end. In the process of purposeful activity, one follows through to the purpose one wants by doing something *with* something, *to* something, or *for* something.[8]

In the adjustment period post-diagnosis of disease or disability, characteristics of the patient's premorbid attitudes, behaviors, and personality become a part of the rehabilitation process. The drive to regain the premorbid lifestyle may become a strong motivation to the patient in setting goals. Careful and sensitive probing by the therapist into professed interests and proven abilities and self-concepts of the patient helps to reveal what the patient was and how he or she views the future.

First gained in the initial contact, this information is reviewed periodically with the patient throughout the rehabilitation process. Insight into the patient's interests with regard to educational and vocational pursuits, homelife, lifestyle, responsibilities, and leisure activities must be gained. Areas to explore include feelings and plans related to family, social contacts, physical and mental potential, life goals for achievement, competitiveness, interest in creative activity, skills, and plans.

Types of activity in which the patient has shown previous interest may become an important part of adjustment to disability. It is important to find out what sort of association and objective the patient had or expects to have with an activity. For example, if one patient is interested in sports, is it in order to compete with skill or ability, to participate socially, to dream of being outstanding, to describe or review, or to enjoy watching a formal game either in person or on television? If another patient's interest is in music, does this person wish to perform well, to perform adequately, to listen, to be knowledgeable in discussions, or to attend performances? Are the patient's favorite leisure activities socializing with friends at home or at community events, camping with family or friends, traveling, or engaging in such solitary outdoor activities as fishing?

The disabled person may never be able to accept the fact of physical or neurological disability. Mourning a loss, the disabled person goes through periods of denial, hope, delusion, hate, guilt, complacence, sadness, depression, hostility, adjustment, and, sometimes, acceptance. The ability to reason aids in passage through these stages, although the person must deal with the disability both emotionally and intellectually.

Diagnostic

Performance in an activity appropriate to the patient's rehabilitation level and goals can show the patient and the therapist what functional level the patient is able to or is willing to achieve. Regardless of negative feelings about the medical condition, the patient is able to experience specific feelings about the current level of achievement. Activity allows a myriad of opportunities for self-expression. Depending upon how it is designed and presented by the therapist, activity provides information regarding quality of performance, level of task completion, skill, talent, insight, strength, tolerance, and ability.

Curative

Activity provides a structure for graded improvement in abilities and gives proof of the level of current achievement. It presents reality to patients with regard to what they are able to do and accomplish. It also aids in bringing them into interaction with both people and tasks. The patient is able to learn about himself or herself and to begin to make a functional link with the environment.

As self-awareness and recognition of the realities of dysfunction grow, the patient becomes able to share in the positive plan for recovery of abilities. Activity provides the patient with the practice of abilities, a sense of continuous accomplishment, a sense of continuity in recovery, and a gradual process of planning. With the development of awareness and an insight into how to begin to determine daily planning of activity, the patient is able to progress with daily feedback concerning performance and to reestablish the human link with peers through social interaction. This aids the patient in establishing an understanding of his or her place in society.

In the process of achieving adaptive behavior through the use of activity, the patient assists in realistic planning through self-staging and gradual accomplishment, and begins to adjust to people and to the environment. The patient begins to see herself or himself as a functioning member of society, regains independent functioning as a person, and begins to reach out to family and peers.

In providing adjustment to disability through the use of therapeutic activities, the occupational therapist assists the patient in learing the following:

1. Physical, mental, and emotional abilities and limitations
2. How to compensate for physical dysfunction
3. The limits of physical and mental tolerance
4. How to compensate for disability by using substitutes for familiar functions
5. How to cope with emotional frustrations caused by lost or decreased independent function
6. The social, economic, interpersonal, and familial implications of dysfunction
7. How to cope with economic problems caused by long-term disability (cost of hospitalization, expense of continuing treatment and assistive devices and equipment, decrease in job opportunities, and the necessity to be dependent on others in previously independent areas of function)
8. How to adapt to a new functional level of achievement
9. How to learn the functional use of leisure time
10. How to organize, adjust to, and accept a new lifestyle

In the rehabilitation process the patient must be encouraged and allowed to function independently at the level of his or her ability in all areas of activity. This approach begins with self-care and ends with vocational independence. If deprived of the experience of doing independently whatever is possible, the patient will lack the opportunity to work and to struggle through the stages of achieving maximum independence. If a therapist or other team member does the job, he or she encourages dependency on the part of the patient. When uninvolved in the treatment plan and implementation, the patient loses commitment to the regaining of self-care skills, self-reliance, identity, and individuality. In assisting the patient to regain these functions, the therapist must put aside his or her own needs and help the patient effectively in the struggle to self-awareness and acceptance.

The patient can do much to make maximum use of remaining physical abilities, adding to them as strength, endurance, and motivation increase. Activity that is specifically and therapeutically directed toward an increase in functional ability can provide important feedback to the patient by showing tangi-

ble proof that she or he *can* perform. Although the level of performance may not reach the patient's former physical or intellectual competence, incentive can be derived from small gains if the activity is directed properly. As the gains increase, so does the motivation, the willingness to try, and the beginnings of acceptance. In the early treatment sessions, the patient must be supported in the forms self-expression may take as she or he experiences the feelings described above.

Environmental Factors

Environment consists of all persons (human environment) and things (nonhuman environment) surrounding an individual. Human performance is greatly affected by environmental influences and by the way a person interprets them. The person encumbered by disability and its accompanying emotions may find on re-entry that a previously known environment becomes unfamiliar and unknown. It may suddenly change from having a safe, familiar, and comforting feeling toward the individual to having an unfriendly, unsafe, unwelcoming, or even hostile aspect. The environment is continually changing during the recuperation of the disabled person; this phenomenon may represent an overwhelming and continuing challenge and may pose an obstacle to adaptation.

In adapting to the familiar environment with a different body and mind, the individual may be in the situation of having to adjust to the old, with decreased adaptive ability, and to adjust to the new with even less ability to adapt. However, the recovering patient may actually be more aware of the adaptive challenges of the environment through a sudden slowing down of all physical and mental adjustment mechanisms.

Dunning suggests that occupational therapists are managers of space (to promote stimulation), people (to encourage social interaction), and tasks (to develop skills).[9] In functioning in this role, the therapist analyzes the effects of the surroundings on a person in terms of the individual's response. Deficits found during the initial interview and evaluation cue the therapist to appropriate changes in the environment, either to stimulate or to inhibit the person's behavior or adaptation. The therapist must assist the patient in gradually adjusting to the challenges of the environment by increasing appropriate performance within it.

The occupational therapy program provides the patient with activities in order to (1) create awareness of self in time and space, (2) develop awareness of the environment, and (3) reveal behavior changes and development of abilities. In the effort to enhance these awareness areas, the occupational therapist should use the following objectives in planning the treatment program: encourage active movement and performance, involve the patient with those nearby and with the environment to provide opportunities, channel abilities, facilitate action, and eliminate barriers to function. Through a program of normal activities in an appropriate environment, the therapist helps the patient to establish a new self-image and to accept changes in physiology, feelings, and appearance. The therapist also aids the adjustment in preparation to re-enter the home and community and to assume healthy attitudes toward self and family.

Environmental influences can have positive or negative effects on the evaluation and treatment of the person with physical or neurological dysfunction. The following elements can structure the environment for success:

1. *Atmosphere:* The area used for evaluation and treatment should have adequate and comfortable space, lighting, and temperature. The therapist initially orients the patient to the meaning of the room, its contents, its location, and its functions, and introduces the patient to the other people in the room. The therapist controls the visual and auditory stimuli in order to relieve anxiety or confusion that the patient may experience.
2. *Sensory bombardment:* Excessive, unexpected sensory impulses (visual, auditory, tactile, proprioceptive, or kinesthetic) can cause the patient to become confused, fatigued, or frightened. Therefore, the therapist controls *all* of the surrounding stimuli.
3. By using voice and body in a supportive, non-threatening way, the therapist becomes a therapeutic tool.
4. An acceptable level of achievement, commensurate with the patient's interests, is necessary to provide positive feedback.
5. In some situations, familiar objects may be threatening during the early stages of treatment. Therefore, unfamiliar activities and exercises may be better for initial evaluation and treatment.

The occupational therapist assists in providing an optimum living environment. Arrangement of furniture in the room, bed location in relation to the door and to other patients, accessibility of personal items, proximity to the emergency call button, and accessibility and ease of use of the bathroom all contribute to mental, physical, and emotional well-being. Where the patient eats and socializes (own room, cafeteria, or dining room) the facilities should be accessible and should encourage independent functioning; the patient should be placed with compatible persons during meal times and for social functions.

In the occupational therapy room, depending on the goals of the treatment program at a given time, the patient should be allowed to work in a secluded area if desired or to work in proximity to others who could have a therapeutic effect on his or her functioning.

Family members and friends can have varying effects on the patient; some may be encouraging and may stimulate functional recovery, while others may be patronizing or pitying and thus may retard progress. The objective of stressing environmental interaction is assisting the patient to adjust to returning home and to use skills to adapt to the environment for maximum function and minimum stress.

Able-bodied persons tend to limit their perception of the environment to what they know or where they are, rather than noticing the conditions to which the disabled person must adapt. In evaluating the needs and the steps to be taken in this area for readaptation, it is important to get a picture of what the patient will be going into. The gradual building of adaptive skills will then aid in the preparation for future environmental changes. Aspects of the environment to be evaluated are: responsibilities of the patient and others sharing the immediate surroundings; expectations of the patient for performance and role; others' expectations and roles; housing design; location of living quarters; type of neighborhood; use of private or public transportation; and location of community resources.

Architectural Considerations

The whole area of housing accessibility for the physically disabled person is complex. The home itself may be difficult to get into and out of, regardless of its inhabitants' limitations. It may also have architectural idiosyncrasies which make it difficult for the disabled person to perform daily activities which were previously done independently.

Checklists to aid in complete evaluation and recommended measurements for access areas (entrance hallways, rooms, and garages) are provided through many resources; some of them are listed at the end of Chapter 22.

Wheelchair users should be instructed about what to look for to determine if a building and its functions are accessible or adaptable. Considerations of the accessibility or challenges presented by any building will become a natural part of planning. National standards, identifying accepted standards of accessibility, are published and available on request from the American National Standards Institute. Federal and state laws have been passed stipulating accessibility regulations and providing enforcement mechanisms for demanding proper construction of public buildings. These are used both in constructing new buildings and in renovating existing ones to assure equal access by all persons, regardless of disability.

Seeing oneself as having less self-worth as a result of disability is a normal reaction to loss. This is confirmed by the social signs of difficulty in acceptance and "forgiveness" of disability by lack of attention to making the physical, man-made environment accessible to the physically disabled. Feelings of anger and helplessness against these attitudes can be channeled positively into working to assist the community to recognize disabled persons as citizens with equal human rights. Community, state, and national organizations of disabled people provide peer support and channels for action for those interested in becoming involved in changing attitudes.

In considering the impact of disability from a social point of view, it is interesting to note Vargo's comment that, although *disability* is regarded as an observable impairment in the functioning of a body part, a *handicap* is a function of the interaction between individuals and their total environment. A society's political and fiscal priorities will determine whether or not people will be able to manage in spite of their disabilities. In a totally accessible society, a disabled person is not handicapped; in a society filled with stairs, curbs, visual identifications of locations, and auditory warning signals, handicapping situations confront every disabled person.[10]

A person's attitude toward his or her own disability affects others as well. For example, a quadriplegic using a wheelchair can diminish the awareness of the wheelchair and a condescending attitude from others by practicing assertive behavior. An upper extremity amputee learns to use his prostheses to perform needed and desired functions in public (putting a coin in a machine, mailing a letter, driving a car, or opening a door for others). A woman who has had an arm amputation as a result of cancer will need to overcome her sensitivity regarding both the use of her prosthesis and the feel of it as a part of her body; by doing this, she can actively engage in social life with her family and friends.

Community

The basic fact that a person has been a part of a neighborhood, school class, or working team prior to disability presents many adjustments in returning to these familiar active friends and formerly comfortable places; residual disabilities may render this person limited in relation to former abilities. How the newly disabled person feels with old friends and in making new friends while using a wheelchair, for example, will depend on the adjustment to accepting the wheelchair as an important part of functioning. The

middle-aged man returning to work as a hemiplegic, recovered enough from his stroke to perform somewhat modified tasks with his fellow workers, may have to accept a slower pace of physical performance and intellectual functioning.

A handicap can be imposed on a disabled person by a society which lacks understanding or information regarding what an individual can or cannot do physically. For example, an employer may focus on the fact that a physical disability exists, rather than on what the person is actually capable of doing with regard to job requirements. Implications for prevocational evaluations and programs are to plan realistic alternatives for the disabled individual that will result in employment which can be performed with success and pride.

Evaluation

The terms *evaluation* and *assessment* have both been used with regard to initial procedures for fact-finding preparatory to treatment of the patient. Generally, both refer to the process of determining, estimating, or assigning values. However, within this section, the term *assessment* refers to the *totality* of results of specific evaluation procedures used, the formation of *an impression of the total composite picture* of the patient's functioning. For example, specific *evaluations* of range of motion, strength, and coordination are used to reach an *assessment* of upper extremity function.

Occupational therapists use a variety of methods and formats to measure and record results of testing in order to provide factual information and for assessment of functional ability. These vary from setting to setting; many forms have been published by treatment facilities and are distributed through the American Occupational Therapy Association (AOTA).

It is important to determine the content and scope of the assessment responsibility within the occupational therapy department and to maintain these limits both in order to avoid unnecessary overlap by team members and to provide the most accurate and effective procedures and data from occupational therapy. Working out role delineations and resultant procedural responsibilities is both a departmental and a team function. The flow sheet pictured in Figure 21-4 shows the general pattern of data gathering, programming, and reporting the therapist uses following the referral of a patient to occupational therapy.

Before beginning the evaluation, the therapist determines the duration of the patient's stay in the setting and how much time will be spent in occupational therapy. This is often determined at the time of

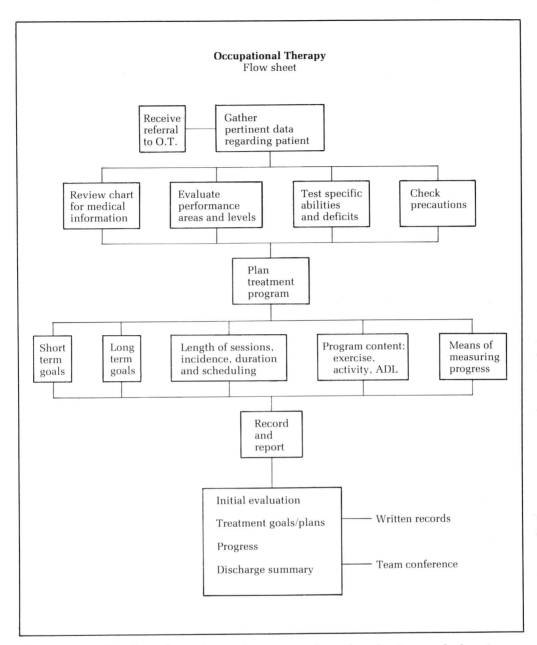

Figure 21-4. The flow sheet shows the progression of evaluation and planning activities that are communicated through written records and team conferences.

referral, but it is usually negotiable according to evaluation information and recommendations. This will be helpful in determining the extent of the evaluation appropriate to the treatment to be provided. In no case should the patient go through hours of evaluation which, while providing the therapist with much information, may not be appropriate to the treatment program, the condition, or the prognosis.

Unfortunately, this imbalance may occur when there is a lack of team effort in setting initial goals, when the evaluation is more extensive than necessary, or when it is poorly organized and overly time-consuming. It is important to remember that the patient does become mentally and physically fatigued during the evaluation process. Therefore, these procedures should include an equal balance of positive feedback and information to the patient and should be accomplished in a realistic amount of time.

Referral

A person may be referred to occupational therapy by anyone recommending evaluation, treatment, or consultation. This is permitted by the American Occupational Therapy Association (AOTA); however, it does not apply in all cases.

For example, in a hospital, rehabilitation center, nursing home, or other medically-oriented setting, a patient usually must have a written and signed referral from a physician in order to be accepted for evaluation or treatment. This ensures eligibility for third-party payment for services where applicable. Lack of third-party reimbursement unfortunately can result in denial of occupational therapy services to the patient, which can mean a loss of valuable assistance in regaining independent functioning.

There are indeed many situations in which an occupational therapist may be able to provide valuable treatment services or recommendations in the absence of a physician. For disabled children, an occupational therapist may be able to recommend specific positioning for schoolwork, assistive devices for eating or writing, or ways for a child to interact with classmates. Often, helpful advice can be given through school/teacher/parent systems.

For the disabled adult, an occupational therapist may be able to assist a factory manager in understanding the ability of an upper extremity amputee to perform the work with a prosthesis, or assist in adapting a work area so that a skilled paraplegic can do the job from a wheelchair.

The *formal request* for occupational therapy is usually designated the *referral*. Unlike the specific treatment prescription request, the referral allows the therapist the freedom to use available evaluation techniques deemed appropriate to provide information about the patient to determine the treatment program recommendations. The physician or other referring party may specify evaluation or treatment techniques, but in order to determine the appropriateness of the referral orders and to provide complete occupational therapy evaluation, treatment, and recommendation reports, it is important for the therapist to perform a full evaluation and develop a complete assessment. This allows the therapist to make further recommendations based on evaluation findings.

The following information may be received within the initial referral: patient identification, diagnosis, precautions or pertinent data, request for service, and physician identification (see Fig. 21-5). If the information is not presented, it may be taken from the patient's chart.

The therapist writes and signs the evaluation report directly below the referral information. Treatment progress notes from the occupational therapy department may be added to the form later. This differs from the problem-oriented system in which team members and physicians reporting on a patient all use the same form and refer to a problem list in reporting information, rather than having each specialist use a separate form.

The following are several methods of referral:
1. Occupational Therapy Department form (Fig. 21-5)
2. Chart order for "O.T.," "O.T. Evaluation," "O.T. Evaluation and Recommendations," "O.T. Treatment," written on the physician's order form on the chart
3. Telephone order from the physician, nurse, or unit clerk
4. Agency order for specific request
5. Verbal order at team case conference

Regardless of the method of referral, it is essential that the order be specific, be dated, and be signed by the referring party. If a telephone order is presented, the therapist can request that the order be made in writing and sent to the therapist, or the therapist can write up the information and send it to the physician for signature and return prior to contact with the patient. This precaution is necessary to insure safety for all concerned with regard to referral practices.

Too often during the evaluation process the therapist designs an ambitious program of testing, often inadvertently draining the patient's physical and emotional strength. The therapist's first concern should be how the patient feels and what attitudes he or she has toward the medical condition, the daily program, personal problems, fears, and ability to cope. In the initial contact, it is good to allow the patient full freedom to express feelings and concerns before beginning the gentle but firm program of evaluation. By getting acquainted with the patient in this manner initially, the therapist is better equipped to elicit cooperation in continuing the evaluation process.

Although it is helpful to have an organized evaluation routine, it is frequently necessary to adjust the routine to meet the specific needs of a patient. For example, if a patient is physically fatigued, the therapist can evaluate an aspect of the condition that will not cause additional fatigue. Similarly, if the patient is anxious because of emotional stress and mental fatigue, the therapist should choose an evaluation area and method that will be acceptable, comfortable, and tolerable. For the most accurate results, it is essential to adjust the chronology of the evaluation procedures to the individual's needs while still trying to complete the evaluation as quickly and as thoroughly as possible.

```
┌─────────────────────────────────────────────────────────┐
│              NAME OF FACILITY                             │
│              OCCUPATIONAL THERAPY REFERRAL                │
│                                                           │
│   Patient Identification                                  │
│   _____        │
│                                                           │
│         REFERRAL FOR EVALUATION AND TREATMENT             │
│   _____        │
│   Diagnosis:                                              │
│   _____        │
│   Precautions or Pertinent Data:                          │
│   _____        │
│   _____        │
│   Request:   a) O.T. evaluation:                          │
│              b) Specific treatment request:               │
│   _____        │
│   _____        │
│   _____ M.D.  _____        │
│         Signature                        Date             │
│   _____        │
│                                                           │
│          REPORT OF EVALUATION AND TREATMENT               │
│   _____        │
│   Date                             OTR Signature          │
│   _____        │
│   _____        │
│   _____        │
│   _____        │
│   _____        │
│   _____        │
│   _____        │
│   _____        │
│   _____        │
│   _____        │
└─────────────────────────────────────────────────────────┘
```

Figure 21-5. Occupational Therapy Referral.

Usually a comprehensive assessment includes enough methods of evaluation to provide the patient with alternatives in performance, thus making the process tolerable and even enjoyable. In creatively adapting the methods to the patient, the therapist can use these different approaches for varying lengths of time and in different order: verbal questioning in the interviewing approach, timed aspect in the speed test, coordination of the performance test under stress, and the quality of the product in the functional test. Throughout the evaluation process it is essential to derive accurate, factual information. The more the patient understands and becomes involved in the procedure, the more progress will be made.

Clinical Approaches

The occupational therapist uses four basic approaches for clinical evaluation:
1. Observation of the patient
2. Interview of the patient
3. Formal evaluation and testing procedures
4. Informal performance evaluation

Each method provides a different approach to gathering information. Therapeutic contact with the patient is initiated and maintained during all the procedures.

Observation of the Patient

The most important approach is observation of the patient. Apart from reading the chart or learning about the patient from other team members, observation is not only the first direct contact but is the one from which the initial impression is formed. How the therapist greets the patient, makes introductions, and involves him or her in the surroundings all convey how acceptable she or he is as a person. The therapist must continually be aware of how she or he, the environment, and the tests are affecting the patient. Signs of the mental and physical condition should be observed closely. Observation requires no previous contact with either the chart or with other people, and can be used effectively in the absence of other information.

By observing the patient's facial expression the

therapist can detect paralysis, drooling, spasticity, confusion, as well as alertness, fatigue, happiness, sadness, or pain. The position of the arms and legs can indicate spasticity, flaccidity, deformity, or pain. The sitting position can give indications of muscle imbalance, discomfort, or lack of voluntary control. Splints or slings also indicate some deficit in normal function. When walking into the room, the patient may display a gait produced by the use of braces, crutches, a prosthetic limb, a cane, or a walker, or reveal a degree of paralysis not necessitating these aids. The skin may exhibit the effects of exertion or anxiety by appearing sweaty or red or becoming pale and clammy. Undue pressure from a splint or brace produces red or ulcerated marks or sores on the skin. If the therapist asks the patient to perform a task, the response can reveal hearing loss, muscle weakness, or incoordination.

Interview with the Patient

The interview is a chance to get to know how the patient feels about what has happened, the resultant effects on life and family, and the crucial priorities of the situation. Little may be known about the patient or the patient's condition. The interview (combined with observation) is the opportunity to find out information helpful to the therapist in planning the therapeutic program. Informal discussion leads to ease with the therapist and with the environment.

Most persons do not tolerate persistent questions about themselves at this point in their rehabilitation, but they may wish to share information regarding their problems in order to try to deal with them. The sincere therapist who observes the patient's reactions during the interview can often pick up valuable information about his or her interests and fears and can regulate the interview according to the reactions, attitudes, and tolerance levels exhibited.

The attitude of the therapist must be acceptable, if trust and confidence are to be inspired. The interview need not be rigidly formal nor need it be completed in a single session. The initial contact marks the beginning of the relationship, which may last a long time, depending on rehabilitation needs. This beginning is crucial to the establishment of a good therapeutic environment, incorporating atmosphere, privacy, duration, acceptance, freedom of expression, and comfort.

Formal Evaluation and Testing Procedures

Formal evaluation procedures provide objective methods with which to judge performance levels. Frequently they are broken down into specific tests to be completed with specific equipment and conforming to specific procedures. Examples of such tests include using a goniometer to measure passive and active range of motion, using a dynamometer to gauge grip strength, using a pinch gauge to register prehension pressure, or using an aesthesiometer to determine two-point discrimination.

Objective tests for coordination include dexterity tests, such as the Crawford Small Parts Dexterity Test (see Fig. 21-6), the Pennsylvania Bimanual Work Sample, the Minnesota Rate of Manipulation Tests (see Fig. 21-7), and the Bennett Hand Tool Test. These tests and many others have norms or standardized measurements for comparing results. At times, however, the norms relate to normal physical performance and thus have selected use for the physically disabled person. Each test has a specific purpose and method of administration. If the norms are to be used in reference to the test score, administration of the test must be according to the instructions. For example, a quadriplegic, lacking a normal level of physical movements and sensory functions of the hands, may perform much lower on a coordination test if speed is an important factor. If the speed factor is removed, however, he may perform with a high level of accuracy and tolerance. Since there are a great many tests available, it is essential to select the test(s) that will reveal the needed information regarding the patient's

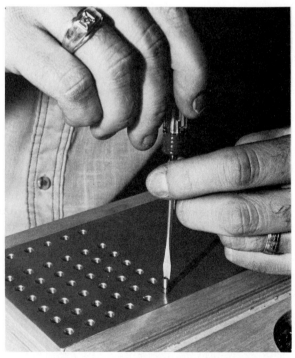

Figure 21-6. Crawford Small Parts Dexterity Test. A timed bimanual coordination test using small screws and a small screwdriver to complete transfer pattern to a metal plate.

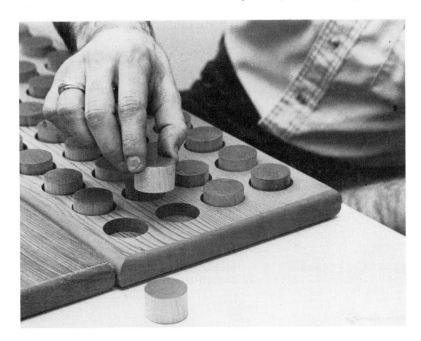

Figure 21-7. Minnesota Rate of Manipulation Test. A five-part timed test using unilateral and bilateral object manipulation patterns for transfer of wooden discs.

performance, so that explicit information can be given to team members as needed.

Tests of perceptual-motor function may include the Ayres Battery and the Frostig Battery, which are not standardized for an adult population, and the Minnesota Spatial Relations Test (Fig. 21-8). Treatment centers use a variety of specific tests to measure performance according to norms; the aforementioned are but a few of those commonly used. Further information on specific tests can be found in the chapter on evaluation by Helen Smith.

Informal Performance Testing

In assessing general performance the therapist evaluates how well the patient accomplishes a specific task. What are limitations of strength, coordination, or range of motion as indicated by ability shown in reaching for, grasping, or placing objects? (see Fig. 21-9A and B). How well is the patient adjusting to limitations? This can be evaluated by observation of the character of social interactions with other patients, mental tolerance of the social context and activity of the occupational therapy room, and ability to work with spouse or the therapist in reviewing self-care abilities in light of eventually going home, where the assistance of a family member may be needed.

Performance testing also involves the assessment of problem-solving ability in accomplishing a task comprising several steps. For example, a woodworking project may be used to test the perceptual-motor abilities of the patient with brain damage. The therapist observes the method of planning the project, signs regarding visual perception, eye-hand coordination, concept of verticality, and proper use of tools.

In performance testing it is essential to set up the task so that, although difficult, it is within the patient's ability range. The use of a familiar task in evaluation may be threatening because it causes the patient to become acutely aware of the loss of ability. Performance testing must include a balance of success along with evaluation of functional deficits. Otherwise, the client may become overly discouraged or negative toward the occupational therapist, and such an attitude can hinder achievement and progress.

Occupational Therapy Worksheet

The worksheet, shown in Figure 21-10, is used to facilitate the recording of information derived from the evaluation procedures. It is called a "worksheet" because it is *not* included in the chart, but rather assists the therapist in noting information that will be included later in the formal summarized chart report. In addition to the documentation of basic information, each functional area is delineated for ease in recording. Additional sheets with detailed information on range of motion, perceptual functions, manual muscle testing, activities of daily living, or homemaking can be used to supplement this information. This depends on the needs of the patient for individualized procedures.

At the end of the worksheet there is space for inclusion of the treatment plan. Following the evaluation, the therapist and the patient design the

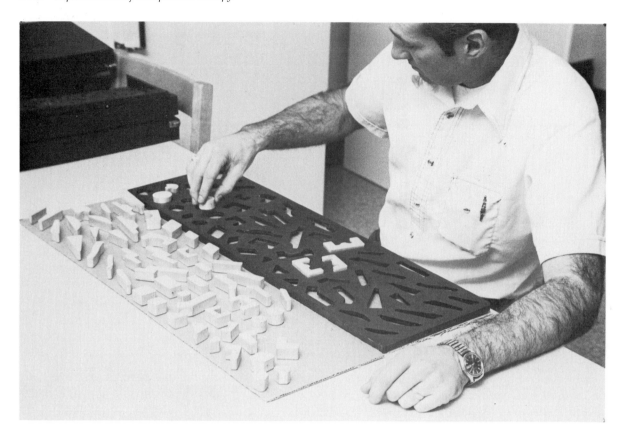

Figure 21-8. Minnesota Spatial Relations Test. A timed standardized unilateral test used to evaluate visual-motor perception and organization as the patient transfers objects one-by-one from one field to another.

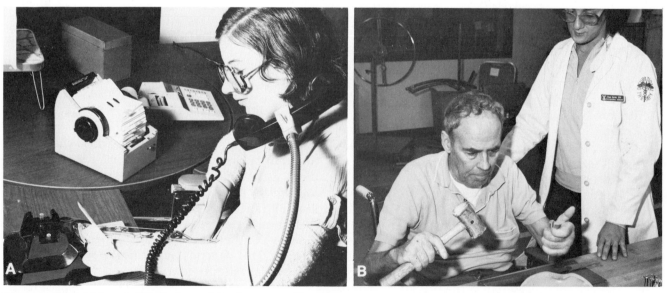

Figures 21-9 (A) and **(B).** Informal Performance Testing.

Discharge Date: _____

Occupational Therapy Worksheet

Name: _____   Admission Date: _____ Room # _____

Address: _____   Diagnosis: _____ Duration: _____

Age: _____ Education: _____   Pertinent History: _____

Occupation: _____   O.T. Referral/Order: _____

Marital Status: _____   Dr.: _____ Date: _____

Children: _____

Other: _____   Precautions: _____

House: Surroundings: _____ Entrance: _____

         # Floors: _____ Bedroom: _____

         Kitchen: _____ Bathroom: _____

         Architectural Barriers: _____

Physical Evaluation:

    Upper Extremities: (ROM, strength, coordination, sensation, muscle tone, movement patterns, endurance)

        RUE: _____

        LUE: _____

        Bilateral: _____

        Functional Deficits: _____

    Trunk and Lower Extremities: (Mobility, sensation, muscle tone, sitting/standing tolerance, balance, gait)

Mental Functioning Evaluation: (attention, awareness, judgment, behavior, retention, reception, abstract reasoning, cognition, problem solving)

Perceptual Functioning Evaluation: (visual, auditory, motor planning, stereognosis, proprioception, perceptual motor correlation)

Functional Activity Evaluation:

    ADL: (position, balance, transfers, mobility, assistive devices used, motivation, perceptual deficits)

        Hygiene/Bathing/Grooming: _____

        Dressing: _____

        Self-feeding: _____

        Writing/Reading: (signature, tracing, copying, spontaneous writing and reading, dominance, field cut, neglect, eyesight)

HOMEMAKING: (food preparation, clean-up, safety, home modifications, assistive devices, positioning, responsibilities, financial management, work simplification, energy conservation)

Figure 21-10. Occupational Therapy Worksheet.

INTERESTS: (vocational, avocational, social skills and abilities)

ORTHOTIC AND ASSISTIVE EQUIPMENT: (type, date given, recommendations)

DATE:

TREATMENT
(equipment, exercise, activity, goal, procedure, positioning, assistive device(s), upgrading, progress)

---

treatment plan. If the therapist uses the evaluation information creatively, it should be possible to formulate goals of treatment and the methods to be used to achieve these goals.

These methods include the positioning of the patient for treatment, adaptations to the equipment used or types of assistive devices provided, and use of splints and other assistive equipment (for example, arm supports). The goals may include unilateral or bilateral improvement in self-care and/or homemaking skills, prevocational readiness, resocialization, functional achievement, and regaining of motivation.

A helpful addition to the worksheet would be notation of progress as well as any conference notes. These sheets not only provide a guideline for the therapist but also can aid a substitute therapist, if necessary.

Checklist

The use of a checklist format is an efficient method for recording objective information. The inclusion of the date on which the measurement was made is essential in order to maintain an accurate record of progress. This is also important for determining at what point a change in the treatment program is necessary. A checklist format can be used efficiently for the following types of evaluations:

1. Range of motion
2. Manual muscle testing
3. Sensory testing
4. Perceptual testing
5. Dynamometer and pinch-gauge testing
6. Activities of daily living
7. Homemaking skills
8. Splint check-out
9. Assistive device check-out

It is helpful to have a variety of these forms, which can be used when needed. Once compiled, the information can be summarized on the worksheet and chart. Checklists are usually considered worksheets, however, they are sometimes included in the chart as primary data. Sometimes a stringent procedure must be followed for approval of the placement of additional sheets in the chart. Also, a short, succinct summary is preferable to lengthy, overly-detailed information; it is more likely to be read. Notes should always be dated and signed, and updated when necessary.

Treatment Principles and Application

It is considered normal to pass through several stages of emotional turmoil between onset and acceptance of disability. A person feels different as a result of disability, and may actually fear what he or she has become. To hold onto the previous known life and self and to struggle to regain them is inherent in all stages of rehabilitation. Heijn refers to "differential motivation" during specific rehabilitation programs to reflect this struggle "to preserve a prior adaptation without accepting the permanent changes imposed."[11]

He further suggests that "motivation is like a vehicle that carries the patient through stressful times in order to achieve potential" and in order to achieve alternatives required by permanent disability.[12] He states that successful rehabilitation depends on "1) the patient's ability to adaptively master the emotional stress which is frequent accompaniment of physical handicap, 2) his ability to renounce or modify highly valued activities, future plans, or relationships, and 3) his ability to implement feasible new plans and actions."[13]

Making the Plan

In developing a treatment plan, the patient needs to be included both in planning and in providing feedback regarding performance. This encourages the patient to take an increasing role in planning the rehabilitation program in preparation for discharge from the structured treatment setting. In taking gradual steps toward responsibility in planning and evaluating, confidence, creativity, and responsibility are developed.

The following are suggested steps to include in treatment planning and implementation:

1. Have the patient participate in initial evaluation procedures, results, and treatment planning.
2. Use factual information from the patient's chart and from the OT evaluation to plan the course of individual treatment.
3. Use the patient's stated interests, major current concerns, abilities, and long-term goals.
4. Plan short-term goals to achieve positive feedback, self-awareness, and satisfaction.
5. Plan long-term goals with regard for implications of disability, financial boundaries, and medical and functional prognosis.
6. Prioritize and change goals according to the areas and growth of self-awareness, acceptance, and motivation.

Implementation

1. Create a therapeutic environment for achievement of treatment objectives.
2. Orient the level of the individual treatment program to both the patient's interest and level of ability.

3. Begin the treatment program with a short-term goal of significance to the patient.
4. Use passive range of motion or demonstration to teach and encourage active patterns of movement.
5. Demonstrate new or adaptive techniques or equipment in the same manner in which the patient is expected to perform or use them.
6. Engage the patient in therapeutic exercise and activity, which provide increased productivity.
7. Engage the patient in problem-solving, planning, and evaluation involved in treatment objectives, implementation, and accomplishment.
8. If appropriate and therapeutic, provide feedback regarding performance to the patient at the end of each session.
9. Relate the completed session to the anticipated session.
10. As appropriate, provide out-of-therapy exercises for independent carry-over.

Functional Areas

Medical treatment consists of specific actions or behaviors directed toward a person in order to relieve or cure. In occupational therapy, the anticipated result of these efforts is the gaining, restoration, or improvement of functional abilities. In establishing the objectives of occupational therapy in the treatment of the patient with physical or neurological conditions, the occupational therapist focuses on five major areas:

1. Awareness of self
2. Maximum level of self-care independence
3. Restoration of functional ability
4. Exploration of vocational and avocational potential
5. Socialization and adjustment to new life patterns

Awareness of Self

In order to seek a defense from the misery of accepting a disabling condition or a long-term progressive illness, the patient may deny its existence. Although physical or intellectual deficits may be an obvious result of the illness, the patient may still either consciously or subconsciously deny the occurrence or implications of the condition. The occupational therapy program provides the patient with the opportunity to see herself or himself as a thinking, doing being. Through the performance of tasks directed toward achievable accomplishments, awareness of abilities and problems is encouraged on a daily basis. The task is directed toward self-accomplishment and self-awareness. In treatment, success and failure are both therapeutic. Failure can be tangible proof to the patient that he or she is denying inability. Although this failure may cause depression, hostility, or discouragement, it is only by knowing both strengths and weaknesses that the patient is able to see abilities currently possessed and abilities to be retained.

Self-care Independence

Self-care represents the most significant aspect of self-awareness and self-acceptance. During the initial stage of denial the patient is effectively able to deny responsibilities, the body, and its functions. Concern is focused on physical sensations such as pain, positioning, and movement. The patient relinquishes responsibility for care of his or her body and may even be afraid of it, since the frightening effects of disease or trauma have made it an "unknown."

During this period it is important for those working with the patient to talk about the body, to reacquaint him or her with it, and to help him or her to accept it. Gradually the patient relearns how to relate to it again through taking responsibility for bathing, grooming, eating, and dressing. Thus, the patient becomes aware of how the body feels and moves, as well as which parts may need more help or experience more pain.

During therapy sessions, movement is incorporated into self-care programs. The responsibility for assistance in independent self-care techniques falls generally to the occupational therapist in collaboration with the nurse. The occupational therapist assesses the self-care problems. For example, inability to distinguish between objects of different shapes or colors or to relate to vertical or horizontal positions, may make the patient unable to determine the front, back, or sleeve of a shirt. A person with a flaccid arm cannot handle eating utensils in the usual manner and thus may have to learn how to cut meat one-handed, switch the fork to the non-dominant extremity, or use a plate guard for control.

The occupational therapist analyzes these problems, determines the approach for handling them, and teaches techniques to be used in performing each activity. These techniques are then used in the patient's daily program.

With the physically disabled person, activities of daily living (ADL) generally comprise those necessary for basic self-care independence: bathing, hygiene, elimination, grooming, dressing, and eating. Consideration is given to such items as eyeglasses, hearing aids, dentures, prostheses, splints, slings, braces, and adapted clothing. The patient's abilities should be evaluated both with and without the adapted equipment in order to accurately assess levels of independence. For example, a patient who is unable to do buttoning without the use of a hand splint is "independent" with the hand splint; he or she is "dependent" without it. This is also true when special utensils or other equipment are required for eating without the assistance of another person.

The disabled person learns how to choose and retrieve clothing from drawers and cabinets, how to apply and secure assistive devices, how to use catheters, tampons, or suppositories as necessary, how to manage such items as soap, washclothes, nail clippers, combs, toothpaste, and make-up. In the process of eating, the patient learns the use of napkins, utensils, glasses, and cups, as well as how to take food from a serving dish and use salt and pepper.

Included in self-care is the use of the telephone, including how to dial the phone, answer it, take a message, and call for help. Those who need special equipment learn how to use it and how to obtain special operator assistance.

In some instances the patient can accomplish self-care and eating tasks by performing them in a different manner rather than by learning how to use special devices or equipment. When devices are necessary (elastic shoe laces, Velcro closures, or elastic thread), or when a new skill must be mastered (one-handed shoe-tying or one-handed meat-cutting), all possibilities should be explored to ensure minimum reliance on, but maximum effectiveness of, the special equipment or the acquired skill. Effectiveness in self-care provides the patient with independence, which aids not only the patient, but also helps in family relationships. The accomplishment of self-care tasks leads to further successes, enhances motivation, and provides daily physical exercise.

Restoration of Functional Ability

Specific restoration of functional ability may precede or follow the development of self-care activity. Body exercise and sensory awareness developed during the accomplishment of daily tasks are correlated with specific activities also directed toward the restoration of functional ability. These activities include specific exercises to improve strength, range of motion, coordination, and function.

The terms *exercise* and *activity* are used here interchangeably, since it is felt that activity provides exercise, and exercise can be provided through activity. An exercise modality may consist of a measured movement or a combination of movements.

Occupational therapy emphasizes active rather than passive exercises and utilizes the abilities of the patient to the maximum. Although assistive equipment (suspension slings, wheelchairs, lapboards, and splints) may help the patient passively, the *pur-*

pose of their use is to achieve the maximum level of independent and active functioning. For example, the suspension sling may facilitate arm movement for a quadriplegic, enabling him or her to bring both hands together, to eat independently, use a button board for practice, write a letter, or type schoolwork. A variety of assistive equipment may be needed to encourage arm and hand function and to prevent fatigue during exercise activities.

The treatment room provides an atmosphere of activity, with emphasis on productive achievement and encouragment to try. Activity is geared toward what is interesting, purposeful, and acceptable to the patient, so that he or she can see its relation to the overall rehabilitation goals. The patient may reject a treatment situation because of not being able to do things done competently in the past. The patient may resent doing familiar tasks in an inferior way, performing the games of a child painfully and laboriously, or being unable to function at an expected or desired standard. For some of these reasons the patient may become belligerent and refuse to participate in the therapy program. The occupational therapist must make every effort to involve the patient in planning appropriate treatment programs and activities.

Exploration of Vocational and Avocational Potential

The occupational therapist discusses future vocational plans with the patient and focuses training objectives on areas related to vocational interests, aptitudes, and goals. For example, a patient who is attending school may wish to spend time improving handwriting and note-taking skills. Job tasks may be simulated in occupational therapy for the individual who can return to work. If new vocational goals are set, such as bookkeeping or mechanical drawing, proficiency in performing these tasks may be gained by using hand splints, special techniques, or adaptations.

Machinery that is available to the occupational therapist for clerical use or for the construction of assistive equipment can serve a dual purpose in providing an evaluation and training tools to the patient with physical or perceptual deficits. After a primary check-out to ensure safety in use, these tools can be used to provide information regarding physical ability, work habits, work skills, and problem-solving abilities.

Avocational interests are explored in order to give the patient an interest in daily activity. Hobbies such as reading, writing, painting, and drawing can be pursued even though physical limitations may require use of adapted equipment.

Socialization

The occupational therapist can assist the patient in making satisfactory adjustment to a disability and in restoring self-confidence by concentrating on accomplishments and capabilities and also by providing opportunities for social interaction. The patient should be encouraged to participate in recreational programs and in the patient-governing bodies that are active in many rehabilitation facilities.

To ease the fear of taking part in outside social activities because of "looking different," the patient should be encouraged to go on outings, such as bowling, baseball games, and movies, while still in the hospital. These activities make the patient begin to function as a member of a community in preparation for discharge into the community. Upon discharge, each person should be encouraged to participate in social and community affairs and to attend functions that were part of his or her life before the injury or onset of disease.

Discharge Planning

With the development of the team approach and the growth of rehabilitation, discharge planning has grown from the concept of placement or referral of a person following discharge to actual preparation for discharge by the patient and the rehabilitation team. The end result of a well-coordinated team effort is effective referral or community re-entry, with all team members contributing to the plan. The most important member of the team is the patient.

Preparation includes medical considerations (continuation of medication, follow-up visits, plans for future treatment procedures), provision of assistive equipment for home exercise functions and independence in daily living, counseling the family on the patient's self-care and general activity, and a home visit to determine the presence of architectural barriers and to evaluate the patient's potential for functioning in the home.

Discharge planning begins with the referral of the person to the treatment setting where the anticipated treatment program is to take place. Thus, the first information regarding discharge questions or expectations will appear in referral materials. The program following referral may diverge from the initial expectations and may result in further discharge planning. Thus, discharge planning becomes a continual process based upon the condition of the patient at any given time, rather than simply a plan of where to go when a given program is completed.

After the referral information is gathered, evaluation occurs. This includes all team members and pertinent information needed for appropriate and optimum treatment of the patient, including information about the patient's home environment, lifestyle, educational level, and occupation. The patient and the team can create a treatment plan that will assist the patient, in preparing to go home. Since the total treatment plan is geared toward meeting the needs of the patient upon discharge, therapy can be seen as important for realistic discharge planning, rather than as a program that bears no relationship to the most crucial problems of returning home.

Publications are available to aid the family and the recovering patient in postdischarge home programs that continue the rehabilitation process. As recovery may continue over a period of years, professional programs are transferred to the patient and family to incorporate into daily routines.

In planning long-range needs and placement, the therapist and the patient must consider such limitations as the following: no home to return to upon discharge; no financial coverage for out-patient services; no transportation available for out-patient services; and no family member to provide attendant care or homemaking services in the home following discharge.

Consumer groups provide many types of support and many opportunities for the disabled individual. National organizations established to benefit victims of disease and to engage in specific relevant research projects publish information for professionals and consumers, hold educational meetings, and provide a forum for discussions. A list of organizations is included at the end of Chapter 22.

Consumer groups, which may include able-bodied friends and professionals, provide initial socialization opportunities at meetings. A person can meet others with the same disability or with similar problems. Discussions focus on common concerns, such as the legal rights of the disabled, architectural and accessibility laws, building codes, transportation needs, housing, employment, and educational opportunities. Attending such meetings can be encouraging and informative for both the patient and the therapist. Such meetings may be held in rehabilitation centers or hospitals, thus making preliminary information and experience available early in the adjustment process.

Correlation With Other Disciplines

The occupational therapist is a member of the treatment team, participating in program planning, patient evaluation and treatment, recommendations regarding referral to other services and programs, report writing, team conferences, student training, and inservice programs.

In the rehabilitation approach there are generally overlaps in evaluation and treatment among such persons as physicians, nurses, occupational therapists, physical therapists, speech therapists, social workers, and vocational rehabilitation counselors. Overlaps can be useful in providing carry-over of activities and exercises and continual monitoring of the patient's progress. Good communication among team members is necessary to encourage coordination rather than antagonism over "who does what." For example, the occupational therapist works with the physician, heeding the medical precautions on correct body positioning, optimal mental and physical tolerance of activity, and progression of pathological symptoms. A coordinated self-care program involves the cooperation of nurses and occupational therapists in planning daily hygiene, grooming, dressing, and eating programs. The occupational therapist coordinates the morning dressing program and general exercise activities with the physical therapy program so that physical gains are maintained throughout the treatment day and fatigue is avoided. The speech therapist aids team members in effective communication skills for patients who have speech deficits. As the social worker deals with the patient and family, he or she needs to know the treatment programs and progress in order to interpret and convey this information to the family, and to assist the patient in understanding the daily program. The vocational rehabilitation counselor relies on the occupational therapist's evaluation of functional ability to determine the need for further education, job return, training, placement, and/or relocation.

A functional delineation of roles among team members is essential for optimal communication and effective rehabilitation. The specific roles of each member of the team may vary in different treatment settings. The following examples illustrate the ways in which team members work together.

Medicine

In the hospital situation it is usually the physician who refers the patient to occupational therapy; therefore, involvement of the therapist in ward rounds and clinics is essential to assist the physician in determining which patients can benefit from which types of programs through occupational therapy. From the physician the therapist learns medical progress, precautions, and preferences regarding therapy as well as treatment priorities and the need for augmentation when necessary. The therapist is the consultant to the physician in terms of activity abilities and tolerance.

Nursing

Since the nurse works in the patient living area of the in-patient treatment setting, a coordinated relationship is necessary with regard to self-care programs and techniques. Since the nurse is aware of the total treatment schedule and program, communication with the occupational therapist ensures the nurse's understanding and follow-through of the OT program. Also, the occupational therapist is likely to learn of the patient's day-to-day behaviors and attitudes by consulting the nurse.

Physical Therapy

Occupational therapists work with physical therapists in the provision of restorative function through exercise and activity. This may, in some instances, be divided according to upper or lower extremity activity, physical tolerance, or exercise and activity, depending on the roles within the treatment setting. Physical therapists and occupational therapists can work well in the same room, providing combined programs in many instances. It is important that the two programs be complementary, rather than contradictory or duplicatory.

Usually the role of the physical therapist is to provide specific exercises and activities related to body movements *per se,* concentrating on the development of coordination, strength, and range of motion. In extending these exercises into activities of daily living and productive functional activities, the occupational therapist must check with the physical therapist regarding specific movement techniques to provide consistency in approach. Specific evaluation tests may be duplicated in each therapy area, however, prime consideration must be given to how the patient performs in each as evaluation data may vary under different conditions. Collaboration is beneficial for scheduling, discussion of the need for splinting and assistive devices, and planning of the time and manner of use of such devices.

Speech Therapy

The speech pathologist and the occupational therapist work together with the patient who has a speech problem in addition to motor, sensory, and/or perceptual deficits. Collaboration occurs in the areas of writing and speech, in choosing exercises for motor writing, and in approaches used during activities where speech is indicated or where reading is used.

The speech pathologist describes the patient's speech program to the therapist and informs the therapist of how to use speech and language in a beneficial way with functional exercises. The occupational therapist can assist the speech pathologist in showing ways to position the patient for therapeutic use of the extremities during speech exercises.

Social Service

The social worker works closely with the patient and family in the social aspects of provision of needed medical care, adjustment to the medical condition and expectations of progress, handling of problems occurring owing to hospitalization, and general understanding and acceptance of the situation. The occupational therapist interprets the patient's functional gains, rehabilitation program, and general reactions and progress for the social workers. Postdischarge needs (home modifications for wheelchair living, funds for assistive devices for independent self-care, acceptance of the fact of disability in effective resocialization) are met by the social worker.

Orthotics

In many institutions and small treatment settings the occupational therapist performs all splinting needs. In others, such service is limited to temporary splinting during acute treatment. In still others, the occupational therapist consults with the orthotist, who provides the orthosis; the occupational therapist then provides check-out and training. The orthotist and the occupational therapist can work well together in planning the design and use of splints. Although both may be trained and adept in fabricating the device, the therapist provides the use training. Splints may be specifically requested or generally suggested at the occupational therapist's recommendation.

In the hospital situation the nurse is informed of the type of splint provided and of its wear and use instructions. The occupational therapist and the nurse check for pressure areas. Splints may be provided for rest or activity, and all should be monitored by the occupational therapist, who will make changes when necessary.

Prosthetics

While the physician or rehabilitation team evaluate and prescribe the prosthesis, it is fabricated by a certified prosthetist who may be either employed within the treatment facility or an outside consultant. Although the occupational therapist may not have been consulted prior to the prescription of the prosthesis, referral is made for prosthetic training in cases of upper extremity amputations. Lower extremity amputees are usually seen for exercises, self-care activities, and functional activities. The occupational therapist can provide pre-prosthetic training if the amputee is referred. If problems occur with the prosthesis, the occupational therapist contacts the prosthetist.

Team Approach

Team members are important sources of information and support for one another. For example, a patient may develop signs of extreme fatigue, such as sweating and difficulty in breathing, while in the occupational therapy area. The occupational therapist contacts the physician or the nurse for assistance in determining the cause and seriousness of the symptoms. The occupational therapist contacts the physical therapist to determine techniques for safe and successful transfer from one chair to another, for information about whether the patient will be safe standing to perform a woodworking project, or whether the patient can safely stand and walk in the kitchen for assessment of homemaking skills.

Both occupational and physical therapists should coordinate muscle testing, range of motion, sensory testing, and assessment of physical tolerance and balance. The speech therapist and occupational therapist work together in designing treatment approaches for the aphasic patient. Realistic vocational planning by the counsellor is aided by the occupational therapist, who assesses the functional abilities of the upper extremities, the intellectual level of functioning in applied tasks, and the general physical tolerance. The physician aids in developing realistic planning in terms of the prognosis and the patient's mental approach to rehabilitation.

The ideal treatment approach to the patient with multiple problem areas, who is cared for by several persons or programs, is the *team approach* in which formal and informal interaction is encouraged among all persons working toward developing and implementing a unified treatment program. This team includes the patient and family as well as team specialists in the health field.

References

1. Daniels, S.: In Disability & sickness: A theory. Project Health 1:1, 4, 1981.
2. Vargo, J. W.: Some psychological effects of physical disability. Am. J. Occup. Ther. 32:32, 1978.
3. Daniels, Project Health, p. 4.
4. Heijn, C., and Granger, C. V.: Understanding motivational patterns: Early identification aids rehabilitation. J. Rehab. 40:26, 1974.
5. Ibid.
6. Reilly, Mary. Occupational Therapy Can Be One of the Great Ideas of 20th Century Medicine, Am J Occup Therapy 16:1–9, Jan/Feb 1962.
7. Ayres, A. J.: Sensory Integration and the Child. Los Angeles: Western Psychological Services, 1979, p. 46.
8. *Ibid.*, p. 64.
9. Dunning, H.: Environmental occupational therapy. Am. J. Occup. Ther. 26:292, 1972.
10. Vargo, Am. J. Occup. Ther. pp. 31–32.
11. Heijn and Granger, J. Rehab. pp. 26–29
12. *Ibid.*
13. *Ibid.*

CHAPTER 22

Functional Restoration—Specific Diagnosis
Elinor Anne Spencer

This chapter is intended to familiarize the therapist with diagnostic and symptom complexes of major disability areas seen in physical rehabilitation programs by the occupational therapist and to provide approaches to evaluation, treatment, and adaptive daily living activity. Although techniques are correlated with specific conditions, they are not limited to those specified.

Beginning with diagnostic distinctions in manifestations of cerebrovascular accident, brain trauma, and spinal cord lesions, more detailed attention is given to specific diagnoses. Neurological conditions are followed by arthritic and orthopedic conditions.

Neurological Considerations

Neurological dysfunction is caused by pathology in the nervous system, often affecting other systems as well. Clinical manifestations are determined by the location, type, and extent of the lesion.

Lesions in the brain are caused by cerebrovascular accident (CVA), head injury, multiple sclerosis (MS), and Parkinson's disease and result in intellectual, personality, physical, and emotional changes. Le-

sions in the spinal cord and nerve roots include spinal cord injury, polio, and the Guillain-Barré syndrome and result in paralysis of the extremities with respiratory, bowel, and bladder involvement. Myasthenia gravis and muscular dystrophy (MD) are primarily diseases of the muscles resulting in dysfunction. Multiple sclerosis, Parkinson's disease, myasthenia gravis, amyotrophic lateral sclerosis (ALS), and MD are progressively debilitating conditions. Depending on the severity of the trauma, there may be significant recovery potential for the person suffering from CVA, head injury, spinal cord injury, the Guillain-Barré syndrome, and peripheral nerve injuries. Although spinal cord injury, polio, and the Guillain-Barré syndrome may show a similar clinical picture during hospitalization, they vary in prognosis. Clinical manifestations of neurological conditions are distinguished by upper motor neuron (UMN) and lower motor neuron (LMN) lesions. The UMN lesion occurs in the corticospinal or pyramidal tract, located in the brain or spinal cord. Resultant conditions are hemiplegia, paraplegia, or quadriplegia. The location and extent of the lesion determines the extent of the paralysis. The clinical signs include loss of voluntary movement, increased muscle tone (spasticity), pathological reflexes in the limbs, and sensory loss.[1] The principle causes of UMN lesions are CVA, brain tumor or trauma, ALS, MS, and spinal cord transection or compression.

UMN conditions resulting in impairment of cerebral functions are CVA (internal brain trauma), head injury (external brain trauma), and MS (disease). UMN conditions *not* resulting in impairment of cerebral functions are spinal cord injury (external trauma), and ALS (disease).

Lesions in the extrapyramidal system result in disorders of muscle tone and involuntary movements, as in Parkinson's disease. Conditions of ataxia resulting from proprioceptive disorders can be caused by lesions in the spinal nerve roots (spinal ataxia) or in the cerebellum and its pathways (cerebellar ataxia).[1] Common causes of ataxia are head injury, brain tumor, and MS.

The LMN lesion occurs in the anterior horn cells, nerve roots, and the peripheral nerve system, causing flaccid conditions of monoplegia, paraplegia, triplegia, and quadriplegia. Diseases contributing to LMN lesions usually are systemic and have symmetrical involvement; an exception to this is polio, which can have widely scattered effects in the limbs. The presence of lesions results in loss of voluntary function, flaccid paralysis, sensory loss, and atrophy. The principle causes are polio, the Guillain-Barré syndrome, ischemia, periphral nerve injuries (see Chapter 25), and brachial plexus injury.

Neurological impairment depends on the location of the lesion (Table 22-1). There is some similarity in the treatment of neurological disorders according to the site of the lesion regardless of the diagnosis. Impairment can involve intellectual functions (perception, organization, problem solving), mental processes (personality, behavior, motivation), motor functions (muscle power, bladder and bowel control), sensory functions (proprioception, sensation, stereognosis, hearing, and sight), coordination (ataxia), and involuntary motions (tremor).

Occupational Therapy Program

The occupational therapy program incorporates three major areas: (1) identification of function through evaluation procedures, (2) development of function through use of specific activities to increase function, and (3) integration of specific functions into daily tasks. The program is determined by consideration of the patient's deficits and abilities as discovered in the assessment and identification of treatment priorities, plans, and methods. The therapist and the patient work out the program together.

Neurological deficits are described here to provide a general clinical awareness of these manifestations for evaluation and treatment procedures. In some cases, the manifestation may be more varied and pronounced at onset (as in trauma); others may appear over a gradual period of time (as in progressive diseases).

Evaluation refers to a specific aspect of function which becomes part of the overall *assessment.* For example, specific evaluation of range of motion (ROM),

Table 22-1 *Correlation of Location of Lesion with Resultant Pathological Condition, Course of Pathology, and Organic Manifestations*

Location of Lesion	Pathological Condition	Course of Pathology	Manifestations
Brain	Cerebrovascular accident	Nonprogressive	Intellectual
	Head injury	Nonprogressive	Personality
	Multiple sclerosis	Progressive	Sensorimotor
	Parkinson's disease	Progressive	Emotional
			Communication
			Physiologic
Spinal cord	Spinal cord injury	Nonprogressive	Sensorimotor
	Guillain-Barré syndrome	Nonprogressive	Physiologic
	Polio	Nonprogressive	
Muscle or myoneural junction	Myasthenia gravis	Progressive	Physical
	Amyotrophic lateral sclerosis	Progressive	Physiologic
	Muscular dystrophy	Progressive	Communication (motor)
Extremity	Peripheral nerve injury	Nonprogressive	Physical

(Note: bracketed manifestations apply to all pathological conditions listed in the group.)

coordination, strength, and sensation contributes to the assessment of physical abilities and deficits.

Functional assessment is incomplete without evaluation of muscle tone, endurance, activity tolerance, cognitive and perceptual abilities, balance, and sensory integration. Specific function of the patient is evaluated by determining or setting the value or amount of function, as shown by standard or modified tests in which the presence, quality, and genuineness of the function demonstrated contribute to the assessment or estimate of overall performance ability and quality.

Progressive Neurological Conditions

The acceptance of a progressive disease and its long-term implications and changes presents many challenges to the patient and his or her family. To learn the nature of intermittent variability of severity or characteristics of deficits requires a clear understanding of the condition by all family members.

Initially, the reality of the disease may be denied, however, long-term care requires involvement of both the patient and the family.

The occupational therapist may see the patient initially during the diagnostic period or further along during the course of rehabilitation or maintenance programs. After careful evaluation of abilities and deficits, the occupational therapist plans a program geared toward assisting the patient to achieve the highest functional level and to utilize assistive equipment as necessary to maintain a program of independent and meaningful daily activity. The therapist assists the patient in adjusting to the chronic nature of the disease and in looking at the disease realistically, anticipating and accepting changes. In knowing how to adapt to symptoms, the patient is better able to cope with the decreasing abilities in a positive way.

Assessment Areas

The assessment of the functional level of the patient with neurological impairment from a brain lesion includes evaluation techniques to assess responses: attitudinal, receptive, expressive, perceptual, passive, active, motor, sensory, intellectual, and integrative. Procedures begin with the choosing and setting up of the therapy environment to elicit maximum response from the patient, who may be highly distractable. Since the use of treatment approaches to augment and vary evaluation techniques can facilitate significant patient response, they are included in this discussion. The length and type of specific techniques used

are determined by the patient's mental and physical tolerance, cooperation, and comprehension. At the beginning of the evaluation the therapist establishes a means of communication with the patient, who may lack speech and/or comprehension of instructions, or who may be disoriented in time and space. As previously mentioned, the chronological order of specific tests of the patient's abilities and functions should be geared to the patient, ability, motivations, fears, and general demeanor.

During evaluation and treatment, optimum body positioning is essential. The biomechanical and functional appropriateness of the patient's position for exercise and activity is vital, whether in bed, in a wheelchair or a regular chair, standing, or walking. The therapist should evaluate the patient's balance and awareness of position and then show the patient different positions that may be used comfortably and safely. If necessary, extremities are passively placed in the optimum position for active motion. Among the devices and concepts which aid the patient are: a mirror for visual feedback, use of gravity for ease of movement, repetition of movement for sensory awareness, sensory contact for reinforcement, bilateral use of the extremities for midline crossing and integration of two sides of the body, and supportive devices to minimize fatigue and maximize function.

Attitude

The patient's attitudes toward his or her medical condition and resultant functional abilities, treatment setting, and the therapist may or may not be revealed on the first contact. Initial observations and evaluations by the therapist reveal information regarding the patient's general affect and behavior, attention span, distractibility, comprehension of verbal, written, or demonstrated instructions, and memory of immediate, recent, sequential, or remote information and events. As mental and physical tolerance may be limited, particularly in the early stages of recovery, attention is focused on facilitating positive performance during evaluation. Techniques are changed or terminated during the session if the patient becomes overly stressed, discouraged, or fatigued. The therapist makes sure that every evaluation period has positive feedback for the patient regarding intact functions and progress.

Receptive/Expressive

The ability of the patient to perceive himself or herself as a total functioning and worthwhile being relates to the ability to receive and use messages from the environment through sensory stimuli and through awareness and integrated interpretation of them. With deficits in auditory, language, and/or intellectual functions, the patient may demonstrate blockage in response to these stimuli. Attention is given to determining what messages the patient does receive, to what extent, and how he or she can use them in applied function. Accurate assessment of this depends on the creativity and skill of the therapist in appropriately using evaluation materials.

The patient may show deficits in the ability to express himself or herself both verbally and behaviorly in accordance with how he or she feels or with actual abilities. Verbal expression may be limited to uncontrolled, repetitive, or meaningless phrases causing poor communication and confusion on the part of the patient and the therapist. Generally, the therapist must speak as if the patient has understood verbal communication, regardless of whether or not the patient appears to not understand. Depending on the amount of control the patient has over physical functions, he or she may use this avenue of expression, particularly if he or she has a language deficit.

Keeping in mind the environmental effects on the neurologically impaired patient, the therapist uses auditory stimulation therapeutically during evaluation and treatment sessions. Verbal cues can be used supportively, as reinforcement, and for orientation. In the same manner, socialization can be used for functional auditory discrimination and localization as well as for providing verbal feedback. Music can be used for relaxation or stimulation during or after effort or as a rhythmic accompaniment to gross motor activity during the use of assistive equipment, such as a support spring suspension sling.

Activities involving movement that changes the plane of the head or body in space can be used to improve position and space concepts. Among these are games involving spatial concepts: shuffleboard (from the wheelchair or while standing), table shuffleboard, catching a ball or beanbag, hitting a ball suspended with the hand, dancing, or marching.

A variety of electronic devices and equipment is available to provide nonverbal communication assistance for persons without expressive language ability (speech) to improve communication and productivity. With the severely physically disabled person in a wheelchair, the first consideration is evaluation of the sitting position and the physical abilities of the head, trunk, and extremities in order to determine options for control of the devices. Scanning equipment can be mounted on wheelchair lapboards or standard tables, can be portables or consoles, and may be equipped with head pointers, strip printers, computers, training aids, and visual systems. Electronic aids can be useful in evaluation, training, and working. Catalog addresses are listed in the appendix for refer-

ence to these useful items, without which many severely physically disabled persons would have no means of communication or would be left to primitive measures lower than their intellectual abilities.

Perceptual

Deficits in awareness of body image, movement patterns, and sensorimotor functions may show evidence in the neglect of intact functions. Awareness of the use of the body, neglect of intact functions, and actual use can be determined by the evaluation of sensory and motor functions. The use of the draw-a-person test, figure assembling tests, identification of body parts, and self-care assessment assists in determination of the function of the total body awareness.

Before giving tests for visual perception, the therapist determines if the patient wears glasses or has a visual acuity deficiency. The patient is then asked to identify familiar objects or printed words. The therapist determines the patient's accuracy in color, size, and shape discrimination. Tests can be used to evaluate the function of figure ground, spatial relations, and form constancy. The patient is asked to read a sentence written in large letters or an advertisement from a magazine; he or she is asked to write his or her name. This identifies the ability to form letters and to interpret them; reading, writing, and block designs can be used to detect the presence of a field cut or neglect of the visual field.

When the patient comes for treatment, he or she should be oriented to the occupational therapy room, with furniture, people, and activities being pointed out and identified. The furniture can be used to relate form constancy and color and shape discrimination.

When denial or neglect of a visual field or extremity is shown, the patient should be encouraged to look at his or her body during exercises and activities. Cutaneous and verbal stimulation can draw attention to the extremity, and the patient should be encouraged to place an arm on the table even though he or she might not be using it actively in a task. Visual tasks such as object assembly, puzzles, reading the newspaper, writing, or copying encourage visual organization.

Intellectual

Ability to write is tested by asking the patient to write his or her name. If the patient is unable to do this, the therapist gives assistance by forming the letters, asking the patient first to trace and then to copy them. Close observation reveals perceptual disorders in spatial relations, directionality, and concepts of form. If the patient is able to write spontaneously, the following activities should be checked: ability to copy letters and numbers, to do simple arithmetical problems, and to answer questions related to a written paragraph. Problem solving and construction abilities can be evaluated by assessing the ability to plan an activity or project and to successfully follow step-by-step procedures to its completion.

Sensory

The therapist touches the patient lightly to determine the patient's perception of the location of tactile stimulus. This can be done either from distal to proximal or vice versa, however, sensory and motor deficits are usually increasingly impaired from proximal to distal. The patient is asked to occlude vision by looking the other way or by closing the eyes. Although a blindfold may be necessary for the patient who is unable to look the other way or does not comprehend the reason for closing the eyes, this may be a frightening technique. The therapist can perform the test by either covering the testing area or by placing the patient's arms under the table while testing, with therapist sitting opposite the patient.

The patient's fingers are touched with rough and smooth objects to determine texture discrimination; familiar objects of varying sizes, shapes, and weights are placed in the hand to determine stereognosis. In the case of hemiplegia the uninvolved extremity should be checked first so that the patient understands what is being asked; then the affected hand and arm should be checked. This provides some positive input and feedback and encourages the patient regarding intact functions.

Sensory Input

Gradual controlled increase of stimuli in all activity should be provided. In all task-oriented activity there is a variety of sensory input: visual, auditory, tactile, proprioceptive, and vestibular. Reinforcement of sensory cues assists memory development and orientation through repetition and familiarity; this increases awareness. Associations should be made between and among activities, for instance, the correlation between vertical–bilateral sanding and pulling up one's pants.

Techniques of Sensorimotor Stimulation and Inhibition

Techniques providing fast, irregular rhythms characterizing stimulation include vibration, pressure, tap-

ping, stretching, joint compression, brushing, icing, resistance, and visual and auditory stimuli.

Techniques of inhibition include warmth, slow stroking, gentle shaking or rocking, pressure on the insertion of a muscle, and joint compression. In addition, cool colors, soft, regular rhythms, and soft, even-speaking tones can be used.

Tactile Stimulation

Application of stimuli to the skin of the involved extremity over flaccid muscles, using touch and moderate pressure, can result in improved sensory response and increased motor function. Passive cutaneous stimulation by the therapist, using stroking, pressure, brushing, and object pressure, stimulates sensation. Manipulation of shapes in both the affected and nonaffected hand encourages feedback from the normal extremity. Pressure over the muscle belly, joint, or tendon stimulates individual muscle response. Cutaneous stimulation from tools adapted with surface textures encourages security of grip and sensory stimulation. Rolling in bed during dressing and bathing stimulates body awareness. Self-stimulation and location of the affected extremity during self-care activities encourage range of motion, bilateral awareness and integration, and increase function.

Motor Ability (Praxia)

The therapist evaluates both sides of the patient's body during motor evaluation. Except in cases of bilateral hemiplegia or accompanying factors such as previous fractures, arthritis, or neurological problems affecting the sound extremity, bilateral evaluation gives an indication of the impairment on the affected side as compared with the sound side. For the confused patient, checking the passive range of motion of both extremities before requesting active movement may help to give a better understanding of the available range, as well as familiarize him or her with the active movement requested. Patients often do not understand technical terms, and therefore, demonstrations of instructions help relieve undesirable anxiety. This technique also helps the apraxic patient, who cannot initiate the voluntary motor act on request, although he or she may have the motor ability to perform the movement.

The therapist checks passive and active range of motion, strength, reflex activity, coordination, proprioceptive and kinesthetic functions, postural reactions, and bilateral coordination. These techniques are modified according to the position of the patient during evaluation.

Safety precautions during motor evaluations are essential. Although the patient may verbally indicate no deficits, the therapist evaluates thoroughly to make certain of the sensorimotor condition. In the assessment of the motor ability, activities can be provided to stimulate strength and coordination and to detect apraxia and more specific motor deficits. The patient's vision should be occluded to evaluate proprioceptive and kinesthetic functions.

The ability to perform the motor act may be more functional when the patient is asked to perform a particular task, such as reaching for an object in the therapist's hand or touching a part of his own body. Return of muscle function in the hemiplegic patient follows the developmental pattern of synergies; therefore, the therapist should observe the *active* movement for signs of synergistic patterns. The therapist should also observe the position of the limbs at rest for signs of spasticity, edema, muscle weakness, or neglect. These can be noted in the posture of the patient while lying in bed or while in a sitting position.

Biofeedback can be used by qualified therapists to provide motivation regarding potential movement, a means of facilitating specific weak muscles, relaxation of spastic muscles, and an awareness of muscle improvement or potential. In using biofeedback with activity, the therapist can combine two media effectively to enable the patient to have a more visual concept of muscle function for task completion.

Biofeedback is particularly meaningful to the patient who has no sensation of muscle contraction, and thus little active input to re-education. Information about which muscles are functioning and how much they are functioning is indicated by the biofeedback machine. Auditory or visual feedback is given in order to indicate muscle contractions. By increasing his or her awareness, the patient is motivated to increase muscle activity, thus increasing the response and motivation. Active exercises used in conjunction with the biofeedback machine encourage understanding of muscular gains.

Feedback devices are available to provide the patient with knowledge of results of muscle contractions not otherwise available to him or her, returning feedback on the performance of an activity. The electrogoniometer is a device which can accurately record joint range of motion while the subject is moving the joint being studied. Another feedback device is a pressure sensitive device which returns a light signal when a programmed amount of pressure is applied and gives a second light signal when a measured, increased amount of pressure is applied. This feedback response may be activation of an electrical appliance rather than a light. Use of these devices provides an objective record of the performance to validate progress.[2]

Self-care

The self-care evaluation is done in the location and manner in which the patient is comfortable. Evaluation is done in privacy to prevent open discouragement if the patient is not independent in a task which he or she previously could perform well. Evaluation of self-feeding skills can be done either in the occupational therapy room or in the patient's room, depending on the patient's desires and mental state. The use of the nondominant, sound extremity may be embarassingly uncoordinated, and practice may be needed to accomplish one-handed self-feeding. It is often desirable for the patient to gain skill in self-feeding before eating in a public place. Evaluation to determine the need for splints, assistive devices, and changes in methods in performing an activity accompanies the assessment of self-care skills. The therapist should observe the performance in self-care activities.

The careful evaluation of all self-care areas is essential to the patient's regaining self-esteem and respect through the retrieval of maximum independent functional ability. Attention to these areas assists the patient in regaining a sense of self-worth as well as regaining his or her family role.

Splinting

The provision of splints and slings for the brain-injured patient remains a controversial subject among physicians, occupational therapists, orthotists, and physical therapists. This controversy is caused by the variety of treatment approaches and settings available. Those using sensorimotor facilitation and inhibition techniques tend to discourage traditional splinting, because it may counteract the use of neurophysiological techniques. Use of *appropriate* splinting design is consistent with neurophysiological treatment techniques used to reduce hypertonicity.

Splinting has four basic options of application: static or dynamic, volar or dorsal. The provision of assistive devices and splints should be carefully assessed and should correlate with other treatments, thereby providing the patient with the maximum advantage of all treatments and modalities available.

When the functional deficits and potentials have been determined through comprehensive physical and sensory evaluation, consideration is given to the need for splinting to assist in restoration of function. Given appropriately, splinting can provide positioning against spasticity and resultant deformity, stimulation to muscle groups, increased sensory awareness, relief of pain or discomfort, and support of weak or malaligned extremities. Splints are generally prescribed to channel or enhance function or to protect nonfunctioning extremities for future functions.

Poorly designed and monitored splints can cause deformities. It is good practice to teach the patient wearing the splint when to wear it and when to take it off or to instruct someone else in this procedure. The patient should know the purpose of the splint, be aware of checking for pressure areas, and know whom to contact if it is not fitting properly.

In the restoration of the upper extremity function, a static cock-up splint may be beneficial to support the weak wrist in a functional position both at rest and during activity. A C bar at the thumb web space to prevent atrophy and tightness provides effective functional positioning. Dynamic splinting using the long opponens with an outrigger system and finger cuffs encourages active use of the fingers during resistive functional exercises to strengthen palmar grasp, opposition, and prehension.

Orthokinetic splinting providing a combination of mobilization and support can be used for (1) relief of pain, (2) increase of muscle strength, (3) increase of range of motion, (4) muscle re-education, and (5) improvement of coordination. This type of splint uses a minimum of static coverage where inhibition is desired and acts as a facilitator of paralyzed extensor muscles through the use of wide elastic straps over the forearm muscle bellies and tendons. The orthokinetic concept is a dynamic one; its purpose is function rather than immobilization.

Slings

An arm sling is commonly used both to support the flaccid arm and to prevent subluxation of the shoulder caused by excess gravitational pull on weak muscles during ambulation. When properly positioned, it also prevents edema of the hand. The patient who uses a wheelchair uses other devices attached to it to support and position his or her arm; an overhead suspension sling, a lapboard, an arm trough, or a padded wedge placed on a lapboard can prevent edema of the hand.

Positioning is very important; every effort must be made, both in bed and chair positioning, to prevent edema, contracture, and subluxation in the hand and shoulder. Although the arm sling is an easily recognizable means of support for the paralyzed arm, care must be taken *not* to use a sling that will cause shoulder pain, increase in adductor or flexor spasticity, or shoulder subluxation, which are results of poor design, application, use, or monitoring.

A balanced forearm orthosis or a suspension sling with an overhead bar can be attached to the wheelchair to support the arm and to facilitate movement. Both of these supports provide mobility to the extremity; therefore, it is important before using special equipment to distinguish whether the need is for static support or dynamic support.

At times a sling and a splint can be combined. However, it must always be remembered that patients can be harmed by the use of inappropriate equipment or by prolonged use, which can impede the return of function and maintain the individual at a dependent level.

Functional Activities

The patient focuses on the activity instead of the goal of specific muscle or extremity function. The goals should be inherent in the activity; thus doing the activity should accomplish the goal.

Sensory stimulus is developed through adapted cutaneous contact with tools, the beater of a loom, or the handle of a sander. Sensory discrimination is stimulated through the adapted tools as well as by the use of materials such as clay, sand, or theraplast. Gross motor reaching and throwing activities to stimulate proprioception and kinesthetic awareness (shuffleboard, beanbag, ball, and dart throwing) are useful. Use of the skateboard attached to the forearm for directed range of motion activities stimulates upper arm active movements. Adaptation can be made for holding a pencil and drawing patterns on paper or on a horizontal blackboard during directed skateboard movement.

Suspension slings and pulley systems incorporating weighted or counterbalanced resistance are both supportive of weak extremities and facilitative to movement. They may be used in conjunction with activities to increase shoulder and elbow function. The addition of a functional hand splint may be used to encourage positioning and grasp. Activities such as weaving, woodworking, and especially sanding, planing, and filing can be adapted to incorporate movements, with gravity assisting for diagonal patterns and to encourage midline crossing.

Trunk stability and correct positioning are encouraged during all activities. Stability of trunk and joints proximal to those being used is necessary for self-directed, goal-oriented, coordinated activity.

Driving

The occupational therapist may not be directly involved in a specific evaluation of a person driving following a debilitating disease or injury. Where there is a definite role, protocols are usually spelled out for each team member.

In the routine performance evaluation the occupational therapist may have pertinent information relevant to the person's safety in driving with a disability. Such signs are: excessive caution, slow reaction time, reduced visual acuity and perception, hearing deficits, tremors, retarded reflexes, and slower adjustment to stimuli. Behavioral changes such as agitation, impatience, impaired memory, spatial disfiguration, or mental confusion can be hazardous in driving. Use of drugs can cause susceptability to the impairments mentioned above, in addition to causing drowsiness or dizziness.

The person who has had a stroke is often anxious to return to driving despite residual deficits from the stroke, which he or she may or may not acknowledge. Inability to accept the resulting dependence on others may prompt the homebound person to resume driving, thus creating a hazard for himself or herself and for other drivers. Deficits in figure ground or color and form discrimination can result in faulty interpretation of signal lights and signs of inability to distinguish these from other visual stimuli. Deficits in auditory discrimination or location can result in lack of pick-up of warning horns or cautioning passengers.

Safe driving is the prime concern. Minor driving aids may be advantageous for the driver with cerebral palsy, a limb amputation, hemiplegia, paraplegia, or quadriplegia. Examples of these include steering devices attached to the steering wheel, change of side for the accelerator or gear shift column, turn signals, lights switches, and other controls.

For the more severely handicapped person, a variety of hand control designs are available, as are other devices necessary for the person lacking lower and/or upper extremity mobility. Special adaptations for cars and vans are available, including ramps and lifts for vans, car-top carriers for wheelchairs, and clamp-downs, which permit a person to drive from his wheelchair.

The upper extremity involved driver may be assisted by hand splints to manipulate controls and to maintain a grip strength.

Physically, a variety of adaptive devices are available to enable the disabled person to resume driving; however, careful assessment is necessary to determine psychological or neurological factors which could preclude safety.

In evaluating the patient's capability to drive, the therapist must consider the following factors:

Physical: Independent wheelchair transfer
Ability to operate all driving controls
Ability to operate steering wheel
Perceptual: Figure ground (road signs)

Spatial relations (angles, curves, left/right)
Ocular pursuit (traffic flow)
Vertical and horizontal perception (turning)
Cognitive: Judgment
Decision making
Analysis of information
Concentration
Psychosocial: Acceptance of disability

Cerebrovascular Accident

The cerebrovascular accident (CVA) is a lesion in the brain commonly referred to as a stroke, an insult, or a shock, because of its sudden onset. It results in paralysis of one side of the body (hemiplegia) or both sides (bilateral hemiplegia). The lesion is characterized by an interruption of the blood supply to the brain tissues in a particular location, caused by thrombus, embolus, anoxia, hemorrhage, or aneurysm. Precipitating factors may include a history of hypertension, arteriosclerosis, or congenital artery wall weakness. Although hypertension and arteriosclerosis contribute to the vessel breakdown or occlusion in the older adult, congenital vascular weakness can result in an aneurysm, a common cause of hemiplegia in the young adult.

Vascular disease can cause a complete CVA with a full picture of hemiplegia or temporary symptoms from a transient ischemic attack (TIA) caused by vascular insufficiency. The TIA may result in brief and spotty impairment of neurological functions; it is frequently a warning of the probability of a more serious CVA in the future. The treatment of the patient with either a complete CVA or a TIA not only should be geared toward rehabilitation of the present problem but also should include prophylactic techniques to prevent further occurrence of TIA or CVA.

Other causes of hemiplegia include external trauma (a blow on the head or striking the head during a fall), heart attack, and brain and spinal tumors. In these cases the character of the condition may vary slightly from the cerebrovascular lesion but, because many of the symptoms are similar, evaluation techniques and treatment procedures used in CVA can be applied.

In this section the role of the occupational therapist in the intensive rehabilitation regimen of a team-oriented approach is discussed. Because of the number and complexity of the manifestations facing the patient, and the impact of these conditions on daily life and family, team members are needed to aid in the rehabilitation process.

Definition

The lesion in the brain that causes hemiplegia usually occurs in one hemisphere and affects the contralateral limbs and face. The result is designated as right or left hemiplegia, *according to the side of the body involved.* In discussing CVA and hemiplegia, it is essential to distinguish between the location of the CVA and the location of the hemiplegia. Should the CVA occur in the left hemisphere, the hemiplegia will be located on the right side of the body and vice versa.

Depending on which side of the brain is involved, there can be, in addition to motor and sensory deficits, impairment of perceptual and cognitive functions, of premorbid personality, of motor planning and problem-solving abilities, and of judgment (see Table 22-2). Urinary continence, motivation, and a sense of social awareness and responsibility may be lost.

A lesion can affect both hemispheres of the brain, causing bilateral clinical signs.

Impact of Hemiplegia

Whether the person is affected by the sudden onset of an internal CVA or by the shock of external head trauma causing hemiplegia, the results of the condition can have a devastating impact on his or her life. The adult patient may be going to school, completing vocational or academic training in preparation for employment, secure in employment, nearing the peak of vocational goals, nearing retirement, or retired. In all of these situations, the patient may suffer

Table 22-2 *Cerebrovascular Accident*

Artery	Areas of Brain Affected	Manifestation
Internal carotid	Frontal lobe	Aphasia (dominant hemisphere)
	Parietal lobe	Contralateral hemiplegia
	Temporal lobe	Homonomous hemianopsia
	Internal capsule	
	Optic nerve	
Anterior cerebral	Anterior part of internal capsule	Contralateral monoplegia (leg)
	Tip of frontal lobe	Sensory loss
	Surface of cerebral hemisphere to parietal-occipital junction	Mental confusion
		Apraxia
		Aphasia (dominant hemisphere)
Middle cerebral	Convolutions of cerebral hemisphere	Contralateral hemiplegia (primarily arm)
	Lateral orbital-frontal region	Contralateral facial weakness
	Internal capsule	Aphasia (dominant hemisphere)
	Anterior thalamus	Homonomous hemianopsia
		Sensory loss
Posterior cerebral	Midbrain	Contralateral hemiplegia
	2/3 Temporal lobe	Hemi-anesthesia
	Middle occipital lobe	Homonomous hemianopsia
	Posterior internal capsule	Ataxia
		Tremor
Basilar	Pons	Symptoms from 3rd to 12th cranial nerves
	Medulla	Loss of proprioception
	Cerebellum	Cerebellar dysfunction
Cerebellar	Midbrain	Cerebellar ataxia
	Pons	Contralateral loss of pain and temperature
	Cerebellum	

the threat of not returning to the previous life style or occupation. The severity of the brain damage, the premorbid health conditions, the patient's attitude toward the condition and rehabilitation, the support of the family, and the restoration of various functions are all factors in rehabilitation.

While the patient's developmental level prior to the CVA was that of an adult, the effect of the CVA may reduce the physical and mental levels to those of a child. The patient may be unable to accept the arduous recuperation of lost functions through specific "childlike" activities, such as strengthening of limbs and development of coordination; learning again to read, write, and speak; or developing independence in self-care and toilet functions. Frequently the patient denies the full implications of self-involvement in the recovery of these functions; the patient may be unable to cope with the multitude of problems facing him or her and his or her family, or the patient may be suffering actual damage to brain tissues that control motivation and adjustment. The adult hemiplegic tends to look back to normal functioning and imposes premorbid standards on present abilities.

Sensorimotor losses are accompanied by changes in body image and personality, which affect both the patient and family and can strain their relationship. Confusion resulting from brain trauma can leave the patient unable to establish self-direction and purposeful motivation or to understand simple conversations. The effects on the patient's personality may result in a change in values, having an effect on level of performance. Because the older adult suffering a CVA has "all that has been gained to lose," one of the most difficult problems for both the patient and the therapist is the belief that the patient has "lived his life" and there is nothing left.

The following factors contribute to disorientation, confusion, malfunction, and lack of progress:

1. Auditory deficit
2. Receptive or expressive aphasia
3. Impairment of verbal or written expression
4. Deficits in learning ability
5. Impairment of previously independent function
6. Denial and neglect of affected extremities and other functional deficits of the condition
7. Distortion of time and place; effect on the individual's ability to perceive and to plan the future realistically
8. Loss of tactile sensation and motor function
9. Loss of proprioceptive and kinesthetic awareness, which hinders integration
10. Impaired bilateral extremity function
11. Apraxia, or loss of voluntary motor activity, which hinders functional ability and motor improvement
12. Visual-perceptual deficits such as field cut, (hemianopsia) visual neglect, or deficits in functional scanning, discrimination of color and form, figure ground

These deficits, although common, may not be present in all hemiplegics or, if present, not to the same extent.

Psychological and Social Implications

Mention has been made of the devastating effect of hemiplegia on the person. Not all persons, of course, react in the same way to catastrophic illnesses or disabilities. Often the reactions will reflect premorbid taboos and fears. The patient's gains from rehabilitation are, to some degree, dependent upon attitudes developed prior to the CVA.

The patient who is lacking in motivation and is depressed is difficult to rehabilitate, and may become a burden to both himself and family. Often the patient is the breadwinner or the homemaker. The loss of ability to carry out these family responsibilities affects both the patient and the family. The family may undergo financial hardships because of the hospitalization, and this may be a further worry for the patient. At times the family finds it difficult to function without the hospitalized member and needs counseling to understand the course of rehabilitation and to solve the seemingly insurmountable problems of daily living.

Social implications for re-entry into the home and community include adjustment to permanent functional deficits, dependence on assistive equipment (braces, slings, and/or a wheelchair), and financial insecurity. The person may no longer be able to drive or to work because of visual and intellectual deficits. Developing a new lifestyle may be necessary.

Initial contact with the patient occurs with the interview and evaluation on a one-to-one basis with the therapist. As disability manifestations are identified, the therapist uses a variety of social techniques to encourage the development of interpersonal skills with other patients. Patient interaction may be facilitated by the therapist during treatment sessions or encouraged through organized group sessions to stimulate peer support and interaction.

Group Activity

The supportive benefits of group activity can be shared by the patient's learning about individual abilities and limitations in physical, communication, and social skills. In structured group activities patients have the opportunity of working together in performing body movement exercises, group pro-

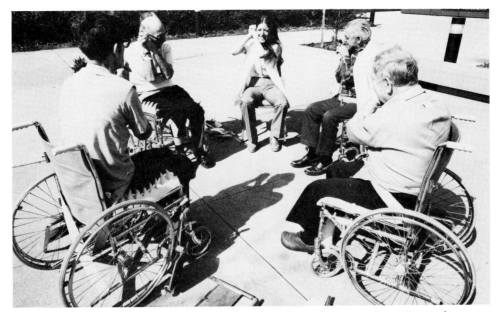

Figure 22-1. Group activity. The therapist demonstrates to patients how to grasp the hemiplegic hand with the sound hand and raise both hands up to touch the right ear. Activity is used for specified body movement and awareness.

jects, recreational activities, or perceptual games, thus stimulating motivation and encouragement.

Group work aids in diminishing fear of personal interaction with family and friends and aids in development of self-awareness and acceptance. Helping team members and receiving help restore self-confidence. In Figure 22-1 the therapist teaches the patient to use bilateral movements to stimulate sensorimotor sensitivity and function, right and left orientation, bilateral use of the arms, and trunk balance. During physical activity, patients talk with each other and the therapist, discuss what they are doing and how, and what they see in the outside environment. Visual perceptual tasks (Fig. 22-2) increase interest in the environment, and the change in atmosphere stimulates new interest and motivation. Group activity aids in integrating sensory, motor, and perceptual skills for improved performance in daily tasks. The peer support gained from group activity is distinct from one-to-one treatment and relates to social skills the patient will need to return home and to the community.

Communication Disorders

Both left and right hemiplegic patients show communication disorders in the early stages following CVA; however, the right hemiplegic tends to retain more severe deficits in speech, verbal reception, and language, because a lesion in the dominant hemisphere (usually the left) affects all language areas to

some degree. Specific problems that occur are impairment in interpretation of the meaning of spoken and written words (receptive aphasia), impairment of the ability to use speech and to write communicatively (expressive aphasia), and impairment of motor function of speech (dysarthria). Distorted auditory reception, loss of hearing, and inability to locate auditory stimuli or to make meaning of them can affect the speech response. Apraxia is the impairment of the voluntary ability to use the speech mechanisms; the patient may possess these functions but is unable to use them. Despite apraxia, the patient may be able to use his tongue, lips, or speech mechanisms for automatic and reflexive actions such as chewing or blowing.

The occupational therapist correlates the use of speech and written language in both instruction giving and writing exercises with the objectives and functional levels recommended by the speech pathologist. Consistency in language development is important for the patient's improvement and self-confidence, as well as for preventing confusion from over-stimulation or expectation of functional ability.

Intellectual and Perceptual Dysfunctions

With the disturbance in sensorimotor reception and expression, the hemiplegic patient frequently demonstrates impairment in abstract reasoning. The severity of this condition depends on the auditory, visual, and tactile abilities that remain intact. Learning

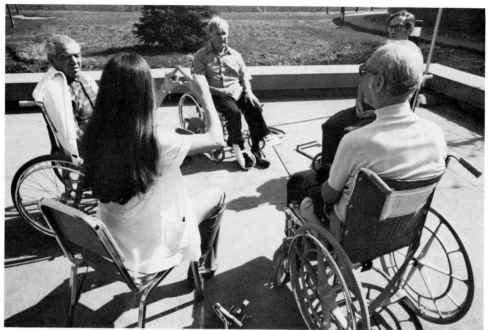

Figure 22-2. Visual perceptual task. The therapist makes the form of a triangle with her fingers and asks the patients to find a similar shape in the environment to stimulate body movement, awareness of the environment, and group interaction.

is affected by sensory deficits that impede learning through the use of auditory instructions, reading, imitation, and demonstration. The prognosis for restoration of independent function depends on the ability to receive and to organize information for learning and implementation. Careful preliminary evaluation of perceptual areas is essential to planning the patient's approaches to learning.

Visual Deficits

Double vision (diplopia), loss of half of the visual field (hemianopsia), and neglect are three common manifestations of visual impairment. Loss of part of the visual field prevents the patients from seeing objects on the right or left side. Patients are unaware of this "cut" in the visual field until they realize that a paragraph makes little sense because they can read only half of it, until they drive their wheelchairs into the side of a doorway, or until they half dress, thinking the task has been completed.

Visual field neglect occurs when the patient ignores visual stimuli on the side of hemiplegia when confronted with simultaneous stimuli from both visual fields (Fig. 22-3). This occurs when visual fields are intact.[3] Distortions in the perception of spatial relations (vertical, horizontal, oblique) result in impairment in deriving meaning from visual stimuli and in using this information in intellectual functions.

Although diplopia can be aided by an eye patch, it is often difficult for the patient to recognize and compensate for a field cut (hemianopsia). Visual cues, practice, and memory of turning the head to the side of the limited field may be helpful.

Sensory Deficits in Extremities

Sensory impairment is manifested in peripheral reception of stimuli, tactile functions in the affected hand, and general sensory awareness. Manifestations of peripheral impairment include lack of sensation of cutaneous stimuli (temperature, touch, pain); inability to locate the area of stimulus; inability to identify the position of the extremity (proprioception); inability to identify a familiar object through tactile sensation (stereognosis); inability to effect the motor act (apraxia); inability to correlate purpose and accomplishment of tasks (ideational apraxia); and inability to carry out new purposeful activities while retaining ability to perform routine activities (ideomotor apraxia). Lack of sensory functions and impairment of sensory receptors in the extremities affect motor functions by causing lack of feedback. Bilateral integrative functions are also affected by sensory deficits.

In all sensorimotor activities it is important to evaluate the status of sensation and sensory function in the extremities before initiating exercises, activities, self-care, or splinting. As one of the objec-

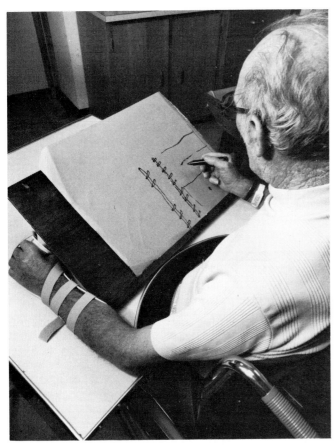

Figure 22-3. Patient with left-sided hemiplegia demonstrates left visual field neglect by drawing only on the right side of the paper.

tives of treatment is sensory integration and total body awareness and adaptation, the patient must be informed of the results of the sensorimotor evaluation.

Physical Manifestations

A lesion in the brain, usually localized in one hemisphere, results in motor impairment in the contralateral side of the body. Complete (-plegia) or partial (-paresis) flaccid paralysis of the upper and lower musculature and facial muscles is manifested in the loss of active mobility of the involved extremities. While passive range of motion is complete initially, gradual onset of spasticity presents the threat of increased muscle tone impeding active range of motion and causing contractures and deformity. The severity of involvement depends on location and extent of the lesion. Some patients begin to gain voluntary muscle power a few days following a CVA. Others may experience no return for months or years. For some, the ability may never be regained. Impairment of the dominant extremity necessitates a change of domi-

nance, and loss of bilateral coordination with a possibility of partial loss of strength and coordination in the sound extremity.

A variety of treatment modalities and approaches is used to aid in the development of isolated and voluntary function of flaccid or spastic extremities. As the development of synergy patterns may occur following a stroke, the patient may have asymmetrical reflexes and sensorimotor behavior. Treatment techniques stemming from neurophysiological approaches to development of volitional extremity function are effectively used in occupational therapy treatment programs or in combined treatment programs with physical therapy. Facilitation and inhibition techniques used appropriately can stimulate independent function.

It is important for therapists to use complementary treatment techniques so that all therapy programs are correlated in common goals and directions. The time of onset, duration, etiology, prognosis, family component, and general medical picture also affect the treatment modalities used in that they affect the length of treatment (one month, several months) and the type of program (inpatient, outpatient). Specific treatment techniques must be correlated with daily programs of therapies, self-care, rest, and recreation. Resource information detailing various specific techniques is available in the bibliography.

Splinting

In the early stage of hemiplegia the extremity tends to be flaccid, and a major concern is the positioning of the extremity to prevent deformity, contractures resulting from spasticity, and edema. If visual neglect and decreased sensation are present, the patient may be unaware of the arm's position or location. Splinting the extremity helps with visual and sensory awareness of the flaccid extremity and contributes toward preventing the above concerns from occuring. A simple cock-up splint can aid in wrist positioning for functional use of the extremity. A static forearm–hand splint can be used at night and during the day when the patient is not actively working with the extremity in therapy, functional activities, or self-regulated range of motion exercises. Snook suggests the use of a spasticity reduction splint, which incorporates the Bobath technique of using a reflex inhibiting posture (RIP) for positioning, using wrist and thumb extension, finger abduction, and extension of the interphalangeal joints.[4] This splint is designed to provide full pan volar support at fingers and thumb, with dorsal coverage on forearm and carpal area of the hand. Finger separators are used to maintain finger abduction, with metacarpal flexion at 45° and wrist extension at 30°. A variation of the static forearm–hand pan splint is to set the wrist and fingers at maximum extension abduction stretch beyond the point of spasticity.

The splint is removed periodically for relaxation, inhibition, and facilitation techniques as appropriate to work toward isolated volitional movements. As the patient begins to regain function, the need for a splint is reassessed to determine wearing time and design alteration, allowing the hand freedom during the day for functional activities, while maintaining or allowing for regained function.

A variety of splint patterns and recommendations are available for use with the patient with spasticity. In some cases, treatment techniques do not include splinting, and hence splinting should not be used. Attention to consistent and collaborative therapy techniques is essential for optimum success in treating the patient. The splint represents a modality which may or may not be desired in the therapeutic regimen.

Self-care Skills and Activities of Daily Living

The level of accomplishment in self-care skills and activities of daily living by the hemiplegic patient is largely dependent on *motivational, perceptual, judgmental,* and *sensory-integrative* factors. While both right and left hemiplegic patients suffer motor paralysis or limitations, there are distinctions in the effects of the locations of the lesions.

Functional areas largely affected by a lesion in the right hemisphere of the brain are those involving motivation, perception, judgment, and sensory integration. Therefore the left hemiplegic patient may deny the affected extremities, have visual or sensory neglect or denial, have distortions in concepts of movement and spatial relations, have lost the concept of the motor act, or lack motivation for self-improvement. These deficits may be more of a hindrance to function than are motor paralysis and physical limitation.

The left hemiplegic patient is more likely to suffer difficulties in tasks such as seeing all the food on the plate or finding eating utensils, grooming the left side of the body, dressing the whole body, or walking than is the right hemiplegic patient.

With the left hemiplegic patient, daily exercises and activities are directed toward increasing sensory awareness and carrying over this awareness into self-care functions. Exercises and activities should include developing visual and proprioceptive awareness of the involved extremity, encouraging turning of the head to the affected side to include the part missing from sight because of field cut or neglect, and increasing the patient's proprioceptive awareness of the involved extremity through developing bilateral functions. Although distortion in body image concepts may hinder self-care independence, the practice of self-care techniques and activities can aid awareness and integration of bilateral functions.

The right hemiplegic person, while also suffering motor paralysis and/or impairment, usually does not incur the problems with judgment encountered by the left hemiplegic person. However, the right hemiplegic person shows varying degrees of communication disability.

The patient whose limitations in function are primarily in the motor areas (flaccid or moderately spastic extremities, for instance) can learn techniques of self-care fairly easily by using the sound extremities to assist the affected ones.

The occupational therapist assists both right and left hemiplegics in self-care feeding, dressing, bathing, and grooming tasks as soon as medically possible and incorporates these skills into the patient's daily program. The patient is also encouraged to use one-handed techniques and assistive devices, such as a rocker knife for cutting meat one-handed, Velcro attachments on clothes for ease of fastening, and elastic shoe laces. Bathing and grooming are assisted by long-handled sponges, bath mitts, and adapted nail clippers for one-handed use.

Use of neurophysiologically-based movement and balance techniques are correlated with self-care activities to encourage developmental patterns of re-education of function, bilateral awareness, and adaptive behavior.

Family education in the patient's ability level and areas of need for assistance is essential. Sessions with the patient and his or her family help to show the latter what the patient has achieved, can do, and needs help in accomplishing. This helps to assure continuation of the patient's ability level upon the return home.

Functional Implications

With sensory and motor loss in the arm and leg on the affected side of the body, the hemiplegic person functionally becomes one-sided. Activities such as rolling over in bed, eating, dressing, bathing, grooming, and two-handed activities are now limited by the paralysis of an arm and a leg. Not only are the specific peripheral functions impaired, but the sense of integration of the body is also affected by the cerebral lesion. The patient may find it difficult to adjust to a necessary change in hand dominance. Activities requiring total sensorimotor awareness are affected. The patient may deny or neglect the functional implications of this condition and may grow to depend on others for assistance in daily functions and responsibilities. The rehabilitation program is geared both toward achievement of maximum independence and toward family awareness and acceptance of the patient's level of function.

Functional activities for development of abilities are geared to the ability level of the patient in all areas previously mentioned: psychological, social, communication, intellectual, perceptual, visual, sensory, physical, splinting, and self-care.

Treatment is directed toward the following goals:
1. Maximum active range of motion, strength, and coordination of the extremities
2. Maximum volitional unilateral and bilateral function of the upper extremities
3. Maximum independence in self-care activities
4. Use of assistive devices for increased function as needed
5. Awareness and acceptance of functional ability
6. Ability to achieve successful social interaction and basic communication (verbal or nonverbal)
7. Prevocational and avocational exploration and planning as appropriate

Vocational Implications

For the young or middle-aged adult suffering hemiplegia, the effect on vocational potential can be serious, depending on skills previously attained and the impairment of intellectual functions. Return to a previous vocation depends in large measure on the type of job the patient was doing, the patient's status in the company, the understanding of the employer, and the patient's ability to regain employable skills. If return to employment is feasible, the occupational therapist includes prevocational assessment and planning in the treatment program and carefully and realistically assists the patient in reviewing alternatives.

Frequently, job competition is too great for re-entry of the worker with permanent hemiplegia. The worker who is no longer able to pursue a vocation suffers a loss in self-esteem, self-image, status in the family, and status in society. Prevocational evaluation for alternative job opportunities and training programs to learn new skills are part of the rehabilitation program.

Head Injury

Head injuries are caused by direct trauma to the skull, with 70% occurring in traffic accidents and falls. Other common causes are industrial accidents, wounds, or direct blows to the head. Resulting trauma includes concussion, contusion, laceration, or compression. Although both skull fracture and brain damage may occur, one can occur without the other.

The resultant state of the brain, rather than the state of the skull, is the most significant effect of a head injury.

A variety of neurological symptoms and manifestations can result from head injury. Depending on the location and extent of the lesion, the symptoms may be of short duration, latent, or extended over a period of years. Outcome of rehabilitation is also related to the length of time the person was in a coma; the longer the coma, the poorer the prognosis.

Post-trauma Manifestations

Post-trauma manifestations include occasional loss of consciousness, dizziness, headache, or vertigo provoked by sudden changes in position; confusion and disorientation about time and place; convulsions; and emotional reactions such as combativeness. Behavior disturbances may be blatant, particularly during the initial recovery period. Personality disorders, amnesia, and delirium may also occur.

These manifestations may be accompanied by intellectual deficits, blindness, diplopia, hemianopsia, olfactory dysfunction, and auditory deficits. Physical symptoms include quadriparesis, unilateral or bilateral hemiparesis, initial decerebrate rigidity, and speech deficits. Restoration of functional, intellectual, social, psychological, and physical manifestations may require a period of years if the injury was severe.

The patient may demonstrate physical and mental deficits similar to those of a person who has suffered CVA: cognitive–perceptual–motor dysfunction, spasticity, disorientation, speech deficits, and disturbance of sensory motor integration. Mental manifestation and personality changes are often more pronounced than those seen in CVA, even though these patients are generally much younger than the stroke victim. These deficits prevent the head-injured person from effectively interacting with the environment and may hinder the progress of rehabilitation. The patient may seem to have actually lost contact with his or her surroundings and able to focus only on the narrow, yet overwhelming feelings, concerns, and behaviors imposed by the sudden traumatic disability.

Functional problems of the patient with brain injury fall into four general categories: (1) cognitive, (2) behavioral and emotional, (3) communication, and (4) physical. The clinical picture represents a pattern of fluctuating symptoms in these areas, subject to frequent change, influenced by internal and external stimuli. This fluctuation is evident throughout the pattern of recovery as the patient tries to adjust to the deficits imposed by the injury, to learn to decrease and eliminate handicapping effects, and to renew self-confidence through awareness and positive acceptance of the immediate and future level of function. In the early stages, therapeutic support during unknown or confusing occurrences is needed to allay anxiety until the patient is gradually able to regain conscious control of feelings, behaviors, motivation, abilities, relationships, and daily activities.

The long-term impact of brain injury may cause interference with learning ability, cognitive integration, social interaction and status, self-esteem, and motivation for personal goal setting and achievement.

Recovery

The rate of recovery and its final outcome of adaptive functional level may vary from patient to patient. Recovery may plateau after 6 months or continue for several years. Recovery scales have been developed in an attempt to determine prognosis and to outline programs appropriate to the patient's abilities. Information from these scales aids in the coordination of goals and methods used by team members involved. There is some tendency to model scales on the developmental patterns of cognitive or intellectual function, behavior, social, motivational, and motor levels.

The DARSHI method (Developmental Assessment of Recovery from Serious Head Injury) uses four chronological segments of development to determine areas and levels of function:

1. 0–4 years, using functions from infant scales
2. 4–8 years, using items from Stanford-Binet Intelligence Scale
3. 8–12 years, using tests for basic information processing, including sequencing, left and right differentiation, and visual perception
4. Mature adaptive function, including concepts, skills, and information processing related to daily activity performance.[5]

The Disability Rating Scale (DR) uses the following six categories from the Glasgow Coma Scale to rate level of head injury according to specific functional area: (1) eye opening, (2) verbalization, (3) motor response, (4) feeding, (5) toileting, (6) grooming, (7) level of functioning, and (8) employability.[6]

The Glasgow Coma Scale indicates eye, motor, and verbal response levels, whereas the Glasgow Outcome Scale consists of five stages relating the ability to work: (1) death, (2) persistent vegetative state, (3) severe physical and mental disability (cannot work), (4) moderate disability, (5) good recovery with continuing emotional problems, but can work.[7,8]

Eson and colleagues state that the quality of neuropsychological recovery is highly variable in rate, pattern, and level of recovery of adaptive function. Levels of adaptive function are defined as follows: *early*—activities of daily living, self-care, and rudimentary social interaction; *middle*—conceptual and information processing skills needed for social interaction, and ability to initiate and carry out sustained, planned activities directed toward a goal; and *complete or near complete*—ability to seek and maintain employment, and ability to participate in normal adult social and recreational activities without supervision.[9]

Treatment

In the effort to plan and implement effective and appropriate successful rehabilitation for the brain-injured person, a variety of approaches have been developed by professional teams and researchers. Whatever the structure or organization of methods of treatment used by the occupational therapist, it is essential that they relate meaningfully to programs and techniques used by others in the daily care of the brain-injured patient.

The program at Loewenstein Hospital Rehabilitation Center identifies three stages relative to the medical picture, based on behavioral characteristics. The first phase is post-coma, characterized by dream-like disorientation in time and space, causing disturbances in establishing order and relationships within environmental stimuli. The second stage is behavioral, characterized by increasing consciousness of the outside world but continuing disturbance in interpreting and handling stimuli, resulting in anxiety and stress fatigue. In the third phase, the patient begins to enter a period of realism and experiences a series of conflicting but realistic changes in self-awareness, which result in a variety of emotional responses. During this stage, the struggle to identify with the external environment satisfactorily and functionally and to integrate external and internal experiences and meanings occurs.[10]

In its approach to rehabilitative management, the Rancho Los Amigos Hospital program describes eight progressive levels of cognitive functioning and behavioral responses based on developmental order: (1) no response (coma), (2) generalized response (inconsistent and non-purposeful), (3) localized response (specific but inconsistent response to stimuli), (4) confused-agitated (heightened state of activity with decreased ability to process information), (5) confused, inappropriate, nonagitated, (6) confused-appropriate, (7) automatic-appropriate, (8) purposeful and appropriate. From the initial assessment the treatment team determines at which level the patient is functioning and then administers treatment in accordance with this developmental pattern.[11]

In working with the patient suffering manifestations of brain injury, it is important to provide an atmosphere free from overwhelming and confusing input and challenges to the sensory systems. Reassurance regarding the program's content, duration, and expectations helps the patient to relax enough to respond to specific treatment techniques. The therapist can limit anxiety by talking about the physical surroundings, what is going on, and feelings about where she or he is, what she or he is doing, and how she or he is doing. This helps with reality orientation, resocialization, and environmental adaptation.

One of the major functions of the occupational therapist is to help the patient to adjust to both symptoms and the general situation in the treatment setting. The patient needs to know why she or he has come to occupational therapy and what is expected. These explanations may need to be repeated for emphasis, clarification, and reminder as the patient improves, to maintain a stabilizing continuity to compensate for fluctuation in moods and abilities. How the therapist uses words and voice tone must be focused on the level of receptivity, but must at the same time show respect. When the lack of spontaneous speech exists, the patient may not respond verbally to questions, comments, or simple requests from the therapist. A code system of communication may be worked out between the therapist and the patient. For example, the patient may be capable of indicating "yes" or "no" by closing his eyes, frowning, moving his head, or lifting an arm. Disorientation and confusion may also result from being unable to communicate.

In preparing for the functional assessment of the brain-injured patient, the therapist must think of the long-term effects of short-term care. This begins with the patient's first contact with the therapist. The initial interview should take place in an area physically comfortable, with few auditory and visual distractions. Input received during early periods may be stored for future use when the patient is more capable of volitional behavior; however, it is important to control the environmental input according to the patient's current level of receptivity. Attention to therapeutic and functional positioning informs the patient of the therapist's concern for comfort, as well as conveying the expectation of active, functional use of his or her body. Repeated abnormal functioning can contribute to later weakness and deformities of both the trunk and the extremities. Having evaluated the effect of the physical environment, the therapist observes the patient's social reactions to the therapist and to other people in the area.

Through discussion with the patient and family, the therapist achieves an indication of what the patient was like premorbidly. This information helps in planning therapeutic programs related to the patient's interests. It is also important to know what accomplishments, failures, dreams, plans, and specific areas of activity had played a significant role in the personal and social life prior to the head injury. Since the patient may suffer amnesia with regard to retrieval of information regarding premorbid life or surrounding the injury, or experience language deficits resulting in reception or expression inadequacies, questions regarding these areas may cause anxiety, irritability, or confusion. Gentle encouragment to discuss the accident assists the patient in clarifying and accepting the medical situation and in understanding why he or she is receiving treatment. This helps prevent the build-up of anxieties regarding the unknowns of the past, present, and future by providing an outlet for self-expression and discussion of changing feelings and concerns. In questioning the patient about the accident, the therapist provides the patient an opportunity to tell "his side," providing a check on the patient's accuracy of information. The patient may experience the following symptoms during initial evaluation and treatment:

1. Postural dizziness: sensation of dizziness or disorientation caused by change of position or quick movements of the head; dizziness may also result from exertion or fatigue.
2. Headache: intermittent or persistent headache, pain, feeling of pressure in the head.
3. Fatigue: related to extent and length of time of physical or mental effort during activity.
4. Eye strain: due to intensive light, contrasting colors, or movement of visual stimuli, weakness in focus or interpretation.
5. Hypersensitivity to sudden, loud, or multiple noises and/or movements in the immediate physical area.

When the patient is seen by the therapist—in the acute stage of trauma, the early rehabilitation phase, the outpatient stage, or during home treatment—will determine the nature and extent of evaluation and treatment programs appropriate. At all levels, continual communication between the therapist and the patient is essential with regard to changes in the treatment goals, progress, and his or her motivation and goals.

The following list is a grouping of specific functional areas which can be used in the assessment to determine the extent of disability demonstrated by the brain-injured patient through specific testing and evaluation procedures common to the particular area.

As noted above, treatment *begins* with assessment of a communication method, of sensorimotor deficits,

Evaluation Areas

COMMUNICA-TION:	Ability to understand and to use speech
	Ability to communicate needs
	Speech
	Writing
	Gestures
	Imitation
BEHAVIOR:	Emotional response
	Self-awareness
	Appropriateness of behavior
	Attention
	Response to testing
	Type of behavior
SOCIAL:	Awareness of self
	Awareness of others
	Appropriateness of behavior
	Reaction to social stimuli
	Reaction to family and therapist
AUDITORY:	Reception of sound
	Discrimination
	Discrepancy of left and right
	Auditory localization
VISUAL:	Acuity
	Response to visual stimulus
	Discrimination of size, color, form
	Spatial relationships
	Figure ground
	Directionality
	Field neglect
	Body image and body parts
SENSORY:	Spatial awareness
	Tactile defensiveness
	Proprioception
	Temperature
	Sharpness and dullness
	Stereognosis
PHYSICAL:	Passive and active joint range of motion

	Contractures
	Deformities
	Skin integrity
	Active response
	Body positioning
	Abnormal tone (spasticity)
	Strength
	Hand dominance
	Developmental level
	Standing, gait, balance
	Reflexes
FUNCTIONAL:	Follow instructions
	Understand instructions
	Initiate movement
	Accomplish task (steps)
	Limitations
	Deviations
	Retention
	Integration
	Self-care carry-over
	Presence of deficits in self-care
	Safety awareness
	Judgment
	Level of independence
EDUCATIONAL:	Premorbid level
	Ability to learn, to retain, to problem-solve
	Concept and use of concrete and abstract
VOCATIONAL:	Premorbid level and skill areas
	Expectations
	Prognosis
	Adjustments
	Job situation
DRIVER EVALUATION:	Visual acuity and perception
	Auditory and visual perception
	Reaction time, physical and perceptual
	Physical coordination, range of motion, strength

orientation, and functional ability. The patient is then treated *symptomatically* with the program directed toward self-awareness, awareness of objects, and toward initiation and accomplishment of purposeful activity. Development of motor strength and coordination is combined with activities to encourage social awareness and interaction with others. Graded intellectual and problem-solving tasks (reading, arithmetic, and writing) aid the patient in regaining function.

Treatment may begin with basic visual and tactile discrimination and sensorimotor activities such as self-care skills, exercise activities, and games. Initially the occupational therapist works with the patient in quiet surroundings, gradually increasing auditory and visual stimuli. The patient is provided with activity simple enough to hold his or her interest. As physical and mental tolerance increase, the therapist can expand the complexity of the environment.

Personal Impact

The trauma of head injury causes significant personal impact. The patient must deal with the residual manifestations with whatever assets can be retrieved from the premorbid life experience. The following areas are common rehabilitation challenges of the brain-injured patient and are described briefly to give a general clinical picture of this patient; it must be remembered that not all patients show the symptoms, nor do they show them to the same extent. Premorbid characteristics of lifestyle, body health and type, achievement, attitudes, and goals may positively or negatively affect the functional outcome.

Since many head injuries are caused by traffic accidents and falls, there may be accompanying physical disabilities, such as amputations, peripheral nerve injuries, paralysis, or fractures that add to the complexity of adequate treatment in all areas. The therapist performs appropriate evaluation and treatment in all areas showing disability; however, attention must be given to the overall priorities and concerns of the team rehabilitation plan.

The treatment approach depends on the levels and areas of function the patient is capable of accomplishing. It begins at the level of the patient's ability and is gradually upgraded as the patient changes. The goals of rehabilitation of the person with a brain injury are:
1. To achieve integration of cognitive and sensorimotor functions
2. To be able to respond to an unstructured environment
3. To be able to participate in productive living
4. To become re-integrated into society

The purpose of occupational therapy with the brain-injured patient is to evaluate the functional assets and deficits with regard to ability to perform self-initiated, purposeful, and productive activity and to assist in developing maximum abilities. Specific objectives are to enable the patient to do the following:
1. Develop perceptual-motor function and sensory integration
2. Refine sensory-motor systems to provide increased volitional motor control
3. Increase attention span and activity tolerance
4. Decrease nonproductive behavior
5. Develop organization and problem-solving abilities for functional activities
6. Improve ability areas and to learn alternative methods of compensation as necessary and appropriate
7. Develop independence in self-care, activities of daily living, and homemaking skills
8. Improve skills for community re-entry and educational or vocational placement

In working with the brain-injured person in specific treatment programs, the therapist uses confidentiality, empathy, stability, consistency, and continuity. Planning, structuring, repetition, and reinforcement are essential. The therapist emphasizes ability and integration by reassuring the patient and by assisting him or her to understand, work with, and accept the condition.

Following evaluation of the specific assets and deficits, assessment of levels of mental and physical endurance, and determination of communication methods to be used, the therapist plans a graded program according to the patient's daily abilities and fluctuations. The patient participates in the planning of this program and is informed of progress.

Environmental Control

Performance may be hindered by general limitations in adjusting to environmental stimuli. Controlling such strong stimuli as the bright light of the sun, loud or sudden noises, or the distracting sounds of people talking is useful. For maximum selective response to the therapist, the patient may initially require an area void of visual and auditory stimuli. As tolerance for stimuli increases, the therapist gives meaning and relevance to gradually increased stimuli and assists the patient in focusing attention while in the presence of distracting sights and sounds.

Social awareness, visual tolerance, concentration, and cognitive functioning and adaptation are stimulated by participating in group discussions and activities, listening to the radio, watching television,

Environment—The patient may exhibit intolerance or incomprehension of the meaning of stimuli. The noise and movements of others may be distracting or fear-producing. If the patient suffers from blurred or double vision, he or she may have low visual tolerance, increased by visual perceptual problems which give inaccurate information regarding objects and relationships in the environment.

Orientation—Basic orientation to objects and properties may be hindered by (1) difficulty in recognition of an object when position or relationship is changed, (2) lack of understanding of relationships between or among tasks, (3) lack of awareness of a picture, concept, or task, (4) difficulty in sequencing of steps to complete a task.

Deficits in orientation to place and time may accompany lack of insight into the present medical condition and resulting situation. Responding to time and space appropriately requires maintenance of a mental representation of material, leading to visual organization and memory.

Cognition—Cognition is knowledge and understanding of the environment gained through the information processing capability of the brain. It involves the mechanisms of perception, memory storage and retrieval of information, organization, and language expression. Cognitive behavior is related to the character and effect of interpersonal relationships. Difficulty in handling input of stimuli (reception, interpretation, organization, order of importance) can hinder ability to store necessary information in the brain for retrieval, resulting in poor concentration for intellectual processing or a deficit in long-term memory.

Language deficits may be evident due to lowered comprehension and thought organization. Personality changes, loss of inhibitions, distortions of judgment, and lack of abstract reasoning combine with memory loss to hinder cognitive function, problem-solving, and learning ability.

Memory—Intellectual changes are manifested in decreased memory, inability to abstract quickly, and lowered attention span. A variety of signs of memory dysfunction may be exhibited, such as (1) shallowness of thought, (2) disorganization or fragmentation of thought, (3) limitation to concrete rather than abstract thinking, (4) difficulty in retrieving information, (5) confabulation, (6) tendency to forget in the middle of a thought, (7) confusion of past and recent events, (8) loss of past and future, with a tendency to live in the moment with general unfamiliarity as to identification and purpose. Memory may show specific decrease in digit span, auditory and visual retention, awareness of routine and current events, retention of previously learned information, and recollection of personal past events and history. The difficulty in following written or verbal instructions may be accompanied by distraction by visual and auditory stimuli affecting accuracy and thoroughness in intellectual functions and resulting in low activity tolerance.

Speech—Dysarthria or disturbances in motor control in language articulation may be present.

Communication—Disturbance in reception or expression of written and spoken language may occur, resulting in speaking, reading, and writing deficits.

Behavior—Clinical response may be characterized by bewilderment, confusion, denial, anger, complacency, or hostility, with fluctuating changes in behavior related to the individual stage of self-awareness and level of adaptation to self and environment. Short-term or chronic personality changes may be experienced, beginning with denial and vagueness in response or with hyperactivity, depending on the level of consciousness and severity of injury to brain tissue. Disturbance in the ability to relate to the environment outside of himself and to time outside of the present may be apparent. Expressed desires and needs may relate to self-concerns and comforts.

Social—The patient may have difficulty in adapting to people and things and may deny reality, forcing others to relate to him or her. Disturbance in self-awareness may allow fantasizing, regarding both condition and behavior, and feelings of unfairness regarding the condition may be expressed. Striving for stability and control, the patient may react poorly to change and time, showing a tendency toward minimal social initiative, occasionally showing suspicion of other people attempting to help. Disorder in judgment may contribute to an emphasis on physical problems rather than on psychological difficulties relating to cognition and behavior.

Physical—The patient may be initially defensive tactually, hypersensitive, apraxic, and/or may demonstrate lack of coordination caused by tremor or ataxia. Spasticity may develop later in the recuperation period. Evaluation of reflex patterns revealing abnormal tone in the brain-injured patient shows three major patterns: (1) decerebrate rigidity or extensor pattern of all extremities, (2) decorticate rigidity flexor pattern in the arms, (3) a mixed pattern of upper extremity flexion and lower extremity extension. Increased muscle tone produces trunk rigidity, which may result in poor sitting balance. Lack of control of trunk muscles may also result in poor sitting patterns. The patient may be sensitive to touch and may lack volitional movement.

playing electronic games, reading books, and reading the newspaper. Gradual increase of responsibility in social and productive activities helps to increase familiarity and function in the environment. In the rehabilitation process, it is important for the patient to be able to adapt to the distractions of the unfamiliar environments in the community in order to be socially adjusted and independent.

Self-Awareness and Behavior

Self-awareness develops through active involvement of the mind and body. Task-oriented individual and group projects can provide opportunities to develop and practice abilities and to reintegrate the positive and negative aspects of functioning. Group projects can extend participation in and responsibility to social activities by demonstrating productivity and skill. Group discussions provide social feedback as to acceptable and non-acceptable behaviors and provide opportunities to change behavior as necessary or desired.

The use of videotaping during activity gives the patient a visual picture of his or her physical and social behavior, which can be viewed privately, critically, and objectively. In viewing the group, the patient is able to distinguish between himself or herself and others and to engage in cognitive development. Working within the group helps the patient to practice social skills useful in developing and maintaining successful contacts with family members, friends, and strangers.

Emotional Adaptations

Working through the stages of denial, anger, and depression to self-awareness and acceptance requires physical and emotional endurance, and often results in fatigue or decreased motivation for continuing the struggle. When the patient is able and ready to begin to deal with the realities of the situation, discussions with the therapist about the injury help to reassure the patient and may clarify what has happened, put present and future goals and concerns into perspective, promote self-understanding, and help the patient adjust to changes. As adjustment occurs, the patient is able to take on more responsibility in decision-making by planning and implementing daily schedules and evaluating progress.

Communication

In using language to communicate with the patient and to stimulate functional response, it is essential that the occupational therapist follow the guidance of the speech pathologist in order to maintain consistency in the aspects and levels of the patient's language development.

Finding a means of response is the initial task of the occupational therapist. Use of physical demonstration followed by imitation by the patient may provide a means of communication for the patient with severe language deficits. Although unable to respond verbally, the patient may be able to read and write words or symbols.

Mental Tolerance

The level of mental tolerance is related to motivation, functional deficits, and amount of adaptation required to carry out instructions. The patient may display a short attention span, distractibility, and fear of insanity, particularly when blindness, disorientation, amnesia, or a combination of physical, psychological, and intellectual manifestations are present.

Techniques to increase mental tolerance include relating a task to an interest area (sports, reading, cooking, or puzzles), using repetition in the task to provide practice of specific skills to reinforce methods of performance, and providing feedback regarding ability. The program should be graded to gradually increase skill and challenge and should use time blocks to increase physical and mental tolerance. Through the therapeutic group experience the patient gains a broader social reality focus, learns coping skills for working with others, and practices assertiveness training for self-confidence.

Memory Development

Memory deficits may prevent the patient from remembering or recognizing people or events from day to day; therefore, continual repetition of tasks and symbols might be necessary until memory is extended. Establishing routines of activity and expecting the patient to perform in consistent patterns may be useful, as may behavior modification techniques.

Memory is needed for mental visualization and learning. In working with a memory deficit, attention is given to determining the number of steps in a task a patient is able to store and retrieve. Exercises can be devised to test and practice memory for past events, types of things remembered, retention time, and carry-over to future planning. Planning and scheduling practice are increased by individual and group exercises in visualization of current events, future events, and carry-over from the day with application to future planning.

Organization of time is improved by the patient's taking responsibility for scheduling daily activities, accepting responsibilities with time limits, achieving carry-over of activities, and reinforcing time and space concepts.

Electronic Devices

The patient who is unable to engage in normal verbal communication is often denied satisfying social interaction and opportunities for personal, educational, and social development. Selection of appropriate equipment for functional communication is preceeded by an evaluation of other equipment being used, cognitive level of function, and optimum body positioning.

Electronic and battery-operated communication aids can assist in evaluation of deficits as well as in retraining programs to develop skills to apply to educational, vocational, and avocational pursuits. These aids are equipped with computer mechanisms providing feedback through a visual or auditory signal, indicating physical and cognitive functional abilities and levels. Devices can be activated by a variety of sources (head turning, mouthstick, light touch, breath control, muscle contractions, and pointing). Use of communication aids by the occupational therapist reinforces the efforts of the speech pathologist in developing physical and cognitive skills and in providing consistency of newly learned techniques. Head sets are useful in minimizing auditory distractions during retraining.

The occupational therapist provides input to the rehabilitation team regarding physical range of motion, strength, coordination, and endurance needed to activate the equipment, as well as with regard to the patient's ability to scan visual input effectively for use of the device. Strip printers or a typewriter may be included to provide additional feedback. With the development of computer systems, electronic aids are increasingly available and adaptable to the disabled person in treatment, at home, or at work. The use of electronic games assists both the child and the adult in adaptation of these systems for practical purposes.

A variety of communication aids is available which can be mounted on a wheelchair or on a desk table and can be powered by rechargeable batteries for practical use. Specific information is available in equipment catalogues. Some are listed in the resource section at the end of this chapter.

Physical/Functional

Before functional activity programs focusing on the upper extremities can be carried out effectively, the patient must be able to achieve and maintain a functional sitting position and balance without using the arms for support. Special equipment may be necessary to achieve this, including aids for position and control. Neurophysiological therapy techniques assist the patient in regaining head control, trunk rota-tion, equilibrium, trunk extension, trunk balance, and arm relaxation for independent isolated control and function. Participation in individual and group physical activities assists the patient in adapting to and overcoming the effects of dizziness. Activities that necessitate changing body position in space (woodworking, gardening, shuffleboard, and ping pong) help in vestibular adaptation.

Specific physical activities provide increased self-awareness and self-worth through the increase in joint range of motion, strength, and coordination. The programs must be correlated with other functional areas such as perception, social interaction, behavior, and tolerance of environmental stimuli. In preparing for discharge, the patient needs to know what he or she can and cannot do with safety and competence. The patient develops and practices physical functions in a compatible, supportive environment, encouraged to learn adaptation when necessary. Decreasing such symptoms as spasticity, contracture, apraxia, tremor, and pain is part of the physical restoration program used to increase functional abilities.

Behavior

The patient may represent a totally new person to his or her family. The therapist learns about the patient *as the person he or she has become* and is challenged to help the family to understand and to accept the person he or she now is. The family helps the therapist to learn what type of person the patient was premorbidly to understand the amount and type of change both the family and the patient are experiencing post-trauma.

The patient may demonstrate loss of inhibitions, distortions in judgment, personality changes, and denial of reality. He or she may lack awareness of the meaning of the present situation. Since the patient may be unable to differentiate between appropriate and nonappropriate social behavior, he or she may benefit from techniques such as behavior modification, group process, reality orientation, and other psychodynamic methods of social adjustment and self-awareness.

Since a patient commonly uses denial to prevent seeing the reality of an imposed traumatic situation, involvement in activity programs not only helps to increase strength, joint range of motion, coordination, and cognitive function, but also provides feedback to the patient regarding his or her actual abilities. Focus is on the *increase of ability*. Activities are chosen to provide the patient the means through which to express feelings of anger and hostility, as well as to assist in the development of speed, accuracy, and competence in productive accomplishment of specific tasks.

Resocialization and Community Re-entry

While in a treatment setting, the patient learns how to live in a controlled and structured environment. In preparation for discharge, the patient must learn how to adapt to other environments as well as how to exercise control over his or her goals and behaviors.

The patient may maintain the delusion that going home will improve the condition or, conversely, that he or she is unwanted or unneeded at home. Family awareness of residual conditions and needs at discharge from the formal rehabilitation program is encouraged in predischarge orientation and guidance sessions. By attending predischarge therapy and group sessions with the patient and the therapists, the family members can see how they can assist with the program and how to welcome the patient back into family life. Sharing in group sessions with other families is helpful to both the family and the patient.

Family orientation to specific problems (memory deficits, tolerance of external stimuli, physical or communications problems) is important before the patient begins resocialization with weekend visits at home. These visits often serve to show the family and the patient both what has been accomplished and how much work remains to be done.

Outpatient follow-up provides physical and psychological support during the transition from hospital or rehabilitation center to family and community re-entry. Through this type of program the patient can continue a therapy program outside of the structured setting. This may help in adjusting to less structured surroundings and aid in developing confidence to plan daily activities and responsibilities. Independent attitudes and functions begin in the treatment setting where, as self-care skills are developed, the patient progresses to being responsible for scheduling time and organizing activities. The patient chooses clothes and retrieves them from drawers and closets, and takes care of grooming and other needs preparatory for daily activities. Independence in the structured treatment setting prepares the person for discharge planning.

Outings from the treatment center or from home help the patient to assume socially appropriate behavior regarding activities and interaction with others. Such activities may include those available through adult programs or church groups. Community activities include such familiar tasks as crossing streets, using money, finding restrooms, reading menus, ordering food, buying things in a store, and paying bills. Trials in doing these things help the patient to communicate and use patience with others.

Other commonly needed skills, including using a pay phone and telephone book, reading a map, listening to and following directions, organizing appointments, applying for a job, and using a newspaper, can be practiced during individual and group outings.

The patient's educational and employment goals depend upon overcoming of intellectual and judgmental deficits as well as developing integrative abilities. Learning, retraining, work adjustment, development of social skills and work habits may be necessary for vocational readiness.

Employment

The level of pretrauma intellectual functioning and achieved educational level help in regaining vocational potential. In regaining the ability to return to work successfully, the brain-injured person is more likely to be hindered by cognitive, behavior, and social difficulties in performance than by physical deficits. Regaining a positive self-image, independence in self-care, physical and mental tolerance, successful social contact and interaction, capability in cognitive and intellectual functioning, and acceptable work habits all contribute to vocational potential for the well-motivated person.

During functional retraining the patient with vocational potential is provided with opportunities to work on familiar skills and those needed for his or her job. Levels of cognitive, social, behavioral, and physical function are determined through prevocational assessment techniques to evaluate the need for retraining or vocational redirection.

Return to work may begin on a part-time basis at first. Retraining and relocating may be necessary to ensure employment of the patient able to work in some capacity but unable to return to a previous occupation at the earlier level of performance. Although premature return to work requiring strenuous physical or mental effort is strongly discouraged, too long a rest from the routine of work may be detrimental to the person capable of employment.

Multiple Sclerosis

Multiple sclerosis (MS), or disseminated sclerosis, is a progressive disease of the nervous system. It begins with the destruction or dissemination of the myelin sheath covering the nerve fibers, which interferes with the transmission of the impulse and results in fatigue. The degenerated sheath is replaced by the eventual formation of multiple sclerotic plaques or patches which affect the white matter of the brain and spinal cord. These plaques may also be found in the gray matter of the cerebral cortex and in the cranial and spinal cord roots.[12]

Characterized by intermittant exacerbations and remissions, the disease may pursue its unpredictable course for many years. It usually affects young adults (ages twenty to forty) during their period of greatest potential and productivity. Although the cause of the disease is unknown, influenza, respiratory infections, pregnancy, surgery, and trauma may be precipitating factors. Change in climate, fatigue from overwork, and poor dietary habits have also been implicated as possible factors. Nervous tension and irritability may precede the onset of physical symptoms, which may vary in intensity, character, duration, and location.

The clinical picture may be hemiplegia, paraplegia, or quadriplegia, and the patient's prognosis and life span are variable. While the average life span of a person with MS may be 20 years, it can vary from 3 months to 40 years; some remissions can last as long as 25 years.[13] There may be long and almost complete remissions in the early stages of the disease. However, after middle age, the course of the disease often progresses.

Symptoms appear in two general modes. The first is characterized by a single lesion or several isolated lesions which result in neuritis, double vision, weakness in a limb, or numbness in a part of the body. The second is insidious and is manifested in a slowly progressive weakness of one or all limbs. Accompanying spinal symptoms include spastic paraplegia, superficial sensory loss in the lower limbs and trunk, impairment of postural sensibility and sense of vibration, and spastic/ataxic gait.[14] Decreased sexuality, loss of self-esteem, and anxiety may be evident.

Common early signs of MS include nystagmus (lateral oscillation of an eye to one or both sides), slight intention tremor in one or both upper limbs, and exaggeration of tendon reflexes. These initial symptoms may disappear over a period of weeks or months, leaving only slight residual physical signs; however, the cumulative effects of multiple lesions later cause permanent changes in personality.[15]

Symptoms of the advanced case of MS include scanning or staccato speech and slurring of syllables, nystagmus, dissociation of conjugate lateral movement of the eyes, weak and grossly ataxic upper limbs, paraplegia, contractures, sensory loss, incontinence, episodes of euphoria, depression, irritability, impairment of postural sensibility, and astereognosis.

Although muscular wasting or atrophy are rare, motor weakness may appear in the extremities, trunk, and face. The patient may experience a feeling of heaviness in the spastic extremities and may lose postural sensibility in limbs and trunk.

Incoordination is a frequent problem for the patient with MS. Intention tremor on involuntary movement is accompanied by muscle imbalance in hands and arms, and the tremor may develop in head movements during the later stages of the disease. When the patient must perform tasks requiring accurate movement, the tremor may increase, resulting in incoordination. Ataxia is evident in the gross movements of both the upper and the lower extremities.

The patient suffers sensory deficits manifested by numbness, impairment of positional and joint sense, fine tactile discrimination, hypersensitivity to contact, postural sensibility and vibration sense, and astereognosis.

The ability to communicate verbally may be hindered by dysarthria caused by spastic weakness or ataxia in muscles of articulation. In some instances the speech impairment may become so severe as to render the patient unintelligible.

In some cases the patient with MS may display only ocular symptoms for many years. Although the patient's vision usually improves within a few weeks of the initial onset of symptoms, residual damage to the optic nerve is manifested in optic atrophy. Sporadic unilateral blindness or diplopia may occur.

The patient may exhibit some reduction in intellectual efficiency and some emotional changes; he or she may suffer wildly contrasting moods, going from euphoria to depression very quickly. Conceptual thinking, memory, attention span, and judgment may be affected. These fluctuations in mental and physical ability are characteristic of the patient with MS and must be considered during evaluation and treatment. The patient is a victim of gradual and intermittent loss of physical and mental control, resulting in emotional reactions and irritability.

Occupational Therapy

During the course of evaluation and treatment, the therapist provides encouragement and support regarding the patient's fluctuating capabilities. Because the patient is prone to anxiety and tension, the occupational therapist emphasizes maintenance of functional abilities and stresses avoidance of becoming chilled or fatigued and of avoidance of situations where injury may occur. The patient may feel good at the start of the day. Energy diminishes in the afternoon, resulting in taking chances that may result in an accident. Decreased sensation, incoordination, transient blindness, and judgment impairment can create life-threatening conditions for the patient with MS.

Evaluation

Evaluation areas include the following:
1. Assessment of physical abilities of the extremities: evaluation of strength, joint range of motion, coordination, and balance
2. Determination of intention tremor: ataxia, paresthesia, sensory function
3. Visual acuity and perception
4. Level of self-care independence
5. Level of functional independence and tolerance
6. Psychological and intellectual functions
7. Behavior characteristics, emotional stability, and adjustment to disabilities

Treatment

General treatment goals include the following:
1. Maintenance of passive and active joint range of motion
2. Prevention of spasticity, contractures, deformities, and decubiti
3. Optimum functional independence
4. Maximum coordination, strength, and function of extremities
5. Understanding and acceptance of the nature and course of the disease
6. Ability to reach maximum functional level of activity
7. Awareness of and use of assistive devices as needed generally and for self-care

Treatment consists in providing the patient with exercises and activities that present graded resistance to weak muscles, prevent substitution patterns from developing, and employ repetition to encourage physical endurance. The occupational therapist must pay close attention to the fatigue factor because the patient may not recognize or admit fatigue.

The patient should be encouraged to engage in exercises and activities that employ all extremities, but he or she may become discouraged with hand activities if sensation and coordination are poor and if intention tremor is prevalent. If the patient has the muscle power and endurance, activities should be performed from both a seated and a standing position.

The patient may need assistive devices and reeducation in ADL; he or she should be encouraged to participate in social functions to maintain the ability to relate to family and friends.

In all activities the patient must be assisted in adjustment to the *progression* of the disability. The patient may deny the gradually worsening condition and become euphoric in an attempt to hide the lack of acceptance and to ward off depression. Euphoria may prevent acceptance of assistive devices and may cause establishment of unrealistic goals. The occupational therapist can aid in the establishment of realistic long-term and short-term goals, maintenance of self-care, and avoidance of anxiety.

Setting a daily schedule of activity that provides rest and productivity within the capability and endurance of the person with MS is essential to maintaining the optimum functional level. Activities, including self-care, homemaking, family responsibilities, education, prevocational exploration, and avocational involvement, can be explored in the treatment program. Education of patient and family can assist all family members in adjustment to fluctuating abilities and acceptance of adaptation for productive and satisfying living. Community agencies such as the Multiple Sclerosis Society provide helpful resources and general support.

Parkinson's Disease

Parkinson's disease is a slowly progressive condition caused by the degeneration of neurons in the *substantia nigra* and *globus pallidus* resulting in damage to the basal ganglia of the brain. This chronic condition may be precipitated by carbon monoxide and manganese poisoning, encephalitis, senile brain changes, and arteriosclerosis. Occurring between the ages of 40 and 80 years, Parkinson's disease causes the gradual loss of physical abilities, resulting in interference with lifestyle, change in appearance and behavior, loss of employment, and depression.

Disturbance in motor function is characterized by slowing of emotional responses and voluntary movement, muscular rigidity and weakness, slowly spreading tumor, and a shuffling gait. Symptoms may appear over a period varying from months to years, with stationary periods of nonprogressive symptoms. The symptom complex may be variable in specific types of Parkinsonism.

Gradually, the person assumes a physical attitude of immobility, with mask-like facial expressions, staring eyes, and loss of free movements of the limbs and rotary movements of the spine. Arms and trunk tend toward flexion, with adduction at the shoulders. Loss of tenodesis action in the distal joints produces a tendency toward stiff wrist extension, finger flexion at the metacarpophalangeal joints and extension at the phalangeal joints. Development of fibrous tissue in the joints causes contractures, with resultant atrophy of muscle due to decreased voluntary movement.

Movements are characteristically slow, demonstrating difficulty in initiating movement, weakness in voluntary movements, and loss of associated movements. Intrinsic movements are awkward and incoordinated, resulting in loss of manual dexterity. General reduction of joint range of motion affects oral articulation, causing slurring of speech, decreased volume, and monotone sound. There is a tendency to drool. Chest excursion may be limited due to muscular rigidity, thus decreasing vital capacity.

Involuntary movements of the extremities are generally described as a jerky, "cogwheel" tremor or a smooth, "leadpipe" rigidity. These common manifestations may be unequal on both sides of the body. Tremor is characterized by rhythmic, alternating movement of the opposing muscle groups simulating a "pill-rolling" motion of the thumb and fingers at the metacarpophalangeal joints. The tremor may shift from one muscle group to another. It is usually present when the patient is at rest and diminishes when he or she voluntarily moves the limb; the tremor increases with emotional excitement, although it can be inhibited temporarily by conscious effort. As the disease progresses, rigidity becomes more pronounced, with resultant limitations in joint range of motion due to contractures and muscle atrophy. The rigidity can cause muscular pain, but does not result in sensory loss.

The typical gait is easily recognized: slow, with shuffling, small steps and a tendency toward lurching. The person shows a flexed or bent position, and the rigid, decreased mobility gives the appearance of the body's moving *en masse*, propelled by momentum and unable to stop quickly. Balance is poor. The patient is described as having a "festinating gait," hurrying with small steps in a bent attitude as if trying to catch up to his center of gravity.[16]

Evaluation

The evaluation begins with complete assessment of the manifestations of the symptoms described in the clinical picture. Degree of involvement is noted, as is the impact upon functional activities. The following areas are included:

1. Passive joint range of motion; presence of contractures
2. Active joint range of motion; characteristics of movement
3. Presence and characteristics of tremor and rigidity
4. Sitting and standing balance, tolerance, and characteristics
5. Presence of pain or other discomfort

6. Functional abilities; self-care, ADL, communication, coordination, strength, reach, grasp
7. Employment status and potential
8. Emotional status
9. Avocational interests and abilities
10. Home situation, lifestyle, social interests, and responsibilities

Treatment

Goals of treatment for the patient with Parkinson's disease are directed toward assisting him or her to achieve a positive attitude toward his or her abilities and toward accepting the gradual decrease in ability. In order to maintain the maximal functional level and to prevent rigidity, it is essential to involve the patient in a daily pattern of continual activity to maintain complete active joint range of motion, strength, and productivity. The course of formalized treatment should be related to a home program so that the patient can continue to do activities which are meaningful. This helps to prevent the patient from becoming immobile owing to depression caused by loss of abilities and skills. The treatment program is developed by both the patient and the therapist to achieve maximum use of movement and to maintain activity tolerance:

1. Maintain maximum independence in functional activities to prevent limitations from rigidity or tremor.
2. Maintain complete reciprocal joint range of motion; prevent contractures.
3. Encourage therapeutic breathing patterns and chest expansion; integrate the breathing patterns with daily activities.
4. Encourage increase of speed and coordination in movement.
5. Encourage independence in self-care; provide adaptive techniques or assistive devices.
6. Develop activity tolerance and increase endurance.
7. Increase activity interests to maintain social, physical, and functional mobility.
8. Provide therapeutic group program for social participation and adaptation.
9. Educate the patient and family regarding the necessity for a home program of good physical habits, exercise, and activity to maintain mobility and motivation.
10. Provide a home program of self-care, homemaking, productive activity, recreation, and community involvement for continued mobility.

Treatment includes graded resistive exercises to increase strength and coordination, gross motor activities to encourage general mobility and to increase chest excursion, fine patterns of movement for maintenance of productive abilities, maximum independence in self-care and ADL, and encouragement of motivation, self-esteem, and socialization.

Because the gradual development of rigidity and immobility are characteristic of Parkinson's disease, auditory stimulation such as music can be used to encourage body mobility through rhythmic marching, dancing, clapping, and singing, either individually or in groups. Participation in groups also provides needed support and encouragement to maintain mobility in spite of continuing symptoms.

Sports can be used for motivation, socialization, and movement; ball-throwing, ping pong, darts, and shuffleboard also increase strength and speed of movement in all extremities. In gross motor activities, balance, coordination, and breathing patterns are emphasized.

Manual activities can be used to maintain gross and fine coordination, strength, and concentration, since these are required for general self-care functions. Activities should be designed so as to encourage good posture, increase mobility, and stimulate successful accomplishment. Manual activities can also be related to assessing and developing vocational skills to enable the patients to keep their jobs. Although patients may experience a change in job activities or responsibilities, it is essential to maintain their daily work status as long as possible.

Broadening of social contact and activity interests helps to provide stimulation in continuing mobility and productivity programs at home. Patient and family education aids in assuring the continuation of these activities. In order to assist the family and the patient in planning daily activity programs, the therapist can guide them to the resources of the National Parkinson Foundation, which is a valuable organization for the consumer, providing helpful information on the disease, on exercise, and on activities to maintain mobility.

Spinal Cord Injury

Injury to the spinal cord results in temporary or permanent paralysis of the muscles of the limbs and the autonomic nervous system, usually manifested *below* the level of the lesion. Symptoms of a temporary nature are caused by compression of the cord without transection or puncture. Permanent paralysis is caused by fractures and dislocations that puncture or transect the spinal cord.

Spinal cord injury is caused by gunshot wounds, stab wounds, falls, automobile accidents, and sports accidents. The most common of these is the automobile accident, when forced flexion and hyperextension of the trunk results in fracture and dislocation of the vertebrae, causing trauma to the spinal cord. Initial symptoms are (1) spinal shock, (2) loss of sensation, (3) flaccid paralysis of the affected extremities, (4) incontinence of bowel and bladder, and (5) decreased reflex activity below the level of the lesion, followed by an increase in reflex activity. In many cases, secondary injury results from improper immediate handling of the injured person at the scene of the accident and during transportation to the treatment facility.

The initial program for the person with spinal cord injury is crucial to his or her total well-being, and the beginning of the rehabilitation process, which may require adjustment to a lifelong disability. It is a gradual, arduous, and sometimes painful progression from total dependence to the maximum level of independence; from the shock of functional loss to the acceptance of achievable abilities. Communication, planning, and coordination among team members are essential to ensure optimum rehabilitation outcomes, medically and functionally, of the spinal cord injured person.

Both the acute care setting and the rehabilitation center provide medical care, carry out rehabilitation measures to prepare the injured person for future life involvement, provide therapy directed toward achievement of maximum levels of bodily movement and function, and implement psychological preparation for self-motivation for daily activity and goal setting. Rehabilitation is the preparation for making and reaching achievable satisfactory goals for the future. The initial rehabilitation period is a mere beginning to the new life the person will lead as a quadriplegic or paraplegic upon re-entry into community living.

In the early care it is essential to prevent the patient from becoming either overly discouraged or overly hopeful. In discussing the medical condition with the patient, doctors may advocate informing the patient, immediately and clearly, of the chances of walking and of the degree of permanent paralysis to expect, in order to avoid false hope by the patient, and family and to facilitate the rehabilitative process. In other cases, the doctor may initially inform the patient that he or she will recover full functions or provide ambiguous answers to questions regarding functional loss, in order to avoid psychological trauma. In the early stages of hospitalization, the patient tends to deny the extent of the injury. At this stage, denial serves as a valuable protective mechanism to avoid seeing the realities that must be faced eventually. In most cases, denial actually helps the patient through the devastating effects of the initial trauma and the long-term implications of disability.

Temporary or permanent implications to the injured person include the following sudden interruption of continuity of the chosen lifestyle; severe loss of familiar bodily sensation, awareness, and volitional functions; loss of bowel, bladder, and sexual controls, physical independence, psychological stability, social effectiveness, sexuality, financial security, educational goals, vocational skills and plans, avocational interests, personal expectations, and hopes of future content and planning.

Common problems which may occur periodically during rehabilitation are denial, anger, hostility, boredom, depression, lack of motivation, dependency, urinary tract infection, decubiti, weakness, atrophy, spasticity, and contractures.

Level of Lesion

Survival, disability, treatment, and function of the spinal cord injured person depend on the level and extent of the lesion. The condition referred to as *quadriplegia* occurs from injury in the cervical and possibly high thoracic areas of the cord and results in sensory deficits and muscular deficiencies of the upper extremities, trunk, and lower extremities. *Paraplegia* occurs from injury to the thoracic and lumbar cord areas and results in sensory deficits and muscular paralysis of the trunk and lower extremities. The terms *quadriplegia* and *paraplegia* refer to paralysis of the limbs, while *quadriparesis* and *paraparesis* refer to weakness of the limbs.

The level of segmental innervation determines the effect of the trauma incurred (Fig. 22-4). The extent of the injury determines the functional outcome.[17] Muscles innervated by segments at and below the level of injury are affected. The sensory and autonomic systems may be involved; functional loss may be asymmetrical, depending on the location of the lesion. Although a functional estimate and expectation can be approximated given the level of the injury, other factors may retard or change the expected rehabilitation prognosis. Among these factors are respiratory complications, head trauma, other accompanying injuries, sensory loss, decubiti, damage to the vertebral column, urinary tract infections, spasm, and lack of motivation for recovery.

General Treatment Considerations

The goals of rehabilitation for the patient with spinal cord injury, regardless of level of lesion, include the following:
1. Attaining the maximum level of self-care
2. Recognizing and developing physical and intellectual capabilities

3. Resuming satisfying relationships with family and friends, and resuming social activities
4. Resuming education and employment activities and plans
5. Understanding the condition and accepting responsibility for continuing the rehabilitation process
6. Learning and following a therapeutic home program
7. Learning and using available community resources
8. Making realistic plans for the future

Planning begins in the acute care facility with protection of the flaccid extremities for future functioning, establishment of short-term and long-term goals, and gradual conditioning to enable the patient to tolerate an upright position. Establishment of maximum use of the upper extremities to perform self-care and productive activities aids the patient in acceptance of permanent paralysis and in preparation for functional wheelchair living. (See Table 22-3) The therapist helps the patient to develop physical and intellectual resources with which to combat the challenges of functional living and social interaction.

Involvement with his or her own plan helps the patient learn to take responsibility in the future and enables the patient to develop an independent attitude toward his or her abilities. This begins during acute care hospitalization, continues during early rehabilitation, and progresses further if treatment continues at a specialized rehabilitation facility.

Positioning

Exercises and activities can be done in almost any position if both the patient and the equipment are properly situated. In preparation for productive activity, the patient should be positioned for optimum biomechanical advantage in function.

Figure 22-4. Segmental innervation of specified ▶ muscles in the cervical spinal cord from C4 through T1. There is commonly a range of innervation from two or three spinal segments, and there is a variation in people as to segmental innervation. In traumatic spinal cord injury, those muscles are affected that are innervated *below* the lesion site. Bilateral symmetry of paralysis depends on the exact location of the lesion and its severity. For example, a transection caused by a fracture dislocation of a vertebra may cause an oblique lesion or an incomplete lesion. Inflammation and swelling can contribute to a higher initial deficit.

C₄	C₅	C₆	C₇	C₈	T₁

Diaphragm, Phrenic Nerve

Trapezius, Spinal accessory nerve

Levator Scapuli

Supraspinatus

Teres Minor

Deltoid

Subscapularis

Infraspinatus

Rhomboids

Brachialis

Brachioradialis

Biceps

Pectoralis Major, Clavicle

Supinator

Teres Major

Extensor Carpi Radialis Longus and Brevis

Serratus Anterior

Pronator Teres

Pectoralis Major, Sternal

Latissimus Dorsi

Triceps

Flexor Carpi Radialis

Palmaris Longus

Abductor Pollicus Longus

Extensor Pollicus Longus

Extensor Digitorum

Extensor Carpi Ulnaris

Flexor Digitorum Superficialis

Flexor Digitorum Profundus

Flexor Pollicus Longus

Abductor Pollicus Brevis

Flexor Carpi Ulnaris

Abductor Pollicus

Lumbricales

Opponens Pollicis

Interossei

KEY: ▯—Reported Range   ▯ Most common innervation, most important segments

Table 22-3 Functional implications of cervical cord lesions. This information represents an average range of capability. Variations can be expected owing to individual spinal innervation and other factors.

Level of cervical lesion	Remaining musculature	Active mobility	Functional loss	Functional implications	Occupational therapy implications
C₄	Sternocleidomastoid Upper trapezius	Neck movements Shoulder elevation	Respiratory endurance Upper extremity functions Trunk sensation and control Lower extremity sensation and control General endurance General independent mobility	Total dependency in self-care Dependency on external devices for upper extremity movement and productive activity Confined to wheelchair Can propel electric wheelchair	Requires assistance in communication skills: tape recorder, electric type-writer (using hand typing sticks, headstick, mouthpiece, electronic communication board), electric page turner for reading, talking books (records) Uses external powered (electric or CO_2) functional hand splints and arm supports for upper extremity activity in the wheelchair Can engage in light recreational and avocational activities for ROM, strength, interest, and motivation
C₅	Sternocleidomastoid Trapezius Rhomboids Partial rotator cuff Partial deltoids Partial biceps	Neck movements Shoulder elevation Scapular rotation, adduction Partial elbow flexion Weak or no sensory function	Ability to change from supine to prone position in bed Ability to achieve sitting position in bed Independent trunk control and sensation Lower extremity sensation and control Wrist and hand functions	Use of externally powered devices for arm and hand functions Assistive devices for self-feeding Dependency in self-care and transfers Can propel electric wheelchair	Devices described above may be necessary Dynamic tenodesis splints for writing, grasping, and other hand functions Mobile arm support, balanced forearm orthosis, or suspension slings for general upper extremity support and mobility Special equipment or devices for telephone, TV operation, eating, drinking Recreational and avocational activities for ROM, strength, interest, motivation

Level	Muscles	Movements/Functions	Weakness	Functional Capabilities	Goals/Assistive Devices
C_6	All muscles of C_4 and C_5 level Partial serratus anterior Partial pectoralis Partial latissimus dorsi Deltoid Biceps Partial extensor carpi radialis	All movements of C_4 and C_5 Scapular adduction, flexion, extension Weak trunk control Shoulder flexion Elbow flexion Wrist extension (tenodesis function for grasp) Weak sensory function in hand	Weakness in trunk control, affecting balance Lower extremity functions Weakness in grasp, release, and prehension	Can achieve sitting position in bed by using trapeze bar (above bed) or rope attached to foot of bed Can assist in wheelchair transfer Can propel regular wheelchair Can use assistive devices for self-care Fairly mobile arm control Weak tenodesis function	Dynamic tenodesis splints for hand functions Assistive devices for independence in self-care: razor holders, utensil holders, pencil holders, extended handles for reaching, dressing loops for pants, sliding board for transfers, devices for toilet needs (catheter and leg bag, suppository management) Friction adaptations to wheelrims or knobs for pushing wheelchair using thenar eminence of hand Typing sticks Push-ups in wheelchair for arm strengthening and prevention of decubiti Independent living skills Driving with hand controls and wheel knobs Vocational goals
C_7	All muscles of C_4, C_5, C_6 level Finger flexors Finger extensors	All movements of C_4, C_5, C_6 Moderate trunk control Functional grasp and release Sensory function of hand	Weakness in trunk control Weakness in intrinsic muscles of the hand and isolated finger functions Limited dexterity and general hand strength	Independent bed and wheelchair mobility Independent bed/wheelchair transfers Strong arm control Has grasp functions and coordination without splints Nonfunctional ambulation for standing and short distances	Assistive devices for toilet activities and lower extremity dressing Upper extremity activities for physical restoration without splinting Can drive with hand controls and do car transfer Independence in daily living and community involvement Vocational and avocational goals

BED. Upper extremity activities can be assisted by the use of an inclined lapboard in the supine and sitting positions with suspension slings attached to traction frames for early arm support.

To avoid the natural tendency of the flaccid extremities to yield to the pull of gravity, they are properly positioned in normal alignment using sandbags, pillows, or footboards to prevent the stretching of unused or weak muscles and the development of contractures of spastic muscles, which would limit future function of the limbs. Undue pressure on flaccid limbs from bed clothes is avoided, and the limbs should be visible to monitor positioning. Prism glasses enable the patient to see his or her extremities and to request repositioning if necessary.

PRONE POSITION ON A CIRCO-ELECTRIC BED. When the patient is prone (face down) on the Circo-electric bed, he or she can use gravity for shoulder flexion and elbow extension. A table is necessary to provide support in elbow flexion if the patient lacks lower arm functions. For the quadriplegic in a prone position, independent eating should be encouraged, using slings, a palmar cuff, a nonskid mat, and positioning the tray under the bed. Plates that have plateguards allow the patient to pick up the food independently.

WHEELCHAIR POSITION. Good position is necessary. The patient is generally seated on a cutout seatboard with a gel, water, or air cushion for hip positioning and prevention of decubiti. The chair should initially have an extended back, adjustable arm, and foot support. A lapboard, suspension slings, or a balanced forearm orthosis can be attached to the wheelchair for the quadriplegic.

STANDING TABLE. This device is used by the patient wearing braces to aid in trunk strengthening and balance, standing tolerance, and upright positioning. Activities done at the standing table may also be accomplished by some patients with sufficient balance by using a belt support to stand at a work table.

SKIN PROTECTION. Protection of the skin and prevention of contractures are essential for the patient with spinal cord injury. Because sensation is lost below the level of lesion, the patient is unable to detect pressure from external objects and is unable to change position easily, because of muscle paralysis. Thus, position changes must be made initially by nurses or attendants. The skin is susceptible to injury from the shearing force of sheets, pressure from footboards used for positioning, and the gravitational effect of the immobile limbs on the mattress. Decubitus ulcers

(pressure sores) develop from local anemia caused by this pressure and appear over bony prominences. Even though air mattresses and water mattresses are used, and routine position changes are followed, decubitus ulcers can still occur.

To avoid pressure sores, the therapist instructs the patient in the importance of turning in bed or shifting weight when seated in the wheelchair. As a patient becomes more mobile, instruction is given on how to check all vulnerable areas of the body, using a long-handled mirror to check the back, buttocks, arms, and lower extremities.

Self-care

The daily accomplishment of self-care and other independent or assisted activities provides the patient with maintenance of joint range of motion, strength, and both physical and psychological endurance. The abilities and progress in these areas should be discussed with the family during the entire hospitalization and rehabilitation process so that they will encourage as much independence as possible.

The person with paraplegia is generally able to regain independent self-care activities and virtually all aspects of daily living. Depending on the level of lesion and manifestations, complications, and motivation for independent function, the person with quadriplegia is challenged with use of electronic assistive equipment, hand splints, and motorized or specially equipped wheelchair to deal with disability in all four extremities.

Assistive Equipment

Use of adaptive equipment may be required for substitution of motion, compensation for decreased trunk balance, assistance for reduced reach and grasp, and for limitation in locomotion. Assistive devices may be needed to perform the self-care activities of personal hygiene, grooming, eating, and dressing. Although assistive equipment may increase functional independence, it may decrease desired sensory and motor function. Some patients refuse all assistive equipment; others want everything, even some that is not needed.

In most cases, the wheelchair becomes a way of life for the spinal cord injured person. Therefore it must be prescribed for individual comfort, safety, maneuverability, and independence. A poorly fitted wheelchair can contribute to deformity, muscle disuse, decubiti, and decreased motivation for function and socialization. The wheelchair needs of the paraplegic and quadriplegic patients are different.

The wheelchair should be ordered as soon as possible in the rehabilitation program to encourage the patient's early association with wheelchair living.

Avocational

Activities that are provided for restoration of specific upper extremity function can become outlets for avocational needs and interests. As the spinal cord injured person works through adjustment to wheelchair living, avocational outlets are needed for venting feelings as well as for providing a sense of accomplishment. As new patterns of movement and skill develop, the patient can apply these to pursuing leisure activity at school or in the community. Many spinal cord injured people have benefitted greatly from participation in organized sports such as basketball, swimming, ping pong, and weightlifting. Competition contributes to resocialization, achievement, and increased sense of self-worth and confidence.

Educational

Vocational goals and discharge plans may include returning to school for the adolescent or young adult with a spinal cord injury. Therapists evaluate the campus for architectural accessibility by the wheelchair to buildings, classrooms, bathrooms, cafeterias, and other areas. A system for carrying books, obtaining optimum work surfaces and heights, and note-taking may be needed by the quadriplegic student. Full involvement of the wheelchair-mobile person in all aspects of the educational environment is essential to acceptance by peers.

Driving

One of the most common social problems facing the wheelchair user is the lack of adequate public transportation. Therefore it is essential that the paraplegic person become independent in using hand controls for driving, car transfers, and placing the wheelchair into the car.

Many quadriplegic individuals can drive with hand controls and a steering knob, although they may need assistance getting in and out of the car, and most need help in getting the wheelchair into the car. For these individuals, a van with a wheelchair lift is recommended for easy access to and from the van. The person may need to transfer from the wheelchair to the driver's seat or passenger's seat once in the van or the van may be equipped with clamps to secure the wheelchair in a position to allow the individual to drive. Predriving evaluation and training programs are available to guide the person in using safe techniques in purchasing an appropriate vehicle and in driving.

Prevocational

The employment potential of the spinal cord injured person is not necessarily correlated with the injury and its residual manifestations. A person with a debilitating injury is able to return to work if he or she is motivated, possesses employable knowledge and skills, is offered reassurance from family and friends, and is able to find a job.

Although the patient may have to change former vocational goals, the occupational therapy program provides the opportunity to learn potential functional levels and to explore feasible vocational areas of interest. Prevocational evaluation determines the employable skills that the person has, can develop, or requires for vocational planning and preparation for appropriate vocational training.

Discharge Planning

The patient and family are included in the rehabilitation program as soon after hospital admission as possible and are fully informed of all of the stages of the rehabilitation process the patient will go through. The process begun in the hospital continues at home, in the rehabilitation facility, and in the community for as long as is necessary. The individual maintains a relationship with the rehabilitation team to achieve planned goals upon discharge through out-patient programs and follow-up.

During hospitalization, the rehabilitation team may encourage the patient to go home on weekends to begin to face the adjustments that will have to be made after discharge and to use skills acquired in the treatment facility in the home environment. These visits alert the family to the patient's capabilities, progress, and general program. It is from these visits that the patient, family, and therapist can work together on home planning and architectural renovations.

The Paraplegic Patient

Evaluation

Evaluation of the paraplegic patient in the initial post-trauma stage may be at the bedside if the patient is immobilized in traction and special equipment or has significant accompanying injuries. In evaluating the paraplegic, the therapist looks for variations in functional ability, which depend on the level of lesion. Although the paraplegic may be initially immobilized, he or she demonstrates full functional use of the upper extremities in active range of motion, sensation, and hand use. While in bed and during the wheelchair phase, the patient will become accustomed to depending on arms and trunk for mobility and function to provide leg positioning.

Specific areas of evaluation during the bed phase include the following:

1. Determine current status, rehabilitation goals, and treatment being provided.
2. Determine medical restrictions of movement as noted in the chart with regard to the status of the spinal cord injury and other accompanying injuries.
3. Note the body position of the patient for proper alignment of the paralyzed trunk and lower extremities.
4. Evaluate the passive and active range of motion and strength of the upper extremities (which should be normal, but may be weak).
5. If not medically restricted, evaluate trunk and lower extremities' movement, noting areas of spasticity, weakness, paralysis, sensory loss, substitution, compensation.
6. Assess need for and ability to use self-care devices to perform daily activities.
7. Interview patient with regard to accident, medical condition and impact, lifestyle, goals, and expectations.
8. Encourage patient to discuss premorbid achievement, avocational and vocational interests and plans.

Treatment

Bed Phase

While confined to bed, the paraplegic patient benefits from an upper extremity activity program to provide strengthening exercise of the arms and hands, to provide initial self-care assistance, to learn body image and self-awareness, to learn the extent of current functions, to provide a sense of self-worth through accomplishment of achievable tasks on a routine daily basis. The longer the patient remains away from productive activity, the more difficult is his or her adjustment to the benefits of the rehabilitative process. The following activities and adaptations are suggested to encourage a positive attitude toward maintenance of restoration of productive abilities:

1. Inclined bed-table, lapboard, and prism glasses for ease in performing upper extremity activity in bed
2. Devices with extended handles for reaching and self-care; long-handled sponge for bathing; reacher for picking up items in proximity
3. Increasing involvement in daily self-care program

4. Low exertion, upper extremity activities for active exercise of the arms while supine; reading, book games, manual activities
5. Activities that offer resistance in hand and arm functions to increase strength and to decrease mental frustration from inactivity; theraplast, leatherwork, making models, copper tooling, macrame, loom weaving and woodcarving.

Self-care for the Mobile Bed Patient and Wheelchair User

Barring the complications of decubiti and excessive spasticity, the paraplegic person is able to learn to be essentially independent in self-care. The high-level paraplegic may have some problems with lower extremity dressing because of trunk instability and loss of muscle strength for balance; however, various assistive devices can help in overcoming these problems.

Self-care activity increases self-awareness, responsibility, and self-esteem. When the restrictions of mobility are removed, the paraplegic patient can begin self-care activities, such as bathing in bed or in the wheelchair using a long-handled sponge to help in reaching the feet.

At this time, if the patient is able to turn in bed and to reach a sitting position, upper extremity dressing can be done in bed as tolerance to the sitting position increases. When the patient can sit for longer periods, lower extremity dressing in bed may be begun. For this, a long-handled reacher may be needed.

Some adjustment time may be required for the patient to regain a sense of balance and body use when first moving from the bed into a wheelchair. When this is accomplished, all bathing and grooming can be done before a mirror and upper extremity dressing can be done in a wheelchair. It is crucial to the rehabilitation of the paraplegic that he or she be encouraged to assume these responsibilities as functional ability is regained. Self-care activities not only provide independent functions but also provide important daily exercise in balance, strength, and coordination. Since fatigue may be experienced in the early accomplishment of these tasks, the treatment program must be coordinated with all other therapies. All rehabilitation team members are informed of the patient's level of accomplishment, so that efforts are coordinated toward the achievement of maximum independence.

Since functioning from a wheelchair will, in most cases, become a way of life for the paraplegic, it is essential that the chair be equipped to meet all physical, personal, and functional needs. The wheelchair should be heavy-duty, but light-weight for ease of lifting in and out of a car; should be as narrow as possible for easy passage through doorways and maneuvering in bathrooms; should have swing-away removable footrests for transfer and proximity to cabinets and work areas; and should have removable desk arms at a comfortable height for arm positioning, transfer, and proximity to tables and counters. A seatboard with a special cushion to prevent decubiti is sometimes used to maintain good positioning of trunk and hips. The foot pedals should clear two inches from the ground for safe travel over bumps and rough ground, the depth of the seat should extend to two inches proximal to the knee bend and the back height should extend no farther than three inches below the axilla to allow free movement of the arms but to provide needed trunk support. Pneumatic tires are often recommended for ease and safety over rough ground and for a comfortable ride. However, because these tires need to be checked for sufficient air pressure and do go flat occasionally, they are contraindicated when the patient is unable to attend to these functions or does not have access to someone who can help. Hard rubber tires may be more practical in this case. In most cases, the paraplegic person will be able to propel a wheelchair both inside and outside on smooth ground with ease, less easily on rough ground.

Assistive Devices

The paraplegic individual needs fewer assistive devices than does the quadriplegic person for independent living. He or she generally uses a seatboard and special cushion for the wheelchair, a transfer board, a long-handled reacher for dressing or retrieving objects from high places or the floor, and wheelchair accessories (drink holder, ashtray, and carrying bag).

Transfers

The patient who is able to transfer with or without a sliding board can practice this skill in occupational therapy by transferring to a regular chair. The chair should have both a firm back and a firm seat. Working from a regular chair increases trunk and upper extremity strength and mobility.

Activities and Skills

In the social and activity-oriented climate of occupational therapy, the paraplegic is able to use his or her arms fully in bilateral strengthening activities, increasing upper extremity coordination, balance, and physical tolerance for performing all productive activity from a wheelchair. Challenges of using cabinets, shelves, electrical outlets, standing electric machinery, and heavy hand tools help in developing skill and self-value in accomplishment. Group activities with peers and other patients (games, projects, discussions, planning) aid in self-awareness, social skills, and responsibility. Construction of assistive equipment such as seat boards, tub boards for transfer, and sliding boards aid in acceptance of their use by the patient and may provide opportunities to gain skills to benefit others as well. (See Fig. 22-5.)

In many cases the paraplegic patient will want to have the opportunity to learn to use braces and crutches to walk; however, the braces are heavy and walking requires much strength. Because of the cost in energy, the patient often resorts to the wheelchair for ease of travel; this occurs after a trial time that may last for months or years.

Life in a wheelchair, however, requires that all activities be done in a sitting position. The patient will be dependent on his arms for mobility, vocation, and avocations. (See Fig. 22-6.) The resourceful paraplegic individual can do virtually anything from a wheelchair—except climb steps, pass through narrow doorways, or reach appliances and counters that are too high.

The occupational therapy program consists of developing upper extremity productivity, which will lead to prevocational and vocational planning. Skills begun in occupational therapy during hospitalization can greatly assist the paraplegic person in accepting limitations and using abilities for developing employable skills and healthy attitudes.

With training the paraplegic person can function independently in self-care from bed and wheelchair, can perform household activities from a wheelchair, can transfer to and from the wheelchair, drive with hand controls, and perform vocational skills. Major problems will be those caused by architectural barriers outside of and within buildings, problems which impair mobility and make job-seeking extremely difficult.

The Quadriplegic Patient

Initial treatment of the person with quadriplegia (paralysis in upper and lower extremities) is immobilization of the vertebral column by skeletal traction, using head tongs or neck bracing. Traction is generally applied for a period of six weeks, following which immobilization is continued with a neck support for two to four months.[18]

The patient's position while in traction is interchangeable (supine and prone) in a completely extended position for optimal protection of the spinal cord and musculature. The injured person may be placed on a Stryker frame bed which rotates horizontally for position change to prone or supine or on a Circo-electric bed, which can be turned from the

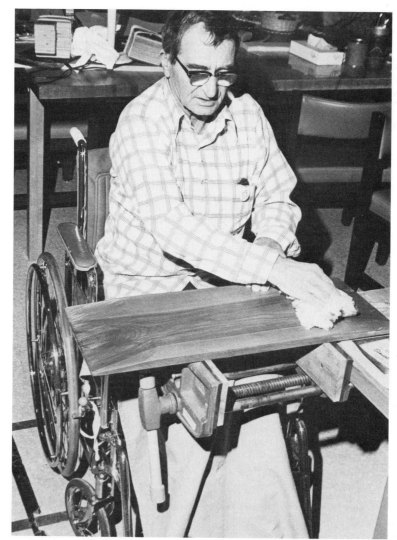

Figure 22-5. Assistive equipment. A paraplegic patient works on his transfer board for upper extremity strengthening and adjustment to wheelchair living.

horizontal to the vertical position on a 180° axis, and stabilized at any angle, allowing placement in supine or prone position. These special beds are used to aid in the essential frequent change in body position for skin and limb protection from decubiti. Change of position is made every two hours. The tilt-table is also used to assist in moving the patient passively from the horizontal to the vertical position. If the patient is not gradually acclimated to changes in space during the initial immobilization, he or she tends to become dizzy when assuming the sitting position following weeks spent in traction.

Early treatment of the quadriplegic patient in the acute stage of trauma consists of turning, massage for circulation and sensory stimulation, and passive range of motion to maintain freedom of joint movement and to prevent muscular contractures and de-

cubiti. Following the traction period, general conditioning exercises are provided, including proper breathing and training in rolling from side to side. Self-care is begun as soon as possible to relieve anxieties regarding nonsensitive and non-moving body parts and to prevent dependency on others for any functions the patient is able to accomplish.

Evaluation

Treatment programs for the quadriplegic patient depend on whether he or she is in the bed phase or the wheelchair phase of rehabilitation.

Bed Phase

During the bed phase, the following steps are recommended for evaluation:

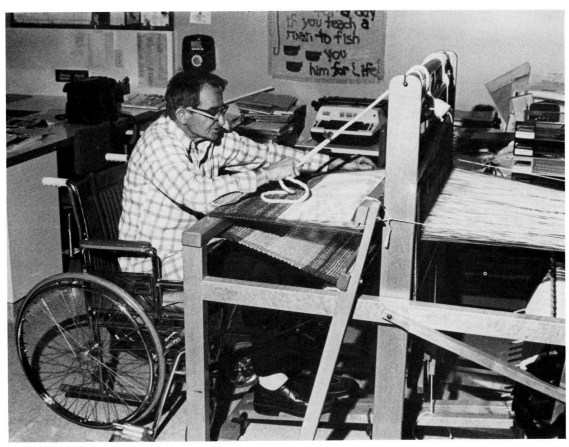

Figure 22-6. Ropes are attached to harnesses on the floor loom to enable the paraplegic individual to change the shed with his arms instead of his paralyzed legs. The addition of weights to the beater and the harnesses provides resistance for arm and trunk strengthening.

1. Review the chart for medical status, treatment prescribed, and bed position restrictions owing to injury to the spinal cord and other areas.
2. Establish non-threatening rapport with the patient on the initial visit, showing empathy and respect. Interview the patient about what happened, the medical situation, treatment plans, and schedule, asking for a description of concerns and priorities.
3. Evaluate active and passive joint range of motion, strength, sensation, coordination, general mobility, and function of extremities and trunk.
4. Evaluate present bed position for alignment of extremities and trunk for prevention of muscle stretching, shortening, and deformity, and for the patient's awareness of position requirements.
5. Examine extremities for reddened areas, which indicate pressure.
6. Determine the functional aspects of upper extremity sensation by requesting the patient to identify the location of and describe sensory stimuli, and identify the location of the extremity during passive positioning.
7. Determine passive and active joint range of motion, identifying restrictions caused by trauma, pain, weakness, spasticity, contractures, or hypersensitivity.
8. Determine the need for hand splints to maintain body alignment for future function to prevent deformity and for sensory awareness and stimulation.
9. Assess the need for arm support to extend the functional positioning of the hands for use; assess the need for arm exercises in a supine position.
10. Talk with the patient about interests, abilities, past achievement, and primary concerns regarding the condition and its implications in his or her personal life.
11. Inform the patient of the results of the evaluation, and discuss his or her personal goals; make treatment plans with the patient for short-term and long-term goals.

Wheelchair Phase

When the patient has progressed to sitting in a wheelchair, guidelines are determined for treatment planning. During all evaluation procedures, assist the patient in movements when necessary. Do not allow fatigue or discouragement. Emphasize what *can* be done and encourage the patient to accomplish it. Be explicit in instructions and demonstrate when necessary. Terminate the evaluation before the patient becomes fatigued and try to end with accomplishment. Talk with the patient regarding his or her interests so that the treatment program can include activities that are related to these interests and aid the patient in setting realistic long-term and short-term goals. The following evaluation areas are examined:

1. Joint range of motion: Move the joints through complete passive range of motion, one at a time, being careful not to cause pain in sensitive joints, particularly in the shoulders and elbows. Give support to the flaccid or weak limbs by holding them carefully during range of motion, always informing the patient of what is to be done. Measure the joint range with the goniometer. Check for spasticity and deformity in the upper extremities.

2. Muscle strength: Provide gravitational assist if necessary to determine how much gravity the patient can resist. Give gentle resistance to joint movement to determine gross muscle strength and presence of spasticity. Use scale gauge to measure gross joint strength against resistance and pinch gauge dynamometer for grip.

3. Sensation: Note the presence of pain in passive movement. Occlude the patient's vision; touch the skin lightly with your finger and determine if the patient responds to the stimulus. Progress from distal to proximal areas. To evaluate two-point discrimination, sharp touch, and localization of stimuli, touch the skin with a sharp object, such as a sharpened dowel stick or a two-point pressure gauge. Determine first whether the patient responds to the stimulus, can localize the stimulus, and can distinguish if there was one or two stimuli. Place an object between the patient's thumb and fingers, move it around in the palmar area, and then ask for recognition of the object by its size, shape, and texture to determine stereognostic function.

4. Position sense (proprioception): Move the body part to be tested gently in reciprocal movements and then ask the patient to identify the position of the limb when stopped. He or she may feel the movement but may be unable to identify the position without seeing it.

5. Patterns of movement: Provide the patient with a reaching or grasping task to perform, for instance, picking up a 2″ × 2″ foam block, reaching to the shoulder, or reaching for an object held in the air. Observe the pattern of movement to determine functioning muscles and presence of spasticity. Observe any substitution patterns the patient may use to the detriment of other muscles which should be strengthened.

6. Functional activities: Determine actual gross grasp, prehension, coordination, strength, and tenodesis function. Determine the ability to perform functional activities, such as picking up an object and placing it, reaching for an object, using two hands, writing, pushing and pulling objects, and turning the pages of a book. Use objects of varied weights, sizes, and textures. Present tasks within the patient's functional ability as determined by joint range of motion, muscle power, sensation, position sense, and patterns of movement already observed and evaluated. Do not ask a patient to do impossible tasks.

7. Determine the trunk control for free movement of the upper extremities in isolated asymmetrical use and use in ADL functions.

8. Evaluate the need for assistive devices or splints for restorative exercises and activities in addition to those needed for positioning and self-care activities.

9. Evaluate self-care and all activities of daily living including self-feeding, grooming, toileting, bathing, dressing, writing, clerical skills, and homemaking skills. The physical plan of the home must also be evaluated.

10. Prevocational evaluation: Evaluate functions for job skills and employment potential when the patient has mastered upper extremity functional activities and ADL within his or her limits.

Treatment

Bed Phase

During all treatment in this phase, the patient should be encouraged to use *all* possible active movement to increase physical endurance, strength, and functional ability. By doing this, the patient becomes involved in his or her program and assumes some responsibility for the rehabilitation process. The therapist provides activities in which the patient is interested and psychological support throughout the treatment regime. The therapist coordinates occupational therapy with nursing and physical therapy personnel and other members of the rehabilitation team in order to aid the patient in gaining maximum function while suffering minimal fatigue and frustration.

Treatment considerations during the bed stage are as follows:

1. Monitor *bed positioning* daily for prevention of decubiti and contractures.
2. Gently *massage* and stimulate sensory receptors of the upper extremities for sensory awareness and tactual localization.
3. Move the upper extremities in gentle, full, *passive range of motion* daily in order to closely monitor changes in range, informing the patient when the extremity is moved, in which direction, and how many times. Encourage the patient to watch the extremity during massage and passive joint range of motion.
4. Preceed active range of motion by gentle *manual resistance* to joints and muscle groups in the hands and arms for sensory stimulation and motor facilitation.

5. Attach *suspension slings* to the traction bar above the bed. These slings serve to support the arms as well as to stimulate available, active movements of the shoulders and elbows. Slings can be modified with springs to facilitate movement and to provide sensory feedback. The use of weights encourages increased muscle power (Fig. 22-7).

Use elbow and wrist straps to support arms for maximum active movement and hand functions; use a palmar cuff with a pocket for insertion of a spoon or a pencil, enabling the patient to use the arms and hands in productive activity.

Facilitate motion of all joints of the upper extremities by using gravitational assist to suspension slings, such as the balanced forearm orthosis adaptations, weights, or a bedtable.

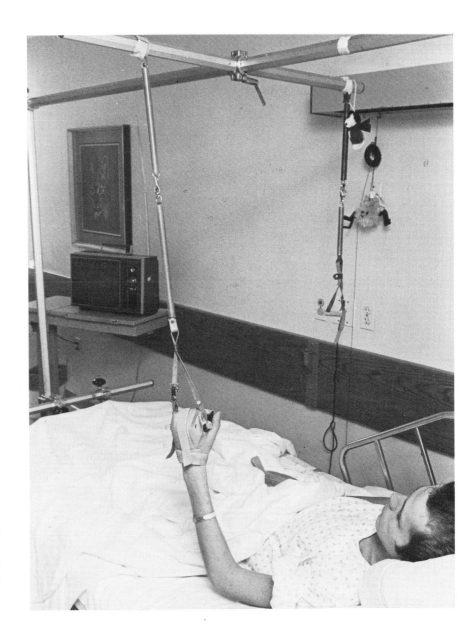

Figure 22-7. Overhead bed traction frame is used for attachment of a spring suspension sling and positioning mitt to facilitate upper arm active exercise against resistance. A pulley system can also be attached to vary and to increase resistance.

6. Use assistive devices to facilitate and support movement; among these devices are a common bath mitt, a universal palmar cuff device to hold a fork for eating, a plate guard to aid in arm control while eating, and arm slings or positioners. These devices encourage exercise through active arm movement, increase body awareness, encourage self-esteem by providing independent function, and decrease dependency.

7. Provide *splinting* to prevent tightening of muscles and deformity. Restriction may be necessary to prevent elbow flexion, wrist flexion, finger flexion, and ankle flexion. It is essential to correlate the use of splints with manual therapeutic techniques. Provide initial static hand splinting progressing to dynamic splinting to stimulate tenodesis function as appropriate. Splinting stimulates sensory awareness and assists in channeling the muscles for function.

8. Set up an electric page turner on the bed-table so that the patient can operate it with palm contact (Fig. 22-8) or with movement of the chin or shoulder if he or she lacks lower arm function.

9. Provide prism glasses to prevent the patient from developing eyestrain while viewing television, reading, seeing and talking with visitors, or watching his or her limbs as the therapist moves them when in a supine position (Fig. 22-9).

During the bed stage, the patient is encouraged to adjust to the vertical position for sitting by using the tilt-table. This adjustment should be accomplished gradually. When cerebral spatial adjustment and physical tolerance increase to a sufficiently functional level, the patient progresses to the semi-reclining wheelchair and then to the fully upright position for continued adaptation to wheelchair mobility, sitting balance, and the use of the upper extremities.

Wheelchair Phase

Wheelchair selection for the quadriplegic is crucial to daily health and function. A variety of chairs, controls, and accessories are available to meet the varied needs of individual capabilities, interests, and lifestyles. For the quadriplegic patient with a high cervi-

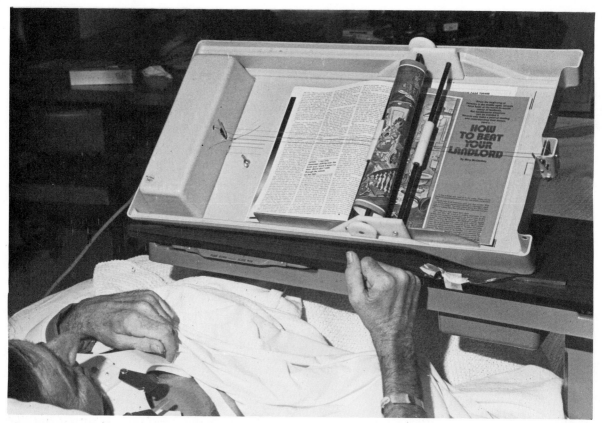

Figure 22-8. Patient with traumatic quadriplegia operates an electric page turner using palm contact with a microswitch attached to the bed table beneath the right corner of the machine. The page turner is inclined for increased ease in visibility from the patient's semisupine position in bed.

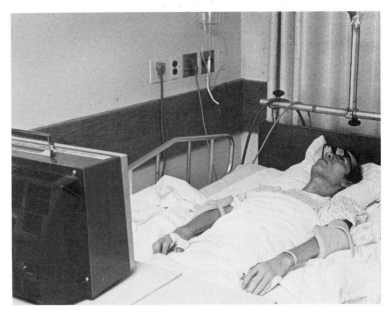

Figure 22-9. Prism glasses prevent eyestrain while viewing television for the quadriplegic patient lying in a supine position in bed. Foam cuff protectors are used to prevent skin breakdown from gravitational pressure of the mattress on the bony prominences of the elbows. Static handsplints provide passive thumb positioning to maintain adductor stretch for position of opposition. Arms are positioned in elbow and wrist extension to prevent flexion contractures.

cal lesion and with severely limited or nonfunctional reach and hand placement, electronic arm or head controls may be necessary. Electronic wheelchair and environmental control systems (Fig. 22-10) enable the severely disabled person to have independent wheelchair mobility and an element of independent function from the wheelchair. With such systems, the disabled person can control appliances such as an electric bed, a call signal, telephone or intercom, television, thermostat, or doors.

Quadriplegics with lower cervical lesion levels benefit from operating electric controls on wheelchairs or by using special accessories on standard, non-electric wheelchairs. For each of maneuvering, the quadriplegic person may require knobs or plastic friction sheaths on the wheel rims for easier propulsion or a motorized chair with touch controls. The back should be higher than that of the paraplegic's chair, since the quadriplegic has loss of trunk control and needs extra support. A brake extension may be necessary for independence in locking brakes. Heel loops and leg rests are needed for foot and leg positioning, and a safety belt may be needed for balance. Although a wheelchair with a reclining back may be used in early treatment to compensate for the quadriplegic's tendency to become dizzy, it is not recommended during later periods. It can increase dependency on the reclined position, which limits upper extremity function.

Adaptations to Activities

When the patient is confined to bed or to the reclining wheelchair, it is often difficult to set up activities that the patient will be able to see and reach. Both the position and the lack of upper extremity mobility place limitations on activity. However, the following are examples of adaptations which can be provided for the quadriplegic patient.

In the bed position the following adaptations are possible:
1. Use the bedtable to position activities (books or visual puzzles) that can be performed by using prism glasses.
2. A table lapboard with a bottom edge can be placed over the patient's chest; this can be inclined and stabilized (using projecting legs) to hold reading materials and other items.
3. Commercial bookholders are useful.
4. Suspension slings can be attached to the traction frames on the bed.
5. Slings, mirrors, and activities can be attached to the Circo-electric bed frame.
6. Activities can be placed on a chair or low table for the patient who is prone on the Circo-electric bed. Feeding trays can also be placed on a chair.

The following adaptations provide for wheelchair activities:
1. An inclined treatment table aids the patient during early treatment when still in a reclining wheelchair.
2. Vises and clamps are used to position and stabilize activities.
3. A lapboard on the wheelchair aids arm positioning and provides an accessible work surface.
4. Controls normally operated by the feet (for instance, a sewing machine control) can be extended and placed on the table so that they can be manipulated by the arms.

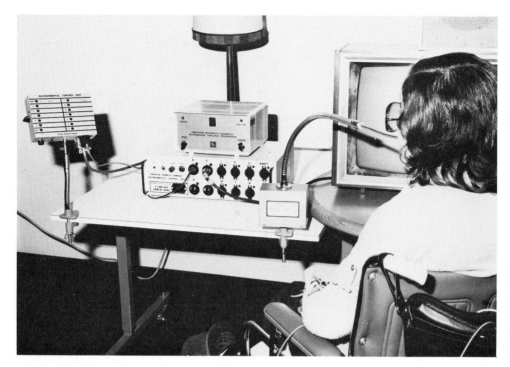

Figure 22-10. Quadriplegic using a mouth-operated environmental control system to activate lamp and television switches independently.

Self-care

Although the quadriplegic patient may have little range of motion and muscle strength with which to accomplish self-care tasks, it is essential for him or her to use available power to accomplish parts of tasks. Limitations in reach, grasp, strength, joint range of motion, respiration, and physical endurance are common. Assistive and substitutive techniques of adaptive body positioning, use of reflexes, and assistance from an attendant help in developing skills.

Long handles to extend reach, palmar cuffs to substitute for hand grip, spring clips to provide sustained grip, loops on clothing, special devices for grooming, soap on a rope, bath mitt, and adapted equipment for grooming and make-up are readily available and often make the difference between ability and handicap. Often, the most limiting factor can be the patient's refusal to participate.

Functional Restoration

All activities should increase upper extremity joint range of motion, strength, physical tolerance, grasp, and psychological adaptation. These activities should include the use of assistive equipment to increase the patient's capacity to function independently and result in the realization of maximum capacities.

Specially designed tables adjusted to the height of the wheelchair, angled for easy access to work surfaces, or on a rotating base (Fig. 22-11) assist the pa-

tient in optimum mechanical advantage for task accomplishment.

Manipulation of pegs and of other objects of varying sizes, weights, and textures improves the grasp, reach, and ability to place objects. These can be presented in the form of peg games (HiQ, checkers or chess) to elicit the patient's interest. The activity teaches isolated arm and hand functions and provides the patient with experience in using assistive equipment.

Constructive activities such as woodworking can be adapted to provide joint range of motion and strengthening of the upper arms and trunk muscles. If the patient has poor grasp, a palmar cuff, bilateral handles, or holding mitts can be used with tools for such tasks as sanding, sawing, planing, or drilling.

Diversional activities are provided for the pure fun of engaging in a game with another person, while at the same time they assist the patient in gaining functional use of the upper extremities. These activities, such as checkers, chess, or Scrabble, can be done in bed or in a wheelchair. Arm support may be needed, as may hand splints, but the patient is able to engage in competitive activity and receive the rewards from it.

Suggestions for adapted activities for the spinal cord injured person, with modifications according to lesion level, include the following:

1. Use of table-based power tools such as small jigsaw, drill press, or printing press, which can have extended handles for easy reach and control

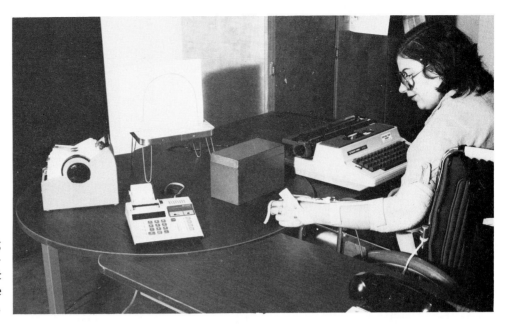

Figure 22-11. A revolving table surface gives easy access to clerical equipment and supplies for effective organization of a work area.

2. Use of handpower equipment, secured if necessary to substitute for the patient's lack of control
3. Vertical and adjustable angled chalkboards for gross arm and writing exercises
4. Use of ropes attached to loom harnesses to enable the patient to change the shed by using the arms, if the lower extremities are paralyzed
5. Special handles on the loom beater to provide supination or pronation exercises
6. Use of a pulley and weight system attached to the loom beater for strengthening upper extremities by providing resistance
7. Use of recreational activities for gross arm exercise: ball throwing, shuffleboard, shooting pool
8. Use of manual activities for sustained upper arm strengthening and light resistive hand use: painting, knitting, hooking
9. Use of activities for sensory stimulus and light resistive hand use: gardening at adapted planters at wheelchair level, forming and painting ceramics
10. Use of homemaking activities: cooking, cleaning, ironing

All activities offer possibilities for adaptation. Some of the activities mentioned are helpful to the paraplegic patient as well as to the quadriplegic patient, because they provide a means to increase strength, endurance, and balance for the trunk and upper extremities. The quadriplegic patient needs these functions for wheelchair manipulation and for performance of all activities. The paraplegic patient needs upper arm strengthening for wheelchair maneuvering over long distances, transferring, standing in braces, and walking with crutches. The build-up of maximum upper extremity strength is essential to the paraplegic. Engagement in an upper extremity activity program is crucial to the beginning of productivity from a wheelchair and leads to independence in daily living tasks, increased responsibility, and, eventually, employment. The paraplegic patient should experience all aspects of functioning from a wheelchair before leaving the rehabilitation setting.

Functional Splints

Early use of appropriate splints benefits the quadriplegic patient in providing muscle exercise, mechanical function for purposeful activity and the assurance that the patient is capable of accomplishing tasks.

The quadriplegic patient is provided with a tenodesis or flexor-hinge hand splint when he or she has achieved active dorsiflexion (hyperextension) of the wrist. It is with active motion against resistance that the patient is able to channel movement through the splint into a strong and functional prehension grip (Fig. 22-12; Fig. 22-13). The tenodesis splint uses the natural function of the finger flexor tendons to tighten in wrist hyperextension and to relax in wrist flexion. Although the patient may be able to effect this function voluntarily with sufficient active wrist extension without the splint, grip sufficient for strong grasp and fine prehension may be lacking in thumb-finger prehension. The splint is applied to give power for the functional needs of prehension.

There are various forms of splints available; some are for trial and training, while others are for permanent use. Trial tenodesis splints may be made by the

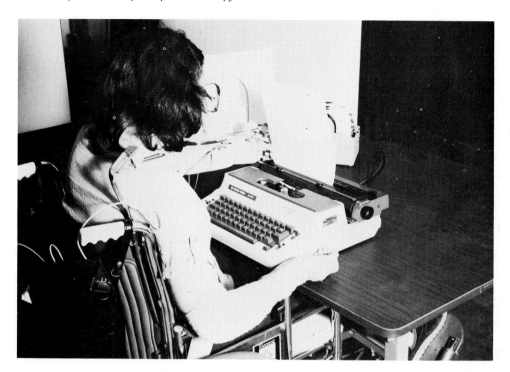

Figure 22-12. Quadriplegic uses a tenodesis splint on her left hand to provide functional prehension to hold and guide paper into her typewriter.

occupational therapist from thermoplastic materials. The patient is taught how to use the splint in active grasping and releasing and in coordination activities. The flexor-hinge hand splint is made by the occupational therapist or the orthotist for permanent use and is usually made of metal or high temperature plastic. The patient may continue to use the splints if they aid in daily activities, or eventually may discard them as muscle power and substitute functions are gained.

If the patient does not have active wrist extension against gravity and resistance, other types of hand-wrist tenodesis splints may be needed to provide the function of grasp. These may be electronically or carbon dioxide (CO_2) controlled to effect an independent grasp. The use of these devices depends on the motivation of the patient, as they require tolerance to noise and the pressure of harnesses and special rigging as well as the acceptance of complicated assistive equipment to substitute for natural functions.

Environmental Control Systems

The high-level quadriplegic who is unable to move his or her upper extremities for functional activity depends on teaching others how to perform needed physical tasks. In spite of this dependence, the severely disabled patient can find independence in environmental control and self-expression in written communication through the aid of environmental control systems. Such systems enable training and practice in functional written communication skills for use in recreational activities, educational needs, or employment functions. Electronically controlled computer systems with typewriter mechanisms, auditory systems, visual feedback, and custom adaptations can be made for positioning and operation.

Community Re-entry

In the occupational therapy program, opportunities for total independence in self-care, activities of daily living, homemaking skills, manual skills, program planning, and evaluation of functional levels and progress assist the patient in developing abilities for successful community re-entry.

The spinal cord injured person benefits from patient and family education sessions, weekend trials of self-care and social skills, group trips into the community during the formal treatment program, and education regarding community resources available following discharge. The patient is able to participate in sports competition, social activities, conferences, workshops, and other functions designed and sponsored by and for disabled people. Due to increased community efforts to eliminate architectural barriers to disabled persons, wheelchair users are finding that, where individual motivations and efforts are demonstrated, they can successfully re-enter communities in fully functioning capacities despite their physical disabilities. In an accepting society, they are disabled, but they are not handicapped.

In suffering a spinal cord injury, the person immediately becomes involved in an interruption of lifestyle content and plans. The loss may be devastating, or adjustment impossible. In accepting assistive equipment, the patient must accept loss of physical

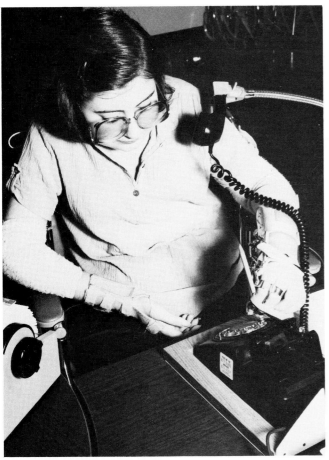

Figure 22-13. Quadriplegic uses tenodesis splint on her left hand to provide sufficient grasp strength to hold pencil used in dialing a telephone. Telephone is held by gooseneck holder attached to the table; it can be positioned easily.

function and use of mechanical substitution. Energy level and motivation determine his or her priorities in the functional use of remaining physical and mental abilities. Whether or not the patient can accept doing part of a task rather than the whole, can accept assistance, and can ask for help when needed are important elements in rehabilitation.

The person who must adjust to permanent spinal cord injury must accept continuing daily personal and social life in a wheelchair. From the onset, he or she begins to make choices which often require compromise:

1. Whether to remain immobile and dependent, or to become mobile and perhaps become partially dependent
2. Whether to use a shiny, metal, electronically operated hand splint to permit handling objects with strength and coordination, or to be dependent on others to pick up objects because he or she lacks hand strength, coordination, and joint range of motion

3. Whether to use limited energy to push the wheelchair independently, or to save energy for other functions and use an electric wheelchair
4. Whether to stay home because many buildings are inaccessible to people using wheelchairs, or to use community resources to determine those that are accessible and to fight to make more of the community barrier-free
5. Whether to make the disability obvious to others by using helpful assistive devices for function, or to remain dependent without independent functions to ensure self-worth through attention-seeking
6. Whether to do part of a task, or to ask someone else to do all of it

These are some of the choices faced by patients in planning for community re-entry. The therapist begins working with patients on adjustment, planning, and practicing new skills, beginning with the evaluation. Early involvement aids patients in learning their capabilities and needs, enabling them to request help and monitor it effectively to strengthen them for the challenges of daily living in the community, where they may find rejection, lack of interest, and lack of help, and where they must be able to use all of their remaining abilities and learned skills to deal with the challenges facing them.

Poliomyelitis

Because of the extensive and effective use of vaccines, poliomyelitis is no longer prevalent in children's hospitals or in adult rehabilitation centers. The occupational therapist occasionally encounters a patient who has had a history of polio which complicates the current admission for treatment. There are times in a prevocational or vocational program when the therapist may need to evaluate the functional ability of the post-polio client.

Polio, a lower motor neuron (LMN) lesion, is an acute infectious disease caused by a virus that affects the anterior horn cells of the gray matter of the spinal cord and the motor nuclei of the brain stem.[19] The result is immediate widespread or localized muscular paralysis with subsequent atrophy. The effect of the paralysis may be asymmetrical and patchy in character, resulting in long-term paralysis in some muscles of one limb and none in others, causing an imbalance. Although the lower limbs are more often affected than the upper limbs, clinical conditions may demonstrate complete or partial monoplegia, hemiplegia, paraplegia, or quadriplegia. Sensation, however, is intact.

Polio results in an immediate and long-term paralysis of muscles, necessitating the eventual use of substitutions for function. In extreme cases the patient may require extensive functional devices and mechanisms for respiration; more commonly the patient may need splints, arm supports, braces, or assistive devices for self-care and other upper extremity functions.

Symptoms include loss of cutaneous and tendon reflexes in the affected muscles, flaccid paralysis of the muscles affected, atrophy, subluxation of adjacent joints, general body weakness, respiratory and circulatory effects, and imbalance of muscle power. Contractures can occur in stronger muscles because of weakness of antagonist muscles. Asymmetrical paralysis of spinal muscles can result in scoliosis. Retarded bone growth can occur in the affected limbs.

Treatment

Early medical treatment begins with immediate and complete bedrest; physical activity increases the risk of further paralysis. Hot packs are provided to relieve muscle pain, and the patient is positioned to protect limbs from contracture and deformity. A tracheotomy may be necessary to provide an airway, and there may be a need for assistance in ventilation for the patient unable to breathe independently because muscles of respiration are weak. Various types of respirators and ventilators are used and might be required throughout the patient's life. During the phase in which the patient is receiving assistance in respiration, a *gentle* program of maintenance of passive and active functions is used.

Massage, passive and active joint range of motion with graded resistance, provision of splinting for prevention of contractures, and functional training follow as the patient regains physical tolerance. Surgical considerations include tendon transfers and arthrodesis to improve function and correct deformities.

The prime precaution in treating the patient with polio is to avoid muscle and body fatigue. Fatigue can result in further weakness and, if the muscles are overworked, loss of function can occur. Aside from this serious problem, it can cause the patient to miss hours of necessary treatment because of the debilitating effects of fatigue in one treatment session. Respiratory and cardiac stress must also be avoided. Signs of labored breathing should be looked for and, if necessary, the treatment should be terminated. The muscle function should be continually evaluated for signs of imbalance.

Treatment sessions should be timed within the span of the physical tolerance in order to avoid general body fatigue. In order to maintain and increase the range of motion, endurance, and coordination, exercises and activities should be progressive and resistive and should be done symmetrically. Preven-

tion of substitution patterns is important in the initial treatment program to encourage strengthening of weak muscles; however, when optimum muscle power has been reached, the patient may have to learn to use substitution patterns to assist in independent functions.

Arm supports and splints can be used both to minimize fatigue and to aid the patient in positioning weak extremities, particularly if there is shoulder girdle involvement. The balanced forearm orthosis (ball bearing feeder) can be used successfully for self-feeding, hygiene, upper extremity dexterity tasks, and other activities. Gravity can be used to assist weak musculature. For the severely involved polio patient, provision of special equipment becomes essential for continuation of upper extremity functions. Devices such as an electric wheelchair, electric page turner, tape recorder, prism glasses, talking books, and special splinting can be helpful. With the proper equipment the severely involved but well-motivated patient can adjust to adaptive functioning for daily activities and employment.

One of the most significant contributions the occupational therapist can make is in providing assistance through adaptive and supportive activities for maximum productivity and social involvement. Because the effect of the disease is permanent, the patient with severe upper extremity involvement must adjust to being assisted by using complicated mechanical and electronic systems to substitute for or assist with arm positioning and hand activities.

Guillain-Barré Syndrome

Guillain-Barré syndrome is an acute distress of the nervous system that involves the spinal nerve roots, peripheral nerves, and, occasionally, the cranial nerves.[20] It is characterized by a hypersensitive response of the peripheral nervous system resulting in polyneuritis or inflammation of the nerves following a viral infection. The disease can affect either sex at any age. The acute phase of this lower motor neuron (LMN) lesion involves rapid onset of paralysis of the limbs with accompanying sensory loss and muscle atrophy.

The initial illness, followed by flaccid paralysis, may affect all four limbs at once or may begin in the legs and spread upward to the arms. It may involve muscles of respiration. Proximal and distal muscles of the limbs are usually affected symmetrically. Reflexes are diminished or lost, sensation is impaired in the extremities and the muscles are tender, but all sensory modalities are not impaired.

The patient with Guillain-Barré syndrome, unlike the patient with polio, has a good prognosis for recovery. Factors affecting recovery are premorbid physical condition, motivation, return of muscle function, and the character of the rehabilitation program.

Prognosis is varied and improvement may be sporadic. Almost complete recovery may be gained within 3 to 6 months or more, or the recovery may be incomplete with slight remissions, serious relapses, or the occurrence of a plateau. The patient may regain independent ambulation but retain some residual weakness and incoordination in all extremities with some atrophy in the intrinsic muscles of the hands. The patient who makes slow progress may develop atrophy which, if unattended, can hinder the effective use of the hands in manipulative tasks. The patient with weakness and incoordination of the legs may require lower extremity braces to substitute for the lack of strong leg muscles.

Rehabilitation Program

The patient with Guillain-Barré syndrome generally benefits from an intensive rehabilitation program. With the initiation of rehabilitation techniques as soon as the medical stability has been reached, activities are introduced to encourage active muscle use in order to prevent atrophy or the wasting of muscles.

A common precaution in the rehabilitation program is the avoidance of fatigue in order to protect future function. Psychological support, practical use of returning musculature in productive activity, and social stimulation are essential for the patients with the disease if they are to become involved in the rehabilitation objectives.

General rehabilitation goals include maintenance of nutrition, prevention of contractures, gradual diminution of the initial rest program, passive and active joint range of motion exercises for affected extremities, activity for muscle strengthening and coordination, restoration of sensation, increase in activity according to the patient's tolerance, splinting to prevent deformity from atrophy and disuse, a self-care program to encourage independent functions, assistive devices to encourage functional use of extremities, and development of work tolerance for pre-vocational preparation.

The occupational therapist designs a program geared to the *gradual* improvement of active functions. Because the patient may be totally paralyzed when first referred to occupational therapy, the first consideration may be to provide splints to maintain the functional position of fingers, thumbs, and wrists to prevent contractures from poor positioning. While on bedrest, the patient can benefit from the stimulation and encouragement of light social activities such as visits from family and friends, watching televi-

sion, and supportive visits from the therapist, who engages the patient in positive conversation regarding his interests, while performing passive range of motion exercises. It is important to maintain free joint motions of the wrist and fingers for grasping activities which use tenodesis function.

Early treatment is similar to that of the spinal cord injured quadriplegic. The therapist must consider maintaining full passive joint range and encouraging active range against gravity. In addition, the therapist provides psychological support and therapeutic social stimulation and encourages the patient to use special devices such as an electric page turner, which can provide the satisfaction of reading independently but requires a minimum of movement to operate.

As the patient improves medically and begins to regain motor power, the occupational therapist provides activities which require increasing ranges of motion, coordination, and strength. The development of strength in specific muscles encourages the strengthening of other muscles.

However, as has been stressed, *care must be taken not to fatigue the patient.* Fatigue can be prevented by the therapist's providing suspension slings or arm supports for positioning and for facilitation of movement for hand functions. As the power begins to return and coordination improves, care should be taken to vary activities between gross and fine, resistive and nonresistive, so that maximum gain can be derived without undue fatigue.

Specific activities of the upper extremities should encourage coordinated movements maintaining good body alignment to minimize the development of substitution patterns. The patient whose recovery is steadily improving needs assistive devices *only* to prevent fatigue and substitution; usually these are not needed permanently. However, the patient whose progress is slower should be encouraged to use assistive equipment to gain strength and function.

From the beginning of treatment, self-care activities can encourage sensory and motor stimulation. Self-feeding and grooming can be started when necessary arm functions begin to return, even if a palmar cuff is used to substitute for grasp. Dressing can be started when physical tolerance increases and the patient has sufficient active joint range of motion.

As the patient regains functions, the program should be upgraded to challenge strength and coordination. The patient should be encouraged to function independently whenever possible and to ask for assistance only when needed. Along with the physical therapist, the occupational therapist monitors the regaining of individual muscle control and checks for muscle atrophy.

Because the prognosis for the return of ambulation and functional upper extremity ability is generally good, the recovering patient is encouraged to participate in an activity program in which abilities for maximum independence can be developed. Recreational activities such as sports serve to improve physical endurance and coordination. (For specific adaptation of activities, assistive devices, and self-care techniques, see the section on spinal cord lesions earlier in this chapter.)

Amyotrophic Lateral Sclerosis

Amyotrophic lateral sclerosis (ALS) is a chronic systemic disease of unknown cause that affects the corticospinal system from the cortex to the periphery. It is characterized by degenerative changes which are most evident in the anterior horn cells of the spinal cord, motor nuclei of the medulla, and corticospinal tracts. The loss of nerve cells causes progressive wasting of the muscles, particularly evident in the upper extremities and in those muscles innervated by the medulla.[21]

The onset of ALS is gradual and steadily progressive, and the disease is generally fatal within 1 to 6 years.[22] It is nonhereditary.

Symptoms may first occur in muscles most used by the patient in his occupation or at the site of an injury.[23] Muscular atrophy usually begins in the intrinsic muscles of the hands and arm musculature; the patient complains of weakness, stiffness, and clumsiness of the fingers. Although the onset usually is centered symmetrically in the upper extremities, it can vary in location and severity. Thenar and finger flexor atrophy generally occur prior to atrophy of the extensors.

Weakness extends proximally from the hands to the shoulders. From the shoulders, the weakness moves to the tongue, where atrophy and paresis of the lips, tongue, and palate cause slurred speech, which eventually becomes unintelligible. The ability to swallow is also affected. As the extensors become involved, weakness in the trunk, loss of head control, and lower extremity paralysis occur; eventually all reflexes are lost.

Treatment

ALS is treated symptomatically to provide maintenance of nutrition, to prevent fatigue, to prevent respiratory infections, and to avoid exposure to cold. Drugs can be used to control problems in swallowing, spasticity, and respiratory and urinary infections.

The rehabilitation program includes moderate activity to maintain strength through muscle re-

education and passive exercises to prevent contractures. The exercise program provides relaxation and alleviation of spasticity. Self-care techniques require the use of assistive devices to substitute for the gradual loss of motor function, including respiratory failure. Gait training, with braces, is used when the patient can tolerate standing.

The occupational therapist provides both physical and psychological assistance in the development of coping skills to the patient with ALS. Therapeutic techniques and activities should be used with care to maximize functional benefit and minimize fatigue. Passive range of motion by the occupational therapist can provide relaxation in addition to maintaining maximum range of motion in the joints. The passive range of motion exercises should be followed by a short, active exercise period determined by the patient's muscle power.

The use of assistive equipment can aid the patient in retaining as much function as possible and to remain active as long as possible. A wheelchair, suspension slings, arm supports, and positioning aids can stimulate the patient to socialize, to care for himself or herself, and to engage in activities which provide a day-to-day enjoyment of life. Environmental control systems or attendant care may be necessary in the later stages of ALS, as the patient loses mobility in his extremities.

Myasthenia Gravis

Myasthenia gravis (MG) is a progressive, degenerative disease that affects the myoneural junction and is characterized by severe muscle weakness. Impairment of conduction of nerve impulses to muscles occurs because of a presynaptic or postsynaptic block at the receptors on the motor endplates caused by a lack of release of the enzyme acetylcholine necessary for conduction.[24] Abnormalities occur in the thymus gland and the body's immune system which block the nerve impulse to the muscle.

Beginning with a gradual onset, this chronic disease is characterized by intermittent, abnormal fatigue of isolated muscle groups. In later stages it results in permanent weakness of some muscles and muscle atrophy in others. Although it can occur at any age, the disease usually affects young adults, with females being more commonly affected than males.

The most common symptom of myasthenia gravis is abnormal muscular fatigue, most frequently observed in the eye muscles; this symptom is accompanied by ptosis (drooping of both upper lids) and diplopia (double vision). In addition the patient may present weakness of the facial muscles; total eye closure; retraction of the angles of the mouth; weakness of the bulbar musculature necessary for chewing, swallowing, and articulation; dyspnea (shortness of breath); weakness in the trunk and limbs causing difficulty in balance and walking; and general fatigue. Initially these symptoms are exacerbated when the patient is fatigued but may disappear following rest. The patient may also have a tendency toward respiratory failure and may demonstrate a high, nasal voice.

In the later stages of the disease the patient experiences difficulty in swallowing and speaking. Eventually he or she becomes bedridden and immobile with severe permanent paralysis.

Remissions (decrease in symptoms) and improvement in general muscle strength and function may be marked and can last for years. However, exacerbation or attacks of weakness caused by physical exertion, infection, or childbirth can occur. These fluctuations can be sudden and of unpredictable severity.

Occupational Therapy

The therapist's prime concern in working with the patient with MG is to aid him or her in regaining muscle power and endurance; the therapist must take care not to cause debilitating fatigue. Because this disease is characterized by remissions, the recuperating patient may be able to regain functional abilities in upper extremities, independence in self-care, and in some instances, may be able to walk. If physical tolerance can be maintained during rehabilitation, the patient might be able to return to a nonexertive form of work. Over-exertion must be avoided and respiratory problems must be prevented. The patient should be encouraged to employ work simplification techniques, therapeutic breathing, and energy conservation during activities.

The therapist should provide gentle, nonresistive activities that are interesting to the patient. These activities should be creative and productive and should provide psychological and intellectual stimulation to maintain a concept of self-worth. During therapy, the patient may use a respirator to maintain breathing.

In the later stages of the disease the bedridden patient may lack ability to use the arms. Should this occur, he or she can benefit from assistive equipment such as arm supports and splints to aid in positioning for function. Electronically controlled devices that substitute for nonfunctioning arms and hands can be activated by micro-switches, minute body movements, chin controls, or breath controls. These devices can enable the patient to operate a tape recorder, record player, television set, radio, or telephone. They have been produced in the United States (Prenke Romich) and in England (POSUM). Although they are expensive to buy and to repair, they enable the severely disabled person with intact intellectual abilities to communicate with the outside world and to have control over his or her immediate environment. For example, systems can be devised for activation of heating systems, windows, doors, lights, and typewriters, in addition to those pieces of machinery mentioned above. A discussion of the social and intellectual stimulation that this equipment can provide to the patient severely disabled with MG appears in Dorothy Clark Wilson's book, *Hilary*.[25]

Muscular Dystrophy

Muscular dystrophy (MD) is a disease of the muscle cell that causes progressive degeneration of specific muscle groups. This disease is of unknown origin and is characterized by variation in the size of individual muscle fibers caused by initial swelling of muscle groups; the result is a pseudohypertrophic (enlarged) appearance of muscles. Although this false enlargement gives the appearance of a very strong extremity, it is caused by an excess of fat in the tissue and is eventually followed by atrophy.

The disease affects children, adolescents, or young adults. The most common type of MD is pseudohypertrophic muscular dystrophy, which normally affects males and is inherited as a sex-linked recessive genetic defect. It may occur sporadically or may affect several siblings.[26]

Symptoms appear during the first decade of life; a previously normal child begins to walk clumsily, tends to fall, and has difficulty getting up after a fall. The characteristic pseudohypertrophy of the muscles manifests itself in the calves, glutei, quadriceps, and deltoids. These muscles are enlarged and firm to the touch but they are usually weak. In some cases this manifestation may appear in the triceps and forearm muscles. The accompanying atrophy usually affects the proximal more than the distal muscles. Muscle impairment can cause weakness of the extensors of the spine, resulting in lordosis, weakness in the knees, and diminished tendon reflexes. While sensation and intelligence are unimpaired, the child with MD may be limited by the rapid onset of severe physical limitations and confinement to a wheelchair. Schooling may be interrupted and the child's capacity to progress with his peers may be diminished.

Early signs of MD are manifested in the sloping appearance of the shoulders; this is caused by weakness in the shoulder girdle. Contractures are common in the later stages of the disease, caused by weakness in muscle groups whose antagonists remain comparatively powerful. An example of the developing contracture is seen in the patient who walks on his toes because of progressive weakness of the anterior tibial muscle and the tendency of the biceps and hamstrings to shorten. When the patient becomes confined to a wheelchair, contractures occur in the trunk, causing postural changes.

Rehabilitation Program

Because MD results in a gradual loss of muscle power and control, the rehabilitation program is directed toward the maintenance of joint range of motion and strength through the continuation of self-care and functional skills. Contractures can be prevented through passive range of motion exercises, proper positioning in the wheelchair for arm function, active exercises and activities for the arms, and assistive devices.

As the weakness increases, assistive equipment such as arm supports are used to assist the patient in reaching, self-feeding, and other arm and hand activities. Special devices may be needed for bathing and dressing and for diversional and productive activities. The therapist should also provide the patient with a home exercise program, which can maintain the existing muscle power and allow participation in various pursuits. Although the life span of the person with MD is shortened, he or she can continue a relatively normal life with the use of adaptive equipment and assistive techniques.

Arthritis

There are many types of arthritis with varying degrees of pathological symptoms that require medical and therapeutic intervention. As the occupational therapist most frequently comes in contact with those suffering from the effects of rheumatoid arthritis, this is the type of arthritis on which this section will concentrate.

Arthritis can affect a person of any age, has a variety of causes and effects, and can be of short duration or a lifelong condition. It can result from local trauma or the aging process (osteoarthritis) or from systemic infection (rheumatoid arthritis). Although it is commonly thought that arthritis is an affliction of the elderly, it may also be a disability of the young.

Degenerative joint disease (DJD) or osteoarthritis is the least feared type of the disease. DJD most commonly affects the fingers at the interphalangeal joints, causing minimal or no pain. Other frequently traumatized joints are the ankles, knees, hips, and elbows. DJD often occurs in people who have been active in sports, those whose jobs have caused strain on their joints, or it accompanies the aging process, affecting the weight-bearing joints. The swelling associated with DJD is in the bony structure, not in the soft tissue as is the case with rheumatoid arthritis.

Treatment of DJD is local, consisting of rest to relieve pain and stress on the affected joints. Heat and therapeutic exercises are provided in a gradual, graded program.

Rheumatoid Arthritis

This is a progressive systemic disease resulting in inflammation, pain, and structural changes in the affected joints. Characterized by remissions and exacerbations, rheumatoid arthritis results in progressive limitation and deformity. Many persons suffering from rheumatoid arthritis are between the ages of 20 and 40 years. They exhibit swollen, reddened, and painful joints during and after excessive use of the affected joints. Because of the limitations imposed by the disease, the person's functional ability, physical appearance, and mental and psychological tolerance are affected. Treatment must be geared toward assisting the patient in combating the debilitating effects of the disease and in maintaining maximum independent functions. The occupational therapist aids the person in learning a self-directed program of joint protection and function to continue at home.

The major clinical focus of rheumatoid arthritis is centered on the joints, where there may be subluxation, dislocation, pain, swelling, stiffness, and deformity. Muscle atrophy can occur owing to limitations in joint movement and decreased muscle activity. Contractures may occur from both decreased muscle activity and prolonged immobilization. Sensory changes and loss of weight are also characteristic. The patient may eventually need leg braces, special shoes, crutches, or a wheelchair for locomotion; hand splints to prevent deformity and to provide function; and a variety of assistive devices to accomplish self-care, ADL, and homemaking tasks.

Precautions

Functional problems caused by arthritis arise from limitations in active and passive joint movement affecting reach, grasp, and coordination. Among the causes are internal joint damage, fear of pain, actual pain, and decreased strength and sensation, and deformity.

During the period of inflammation, the joint is vulnerable to deformity produced by repetitive stress causing a malalignment of the part. Muscles are strained and weakened during this time, giving less resistance to the development of deforming positions. If muscles become overstretched and shift position, they can actually maintain and strengthen the deformity. This is frequently seen in the ulnar deviation of the MP joints due to lateral slippage of the long finger tendons. When this realignment occurs, continuous finger flexion encourages the deformity rather than counteracting it.

The following precautions should be used while performing physical evaluations and during treatment of the patient with arthritis:

1. In the presence of dislocation and subluxation:
   (a) Avoid over-activity of the affected joints.
   (b) Avoid resistive exercises.
2. In the presence of pain and swelling:
   (a) Limit passive range of motion of the extremity during the acute stage of the disease.
   (b) Encourage active range of motion with resistance (as tolerated).
   (c) Do not allow fear to develop.
   (d) Minimize strenuous activity and alternate activity with rest periods.
3. Avoid over-exercise; work within the limits of joint pain, exertion, swelling, and general tolerance.
4. Prevent muscle atrophy:
   (a) Limit exercise to the maximum range of motion with regard to specific joint range.
   (b) Provide an activity in which the patient can work on strengthening muscles when he or she can work against resistance.

Surgical Considerations

One of the preventive surgical procedures performed to combat the symptoms of rheumatoid arthritis is synovectomy. This procedure is performed early in the course of the disease to relieve pain and swelling of the joint, to release contractures, and to prevent arthrodesis of joints. Other surgical procedures include arthroplasty and joint replacement. These surgical procedures are directed toward relieving pain, aligning joints, establishing function, and increasing range of motion. When a surgical procedure is considered, the occupational therapist should inform the surgeon of the patient's functional ability so that function is retained after surgery. The patient's attitude and expectations regarding surgery are crucial to rehabilitation.

Through careful evaluation of functional activities, the occupational therapist is able to determine an accurate picture of what the patient is incapable of doing because of deformity, pain, or muscle imbalance. It is important to communicate this information to the surgeon prior to surgery.

Evaluation Approach

The occupational therapist assesses the mental and physical tolerance by chart review, observation, and discussion of the patient's progress with members of the rehabilitation team. Evaluation sessions should not be prolonged beyond the effectiveness of both the patient and the therapist.

During the session, the therapist provides encouragement and support; particular areas for consideration are the patient's stated concerns and apprehensions, medical condition, and resultant functional challenges.

The occupation therapist varies the tests and activities so the patient can complete them without unnecessary pain, frustration, or joint stress. It is important that the therapist emphasize the patient's abilities realistically.

Specific Evaluation Techniques

1. Examine the extremities for signs of redness, swelling, atrophy, discoloration, surgical scars, malalignment, joint deformities, hyperflexion, hyperextension, abduction, adduction, and ulnar deviation.
2. Examine the relaxed limbs for signs of atrophy, joint limitation, and discomfort.
3. Examine splints, braces, or other special equipment. Determine the patient's ability to use and care for the devices and evaluate their effectiveness.
4. Gently move the extremities through the passive joint range of motion, noting the presence of subluxation, limitation, muscle tightness, or pain.
5. Ask the patient to move his or her extremities through all ranges of motion actively and to indicate if there is pain.
6. Check the muscle strength by providing resistance to active range of motion.
7. Provide activities that demonstrate the functional use of hands and arms:
   (a) *Grasping* small objects such as coins, paper clips, a pencil, or a key
   (b) *Lifting* heavy objects such as a hammer, using one hand, and a large can of sugar, using two hands
   (c) *Reaching,* by placing a book on a shelf, turning on a faucet, or opening a drawer
8. Observe the use of the hands in task activities such as writing, removing a letter from an envelope, counting money (either change or bills), and finding a page in a book.
9. Evaluate self-care: active bathing, grooming, eating, transferring from one position to another, walking, and carrying needed items.

The therapist should remain alert for signs of mental, psychological, or physical fatigue. The patient's confidence is gained by asking him or her to describe present needs, interests, and concerns and to discuss future plans.

Principles of Treatment

The following are basic principles of treatment of the patient with rheumatoid arthritis:

CONTROL OF THE RHEUMATOID PROCESS. Anti-inflammatory and analgesic drugs are used to control the disease. Bedrest is essential during the acute phase and following surgery in instances of severe destruction of the joints. Although procedures may succeed in retarding the rheumatoid process for a period of time, the patient may continue to have exacerbations of the disease. When the joints show a reduction of swelling and inflammation, the rehabilitation program can begin.

JOINT MOBILITY THROUGH RANGE OF MOTION (Fig. 22-14) Passive and active joint range of motion of all extremities are essential for functional restoration. Passive and active joint range of motion techniques should be employed to determine the presence of pain and limitation. Active range of motion with resistance should be encouraged only after pain, swelling, and inflammation have been sufficiently reduced to prevent a chance of deformity.

FUNCTIONAL TRAINING. The occupational therapist uses a functional training program to make the patient aware of both limitations and abilities. Analyzing the patient's daily activities can assist the therapist in providing specific self-care techniques, and appropriate, productive avocational activities in conjunction with joint protection.

MAINTENANCE OF MUSCLE POWER. The patient with rheumatoid arthritis may exhibit weakness. Defor-

mities may prevent functional use of muscles and joint alignment may be continually challenged. Without adequate joint function, muscle power is reduced, but the use of a functional hand splint can properly align muscles, joints, and tendons. Activities requiring strength must be used carefully in the therapeutic program (Fig. 22-15). Too much resistance can cause joint pain. The occupational therapist must avoid activity that will cause fatigue and must make the patient aware of limitations in strength.

INDEPENDENCE IN SELF-CARE. Because of the existence of pain and joint limitations characteristic of arthritis, the patient may suffer deficiencies in self-care, may avoid dressing, or may request assistance in basic activities of daily living. The therapist should encourage the use of self-care techniques as therapeutic exercises, employing assistive devices and special equipment to conserve energy and avoid further joint destruction.

INCREASE PHYSICAL AND MENTAL ENDURANCE. The person with rheumatoid arthritis is subjected to frequent hospitalizations. Exacerbations and remissions are common, and the patient displays frustration caused by the inability to cope with family or job responsibilities.

The therapist should encourage the patient to develop a regime of alternate rest and work which will

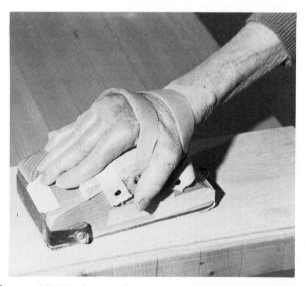

Figure 22-15. Strengthening Activity. This patient with rheumatoid arthritis has had surgical replacement of the metacarpophalangeal joints. She uses a sanding block for resistive activity to achieve range of muscle functions of the arm. The patient's hand is positioned in maximum extension of the metacarpophalangeal joints to provide passive stretching during exercise of the arm.

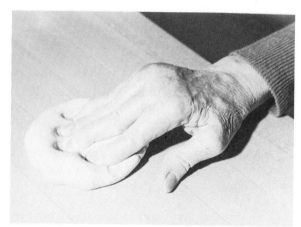

Figure 22-14. Range of motion strengthening. Use of a soft, resistive plastic material provides a medium for specific finger and hand exercises that the patient can be taught to do alone, after treatment or at home.

protect joints and conserve energy. The patient should also be instructed in the principles and use of joint protection techniques. The development of awareness of the nature of the disease can help both the patient and family cope with physical limitations that result from tension, overwork, or pain.

ASSISTIVE DEVICES. These devices should be used only to increase function or to protect impaired joints. They should be lightweight, simple to operate, and acceptable to the patient. They should encourage independent function. If the patient cannot use the device easily, he or she will discard it.

HOME PROGRAM. The occupational therapist must stress the need for the patient with arthritis to continue the therapeutic program at home. Among the elements of discharge planning are a home visit to determine architectural barriers, necessary rearrangement of furniture and toilet facilities, assistance with work space and appliances, and development of specific devices.

Specific Approaches

The approaches to treatment must be individualized to meet the needs of various patients. The outpatient may be seen for the first time at the request of a physician for the construction of resting splints or splints to protect joints and to provide improvement of function, for energy conservation orientation, and for the provision of assistive devices. The outpatient often has a family to care for, a job to perform, or school to attend. With the implementation of various aids and programs, the patient can perform tasks with greater ease and comfort, and can gain the satisfaction of accomplishing chosen activities with less pain and stress. Following the remission of painful symptoms requiring medical treatment, the patient may need only a few treatment sessions. The homemaker can be assisted in organizing time and tasks to minimize tension. The employed arthritic person can be assisted in self-evaluation of job activities and can learn how to adapt equipment or arrange the work schedule. The student can learn ways to ease the strain of note-taking in class and of carrying books and equipment. The student should also be encouraged to participate in social activities and engage in recreation.

The inpatient is likely to be on bedrest during the acute stage of arthritis. Evaluation and initial treatment may be accomplished during this time. During the period of inflammation, there should be little stress on joints, and daily activities of bathing and feeding should be assisted. Bathing can be simplified with the use of a bath mitt or a long-handled sponge.

For meals the patient can be provided with a fork with a built-up handle, a serrated knife, a large-handled plastic mug, easily-managed food containers, and a rubber mat upon which to place plates.

Bed positioning is extremely important to prevent deformities and to encourage the most beneficial, comfortable, and successful means of functioning. The patient should use a firm mattress and should lie flat in the supine position with arms and hands straight at the sides. A small pillow may be used if necessary. Light covers should be used to minimize weight on sensitive limbs.

Prism glasses for television viewing or seeing visitors can minimize fatigue and eyestrain during this period. A book holder that can be angled for bed use, and a lapboard placed in a comfortable position, can be used for reading and writing. All items should be placed within easy reach.

During the period of bedrest the patient often suffers pain from inflammation of the joints and requires encouragement and diversion more than active exercise. Exercise, when used, should *not* include resistance at this time.

Poor positioning of the extremities may cause pain, poor alignment, stiff joints, deformity, and general discomfort. Thus, splints may be indicated during the acute inflammatory stage of rheumatoid arthritis.

The importance of positioning continues when the patient is sitting in a chair, using a wheelchair, or walking. When the patient is able to sit in a chair for activity, attention should be given to proper alignment of the body. A high-backed chair should be used for trunk and head support. Feet should be placed firmly on the floor and firm cushions should be used to raise the patient to a comfortable position. Good positioning minimizes strain, encourages mechanical advantages in function, and prevents deformities.

When the patient is in a wheelchair or is ambulatory, the occupational therapy program becomes more intensive. As soon as medically feasible, the patient can engage in light activities which employ maximum active range of motion. Needlework, Turkish knotting, light weaving, and painting can be used to strengthen the upper extremities and to increase joint range of motion and coordination.

The occupational therapist is responsible for teaching the patient the use of assistive devices and techniques that can aid in self-care and homemaking activities. For example, built-up handles, mitts, and rubber mats for cooking utensils aid the homemaker. Dressing can be assisted by the use of long-handled implements, and reachers can be used to grasp objects from the floor or from high places.

The arthritic patient's home can be made safe by

the addition of railings at stairways, removal of heavy doors and scatter rugs, provision of easily managed latches on doors and cabinets, and arrangement of furniture and work areas for ease of movement and function. The occupational therapist can advise the patient in these labor-saving and safety factors.

In order to maintain muscle power and prevent deformity, the patient learns methods of using the muscles that maintain joint range of motion, strength, coordination, and body alignment. Therapeutic use of joints keeps the patient functioning with maximum use of muscles and prevention of deformity. The most effective way of performing protective exercises for preservation of joints and prevention of deformity is to incorporate these therapeutic positions and movements into daily living activities.

Making a daily plan of activities serves to schedule them according to degree of physical stress, enabling the patient to alternate work and rest activities, gross and fine motor functions, sitting and standing, to provide therapeutic change to maintain activity tolerance and realistic productivity according to the individual's needs, desires, and abilities.

Splinting

The provision of splinting for the patient with rheumatoid arthritis is both crucial and controversial. As Hollander wrote, "It is usually much easier to prevent a deformity in arthritis than to correct one."[27] Some experts believe that no splint at all is preferable to a splint that causes decreased function or deformity.

The purposes of splinting the arthritic are provision of support to diseased joints, alleviation of pain, prevention of deformity, maintenance and promotion of function, and establishment of functional alignment.

Splints are used at night to maintain the extremity in a static position, providing proper alignment of the joints without undue stress on them, and establishing a functional position for daily activities. Because the wrist is the key joint for hand function, stabilization and alignment of the wrist joint must be done prior to splinting of the fingers. The splint used at night can be a volar splint extending from the distal third of the forearm to the fingertips, with abduction and extension of the thumb. In some cases the thumb may be left free, and the splint may terminate at the distal portion of the metacarpophalangeal joints. This construction may be necessary to prevent stiffening of the phalangeal joints in extension, since they should be slightly flexed.

Daytime splints also maintain functional align-

ment of the arthritic patient's wrist and fingers; however, the splints must be of different types from those used at night. If the pain is at the wrist, static positioning can stiffen the joints and thus the splint must be removed and the joints allowed full range of motion several times during the day. Dynamic splinting must be controlled to prevent both pain from movement and deformity from poor positioning. The palmar aspect of the splint can terminate at the palm. Finger cuffs and rubberbands can be used to provide finger mobility with an outrigger for positioning and resistive activity. With this type of positioning, it is essential that the wrist be stabilized to minimize trauma to the finger joints.

After the occupational therapist has constructed the splint(s), they should be inspected to ensure that they provide proper support and comfort. Splints should be lightweight, cover a minimum amount of skin, and be easily applied or removed (Fig. 22-16). The patient must be advised to inform the therapist of areas of irritation and to use both passive and active range of motion exercises in conjunction with the use of the splint.

Water

In occupational therapy, water can be used as a therapeutic medium to relax and soothe the painful extremity in preparation for passive and active joint range of motion exercise and activity. Careful massage of joint and tendon areas by the therapist, as shown in Figure 22-17, helps to loosen up stiff areas for active movements.

This limbering-up may be provided in the physical therapy session and is particularly beneficial if scheduled just before the occupational therapy session. In preparation for functional activity, the patient benefits from warmth and from the desensitizing, flotation effect of this exercise. Doing grasping exercises of increasing resistance and coordination uses the warmth and flotation to an advantage.

Principles of Joint Protection

Education of joint protection is an essential part of the occupational therapist's work in rehabilitation. Because of pain and instability, some arthritic patients fear further damage to the joints and therefore avoid using them. On the other hand, an arthritic patient may deny the disability, avoid preventive precautions, and actually cause destruction and deformity.

Adopting the joint protection attitude and techniques can benefit the school-aged child with arthritis; he or she can endure writing exercises by using custom-made hand, wrist, or finger splints and

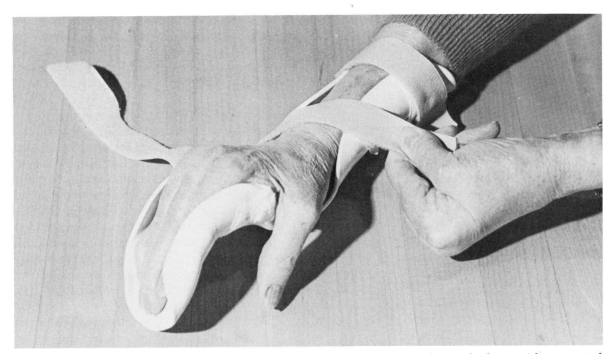

Figure 22-16. A patient with rheumatoid arthritis puts on her volar splint, which provides rest and functional positioning of the hand and wrist at night or during the day.

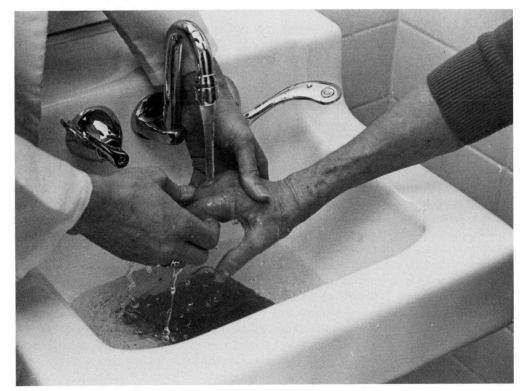

Figure 22-17. Warm water and percussion both stimulate and soothe painful arthritic joints during massage and passive range of motion in preparation of functional activity by the patient.

large square or rough-textured pencils for traction. Work surfaces, chair contour and height should fit the child comfortably and therapeutically to maintain stable, pain-free positioning for maximum performance.

The patient must become involved in the rehabilitation process, carrying over program principles learned during hospitalization. Among these principles of joint protection are the following.

1. Avoid positions that cause deformity. The therapist should encourage the patient to look carefully at the affected extremities to determine whether or not natural positions are resulting in redness, swelling, or pain. Tests for both passive and active joint range of motion should be discussed with the patient so that he or she recognizes how to avoid excessive strain during daily activities.

2. Avoid sustained positions. The occupational therapist should teach the patient that maintaining a fixed position places stress on specific joints. For example, the longer a person grasps an object, the greater the likelihood of pain and stiffness upon release of the object. The arthritic must be encouraged to change position or activities frequently, encouraging the reciprocal muscle movement to stretch tightened muscles and to relieve pressure on the joints.

3. Use the strongest joints for heavy work. Patients with arthritis must be taught to compensate for weakened joints and to try to develop bilateral capacity.

4. Do not start what you cannot stop. Arthritic patients are often characterized by ambition and a strong work ethic. These traits impair the ability to create a pace compatible with the disease. The occupational therapist must instruct the patient in energy conservation, organization of tasks, and awareness of fatigue.

5. Use joints to the greatest mechanical advantage. Certain activities can be done more easily in a standing position; among them are mopping a floor, mixing a cake, or washing one's hair. Among activities which are more easily done while seated are reading a book, working on a puzzle, doing needlework, or sewing. The crucial element here is not only putting the body in the most advantageous position of function but also preventing stress on other joints. If the mechanical aspects of different positioning for different activities are analyzed thoroughly by the therapist, the findings can be valuable in assisting the therapist in adapting positions and activities to increase function. Not using the body in a position that utilizes strong muscles and joints effectively may cause strain and even present a safety hazard.

6. The patient must be taught to respect pain. Although one can sometimes detect the signs of pain on someone's face or can learn of pain through the patient's complaint, pain itself is highly subjective. Tolerance levels of pain vary and, when there is a sensory deficit, the perception of pain may be entirely lacking. In periods when the arthritis is active, the patient may complain of severe pain, and there may be visible inflammation of joints. In the stages following acute attacks of arthritis, the pain must be considered when planning activity programs. It must be conveyed to the patient that joint protection is for the purpose of improving and maintaining function rather than restricting function. This is often misinterpreted and the patient ignores the suggestions for optimal bodily functions in the presence of arthritis. Improper use of joints can increase pain. Lack of attention to position changes and activity changes can cause pain. Mental denial, frustration, or tension can cause improper use of joints and put undue strain on them. The patient must plan activities to maximize function and range of motion.

Orthopedic Considerations

Among patients referred to occupational therapy are those with hand injuries and persons with hip, back, upper or lower extremity fractures which confine them to bed or cause them to be placed in traction. For persons with upper extremity injuries, the surgeon may request functional training for increasing joint range of motion, strength, and coordination; provision of assistive devices for self-care; static and dynamic splinting for upper extremity injuries; and supportive activities for those in traction. The number of patients with orthopedic conditions seen and treated by the occupational therapist depends on the recognition of the value of occupational therapy by the orthopedic surgeon.

The patient with brain or spinal cord injury may also have sustained one or more fractures of the extremities because of the type of accident in which he or she was involved. In this case, the more severe injury may complicate the healing and general care of the fractured limbs. If the patient exhibits communication deficits, behavior disturbances, or decreased sensation, it is important that he or she understand what the therapist is doing and why. Sensitivity may be increased or decreased owing to neurological signs. If splinting or assistive devices are used in the presence of a sensory deficit, the pressure on the affected extremity or extremities should be well monitored for fit, function and pressure areas. Alternate therapeutic approaches may be necessary to facilitate passive and active joint range of motion in the presence of traction or additional therapeutic equipment.

Evaluation

The evaluation varies depending on the type of injury and the extent of the immobilization. For example, a patient with a neck injury may be seen initially while he or she is in neck traction. If the spinal cord has not been injured, there may be weakness but not paralysis in the extremities. The patient with a lower back injury may have full upper extremity function but be confined to the supine position in bed and may have restrictions on back movements with or without lower extremity dysfunction. The patient with a lower extremity fracture may have full use of the arms but be confined to bed in leg traction, or there may be precautions against hip flexion. A person with an upper extremity orthopedic injury may be in bed, in a wheelchair, or ambulatory.

In preparing to evaluate the patient, the occupational therapist should review the medical factors pertinent to the injury and the present medical condition. These factors include the type of fracture, length of time and type of immobilization, alignment and progress of bony union, presence and extent of nerve involvement, presence of infection, precautions of mobility, safe joint movement, and muscle stretching, and consideration of removal of supporting casts, braces, or splints during activity or exercise.

Evaluation includes passive and active range of motion of the joints proximal and distal to the immobilized joint(s): general mobility of all extremities; positioning alternatives; feasibility of the use of a wheelchair or of walking; and the existence of accompanying factors such as paralysis, trophic changes, edema, pain, fatigue, contractures, scar tissue, and psychological problems. The occupational therapist evaluates the level of functional ability and independence in activities of daily living.

General principles of treatment for the affected limb include the following:

1. Support the injured part to relieve trauma, to prevent further destruction of tissue, to ensure proper alignment of the extremity, and to prevent pain from joint limitation.
2. Prevent disuse atrophy in the musculature surrounding the traumatized area by encouraging the patient to maintain strength, range of motion, and function.
3. Provide a therapeutic exercise program for reeducation of muscles and joints.
4. Encourage normal functional return following immobilization through gradual use of the extremity in unilateral and bilateral activities.
5. Assist the patient's adjustment to cosmetic and functional changes caused by trauma.

A patient may have pain in the extremity caused by the trauma itself or by immobilization; such a patient may not be motivated to participate in a full program of exercise and activity. The therapist encourages the patient to become involved in rehabilitation in order to prevent deformities, pain, and substitution of motor patterns in the weakened limb.

The patient with upper extremity trauma may remain in the acute care setting for a relatively short period of time, but long enough for adequate setting of the fracture, healing of surgical sites, and stabilization of medical complications. Initial casting is usually done by the physician, but the occupational therapist may be requested to assist in preparing for future adjustment by splinting in coordination with a functional exercise and activity program.

Treatment

Upper Extremity

Shoulder disabilities can occur postoperatively in cases involving tumor, traction, immobilization, fracture, or periarthritis. Clinical signs include pain, muscle atrophy, shoulder weakness, contracture of the adductors with the inability to rotate externally, fear of movement, and stiffness. Following heat, massage, and whirlpool activity in physical therapy, the occupational therapy program includes graded activities to increase strength, joint range of motion, and function by using such activities as the floor loom, printing press, woodworking, macrame, and basketry. The patient should be encouraged to participate in recreational activities such as shuffleboard, darts, bowling, and ball games to develop full use and integration of the injured extremity. The physical tolerance and fatigue level should be the gauge used for gradation of the program. Prevocational evaluation becomes part of the treatment program for the patient who will be able to return to work. The occupational therapist works closely with the vocational rehabilitation counsellor in identifying specific job-related abilities. The industrially oriented program is basically one of regaining work tolerance in a graded conditioning program.

For upper extremity injuries, activities such as using hand tools and power machinery, painting, and shoveling are used. The conditioning program should utilize productive work tasks, and activity time should be increased as endurance develops. However, the patient should be monitored for signs of pain, swelling, or fatigue. Home activity programs should be developed to encourage the patient to maintain a general conditioning program.

Patients who have a fractured *forearm or hand* may require a splint as a supportive device for strenuous activity. Unless there is a peripheral nerve involvement from the injury, the orthopedic surgeon usually provides the initial splint. However, the occupational therapist may be asked later to provide a dynamic splint to encourage finger function. The most useful treatment is functional training in the use of the injured extremity. Productive activity is essential to the achievement of this goal. Graded manual activity and specific dexterity training in the affected hand are essential for the regaining of functional abilities. If the patient cannot regain adequate use of the hand through functional activity, counselling for alternative job training and placement may be required.

Patients who suffer residual effects from surgery (scarring or amputation) may need cosmetic adjustments. The occupational therapist counsels the patient, pointing out assets and helping him or her accept the additional trauma of cosmetic disfigurement.

Lower Extremity

When a patient has suffered a fracture of a lower extremity, the occupational therapy program begins with activities to provide support while the patient is confined to bed. When able to stand and bear weight on the injured extremity, the patient can begin a program of standing tolerance and general reconditioning. Lower extremity active exercises include graded, resistive exercises of the extremity, coordination exercises, and use of the extremity involving the entire body.

Adaptations to the floor loom, printing press, bicycle, and woodworking equipment can aid in gradual increase in strength and coordination. Work-simulated tasks designed for the injured worker offer preparation for the demands of the job.

For the patient who has had a *back or leg injury,* work activities include weight bearing, lifting, carrying, climbing, and bending. Activities such as lifting, carrying weights, climbing ladders, shoveling, chopping wood, pushing a wheelbarrow, and pulling heavy objects are given and upgraded according to the patient's tolerance. Specific activities for strengthening a limb and increasing tolerance that are used for the patient having a lower extremity injury include balancing and exercising using adapted equipment such as a bicycle saw, or treadle sander, lathe, or printing press.

Fractured Hip—Hip Replacement

The patient with a fractured hip or with a hip replacement is commonly referred to the occupational therapist by the orthopedic surgeon, rheumatologist, or physiatrist. The patient benefits from supportive activities, self-care training, assistive devices, home evaluation, and home adaptation.

During the bedrest stage following surgery the

patient may benefit from supportive activities that assist in psychological adjustment and divert attention from pain. When there is medical clearance for the patient to move around in bed, he or she should be encouraged to participate in morning hygiene and self-care. Because the patient may be restricted in the use of the hip joint in flexion and resistive movements, long-handled reachers and special hooks can provide assistance in dressing. When the physician concurs, joint range of motion of the hip should be encouraged during activity. However, the rehabilitation process must be gradual.

The patient may be discharged from the hospital before he or she has fully recovered from the injury or surgery; therefore, a home program should be established to protect the hip from further injury and to encourage participation in exercise and self-care activities. The occupational therapist instructs the patient in both protective precautions and the use of various devices that can assist in self-care. The patient should avoid bending the hip more than 90° and crossing the legs at the knees or ankles. A firm, knee-height, straight-backed chair with arm rests should be used. Reclining chairs are very difficult for the patient to get into or out of, can cause him to fall, and thus should be avoided. Toilet seat extensions and firm pillows in low chairs can ensure proper height for adequate transfer and comfort.

The patient should be advised to sleep in a supine position to promote good alignment of the hip joints. If the patient is accustomed to turning in bed, a pillow should be placed between the legs to inhibit movement.

Other aspects of the home program include instruction and advice in the use of assistive devices for bathing (long-handled sponges, soap on a rope, and nonskid safety strips in the shower), for dressing (long-handled shoehorn, stocking aids, elastic shoe laces, and reachers), and for other activities of daily living. A "walker bag" attached to the crutch may be used to carry small objects. Cars with low reclining seats should be avoided when possible, but a cushion may be used to raise the seat to a comfortable height.

Peripheral Nerve Injuries

Peripheral nerve injuries result from direct trauma to the extremity and affect all muscles innervated below the point of injury. Common causes include fractures, dislocations, crush injuries, compression, and lacerations. Primary impairments include sensory and motor dysfunction, contractures, deformity, and swelling. Continuing malfunction of the nerves can cause long-term or permanent muscle dysfunction, deformities of the hand, sensory loss, and trophic changes.

Rehabilitation Program

The general rehabilitation goal is to return the patient to a maximum level of function and independence. The injury may have caused serious damage to the sensorimotor system, resulting in the loss of extremity function caused by blocking of the conduction of nerve impulses. Depending upon the location and severity of the injury, the patient may suffer a long-term disability. The rehabilitation program focuses on return of the capacity to use the extremity and development of sensory and motor function. Physical and cosmetic changes in the extremity may cause difficulties in the patient's psychological adjustment to disability.

From the initial immobilization in a cast to later dynamic splinting by the occupational therapist, treatment must be carefully monitored. Specific forms of splinting are used protectively and as a forerunner and stimulus to function. The design of the dynamic splint provides minimal coverage of the extremity but allows flexible, controlled use of the hand. Elastic or spring finger cuffs facilitate movement. The affected extremity needs to be exercised to prevent disuse atrophy. Because there may be muscle imbalance following nerve injury, the splint should prevent overstretching of the strong, unaffected muscles. Correct alignment is essential to provide the patient with mechanical advantage and to preserve functional potential.

Skin changes and sensory deficits may be caused by poor circulation. Therefore, a concern of the occupational therapist is to maintain the integrity of the skin.[28] The therapist checks the effect of splinting and other devices on the affected extremity, uses cutaneous stimulation to encourage functional return of sensation, and helps the patient to develop an awareness of pain, temperature, and tactile discrimination. With these supportive concepts, the patient can avoid further injury to the desensitized limb.

Passive and assisted movements of the limb restore the flexibility of the joints. Gentle, passive joint range of motion, accompanied by heat and warm water, facilitates movement. As strength increases, the occupational therapist increases the resistance provided by various exercises or activities. However, care must be taken not to fatigue the patient or overstretch weakened muscles. The therapist's observation should include checking to make sure that the patient is not using substitution patterns that impair the development of function. Sensory stimulation includes manipulation of objects of different sizes, textures, weights, and shapes.

Contractures impede rehabilitation. Once they occur, they are difficult to release through passive stretching, which may cause joint damage if done improperly. Splints can be useful in preventing contractures in the early phase of treatment.

The therapist may use static or dynamic positioning to support the joints in normal alignment and muscle balance. Specific designs for splints will depend on the patient's functional capacity.

The occupational therapist encourages the patient to develop maximum functional use of the impaired extremity. Total body use is important in reintegrating the disabled extremity with the rest of the body; activities which are gradually upgraded in resistance encourage coordination, increase function, and augment general physical and mental tolerance of the condition. However, the occupational therapist must be careful not to overwork the patient; excessive exercise can cause edema in the affected extremity, creating stiffness in the joints, thus hindering range of motion. (For additional information, see Chapter 25 on Hand Rehabilitation.)

Carpal Tunnel Syndrome

The carpal tunnel syndrome results from compression of the median nerve at the wrist's transverse carpal ligament, resulting in paresthesia and pain involving the first three fingers of the hand, the forearm, and the wrist. Usually the symptoms are worse at night than during the day. Forces and sustained positions of the wrist can cause pain. Driving for long periods, knitting, typing, or carrying packages can exacerbate the symptoms.

The syndrome is characterized by joint swelling, sensitivity on joint flexion and extension, and pain caused by maintenance of a fixed position. There is a sensory loss in the median nerve distribution and the thenar eminence may display atrophy. Carpal tunnel syndrome is caused by rheumatoid arthritis, malunion of the wrist fracture, tumors, diabetes mellitus, and occupational stress.

Steroid injections may be used for local treatment; however, these can cause additional trauma to the joint and require surgical intervention for release of pressure. Immobilization of the wrist in a neutral position may provide relief during the day. It is important to advise the patient to avoid activities that cause stress.

Volkmann's Ischemic Contracture

This debilitating condition of the upper extremity can occur directly after trauma or can result from swelling within restricting bandages or casts. Two thirds of the patients with Volkmann's ischemic contractures are under 30 years of age, and most are between the ages of 2 and 16 years.[29] The condition usually results from fractures of the humerus. Other causes include damage to the brachial or the axillary artery from gunshot wounds or from embolus, rupture, trauma, or pressure involving the forearm.

Ischemia is caused by swelling in the arm. Interference with circulation in the lower arm deprives all involved tissues of their blood supply. The rapid onset results in initial necrosis of tissue and progresses to fibrosis and contracture. The intrinsic muscles of the hand are affected by "glove anesthesia," and there is impaired nutrition of hand and forearm.[30]

The clinical picture reveals an adematous, cold, numb forearm; the hand is blanched and has a smooth, glossy appearance. The patient has difficulty moving his hand and has paralysis of the flexor, extensor, and intrinsic muscles of the hand along with loss of sensation. The arm muscles are tender, swollen, and hard over the forearm. Contractures may be present with flexion in the distal joints and extension in the proximal joints of the fingers. Extensors of the fingers may be functional; however, the patient may be limited to extending the fingers with wrist flexion because of tight flexor tendons. Median, ulnar, and radial nerves are involved, with the median nerve being most affected. Muscle atrophy occurs and the bones become osteoporotic. In children, bone growth is retarded and deformity is increased.

Medical treatment involves immediate removal of the restricting cast or bandages, reduction of the fracture, and release of the pressure causing the ischemia. Release of the nerves, nerve repair, and tendon and nerve transfers may be done along with excision of the necrotic areas and skin grafting. Because of the continuous initial progressive contracture, a splint is provided to maintain extension of the wrist and fingers.

Occupational Therapy

The role of the occupational therapist is to provide specific passive and active joint range of motion and strengthening exercises to aid the patient in regaining maximum use of the extremity. The therapist uses techniques to provide positioning to prevent deformity, to support maximum use of the hand and arm, and to encourage use of both extremities in assisted bimanual activity, and to offer counselling regarding acceptance of the appearance of the arm. The prognosis for restoration of function of the hand depends on the severity of the condition, the availability and feasibility of surgical procedures, and the motivation of the patient. He or she may be required to change hand dominance and to adapt to the functional and cosmetic aspects of the disability.

The activity program stresses maximum use of the involved extremity with specific grasping exercises to utilize the functional gains of surgery. In providing splints for finger traction, the therapist must pay attention to preventing cutaneous pressure areas because of decreased sensation.

The occupational therapist assists the patient in adapting to the use of one-handed activities, giving instructions in using the involved extremity as an assist in holding or carrying items, and in using gross arm motions in bilateral movements. The patient is also trained in coordination and use of the unaffected arm.

If surgical repair has been done to the tendons or nerves, the patient may require reeducation in functional movements, and splinting may be necessary to maintain the capacity to use the injured extremity. The occupational therapist must also encourage the patient to accept the condition and to deal with both the limited function and the appearance of the arm.

Summary

This chapter is designed to present an introduction to clinical occupational therapy principles, theories, approaches, and techniques used to provide functional restoration of persons disabled from disease or trauma. Beginning with the impact of disability on the individual lifestyle, material relates to the therapeutic use of activity, implications of physical, sensory, and perceptual deficits, and the effect of human and nonhuman environmental factors.

The value and effectiveness of the occupational therapy program depend on the ability of the therapist to determine the unique premorbid lifestyle and its meaning to the patient and to design the treatment program in collaboration with the patient, his or her level of ability, and his or her level of adjustment to temporary or permanent disability and its impact on the patient's goals.

Our ultimate proof of the level, value, and meaning of function in any of these areas is through the accomplishment of a task requiring the use of occupation or the engagement in functional activity. The value of the use of activity in occupational therapy depends on the therapist's knowledge of and ability to use activity and to use it therapeutically.

We can test and train for individual measures of specific needs for task accomplishments through repetitious drills restoring specific functions, but *a task is accomplished according to the integration of all functions involved.* Specific methods and chronology of evaluation and treatment are related to everyday activities such as self-care, educational, vocational, and avocational interests and needs. Attention is given to the developmental age and achievements of the patient at the time of trauma or the onset of disease;

these are important to both premorbid lifestyle and future planning.

Crucial to working with the patient with a physical disability is the recognition of psychological factors and their implications in intellectual, perceptual, social, and cognitive functioning. These aspects are included in the discussion of specific disabilities as recognized by the clinical signs while observing performance during the evaluation and treatment programs.

The patient knows the meaning of "ability to function," but as a disabled person, he or she must learn the meaning of "disability to function." As the patient learns both what he or she was and what he or she will become, the therapist sets the stage for attitudes by setting the environment to be conducive to functional performance. The patient makes choices regarding abilities and regarding the help he or she needs; these choices are based on lifestyle and priorities.

Occupational therapy theory and practice are based on *performance* as the major indicator of functional ability through evaluation and treatment procedures. Exercise should be correlated with activities of daily living, which then provide exercise in the accomplishment of the activity. A transition is made from the exercise to self-directed, purposeful activity.

In order to reach independence at any level, the disabled person must achieve enough control over the natural and the man-made environment to be able to achieve his or her goals with self-respect and satisfying achievement. Environmental factors play a large role in the new lifestyle the person may realistically plan; they must be a part of treatment goals and the program for appropriate discharge planning.

In the rehabilitation of a person with a permanent physical disability, the therapist aids him or her in progressing from "the sick role" to "the disabled role" in order to work toward functional, independent adjustment to the permanent disability.

Basic evaluation and treatment approaches should be supplemented with more specific techniques outlined both within this chapter and elsewhere in this text.

Whether or not the occupational therapist is a member of a formal team, collaboration with other programs and professionals is to the advantage of both the patient and the treatment personnel. To provide service to the patient with functional deficits of either a temporary or a permanent nature, the occupational therapist needs a variety of resources to gain comprehensive awareness of medical aspects, rehabilitation programs, settings, equipment, and personnel, organizations, and publications by and for consumers. In addition to gaining familiarity with medical publications, the therapist also gains valuable insight into the needs, concerns, interests, and activities of the patient (consumer) by participating in community programs designed by and for disabled people.

References

1. Rusk, H. A.: Rehabilitation Medicine, ed. 3. St. Louis: C. V. Mosby, 1971, p. 449.
2. Morris, A. F., and Brown, M.: Electronic training devices for hand rehabilitation. Am. J. Occup. Ther. 30:379, 1976.
3. Mossman, P. L.: A Problem-Oriented Approach to Stroke. Springfield IL: Charles C Thomas, 1976, p. 188.
4. Snook, J. H.: Spasticity reduction splint. Am. J. Occup. Ther. 33:648, 1979.
5. Eson, M. E., Yen, J. K., and Bourke, R. S.: Assessment of recovery from serious head injury. J. Neurol. Neurosurg. Psychiatry. 41:1036, 1978.
6. Rappaport, et al.: Disability rating scale for severe head trauma patients. Coma To Community—Third Annual Conference. Head Trauma Rehabilitation, 1980.
7. Jennett, B. and Teasdale, G.: Aspects of coma after severe head injury. Lancet. 23 April 1977:878.
8. Jennett, B. and Bond, M.: Assessment of outcome after severe brain damage: A practical scale. Lancet. 1 March 1975:482.
9. Eson, M. E., Yen, J. K., and Bourke, R. S.: Assessment of recovery from serious head injury. J. Neurol. Neurosurg. Psychiatry. 41:1036, 1978.
10. Stern, J. M.: Cranio-cerebral injured patients: Psychiatric clinical description. Proceedings of the Seventh International Congress of the World Federation of Occupational Therapists. Jerusalem, Israel: 1978, pp. 81–84.
11. Hagan, C., Malkmus, D., and Durham, P.: Communication Disorders Service: Rancho Los Amigos Hospital. Revised 11/15/74 by Malkmus, D., and Stenderup, K. Downey CA, 1972.
12. Brain, B., and Walton, J. N.: Brain's Diseases of the Nervous System. London: Oxford, 1969, p. 494.
13. Bannister, R.: Brain's Clinical Neurology, ed. 4. London: Oxford, 1973, p. 394.
14. *Ibid.*, pp. 392, 393.
15. *Ibid.*, p. 392.
16. Brain: Brain's Diseases, p. 525.
17. Long, C., and Lawton, E. B.: Functional significance of spinal cord lesion level. Arch. Phys. Med. Rehabil. 36:249, 1955.
18. Rusk: Rehabilitation Medicine, p. 321.
19. Bannister: Brain's Clinical Neurology, p. 347.
20. Brain: Brain's Disease, p. 814.
21. *Ibid.*, p. 595.
22. Alpers, B. J., and Mancall, E. L.: Clinical Neurology, ed. 6. Philadelphia: F. A. Davis, 1971, p. 598.
23. Brain: Brain's Diseases, p. 598.
24. Bannister: Brain's Clinical Neurology, p. 329.
25. Wilson, D. C.: Hilary. New York: McGraw-Hill, 1973.

26. Bannister: Brain's Clinical Neurology, p. 323.
27. Hollander, J. L., and McCarthy, D. J., Jr.: Arthritis and Allied Conditions. Philadelphia: Lea & Febiger, 1972, p. 603.
28. Licht, S. (ed.): Rehabilitation and Medicine. Baltimore: Waverly Press, 1968.
29. Boyes, J. H.: Bunnell's Surgery of the Hand, ed. 5. Philadelphia: J. B. Lippincott, 1970, p. 240.
30. *Ibid.*

Bibliography

A Guidebook to: The Minimum Federal Guidelines and Requirements for Accessible Design. U.S. Architectural and Transportation Barriers Compliance Board, 330 C Street, S.W., Room 1010, Washington DC 20202, 1981.

Abreu, B. C. (ed.): Physical Disabilities Manual. New York: Raven Press, 1981.

AOTA Publications Mart Catalog. Rockville MD, 1980.

Ayres, A. J.: Sensory Integration and the Child. Los Angeles: Western Psychological Services, 1979.

Basmajian, J. V. (ed.): Biofeedback: Principles and Practice for Clinicians. Baltimore: Williams & Wilkins, 1979.

Basmajian, J. V.: Therapeutic Exercise, ed. 3. Baltimore: Williams & Wilkins Co., 1978.

Blakiston's Gould Medical Dictionary, ed. 4. New York: McGraw-Hill, 1979.

Bobath, B.: Adult Hemiplegia: Evaluation and Treatment, ed. 2. London: Heinemann, 1978.

Brunnstrom, S.: Movement Therapy in Hemiplegia. New York: Harper & Row Publishers, 1970.

Buckwald, E.: Physical Rehabilitation for Daily Living. New York: McGraw-Hill, 1952.

Cave, E. F., Burke, J. F., and Boyd, R. J.: Trauma Management, Chicago: Year Book Medical Publishers, 1974, p. 269.

Critchley, M.: The Parietal Lobes. New York: Hafner Press, 1953.

CVA (Bibliography, standards of practice, resources). Rockville MD: AOTA.

Cynkin, S.: Occupational Therapy toward Health through Activities. Boston: Little Brown and Company, 1979.

DePalma, A. F.: The Management of Fractures and Dislocations, Vol. 1, ed. 2. Philadelphia: W. B. Saunders, 1970.

Dorland's Illustrated Medical Dictionary, ed. 26. Philadelphia: W. B. Saunders, 1981.

Diller, L., and Ben-Yishay, Y.: Studies in Cognition and Rehabilitation in Hemiplegia. Rehabilitation Monograph #50. New York: Behavioral Science, Institute of Rehabilitation Medicine, New York University Medical Centers, 1974.

Electronic Aids for the Severely Handicapped: Wheelchair Control Systems. Shreve OH: Prentke Romich Company, R.D. 2, Box 191.

Ehrlich, G. E. (ed.): Total Management of the Arthritis Patient. Philadelphia: J. B. Lippincott, 1975.

Farber, S. D., and Huss, J. A.: Sensorimotor Evaluation and Treatment Procedures, ed. 2. Indianapolis: Indiana University-Purdue University, 1974.

Field, E. V. (ed.): Multiple Sclerosis. Baltimore: University Park Press, 1977.

Flower, A., Naxon, E., Jones, R. E., and Mooney, V.: An occupational therapy program for chronic back pain. Am. J. Occup. Ther. 35:243, 1981.

Friedman, L. W.: The Psychological Rehabilitation of the Amputee. Springfield IL: Charles C Thomas, 1978.

Ford, J. R., and Duckworth, B.: Physical Management for the Quadriplegic Patient. Philadelphia: F. A. Davis, 1974.

Galbreaith, P.: What You Can Do for Yourself. New York: Drake, 1974.

Garrett, J. F., and Levine, E. S.: Psychological Practices with the Physically Disabled. New York: Columbia, 1973.

Gilbert, A. E.: You Can Do It From a Wheelchair. New Rochelle NY: Arlington House Publishers, 1974.

Gilfoyle, E. M., Grady, A. P., and Moore, J. C.: Children Adapt. New Jersey: Charles B. Slack, 1981.

Golden, Charles J.: Diagnosis and Rehabilitation in Clinical Neuropsychology. Springfield IL: Charles C Thomas, 1981.

Gruen, H., Medsger, T. A., and White, J. F.: Joint Protection Training for the Patient with Early Rheumatoid Arthritis. Basle, Switzerland: CIBA-GEIGY Ltd., 1980.

Gurgold, G. D., and Harden, D. M.: Assessing the driving potential of the handicapped. Am. J. Occup. Ther. 32:41, 1978.

Heilman, K. M., and Valenstein, E.: Clinical Neuropsychology. New York/Oxford: Oxford University Press, 1979.

Heiniger, M. C., and Randolph, S. L.: Neurophysiological Concepts in Human Behavior: The Tree of Learning. St. Louis MO: C. V. Mosby, 1981.

Jebsen, R. H., Taylor, N., Trieschmann, R. B., Trotter, M. J., and Howard, L. A.: An objective and standardized test of hand function. Arch. Phys. Med. Rehabil. June: 311, 1969.

Jennett, B., and Teasdale, G.: Aspects of coma after severe head injury. Lancet. April 23, 1977, 878.

Jennett, B., and Teasdale, G.: Management of Head Injuries. Philadelphia: F. A. Davis, 1981.

Jones, M. S.: An Approach to Occupational Therapy, ed. 3. Boston: Butterworths, 1977.

Kessler, H. H.: Disability—Determination and Evaluation. Philadelphia: Lea & Febiger, 1970.

Krusen, F. H., Kottke, F., and Ellwood, P. M.: Handbook of Physical Medicine and Rehabilitation, ed. 2. Philadelphia: W. B. Saunders, 1971.

Lucci, J. A.: Occupational Therapy Case Studies. Flushing NY: Medical Examination Publishing Company, Inc., 1977.

Marquit, S.: Psychological Factors in the Management of Parkinson's Disease. Miami FL: National Parkinson Foundation, Inc.

Licht, S. (ed.): Stroke and its Rehabilitation. Baltimore: Waverly Press, 1975.

MacDonald, E. M.: Occupational Therapy in Rehabilitation, ed. 2. London: Bailliere, Tindall, and Cox, 1976.

Malick, M. H., and Meyer, C. M. H.: Manual on Management of the Quadriplegic Upper Extremity. Pittsburgh: Harmarville Rehabilitation Center, 1978.

May, E. E., Waggoner, N. R., and Hotte, E. B.: Independent Living for the Handicapped and the Elderly. Boston: Houghton Mifflin, 1974.

Morris, A. F., and Brown, M.: Electronic training devices for hand rehabilitation. Am. J. Occup. Ther. 30:376, 1976.

Moskowitz, R. W.: Clinical Rheumatology. Philadelphia: Lea & Febiger, 1975.

Najenson, T., Groswasser, Z., Mendelson, L., and Hackett, P.: Rehabilitation outcome of brain damaged patients after severe head injury. International Rehabil. Med. 2:17, 1980.

Newcombe, F., Brooks, N., and Baddley, A.: Rehabilitation after brain damage: An overview. International Rehabil. Med. 2:133, 1980.

Nichols, P. J. R.: Rehabilitation Medicine: The Management of Physical Disabilities, ed. 2. Woburn MA: Butterworth, 1980.

O'Brien, M. T., and Pallett, P. J.: Total Care of the Stroke Patient. Boston: Little, Brown and Company, 1978.

O'Sullivan, S. B., Cullen, K. E., and Schmitz, T. J.: Physical Rehabilitation: Evaluation and Treatment Procedures. Philadelphia: F. A. Davis, 1981.

Occupational Therapy in the Care of Spinal Pain Patients. Downey CA: Professional Staff Association, Rancho Los Amigos Hospital, Inc.

Olszowy, D. R.: Horticulture for the Disabled and Disadvantaged. Springfield IL: Charles C Thomas, 1978.

Palmer, M. L.: Manual for Functional Training. Philadelphia: F. A. Davis, 1980.

Payton, O. D., Hirt, S., and Newton, R. A.: Scientific Bases for Neurophysiological Approaches to Therapeutic Exercise. Philadelphia: F. A. Davis, 1977.

Pedretti, L. W.: Occupational Therapy Practice Skills for Physical Dysfunction. St. Louis MO: C. V. Mosby, 1981.

Proceedings of the Seventh International Congress of the World Federation of Occupational Therapists. "Occupational therapists in a changing world." Jerusalem, Israel, 1979.

Product Inventory of Hardware, Equipment and Appliances for Barrier-Free Design, ed. 2. Minneapolis MN: National Handicap Housing Institute, Inc., 1981.

Reed, K., and Sanderson, S. R.: Concepts of Occupational Therapy. Baltimore: Williams & Wilkins, 1980.

Redford, J. B. (ed.): Orthotics Etcetera, ed. 2. Baltimore: Williams & Wilkins, 1980.

Report on Neuromuscular Re-education (biofeedback). Minneapolis: Medgeneral (Dave Howson), 1976.

Rogers, J. C., and Figone, J. J.: The avocational pursuits of rehabilitants with traumatic quadriplegia. Am. J. Occup. Ther. 32:571, 1978.

Shafer, R.: Occupational therapy for lower extremity problems. Am. J. Occup. Ther. 28:99, 1974.

Simon, J. I.: Emotional aspects of physical disability. Am. J. Occup. Ther. 25:408, 1971.

Trombly, C., and Scott, A.: Occupational Therapy for Physical Dysfunction. Baltimore: Williams & Wilkins, 1977.

Uniform Terminology System for Reporting Occupational Therapy Services. Rockville MD: American Occupational Therapy Association.

Wilson, D. J., McKenzie, M. W., and Barber, L. M.: Spinal Cord Injury: A Treatment Guide for Occupational Therapists. Thorofare NJ: Charles B. Slack, 1974.

Wittmeyer, M., and Barrett, J. E.: Housing Accessibility Checklist. Seattle WA: Univeristy of Washington, 1980.

Wittmeyer, M. B., and Stolov, W. C.: Educating wheelchair patients on home architectural barriers. Am. J. Occup. Ther. 32:557, 1978.

Wright, B. A.: Physical Disability—A Psychological Approach. New York: Harper & Row, 1960.

Wright, G. N.: Total Rehabilitation. Boston: Little Brown & Co., 1980.

Consumer Education

A Source Book: Rehabilitating the Person with Spinal Cord Injury (Superintendent of Documents, United States Printing Office, Washington DC 20402)

Accent on Living (Accent on Living, Inc., P.O. Box 726, Gillum Road and High Drive, Bloomington IL 61701)

Active Handicapped (The Active Handicapped, Inc., 526 Aurora Avenue, Metairie LA 70005)

After a Stroke . . . Patient and Family Guide (Harmarville Rehabilitation Center, P.O. 11460, Guys Run Road, Pittsburgh PA 15238)

Brooks, J. S., Dasher, C. W., and Kelly, P. A.: Low Back Pain: An Instructional Guide for Patients with Low Back Pain. Birmingham AL: University of Alabama Hospitals.

Corbet, B.: Options: Spinal Cord Injury and the Future. Newton Upper Falls MA 02164: National Spinal Cord Injury Foundation, 1980.

Cousins, N.: Anatomy of an Illness as Perceived by the Patient. New York: W. W. Norton and Company, 1979.

Disabled USA (The President's Committee on Employment of the Handicapped, Washington DC 20210)

Do It Yourself Again. Self-help Devices for the Stroke Patient (American Heart Association, New York NY 10010)

Duvoisin, R. C.: Parkinson's Disease: A Guide for Patient and Family. New York: Raven Press, 1978.

Forsythe, E.: Living with Multiple Sclerosis. Salem NH: Faber & Faber, 1979.

Handbook of Care for Paraplegics and Quadriplegics (English and Spanish. National Spinal Cord Injury Foundation, Newton Upper Falls MA 02164)

Haviland, N., Kamil-Miller, L., and Sliwa, J.: A Workbook for Consumers with Rheumatoid Arthritis. Rockville MD: American Occupational Therapy Association, 1978.

Home Care Programs in Arthritis: A Manual for Patients (Allied Health Professions of The Arthritis Foundation, Suite 1101, 3400 Peachtree Street, N.E., Atlanta GA 30326)

Jay, P.: Help Yourselves: A Handbook for Hemiplegics and Their Families. New York NY: State Mutual Books & Periodical Service Ltd., 1979.

Laurie, G. (ed.): Respiratory Rehabilitation and Post-Polio Aging Problems. Rehabil. Gaz. (1980) 23:3–15.

Lear, M. W.: Heartsounds. New York: Simon and Schuster, 1980.

Paraplegia Life (National Spinal Cord Injury Foundation, Newton Upper Falls MA 02164)

Paraplegia News (Paralyzed Veterans of America, 4350 East-West Highway, Suite 9001, Bethesda MD 20814)

Principles of Joint Protection and Work Simplification for Persons with Rheumatoid Arthritis. Judy Feinberg: Occupational Therapy Department, Indiana University School of Medicine and The Indiana University Arthritis Center, Bloomington IN

Rehabilitation of Head Injured Adult—A Family Guide. (Professional Staff Association, Rancho Los Amigos Hospital, Inc., 7413 Golondrinas Street, Downey CA 90242)

Report. (National Center for a Barrier Free Environment, 8401 Connecticut Avenue, Washington DC 20015)

Russell, H.: The Best Years of My Life. Middlebury VT: Paul S. Eriksson, 1981.

Rehabilitation Gazette (Rehabilitation Gazette, 4502 Maryland Avenue, St. Louis MO 63108)

Rehabilitation Guide. (Rehabilitation Institute of Chicago, Research Dissemination, 345 East Superior Street, Chicago IL 60611)

Rehabilitation World. (U.S. J. International Rehab. Information, 20 West 40th Street, New York NY 10018)

Self-Help Manual for Patients with Arthritis (Allied Health Professions of The Arthritis Foundation, Suite 1101, 3400 Peachtree Road, N.E., Atlanta GA 30326)

The Source Book for the Disabled. Hale, G. (ed.) New York: Paddington Press Ltd., 1979.

The Squeaky Wheel (National Paraplegia Foundation, 333 North Michigan Avenue, Chicago IL 60601)

Watkins, R. A., and Robinson, D.: Joint Preservation Techniques for Patients with Rheumatoid Arthritis. Chicago IL: Rehabilitation Institute of Chicago.

What the Patient Should Know about Parkinson's Disease: General Exercise Program and Suggestions for the Parkinson Patient. (National Parkinson's Foundation, Inc., Miami, FL 33136)

Wilson, D. C. Hilary. New York: McGraw-Hill, 1975.

Work Simplification. (Occupational Therapy Department, Bellin Memorial Hospital, 744 South Webster Avenue, Green Bay, WI 54305)

You and Your New Hip (Occupational Therapy Department, University Hospitals of Cleveland, Cleveland OH)

Journals and Periodicals

Access Information Bulletin. National Center for a Barrier Free Environment.

American Journal of Occupational Therapy.

American Journal of Physical Medicine.

American Rehabilitation.

Archives of Physical Medicine and Rehabilitation.

Arthritis and Rheumatism.

Bulletin of Prosthetics Research.

Inter-clinic Information Bulletin.

International Rehabilitation Medicine.

Journal of Rehabilitation.

Orthotics and Prosthetics.

Prosthetics and Orthotics International.

Organizations

American Academy of Physical Medicine and Rehabilitation
30 North Michigan Avenue
Suite 922
Chicago, Illinois 60602

American Congress of Rehabilitation Medicine
30 North Michigan Avenue
Chicago, Illinois 60602

American Heart Association
7320 Greenville Avenue
Dallas, Texas 75231

American Physical Therapy Association
1156 15th Street, N.W.
Washington, DC 20005

American Speech and Hearing Association
10801 Rockville Pike
Rockville, Maryland 20852

Architectural and Transportation Barriers
Compliance Board
330 C Street, S.W.
Washington DC 20201

Arthritis Foundation
Suite 1101
3400 Peachtree Road, N.E.
Atlanta, Georgia 30326

Association for the Severely Handicapped
7010 Roosevelt Way, N.E.
Seattle, Washington 98115

Careers for the Disabled
261 Madison Avenue
Suite 1102
New York, New York 10016

Clearinghouse on the Handicapped
Office of Special Education and Rehabilitative Services
U.S. Department of Education
Room 3106 Switzer Building
Washington, DC 20202

Disability Rights Center, Inc.
1346 Connecticut Avenue
Room 1124
Washington, DC 20036

Georgia Warm Springs Foundation
122 East 42nd Street
New York, New York 10017

Goodwill Industries of America, Inc.
9200 Wisconsin Avenue
Washington, DC 20014

Housing and Urban Development Programs
Housing and Urban Development Building
451 Seventh Street, S.W.
Washington, DC 20410

International Center for the Disabled
340 East 24th Street
New York, New York 10010

International Rehabilitation Medicine Association
Administration Secretariat
P.O. Box 146
CH-4011 Basle, Switzerland
Muscular Dystrophy Association of America, Inc.
810 Seventh Avenue
New York, New York 10019
Myasthenia Gravis Foundation, Inc.
15 East 26th Street
New York, New York 10010
National Amputee Foundation
12-45 150th Street
Whitestone, New York 11357
National Center for Law and the Handicapped
1235 North Eddy Street
South Bend, Indiana 46617
National Easter Seal Society
2023 West Ogden Avenue
Chicago, Illinois 60612
National Handicapped Sports and Recreation Association
Capitol Hill Station
P.O. Box 18664
Denver, Colorado 80218
National Head Injury Foundation
280 Singletary Lane
Framingham, Massachusetts 01701
National Library Service for the Blind and Physically
Handicapped
Library of Congress
1291 Taylor Street, N.W.
Washington, DC 20542
National Multiple Sclerosis Society
205 East 42nd Street
New York, New York 10017
National Parkinson Foundation, Inc.
1501 Northwest 9th Avenue
Miami, Florida 33136
National Recreation and Park Association
1601 North Kent Street
Arlington, Virginia 22209

National Rehabilitation Association
1522 K Street, N.W.
Washington, DC 20005
National Rehabilitation Information Center
4407 Eighth Street, N.E.
The Catholic University of America
Washington, DC 20017
National Spinal Cord Injury Foundation
369 Elliot Street
Newton Upper Falls, Massachusetts 02164
Office for Handicapped Individuals
200 Independence Avenue, S.W.
Room 338D
Washington, DC
Paralyzed Veterans of America
4350 East-West Highway
Suite 900
Bethesda, Maryland 20814
President's Committee on Employment of the
Handicapped
Washington, DC 20210
Rehabilitation International
432 Park Avenue South
New York, New York 10016
World Health Organization
Geneva 27 Switzerland

Acknowledgments

Sincere appreciation to the administration and staff of Harmarville Rehabilitation Center, and particular thanks to the members of the Occupational Therapy Department for their patience and encouragement during this writing. My thanks also go to Ed Collins and Ron Gregory for taking photographs and to the patients who were willing to be photographed. Alice Kuller, Librarian at Harmarville Rehabilitation Center, provided immeasureable assistance with the references for this chapter, and Evelyn Barto, Pat Curran, and Elinor G. Spencer have my thanks for their assistance with editing and typing the manuscript.

CHAPTER 23

Functional Restoration— Human Sexuality

Marianne Rozycka Dahl

Sexuality is becoming increasingly recognized and accepted as a major component of the human personality. This recognition has led to an acute awareness by health professionals of their responsibility to deal directly with the sexuality of their clients.

The subject of human sexuality encompasses a complex and subtle blend of the biological, psychological, social, and interpersonal aspects of being either a man or a woman. Some physiological function and anatomical structure distinguish male from female (Tables 23-1 and 23-2).

Family responsibilities and other life-roles are influenced by sex. Clothing and the way it is worn reflects sexuality. Even the choice of friends and leisure time activity may be affected by one's sex.

The way we choose to communicate, satisfy, and deal with our sexuality is based upon development of a sexual identity. Freud explored the role and significance of sex in human life.[1] His concept of progression through psychosexual stages was broadened by Erikson in his theories of ego development.[2] Psychosexual theory can be a useful guide in better understanding the subtle interplay of sexuality and

Table 23-1 *Female Sexual Response Cycle*

	Able-Bodied Female	*Disabled Female*
Wall of vagina	Moistens	±
Clitoris	Swells	Swells ±
Labia	Swells and opens	Swells ±
Uterus	Contracts	±
Inner $^2/_3$ of vagina	Expands	±
Outer $^1/_3$ of vagina	Contracts	±
Nipples	Erect	Erect
Muscles	Tense, spasms	Tense, spasms
Breasts	Swell	Swell
Breathing	Increases	Increases
Pulse	Increases	Increases
Blood pressure	Increases	Increases
Skin of trunk, neck face	Sex flush	Sex flush

Adapted from Cole, T., by Glass, D. D.: Sexuality and the spinal cord injured patient. In Oaks, W. W., Melchiode, G. A., and Fisher, I. (eds.): Sex and the Life Cycle. New York: Grune & Stratton, 1976, p. 187. Reprinted with permission.

Table 23-2 *Male Sexual Response Cycle*

	Able-Bodied Male	Disabled Male
Penis	Erects	Erects ±
Skin of scrotum	Tenses	Tenses ±
Testes	Elevate in scrotum	Elevate in scrotum ±
Emission	Yes	No ±
Ejaculation	Yes	No ±
Nipples	Erect	Erect
Muscles	Tense, spasms	Tense, spasms
Breathing rate	Increases	Increases
Pulse	Increases	Increases
Blood pressure	Increases	Increases
Skin of trunk, neck, face	Sex flush	Sex flush

Adapted from Cole, T., by Glass, D. D.: Sexuality and the spinal cord injured patient. In Oaks, W. W., Melchiode, G. A., and Fisher, I. (eds.): Sex and the Life Cycle. New York: Grune & Stratton, 1976, p. 187. Reprinted with permission.

personality development. Belmont states "The particular nature and quality of adult sexual behavior will be heavily determined by what happens during the child's progression through the psychosexual stages."[3]

The Masters and Johnson studies and those of Kinsey highlighted the impact of human feelings on adequacy of sexual expression and communication.[4,5,6] Until recently the professional who worked with the disabled person tended to avoid dealing with the client's sexuality because the professional was inhibited by lack of knowledge, by personal uneasiness with his or her own sexuality, or by myths and taboos concerning the sexuality of the disabled.[7] Religious beliefs and socioeconomic and ethnic influences also have an impact on a person's sexual attitudes and knowledge.

Based on work done at the University of Min-

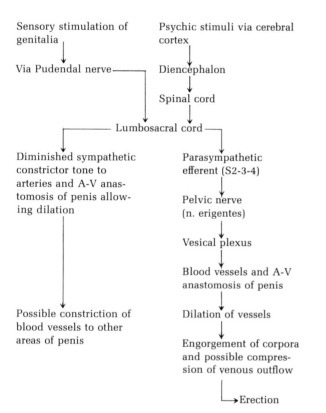

Figure 23-1. Multisystems involved in the physiological mechanism of erection. From Glass, D. D.: Sexuality and the spinal cord injured patient. In Oaks, W. W., Melchiode, G. A., and Fisher, I. (eds.): Sex and the Life Cycle. New York: Grune & Stratton, 1976, p. 185. Reprinted with permission.

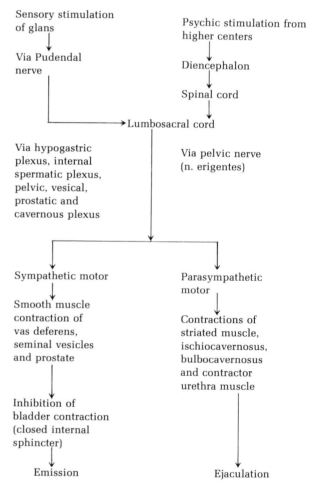

Figure 23-2. Multisystems involved in the physiological mechanism of ejaculation. From Glass, D. D.: Sexuality and the spinal cord injured patient. In Oaks, W. W., Melchiode, G. A., and Fisher, I. (eds.): Sex and the Life Cycle. New York: Grune & Stratton, 1976, p. 186. Reprinted with permission.

Table 23-3 Suggested approach in dealing with the client's sexual problems.

A traditional approach	because	but	An approach for the occupational therapist	because
My responsibility is to help people achieve a better state of health. I'll concentrate on that.	Sex is separate from health. If the disabled person wants to know about sex he/she will find out himself/herself.	Perhaps no one will inform the disabled person about his/her sexual potential.	Initiate discussion and endorse sexuality. Be aware of physiological mechanisms of sex (see Tables 23-1 and 23-2 and Figs. 23-1 and 23-2). Recognize that it is difficult for many people to deal directly with explicit sexuality. Know when to refer a client to an appropriate team member for specific sexual information.	Healthy sexuality is a part of total rehabilitation and all team members are responsible for helping the client achieve a better state of health.
Rehabilitation facilities are designed to promote constant interaction sometimes with loss of privacy.	Most learning is done better by interacting with others rather than alone.	Some activities require privacy for learning to occur.	Be sensitive to privacy needs. Don't overreact to human sexual behavior should it occur, e.g., erection during ADL training. When appropriate, recommend opportunity for aloneness, e.g., hospital pass for home visit.	Anxiety-free practice promotes integration.
Sex can be distracting—concentrating a disabled person's attention on rehabilitation activity will avoid these distractions.	Sexuality is not important to the rehabilitation process anyway. If sexuality is recognized, it may become unmanageable.	Sex is a natural part of life and awareness of sexuality belongs in the rehabilitation process.	Encourage sexual awareness and responsibility as part of ADL. Teach skills in attractive dressing and grooming techniques including application of cosmetics, after-shave, and so forth. Teach skills in relating to others as appropriate to the client's need and lifestyle, e.g., role-playing slow dancing with a client with loss of coordination who plans to attend school dance on weekend with his girlfriend.	Learning of social sexual skill should be expected and encouraged just as people are expected to learn other ADL.

Table 23-3 (continued)

A traditional approach	because	but	An approach for the occupational therapist	because
Should a disabled person demonstrate socially unacceptable sexual behaviors according to hospital standards he/she may be reprimanded or shunned. If it continues he/she may even be discharged.	Hospital personnel should maintain "proper" sex model.	Ignoring or reprimanding a disabled person for testing a self-image of a whole person may communicate that he/she is incompetent and not okay.	Avoid overreacting to behavior with sexual content. Objectively share information with team members so that the behavior can be understood. Deal with the client as you would like to be dealt with. Encourage the client to discuss feelings with appropriate team members.	Methods of expressing sexuality can be developed by problem solving rather than punishment.
Many medical, nursing, and therapy procedures must be done no matter how personal they may seem to me.	In a professional relationship objectivity is ensured and I really don't have sexual feelings toward my clients.	Denying our own sexual feelings could inhibit them in our clients.	Deal with personal aspects of therapy openly and sincerely. Be aware of your effect on a client especially during dressing or bathing training. Acknowledge your client's effect on you. Realize that nonverbal communication can give the client input as to his/her own sexuality.	Sexuality is an early concern of many disabled people. Acknowledging feelings will endorse honesty and responsibility.
When appropriate I answer questions about sexual capacity or sexual attrativeness.	If I initiate an awareness of sexuality, the client may get the wrong idea and will get hurt.	Some people are shy and need "permission" to speak freely about sexuality.	Recognize that we are all sexual beings. Be aware of the possibility of sexual response for the disabled (see Tables 23-1, 23-2, and 23-4). Anticipate sexual concerns and be prepared either to deal directly or to refer to another for help. Take the responsibility to become comfortable with your own sexuality.	The disabled person will appreciate your sensitivity and concern. When sexuality is discussed, new disability may be avoided.

Adapted from Cole, T. M.: Mimeographed material from Program in Human Sexuality. University of Minnesota Medical Center, Minneapolis.

Table 23-4 *Diagnostic significance of sexual functions.*

Type of lesion	Erection	Ejaculation	Orgasm
Complete upper motor neuron lesion	Frequent (93%) Always only reflexogenic	Extremely rare (4%) Always following reflexogenic erection	Absent
Incomplete upper motor neuron lesion	Most frequent (99%) Reflexogenic (80%) Combined with psychogenic (19%)	Less infrequent (32%) More often following reflexogenic erections (74%) than psychogenic erections (26%)	Present with ejaculation
Complete lower motor neuron lesion	Infrequent (26%) Always only psychogenic	Infrequent (18%) Always following psychogenic erections	Present with emission
Incomplete lower motor neuron lesion	Frequent (90%) Psychogenic combined with reflexogenic	Frequent (70%) Following psychogenic and reflexogenic erections	Present with ejaculation

Adapted from Bors, E., and Comaar, A. E., by Glass, D. D.: Sexuality and the spinal cord injured patient. In Oaks, W. W., Melchoide, G. A., and Fisher, I. (eds.): Sex and the Life Cycle. New York: Grune & Stratton, 1976, p. 184. Reprinted with permission.

nesota School of Medicine, Cole has made the following assumptions:[8]

1. Sexual concerns do exist for the disabled person.

2. It may require more than personal experience or opinion to deal with these concerns.

3. A person's ability to solve sexual problems is often hindred by biases, myths, taboos, and overreaction to sexual information or by the same attitudes on the part of the professional.

Many people, including health professionals, find difficulty in dealing directly with explicit sexuality. It is important, however, that the occupational therapist foster a recognition of the fact that all have sexuality and initiate discussion of these aspects of life. By recognizing the sexual components of medical, social, psychological, and vocational aspects of physical disability, the occupational therapist becomes better prepared to assist the disabled with sexual adaptation. Table 23-3 suggests an approach for the occupational therapist in dealing with patients with sexual problems.

There are many resources available to the therapist who wishes to develop an increased understanding of his or her own attitudes and sexuality, and by accepting one's own sexual self be able to deal more effectively with the sexual self of the client. The bibliography is designed to be a guide and reference source for those concerned with obtaining more information regarding sexuality.

References

1. Freud, S.: Three essays on the theory of sexuality, 1905. In Strachey, J. (ed.): The Standard Edition of the Complete Psychological Works of Sigmund Freud. London: Hogarth Press, 1953, Vol. 7, pp. 125–245.
2. Erikson, E.: Childhood and Society, ed. 2. New York: W. W. Norton Co., 1963, p. 445.
3. Belmont, H. S.: Psychodynamic understanding of sexual development in childhood. In Oaks, W. W., Melchiode, G. A., and Fisher, I. (eds.): Sex and the Life Cycle. New York: Grune & Stratton, Inc., 1976, pp. 29–37.
4. Masters, W. H., and Johnson, V. E.: Human Sexual Response. Boston: Little, Brown, Co., 1966, p. 366.
5. Kinsey, A. C., et al.: Sexual Behavior in Human Female. Philadelphia: W. B. Saunders Co., 1953, p. 842.
6. Kinsey, A. C., et al.: Sexual Behavior in Human Male. Philadelphia: W. B. Saunders Co., 1948, p. 804.
7. Cole, T. M., Chilgren, R., and Rosenberg, P.: A new programme of sex education and counselling for spinal cord injured adults and health care professionals. Paraplegia 11:111–124, 1973.
8. Cole, T. M.: Mimeograph outline. Program in Human Sexuality, University of Minnesota Medical School. Sexual Attitude Reassessment Workshop: Moss Rehabilitation Hospital, Philadelphia, 1972.

Bibliography

Abram, H. S., et al.: Sexual function in patients with chronic renal failure. J. Nerv. Ment. Dis. 160:220–226, 1975.
Andreason, N. J., et al.: Long-term adjustment and adaptation mechanisms in severely burned adults. J. Nerv. Ment. Dis. 154:352–362, 1972.
Birnbaum, M. D., et al.: Psychosexual aspects of endocrine disorders. Med. Aspects Hum. Sexuality 7:134–150, 1973.
Chipouras, S., et al.: Who Cares? A Handbook on Sex Education and Counseling Services for Disabled People. Washington, DC: George Washington University, 1979.

Cole, T.: Touching. Sound film available through Multimedia Resource Center, P.O. Box 439, San Francisco CA 94102. 1971.

Cole, T.: Just What Can You Do? Sound film available through Multimedia Center, P.O. Box 439, San Francisco CA 94102. 1971.

Comfort, A.: Sexuality in old age. J. Am. Geriatr. Soc. 22:440–442, 1974.

De Leon, G., et al.: Heroin addiction—its relation to sexual behavior and sexual experience. J. Abnorm. Psychol. 81:36–38, 1973.

Dlin, D. M., and Pertman, A.: Sex after ileostomy and colostomy. Med. Aspects Hum. Sexuality 6:32, 1972.

Johnson, W.: Sex Education and Counseling of Special Groups: The Mentally and Physically Handicapped, Ill and Elderly, Springfield IL: Charles C Thomas, 1975.

Lemere, F., et al.: Alcohol induced sexual impotence. Am. J. Psychiatry 130:212–213, 1973.

Manson, M. P., et al.: Some psychological findings in the rehabilitation of amputees. J. Clin. Psychol. 9:65–66, 1953.

Masur, F. T.: Resumption of Sexual Activity Following Myocardial Infarction. Sexuality and Disability 2:98–114, Summer 1979.

Meyerowitz, J. H.: Sex and the mentally retarded. Med. Aspects Hum. Sexuality 5:94–118, 1971.

Mooney, T. O., et al: Sexual options for paraplegics and quadriplegics. Boston: Little, Brown, Co., 1975.

Rosenblum, J. A.: Human sexuality and the cerebral cortex. Fid. Nerv. Sys. 35:268–271, 1974.

Sexuality Today Newsletter, Atcom, Inc., New York, 1981.

Sidman, J. M.: Sexual functioning and the physically disabled adult. Am. J. Occup. Ther. 31:81–85, 1977.

Wagner, N.: Sexual activity and the cardiac patient. In Green, R. (ed.): Human Sexuality: A Healthy Practitioner's Text. Baltimore: Williams & Wilkins, 1975.

Weiss, A. J., et al.: Sexual adjustment, identification and attitudes of patients with myelopathy. Arch. Phys. Med. 47:245–250, 1966.

Wlig, E. H.: Counseling the adult aphasic for sexual readjustment. Rehabil. Counsel. Bull. 17:110–119, 1973.

CHAPTER 24

Functional Restoration—
Upper Extremity
Orthotics *Maude H. Malick*

Great strides have been made in the construction of orthotics for the upper extremities using plastic materials as a result of the NASA (National Aeronautics and Space Administration) programs. Reliability in dynamic splinting has increased as a result of the greater sophistication in electronics and external power sources. This is true not only in the United States but also in Europe, South Africa, and Australia. Since low temperature plastic materials are remoldable, splints can be easily constructed or adjusted while the patient waits. Many splints can be custom designed, constructed, fitted, and applied within an hour. Orthoplast, a transpolyisoprene material, allows the therapist to fabricate temporary progressive splinting with minimal effort. Orthotic principles that apply to the low temperature materials are the same as those applying to the metal or high temperature materials. Low temperature materials require more contour or reinforcement when rigidity is required.

A series of polycaprolactone materials, such as Polyform, Kay-Splint, Aquaplast, and Varioplast, are effective low-temperature materials. These materials can be handled easily if the molding temperature requirements are strictly adhered to. Static and dynamic splints can be constructed readily but should only be considered for 3 to 6 months of use. Laminated plastic, high temperature materials, and metal are indicated if splint (orthotic) requirements indicate longer wear. Where moving parts such as metal joints, hinges, and telescopic units are needed in the wrist-driven orthosis, they should be constructed and assembled by a qualified orthotist. A good example of this is the Engen telescopic reciprocal wrist orthosis which, in a modular fashion, utilizes laminated plastic, metal, and rods to make an effective orthosis for the quadriplegic patient.

When evaluating the orthotic requirements of the patient, careful analysis should be made of the forearm and hand to evaluate what stability is lacking and what motion is needed in order to perform functional tasks. Range of motion tests and functional motion tests should be used to evaluate strength, range, coordination, and sensory deficiencies, noting whether and where spasticity is present. When orthotic devices are indicated it is important to do the following:

1. Fully explain the forearm and hand evaluation to the patient and involve the patient in the design and selection of the orthosis.

453

2. Fabricate the orthosis so that it will be well fitted, designed, and constructed.
3. Begin use of the splint early in the treatment program and then discard the splint if it is no longer useful.

The therapist must always consider the psychological aspects of splinting. Patient acceptance may vary, but ease of acceptance can be greatly influenced by proper explanation of its necessity. The orthosis should meet functional requirements and be cosmetically acceptable. Comfort, stability, and value of the orthosis are probably the greatest factors in patient acceptance.

Initially the splint should be worn only under the therapist's supervision for short periods to be sure no pressure areas exist. Straps must be adequate and secure so that the orthosis retains its correct position. Slipping distally, with its accompanying misfit, is the greatest cause of pressure areas.

Most ADL activities are performed more usefully when the forearm and hand are in the best functional position. An orthosis provides the proper position, supports weakened muscles, and stabilizes joints. In most cases, the dominant hand, when affected, is splinted, but if both upper extremities are affected, bilateral orthoses may be considered. When shoulder and elbow function are impaired, overhead slings and balanced forearm orthosis (mobile arm supports) should be considered. The patient should be carefully trained with the orthosis and should be given written detailed instructions. The patient should be trained to put on and take off the orthosis and instructed about its proper fit and mechanics. Many simple assistive devices can be quickly constructed with the low temperature plastics on a temporary basis before those of a permanent nature are considered.

Orthotics of the Hand

Orthotics and splinting are often used interchangeably, especially in reference to the upper extremity. With the availability of low temperature plastics, the occupational therapist can readily make nearly any splint to meet the splint requirements of patients. Since the number of occupational therapists outnumber the orthotists 15 to 1, the responsibility for hand splinting largely falls to the occupational therapist.

The occupational therapist must assess or evaluate both the patient's affected hand and unaffected hand in order to determine the specific purpose of the splint and the parts to be splinted. The purpose of the splint determines whether the splint should be static or dynamic as well as the regimen in which it is to be used. All splints are a part of an overall patient management program.

Static splints may be protective, supportive, or corrective in their design. A static splint may be indicated to protect weak muscles from being stretched by providing the force to counteract a strong muscle group and in this way provide a functional balance while healing is taking place. The splint can support the hand, joint, or arch as a substitute for weak muscles, as in the case of arthritis. Corrective splinting can specifically position or force an involved joint or bone into correct or near correct alignment. Static splints have no movable parts and wherever possible should hold the involved forearm and hand in functional position.

All splints must be taken off at intervals and be a part of a maintenance exercise program. The splint and the patient's hand should be washed and dried, and the hand carefully replaced in the splint in the correct position. The therapist must always be aware of swelling or edema. Edema can be due to constriction of the splint or its strap. Prolonged static splinting can cause immobility of joints. The patient should be encouraged to use the splinted extremity as much as possible to maintain muscle tone and joint mobility. No splint should immobilize more joints in the hand than are specifically indicated by the evaluations.

All splints should be neat and constructed with careful craftsmanship. They should be lightweight, durable, cosmetically acceptable, washable, and carefully designed to avoid loss of the special properties of the thermoplastic material.

Choice of Splinting Materials

There is a wide variety of splinting materials available. Their varying properties must be understood in order to use them properly. They can be classified in four groups:
1. High temperature materials
2. Moderate temperature materials
3. Low temperature materials
4. No heat, or layered materials

In general, high temperature materials are best cut flat with hand or power tools such as a jigsaw; they should be formed on a plaster positive mold to avoid burning the patient. Low temperature and layered materials may be cut with a scissors; they do not require a mold and can be molded directly on a patient. All materials listed except the layered materials come in sheet form of various thicknesses. Application of the various materials is dependent upon their thickness and rigidity and the design of the splint. The less rigid materials will require more area and contour for support.

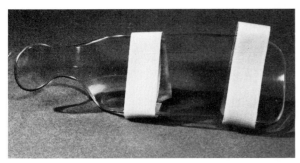

Figure 24-1. A simple palmar wrist cock-up splint made of Nyloplex provides an aesthetically appealing rigid wrist support. Nyloplex is a high temperature plastic that must be formed over a plaster mold.

High temperature materials include Nyloplex, Royalite, and Kydex. A splint of this type is shown in Figure 24-1. A moderate temperature material is high impact vinyl. Low temperature materials include Orthoplast, Polyform, San-Splint, Kay-Splint, SOS Plastazote, and Aquaplast. An example of no heat or layered material is Plaster of Paris bandage. In general, low temperature plastic materials are used for temporary progressive splinting and the high temperature plastic materials for long-term splint requirements.

Construction of the splint requires a thorough knowledge of the properties of the materials and the imagination of the occupational therapist. Patterns and models are guidelines only and should be modified to meet each patient's special requirements. Static splints should never be used longer than is physiologically indicated and should never be used if a dynamic splint would be equally effective. Splints should immobilize only the intended joints, leaving all the adjacent joints free to move. Static splints can do the following:

1. Prevent unwanted motion
2. Relieve pain
3. Prevent deformity and contractures
4. Substitute for weak or lost muscle function
5. Maintain a functional position for bone, muscle, tendon, or ligaments during a healing process

Physiological Considerations

It is requisite that each occupational therapist understand the bony skeleton, joint locations, and muscle insertions and functions of the forearm, wrist, and hand. The versatility of motion in the hand depends on the amount of motion in every joint above it. The shoulder, elbow, and wrist must be stable and functional in order to use the hand. Without shoulder motion, the hand is limited to the arc of motion in front of the body allowed by elbow motion. Without elbow motion, the hand is limited to the small arc in which the hand is placed by the wrist.

No matter what splint is used, the hand must be kept in functional position (Fig. 24-2). The functional position of the hand is as follows:

1. Wrist in 30 degree dorsiflexion
2. Normal transverse arch
3. Thumb in abduction and opposition with the pads of the four other fingers
4. Metacarpal and proximal interphalangeal joints in 45 degree flexion

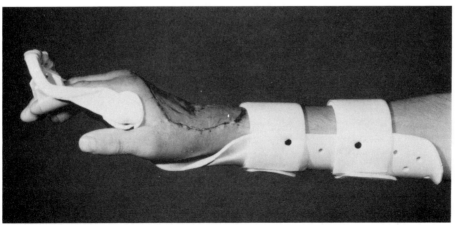

Figure 24-2. An orthoplast palmar splint used to maintain the wrist and interphalangeal joints in a functional position. A low profile dynamic outrigger was made to support the fingers. The straps were placed to avoid crossing the dorsum of the metacarpals.

Palmar Creases

The palmar surface of the hand is covered with thick, tough, and not very pliable skin. This lack of pliability accounts for a system of palmar creases, which allow for flexion and motion. These creases vary slightly on each individual and should act as guidelines for the designing and fitting of each splint. The distal palmar crease must not be impinged upon if full metacarpophalangeal (MCP) flexion is required. Likewise, the thenar crease must not be impinged upon if opposition is required. The wrist creases indicate the best location for a splint strap to stabilize the splint and prevent it from sliding forward.

Arches of the Hand

The palm of the hand is concave from side to side and also in its length. This shape is formed by three arches (see Fig. 24-3), which are of prime consideration when constructing a splint.

TRANSVERSE ARCH. The distal transverse arch is also called the metacarpal transverse arch. When the hand is at rest, the arch is slightly oblique. This arch is deepened when the hand is used functionally. The mobility of the fourth and fifth metacarpal within the arch contributes directly to the dexterity of all the fingers. If this metacarpal mobility is constricted, the functional motion of the fingers is directly impaired. Therefore the ability of the arch to deepen should always be considered when designing a splint. There should be freedom and some excursion considered if a palmar bar or support is designed into a splint.

The proper functioning of the thumb depends on the integrity of the transverse arch also. If the arch is depressed, the hand becomes flat and the thumb is unable to oppose the fingers. This opposition is only possible when there is some cupping of the palm, and when the curve of this arch is able to be increased voluntarily. Any weakness or damage to this arch

will impair the strength, mobility, and precision of the motion of the thumb.

LONGITUDINAL ARCH. The longitudinal arch follows the long lines of the phalanges and metacarpal and carpal bones at a slightly oblique angle and primarily involves the third finger. The mobility of the phalanges (fingers) directly affects the efficiency of the hand grasp.

PROXIMAL TRANSVERSE ARCH. The proximal tranverse (or carpal) arch is located at the wrist and is troughlike. It is formed by the annular ligaments and the carpal bones. It is this arch that provides the mechanical advantage to the tendons of the finger flexors by providing the fulcrum.

THE "BALL" AND FUNCTIONAL POSITION. The "ball" is the result of the combination of the three aches. It is located directly over the metacarpals which the three arches form. Often the ball is the best pivotal position of support for the hand in a splint. It can be noted when grasping an object. The splint must conform to this ball if it is to fit properly and allow normal function.

When the hand is in the position of function it maintains its arches, slight dorsiflexion of the wrist, and moderate flexion of all the joints of the fingers with the thumb in opposition. This position is maintained primarily by two key sets of joints: the wrist for the hand and the metacarpophalangeal joints for the fingers.

Requirements of a Well-Designed Splint

A well-designed and fitted splint should be individually constructed to support, reestablish, or facilitate normal coordinate movement, preserve normal physiological status of muscles, and prevent deformities. The splint should provide the patient with as func-

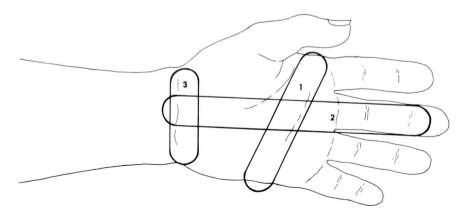

Figure 24-3. The three arches of the hand are of primary importance to hand function. (*1*) The transverse arch; (*2*) the longitudinal arch; and (*3*) the proximal transverse arch can be identified easily by the creases of the hand.

tional a hand as possible for performing as many activities as possible. This is best done when the splint conforms to the following characteristics:
1. Maintains normal arches
2. Retains normal axis of motion
3. Permits balanced function of unaffected muscles
4. Provides most practical prehension pattern
5. Allows maximal mobility with optimal stability
6. Frees palmar surface of hand and digits for greatest sensory perception.

Precautions Regarding Pressure Areas

Pressure areas can be created in splinting by the force placed on hand areas for correct positioning. Certain areas are prone to pressure, including the following:
1. Dorsum metacarpophalangeal joints with dorsal splint
2. Palmar (volar) surface of metacarpophalangeal joint of thumb and index finger with C-bar of opponens cuff
3. Palmar (volar) surface of distal joints of fingers with palmar resting-pan splints, especially with flexion contractures
4. Dorsal surface of the first phalanx of each finger with lumbrical bar
5. Head of ulna with the wrist strap of the dorsal opponens splint or the forearm section bar of the long opponens splint
6. Metacarpal joint of the thumb just distal to the head of the radius with the opponens bar
7. The center of the palm with the palmar (volar) surface of a wrist cock-up, especially when there is wrist flexion contracture

Pressure areas can be avoided by correct splint designs which include the following:
1. Following contours of the normal hand and forearm
2. Placing minimal stretch on joints or muscles in deformed positions over a longer period rather than striving for immediate correction
3. Increasing splint surface area to distribute pressure and by using padding

General precautions include the following:
1. Design and modify splints individually in order to meet the needs and changes in each patient's extremity. The splint should be viewed systematically and reevaluated according to need, fit, and purpose.
2. Wear splints intermittently. The length of time is determined by the physician or therapist and usually is not more than 10 to 12 hours daily. Splints should be worn only as long as they are performing a function.

3. Avoid tight encircling straps to prevent constrictions. There should be no blanched areas where circulation is decreased.
4. Avoid pressure areas over bony prominences.
5. Avoid making too short a forearm section because this will provide inadequate leverage. Conversely, too long a forearm section will impinge on elbow joint (and limit flexion). A good general rule is for the forearm section to be two thirds the length of the forearm. The splint should be checked when the patient is seated.
6. Fit the palmar piece over the metacarpal transverse arch accurately and allow the metacarpal joints to flex to a right angle.
7. Contour sides of finger, thumb, and platform splints to follow the natural curve of the digits. Metacarpal and proximal interphalangeal joints should be flexed to about 15 to 45 degrees. Avoid positions which would lead to hyperextension of finger joints. The thumb should be held in a functional position of 45 degrees abduction and opposition.

Dynamic Splints
Purpose of Dynamic Splinting

Dynamic splinting is the application of a force on a moving part, which remains nearly constant as the part moves. Often it is called active splinting; this refers to the specific and directional mobility that the splint gives the joints by providing forces that substitute for absent muscle power. This joint mobility decreases adhesions, maintains joint function, and prevents ankylosis of the joint.

Dynamic splints must be designed and constructed carefully to provide specific traction with good directional control. Outriggers, which must be placed accurately and secured firmly to the body of the splint, often can be used (see Fig. 24-4). The stability and maintenance of splint position on the hand are of prime importance.

A large percentage of patients requiring dynamic splinting are seen in acute care hospitals following surgery or trauma to the forearm and hand and, subsequently, are seen as outpatients and in rehabilitation centers. Dynamic splints frequently are used to substitute for absent muscle power, to prevent contractures or impending contractures, to maintain balance, to promote rest, or to mobilize specific joints.

Splints may be required for the following reasons:
1. Skeletal substitution
   a. To aid in fracture alignment
   b. To support bones and joints having pathology
2. Muscle balance
   a. For paralyzed muscles

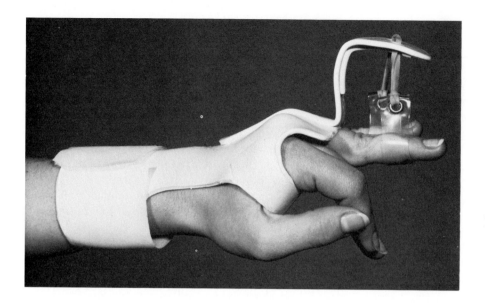

Figure 24-4. A dorsal splint with a lumbrical bar incorporating an outrigger. This applies an extension assist to the PIP joints by stabilizing the proximal phalanx.

b. For divided tendons or muscles
3. Joint motion
   a. To preserve joint motion
   b. To increase joint motion
4. Rest
   a. To promote wound healing of newly repaired structures
   b. To treat infection
   c. To relieve pain

The patient should be under close supervision of the physician and the occupational therapist. He or she should be encouraged to maintain and restore joint motion, follow the exercise program, and have the splint checked and adjusted regularly. The therapist must maintain an accurate joint measurement progress record.

Medical Principles

Good general medical principles must be considered in dynamic splinting. These principles include the following:
1. Moving muscles must be given an opposing, balancing force in order to maintain joint mobility and freely gliding tendons. A corrective force, often in the form of a finger cuff and rubber band, is necessary.
2. Movement prevents joint limitation, muscular atrophy, and deformity such as ankylosis.
3. Joints never should be immobilized needlessly.
4. Where there are injuries on the *flexor* surface, the wrist and fingers should be placed in flexion.
5. Where there are injuries in the *extensor* surface, the wrist and fingers should be placed in a neutral (resting) position.

6. Whenever possible, the position of function should be maintained prior to the application of any dynamic unit.
7. The hand should be elevated in the presence of edema since edema causes fibrosis and prevents function. The edema should be reduced as quickly as possible so that early motion can be encouraged and the movement in the uninvolved parts of the hand maintained.
8. Construction of straps that constrict venous return should not be used. Excessive tension of circular straps causes edema and increases the danger of ischemic contractures.

Static Base of the Dynamic Splint

The static base of the dynamic splint is of primary importance in all splinting. This base is the secured (anchored) foundation upon which all the support and moving parts rely. The static base of the splint does the following:
1. Provides foundation for proper (functional) alignment of joints
2. Provides a foundation to which the outrigger is attached with its traction components
3. Provides the foundation for a hinge joint
4. Aids in the relaxation of any spastic muscle
5. Allows tissues to adapt to their new position
6. Protects a newly repaired structure
7. Provides the support for proximal parts to allow increased function in distal joints or uninvolved parts
8. Aids in the positioning for edema control

Immobilization leads to joint stiffness; this must be remembered when constructing the static base of a splint.

Forces

Dynamic splinting should provide constant force over a long period of time in contrast to strong, short-term pressure. It operates according to a principle similar to the one an orthodontist uses in straightening teeth. Active motion can be encouraged, for the pumping effect of muscle contraction helps relieve edema and increases joint range of motion. Eight hours of light, steady tension are more successful than vigorous passive exercise for 20 minutes, especially where contractures are present. Progressive alteration to a static splint can draw out a contracture, and active dynamic splinting can aid in maintaining the correction.

Active dynamic splinting has a physiological effect as well, for when the muscles are moving they pump away stagnant fluids that wash out the toxins, and the tendons keep gliding and the joints keep moving. Thus, the formation of adhesions is prevented and the good mobility of joints can be maintained.

Directional Pull

In splinting when applying flexion traction to the fingers, the direction of the pull is of paramount importance. The pull on the fingers must not draw them straight down to the palm of the hand but rather obliquely aim them at the scaphoid bone or the base of the third metacarpal. In normal opening of the hands, fingers abduct; in normal closing of the hand, fingers adduct moving in an oblique arc of motion (see Fig. 24-5).

All the fingers, except the middle one (which may flex straight down), cross the palm obliquely from 10 to 30 degrees. The same line of pull or of direction should be maintained when finger traction is used. If the splint is incorrectly designed with the finger pul-

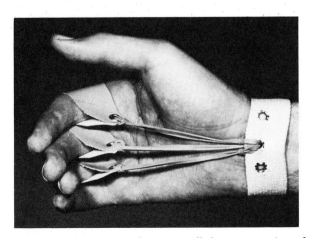

Figure 24-5. Dynamic flexion cuff demonstrating the correct line of pull.

led straight down in flexion, a serious ulnar deviation will appear when the patient tries to extend the fingers. If bone callus has formed, the deformity may need surgical intervention.

Exercise Program

Dynamic splints are used to maintain forces and position as well as to be a part of a graduated exercise and activity program. The combination of good dynamic splinting and an exercise program aids in good hand rehabilitation.

The exercise and activity program aids in the excursion of the joint and is good for maintaining the tone of the skin and improving the circulation to the injured part. A patient also can gain confidence by seeing to what degree the hand can be moved safely. Exercises are best performed by the patient following instructions from the therapist so as not to go beyond the point of pain.

When there is lack of sensation, one must be extremely careful to avoid pressure or increase resistance too rapidly in a traction program. Applying heat prior to the exercise program is often a great help in relaxation and facilitation of movement.

Instructions for the Patient

A patient should understand the purpose of the splint, its accurate positioning, and exactly what motion or movement or range is being sought. The therapist should explain functional anatomy of the hand to the patient. The therapist could demonstrate his or her own hand movement and range of motion so that the patient can understand the regimen more clearly and have confidence in it. The patient can use the unaffected hand to explore normal ranges of motion.

Careful instructions in the use of the dynamic splint are absolutely necessary and written instructions are imperative when a splint is given to the patient on an outpatient basis. The patient should be seen at least once a week to measure range of motion of hand joints. Adjustments must be made as gains are made in the mobilization of joints and as muscle power increases. The regimen is successful when there is improvement, little or no pain, and minimal edema. One must be careful in the follow-up program to make sure that the hand does not begin to shift back into its old or nonfunctional position as soon as the dynamic splint has been removed.

Bibliography

Anderson, M. H.: Upper Extremities Orthotics. Springfield IL: Charles C Thomas, 1979.

Barr, N. R.: The Hand. Principles and Techniques of Simple Splint Making in Rehabilitiation. London: Butterworths, 1975.

Bunch, W. H., and Keagy, R. D.: Principles of Orthotic Treatment. St. Louis: C. V. Mosby, 1976.

Cailliet, R.: Hand Pain and Impairment. Philadelphia: F. A. Davis, 1975.

Fess, E., et al.: Hand Splinting: Principles and Methods. St. Louis: C. V. Mosby, 1981.

Hunter, J. M.: Rehabilitation of the Hand. St. Louis: Mosby, 1978.

Johnson, M. K.: The Hand Atlas. Springfield IL: Charles C Thomas, 1975.

Malick, M. H.: Manual on Dynamic Hand Splinting. Pittsburgh: Harmarville Rehabilitation Center, 1978.

Malick, M. H.: Manual on Static Hand Splinting. Pittsburgh: Harmarville Rehabilitation Center, 1980.

Redford, J. B.: Orthotics, Etc. ed. 2. Baltimore: Williams & Wilkins, 1980.

Robertson, E.: Rehabilitation of Arm Amputees and Limb Deficient Children. London: Bailliere-Tindall, 1978.

Wolfort, F. G.: Acute Hand Injuries: A Multispecialty Approach. Boston: Little, Brown, 1980.

Wynn-Parry, C. B.: Rehabilitation of the Hand, rev. ed. 4. London: Butterworths, 1981.

CHAPTER 25

Functional Restoration— Hand Rehabilitation *L. Irene Hollis*

Rehabilitation of the hand is not only a specialty area in its own right, but it is also touched upon in all aspects of occupational therapy. Patients with physical disabilities of the upper extremities are treated through the use of manual tasks, as are those with psychosocial problems. The often quoted statement from Reilly's Eleanor Clarke Slagle lecture: "Man, through the use of his hands, can influence the state of his health," is borne out in clinical practice.[1] The blind become dependent upon the use of their hands and latent skills must be fully developed. The deaf communicate with sign language which requires finger agility. From pediatrics to geriatrics hand activities are utilized in treatment because the individual becomes involved in "doing" rather than "having things done to."

Anatomy of the Hand

Basic to the therapist's most effective utilization of hand activities is the understanding of the anatomy of the hand and arm. The usual course in anatomy at school is geared to cover general information, so special effort must be made to learn the details of hand anatomy. This can be done in several ways. There is no better way to do this than to dissect a fresh specimen, but this is not always available. Another avenue for learning is observation of surgical procedures of the hand, which is quite beneficial. There are also well done audiovisual aids. The 16 millimeter movie *Functional Anatomy of the Hand*, made by a plastic surgeon, is a classic in this field.[2] Another classic is the December 1951 issue of the Ciba Clinical Symposia *Surgical Anatomy of the Hand*.[3] This small booklet has a fine text and the drawings by Frank Netter are of special benefit. This issue has been reprinted several times.

Not only should the therapist be knowledgeable concerning specifics of hand anatomy, but he or she should also inform patients of their condition. The Ciba booklet provides schematic drawings which can be shown to the patient to illustrate involved structures. The more the patient knows and understands about the injury or condition, the more cooperative the patient may be in carrying out the treatment program. It has been said that patients have to rehabilitate themselves. The therapist can lay out a course but it is the patient who must direct efforts so that maximal improvement will ensue. The patient's comprehension of the extent of injury to the structures and the value of the diverse therapy routines is fundamental to the treatment. The hand surgeon usually explains details to the patient, but it is not until the therapy program gets underway that the average patient starts asking questions and really understands the scope of the problem. The time spent in informing the patient of pertinent details is well invested. Various models of hand anatomy can be used, but demonstrations of surface anatomy (directions of muscle pull and bulk of contracting muscles) on yourself or another patient are especially valuable.

A clinic in which a number of people are undergoing hand rehabilitation serves as an excellent laboratory. Usually there is more than one person with a similar injury. The therapist needs to be available to clarify points at times, but the value of having patients with similar problems at different stages of their recovery being exposed to one another is inestimable. Colored photographs need to be taken from time to time since these can be used for demonstrations in the event no similar case is available.

Referral Criteria

When setting up a specialty hand rehabilitation program, just what categories of patients the program will accept should be spelled out. As a general rule any person may be referred to occupational therapy for hand rehabilitation who exhibits one or more of the following conditions of the hand or arm as a result of congenital, traumatic, pathological, or psychological causes:
1. Limited joint range of motion
2. Limited strength or endurance
3. Incoordination and limited dexterity
4. Sensory impairment
5. Physiological amputation of the entire hand or any part thereof
6. Edema
7. Impairment resulting from disfigurement
8. Definite potential for developing any of the above conditions

The Hand Rehabilitation Center at Chapel Hill, N.C. was the first such specialty center in the United States. It had limited space so it was decided to concentrate on the traumatically injured hand. The Hand Center did not accept hemiplegic patients nor those with cord injuries; there was a program available for them at the general hospital adjacent to the Hand Rehabilitation Center. More than half of the patients were injured on the job. About a fourth were referred by Vocational Rehabilitation. The remainder were children with congenital conditions or private patients who had been involved in auto or home accidents.

Evaluation Procedures

The moment a person appears in the occupational therapy clinic the therapist can start evaluating by *observing* the patient's use of his or her hands. To understand the disabled hand one must know the normal one. There are individual variations, but the position of function is one that calls for wrist dorsiflexion or extension so that (1) the opposed thumb is in line with the radius and (2) the second and third metacarpals, under control of the extensor carpi radialis longus and brevis muscles, are extended about 45 degrees. The two ulnar metacarpals are not extended as much, and this is one reason there is a transverse arch of the hand (Fig. 25-1).

The injured hand is frequently held with the thumb and the two ulnar metacarpals in as much extension as the stable second and third ones. The common digital extensor tendons are called into action to lift the two ulnar metacarpals. These tendons also extend the fourth and fifth metacarpophalangeal (MP) joints, and, as a result, the palmar arch is flattened and a clawhand results. This position (Fig. 25-2) is nonfunctional and should be brought to the attention of the patient so that he or she can relax the thumb and the ulnar extensors and let the fingers fall into the amount of flexion that occurs when the viscoelastic quality of the flexor profundus tendons is unopposed by active extensor pull.

The patient may hold the injured hand motionless. This is unnatural and suggests that the patient may experience pain on motion or has "psychologically amputated" the hand. Hands are connected intimately with our mental processes. Normally a constant stream of sensory impulses passes from the hand to the brain and coordinated motor impulses are transmitted from the brain to the hand in response. At times a particular injury or disease process

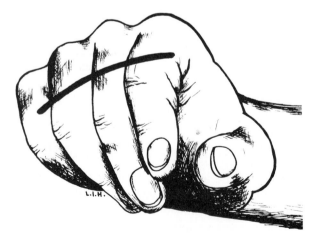

Figure 25-1. The functional position of a hand. Note the transverse metacarpal or palmar arch.

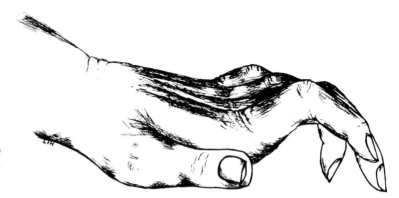

Figure 25-2. A nonfunctional position of the hand. The transverse metacarpal arch is flattened.

interrupts this pathway so that no impulses are transmitted. This is a physiological state. However, in numerous cases, there is no obvious pathology to account for the lack of transmission of impulses. Instead it may be due to inhibition, usually at a subconscious level, on the part of the patient who has disassociated the injured hand from control by the brain. Such a disassociation can be overcome through purposeful activities in the occupational therapy, and the sooner a program is initiated the easier it is to reverse this unhealthy state. One may start with something as simple as having the patient repetitively hit a piece of sponge suspended at eye level. This gross activity serves to help the patient begin to motor plan and re-orient the injured part.

If the protective position is a result of pain the therapy program should be directed toward decreasing the pain or increasing tolerance toward it. Application of a supportive splint is sometimes effective or the use of heat or cold might help. Both thermal modalities are effective in many cases. The therapist must find the process most beneficial to the patient and instruct in the application of it or, better, suggest daily activities that will incorporate use of one or the other. A patient with arthritis may work in more comfort if hot air from a hair dryer is directed toward the hands. How often washing dishes in warm soapy water is therapeutic! In others, application of ice is more effective.

The therapist may also have to institute a program of sensory bombardment to alter the threshold at which one is able to tolerate stimuli. Very often a patient who has had a crushing injury may have hypersensitivity throughout the hand. Small sensory nerves are involved and, when the bandage is first removed, the initial response to touch or contact is one of pain. As long as the injured hand is wrapped in a bulky bandage there is little or no sensory input and this period of sensory deprivation may lower the patient's pain threshold to the extent that he or she is

unable to tolerate having a therapist evaluate joint range of motion. The therapist should start the bombardment by using a fast brush, by having the patient rub gently over the entire surface of his or her own hand with a soft material, then rub more vigorously and introduce rougher textures. Sensory bombardment may progress to use of a tool that vibrates or a tapper. The patient can respond very rapidly to such stimuli and even during the first treatment session there may be enough improvement that the initial evaluation can be tolerated.

The hour invested in a thorough evaluation is time well spent.[4] A formal study should be done initially and this can serve as a baseline. The sample Hand Evaluation is used at the Hand Rehabilitation Center, Chapel Hill, N.C. All or portions of the evaluation should be repeated at intervals to document losses, gains, or areas in which no changes are measurable. Such evaluations are time-consuming but they provide the opportunity to become better acquainted with the patient and to learn as much as possible about the type of condition and the resultant decreases in active as well as passive ranges of motion and strength of pinch and grasp. An assessment should be made concerning the areas on the skin of the hand where there is total absence of sensibility and areas that are near normal or hypersensitive to touch. These areas are recorded on the outlines of the hands on the Hand Evaluation Chart.

During the evaluation period the occupational therapist keeps in mind the splinting requirements that will need to be met. The therapist should check for extrinsic, intrinsic, and Landsmeer's ligament tightness. Bunnell introduced these tests many years ago, and they help to determine some of the reasons for poor hand function.[5] Considering what motion the muscle group being evaluated performs, the evaluator, in administering these tests, starts with the proximal joint affected and moves that joint in the opposite direction. The evaluator then attempts to

HAND EVALUATION*

NCMH Unit Number: _____   Patient Name _____

y = yes; n = no

I. Functional Activity	Date: Eval. by:				Date: Eval. by:				Date: Eval. by:				Date: Eval. by:				Date: Eval. by:			
	I	L	R	F	I	L	R	F	I	L	R	F	I	L	R	F	I	L	R	F
A. Key pinch by digit																				
B. Pulp to pulp pinch by digit																				
C. Gross grip FN–PPC (cm)																				
D. Gross grip (mm Hg)																				
E. Pinch grip (lb)																				
F. Pick up a pencil																				
G. Write with a pencil																				
H. Button the button																				
I. Open, close safety pin																				
J. Comb hair																				
K. Use a drinking glass																				

II. Volume Measurement	Norm = Invol. =	Norm = Invol. =	Norm = Invol. =	Norm = Invol. =	Norm = Invol. =

III. Pain: Ask the patient to describe the pain and record area, resting or in motion, severity (none, mild, moderate, severe)

IV. Sensory Evaluation
   A. Using light touch. Record yes or no in each of the areas.
   B. Coin identification.
   C. If sensory deficit is evident, do ninhydrin test and attach record

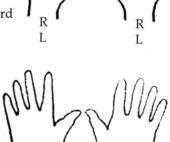

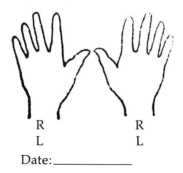

* Printed with permission of Hand Rehabilitation Center, Chapel Hill, N.C.

HAND EVALUATION (*Continued*)

V. Joint range of motion

			Act.	Pass.	Act.	Pass.	Act.	Pass.	Act.	Pass.	Act.	Pass.	Act.	Pass.
		Date:												
Index:	MP	Ext.												
		Flex.												
	PIP	Ext.												
		Flex.												
	DIP	Ext.												
		Flex.												
Long:	MP	Ext.												
		Flex.												
	PIP	Ext.												
		Flex.												
	DIP	Ext.												
		Flex.												
Ring:	MP	Ext.												
		Flex.												
	PIP	Ext.												
		Flex.												
	DIP	Ext.												
		Flex.												
Fifth:	MP	Ext.												
		Flex.												
	PIP	Ext.												
		Flex.												
	DIP	Ext.												
		Flex.												
Thumb:	MP	Ext.												
		Flex.												
	IP	Ext.												
		Flex.												
	MC	Abd.												
Wrist:		Ext.												
		Flex.												
Forearm:		Sup.												
		Pro.												
Elbow:		Ext.												
		Flex.												

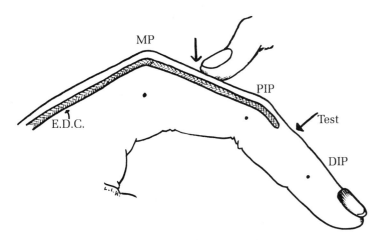

Figure 25-3. Test position for extrinsic tightness.

move the next more distal joint into the position opposite that which muscle action would be expected to produce.

In testing for extrinsic tightness (Fig. 25-3) the evaluator desires to find out whether the patient's inability to flex the metacarpophalangeal (MP) and interphalangeal (IP) joints simultaneously is due to adhesions along the finger extensor tendons on the dorsum of the hand or whether it is due to limitations within the joints. As the test is administered the MP joint is passively flexed and attempt is made to move the proximal interphalangeal (PIP) joint into flexion. If the PIP joint will not passively flex, the pressure on the MP joint is relaxed and the evaluator again attempts to flex the PIP joint. If this can be done easily the extensor tendon must be adherent along its course on the dorsum of the hand, and it is only when slack is allowed in the tendon across the MP joint that the PIP joint can flex. If one is unable to flex the PIP joint regardless of the position of the MP joint, then one surmises that the problem is one of PIP joint stiffness resulting from articular pathology rather than extrinsic tightness.

Intrinsic tightness results in an "intrinsic plus" deformity with the MP joints in flexion and the PIP joints in extension. In the early stages of intrinsic tightness the evaluator can detect evidence of it by moving the finger into extension at the MP joint and

then attempting to flex the PIP joint (Fig. 25-4). If there is more resistance when the finger is in this test position than when the MP joint is flexed and the PIP joint is also flexed, intrinsic muscle tightness is suspected. This would influence decisions regarding splinting the hand structures.

The third in this series of tests is one called Landsmeer's ligament tightness testing (Fig. 25-5). Milford, in his book on the ligaments of the hand, shows excellent photographs of Landsmeer's ligament (oblique retinacular ligament).[6] This is only a ligament, not a tendon; it is the sole identified structure which crosses *only* the PIP and distal interphalangeal (DIP) joints. It does not cross the MP joint, and so the position of the MP joint has no direct effect upon the test. A finger that has had disruption of the extensor hood and tendon over the PIP joint goes into a boutonnière deformity (Fig. 25-6). The lateral bands slip down volar to the axis of rotation at the PIP joint and when the intrinsic muscles contract to put tension on these lateral bands they pull the joint into more flexion rather than extending it, and the DIP joint goes into more hyperextension. This can be accounted for in two ways since the patient frequently rests his or her fingertips on a flat surface and attempts to pull the finger into an extended position. The patient does not accomplish PIP extension but does force the DIP joint into hyperextension. Once the DIP joint goes beyond

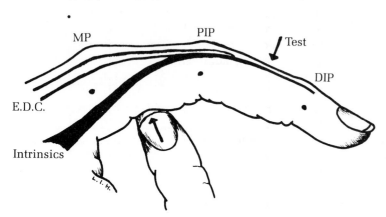

Figure 25-4. Test for intrinsic muscle tightness.

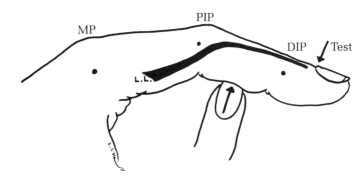

Figure 25-5. Test for Landsmeer's ligament tightness.

zero degrees or into some hyperextension, the lateral band has a more direct pull on its insertion on the distal phalanx and, as a result, the finger goes into even more hyperextension at the DIP joint. Landsmeer's ligament originates on the volar-lateral aspect of the proximal phalanx, runs volar to the axis of rotation at the PIP joint, but joins the lateral bands as they cross the middle phalanx and run dorsal to the axis of rotation of the DIP joint. The ligament joins the lateral bands as they insert on the dorsum of the distal phalanx. The presence of Landsmeer's ligament tightness complicates a boutonnière deformity since it may become fibrotic in a relaxed, shortened position and there is inability to flex the DIP joint when attempting to extend the PIP joint fully. In fact the patient may be unable to get the DIP joint down to neutral when the PIP joint is in extension. In treating any boutonnière deformity one should check for Landsmeer's ligament tightness and initiate a splinting program if there is any evidence that the DIP joint cannot be flexed when the PIP joint is in extension but can be flexed when the PIP joint is flexed. The position of the MP joint is immaterial since the ligament does not cross that joint. The test position can be compared to the position for intrinsic tightness (Fig. 25-4) if one moves distal one joint so as to move the PIP joint into extension and attempts are made to place the DIP joint into flexion.

One other important evaluation procedure is measurement of edema. One can compare the normal to the injured hand and either a water displacement method can be applied or a tape can be used to check the circumference of a finger or arm.[7] Edema can be quite pernicious when it accumulates in the hand since the serous fluid, rich in fibrin, can cause the small finger joints to stiffen very rapidly. One has to consider the reduction of edema a high-priority goal.

Goals in Rehabilitation

The most practical goal that can be set is that of achieving a functional hand for the patient. The patient must be involved in the setting of goals since he or she knows what range of motion, strength and coordination vocational and avocational pursuits require. The patient must put forth the most effort to reach the goals, and is the one who has to live with the results of rehabilitation efforts. The therapy and medical members of the team must add input to help keep the goals in line with the reality of the situation. Surgery is not indicated in many instances, so the burden of restoration of adequate joint motion falls to the therapists who apply conservative approaches to get improved flexion, extension, abduction, adduction, as the case demands.

One important way in which occupational therapists have contributed to the conservative approach is by designing and fabricating splints. Many of the splints are small, for one finger only, and need to be modified frequently to keep up with the progress being made in range of motion. The therapists are best suited to supply these small splints since they are in daily contact with the patient. An orthotist may be called upon to provide a splint for long-term use as in a brachial plexus injury, hemiplegia, polio, or quadriplegia, but most of the orthotists readily admit that the occupational therapist is in a better position to provide short-term splints.

Many of the splints are *supportive* in design since some joints need to be held in a certain position to allow healing to take place in the soft tissues about the joints, or to allow a fracture to be immobilized. In some instances painful hands are made more comfortable with supportive splints. The patient must be taught to relax in the splint and not "fight" it.

Corrective splints can be static or dynamic.

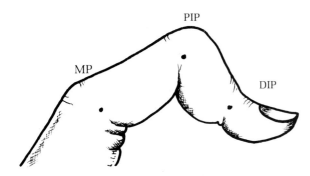

Figure 25-6. Boutonnière deformity.

Usually dynamic splints are more effective since a small amount of force can be exerted by rubber bands or springs over a long period of time similar to the way orthodontic appliances can accomplish so much. Dr. Paul Brand's philosophy concerning the inevitability of gradualness is applicable here. Such dynamic splints can be made to get wrists back into an extended position so that finger flexors can work more advantageously. Gradual force from a specifically designed splint can gain flexion or extension of an elbow or supination or pronation of a forearm. The amount of force required to move the large joints may be great, but for the small joints of the fingers it is minmal. Caution should be emphasized here since this small force must be applied quite close to the joint axis of rotation to avoid damaging the joint surfaces in the event there are adhesions causing compromise of the gliding motion of the joint.

Some dynamic splints are *resistive* to the pull of the tendons. Such can be applied when one wishes to strengthen muscles that have the potential for developing a more powerful pull. A small amount of resistance often enables a patient to get a better sense of muscle action. Flexor motion, for instance, may be initiated if a dynamic splint supplies a very gentle extension pull on the fingers. The dynamic force can be *assistive* to aid a patient by augmenting a small amount of active motion. The therapist must closely supervise the patient in the use of dynamic splints since he or she may "fight" the pull of the splint and increase the imbalance between the weak muscle that should be assisted and the stronger muscle that already overpowers the weak one.

The patient may need modifications of the devices used in activities of daily living as well as tools used at work. The occupational therapist can supply these *adaptive* devices. Many of them must be individually designed and can be fabricated in the clinic. The patient may be involved in fabricating his or her own devices. This approach pays double dividends since the patient has more pride in something he makes, and will be able to repair it after he or she gets home.

Specific Involvement

Peripheral Nerve Injuries

Most peripheral nerves have two components: sensory and motor.

Median Nerve Involvement

Of the three major nerves influencing the hand, wrist, and forearm the *median nerve* usually is considered to be the most important one. Its importance is due to the sensory component and its motor function on the intrinsic muscles of the thumb. Specialists who have worked out the physical impairment ratings, which are used in practice to determine what monetary compensation is due a person who was injured on the job, declare that a hand that lacks median sensibility has a 75% disability. This is based on sensory loss alone. The hand that lacks tactile sensibility in the thumb and index finger does not function normally. Patients do not know without looking when they hold an article between these numb fingertips, and so they often drop the items. They lack coordination since they have no position sense. They are unaware of sharp edges and hot surfaces and may inadvertently injure the hand. A burn or cut on such a patient does not heal easily since the circulation to an insensitive finger is compromised.

One responsibility of the occupational therapist is to instruct the patient in protective measures so eyes will be used to substitute for the absent sense of touch. People who lose their sense of touch gradually, due to a disease process such as diabetes or leprosy, adjust to this loss and can continue to function quite normally. It is the person who suffers a total loss instantly from trauma who is unable to adjust. Surgeons repair the severed nerve but seldom does the patient regain perfect cutaneous sensibility. Sensory nerves are so complex in function that with an average repair, the patient may get return of protective sensation only. The patient can avoid burning or cutting the hand but lacks the highly discriminatory sensibility that enables him or her to perform finely coordinated activities. A good program of sensory reeducation does improve the ability to function and thus should be instituted as early as possible.[8] Such a program is frequently overlooked, but is as important as the muscle reeducation program.

If the motor component of the median nerve is cut at or near the wrist, the result is loss of ability to abduct and oppose the thumb. Without these movements the thumb is held close to the palm and when one attempts to circumduct the thumb across the palm so that it can touch the small finger tip-to-tip it slides instead flatly across the palm and the thumb and small fingernails touch. One is unable to position the thumb so as to reach around a glass, for instance. If the nerve is repaired successfully at the wrist level, nerve regrowth will take place at about 1 millimeter a day or an inch each month. Therefore, within 3 to 6 months the thenar muscles should be showing some signs of reinnervation.

During this period of waiting for evidence of regeneration of the nerve, the occupational therapist should apply a splint to hold the thumb in the functional position described previously. If the thumb is permitted to be pulled into extension by the muscles innervated by the intact radial nerve, the small muscles which make up the thenar group will be on stretch and will not function well even if the median nerve does regenerate. If the hand is splinted so that the thumb is in front of the index finger and some type of C-shaped spacer or dynamic pull is used to hold the first and second metacarpals apart, the thenar muscles are not stretched, and the patient can make functional use of the index and long fingers to pinch against the thumb. Any number of activities are then possible for the patient and a somewhat normal pattern of hand use can be maintained.

This preservation of purposeful use of the hand during recovery is a significant contribution in itself. Habit pattern pathways account for one's ability to automatically maneuver items between the fingers and perform coordinated tasks. Some of this automaticity is compromised because of the decrease in tactile sensibility but, by supplying the patient with a carefully designed splint which positions the thumb without interfering with the active motion in the index and long finger, one can expect a far better outcome from a median nerve injury. The therapist should be alert to any poor habit patterns or positions of the thumb that will be detrimental.

Ulnar Nerve Involvement

An ulnar nerve involvement is not as important in the areas of sensibility of the hand as a median nerve injury, but the motor loss is far greater. The sensory status of the surface of the ulnar palm plus the volar small finger and half of the ring finger is involved when the volar digital branch of the ulnar nerve is severed. If the dorsal branch of the ulnar nerve, which takes a separate path proximal to the wrist, is severed the entire dorsum of the ulnar half of the hand plus the dorsum of the entire small finger and half of the ring finger are anesthetic. The dorsal branch is injured less often than the volar branch and the presence of adequate sensation on the back and side of the small finger helps to serve as protection against burns and cuts on that side, even though the volar sensory branch may be severed.

The major involvement in the hand from an ulnar nerve injury is the result of the motor loss. Muscles that originate distal to the wrist are called intrinsic muscles. Three fourths of the intrinsic muscles of the hand are innervated by the ulnar nerve. Not only are the intrinsic muscles that make up the hypothenar group on the ulnar side of the palm innervated by the ulnar nerve but also the four dorsal interossei, the three palmar interossei, and the lumbricals to the ring and small fingers. The huge thumb adductor which originates on the third metacarpal and inserts on the proximal phalanx of the thumb has ulnar nerve supply as well as the deep belly of the flexor pollicis

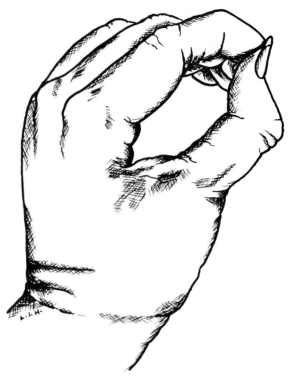

Figure 25-7. Froment's sign in the thumb.

brevis muscle. Every digit suffers from loss of the ulnar motor supply. Loss of the adductor power of the thumb is quite disabling to an individual, and the thumb often collapses at the MP joint into what is known as Froment's position (Fig. 25-7). Without the mediating influence of the interossei the fingers are at the mercy of the extrinsic flexors and extensors (those that have their muscle bellies in the forearm with only the tendons running across the wrist and inserting on various phalanges). Without the regulating pull of the interossei, the fingers collapse into a claw position (Fig. 25-2). Without early intervention through splinting, this dysfunctional position results in harmful contractures. The hyperextended MP joints allow the collateral ligaments on each side of the joints to become fibrotic in a shortened position so that it becomes impossible, through passive or active motion, to have the proximal phalanx glide around the head of its metacarpal. Early application of a simple MP flexion splint (Fig. 25-8) keeps the collateral ligaments elongated and provides an additional force, even though it is an outside force, that enables the central slips of the common extensor tendons to act on the proximal interphalangeal joints rather than having all of their power exerted to extend or hyperextend the MP joints.

Throughout the waiting period to see whether the repair of the ulnar nerve has been successful and whether the interossei will be reinnervated, the occupational therapist should examine the patient at regu-

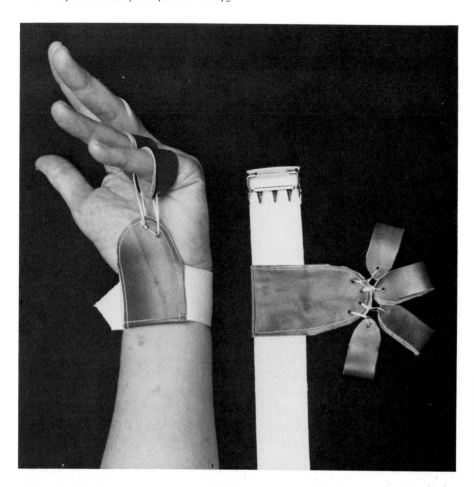

Figure 25-8. Simple anti-claw splint. It is used on only two fingers when there is an ulnar nerve injury but on all four when both the median and ulnar nerves are involved.

lar times from 2 to 4 weeks apart to check on progress, to repair the splints and modify them if necessary, and to reinforce functional patterns. Sensory reeducation can be applied as well as neuromuscular facilitation techniques. When there is evidence of return of some motor activity the patient should be examined by the therapist more often and provided with meaningful activities which will reinforce use of the minimal motion as it becomes available to the patient. At this time the significance of not over-using and abusing the returning motor functions is just as important as the carefully guided use of these functions. The skills of the therapist are very important in this phase of therapy. For example, there may be a need to devise specific pieces of equipment which the patient can use to strengthen the interossei by flexing the MP joints so the proximal phalanges contact a surface without having the PIP and DIP joints flex. The patient might participate in a leather–lacing project and hold the lacing between proximal phalanges and the platform portion of the device worn (Fig. 25-9). Repetitive actions involving simultaneous MP flexion and IP joint extension are beneficial to the patient who is trying to strengthen the intrinsic muscles as they are being reinnervated.

Combined Median and Ulnar Nerve Involvement

When both median and ulnar nerves are lost the resultant condition is difficult for the patient to tolerate. The total loss of sensibility discourages use of the hand and the motor deficits make it impossible to pinch or grasp. With the thumb and fingers going into hyperextension at the proximal joints and full flexion at the distal joints it is impossible for the thumb to contact the fingertips to pinch. Some lateral pinch or "key pinch" is possible with the thumb contacting the side of the index finger, but this is ineffective except for turning a key in a lock. It can be used for some dressing activities but should be discouraged since it increases the possibility of adduction contracture of the thumb. A splint similar to the one shown in Figure 25-10 holds the thumb in abduction and maintains the MP joints of the fingers in enough flexion to permit the use of the common extensors to extend the IP joints. The position of pinch is reestablished but, since there is no cutaneous sensibility, the patient must be taught to watch closely to avoid damaging the fingertips. In some cases rubber finger stalls may need to be applied to protect the insensi-

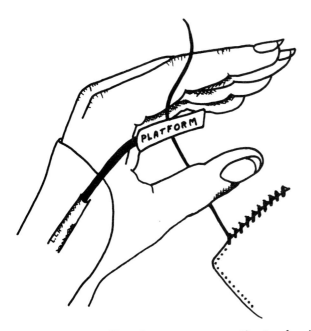

Figure 25-9. A splint for use on a patient who is learning to contract the intrinsic muscles to flex the metacarpophalangeal joint and extend the interphalangeal joints. The patient can do leather lacing by having the proximal phalanges contact the platform and hold the lacing.

tive tips and to provide traction. Joint mobility can be maintained and the patient will have a more useful hand when the nerve regeneration restores sensibility and muscle function or when tendon transfers are done surgically in the event motor nerve regeneration is insufficient.

Radial Nerve Involvement

The radial nerve must be injured at or above the elbow to have its injury totally affect the hand in the motor realm. There is a branch of the radial sensory nerve which traverses the forearm and is superficial along the distal dorsal border of the radius. This sensory nerve supplies about half of the dorsum of the hand and as far as the PIP joint on the dorsum of the radial digits. Loss of sensation over this area is not disabling; however, an injury to this dorsal sensory branch can cause a pain syndrome that is devastating. Particular attention should be paid to this trigger area and efforts should be made to relieve the discomfort if possible by desensitizing techniques before it reaches a proportion that interferes with functional use of the forearm and hand.

The motor branch of the radial nerve spirals around the lateral, distal third of the humerus and is

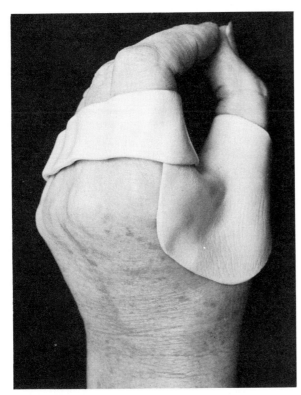
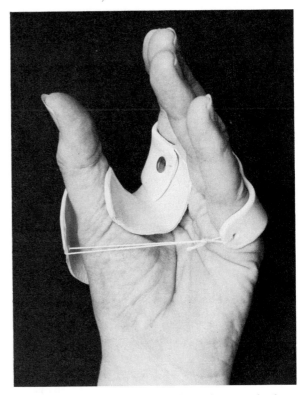

Figure 25-10. Two views of a splint for use on a patient who has combined median and ulnar palsy. This splint provides support for the thumb and keeps the fingers from going into a claw position.

frequently involved in "Saturday night paralysis" or other compression injuries in this area. As a result of the radially innervated wrist, finger, and thumb extensors being at least temporarily denervated, the ability to hold the wrist in an extended position is lost so that the grip strength is greaty diminished. There is no way for an individual with such a radial nerve injury to actively extend the fingers at the MP joint, and therefore, in order to open the hand, he or she resorts to use of the intrinsic muscles which flex the MP joints even though they do extend the IP joints. A simple splint made from brass welding rod with leather finger cuffs and a wrist and forearm strap (Fig. 25-11) can give support to the hand by suspending the fingers from the proximal phalanges. No palmar cuff is necessary so there is nothing to interfere with grasping tool handles. When using the splint, the wrist flexors are actively contracted to get passive extension of the fingers in order to reach around a large

article. One joint, either the wrist or the MP joints of the fingers, must give in order for the other one to assume a new position. The splint on the left in Figure 25-11 is the original design and was based upon the use of nylon cords to simulate external finger extensor tendons which were "tenodesed" or secured at the wrist. As long as the patient has mobile joints and active use of wrist and finger flexors, he or she can use this type of splint to control wrist drop. The wire is bent to provide built-in wrist extension. The splint may be simplified, as seen on the right in Figure 25-11, by eliminating the nylon cord and placing the leather finger cuffs directly on the brass wire which rests above the proximal phalanges. One does need to apply some material at each side of the wire to block the finger cuffs from slipping around the bend. As shown in the illustration, small pieces of Kay splint have been heated and shaped around the wire to serve as stops. A small stop can also be sol-

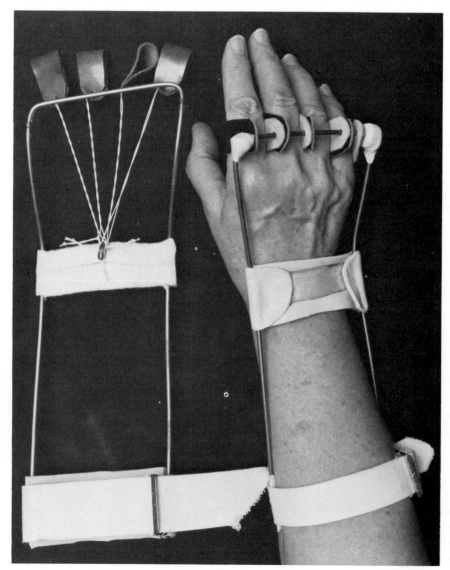

Figure 25-11. A radial palsy splint. The splint on the left has nylon cord to simulate the extensor tendons. These are attached to each leather finger cuff. The cord runs through a small wire loop soldered to the wire frame directly above each finger. The cord is then fastened to a hook on the wrist cuff and serves to provide a tenodesis effect. The splint on the right is simplified and has the finger cuffs slipped onto the wire frame.

dered on the wire. This splint is very effective and permits nearly normal use of the hand during the waiting period to see if a compressed radial nerve will have return of function or while awaiting surgical tendon transfers in the event the nerve has been irreparably damaged.

Tendon Injuries

There are controversies among hand surgeons concerning all aspects of reconstructive surgery, but disagreement is perhaps most evident concerning management of flexor and extensor tendon injuries. The therapist must adjust his or her program to be consistent with the philosophy of the surgeon supervising the cases referred for therapy.

One point of agreement among all surgeons is that finger joints must be mobilized as thoroughly as possible prior to surgical intervention. Occupational therapists should participate and innovate in the mobilization phase. One can attach a finger in which the flexor tendons have been severed to an adjacent, mobile one by using Velcro to make a fellow traveller (Fig. 25-12). This is preferable to taping two fingers together since the Velcro is double thick between the fingers and keeps them slightly apart, thus avoiding maceration of the skin. If three or four fingers have severed flexor tendons one may resort to using a pair of cotton work gloves and sewing nylon fishing line up each glove finger on the palmar side to serve as "external" flexor tendons. These lines are tied to rubber bands in the distal palm and the rubber bands are stretched down to hook on a wrist strap. The tension of the rubber bands maintains the fingers in some flexion but the patient can extend actively to open the hand. Both of these methods enable a patient to hold a steering wheel or broom handle without resorting to activating the intrinsic muscles of the injured

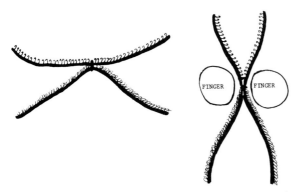

Figure 25-12. A fellow traveller made from Velcro. The soft side of the Velcro faces the back of the hook piece when it is sewn together in the middle. Each piece is then turned back upon itself and sewn again.

finger or fingers. Without the aid of the glove or fellow traveller the patient is apt to recruit the intrinsics (which flex the MP joint but extend the IP joints) and the stage is set for development of a very poor habit pattern as well as debilitating intrinsic tightness. The poor habit pattern is referred to as "extensor habitus" or "paradoxical extension." Avoid letting it develop since it is difficult to eliminate in the presurgical phase. Should a patient overuse the intrinsics following flexor tendon grafting, he or she is apt to have an inadequate result from tendon surgery.

In some commonly followed treatment schedules, on the twenty-first to the twenty-fifth day after surgery when the occlusive dressing is removed (which was applied to control edema and position the hand to put slack on the repaired flexor tendon), a protective splint should be used to eliminate the possibility of inadvertently disrupting the tendon repair. This splint should be worn at all times except when the patient is being supervised in an exercise routine. During this period, a padded banding metal splint can be applied on the dorsum of the hand so a distal Velcro strap can be secured around the proximal phalanx without blocking the PIP joint. The MP joint is held in extension and the patient is asked to actively flex the PIP joint. Even though both flexor tendons are cut (the profundus and superficialis), the surgeon frequently prefers to repair only the profundus tendon. When the patient is asked to flex the PIP joint, it may seem to be an incorrect order in view of the fact that he or she will use the profundus muscle belly to accomplish this motion. We have found that a better result can be attained early if one concentrates on the PIP joint motion rather than MP or DIP joint motion. One can fabricate a calibrated gauge for the patient to measure active, unresisted PIP motion. Passive flexion but no passive extension is used during the first 2 weeks out of dressing. In the third week of therapy one may introduce passive extension of only one joint at a time. The MP and DIP joints should be positioned in flexion while gently extending the PIP joint passively. The MP and PIP joints should be flexed while the DIP joint is extended. This method affects the joint tightness, not the tendon anastomosis. By the fifth week of rehabilitation (8 weeks after surgery) one can be aggressive with resistive flexion and passive extension. This time schedule may be altered some according to the philosophy of the surgeon but will be consistent with most programs.

A repaired extensor tendon must be protected for 28 days, at least one week longer than a repaired flexor tendon. The reason for this difference is that flexor tendons and muscles are powerful and can exert too much force if they are permitted to actively pull against the thin weak extensors. The extensors are not designed for power, but for range of motion. If adequate flexor range is not obtained by the tenth week after surgery on an extensor mechanism, the therapist should plan to apply a proper splint of the dynamic type to get further wrist and finger flexion range simultaneously. At this late stage the extensor tendons may be able to extend the wrist and MP joints effectively, but there may be adhesions which limit the patient from achieving an adequate grip. Through use of the extrinsic tightness test as shown in Figure 25-3, one can evaluate this problem. The test can be modified also to passively flex the wrist then test for MP flexion in order to locate just where the adhesions are. Priorities may need to be altered and flexion range must receive added emphasis.

Occupational Therapy Activities

The therapist should choose wisely when selecting the variety of activities that will be used in a specialty program for hand rehabilitation. If the budget is limited, one can concentrate on a few activities rather than investing in equipment and supplies for a wide variety. The main guideline is to select activities that can be adapted readily to provide the motions required in treatment and which permit themselves to be graded as to demands on strength, range of motion and coordination.

Games that Provide Specific Activity

Games provide an endless variety of demands. Many peg games that are available commercially in miniature sizes can be reproduced in larger sizes so that the pegs can be more easily manipulated. The holes in these games can be placed farther apart and early attempts on the part of the patient can lead to success rather than frustration. Some games can be played by one person and several of these should be available, but those that require two or more players are also needed to aid with socialization. A peg game can be used as an early modality for a patient who has had nerve and flexor tendon damage. In the absence of sensation there is no danger of the patient harming the hand, and the fingers can be supported with small splints to channel flexor motion to the joints which must be exercised. For more strengthening the patient can use self-closing, spring-loaded clamps to move the pegs or, for sustained grasp, a pair of pliers can be modified by adding a spring opener made from steel banding metal (Fig. 25-13). The patient has

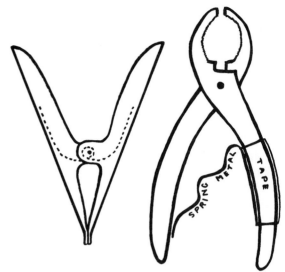

Figure 25-13. Self-closing clamps and self-opening pliers for use in playing peg games and doing leather lacing.

to hold firmly or the pliers will release and the peg will fall.

Marbles can be used to play the games if one has a reamed out hole for the marble to fit into as well as a drilled hole in the center of each depression deep enough and of the correct size to hold the peg. The marbles provide another challenge to the patient since they are more difficult to handle.

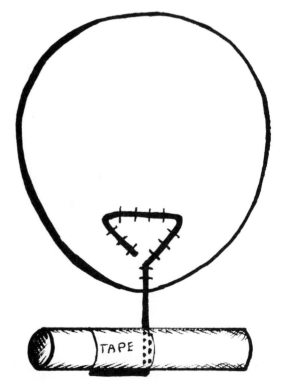

Figure 25-14. An adapted Ping-Pong paddle for use in improving balanced wrist extension.

A suspended golf practice ball, a small basket made by cord knotting with a light string around a 4-inch wire loop, and a modified Ping-Pong paddle (Fig. 25-14) can provide a challenging activity to aid in gaining wrist extension. The hand grip is at a right angle to the paddle and encourages balanced wrist extension. An upright post can be attached to a chair back to enable one to strap the forearm in a perpendicular position to ensure use of wrist extension when the patient bats backhand at the ball. A different paddle can be made for use when trying to gain pronation or supination (Fig. 25-15). A file handle or dowel can be provided for the patient to grip. Aluminum clothesline wire can be inserted into the handle and attached to the paddle so that the angle can be changed to meet various needs. For supination or pronation the patient should sit with the forearm resting on a padded shelf which is horizontal to the chair back and with a strap around the forearm close to the flexed elbow. A strap in this location does not interfere with supination or pronation. The wire in

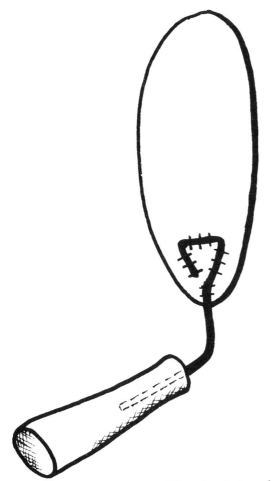

Figure 25-15. A Ping-Pong paddle adapted so that a patient can work towards active supination and pronation.

the paddle handle can be bent so that even limited range of motion of the arm can result in contact with the suspended ball.

Adapted Craft Activities

Leather-lacing projects provide opportunities to vary the ways in which a patient will pull the lacing through. A specially designed palmar device provides a platform placed in the exact position necessary for the damaged finger to contact it. Such a device is appropriate for use for the small finger if one is trying to get a patient to use the flexors of that finger. A lacing platform as shown in Figure 25-9 is designed to encourage MP flexion through use of intrinsic muscle action. A variety of spring-loaded clamps (see Fig. 25-13) can be collected so that the patient can progress from one requiring very weak grip strength to stronger clamps as strength increases. The self-opening pliers depicted in Figure 25-13 require sustained grip or the pliers will open and the lacing will drop out of the jaws.

Stippling of leather belts is a useful therapeutic project. One can take 6 inches of a ¾ inch dowel and drive a small nail into one end. The head of the nail can be clipped off and the end of the nail filed to make a modified point. Sponge rubber can be placed around the dowel handle to build up the size enough to permit the patient to grip the tool firmly and push the nail point into dampened belt leather far enough to make a depression. This is a repetitive task and can result in a rewarding finished product. Stipplers can be modified in design in order to meet the treatment requirements of a variety of patients (Fig. 25-16).

When a patient with rheumatoid arthritis has the common problem of ulnar drift of the fingers, a stippler handle can be adapted to provide projections which fit to the ulnar side of each finger when the dowel is grasped. With each use of the stippler the fingers are forced into radial deviation.

Another useful variation of the stippler depicted is one inspired by the brake lever on a Volkswagen. The aluminum tube is grasped with the fingers; the thumb, through the use of the long flexor, plunges the wooden dowel down so the point contacts the leather. The rubber band offers resistance to the thumb flexion and will return the dowel to its original position. This stippler is good for strengthening grasp in general as well as thumb flexion.

Woodworking projects also offer a variety of adaptations. Many patients work in furniture factories and have introduced therapists to salvage materials that their companies are happy to provide. Table and chair legs that have flaws may often be supplied by some firms. Projects such as foot stools, plant stands, and small tables can be made from the legs in combi-

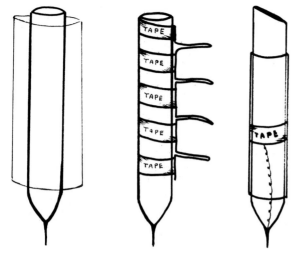

Figure 25-16. Leather stippling tools made from wooden dowels with nails driven in the ends. The heads are cut off and the nails are filed to modified points. (*Left*) Sponge rubber wrapped to build up the dowel. (*Center*) Projections formed from Kay splint and taped to the dowel to make a tool for use by a patient who has ulnar drift of the fingers. (*Right*) A plunger type stippler inspired by a Volkswagen brake lever. The dowel is slipped through an aluminum tube and a rubber band is taped to the tube and tied to the nail. This stippler is useful when one needs an exerciser for the flexor pollicis longus muscle.

nation with Formica-covered sink cutouts from cabinet makers. In order to sandpaper the round legs a different type of sander has been designed (Fig. 25-17). If the table leg is positioned high on a surface, this strip sander can be used by alternately flexing and extending the arms. The adapted handle encourages use of finger flexors. This activity is also useful for reducing edema since the hand is in an elevated position and all of the hand and arm muscles are actively contracting and relaxing.

Job Simulation

In goal setting for occupational therapy one frequently needs to find out exactly what strengths and ranges of motion are required of patients on their jobs. These conditions can be simulated as much as possible in the clinic to help in determining whether a patient will be able to return to work. One can use spring scales and attach fabrics or dowels to have patients pull in the manner required to see whether they can pinch firmly enough to hold the material related to their job requirements. Leather, fabric, yarn, sheet metal and a variety of tubing sizes have been materials patients may hold or pull. As a therapist works with a patient and realizes what he or

she is going to need to hold or maneuver in order to get back on the job, the therapy activities can involve materials similar to those that will be expected to be handled later. Instead of always relying on the routine evaluation forms, the therapist must innovate and add items to fit the evaluation to the individual patient. For a truck driver one might use the round metal frame over which a laundry bag is stretched. The patient sits and places his feet on the braces near the floor and resists the pull of his hands which are using the open circular frame at the top to simulate the steering wheel. A truck steering wheel is usually relatively horizontal rather than vertical, and this simulation can aid the therapist in finding out whether the arm and hand can function adequately to allow returning to employment. Of course, this is only a job simulation, but it does serve to indicate to the patient and therapist how strength is improving.

A torque wrench can provide feedback as to how much force a patient can exert in pulling or pushing levers. Employers will supply information concerning the number of inch-pounds required to shift the levers in a plant so a patient has a realistic goal toward which to aim.

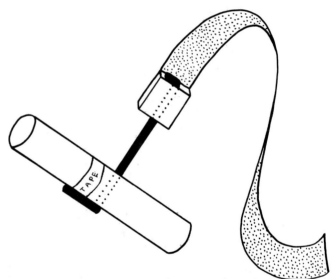

Figure 25-17. An adapted strip sander. A hole can be drilled through the center of a wooden dowel and a piece of wire run through and bent at a right angle so it can be taped to the dowel. At the other end the wire runs through a small wooden block to which is tacked and taped a long strip of sandpaper. The strip of sandpaper can be cut from a sanding belt since belts are reinforced with fabric and will not tear easily, or several sheets of sandpaper can be laid edge to edge with a continuous strip of reinforced tape applied across the back of several and then cut into strips.

Patients who live in the country may complain that they are unable to carry a bucket of water from the well. As part of such a person's occupational therapy program, one can make use of a bucket containing sandbags rather than water. The patient carries it with increasing weight and for longer distances as grip strength and upper extremity function improve.

There are limitless possibilities of devising job simulations. An industrial nurse or vocational counsellor, willing to work closely with the occupational therapist, can obtain job descriptions and borrow tools used in patients' occupations. Such coordinated efforts help to make a rehabilitation program more realistic and aid in returning a patient to employment sooner.

Outcome Criteria

To ensure that a patient referred to an occupational therapy program for hand rehabilitation receives optimum benefits, one must examine the records to see the condition of the patient when he or she entered the program and screen the documented evidence to find indications that the treatment processes applied contribute to the patient's overall benefit.

Surgeons frequently refer people to occupational therapy for assistance in diagnosis. After a massive hand injury it is not always easy to make a decision regarding which structures have been damaged and are in need of repair. The therapist should explore various possibilities and administer specific tests or place the hand in test positions consistent with the nature of the condition to determine response. All findings should be recorded carefully so the surgeon has the benefit of all data on which to base clinical and therapeutic decisions.

After a person has been treated by an occupational therapist, the records should reveal the measurable improvement in the range of joint motion, strength, and endurance. Improvement of functional ability, coordination, and dexterity should also be documented. If a patient has been referred because of sensory impairment, the therapist's notes and records should indicate the status at the time of entry into the program. Subsequent notes must indicate the decrease in areas that are totally without response to sensory stimuli with the notes showing improvement delineated carefully. In some cases no improvement is evident but the therapist should indicate in the chart how the patient has been helped to cope with insensitive fingers by teaching protective measures.

Since edema has a detrimental effect on the joints of the hand, records should show clearly how successful the efforts toward reducing edema have been.

Hand volume measurements can be graphed. This will enable noting when edema is decreased and, if it has been recorded regarding what activity preceded each measurement, conclusions can be drawn regarding which of the activities have been the most beneficial in reducing edema.

The records for amputees who have been referred for treatment should indicate how consistently their full or partial prostheses have been worn and how many activities of daily living they perform using the prostheses. Many amputees and those with severely mangled hands suffer from the trauma imposed upon their self-images. It is difficult to measure the effectiveness of one's input into solution of this problem, but the progress notes should indicate changes in the behavior patterns related to self-image.

As the records are reviewed to determine whether improvement continues or whether a plateau has been reached, one is made acutely aware of the importance of well-documented progress notes. People are referred to occupational therapy for treatment of a variety of conditions and the professional skills of the therapist bring about results that should be documented sufficiently to justify physicians' continued referral of patients to the service.

Conclusion

The technical skills of the occupational therapist are important, but even more important are the judgmental skills. These help to raise our profession into a realm which we all aspire to reach. Professional judgment is increased through a series of experiences entered into with an inquiring mind and through continuing study of the literature within the field.

The following list of books and articles is dated, but contains some of the classics which still serve as important basic references. No list will be adequate by the time it appears in print.

The author urges the reader to keep up by reading monthly publications and following this by studying the references listed at the end of the articles read. One should not depend on the interpretation of someone else. It is far better for each individual to read widely in the specific area in which he or she is interested. Each person brings a new light to the material referred to in an article. Improved understanding may result which will contribute to the overall rehabilitation procedures found to be effective. Each therapist must assume responsibility for advancing our knowledge in this specialty area.

References

1. Reilly, M.: Eleanor Clarke Slagle Lecture. Occupational Therapy Can Be One of the Great Ideas of 20th Century Medicine. Am. J. Occup. Ther. 16:1, 1962.

2. *Functional Anatomy of the Hand,* 16 mm movie. Davis and Geck, American Cyanamid Co., Danbury CT 06810.
3. Lampe, E. W.: Surgical Anatomy of the Hand. Ciba Clinical Symposia, Ciba Pharmaceutical Products, Inc., Summit NJ, 1951.
4. Perry, J. F., and Bevin, A. G.: Evaluation procedures for patients with hand injuries. Phys. Ther. 54:6, 1974.
5. Boyes, J. H.: Bunnell's Surgery of the Hand, ed. 5. Philadelphia: J. B. Lippincott Co., 1970.
6. Milford, L.: Retaining Ligaments of the Digits of the Hand. Philadelphia: W. B. Saunders Co., 1968.
7. DeVore, G. L.; and Hamilton, G. F.: Volume measuring of the severely injured hand. Am. J. Occup. Ther. 22:16, 1968.
8. Dellon, A. L., Curtis, R. M., and Edgerton, M. T.: Reeducation of sensation in the hand after nerve injury and repair. Plastic Reconstr. Surg. 53:3, 1974.

Bibliography

American Academy of Orthopedic Surgeons: Symposium on Tendon Surgery in the Hand. St. Louis MO: C.V. Mosby, 1975.

Barr, N. R.: The Hand: Principles and Techniques of Simple Splintmaking in Rehabilitation. London: Butterworths, 1975.

Bunnell, S.: Surgery in World War II, Hand Surgery. Department of the Army, Washington, DC, 1955.

Chase, R. A.: Surgery of the Hand, The New England Journal of Medicine, Part I, December 7, 1972, Part II, December 14, 1972.

Flynn, E. J.: Hand Surgery. Baltimore: Williams & Wilkins, 1966.

Hollis, L. I.: Splint Substitutes, Amer. J. Occup. Ther., vol. 21, 139–145, 1967.

Hollis, L. I.: Letters to the Editor, Amer. J. Occup. Ther., Vol. 21, 396–397, 1967.

Hunter, J. M. et al.: (eds.): Rehabilitation of the Hand. 72 Contributing Authors. St. Louis, MO.: C.V. Mosby, 1978.

Kaplan, E. G.: Functional and Surgical Anatomy of the Hand. Philadelphia: J.B. Lippincott, 1965.

Leont'ev, A. N., and Zaporozhets: Rehabilitation of Hand Function. N.Y.: Pergamon Press, 1960.

Moberg, Erik: Objective Methods for Determining the Functional Value of Sensibility in the Hand, J. Bone Joint Surgery, 40-B:454–476, 1958.

Moberg, E.: Criticism and Study of Methods of Examining Sensibility in the Hand, Neurology 12:8–19, 1962.

Peacock, E. E., Jr.: Dynamic Splinting for the Prevention and Correction of Hand Deformities, J. Bone Joint Surgery, October, 1952.

Seddon, H.: Surgical Disorders of the Peripheral Nerves. Baltimore: Williams & Wilkins, 1972.

Spinner, M.: Injuries to the Major Branches of Peripheral Nerves of the Forearm. Philadelphia: W.B. Saunders, 1972.

Surgery of the Hand, Surgical Clinics of North America, Vol. 40, No. 2, 1960.

Weeks, P. M., and Wray, C. R.: Management of Acute Hand Injuries: A Biological Approach. St. Louis MO: C.V. Mosby, 1978.

Wynn-Parry, C. B.: Rehabilitation of the Hand. London: Butterworths, 1973.

Zancolli, E.: Structural and Dynamic Bases of Hand Surgery. Philadelphia: J. B. Lippincott, 1968.

Resources

American Occupational Therapy Association
    American Journal of Occupational Therapy
    Packet on Hand Rehabilitation
    Newsletter of Specialty Section, Physical Disabilities
    A.O.T.A. Newspaper
    Slides, Movies and Video Tapes (by Irene Hollis and others)
    Continuing Education Courses
    Research Papers
American Society of Hand Therapists
    Publications
    Meetings
    Continuing Education
The Journal of Hand Surgery, American Society for Surgery of the Hand
The Hand, British Society for Surgery of the Hand
Commercial distributors of splinting materials and adapted equipment
NASA Biomedical Application Teams
Pioneers (Retired Engineers with Western Electric)

CHAPTER 26

Functional Restoration—
Burns *Maude H. Malick*

The United States has one of the highest fire death rates of the five major industrialized nations in the world.* Over 15,000 persons die each year in fires or as a result of thermal injuries. Over one million adults and children are burned annually, requiring admission to a hospital or limiting their activity for more than a day. One hundred thousand of these burned individuals require hospitalization either in burn-care centers or in community hospital facilities. However, only 10% of these burn patients are cared for in specialized burn-care units. Of the approximately 6000 children burned, 50% stay in a hospital facility for 1 month or less, 25% for 2 months, and the remainder for 3 months or more. Yet, at the same time, youth promotes a higher survival rate. Studies have shown that approximately 50% of all burns occur to individuals under 20 years of age, making this a crucial problem for the young. Eighty percent of the burns occur in the home.

Types of Burns and Initial Treatment

The most common cause of flame burns is clothing ignited from uncontrolled fires, while hot liquids, primarily coffee or boiling water, cause the majority of scald burns in the home. The mortality rate associated with flame burns in children is approximately 25% as opposed to 5% from liquid burns. Twenty-five percent of all burns among children result from heating units, hot liquids or vapors, stoves, electrical appliances, and matches. The inappropriate use of matches or lighters remains the leading cause of clothing ignition in children, with 86% of these accidents involving children under 10 years of age.

Statistics from the National Burn Information Exchange* indicate that the mortality rate is four times higher in the groups of patients in which burns are

---

* Facts on pages 479–483 are from MacMillan, B. G.: Burns in children. Clin Surg. 1:633–643, 1974.

---

* The National Burn Information Exchange is a service of the American Burn Association. The current address is given at the end of the chapter.

associated with clothing. Twenty-four percent of the patients sustaining clothing-related burns die in the hospital as compared with only 6% of patients whose clothing had not burned. The National Consumers Bureau has now made it mandatory for children's clothing to be made of nonflammable fibers.

The electrical burn is seen more in males than in females, and the extent of injury is dependent upon the number of volts to which the body has been subjected. In over 75% of electrical burns, the upper extremity has been injured or involved. The number of amputations from electrical burns is extremely high, with accompanying increased morbidity. The mortality is highest in those suffering severe electrical injury, and it is caused primarily by respiratory and cardiac arrest rather than by the burn.

The primary objective for all thermal burns is to extinguish all flames, remove smoldering clothing, and position the patient horizontally. Standing often results in smoke inhalation. In chemical burns, the area should be immersed or washed with large amounts of water to dilute the chemical agent.

The initial application of cold to minor burns is extremely helpful in reducing pain and edema, provided it is applied soon after the injury. Care should be taken not to use large cold compresses when transporting patients for prolonged periods of time, since severe hypothermia may result, interfering with capillary profusion and viability of the injured areas.

The burned areas should be covered with a clean material. Ointment or any other remedies should not be applied, so that an accurate assessment of the injury can be made at the initial medical facility. The extensively burned patient should not be given water, because the dangers of aspiration and water intoxication may jeopardize the future course of the patient.

Anatomy and Physiology of the Skin

The skin is the largest organ of the body. It is made up of three layers. The outer layer, which is called the *epidermis,* is approximately 60μ to 120μ thick, except on the palms and soles of the feet, which are from 0.5 mm to 0.8 mm. There are no blood vessels, capillaries, nerve endings, or lymphatics in the epidermis. Directly beneath the epidermis is the *dermis,* which is five to ten times thicker than the epidermis. This layer contains lymphatics, blood capillaries, nerve endings, hair follicles, sweat glands, and sebaceous glands. These are embedded in a ground substance that also contains collagen fibers, fibroblasts, reticulin, and elastin fibers lying in smooth parallel forma-

tions. The subcutaneous tissue lies directly beneath the dermis and epidermis.

In addition to providing a covering for the bony framework of the body and the life-sustaining organs, the skin serves the following purposes:

1. It protects against infection. It maintains a physical barrier that keeps out organisms and other bacteria. It has a bacteriostatic and bactericidal capability that can destroy small numbers of bacteria that penetrate the skin.
2. It prevents loss of body fluids. The structure of the skin is such that it can assist in maintaining the delicate fluid balance that is required by the body and functions to avoid dehydration.
3. It controls body temperature. The increase and decrease of evaporation of water from the sweat glands act as a temperature control. The sweat glands excrete excess water in small amounts of sodium chloride, cholesterin, and traces of albumin and urea.
4. It is an organ of sensation. The nerve endings within the dermis distinguish light or excessive pressure, pain, and low or high temperatures, thus allowing the individual to modify what he is doing in order to avoid damage or pain. The sebaceous glands protect the skin by the secretion of oils that soften and lubricate the skin. Vitamin D is made when the sunlight reacts with the cholesterol compounds within the skin.
5. It is cosmetic. The skin varies in pigment, texture, and whirls and patterns. This variation from one race to another and from one individual to another serves as a means of identification.

All of these purposes should be taken into consideration in determining the extent of the burn and its trauma to the patient both in its physical management and in its psychological components.

Classification of Burns

The extent of the total body burn should serve as the basis for the selection of the treatment facility. Burns of up to 15% of the total body surface can be adequately handled in community hospitals and those up to 25% in general hospitals. If more than 30% of the body area is burned, the patient should be taken to a burn center. Minor burns include partial-thickness burns of less than 20% of the total body surface and full-thickness burns of less than 10%. If the patient is to be transferred to a facility with more advanced services, the evacuation should be carried out as early in the immediate postburn course as possible. All patients with burns of the hands, perineum, and face should be admitted to the hospital.

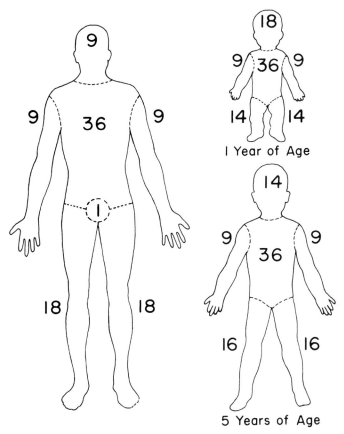

Figure 26-1. Rule of Nines.

I Year of Age

5 Years of Age

ified. A detailed diagram should be completed only after the blisters and dirt have been removed, because dirt and debris of normal skin often have the appearance of burned skin.

The Rule of Nines aids in estimating the percentage of burn, for it divides the body surface into areas of approximately 9% or multiples of 9%. The head, the neck, and the upper extremity each represent 9%; the lower extremity and the front and the back of the torso each represents 18%; and the perineum represents 1%. The rule is modified for children from birth to 1 year of age, allowing from 18 to 19% for the head and neck and 13% for the lower extremities. One percent is subtracted from the head and neck and added to the lower extremity for each year in ages one to ten. At the time of definitive care, more accurate estimate of the extent of burn is made by using a table that more precisely relates to the changes of body proportion to maturation.

Burn injuries are arbitrarily classified as minor, moderate, and severe (Table 26-1). Minor burns rarely require hospitalization. Patients with full-thickness burns of less than 2%, not involving critical areas, may be treated as outpatients until they require hospitalization for skin grafting. Noting that a patient's hand is about 1% of the total body surface can be useful in estimating the area of the burn on admission. The following criteria can be used to determine the degree of the burn:

Superficial first degree burns (Fig. 26-2) are confined to the epidermis, and they are characterized by erythema that blanches under pressure. There can be slight pain and edema but no blistering. The superficial burn can heal in a week because enough epithelial cells remain in the skin to provide new dermis.

Partial-thickness second degree burns involve the dermis, and they are characteristically more painful and sensitive to pinprick, with blisters and considerable subcutaneous edema. The treatment of partial-thickness burns is entirely directed toward

The severity of the burn is determined by the size and depth of the burn, the age of the patient, past medical history, and the part of the body burned. Only after these factors are determined can the proper decisions be made about disposition, treatment, and prognosis of the patient.

The area of the body burned can be determined in several ways. In adults of 16 years or more the Rule of Nines applies, and it is adequate for most clinical purposes (Fig. 26-1). For infants and children the burn estimate diagram and table have been mod-

Table 26-1 *Means of classifying severity of burns.*

	Minor	*Moderate*	*Severe*
Percent partial thickness	Less than 15%	15% to 30%	More than 30%
Percent full thickness	Less than 2%	2% to 10%	More than 10%
Hand, face, feet, and perineum	Not involved	Not involved	Involved
Age	Of little significance	Of little significance	Less than 18 months, more than 65 years
Etiology	Of little significance	Minor chemical and electrical burns	Major chemical and electrical burns
Complicating illnesses	Of little significance	Of little significance	Cardiac, renal, and metabolic involvement

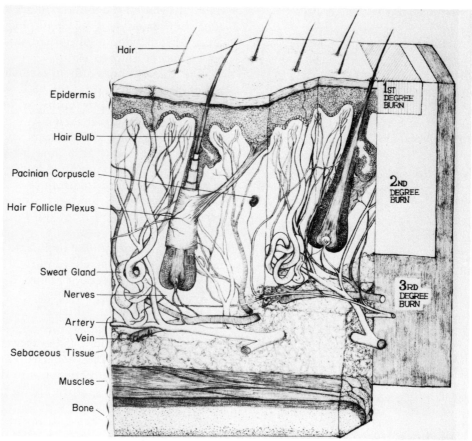

Figure 26-2. Cross section of the skin showing the depth of burn in relation to skin damage.

the prevention of infection. Bacterial infection can seriously interfere with healing and can change a partial-thickness burn into a full-thickness burn.

Deep partial-thickness burns are burns in which the epidermis and part of the dermis are dead. The deep dermis is injured but alive, and it will provide tissue for spontaneous healing. The hair follicles and sebaceous glands are destroyed. Only the deepest parts of the sweat glands in the epithelium will survive. Small bits of epithelium will suffice for re-epithelianization on the surface, although it occurs more slowly than in the superficial partial-thickness burn. This type of burn is sometimes referred to as deep thermal burn.

Full-thickness third degree burns involve the destruction of the full thickness of the skin with possible muscle, tendon, and bone damage. Spontaneous healing is not possible. Grafting is usually necessary after the necrotic eschar has been removed. The area of third degree burn is usually dry and unblistered; it is depressed below the surface of the surrounding burns; and it is transparent with thrombosed vessels in its depth. The burn is painfree and insensitive to pinprick. Deep flame burns and some electrical burns may appear charred or black. Doubtful depth areas are leathery, waxy-white or red, and nonblanching with subcutaneous edema. Occasionally blisters occur. Pinprick sensation can be absent. These burns usually destroy the full thickness of skin in children and areas of thin skin such as ears, eyelids, and inner forearm in adults. The swelling and pain associated with burns of the preorbital area, perineum, and both hands and feet frequently make outpatient nursing difficult.

Other Major Burn Damage

Respiratory Tract

Respiratory-tract injuries are one of the major causes of mortality in burn patients. In considering causes of respiratory distress in the acute burn, keep in mind that only a few patients with facial burns require an artificial airway or ventilatory assistance and then only rarely during the first 24 hours. The oral airway is necessary if the patient is comatose, and close observation is necessary for signs of airway obstruction. If the patient has evidence of facial burns with singed nasal hairs and soot about the nose and mouth, careful monitoring is required. A tracheostomy should be performed only if absolutely necessary.

Body Fluid

When the burn occurs, there are changes in the distribution of the body fluid. Depending on the temperature and the duration of heat causing the burn wound, a certain depth of injury or tissue death occurs. In minor burns where a thin layer of epidermis and dermis are exposed to heat for a short time, the changes will be minimal, and they may include redness with a separation of the outer layer of epidermis, caused by blistering or slight edema. With prolonged exposure to heat, the capillary bed and the deeper tissues are traumatized and destroyed. This trauma takes the form of increased capillary permeability or a thrombosis in severe wounds. As capillary permeability increases, the capillaries leak fluid into the interstitial spaces, and interspatial fluid is increased. This is called *edema*. The lymphatic system would normally carry away the increased tissue fluid, but when the burn is large there is a great deal of plasma leak, and the lymph system is rapidly overloaded. The lymphatic system may also have been damaged by the heat.

In minor burns the reabsorption occurs at the same rate as accumulation of fluid, so edema does not occur. When massive edema does occur, immediate surgical measures may be needed to avoid vascular constriction.

Limb Ischemia

Escharotomies may need to be performed both to relieve pressure and to prevent limb ischemia. Edema developing under circumferential full-thickness burns in an extremity may produce a rise in interstitial pressure sufficient to cause cyanosis of the distal unburned skin, impairing capillary filling and producing progressive neurologic deficits. Medial and lateral incisions of the eschar only to relieve pressure are painless when made through third degree burns, and they should be performed promptly if the signs of ischemia develop. In electrical burns, even fasciotomy is necessary occasionally to relieve pressure. With increasing burn edema, a circumferential full-thickness chest burn may significantly restrict the motion of the thoracic cage, requiring an escharotomy for relief. This is especially likely in children who may become exhausted by the increased ventilatory effort.

Role of the Occupational Therapist

During the first 72 hours after a severe burn injury, the patient is in burn shock. During this period the burn team's duty is to stabilize the many internal and external changes caused by the thermal insult. As a result of the burn and loss of skin, the body has lost its ability to protect itself against infection, to maintain a balance in body fluid, and to prevent heat loss. Although most burn units maintain approximately 80°F room temperature, heat shields are also often used to maintain body heat.

The occupational therapist plays an important role in the initial phase of burn management by preventing soft-tissue contractures, which are the major cause of loss in joint function and distorted skeletal positioning. Because of burn trauma and heat loss, the patient quickly assumes the flexed, adducted fetal position for comfort and warmth. This position directly causes contracture deformities resulting from the shortening of healing tissues across and around the joints of the burned parts of the body. These contractures restrict full range of motion, and their strong flexor pull can cause grotesque distortions of the extremities, most notably around the face and neck, especially when anterior neck and face burns exist. The impending contractures can be prevented by careful early positioning at the time of admission, daily monitoring of positioning and splinting, and active exercises.

Positioning and Splinting

Proper bed positioning must be initiated immediately on admission in order to prevent deformity (Fig. 26-3). In general, the position of extension must be maintained, accompanied by frequent short periods of active exercise as is practical during dressing changes and tubbing. By placing the joints in extension, the overlying burn scar is maintained at its maximum length, and contractures can be prevented. This extended position must often be accomplished by the use of extension splints across the major joints of the body. These apply traction to the healing tissue in the form of an opposing force (Table 26-2). When evaluating the need for splinting, consideration should be given to areas where the burns involve a joint or where they are lateral to the flexor surface of a joint. Uninvolved joints should be free to prevent tendon shortening and stiffness.

Exercising

All of the joints should be exercised daily, preferably using active motion rather than passive motion to prevent joint stiffness. Active motion contributes to the maintenance of muscle mass and strength, while passive motion prevents tendon adherence as well as the tightening and shortening of the joint capsules. Passive motion should be gently executed and never pressed beyond tissue resistance.

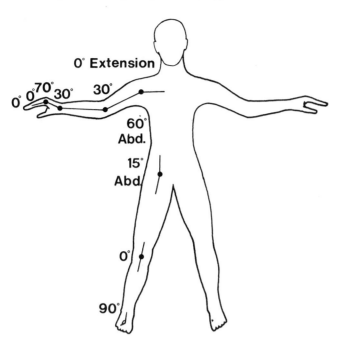

Figure 26-3. Initial burn position.

All wounds should be carefully cleaned, debrided, and dressed at least twice daily. Splints must be thoroughly washed and dried before reapplying. Low-temperature splints such as those made of Orthoplast, Kay-Splint, and Polyform can be gas autoclaved. Exercise, self-care activities, and night splint regimen must be followed until the burned areas spontaneously heal and, in third degree burns, until the grafted areas have set, which usually is 7 to 10 days postgraft.

Pressure Stretch Techniques

A research study conducted at the Shriners' Burns Institute in Galveston, Texas, has indicated that more than 80% of patients who have suffered second and third degree burns will develop hypertrophic scarring throughout the burned areas after new skin and grafts have healed (Fig. 26-8). If the development of scar hypertrophy is not controlled, crippling disfigurement is likely as a result of severe contractures and the unchecked formation of thickened, knobby red scar tissue. In normal burn wound healing there is a great increase in vascularity to form the granulation tissue that the body uses to restore the damaged skin site. Studies conducted by Dr. Hugo Linares at the Shriners' Burns Institute indicate that the granulation tissue shows an increase of *fibroblasts*. Fibroblasts are the cells that synthesize mucopolysaccharides and collagen fibers necessary for the development of new connective tissue.

In the development of normal skin dermis, fibroblasts appear to be irregular in shape and flat with a

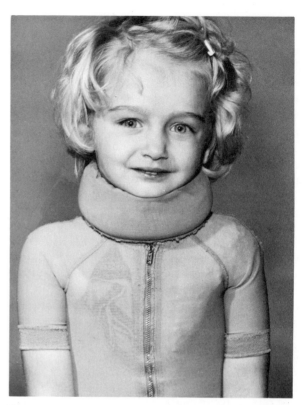

Figure 26-4. Soft cervical collar.

lumpy surface. But the fibroblasts that develop within the reticular layer of a hypertrophic scar are spider-shaped with rounded nodular bodies. These fibroblasts produce an excessive amount of collagen fibers that adhere to one another in an irregular pat-

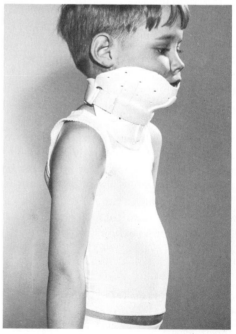

Figure 26-5. A rigid low-temperature thermoplastic cervical collar.

Table 26-2 *Directions for positioning and splinting.*

Body Part	Positioning	Splinting
Neck	Slight extension No pillows should be used Mouth of patient should be able to be closed	Soft cervical collar (Fig. 26-4) Rigid (low-temperature thermoplastic neck conformer) (Fig. 26-5)
Shoulders	Arms abducted 60° to 90° with slight internal rotation	Traction or axillary splints may be used Small pillow between scapulae will encourage external rotation
Elbow	Full extension when anterior surface of arm is involved Elbow should be ranged with exercise and/or activity during the day and positioned at night in full extension	Three-point extension splint can be worn over dressings (Fig. 26-6)
Hips	Whether prone or supine—neutral extended position Legs should be abducted 15° from the midline	Abduction position can be accomplished by positioning drop foot splints approximately 12 in. apart A bar placed between the knees attached to the three-point extension splints will maintain abduction
Knee	Full extension	Three-point extension splints for night use (Fig. 26-6)
Ankle	90° (which is normal standing position) prevents the shortening of the Achilles tendon	Foot board—drop foot splints When using a posterior splint, the heel must be suspended to prevent pressures sores. When prone, position patient so that foot hangs over edge of the mattress. Extension splints can be attached to tennis shoes to aid in positioning.
Spine	A straight-line position to prevent scoliosis, especially with lateral body burns.	
Hands	Wrist 30° extension or dorsiflexion Metacarpophalangeal joint 70° flexion Proximal and distal interphalangeal joints full extension Thumb abducted and extended to maintain web space (Fig. 26-7)	Functional pan splint placing interphalangeal joints in full extension maintaining "burn" position

tern. The nodules of compact collagen permit little or no interstitial spacing because they fill the middle and lower reticular layers of the dermis. The collagen filaments entwine with each other in ropelike fashion (Fig. 26-9). In addition to the irregular shape of the nodules, a hypertrophic scar will synthesize collagen at more than four times the rate of normal skin. It is this pile-up of collagen-filled nodules that gives rise to the rigid, thickened hypertrophic scar that later can cause contractures.

It has been known for some years that the application of controlled, consistent pressure to the surface of an immature hypertrophic scar will, in time, reduce the scar and leave a smooth, pliable skin surface. But the problem of how pressure could be applied and maintained throughout the maturation

of the scar persisted. Pressure dressings and elastic Ace wraps were tried, but all of these materials slipped, bunched up, constricted, or fell off.

The Jobst Institute in Toledo, Ohio, developed a special Dacron Spandex elastic fabric to be used in the construction of carefully fitted pressure gradient garments. Garments constructed from the new fabric, when accurately measured, fitted, and consistently worn by burn patients, provide and maintain adequate pressure to prevent hypertrophic scar formation. In addition, the multidirectional stretch of the fabric allows any normal movement of the body. The garments are custom engineered and constructed for each patient to provide a consistent gradient pressure over the burn scar areas.

The garment can be engineered to apply specific

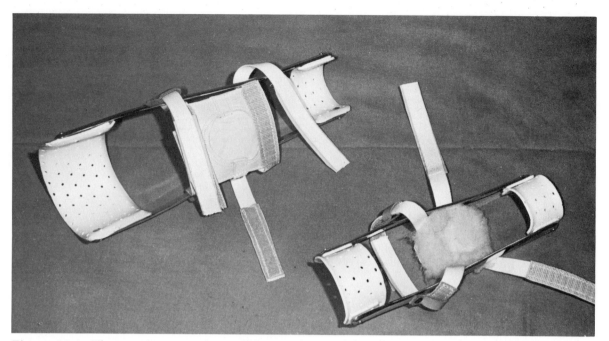

Figure 26-6. Three-point extension splints can be used for elbow and knee extension.

pressure directly over the burned areas, including the entire body (Fig. 26-10). Often one body area will be grafted or will heal several weeks before the rest of the body is ready for measuring. These areas should be measured and garments should be ordered as early as possible (Fig. 26-11), leaving large unhealed areas for measurement later. Compression dressing such as Tubigrip can be used in the interim.

Healed burns that are ready for measurement can vary greatly in color from a deep purple to a pink. The measurement and fitting of pressure gradient garments may begin as soon as these open areas of newly healed scar tissue are reduced to the size of a dime. In other words, any graft site, whether it is a patch or mesh, should be almost completely healed before measurement. In fact, a minimum of 7 days postgraft should be allowed before measurement is considered. Donor sites should also be dry and well healed before garments are fitted.

The pressure garments must be carefully measured and designed in order to provide adequate pressure over the burned areas and still allow normal

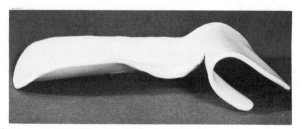

Figure 26-7. Functional position splint for the thumb.

body mobility. Full-length zippers should be designated whenever a burned extremity is involved. In this way all shearing effects can be eliminated when the garments are donned. In order to be wholly effective, the pressure garments must be worn consistently 24 hours a day for 12 to 18 months or until full-scar maturation. The patient and his or her garments and splinting should be followed on a regular outpatient basis (every 2 weeks and later monthly) in order to monitor the pressure and position management.

Even with the success of pressure techniques, certain body areas have additional needs. The areas around the nose and mouth of the face and the concave body areas require interface molds to maintain consistent pressure. Rivers has written about the use of Uvex face molds to apply definitive pressure to remodel the facial scars.* Silastic Elastomer can be used as a flexible mold worn under the pressure garments to apply adequate pressure to specific areas such as the face, anterior chest, feet, and axilla. This Dow Corning product fills the concave gapping that occurs with normal movements when wearing pressure garments. Both have proven highly successful.

The pressure stretch techniques are essential to soften, smooth, and maintain elastic skin during the maturation process and to prevent hypertrophic scarring and subsequent contractures. The pressure

---

* Rivers, E. A., Strate, R. G., and Solem, L. D.: The transparent face mask. Am. J. Occup. Ther. 33:108–113, 1979.

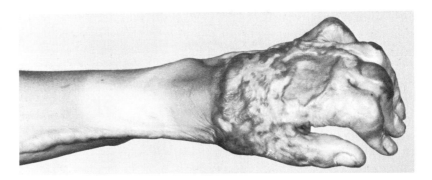

Figure 26-8. Scar hypertrophy on a burned hand.

techniques are also effective after scar hypertrophies. Adequate pressure can reduce the scarring, soften the hypertrophies, and gain elasticity. In this way joint mobility is gained, and severe contractures can be avoided.

The Burned Hand

The burned hand is of major concern to the occupational therapist. The hand burn occurs most frequently because the hand is used to extinguish the fire. Dorsal hand burns are the most frequent and the most disabling of hand burns. Dorsal burns of the hand tend to produce a deformity that consists of hyperextension of the metacarpophalangeal joints, flexion of the interphalangeal joints, adduction and extension of the thumb, radial deviation to the wrist,

and wrist flexion. The resulting flattening of the transverse and longitudinal palmar arches renders the hand nonfunctional. All of these deforming positions will develop into contractures unless the hand is appropriately exercised, splinted, and treated.

The basic burn splint should be designed individually to prevent the development of hand deformities. In addition to preventing wrist flexion, the splint prevents metacarpophalangeal joint extension deformity and proximal interphalangeal joint flexion contracture commonly called the "claw" deformity (Fig. 26-12). The extensor tendons that lie on the dorsum of the hand are so poorly protected that they are extremely vulnerable to injury as they cross the proximal interphalangeal joint. The classic boutonnière deformity is seen all too frequently. When the wrist is held properly in extension, the metacarpophalangeal

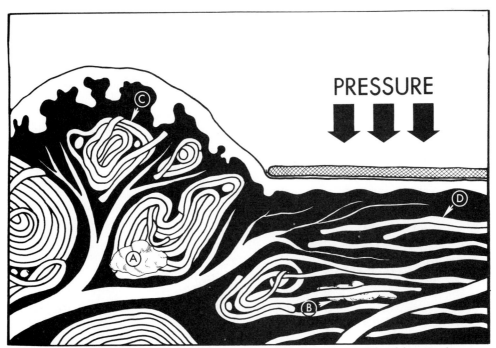

Figure 26-9. Effect of pressure on healing scar tissue: *A*, Fibroblast in hypertrophic scar; *B*, Fibroblast in nonhypertrophic scar; *C*, Ropelike collagen filament in hypertrophic scar; *D*, Linear parallel arrangement of collagen filament in nonhypertrophic scar.

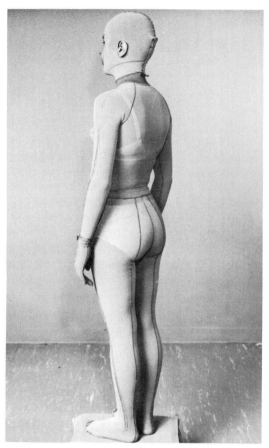

Figure 26-10. Jobst pressure gradient burn garment.

joints tend to flex because of the effects of gravity and the tension on the intrinsic muscles. This position allows the intrinsic muscles to act on the interphalangeal extension. However, the most vulnerable joint in the hand is the proximal interphalangeal joint.

If direct burn damage to the extensor mechanism or through proximal interphalangeal joint flexion causes the middle extensor slip to be caught between the unyielding eschar and the underlying heads of the proximal and middle phalanges, partial destruction of the extensor mechanism will result. The lateral bands of the joint can be shredded or can slip volarly, thus causing the hand to assume the typical burn hand deformity. For this reason careful positioning of these two sets of joints is mandatory, and no fist clenching is permitted until the stability of the extensor mechanism is assured. Internal splints with Kirschner wires can be used to prevent the development of metacarpophalangeal, interphalangeal, and thumb deformities as well.

The main indication for internal splinting is destruction of a tendon from the burn or bacterial invasion. This most frequently occurs to the extensor mechanism over or just proximal to the proximal interphalangeal joint. Careful external splinting judiciously monitored can prevent the flexion deformity. If the flexion deformity is not corrected, the pull of the flexors, mainly the strong sublimis, will cause the

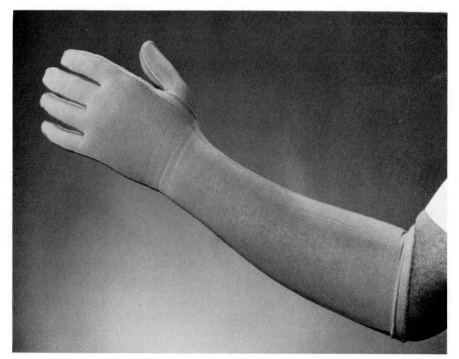

Figure 26-11. Pressure gradient gloves.

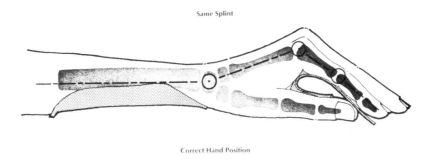

Same Splint

Correct Hand Position

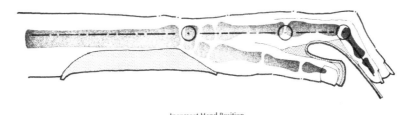

Incorrect Hand Position

Figure 26-12. Burn functional hand splint. If the splint is allowed to slip forward a claw deformity can result.

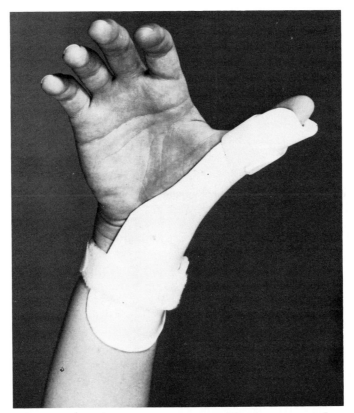

Figure 26-13. A pressure contour splint can correct deformity.

proximal interphalangeal joint to flex often beyond the 90 degrees of flexion. Thumb adduction will also occur unless the thenar web space is maintained and the thumb placed in the position of abduction and opposition. Often direct-pressure contour-pan splinting is required to soften, stretch out, and oppose existing contractures (Fig. 26-13). Progressive contour pan splinting can stretch out an immature (pink) scar in order to reach maximum extension and motion in a joint.

Treatment Plan

When the course of occupational therapy is planned, the following factors must be considered: the depth of burn, location of burns, associated injuries, extent of total body injury, extent of injury to the hands, the age of the patient, and patient cooperation. Age is of particular importance. Most children are unable to understand or cooperate in a program of active motion, but they can understand carefully planned play and self-care activities. The hands of children can be splinted for prolonged periods without producing undue stiffness. Within a few days the full active range of motion can be reached even after numerous days of static splinting. Elderly patients often lack the strength or comprehension to carry out exercises for active motion, so careful splinting and monitoring must be instituted. Early self-care activities can provide the motivation for movement. The members of the burn team or hospital staff should encourage cooperation and should repeatedly emphasize correct positioning and active motion. Staff and patient education must be ongoing to aid in the prevention of deformity and to encourage early functional return.

Palmar burns to the hand produce contractures and deformity pulling toward the location of the injury. Dorsal splinting or contoured palmar-pan splints (Fig. 26-14) that hold the hand in full exten-

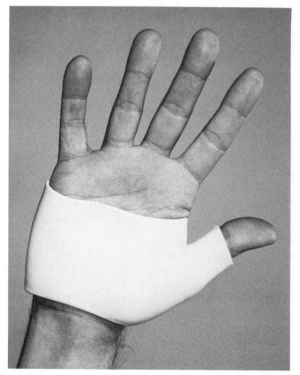

Figure 26-14. A palmar extension pan splint can be used to soften scar tissue and correct web space contractures.

sion should be considered. Wrist-flexion contractures and deformities can easily arise with accompanying adduction and flexion contractures of the thumb.

Early self-care activities such as eating and personal hygiene should be started as soon as the patient is medically stable. Sometimes adaptive devices may be needed, but they should not be used unless absolutely necessary. Many problems related to functional loss of joint motion and anatomical deformities can be alleviated through normal use of the extremities and activity. Strength will return in weakened and atrophic muscles, especially with early ambulation and normal daily movements of the body. Adhesions of tendons and surrounding structures will also be freed through continuing activities of daily living. Time is an important factor. Capsular structures, shortened by poor positioning or inactivity, can be stretched when appropriate activities are planned.

The occupational therapist should work toward full self-care independence and increase in extremity function, physical endurance, and muscle strength. A homemaker checkout should be required to see if any additional training is required such as work simplification and energy-conservation techniques. Bilateral activities should be stressed, and easy-flow work patterns should be established. Self-care activities can be used as a form for therapeutic exercise.

Early ambulation with good posture should be encouraged. If extensive leg burns exist, wrapping with Ace bandages using the figure-eight technique may be indicated to alleviate pain caused by blood rushing to the lower extremities. If the patient has had skin grafts to the legs, bedrest must be maintained for 10 days postgraft. Even though venous circulation has returned to the graft site and the graft appears stable, adequate arterial blood flow will take longer to become established. The patient may be allowed to stand and move about with Ace wraps after 10 days to encourage ambulation and proper foot positioning to eliminate heel cord contractures. Pressure leg garments should be considered. Active motion in the form of exercise, self-care activities, planned activities, and ambulation will improve muscle strength, free adhesions, and stretch skin and joint contractures.

Dynamic splinting may be required to do corrective positioning, to counterbalance flexion contractures, and to apply a slow traction pull. Splints are indicated for a metacarpophalangeal flexion deformity. Early adduction contracture of the thumb may be an indication for dynamic splinting. If the thumb contracture persists, resulting in the adduction deformity, early surgical intervention is often employed.

Contact axillary splinting in the form of an airplane splint is frequently indicated for anterior chest and shoulder burns. The airplane splint can be constructed out of shaped aluminum cuffs and rods or contoured low-temperature plastics. The shoulder should be maintained in 90 to 100 degrees abduction. Strapping will be required to maintain this position.

A variety of graded work and recreational activities that include leatherwork, weaving, and woodwork projects can be programmed to increase range of motion, to develop work tolerance, and to increase personal independence.

Psychological Considerations

The emotional aspects of burn care deserve careful consideration, because the patient suffers not only devastating physical trauma but also overwhelming psychological stress. The occupational therapist, as an active member of the burn team, will need to aid in the identification and management of these psychological problems. Age, personality, family support, and social and economic factors influence the manner in which the patient can handle his or her problems.

The fear of death is real for the burn patient in the face of immobility, prolonged and intense pain, separation and isolation, loss of control over one's fate, and association with dying patients. The fear of mutilation and disfigurement can be traumatic, especially as body changes occur throughout the treatment process. Especially threatening are fears of disfigurement experienced by patients with facial burns. Genuine grief must be recognized as the patient faces discharge with the loss of an acceptable body image and fear of nonacceptance by the outside world.

The patient's self-perception has impact on the individual's personality, and feelings of hostility and grief can develop. The patient must also be able to cope with emotional stress, not only in relation to feelings towards self, but also in relation to feelings toward individuals and circumstances concerned with the accident.

Disruption of life cycle and separation from the family circle can cause complex problems, especially if hospitalization is for any length of time. The patient may develop, as a substitute for familial emotional support, new methods for gaining gratification and reward. The severely burned patient frequently is in conflict over dependency versus independency. Some patients find it difficult to accept forced dependency and to develop necessary trust relationships with others.

Prolonged hospitalization and convalescence put a strain not only on the patient but also on the attending medical team. Each surgical procedure must be interpreted carefully. Strong anxiety in the patient must be recognized, especially in relation to the patient's perception and interpretation of the injuries in light of plans and goals.

When massive burns exist, the patient often has a hospital stay of more than 90 days and he or she faces a longer term of continuing medical procedures. Many times these procedures are carried out in a rehabilitation unit or center. The rehabilitation facility is appropriate for aggressive rehabilitation. Transfer to a rehabilitation area also gives the patient a feeling of progress. A physical medicine evaluation should be made early in the acute-care stage; management by a physiatrist in a rehabilitation center then can be recommended and planned.

Initially, the therapist is involved as part of the burn team in the identification of physical and psychological problems and in planning management of those problems. Development of rapport and an interpersonal relationship between the therapist and the patient is of vital importance in the management of the patient. A kind but realistic approach will be most helpful to the patient in coping with numerous problems as they become apparent. The therapist can be effective by interpreting the problem realistically and reducing the patient's stress by providing sound emotional support. Much of the ongoing anxiety can be alleviated by giving the patient a sense of worth and by maintaining interpersonal relationships.

At the first encounter the therapist should introduce himself or herself to the patient, orient the patient to his or her environment, and interpret the therapist's role. During treatment the therapist aids the patient by explaining what procedures and treatments are necessary and by defining medical terms in lay terminology. In this way a sound rapport and respect can be developed between the patient and the therapist. Thus, the patient can more easily express feelings and he or she will be more amenable to re-establishing personal independence and cooperation throughout the longer phase of rehabilitation and scar maturation.

Counseling should be directed toward a return to normal activity as quickly as possible, with the importance of follow-up visits stressed. Often the family and friends must be counseled to aid in interpreting and understanding the patient's reactions and feelings. This is especially important when there are feelings of grief or hostility. Group therapy sessions are important for the psychological rehabilitation of the patient. In these sessions the patient should be allowed to express fears and anxieties openly. Here he or she can discuss possible solutions with others in the same situation. The social worker and psychologist should be members of group therapy sessions. The family should be included in discussions with the patient in order to discern ways of handling situations that they will encounter after the patient returns to the home, job, or school.

Nutrition

Nutrition must be carefully monitored and modified so that the catabolic phase of metabolism is corrected. The patient should be in positive nitrogen balance or anabolism, which promotes healing. This positive nitrogen balance is necessary, and it must be maintained through a high-caloric, high-protein diet. The patient must recognize that good nutrition with a well-balanced diet is necessary for tissue repair and maintenance of strength during the rehabilitation period.

Follow-Up Program

A schedule for close outpatient follow-up is necessary to check and to maintain a good outpatient protocol. In this way scar maturation, joint problems, pressure garments, and need for reconstructive procedures can be monitored (Fig. 26-15). The social worker should

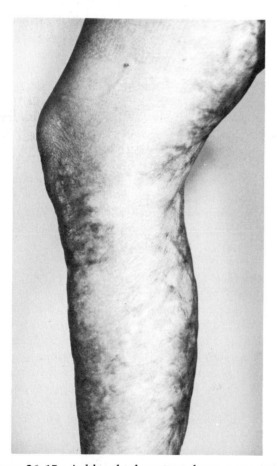

Figure 26-15. A blanched mature burn scar can be attained with proper pressure techniques on the burn scar areas. Close outpatient follow up is necessary to maintain the schedule.

be active in the outpatient program to monitor the home situation, to provide home-care services as needed, to give emotional support, and to provide for equipment and transportation needs. Should reconstructive surgery be indicated, whether it be functional or cosmetic, the patient must understand the need for the procedures and the need for time to pass before many of these procedures can be accomplished. The surgeon and the physiatrist should work together to correct deformities in order that the patient may gain maximum function.

The most frequent areas of reconstruction are the webbing of the hands, thumb adduction, wrist flexion, axillary contractures, facial contracture, and posterior knee contractures. Children require the most reconstruction because their scar tissue may not grow as rapidly as developing bone.

The American Society for Burns Recovered, Inc., is a national organization formed to aid burned individuals and their families to cope with ongoing problems. The national office is in Orange, New Jersey. Local chapters have been formed in most major cities in which active burn units are located.

Bibliography

Artz, C. P., Moncrief, J. A., and Pruitt, B. A.: Burns—A Team Approach. Philadelphia: W. B. Saunders, 1979, pp. 466–478.

Baebel, S., Bulkley, A. L., and Shuck, J. M.: Physical therapy for burned patients. J. Phys. Ther. 53:1289–1293, 1973.

Boswick, J. A., Jr.: The management of fresh burns of the hand and deformities resulting from burn injuries. Clin. Plast. Surg. 1:621–631, 1974.

Evans, E. B.: Orthopedic measures in the treatment of severe burns. J. Bone Joint Surg. 48:643–699, 1968.

Evans, E. B.: Preservation and restoration of joint function in patients with severe burns. J.A.M.A. 204:843–848, 1968.

Evans, E. B.: Prevention and correction of deformity after severe burns. Surg. Clin. N. Am. 50:1361, 1970.

Evans, E. B., et al.: Prevention and correction of deformity after severe burns. Surg. Clin. N. Am. 50:1361–1375, 1970.

Fujimori, R., Hiramoto, M., and Ofuji, S.: Sponge fixation method for treatment of early scars. Plast. Reconst. Surg. 42:322–327, 1968.

Goldberg, R. T.: Rehabilitation of the burned patient. Rehab. Lit. 35:73–77, 1974.

Jaeger, D. L.: Maintenance and function of the burned patient. J Phys. Ther. 52:627–633, 1972.

Kischer, C. W.: Fibroblasts of the hypertrophic scar, mature scar and normal skin: A study by scanning and transmission electron microscopy. Texas Rep. Biol. Med. 32:3–4, 1974.

Kischer, C. W., Shetlar, M. R., and Shetlar, C. L.: Alteration of hypertrophic scars induced by mechanical pressure. Arch. Dermatol. 111:60–64, 1975.

Larson, D. L.: The Prevention and Correction of Burn Scar Contracture and Hypertrophy. Pamphlet, Shriners Burns Institute, Galveston Unit, Texas, 1973.

Larson, D. L.: Repair of the boutonniere deformity of the burned hand. J. Trauma 10:6, 1970.

Larson, D. L., et al.: Development and correction of burn scar contracture. In Matter, P. (ed.): Transaction of the Third International Congress on Research in Burns. Prague, 1970.

Larson, D. L., et al.: Skeletal suspension and traction in the treatment of burns. Ann. Surg. 168:981–985, 1968.

Larson, D. L., et al.: Techniques for decreasing scar formation and contractures in the burned patient. J. Trauma 11:807–823, 1971.

Larson, D. L., Abston, S., Willis, B., et al.: Contracture and scar formation in the burn patient. Clin. Surg. 1:653, 1974.

Lavore, J. S., and Marshalls, J. H.: Expedient splint of the burn patient. J. Phys. Ther. 52:1036–1042, 1972.

Linares, H. A.: Granulation tissue and hypertrophic scars. An International Symposium and Workshop on the Relations of Ultrastruction of Collagen to the Healing of Wounds and the Surgical Management of Hypertrophic Scars. Cincinnatti OH, 1973.

Linares, H. A., et al.: The histiocytic organization of hypertrophic scar in humans. J. Invest. Derm. 59:323–331, 1972.

Linares, H. A., et al.: On the origin of the hypertrophic scar. J. Trauma 13:70–75, 1973.

MacMillan, B. G.: Burns in children. Clin. Plast. Surg. 1:633–643, 1974.

Malick, M. H., and Carr, J.: Manual on the Management of the Burn Patient. Pittsburgh, PA: Harmarville Rehabilitation Center, 1982.

Malick, M.: Manual on Dyanmic Hand Splinting. Pittsburgh, PA: Harmarville Rehabilitation Center, 1978.

Malick, M., and Carr, J.: Flexible elastomer molds in burn scar control. Am. J. Occup. Ther. 34:9, 1980.

Rivers, E. A., Strate, R. G., Solem, L. D.: The transparent face mask. Am. J. Occup. Ther. 33:108–113, 1979.

Shetlar, M. E., et al.: The hypertrophic scar, hexosamine containing components of burn scars. Proc. Soc. Exp. Biol. Med. 139:544–547, 1972.

Shetlar, M. E. et al.: The hypertrophic scar, glycoprotein, and collagen components of burn scars. Proc. Soc. Exp. Biol. Med. 138:298–300, 1971.

Tanigawa, M. P. C., O'Donnell, O. K., and Graham, P. L.: The burned hand—a physical therapy protocol. J. Phys. Ther. 54:953–958, 1974.

Von Prince, K. M. P., Currerri, P. W., and Pruitt, B. A.: The application of finger nail hooks in splinting of burned hands. Am. J. Occup. Ther. 24:156–159, 1970.

Von Prince, K. M. P., and Yeakel, M. H.: The Splinting of Burn Patients. Springfield IL: Charles C. Thomas, 1974.

Willis, B.: Burn Scar Therapy—A Treatment Method. Pamphlet from Toledo OH: Jobst Institute Inc., 1973.

Willis, B.: Custom splinting the burn patient. In Lynch, J. P., and Lewis, S. R. (eds.): Symposium on the Treatment of Burns. St. Louis: C. V. Mosby, 1973, pp. 93–97.

Willis, B.: Splinting the Burned Patient. Galveston: Shriners Burns Institute. Pamphlet distributed by Johnson & Johnson, New Brunswick NJ, 1971.

Willis, B.: The use of orthoplast isoprene splints in the treatment of the acutely burned child: A follow-up. Am. J. Occup. Ther. 24:3, 1970.

Resources

American Burn Association
Frances C. Nance, M.D.
Louisiana State University
Medical Center
Department of Surgery
1542 Tulane Avenue
New Orleans, Louisiana 70112
(maintains an active office providing a full range of educational, medical, research, and patient referral services)
American Society for Burns Recovered, Inc.
439 Main Street
Orange, New Jersey 07050
Dow Corning/Wright
P.O. Box 100
Arlington, Tennessee 38002
Jobst Institute
653 Miami Street
Toledo, Ohio 43694
(visual aids and educational material)

CHAPTER 27

Functional Restoration—
Amputations and
Prosthetic Replacement *Elinor Anne Spencer*

It's not what you've lost that counts, it's what you do with what's left.[1]

McGonegal/Russell

To be an amputee is to be without a limb or limbs as a result of injury, disease, or congenital deformity. Bodily functions develop in the presence of anomalies in children with congenital deformities or early postbirth amputations, but postadolescent amputees suffer the loss of a part of the body that had previously been integrated into the total body image. Function, sensation, and appearance of the involved extremity are affected, and the amputee must rely on an insensitive mechanical device as a replacement for the natural limb. Since the traumatic amputee has usually matured physically, the circumstances of the amputation, its meaning, and its consequences are different from those of the congenital or very young amputee. This chapter emphasizes the rehabilitation team's work with a person who has suffered traumatic amputation after adolescence.

There are many causes of amputations: trauma, peripheral vascular disease, thrombosis, embolism, malignancy, and trophic changes. The most common cause of upper extremity (UE) amputations is trauma resulting from industrial accidents, which are usually connected with the use of high speed power tools. The most common cause of lower extremity (LE) amputations is peripheral vascular disease.

Generally the physical therapy service is responsible for prosthetic training of the LE amputee but, since LE amputees are frequently referred to the occupational therapy service for assistance in motivation, physical restoration, self-care independence (ADL), and prevocational assessment, this chapter discusses some appropriate treatment objectives and activities. However, because the occupational therapist participates actively in the prosthetic training program of the UE amputee, this will be the main focus of the chapter.

The patient's reactions to the loss of a limb vary depending on age when the amputation occurred, intelligence, physical development, sex, vocation, avocational interests, social status, and finances. The amputee may also have problems in function because of the presence of phantom sensations, a phenomenon in which the amputee actually feels the presence of part of the limb that has been amputated. This can lead to difficulties in his or her accepting, tolerating, and learning to use the prosthesis (the artificial limb).

The amputee rehabilitation program begins with the decision to amputate, and it ends with the successful functional and cosmetic integration of the prosthesis into the body schema. Whether the cause of the amputation is trauma or disease, the first step in the total program is the consideration of the type and level of surgery and the psychological and physical preparation of the patient.

Surgical Considerations

During the surgical procedure of amputation the physicians try to save as much tissue as possible. The importance of structural length and support of the bone, length and strength of the cut or damaged muscles, and sensation through adequate skin coverage bear out the practicality and necessity of preserving tissue. Regardless of the level of the amputation, the muscles involved directly or indirectly in the function of the amputated part are affected by the loss.

Prior to the operation, the necessity of the amputation, the expected result, the postoperative conditioning program, the possibility of difficulties in adjustment, and the prosthetic training program are explained to the patient. He or she must be prepared both medically and psychologically for the problems which he or she may encounter as he or she prepares to use the prosthesis.

Both during and after surgery, effort is made to form the stump in such a way as to maintain maximum function of the remaining tissue and to provide maximum use of the prosthesis. Blood vessels and nerves are pulled down, cut, and allowed to retract so that they do not interfere with the amputee's use of the prosthesis by causing pain in the stump when the device is used.

Either a *closed* or an *open* amputation may be done by the surgeon. The open amputation allows free drainage of affected material, minimizing the possibility of infection before closure. The immediate closed amputation may reduce the period of hospitalization, but it also reduces free drainage and introduces the danger of bacterial growth. When the closed amputation is performed, either immediately or following sufficient drainage, the maximum amount of tissue is saved. However, regardless of the surgical method used, the stump must be strong and resilient and must have a snug, comfortable contact with the socket of the prosthesis, for the amputee will exert much pressure on the stump while using the device.

Special Considerations and Problems

Physical problems may affect or hinder the prosthetic training program with either the UE or the LE amputee. Such problems are the length of the stump, its skin coverage, its sensitivity (*i.e.*, presence of hypersensitivity and/or edema), its healing, the condition of the skin, and the presence of infection. For example, an amputee with either a very long stump or a very short one may find the design of the various components of the prosthesis unsatisfactory either cosmetically or functionally. Perspiration, the natural result of physical effort, may result from excessive confinement of the stump in the prosthesis' socket, for the stump lacks ventilation. The occupational therapist must also be aware of the possibility of the amputee's being allergic to plastics and resins from which the socket is made.

The sensation of the stump is important to the rehabilitation of the amputee. If a hand has been amputated and the patient has been fitted with a prosthetic prehension device, he or she no longer experiences functional sensation in the area that has been amputated. Although he or she has sensation in the stump, it is functionally lost when he or she puts on the prosthesis. Therefore, he or she will have to depend on visual cues in order to use the terminal device to handle objects. Sensation can also be a problem if the socket is ill-fitting or if the stump is not well-formed at the distal end. Therefore, the amputee must become adjusted to the pressure of the socket on the stump. He or she also must become used to the pressure of the harness on his or her shoulders and to the weight of the prosthesis.

Levels of Amputations of the Upper Extremity

The higher the level of amputation, the more the amputee must depend on the prosthesis for replacement of bodily function and the more extensive the prosthesis must be. Generally accepted levels of amputation are indicated in Figure 27-1.

Amputations at the joints are referred to as *disarticulations* (*i.e.*, finger, wrist, elbow, or shoulder disarticulation). Amputations below the wrist across the metacarpal bones are referred to as *transmetacarpal*. At this level and below, amputations are referred to as *partial hand*. Should the amputation occur between the wrist and the elbow, the level is referred to as *below elbow* (BE), and amputation between the elbow and the shoulder is referred to as *above elbow* (AE). Amputations at the surgical neck of the humerus (dis-

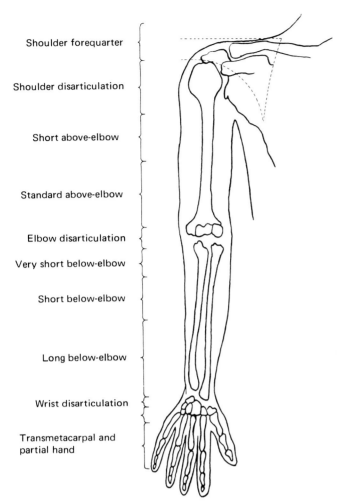

Shoulder forequarter

Shoulder disarticulation

Short above-elbow

Standard above-elbow

Elbow disarticulation

Very short below-elbow

Short below-elbow

Long below-elbow

Wrist disarticulation

Transmetacarpal and partial hand

Figure 27-1. Amputation levels of the upper extremity.

tal to the humeral head) to the shoulder articulation are referred to as *shoulder disarticulations*. Amputations above the shoulder joint involving the clavicle and scapula are referred to as *forequarter*.

Although there are general types of prostheses for each level of amputation, each prosthesis is medically prescribed for the person's individual needs, and the artificial limb is custom-made and individually fitted.

Phantom Sensations

Phantom sensations are common among amputees. Frequently, crush injuries, with their accompanying sensations of burning or cramping, are the most prevalent causes of phantom sensations. The sensation is that the limb remains a part of the person in spite of the amputation. Although, in most cases, this awareness is painless, at times it can become intolerable to the patient, and actual pain may result. In

such a case, a revision of the stump through surgical methods may be necessary.

The phantom sensations are usually felt as the distal parts of the extremity (*i.e.,* the amputee senses the existence of a nonexistent hand or foot). These phantom sensations seldom involve the total extremity.

Usually the patient describes the feeling of a presence, perhaps a tingling sensation. In addition to supportive counselling, the most effective compensation for the phantom sensation is the early use of the stump combined with either a temporary or a permanent prosthesis. The distal contact of the stump with the socket can have a desensitizing effect on the stump and can thus minimize phantom or painful sensations.

The amputee may also have to accept a new body image; this is difficult for some amputees because major changes in their body images will occur with the loss. Some amputees may be disturbed by this change in body concept and may have subsequent difficulties in prosthetic training. To be functionally useful, the prosthesis must be integrated into the body schema and must become a part of the individual.

Cineplasty

Under most circumstances a conventional prosthesis, using shoulder harnessing for suspension and control of prosthetic function that is channeled through a control cable, is provided for the amputee.

However, if the rehabilitation team and the patient wish, a second surgical procedure can be done after the initial procedure is well-healed. The biceps or pectoral cineplasty is done occasionally in order to eliminate the shoulder harnessing and to increase sensory feedback from the terminal device. The more common of the two sites for cineplasty is the biceps muscle. A surgical tunnel is made through the muscle into which a plastic pin is inserted and the control cable is attached to both ends of this pin. The prosthesis is then controlled by the contraction and relaxation of the biceps muscle (Fig. 27-2).

Because the tunnel must be kept clean consistently, there is considerable chance of infection if the amputee does not take sufficient care of his or her hygiene. Additionally, the amputee who has had a cineplasty procedure must be able to accept the cosmetic effect of the tunnel through the biceps muscle.

Cineplasty is no longer a common surgical procedure in UE amputation. Modern myoelectric systems are providing the patient with increased functional and cosmetic prosthetic integration. Improvement in harness and socket design have increased the effi-

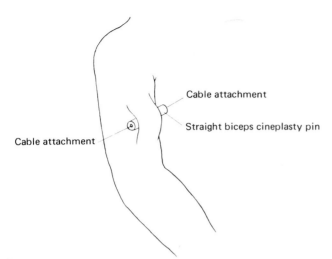

Cable attachment

Straight biceps cineplasty pin

Cable attachment

Figure 27-2. Biceps cineplasty tunnel with straight cineplasty pin.

ciency of prosthetic suspension. Elimination of the conventional harness for general use of the BE prosthesis is feasible with the myoelectric components as with the cineplasty prosthesis. With heavy work, a conventional harness is still used, even with the cineplasty prosthesis.

Limb Replantation

Limb replantation, or the rejoining of the amputated part following direct trauma, has been done with varying success. It is generally accepted that prosthetic replacement is limited as an acceptable substitute for natural appearance and function of the lost part and that it will always remain a substitute. Dis-advantages of prosthetic replacement include the necessity of achieving replacement of normal function through mechanical means, loss of functional sensation, periodic breakdown of devices, psychological reactions to loss, and the effects on the concept of self-image. In the effort to provide the amputee with a natural replacement, replantation has been done when immediate medical attention is available and when the amputated part of the limb can be adequately salvaged and replaced safely. Success depends on vascular continuity and nerve and tendon repair. Fibrosis and atrophy can occur, however, and the replanted part may be limited in function and sensation.

Figure 27-3 shows an amputee who has functional amputated digits of her right hand and a hand replantation of her left arm. This was done at the wrist. In this case a 1-inch prehension range was achieved; however, digital sensation is minimal. The amputee shown here uses her hand as a functional assist, and she enjoys the relatively normal cosmetic look. Since amputees are likely to have different opinions regarding cosmetic value and function, it is important to find out how the amputee feels in regard to the replacement alternatives for both.

Parts of the Conventional Upper Extremity Prosthesis

Terminal Devices

The most significant component of the prosthesis is the terminal device (TD), which provides either function or cosmesis.

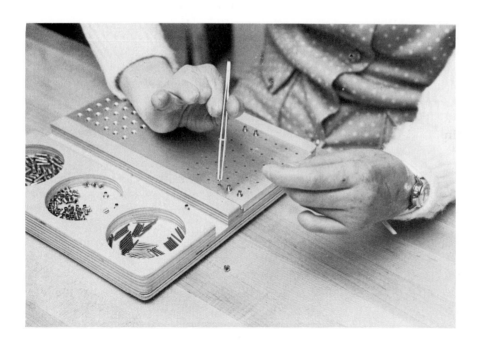

Figure 27-3. Bilateral amputee uses right partially amputated fingers to grasp tweezers. The left hand is a replantation and has limited pinch function and acceptable cosmetic value but lacks functional sensation.

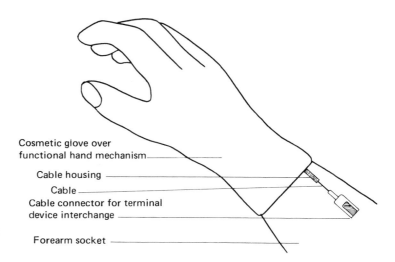

Figure 27-4. Functional hand with cosmetic glove and cable attachment.

A cosmetic terminal device, used principally for appearance, may be as simple as a flesh-colored glove used to cover a partial hand. Aside from being used to hold light objects or to position objects by pushing or pulling, this cosmetic device may have little functional value for the amputee. However, its psychological value is unquestioned.

A second type of cosmetic terminal device is the functional hand that can be attached to the wrist unit of most UE prostheses (Fig. 27-4), and it is operated by cable control. The functional hand consists of a plastic spring-controlled device with fingers that are controlled in flexion and extension at the metacarpophalangeal joints by the control cable of the prosthesis. The thumb of the hand can be placed manually in either of two positions: to grasp small objects or to grasp large ones. A plastic glove fits over the hand, presenting a natural appearance. The gloves are available in a variety of skin tones.

Functional hands have either voluntary opening or voluntary closing mechanisms activated by cable control, and they may either lock in position or be free-wheeling or nonlocking.

The hook is the most functional of the terminal devices. It is made of either steel or aluminum, and it is canted or lyre-shaped. It is either locking or nonlocking, with either voluntary opening or voluntary closing capacity (Fig. 27-5). The hook may be lined with neoprene, to protect objects while the amputee is grasping them, or serrated, to improve grasp. The needs of the amputee determine the weight, length, design, and function of the hook device chosen by the rehabilitation team.

Many kinds of hooks are available to provide for the diverse needs of the amputee. Among them are aluminum hooks required for above-elbow and shoulder disarticulation amputees who need minimum weight of the prosthesis, steel hooks for below-elbow amputees requiring durability, farm-ers' or carpenters' hooks for ease and safety in tool handling, and narrow opening hooks for use in laboratory or office work. Special hooks are available for bowling and for holding a baseball mitt. Special adaptations are available for ease in grasping tools or in driving.

A series of children's hooks are available with rubber or plastic parts to increase cosmesis and to prevent harm to objects while the child is using the prosthesis to play.

Hooks and functional or cosmetic hands are generally interchangeable through the common wrist unit attachment that is laminated onto the forearm socket.

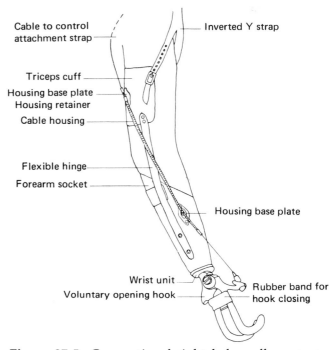

Figure 27-5. Conventional right below-elbow prosthesis.

Wrist Unit

The terminal device (either cosmetic or functional) is connected to the forearm socket (or shell) by the wrist unit. The three basic wrist units are locking, friction, and oval.

The advantage of the *locking unit* is that it prevents the hook from rotating during heavy industrial work. By pushing a button on it, the amputee manually operates the wrist unit, which allows the position of the hook to be changed by rotation. The hook can easily be ejected for interchange of hook and hand.

The *friction unit* has threads, and the hook must be screwed into the unit. Although this procedure is more time-consuming than that of the locking unit, the hook can be more easily positioned for specific tasks. Either the locking or the friction unit can be used with both BE and AE prostheses.

The *oval unit* is a special, thin unit for a wrist disarticulation prosthesis; it is used where the length of the components must be minimal in order to make the length of the amputated arm conform to that of the sound extremity.

A wrist flexion unit is available for placement of the hook in three wrist flexion positions for increased function. It is a manually operated device, and it is usually prescribed for the bilateral amputee for added versatility in terminal device positioning. One activity that is aided by this device is shaving; it helps as well in other activities close to the body.

Terminal devices and wrist units have standard connections. When the desired type of terminal device is chosen, one needs simply to determine the type and size of the wrist unit to accompany it. Usually the wrist unit is chosen according to the way in which the amputee will use the prosthesis in activities of daily living and at work.

The Socket

The plastic laminate socket may be either single- or double-walled. A BE amputee has a double-walled socket consisting of an inner wall that conforms to the stump and an outer wall that provides length and contour to the forearm replacement.

The wrist unit is laminated onto the distal end of the forearm socket. Since the forearm socket can be used by both the AE and the BE amputee to carry objects (*i.e.*, a coat, a handbag, or packages) as well as to push or to pull large or heavy objects, it is made of strong plastic resins that provide lightness and durability.

Since overall weight and bulk must be minimized for the AE and shoulder disarticulation amputees, a single-walled forearm socket, or shell, is used for these prostheses. The socket provides length and con-

tour to the forearm replacement. A double-walled socket is provided for the upper arm stump.

The Munster-type socket was devised mainly for the short stump of the BE amputee to eliminate problems of fit, security, and poor leverage that were prevalent with the conventional split-sockets, difficult to fit on this type of amputee. It consists of a single double-walled forearm socket that extends just proximal to the olecranon process posteriorly and that fits around the biceps tendon anteriorly. The socket is preflexed at approximately 35 degrees, thus limiting complete flexion and extension of the elbow. However, even with this disadvantage in range of motion, the fit is adequate for lifting and holding.

The more distal the socket coverage on the forearm, the more active supination and pronation the amputee will have with the prosthesis on. Extending the socket length proximally increases stability of the prosthesis for functional use.

Upper-Arm Unit

The upper-arm unit of the AE prosthesis is a double-walled socket with the locking elbow unit laminated onto the socket. Since the AE amputee lacks independent elbow flexion and extension, these are provided mechanically by an elbow unit which is activated, locked, and unlocked by the cable control system. A turntable at the joining of the locking elbow unit and the upper arm socket can be manually moved for internal and external rotation of the forearm, enabling the amputee to work with the hook directly in front of the body or out towards the side. The forearm shell is attached to the locking elbow unit and the upper arm socket (Fig. 27-6).

Shoulder Disarticulation Prosthesis

The shoulder disarticulation prosthesis has a supporting socket portion which sometimes extends to the anterior and posterior aspects of the shoulder, depending on the level of the amputation. Frequently, a passive abduction hinge joint is added at the shoulder for ease in manually positioning the arm and donning clothing.

Hinges

Hinges provide functional alignment and positioning between the forearm and the upper-arm socket or the harness. In addition, the flexible dacron or leather hinges used in the BE prosthesis allow active rotation of the forearm with a minimum of restriction. In the AE prosthesis the steel hinges provide rigidity to the

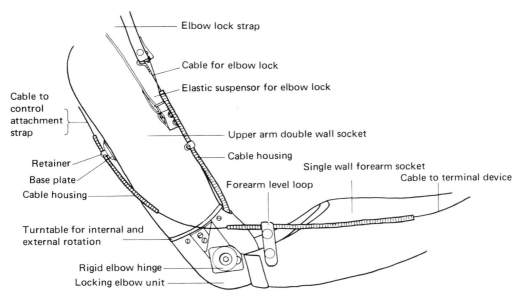

Figure 27-6. Conventional right above-elbow prosthesis with locking elbow unit.

mechanical elbow joint to ensure strength, durability, and dependability.

Harness

The function of the harness is to provide stable support of the prosthesis to facilitate the amputee's wearing and using of it, to provide attachment for the control cables, and to assist the cables in the operation of the prosthesis. Basically, the Dacron straps are formed in a figure-eight pattern with extra straps added as needed for better support or additional control function. For ease in use, the figure-nine harness is used with the below elbow Munster prosthesis. For the wrist disarticulation amputee, a simple cuff socket and a figure-nine harness may suffice.

The shoulder saddle harness (Fig. 27-7) is used for the BE amputee to minimize stress from the axillary loop used in the figure-eight harness; this stress occurs on the sound arm during heavy work. The shoulder saddle is fabricated of leather, dacron, or polyethylene. Shaped like a saddle, it rests over the shoulder of the amputated side, and it is attached to the prosthesis anteriorly and posteriorly, bearing the weight of the axial load rather than transmitting the pull to the sound axilla.[2] A chest strap is used to secure the saddle in position and to attach control cables.

Use of the saddle harness enables the amputee to lift heavier loads with the prosthesis and to gain complete range of motion. There is less discomfort for the amputee because the saddle covers larger and stronger weight-bearing areas over the shoulder. The chest strap also distributes pressure over a larger body surface, thus preventing problems from tight

pull of the axillary loop in the sensitive axillary area of the sound arm.

Stump Sock

A stump sock is worn by the amputee to aid in absorption of perspiration, to provide warmth to the stump, and as padding for comfort and fit of the socket. An AE amputee frequently uses the short sleeve of a T-shirt in place of the stump sock. Use of an under-blouse or T-shirt can alleviate discomfort from the harness straps in beginning training sessions.

Control System

The control system determines the functional value of the prosthesis for the amputee. The control cable of the terminal device is attached to the device and to the harness. This cable is guided along the socket and cuff or the upper-arm socket by retainers that hold it in the most advantageous position for ease of function. Terminal device operation is generally accomplished by foward flexion of the shoulder. During the training period, the amputee practices this isolated motion, and eventually he or she is able to operate the hook or hand with minimal physical strain.

For the AE amputee this basic terminal device control cable also serves in flexion and extension of the mechanical elbow when the elbow unit is unlocked. It is activated by forward shoulder flexion. At times, additional joint motions are used in this cable operation: (1) because of limitation of shoulder control or strength; (2) to provide smooth operation of the prosthesis; (3) to enable the wearer to achieve maximum

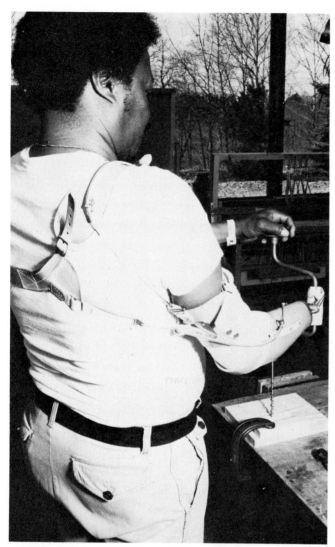

Figure 27-7. Right below-elbow amputee uses conventional below-elbow prosthesis with shoulder saddle harness over the right shoulder to assist in freedom of movement for bilateral wood-working procedure.

function of the mechanical arm and hand in reach, grasp, release, and hold. These motions may be shoulder abduction and adduction, scapular abduction and adduction, or shoulder flexion of the unamputated arm.

The second basic cable operates the elbow lock. It is attached internally or externally to the elbow unit, and it extends to the anterior deltoid-pectoral strap of the harness. A combination of shoulder elevation, depression, external rotation, and extension is used both to lock and unlock the elbow unit.

Control cables for the shoulder disarticulation and forequarter prostheses are attached to the humeral or scapular part of the upper-arm socket, and their exact design and function are determined by the needs of the individual amputee.

During the training period, the amputee is carefully instructed to isolate the patterns of joint and muscle movement that control the operation of the prosthesis. (The instruction process will be discussed in the section on prosthetic training.) The extent to which the prosthesis provides the amputee with increased function depends on the quality of the fabrication of the prosthesis, its fit, the comfort and limitations of the wearer, and the range of mechanical function. The amputee's limitations may be physical, psychological, and/or social. The range of mechanical function of the prosthesis includes grasp, release, hold, push, pull, and reach, which, depending upon the control by the wearer and the types of prescription components, can be extensive for the amputee.

Cineplasty Prosthesis

As mentioned earlier, the cineplasty prosthesis is a special form of prosthetic device. In this case, the harness functions as additional support and comfort for the wearer, but it is not necessary for the actual function of the prosthesis. The same terminal devices, wrist units, and socket design described earlier can be used. However, the control system is different because the surgical procedure consists of forming a tunnel through the biceps muscle (see Fig. 27-2).

This procedure is undertaken following the standard amputation. A plastic pin is inserted through the tunnel. At each end of the pin is a cable attachment from which a cable extends. These cables eventually join in a common adjustment plate, and another cable extends from this point to the terminal device (Fig. 27-8).

For added security, a triceps cuff may be strapped around the upper arm (Fig. 27-9). This cuff is attached to the forearm shell with flexible hinges.

In addition to eliminating the necessity of binding harnessing, the cineplasty control system approximates normal isolated muscle function. Rather than joint motion or muscle expansion for control, the cineplasty prosthesis is operated by the biceps muscle. With biceps control there is some simulation in sensation in the terminal device.

A person who has a cineplastic procedure generally has undergone preprosthetic training and has learned to use a harness-controlled prosthesis prior to cineplastic surgery and thus, if necessary, can revert to the use of a standard control system.

Bilateral Amputee

The bilateral amputee faces not only the functional and cosmetic adjustments of the unilateral amputee but also the complete loss of sensory contact with objects while using the prostheses. Prosthetic replacement is prescribed according to the level of am-

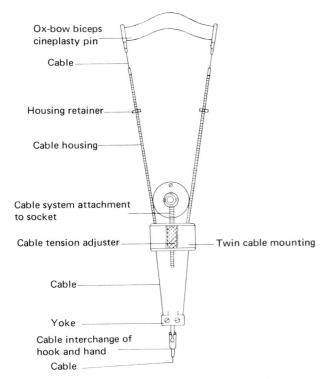

Figure 27-8. Biceps cineplasty cable control system.

putation. Particular attention is given to minimizing weight and to providing ease of bilateral operation of the elbows and terminal devices through the control system. For ease in putting on and removing of the prosthesis by the amputee, as well as for its security and adjustment, the two prostheses are secured to a common harness system. A wrist flexion unit is helpful on one side for added mechanical positioning.

Because sensation is essential to the *blind* bilateral amputee, the Krukenberg surgical procedure may be done if the individual has a long below-elbow amputation of either or both arms. This procedure involves the separating of the radius and ulna and accompanying musculature to enable the amputee to achieve a grasp and release function through supination and pronation of the forearm. Sensation is maintained as grasp is achieved without an external prosthesis. Some amputees can achieve independence with this procedure.

Partial Hand Amputee

A major consideration in the partial hand traumatic amputation is whether to leave remaining healthy hand tissue or to amputate for optimal prosthetic use and cosmetic coverage. This area of consideration demands individual and creative design and application of functional and cosmetic components. Options involving surgery, prosthetics, and orthotics are reviewed.

The amputee with a partial hand amputation may or may not need or use a prosthesis. In the effort to save as much tissue as possible, the surgeon can often save parts of the hand for motor function and sensation. As shown in Figures 27-10, 27-11, and 27-12 full function can be maintained for the grasping of tools and general coordination and sensation with partial amputation of the fingers. In this case, there is complete function of the metacarpophalangeal joints for adequate positioning of the fingers, and strength is preserved in the muscle tendons as in fingertip sensa-

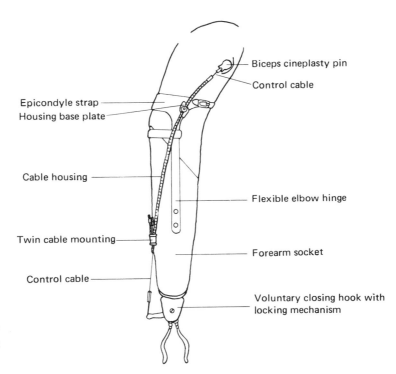

Figure 27-9. Right below-elbow cineplasty with voluntary closing hook.

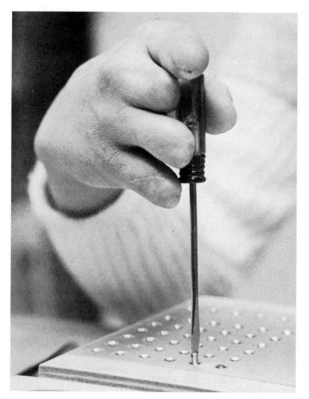

Figure 27-10. The amputee grasps a small screwdriver between the partially amputated fingers and the remaining thumb.

tion. Complete amputation of the fingers necessitates prosthetic replacement to provide grasp and prehension. Figures 27-13, 27-14, and 27-15 show the use of a functional replacement to enable the amputee to use tools. The amputee shown here has normal function

and sensation in the thumb. Cosmetic replacement can also be provided by a glove with soft or firm fingers that can be manually positioned for function and appearance.

A custom glove may fit over a passive partial hand replacement, molded from the sound hand, and fabricated as desired. It may be supplied with or without a zipper for ease in wearing; it can also be designed with freckles, veins, and hair to provide a natural appearance.

Levels of amputation are generally classified as transphalangeal, thenar, transthenar, or transmetacarpal, with or without the thumb. Surgical reconstruction of the hand or part of it may be feasible to maintain functional structure and sensation and to avoid prosthetic or orthotic replacement.

Occupational Therapy and the Upper Extremity Amputee

Physical Considerations

Generally speaking, the longer the stump, the more the amputee can do both in the preprosthetic program and in the prosthetic training program. With a well-healed, healthy stump, the amputee has a good purchase power on the socket and security in its fit. In the case of a BE amputation, the longer the stump, the more active supination and pronation the patient is likely to have. This situation will assist him or her in positioning the hook for grasp and placement of objects. Also, if the stump is long, either AE or BE, it is more useful to the amputee; he or she has a ten-

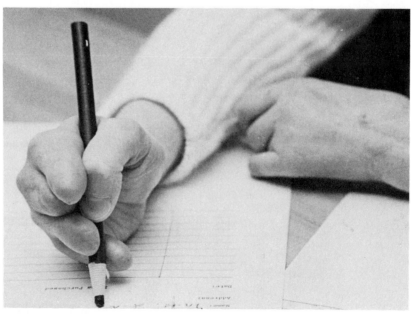

Figure 27-11. The amputee with full use of the thumb is able to write normally with adaptive grasp by the partially amputated fingers.

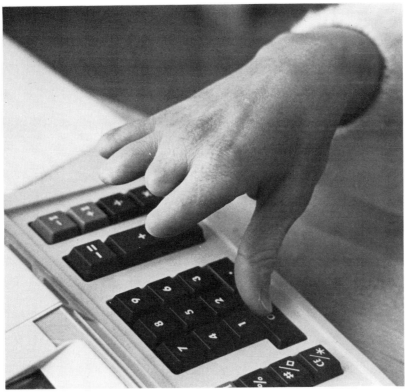

Figure 27-12. This individual had partial finger amputation caused by an industrial machine. Full mobility at the metacarpophalangeal joints and complete sensation enable the amputee to use a calculator effectively.

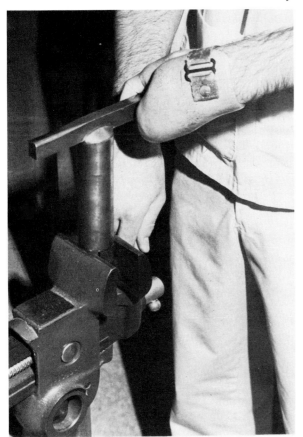

Figure 27-13. This partial hand amputee uses a prosthesis to replace the fingers and to provide opposition to the remaining thumb for grasping.

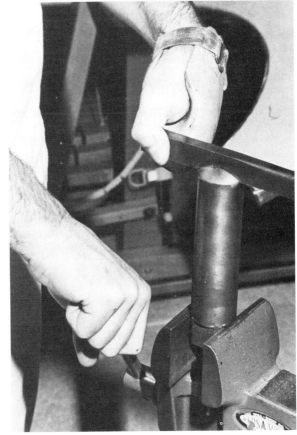

Figure 27-14. This finger replacement prosthesis provides opposition to the thumb for grasping.

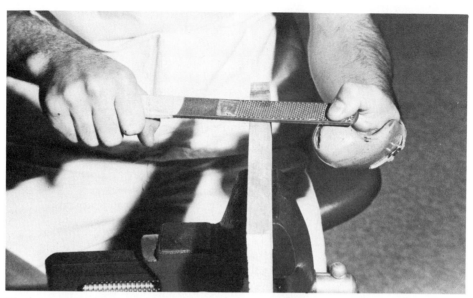

Figure 27-15. This patient wears a partial hand prosthesis to hold tool for bimanual wood filing.

dency to use it more frequently, thus maintaining normal range of motion and strength.

During the postoperative and preprosthetic periods, the patient will usually automatically change dominance to the sound extremity. If the dominant extremity has been amputated and the patient is forced to use the nondominant extremity for grasp and placement of objects, he or she may have some incoordination. In this case, he or she can benefit from activities with the sound extremity to improve the fine coordination of the previously nondominant arm. The amputee who has suffered loss of the nondominant extremity may be less motivated to use the prosthesis, for he or she will depend on the dominant extremity to compensate for the other arm.

It is important to stress bilateral activities to help the patient adjust to limitations in reaching and in holding large objects as well as to aid the development of bimanual coordination. Involvement in activities aids in the healing of the stump and in learning to use the prosthesis.

The bilateral amputee usually chooses the side with the longer stump to become the dominant side. Sometimes he or she is trained in the use of one prosthesis at a time. However, since the two prostheses have a common harness and the body must adjust to the weight and balance of the mechanical devices, the bilateral amputee may start the training program with both limbs, concentrating on one at a time.

Immediate and Early Postsurgical Fitting

It is commonly recognized that early fitting of the prosthesis aids the training program. Some doctors

and therapists think that it is more desirable to fit several temporary prostheses rather than to wait for several months for the arrival of the permanent one. This technique provides early prosthetic training while the permanent limb is being fabricated. There are four approaches to shortening the time between the amputation and the fitting of the permanent prosthesis.

1. In some cases, particularly if the patient has a long stump, utensils can be fitted into the Ace bandage, which is applied to the stump to facilitate shrinkage.

2. Utensils can be fitted into the pocket of a strap and wrapped around the stump with a Velcro fastening. A temporary prosthetic cuff can be devised from plaster or leather to which either utensils or the terminal device and controls can be attached.

3. Early fitting, several weeks postoperatively, has met with success. This temporary prosthesis consists of a plaster cuff with components and a control system similar to the ones the permanent prosthesis will have.

4. The immediate postsurgical fitting is being done with upper extremity amputees. It has been found that immediate fitting, in addition to shortening the time between amputation and the wearing of the prosthesis, has hastened control of edema, lessened postsurgical pain, encouraged conditioning of the stump, and provided more rapid use of the controls and the prosthesis. The plaster dressing with conventional harness and controls is applied at the time of surgery or during the immediate postoperative period. The plaster casts are

changed as the stump shrinks. Provision of this type of immediate prosthesis encourages a positive approach from the patient and early learning of prosthetic use; thus, when the amputee receives the permanent prosthesis, he or she has developed appropriate muscle use and has learned controls.

Psychological Reactions

In assisting the amputee in adjusting to his or her condition and in becoming motivated to learn the function and care of the prosthesis, the occupational therapist must recognize the amputee's psychological reactions to his or her situation. If the patient feels guilt or shame regarding the amputation, his or her relationships with family and friends may be affected, presenting difficulties. He or she may be depressed and may refuse to cooperate with the training program. On the other hand, the amputee may be interested in compensating for the loss by learning as much as he or she can about the prosthesis, by accepting change, and by demonstrating eagerness to learn.

It is very important to consider the patient's feelings and useful attitudes. The prosthesis should be presented in a way that is meaningful to the amputee. For some persons, function is most important; for others, appearance is the greatest concern. For either, prosthetic replacement can help the amputee by providing function and cosmetic value.

Becoming familiar with the prime concerns of the amputee with regard to vocational and social needs as well as self-esteem begins with the initial contact between the patient and the therapist. Careful attention is given to combining the components needed and desired by the individual. Careful initial evaluation, preprosthetic preparation, and prosthetic training in all areas of function are necessary for adequate acceptance and use of the prosthesis by the amputee. The therapist's positive attitude toward the amputee, his or her stump, his or her fears, achievement of lost function, and cosmesis through prosthetic replacement reinforce the patient's attitude. Most important is the provision of opportunities for the patient to use the prosthesis in all appropriate activities and to socialize with others in the process. Involvement of family members in the training program may also be helpful.

Preprosthetic Period

The preprosthetic period is the time between the amputation and the fitting of the prosthesis. This is the period of "getting ready" for the prosthesis. The patient should be confronted with the importance of the preprosthetic program as preparation for prosthetic replacement. A successful preprosthetic program hastens physical and psychological adjustment to the prosthesis and minimizes problems in wearing and using the permanent prosthesis. In this period it is important to counsel and guide the amputee regarding both the acceptance of his or her condition and the acceptance of the mechanical device which must substitute for natural motor power, sensation, and physical appearance. Counseling sessions with the amputee should also include his or her family and friends in order to involve them in the training program.

When medically approved, passive and active strengthening activities are started by the physical therapist and the occupational therapist to encourage maximum use of the stump, maximum range of motion (ROM), and maximum use of muscles, especially those of the arm and shoulder. A well-planned preprosthetic exercise program contributes to successful adaptation and provides strong muscles for the training in isolated motions for control and use of the prosthesis.

Following the amputation, the loss of the weight of the missing part causes a shift in the amputee's center of gravity. Atrophy of the musculature on the side of the amputation, scoliosis, and compensatory curves may occur if the patient does not have proper exercise. Therefore, the beginning exercise program is geared toward correcting faulty body mechanics and providing the amputee with sufficient ROM and strength to operate the prosthesis.

The first step is to establish good rapport with the patient so that it will be possible to help him or her in working through his or her necessary adjustments and in learning independence in daily living with the aid of an artificial limb. The relationship between the training therapist and the patient is a very important one, for the therapist must understand the patient's attitudes toward the prosthesis in order to help him accept and use it. The amputee may have fears of being different, may question the attitudes of others toward himself, and may even question himself about possible inadequacies.

Before the amputee receives the prosthesis, he or she must develop strength and tolerance in the stump. As soon as possible following the amputation, exercises are begun to maintain and, if necessary, to regain normal passive and active ROM in the joints proximal to the amputation (Figure 27-16). Since the hospital stay may be short, these exercises are designed so that they can be done in outpatient situations in the clinic. Although this may be painful to the patient, it is important to maintain and encourage maximum movement and use of the extremity during the healing period in order to prepare the amputee for the prosthesis, to prevent weakening of

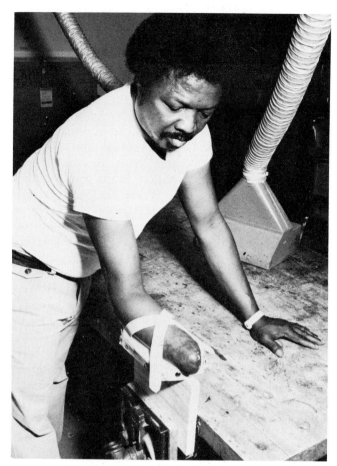

Figure 27-16. Below-elbow amputee benefits by early active use of the amputated extremity by sanding with an adapted sanding block. The patient gains early awareness of the use of his arm, and pressure on the sanding block helps to desensitize his stump.

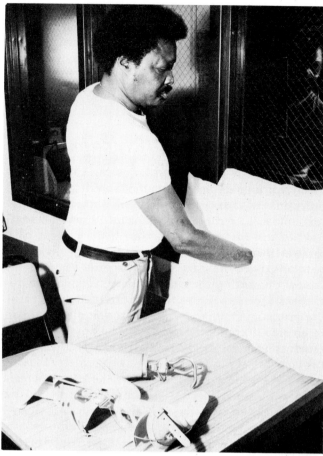

Figure 27-17. To desensitize and improve pressure tolerance of the distal stump in preparation for socket contact, the amputee punches a soft pillow with increasing arm force.

muscles through disuse, and to encourage shrinkage of the stump.

After complete healing, the stump is massaged to encourage circulation, to prevent adhesions from scar tissue, to reduce swelling, to encourage desensitization, and to prevent the patient from fearing to handle the stump (Figure 27-17). Bandaging with an elastic Ace bandage or "shrinker" is done several times per day to encourage shrinkage and shaping. Wrapping should be done carefully with attention to tightness, unnecessary folds in the bandage, and complete, even coverage of the stump to ensure comfort to the patient. Bandaging should be done from the distal to the proximal end. Care must be taken not to bandage so tightly as to produce muscle atrophy.

To encourage the use of the stump, the occupational therapist may strap utensils to it which are used in ADL. Such utensils may include a knife, fork, or toothbrush. The amputee should be encouraged to use the individual implements in ADL.

The shrinking and shaping are also hastened by provision of a temporary prosthesis in the form of either a leather or a plaster cuff to which utensils can be attached for functional use of the extremity.

In this period, maximum use of the arms should be encouraged in both unilateral and bilateral exercise and functional activities. Additionally, since posture can be affected by the loss of a part, balance and posture exercises are necessary to prevent substitution patterns; these exercises help to make the amputee aware of his or her new body image.

Although the preprosthetic program can be enhanced by the use of a temporary prosthesis, the amputee's tolerance determines when it may be applied. The temporary prosthesis aids the amputee in overcoming the initial psychological shock of amputation in the following ways—it provides a temporary replacement for the length of the missing arm; it provides him or her with a degree of independence, since a fork or a tool or other utensils may be attached to it to provide functional use of the amputated extremity. Additionally, a temporary prosthesis aids in cosmetic lengthening of the stump and, most significantly, is a device with which the amputee can perform bimanual and bilateral activities. One of the most important parts of the training program lies in the amputee's early involvement in activities which show results (Fig. 27-18).

At this time, the amputee should be encouraged to use the sound arm in one-handed activities, even though he or she may not be naturally motivated to do so. If the amputated arm had been the dominant one, he or she may have temporary difficulties in accepting the loss and in using the nondominant arm. In this case, he or she may need exercises to develop coordination patterns in the remaining limb. Activities such as eating, dressing, writing, and bathing may be difficult with the nondominant hand. It is important at this time to provide a program to encourage successful one-handed use in daily activities.

For the amputee with a cineplasty, the biceps muscle becomes the motor for the prosthesis, thus providing the link between the muscle and the prosthetic mechanism. Because the cineplasty pro-

vides increased arm ROM and the amputee is free of a harness, it allows the amputee to hold the prosthesis in any position without affecting the operation of the terminal device. For maximum use of the cineplasty prosthesis, it is necessary to have a 1½- to 2-inch excursion of the surgical tunnel. Routine exercises to maintain this excursion include isolated muscle exercise of the biceps, isometric contractions and holds, and sufficient relaxation for the excursion and the opening of the terminal device. The cineplasty prosthesis is reported to provide improved dexterity and sensitivity to the amputated limb by the physiological use of the stump muscles.

In preparing the patient for prosthetic wear and in providing the prosthesis appropriate to the patient's needs and expectations, the occupational therapist must consider several important questions. First, does the patient need it? This will depend on the patient's limitations as a result of the amputation, his or her vocational and avocational needs and interests, and his or her attitude towards the value of the prosthesis. Another question relevant to the prescription is what does the amputee need it for, and will he or she wear it? This depends largely upon attitude towards the loss of the limb, loss of function, and relationships of the amputee with other people. Does he or she need and want function or cosmetic acceptance or both? What is most important to him or her in homelife, at work, in hobbies, and in social life?

Following the preprosthetic program, or near its end, these questions are taken into serious consideration in order to prescribe the appropriate prosthetic components for the maximum benefit to the amputee. At this point the rehabilitation team comes together for consultation.

Prior to the prescription the physiatrist measures the stump and examines the patient. The parts and controls of the prosthesis are determined by many factors: range of motion, strength, length, skin coverage and appearance, incision site, shoulder strength, and job requirements. Ideally, the physiatrist prescribes the prosthesis at the amputee clinic in the presence of the rehabilitation team and the patient and with the consultation of those who will be training the patient to adjust to and to use the prosthesis. At this time, if not before, the occupational therapist can acquaint the new amputee with the various components and harnessing that he or she is likely to have and perhaps can introduce him or her to another amputee who has completed the training program and is using the prosthesis successfully.

The accompanying preprosthetic evaluation form can be used by the occupational therapist as a guide to determine what are appropriate components (hook and hand) for the amputee (Fig. 27-19). If the patient has not remained in the hospital during the post-

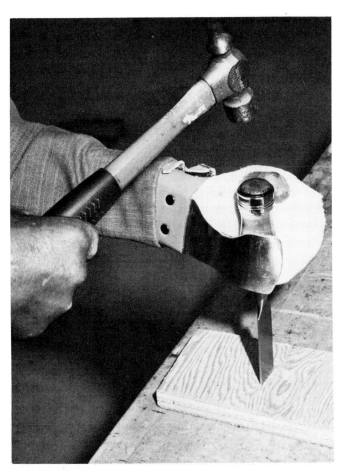

Figure 27-18. Partial hand amputee uses an orthotic post to assist firm grasp of the chisel.

Occupational Therapy Pre-prosthetic Evaluation

Name: _____ Date: _____
Address: _____ Telephone No. _____
Age: _____ Dominance: _____
Date, cause, and type of amputation: _____
_____

Level of amputation: _____ Length of stump: _____
Prosthesis: #1 _____ #2 _____ #3 _____ #4 _____
Type of present prosthesis: _____
Occupation: _____
_____

Date last worked: _____
R.O.M. in shoulder: _____ elbow: _____ wrist: _____
    supination-pronation: _____
Strength in shoulder: _____ elbow: _____
Pain in stump: _____
Phantom sensations: _____
Current use of limb without prosthesis: _____
Use of previous prosthesis: _____
Attitude toward new prosthesis: _____
    a) function: _____
    b) cosmesis: _____
Additional remarks: _____
_____
_____

Prescription at clinic: _____
_____

Prosthetist: _____ #Training sessions: _____
                              Signed: _____

Figure 27-19. Sample preprosthetic evaluation form.

operative, preprosthetic period, the evaluation form is helpful in determining his or her limitations and needs in terms of strengthening the extremity and trunk for prosthetic wear and use. Should an amputee return to the hospital's amputee clinic for prescription of a new prosthesis, this form is helpful in evaluating whether he or she should be given the same type of prosthesis or if different components would be more helpful. The occupational therapist can also assess the amputee's needs for further training, especially if he or she has not used the prosthesis extensively in daily activities.

Check-out of the Prosthesis

Before the amputee begins his or her training program, members of the rehabilitation team examine the prosthesis to make sure that it conforms to the prescription and that it is mechanically sound. In performing the check-out of the prosthesis, the occupational therapist evaluates its fit and comfort for the wearer and checks the motion and function of the components. Should adjustments need to be made in any part of the prosthesis, the rehabilitation team

makes recommendations to the prosthetist in order to ensure that the amputee does not begin the training program with an uncomfortable or mechanically mediocre device. The physician makes the final approval of the prosthesis.

At the time of the check-out, which occurs during the first training session, the occupational therapist begins to acquaint the amputee with prosthetic terminology. The amputee learns the names of the parts and their functions, and learns the proper attachment of the harness and the components so that he can keep the prosthesis clean and can interchange the terminal devices efficiently.

In instructing the patient in the care of the prosthesis, the occupational therapist teaches the amputee the proper use of the hook, wrist unit, and cable system. The amputee is instructed to use just enough motion to open or close the hook, to watch for worn rubberbands, to avoid putting unnecessary strain on the cable, and to watch for spreading of the housing and excessive friction between the cable and the housing.

The socket should be kept clean with soap and water; the stump socks should be washed daily; and the harness should be washed at least once per week.

Leather parts can be cleaned with saddle soap. If the tips of the Dacron harness straps begin to fray, they can be sealed at the edge by singeing with a match.

The amputee should be instructed to use only cable control to operate the functional hooks and hands. Manual operation may damage the mechanism. The amputee should also be warned never to use the terminal device in such activities as hammering nails or removing screws, because this can tear threads and damage hook neoprene.

The cosmetic gloves on the functional hand are perishable. It is important to guard the glove against tearing, since it functions as a protection of the hand mechanism from dirt and wetness. Also, these gloves soil easily, can be stained or marked if laid on dirty surfaces, and darken with age. Substances such as certain foods, ink, newsprint, and chemicals can damage the glove and lessen its cosmetic effect. The occupational therapist should recommend that the amputee keep the hand in a plastic bag when it is not in use. The amputee should be warned against oiling parts of the prosthesis or removing the glove from the hand, and he should be counseled to return to the prosthetist for any assistance needed.

Training Program

A successful training program for an amputee requires the coordinated efforts of a rehabilitation team. This team includes the surgeon, nurse, physiatrist, physical therapist, occupational therapist, social worker, prosthetist, rehabilitation counsellor, and psychiatrist or psychologist. A coordinated effort of these persons is necessary for the provision of appropriate prosthetic replacement and training in the use of the prosthesis.

At the beginning of the training program, the prosthesis should be put on over a light-weight shirt so that the occupational therapist and the amputee can see the prosthesis function and so that it is not hindered by tight clothing. The amputee should become accustomed to using the mirror as a guide to learning the correct positioning of the harness straps in back and in learning the control motions.

Loose clothing is recommended for the amputee to facilitate putting on, wearing, and using the prosthesis. Clothing with front fastenings, Velcro closures, and wide shirt cuffs are helpful. The use of a buttonhook (Fig. 27-20) designed especially for the amputee can assist him or her with the problem of fastening the sleeve button on the sound side. Sewing the buttons on with elastic thread enables the amputee to leave the button fastened when removing the shirt, even if the cuffs are narrow, for the cuff will then stretch enough to allow the hand and arm to be removed from the sleeve. When putting on the shirt,

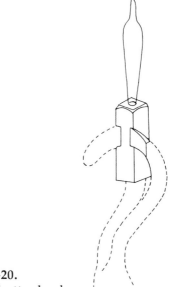

Figure 27-20.
Amputee buttonhook.

the amputee should remember to put it on the amputated side first. One-handed shoe tying and special closures can simplify dressing procedures.

There are two approaches commonly used in training amputees. In one, the training program is directed toward developing the potential level of the amputee's performance. With this approach a unilateral amputee learns to develop fine coordination with the prosthesis, so that he or she can have maximum use of it even in case of an injury to the remaining extremity. The other approach varies from the potential approach in that the amputee is trained in the use of the prosthesis only as an aid in bimanual activities. Regardless of the approach, activities should be chosen that are suitable to the amputee's needs. The occupational therapist should encourage the amputee to indicate any additional and special training that he or she desires.

The training period serves as a "try out" period to check the efficiency of the prosthesis and the practicality of the components to suit the amputee's individual needs as well as to make adjustments of malfunctions of the device.

The length of the training sessions should be increased as the amputee's tolerance and adaptation increase. He or she must master its use in training before combining the prosthesis and remaining extremity in bimanual activities and before wearing the prosthesis outside the clinic. Wearing it outside the clinic for an overnight period is advised for the first out-of-clinic experience. This is preferable to having the amputee wear it at home for an entire weekend. Training with the hand should be delayed until use of the hook has been mastered, unless the amputee has only a hand provided.

The general goals of training include (1) independence in self-care and ADL, (2) return to former work or to a better job, (3) improved appearance, (4) return to hobbies and recreation, and (5) mastery of new skills.

Certain factors affecting the amputee's capacity to learn may, unfortunately, be detrimental. They include poor habits uncorrected in preprosthetic training, lack of motivation, lack of sensory feedback from the nonsensory prosthesis, time needed for training, age, inability to learn, and lack of a sense of accomplishment. The occupational therapist must attempt to minimize an amputee's negative attitude toward any or all of these factors.

The positive attitude of the amputee is important; he or she must want to learn. The occupational therapist must encourage the amputee to have varying positive attitudes toward the prosthesis, such as considering it as a tool, a device to conceal his or her disability, an improvement of his or her body image, and/or a substitute for loss. Since it is important for the amputee to eventually integrate the prosthesis into his or her bodily function, he or she must become acquainted with it as a potential part of self, both functionally and cosmetically. The amputee should have a feeling of success after each training session.

Early training in successful use of control motions can enable the amputee to feel that he or she will be successful in future training activities. He or she should be cautioned against using the opposite shoulder to control the device and should be taught to operate the prosthesis with the amputated extremity as much as possible. Control motions should be minimal to save strength and, thus, to extend the time during which the amputee can wear and use the prosthesis.

In the first training session, the amputee should be taught the use and care of the stump sock (mentioned earlier).

Sensation is a natural guide to motor control. We recognize objects by shape, texture, size, and movement. But the amputee must often substitute vision for sensation (*e.g.*, using visual cues in observing the amount of hook opening). He or she combines this with the sensation of cable tension to provide visual-sensory training, using the perception of both position and force. The proprioceptive sensation in the stump and the arm can aid here. He or she also uses auditory cues, such as the clicks in the elbow lock, hand, and hook for efficient operation of the prosthesis.

During the first session it is important to acquaint the amputee with the actual function of the hook by teaching exercises for opening and closing it. Since many voluntary opening hooks are prescribed for amputees, let us use them as an example.

Following the cable pull by shoulder flexion, the cable tension is released by shoulder extension and the hook is pulled closed by its rubberbands, which yield 1 pound of pressure each. The standard number of rubberbands employed is usually three or four, although up to eight and more may be used for the BE amputee for added grip strength. (Fig. 27-21 shows a device for applying rubberbands.) The amputee begins his or her training by learning to isolate the control motions needed to activate the hook. Then, using visual cues and sensing in his or her shoulder the resistance of the rubberbands, the amputee learns how to control the exact opening of the hook. In order to minimize the energy expenditure needed to use the hook, the amputee should be encouraged to open the hook only slightly more than the size of the object he or she wishes to pick up—just enough to grasp the object. The amputee should practice with objects of different sizes and weights in order to achieve control. Additionally, drills requiring the grasp of objects of different forms, textures, and materials are necessary for the amputee to learn the basic motions used in operating the hook (Fig. 27-22). Since some materials are light, breakable, or easily crushed (*i.e.*, a paper or plastic cup), it is important to teach the amputee to employ a minimum of pressure by maintaining tension on the cable during grasp. The amputee should also learn to operate the hook in different planes of arm movements, so that he or she will achieve maximum functional use.

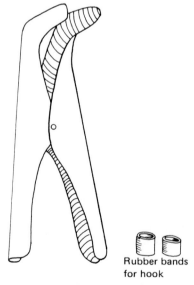

Figure 27-21. Band applier for voluntary opening hook.

These drills for grip control should be extended to other components of the prosthesis. The amputee must learn how to preposition the terminal device at the wrist unit, how to operate the elbow unit, how to use the turntable, how to coordinate the elbow lock and elbow flexion and extension, and how to preposition the shoulder. In these drills the use of the terminal device is combined with a number of gross arm functions. The amputee learns the grasp, placement, and release of objects on shelves, tables, and the floor and learns to depend on the grip of the hook or functional hand (Fig. 27-23).

During this early drill period, use of the sound extremity should be encouraged. During the rest periods the amputee should be encouraged to practice unilateral activities as well as bilateral ones. It is through these more complicated coordination activities that the prosthesis begins to be functionally integrated into the bilateral UE activities of the amputee. Although the unilateral amputee may already have become independent in ADL during the preprosthetic period, there are many things that we are accustomed to doing with two hands. For example, the amputee may find it difficult to cut meat, button a shirt sleeve, tie shoes, or wrap a package with one hand. The prosthesis may help him or her to accomplish these things, or the occupational therapist may discover that additional adaptive devices are needed.

Whatever the problem, the occupational therapist should encourage the amputee to become skillful in the use of the hook and to devise ways to increase independence in function. Participation in woodworking, sewing, weaving, or other avocational activities can be motivating for the amputee, can pro-

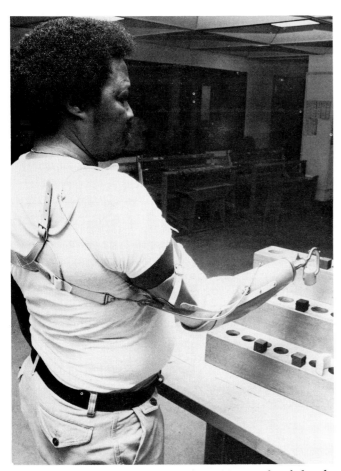

Figure 27-22. Amputee practices control of hook opening and closing in grasp, release, and placement of blocks of varying shapes.

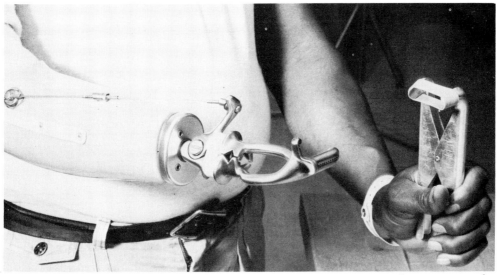

Figure 27-23. During initial prosthetic training, the amputee learns to apply bands to the voluntary opening hook to increase grip pressure of the hook.

vide coordination and strength, can show how his or her prosthesis can help in doing things, and can aid in integrating the prosthesis into bodily function (Fig. 27-24).

Using a worksheet checklist of activities accomplished can be helpful in recording the amputee's progress of training in both the clinic and the home. Since there are many activities that the patient will do at home that cannot be simulated in the clinic, the therapist should continue to encourage the amputee to do new things at home following each training session and to report successes or difficulties with new tasks. In this way, the therapist is able to assist the patient not only in controls, training drills, and activities, but also in tasks and responsibilities in the routine of daily living. Thus, the program becomes relevant to each amputee's needs.

Activity categories on the worksheet should include basic prehension activities, dressing and grooming (including putting on and taking off the prosthesis), eating and social skills (using keys and opening an umbrella), homemaking, clerical activities, and activities related to vocational and avocational interests.

Another training aid is a prosthetic training board with common objects (locks, light switches, pencil sharpener) attached to it.

Recreational activities during the preprosthetic and prosthetic training periods provide general body conditioning and development of a new image for the amputee.

Prevocational Training

Because industrial accidents are a frequent cause of UE amputations, a prevocational assessment should be included in the training program to assist the amputee in recognizing capabilities in prosthetic function and whether or not he or she, as an amputee, can safely return to a former occupation or whether he or

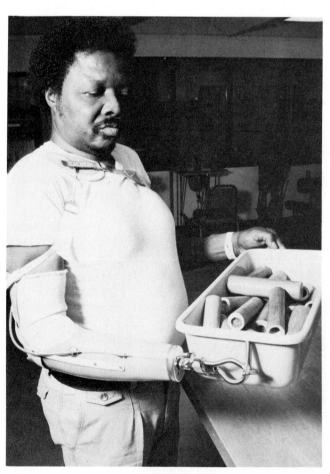

Figure 27-24. The unilateral amputee practices bimanual activities to learn how to use the prosthesis as a functional assist. Here it is not necessary to open the hook, but it must be positioned properly on the object for assist in carrying a heavy load.

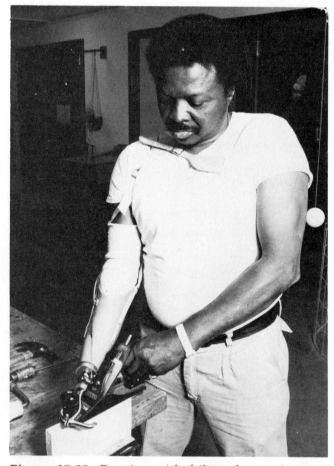

Figure 27-25. Practice with bilateral grasping and use of common construction tools improves coordination and bilateral integration. Here the amputee uses a steel carpenter's hook with serrated edges for firm grasp.

she needs to consider a change of occupation and additional vocational training. Specific tasks related to the individual's type of work should be included in the prosthetic training program to assess his or her safe and efficient handling of tools, power equipment, and heavy and light materials. Work tolerance can be assessed by the use of timed job-simulated tasks (Fig. 27-25, 27-26).

Prevocational considerations include training in general household activities. Training in the accomplishment of homemaking tasks such as meal preparation, cleaning, and household repairs are included. Child care is also included in the prevocational program.

In assisting the amputee to return to his former job or to redirect his vocational goals, the occupational therapist works closely with the vocational counselor and the employer. Use of standardized testing procedures and work simulated activities are an important part of the program to provide data for assessment of attitudes, aptitudes, work habits, and skills.

The Child Amputee

"The goal of pediatric (re)habilitation is to facilitate a developmental process by which the child can hopefully achieve his potential for functioning."[3] If this is not carefully considered in the functional development of the child, "the child with impaired movement experiences dysfunction in performance and develops purposeless behaviors and activities."[4] "Movement puts the child in relationship with his surroundings so that through this relationship the child can have an effect upon his environment as well as be affected by his environment."[5]

Depending on the nature of the condition, a child with congenital skeletal deficiency develops adaptively without prosthetic replacement of missing parts and often without the need of symmetry. Although lack of a prosthesis may be less of a concern for the child and the parents in early development, it may seem more necessary or desirable in adolescence or young adulthood; at this point, preparing to wear a prosthesis often requires a tremendous physical and psychological adjustment.

Ideally, the prosthesis is prescribed within 6 months or 1 year of age or as soon as possible after a traumatic amputation. This is essential for the young child to prevent the natural development of habits that might be detrimental to early adaptation and integration of prosthetic replacement for optimum present and future function.

The training program of the child amputee must relate to activities natural to his or her level of development. Early fitting during the prewalking period

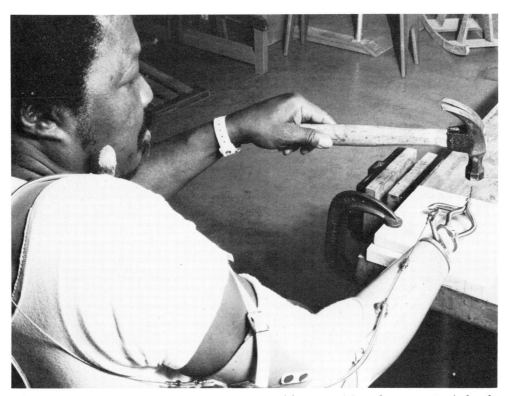

Figure 27-26. The below-elbow amputee is able to position the carpenter's hook to hold a nail for hammering.

aids the child in developing gross bilateral coordination and balance in integrated trunk and extremity activity.

During the first year of development from the horizontal to the vertical position in bodily reflexes, the child learns his body parts, their extent, and their use through imitation, trial, adaptation, and accomplishment.

Education and training are vital for the family to encourage psychological adjustment to the prosthesis and to teach the importance of putting on, removing the prosthesis, checking skin areas for irritation, and encouraging positive play activities for the child using the prosthesis. Children are often hindered by parental distractions during training sessions, so times should be scheduled for the child alone and for the child and parent together. This results in effective training for prosthetic function and for family education. The most successful method of teaching a child prosthetic function is through the medium of play; consideration of the age and attitude of the child is essential to effective planning.

The child with congenital limb deficiency is considered for prosthetic replacement within the first year, generally by 6 months of age. He may first be fitted with a semirigid passive Robin-Aids mitt with a Munster-type socket with preflexed elbow and figure-eight harness control. This prosthesis can be used for gross bilateral use and initial balance activities. This cosmetic device is preparatory to the functional one.

At 6 months a mechanical element is added to the prosthesis. Natural development of movement in time and space, supplemented by guidance in use of appropriate components, can be incorporated into the child's body image and can assist functional use in further development. From 12 to 18 months, the child becomes ready for a functional terminal device with cable control.

A CAPP (Child Amputee Prosthetics Project) device may be provided. This is a voluntary opening terminal device made of nylon and Kraton that provides function and cosmesis and can be used until the child is 8 years old. An alternative to this is the voluntary opening, covered child's split hook with a protective plastisol covering. The above-elbow amputee may use a preflexed socket until 2 years of age for ease in using the terminal device and for bilateral proximity in holding objects and body balance while using the prosthesis.

As the child plays wearing the cable-operated prosthesis and notices the hook opening and closing, he learns to control this action. With early fitting, the child generally has a hook by 2 years of age. The smallest hand is for a 5-year-old. "Children become aware of the purpose for changing the position of the forearm during the third year of life. They learn to operate the prosthetic controls and apply them to functional activities during the fourth year of life."[6]

In her discussion of AE prosthetic training of the young child, Shaperman notes five developmental factors related to learning control use:
1. ability to see some purpose for positioning the forearm and willingness to explore new uses for this positioning;
2. ability to follow verbal instructions and perform drills;
3. ability to meet the physical requirements for consistent operation of the dual control system;
4. possession of a well-fitting, well-functioning prosthesis and availability for therapy;
5. experience of some previous success in using the prosthesis.[7]

Principles of training the child amputee include the following:
1. Begin with early minimal and simple prosthetic coverage.
2. Engage the child in gross sensorimotor activities to develop body awareness and use of the prosthesis.
3. Correlate training activity with prosthetic skill and developmental level.
4. Provide and train in control use as appropriate to the child's development, level of reception, comprehension, and physical functional ability.
5. Involve the family in the training program.

Whether or not the child benefits from prosthetic replacement depends on functional capacity, ingenuity, integration, and family support. It is important that the child with congenital deficiency be provided a prosthesis before starting school. Generally a new prosthesis is provided every 4 years to accommodate growth and functional development.[8]

Myoelectric Control

Developments in the use of myoelectric controls for prosthetic and orthotic replacements of lost limb functions have been steadily increasing in clinical application. A major significance of myoelectric prosthetic control is the use of signals from the neuromuscular system to activate specific component functions.

By approaching the amputee and prosthetic replacement as a complete unit or system, research and clinical teams are integrating natural and artificial elements.[9] In the effort to assist the amputee in achieving both efficient and natural function and appearance, combinations of both conventional and myoelectric components may be considered within the same prosthesis, particularly for amputation or skeletal deficiencies above the elbow. Myoelectric components and controls are available for operation of cosmetic/functional hand, wrist rotation, and elbow flexion and extension. These are available for unilateral, bilateral, below-elbow, and above-elbow amputees.

A myoelectrically controlled prosthesis or component operates by using the electric potential produced by a contracting muscle to activate a battery-driven motor to operate a prosthetic component. Proportional control of the motor by regulating the extent or speed of muscle contraction can affect the force or speed of the movement of the component.[10]

Myoelectric prostheses are provided to children and adults both experimentally and clinically. In both cases the candidates for myoelectric fitting are chosen for optimum success in myoelectric wear and use. Since the myoelectric prosthesis is expensive, both in initial provision and in maintenance, proximity of the amputee to the prosthetist, adequate funding resources, vocational appropriateness, and available prosthetic check-out and training are essential considerations. During the initial prosthetic prescription, factors such as the level of amputation, condition of the limb, number of limbs involved, extent of power, and control in the remaining limb and body are assessed.

Positive aspects of the myoelectric approach are listed:
1. utilization of natural muscle stimuli to activate component operation;
2. more accurate control with less energy output from the amputee;
3. elimination of the shoulder harness for operation;
4. ease in full-range of isolated extremity movements;
5. improved natural control and cosmesis of the prosthesis;
6. decreased body movement to control prosthesis.

Negative aspects of the myoelectric approach are listed:
1. high expense of controls, components, and repairs;
2. required skilled repair with breakdown of parts;
3. limited number of candidates for myoelectric wear and use;
4. noise of component operation;
5. daily battery charge required;
6. lack of proprioceptive feedback from harness;
7. added weight;
8. efficient control sites necessary;
9. muscle fatigue.

Good candidates for myoelectric replacement have the following attributes:
1. a healthy attitude toward the disability;
2. a desire for myoelectric control;
3. committment toward following procedures and responsibilities for myoelectric wear and care;
4. healthy skin and stump for effective socket and electrode contact;
5. fair muscle function in the arm to produce electrode signals for component operation.

During the process of evaluation and prescription, the amputee is introduced to the advantages and disadvantages of conventional and myoelectric control relative to his capabilities, interests, objectives, and readiness for prosthetic replacement.

Preprosthetic Considerations

Ability to isolate and control the muscle sites and to develop strength and speed of muscle contraction determines effective prosthetic use by the amputee. Assessment of surface EMG muscle sites to control a prosthesis is made using the myotester. Further training with the myotester helps the amputee to develop signal levels and reliable isolation of potential myoelectric control sites. This may be done using bench-mounted units such as the terminal device and the wrist unit.[11] A temporary plaster prosthesis may be used to determine the preliminary ability of the amputee to use myoelectric controls implanted in the socket. Efficiency of muscle control is established through use of the temporary prosthesis until the permanent one is ready for fitting and training. Preprosthetic activities also include practice in unilateral functional activities with the sound or remaining extremity, particularly if it is nondominant. Assistive devices for independent living skills may be beneficial during this period.

Identification of muscle sites and the number required for prosthetic operation depend on the level of the amputation and the ability of the amputee to isolate and use the muscle contractions. For example, a below-elbow amputee may use either a single site or two sites for terminal device operation. In the dual control, extensor muscle contraction may be used to open the terminal device, and flexor muscle contraction may be used to close the terminal device, thus simulating normal body associations. The above-elbow amputee may use biceps contraction for prosthetic elbow flexion and triceps contraction for prosthetic elbow extension, with co-contraction of these muscles to open and close the hand.

Passive, manually operated shoulder, elbow, and wrist components may be used. Cosmetic and functional electric hooks, hands, and elbows are commercially available. Electronic controls and batteries are stored within the sockets, or the hand of the prosthesis, or externally (Fig. 27-27).

Sockets are single or double-walled, depending on the level of amputation. Generally, the harness is

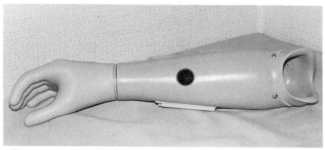

Figure 27-27. Complete below-elbow myoelectric prosthesis with cosmetic/functional terminal device, external battery pack, and double-walled forearm socket.

eliminated and the prosthesis is self-suspended on the extremity. In the below-elbow prosthesis, a supracondylar suspension, using bony prominences, or a Munster-type socket high on the forearm, is used for secure fit and comfort. In the Munster-type socket there is no supination and pronation available in active movement, and elbow flexion and extension are limited. The above-elbow socket or APS uses atmospheric pressure suspension.

Fitting

Ideally, a prosthesis is provided for the amputee as early as possible following healing and relief of swelling in the stump. Bender states that, in most cases, application of the prosthesis soon after the amputation reduces pain and edema in the stump, facilitates healing, and ensures minimum waiting time until a permanent one can be fitted.[12] In keeping with these findings, immediate postsurgical fitting of a prosthesis is provided by using a rigid cast socket to which controls and components are attached. Prosthetic replacement is referred to as *immediate fitting* if done before the sutures are removed, and as *early fitting* if done following removal of the sutures but before the permanent prosthesis is fabricated and fitted.

These preliminary temporary fittings assist the amputee in adjusting to prosthetic replacement and use. Early and permanent fitting of myoelectric controls involves locating suitable control sites for electrodes, casting for electrode placement locations, provision of the permanent socket with electrode emplacements, provision of the component system, controls, battery pack, on/off switch, and pigmenting. Since provision and maintenance of myoelectric controls and components are expensive, the amputee may first be provided with a conventional prosthesis with harness control to determine individual feasibility for myoelectric wear and function. In order to best meet the individual needs of the amputee, combina-

tions of cable-driven and myoelectric components can be used as feasible and appropriate to provide optimum functional and cosmetic aspects.

It may be recommended that the amputee have two prostheses so that one is available should one be in need of repair. This is to prevent the efficient prosthesis wearer and user from the inconvenience of not having the functional and cosmetic benefits of the prosthesis available to him or her at all times. As with the standard prosthesis, there is a big difference between learning the control system of the myoelectric prosthesis and the application of bodily use of the control system to perform functional activities. Prosthetic wear requires a gradual adjustment, acceptance, tolerance, and use.

Training

Prosthetic training is done on either an inpatient or an outpatient basis, and it progresses from the initial preprosthetic program of isolating muscle contractions to produce signals for specific training in component operation. The prosthetic training program includes the following:

1. check-out of the fabrication, fit, and efficiency of the prosthesis;
2. evaluation of the amputee's ability to effectively control the prosthesis;
3. specific training in general component use and coordination;
4. instruction in the care and operation of the prosthesis;
5. training in self-care activites;
6. use of prosthetic and natural upper extremity components in bimanual and bilateral functional activities.

During all stages of training, the therapist monitors and discusses progress and problems with the patient to insure optimum success in prosthetic wear and use by the amputee. Social interaction with other amputees assists him in adjusting and problem-solving.

The extent of daily use of myoelectric controls is dependent on conservation of the battery's energy during nonuse. This is accomplished by a manual switch that is turned on to use the controls and turned off when the amputee removes the prosthesis or during long periods when the control use is not necessary. To avoid blockage between the electrode contact and the muscles, a stump sock is not worn. The amputee is taught to examine skin areas on removal of the prosthesis to monitor skin irritation from the socket, as well as to keep the socket and parts clean.

Wear and successful use of the prosthesis depend

on an appropriate prescription and effective training program with adequate periodic follow-up and monitoring of the function of the prosthesis. In some cases, a spare prosthesis may be provided after the first 6 months to assure continued prosthetic use by the amputee during necessary repairs.

During the training program, patients share experiences and meet individual needs through group discussions. As prosthetic replacement of function is a personal and individual adjustment, patients are encouraged to take part in planning the program by talking about individual expectations, goals, problems, and ideas regarding their prosthetic replacement.

Pediatric Considerations

In providing prosthetic components to the child with either a congenital deficiency or a traumatic amputation, it is essential to consider his developmental level. The sooner the prosthesis can be fitted, the better. Sorbye reports that children between the ages of 2½ and 4 years are the most suitable for the below-elbow myoelectric prosthesis and that all children should be able to learn to use one.[13] He advises that a change from the standard or split hook prosthesis should be made before the child is 4 years old to avoid problems of adjusting to a change in the prosthesis and the prosthetic control system.

Candidacy for myoelectric replacement in children depends on personality, maturity, and interest of the child and his family, since all will be involved in learning the system and in monitoring prosthetic wear and use with regard to training. Sorbye states, "The children teach themselves how to open and close the prosthetic hand within a few minutes from the initial application, over 2½ years of age."[14] Training programs emphasize two-handed activities and involvement in developmental activities appropriate to the age and maturation of the child. Whether or not the child amputee benefits from the prosthesis depends on the functional capacity and ingenuity of the child.

Endoskeletal Modular System

The endoskeletal modular prosthetic system is designed primarily for cosmesis provided by a central inner tubular (pylon) support covered with a soft, pigmented polyurethane foam to give natural contour and soft appearance. A nylon stocking covering is stretched over the foam. A variety of interchangeable components are available to meet the needs of the amputee. The modular arm includes a nonfunctional cosmetic hand, passively activated elbow, and shoulder units. Harness and control cables can be eliminated, because the components are operated manually with the sound hand.

Occupational Therapy and the Lower Extremity Amputee

Amputations of the lower extremities are generally more common than those of the upper extremities because of the high incidence of peripheral vascular disease and traumatic injuries to the lower limbs. Psychological reactions mentioned earlier concerning the upper extremity amputee pertain also to the lower extremity amputee. Since age, body build, physical and medical condition, vascular supply, and motivation are factors in the rehabilitation of the lower extremity amputee, there are some patients for whom provision of a prosthesis is contraindicated. These persons are encouraged to maintain maximum independence and mobility with the aid of a wheelchair, crutches, and other necessary assistive devices. The amputee for whom a prosthesis is appropriately prescribed can usually look forward to partial restoration of basic functions, independence in self-care, and the opportunity of returning to work of some kind.

Basically, the detailed study of lower extremity (LE) function, preprosthetic preparation, prosthetic prescription, check-out and training, and the management of problems encountered by the LE amputee are handled by the physician and the physical therapist. However, there are many ways in which the occupational therapist can also contribute to the functional rehabilitation of the LE amputee. In a general hospital or a rehabilitation center, the occupational therapist may actually work with as many or more LE amputees as UE amputees.

Preprosthetic Period

Passive and active exercises of the lower extremities are performed or supervised by the physical therapist during the early postoperative period of healing. The nurse or physical therapist teaches the amputee to bandage the stump to encourage shrinkage and forming of the stump for prosthetic fitting. Proper positioning of the body in the wheelchair is important to prevent contractures in the joints proximal to the amputation, scoliosis of the spinal column, and edema—all of which could hinder successful prosthetic function. In the case of below-knee (BK) amputation, the use of a seat-board adapted for the individual amputee can be used in a regular chair or a wheelchair to maintain the knee in passive extension with knee flexors stretched while the amputee is performing activities in a sitting position.

The LE amputee may be referred to occupational

therapy in the preprosthetic or the prosthetic phase of training or both. In either case, the occupational therapist should become familiar with the medical aspects of the patient's care and the goals of the rehabilitation program. Pertinent information the occupational therapist should learn from the chart or from the staff members should include the following:

1. location, type, level, and cause of amputation;
2. condition of the stump and amputated extremity;
3. general body condition;
4. precautions and complicating conditions;
5. previous prosthetic replacement, if any;
6. recommendations for passive and active positioning of the joints of the amputated extremity;
7. the appropriate amount of standing and walking and the degree of safe support needed by the amputee.

Throughout the preprosthetic and prosthetic stages of training, the amputee may go through changes in attitude and behavior as he or she gradually realizes the extent of the loss and its effect on his or her life. Continual counseling is often necessary to help the amputee to adjust to the amputation, the change in body image, and the wear and use of the mechanical device to substitute for natural function. He or she must also adjust to working with his or her arms, gearing himself or herself to abilities rather than disability, finding new interests, and socializing in the new situation.

The seat-board mentioned previously can be made by the amputee as part of an upper extremity exercise program. It can be made of ½ or ¾ inch plywood that conforms to the measurement of the inside of the chair seat; one side extends to the end of the amputee's stump. The extended side should be narrow enough to prevent interference with the comfort of the sound leg in a sitting position, and at the same time should provide passive extension to the knee of the amputated leg. The seat-board should be padded sufficiently for comfort, and particular attention should be paid to such sensitive areas as the end of the stump.

In this preprosthetic phase the amputee may come to occupational therapy either in a wheelchair or walking with crutches. A variety of treatment techniques can be used. Since balance and upper extremity and trunk strength will be important in prosthetic use, maximum function of these areas is encouraged. Insofar as the amputee can tolerate the exercise, his or her sitting tolerance and balance is challenged by the use of upper extremity activities. Although at first an amputee with a high above-knee (AK) amputation or bilateral leg amputations may need to hold onto the chair with one hand to support himself or herself in a sitting position while using the

other hand, he or she should be encouraged to depend on the trunk for balance to leave both arms free for UE activities. As upper extremity strength and confidence in balance increase, ROM and resistance required in performing manual activities should be increased to further challenge trunk balance. Activities such as woodworking, weaving, and printing may be adapted to the amputee's individual needs. An activity in which the patient has a vocational or avocational interest may provide motivation in the activity so that he or she can increase tolerance of the given position and redirect energies from anxieties regarding his or her condition toward purposeful activity. Activities at this stage are directed toward the amputee's achieving independent function of arms and trunk while seated in a wheelchair.

Another aspect of independence regards self-care tasks. These include bathing and care of the stump, transfers, and dressing. A unilateral amputee should have little or no difficulty in this area. However, aids such as grab bars for bath and toilet, a transfer board or tub seat for bathing, and a raised toilet seat can be helpful as the amputee adjusts to a new body image and copes with the problems of balance. Phantom limb sensations can be a complicating factor if the amputee suddenly moves to get up and forgets that he or she cannot stand on the amputated limb, even though feeling is there. Continued physical and psychological support in these instances is necessary to minimize fear and to encourage confidence. Dressing is usually easier from a sitting position on the bed. Front fastenings and loose clothing also help to minimize frustrations.

Maximum independent function should be encouraged both with and without the prosthesis. For example, the amputee should be encouraged to stand on the sound leg in front of a table for short periods of time. This will encourage hip extension of the amputated side, and it will develop balance. However, attention must be paid to the amount of standing time so as not to encourage scoliosis of the spine.

Therapists have found that immediate postoperative fitting of a prosthesis or the use of a temporary pylon and the working prosthesis after the amputee's scar tissue has healed is beneficial to the LE amputee training program. The temporary pylon provides the amputee with early replacement of the amputated limb to encourage functional activity while the stump is being conditioned and the permanent prosthesis is being made.* The pylon consists of a plaster stump socket to which a pylon is attached to provide length and base support to the amputated leg. With the

---

* For specific designs of the pylon, see M. S. Jones: *An Approach to Occupational Therapy.* London: Butterworths, 1964, Chapter 6.

pylon the amputee can stand and ambulate soon after the amputation.

A working prosthesis is permanently attached to the machine that the amputee will use for exercise (*i.e.*, to the foot-powered lathe or the bicycle jigsaw). It also consists of a stump cuff that is laced up the sides for east in putting on and that provides a comfortable fit for different persons. It is open at the distal end to eliminate pressure on the end of the stump.

When the patient has put the cuff on the stump, he or she fits the pylon shafts into the cuff. As the base is attached to the bicycle jigsaw or the lathe, the amputee is then able to operate these machines and thus engage in active LE exercise of the amputated limb. The working prosthesis could be used with a foot-powered floor press, treadle sewing machine, or loom if properly adapted to the needs of the amputee. ROM and resistance can be graded, and the amputee can engage in an activity requiring coordination, balance, and strength of all four extremities and the trunk.

It must be remembered that at first the amputee fatigues more rapidly, even in the activity of maintaining sitting and standing positions, and that until tolerance increases, energy is directed toward these basic functions.

Prosthetic Training Program

The LE amputee depends on the prosthesis for support of the body in standing and walking. It is important that the prosthesis be appropriately prescribed, that it fit comfortably, and that it provide adequate functional assistance. The prescription and mechanical function of the prosthesis are checked thoroughly by the physical therapist. Function of the parts, how the amputee should put on the prosthesis, and how he or she should use it are taught by the physical therapist.

Independent locomotion depends on the fit and comfort of the prosthesis as well as on the general condition and tolerance of the amputee. Some may be able to discard their wheelchairs fairly soon. However, the amputee with poor tolerance of the prosthesis or a poorly fitting one may need the security of the wheelchair for a long time. In either case, the occupational therapy program can benefit the amputee by encouraging work in the treatment room doing activities in a standing position when he or she can tolerate it. Even if the amputee is still dependent on the wheelchair early in prosthetic training, he or she must eventually adjust to the mechanical, insensitive prosthesis by learning to judge where it is relative to the rest of the body, and he or she must learn how to function with it.

When the amputee receives the prosthesis, most

of his or her attention will be on the fit and use of it. Since he or she needs rest periods from ambulation training, he or she continues in an occupational therapy program for upper extremity strengthening and prosthetic tolerance. The activities outlined in the preprosthetic period are continued. At this point, they are done with the prosthesis on unless the amputee is resting the stump or has been irritated by the prosthesis. His or her program is geared toward encouraging acceptance of the prosthesis (to function in activities challenging UE and LE coordination and function), prosthetic tolerance, development of ADL independence, UE and LE activity exercise program, realization of his or her capacities, and vocational and avocational guidance.

Wearing time of the prosthesis is gradually increased according to the comfort and tolerance of the socket in sitting and standing positions. As the amputee will be weightbearing in the standing position, he or she must adjust to the sensation of bilateral weightbearing and the sensitivity of the stump to the hard edges and base of the socket. According to his or her tolerance and balance, the amputee can decrease the support he or she uses while standing. Engagement in UE activities in a standing position, which provides a wide range of motion and resistance, helps to challenge and to increase standing balance. Walking to cabinets to get and replace materials or tools and walking around tables and machines should be encouraged to increase functional independence. Carrying articles from place to place also further challenges balance and independent function. Aids such as a cart with wheels or a tray can minimize the stress of carrying items.

In ADL, the patient now learns to incorporate the prosthesis into bodily activites. He or she learns at what point in dressing activities to put on the prosthesis so that it will aid, rather than interfere with, ease and speed in dressing.

An important part of the prosthetic training program is aiding the amputee to realize his or her capabilities. In the occupational therapy environment, tasks may be set up both to improve the amputee's tolerance and function with the prosthesis and to relate to the requirements of his or her job.

Prevocational Exploration

Amputation may prevent a person from returning to a former line of work, and it may be a great source of anxiety. When the amputation prevents the individual from returning to a former occupation, the occupational therapist can provide valuable information to the vocational rehabilitation counsellor regarding the functional capabilities of the amputee. Information regarding interests, intelligence, physical abilities and skills, work tolerance, work habits, and general motivation for achieving new skills assists the counsellor in investigating new possibilities for the employable amputee in vocational planning.

Through formal prevocational performance evaluation using standardized dexterity tests, interest tests, and work-simulated tasks, the occupational therapist is able to provide an indication of motivation and readiness for vocational exploration. Through simulated work activities, the therapist is able to assess general work habits, comprehension, problem-solving ability, social compability, quality of work, and work tolerance.

Future Considerations

Research is continuing into more effective control systems and sites and for the development of improved components to simulate natural movements and functions. Efforts are being made to lessen weight, to improve locking and grasping mechanisms in the hand and the hook, to improve the glove material, and to increase the overall cosmesis of the prosthesis. Specific considerations are development of a more efficient elbow unit, rerouting of the cables to the inside of the arm instead of the outside, improved cosmetic appearance, higher operating efficiencies, and decreased wear on clothing. There is also research interest in providing active wrist rotation.

The experimentation in electric control is directed toward providing the amputee with a total coordination pattern and better integration of the total body system. The aim is to provide a link between the person and the prosthetic device by using a stimulus from the person's energy to activate the prosthesis.

Another idea is the use of phantom sensations to aid in the control of the BE prosthesis, using the signals from the forearm muscles for prehension and forearm rotation (pronation and supination). This method does not apply to the AE amputee, since the forearm muscles are gone and the power source muscles are removed from the terminal device.

Sensory Feedback

In spite of the advance in the development of mechanical and electronic prosthetic components and control systems, development of prosthetic replacement of lost sensory functions have been much slower, forcing the amputee to depend on visual and auditory monitoring for effective operation of standard cable-operated and myoelectric prosthesis.

With the loss of sensation caused by prosthetic replacement of a limb part, there is much effort toward the provision of sensory feedback to the amputee regarding prosthetic hand functions such as perception of grip strength and stability, kinesthetic information regarding hand and arm position, or movement and perception of the actual force in the joints of the prosthesis. Gross sense of the extremity in space exists, but there is poor sense of hook pressure for grip. Harness and cable stress and movement give a gross indication at times for hook opening and closing.

The harness system used in controlling the components of the conventional "body movement" or "joint-operated" prosthesis provides the amputee with proprioceptive awareness or feedback regarding the function of the prosthesis; this is lacking in the myoelectric prosthesis, which is not suspended or operated through a body harness. Although visual cues are necessary to guide in the accurate manipulation of objects with the terminal device, the amputee learns to perceive hook operation to some degree by harness and socket tension, weight of the prosthesis, material coverage of fabrication, sound of the control, and components in operation. When an external power source is provided, this information from the control cable is unavailable, because a much smaller and delicate movement is required to open a valve or trigger a microswitch, providing less feedback of information from the controlling mechanism.[15] Findings such as these have led to development of artificial feedback systems.[16]

Ongoing research continues to be directed toward incorporation of artificial feedback mechanisms within myoelectric prostheses to provide increased sensory integration of the prosthesis and the remaining arm, proprioceptive awareness of position and movement, and perception of the degree of force in joints of the prosthesis and detection of change in the grip of the terminal device. In addition to myoelectric electrodes, strain gauges or stimulating signals have been used to cause a tingling sensation in the stump relative to the force in the prosthetic grip, changing as the pressure changes to provide controls information through sensory feedback.[17]

Shannon and Agnew state that the presence of the sensory feedback is appreciated (by subjects) and enables them to hold objects confidently—even when the object held is obscured from vision.[18] Other considerations in providing sensory feedback include vibrations within electric systems, electric currents indicating magnitude of the force applied, information regarding the speed of the prosthetic hand closure, and tactile and joint position information.

In addition to the prohibitive cost of these experimental devices, another problem with an external power source is the replenishment of power. But efforts to produce designs that will simulate characteristics of normal muscle functions continue in hopes of achieving the goal of successful integration of the device and the person.

With the continuing research into the use and application of external power, the concept of "man-machine," or the integration of the person and the assistive device, is often cited. Since the physician and prosthetist recognize the need for an engineer who can provide devices operated with external power, the engineer or specialist in bioengineering has become a new member of the rehabilitation team.

Summary

The most important factor in prosthetic replacement is the choice of the right components and control system to suit the functional and emotional needs of the amputee. Patient and family education are as essential as a therapeutic prosthetic training program directed toward return to school or employment, family, home, and community.

The occupational therapist is a principal team member in the prosthetic training program of the amputee; with sufficient expertise, the occupational therapist can recommend the type of prosthesis appropriate for the amputee through preprosthetic evaluation and preparation of the patient for effective prosthetic wear and use.

In order to assist the child with a congenital skeletal deficiency or the child or adult with a traumatic amputation and resultant prosthetic replacement, the occupational therapist must become familiar with the following: (1) surgical procedures, precautions, and complications commonly incurred; (2) psychological aspects of limb loss; (3) prosthetic components, systems, and considerations; (4) preprosthetic conditioning programs; (5) prosthetic training; and (6) research and development with regard to components and systems.

Successful adjustment of the amputee for prosthetic wear and use depends on the following:
1. site and character of the amputation;
2. nature of surgical repair;
3. adequacy of prosthetic prescription, fabrication, and fit;
4. efficiency of check-out, training, and follow-up;
5. attention to the amputee's concerns, desires, and goals;
6. appropriateness of the prosthetic replacement and training.

Movement ranges, grips, reach, and force mechanisms have been provided by conventional prostheses through a variety of components and harnessing systems. It is an accepted view that the sooner the prosthesis is applied, the greater the chance of limiting problems in wear and function caused by phantom sensation or pain, and that early functional use is of psychological benefit to the amputee.

Early prosthetic fitting is important for both the congenital amputee and the traumatic amputee. The earlier a child is fitted with a prosthesis, the sooner he or she is able to incorporate it into his or her developmental activities, daily activities, and eventually school activities. The child is initially fitted with a simple prosthesis with a mitt hand and a Munster-type socket.

The occupational therapist monitors the amputee's adaptation through the preprosthetic and prosthetic period, checking the prosthesis for fit, comfort, and optimal function.

Principles of Effective Prosthetic Replacement

1. The amputee must be able to tolerate a prosthesis physically for functional wear and use.
2. The amputee must be able to accept the use and appearance of the prosthetic replacement feasible for him or her in relation to his or her lifestyle and daily needs.
3. The prescribed prosthesis components and design must be appropriate to the needs and expectations of the patient.
4. The prosthesis must fit properly before functional training and use is begun.
5. Essentials of prosthetic provision are evaluation, preprosthetic training, check-out of prosthesis, prosthetic training, and follow-up.

Technological advances in design and fabrication have resulted in rapid changes in the field of prosthetic replacement. New developments in endoskeletal modular prosthetic components allow increased versatility in replacement of lost lower extremity cosmesis, body support, and functions. The trend toward a more natural and comfortable gait has resulted in advances in hydraulic systems and socket design. As components become more adaptable, the effort toward saving as much tissue as possible results in increased feasibility of effective prosthetic replacement.

There have been significant gains in myoelectrically controlled systems and components now available clinically. Current research into sensory feedback from prosthetic functions activated through the neuromuscular system is carried out in the laboratory, as is the use of phantom sensations to aid in prosthetic control. Research continues on provision of sensory feedback, implanted electrodes, the function/cosmesis relationship, how to decrease the weight of the prosthesis, and how to make prosthetic movements more quickly.

Occupational therapists need to keep abreast of research and development in surgical techniques, myoelectric components, and other technologies.

References

1. Russell, H.: The Best Years of My Life. Middlebury VT: Paul S. Erikson, 1981, p. 17.
2. Bender, L. F.: Prosthesis and Rehabilitation after Arm Amputation. Springfield IL: Charles C. Thomas, 1974, p. 57.
3. Gilfoyle, E. M., Grady, A. P., and Moore, J. C.: Children Adapt. Thorofare NJ: Charles B. Slack, 1981, p. 3.
4. Ibid., p. 2.
5. Ibid., p. 1.
6. Shaperman, J.: Learning patterns of young children with above-elbow prostheses. Am. J. Occup. Ther. 33:305, 1979.
7. Ibid., p. 304.
8. Bender, L. F.: Prostheses and Rehabilitation after Arm Amputation, p. 157.
9. Childress, D. S., Holmes, D. W., and Billock, J. N.: Ideas on myoelectric prosthetic systems for upper-extremity amputees. In Herberts, P., Kadefors, R., Magnusson, R., and Petersen, I.: The Control of Upper-Extremity Prostheses and Orthoses. Springfield IL: Charles C. Thomas, 1974, p. 87.
10. Robertson, E.: Rehabilitation of Arm Amputees and Limb-Deficient Children. London: Bailliere Tindall, 1978, p. 44.
11. Stein, R. B., Charles, P. D., Hoffer, J. A., et al.: New approaches for the control of powered prostheses particularly by high-level amputees. Bull. Prosthetic Res. 17:10, 1980, p. 52.
12. Bender, L. F.: Prostheses and Rehabilitation after Arm Amputation, p. 34.
13. Sorbye, R.: Myoelectric prosthetic fitting in young children. J. Clin. Orthop. Rel. Res. 148:36, 1980.
14. Ibid., p. 36.
15. Robertson, E.: Rehabilitation of Arm Amputees and Limb-Deficient Children, p. 42.
16. Herberts, P., and Korner, L.: Ideas on Sensory feedback in hand prostheses. Prosthet. Orthot. Internat. 3:157, 1979.
17. Brittain, R. H., Santes, W. F., and Gibson, D. A.: Sensory feedback in a myoelectric upper limb prosthesis: A preliminary report. Can. J. Surg. 22:481, 1979.
18. Shannon, G. F., and Agnew, P. J.: Fitting below-elbow prostheses which convey a sense of touch. Med. J. Austral. 1:243, 1979.

Bibliography

Agnew, P. J., and Shannon, G. F.: Training program for a myoelectrically controlled prosthesis with sensory feedback system. Am. J. Occup. Ther. 35:722, 1981.

Blakeslee, B.: The Limb-Deficient Child. Berkeley and Los Angeles: University of California Press, 1963.
D'astous, J. (ed.): Orthotics and Prosthetics Digest Reference Manual. Ottawa: Edahl Productions Ltd., 1981.
Dickey, R. E., and Stieritz, L.: Amputation and impaired independence. In Abreu, B. C. (ed.): Physical Disabilities Manual. New York: Raven Press, 1981.
Ey, M. C.: Experiences with myoelectric prostheses: A preliminary report. Inter-Clinic Information Bull. 17:15, 1978.
Ey, M. C., and Helfgott, S.: A temporary thumb prosthesis. Inter-Clinic Information Bull. 17:9, 1978.
Fishman, S., and Kay, H. W.: The Munster-type below-elbow socket, an evaluation. Artif. Limbs 8:4, 1964.
Friedman, L. W.: The Psychological Rehabilitation of the Amputee. Springfield IL: Charles C. Thomas, 1978.
Garrett, J. F., and Levine, E. S. (eds.): Rehabilitation Practices with the Physically Disabled. New York: Columbia University Press, 1973.
Gerhardt, J. J., et al.: Immediate post-surgical prosthetics: Rehabilitation aspects. Am. J. Phys. Med. 49:3, 1970.
Herberts, P., Korner, L., Caine, K., and Wensby, L.: Rehabilitation of unilateral below-elbow amputees with myoelectric prostheses. Scand. J. Rehabil. Med. 12:123, 1980.
Hunter, J. M., Schneider, L. H., Mackin, E. J., and Bell, J. A.: Rehabilitation of the Hand. St. Louis: C. V. Mosby, 1978.
Jones, M. S.: An Approach to Occupational Therapy. London: Butterworths, 1977.
Kay, H. W., et. al.: The Munster-type below-elbow socket, a fabrication technique. Artif. Limbs 9:4, 1965.
Lehneis, H. R., Frisina, W., Susman, W., and Cohen, J.: A universal terminal device: Preliminary report. Inter-Clinic Information Bull. 17:1, 1978.
Loughlin, E., Stanford, J. W., and Phelps, M.: Immediate post-surgical prosthetics fitting of a bilateral, below-elbow amputee, a report. Artif. Limbs 12:17, 1968.
Madruga, L.: One Step at a Time: A Young Woman's Inspiring Struggle to Walk Again. New York: McGraw-Hill, 1979.
Mastro, B. A. and Mastro, R. T. (eds.): A Review of Orthotics and Prosthetics. Washington DC: American Orthotic and Prosthetic Association, 1980.
Mulhern, F. P.: Biceps cineplasty exercise. Am. J. Occup. Ther. 11:322, 1957.
Munroe, B., and Nasca, R. J.: Rehabilitation of the upper extremity amputee. Military Med. 140:6, 1975.
Murphy, E. F., and Horn, L. W.: Myoelectric control systems—a slected bibliography. Orthotics and Prosthetics 35:34, 1981.
Orthotics/Prosthetics (information packet). Rockville MD: American Occupational Therapy Association Division of Professional Development, 1979.
Pedretti, L. W.: Occupational Therapy Practice Skills for Physical Dysfunction. St. Louis: C. V. Mosby, 1981.
Prosthetics Yes . . . Bionics Maybe ??? (review of Third World Congress of International Society of Prosthetics and Orthotics, NYC, 1977). Whitestone NY: National Amputation Foundation.
Reilly, G. V.: Pre-prosthetic exercises for upper extremity

amputee with special reference to cineplasty. Phys. Ther. Rev. 31:183, 1951.

Review of Visual Aids for Prosthetics and Orthotics. Committee on Prosthetic-Orthotic Education, Division of Medical Sciences, National Academy of Sciences, National Research Council, Washington DC.

Rosenfelder, R.: Infant amputee: Early growth and care. J. Clin. Orthop. Rel. Res. 148:41, 1980.

Santschi, W. R.: Manual of Upper Extremity Prosthetics, ed. 2. Los Angeles: Department of Engineering, UCLA, 1965.

Sarmiento, A., et. al.: Immediate postsurgical prosthetics fitting in the management of upper-extremity amputees. Artif. Limbs 12:14, 1968.

Shaperman, J., and Sumida, C. T.: Recent advances in research in prosthetics for children. J. Clin. Orthop. Rel. Res. 148:26, 1980.

Talbot, D.: The Child with a Limb Deficiency, A Guide for Parents. Los Angeles: UCLA Child Amputee Prosthetics Project, 1979.

Taylor, C. L.: The biomechanics of control in upper-extremity prostheses. Orthot. Prosthet. 35:7, 1981.

Tohen, Z., and Alfonso, M. D.: Manual of Mechanical Orthopaedics. Springfield IL: Charles C. Thomas, 1973.

Trombly, C. A., and Scott, A. D.: Occupational Therapy for Physical Dysfunction. Baltimore: Williams & Wilkins, 1977.

Wellerson, T. L.: A Manual for Occupational Therapist on the Rehabilitation of Upper Extremity Amputees. New York, published under the auspices of the American Occupational Therapy Association, 1958.

Whipple, L.: Whole Again. Ottawa: Caroline House Publishing, Inc., 1980.

Journals

Artifical Limbs: A Review of Current Developments. Committee on Prosthetics Research and Development, Division of Engineering and Committee on Prosthetic-Orthotic Education, Division of Medical Sciences of the National Research Council, National Academy of Sciences, Washington DC.

Bulletin of Prosthetics Research. Veterans Administration, Department of Medicine and Surgery, Washington DC 20420.

The Canadian Journal of Surgery. Canadian Medical Association, 1867 Alta Vista Drive, Box 8650, Ottawa, Ontario, KIG OG8, Canada.

Inter-Clinic Information Bulletin. Prosthetics and Orthotics. New York University Post-Graduate Medical School, 317 East 34th Street, New York NY 10016.

The Medical Journal of Australia. Australian Medical Publishing Co., 71-79 Arundel Street, Glebe, N. SW. 2037 Australia.

Orthotics and Prosthetics. Journal of the American Orthotic and Prosthetic Association, 717 Pendelton Street, Alexandria VA 22314.

Prosthetics International. Journal of the International Society on Prosthetics and Orthotics, Secretariate: I.S.P.O., P.O. Box 42, DK 2900 Hellerup, Denmark.

Scandinavian Journal of Rehabilitation Medicine. Stockholm, Sweden: The Almqvist & Wiksell Periodical Company.

Resources

American Orthotic and Prosthetic Association
717 Pendelton Street
Alexandria VA 22314
Child Amputee Prosthetic Project
(CAPP prosthesis and components)
University of California at Los Angeles
Los Angeles CA
Fidelity VA-NU Myoelectric Hand System and Cosmetic Components
Fidelity Electronics, Ltd.
5245 West Diversey Avenue
Chicago IL 60639
Hosmer Dorrance Corporation
(conventional, modular, and external power components)
P.O. Box 37
561 Division Street
Campbell CA 95008
Motion Control
(Utah Artificial Arm; myoelectric elbow)
1005 South 300 West
Salt Lake City UT 84101
National Amputation Foundation, Inc.
12-45 150th Street
Whitestone NY 11357
Northwestern University Medical School Prosthetic-Orthotic Center
345 East Superior Street
Chicago IL 60611
Otto Bock Orthopedic Industry, Inc.
(conventional, myoelectric, and endoskeletal components)
610 Indiana Avenue North
Minneapolis MN 55422
Pope Brace
(Accru-Hook system)
197 South West Avenue
Kankakee IL 60901
Prosthetics and Orthotics
New York University Post-Graduate Medical School
317 East 34th Street
New York NY 10016
Prosthetic Research Laboratory at Northwestern University Medical School
Michigan Department of Public Health
Area Child Amputee Center
Grand Rapids MI
Realistic Industries
(cosmetic components)
3010 Lyons Road
P.O. Box 6158
Austin TX 78702

Therapeutic Recreation Systems
   (prehensile hook terminal device)
   2860 Pennsylvania Avenue
   Boulder CO 80303
Variety Village Electro Limb Production Centre
   (myoelectric and cosmetic components)
   3701 Danforth Avenue
   Scarborough (Toronto) Ontario
   Canada M1N 2G2

Acknowledgments

The author wishes to thank the administration, staff, and patients of Harmarville Rehabilitation Center for their cooperation with the writing of this chapter. In addition, thanks to Ed Collins, Ron Gregory, and Patricia Marvin for photographs, and to Patricia Marvin again for references and general assistance. Alice Kuller, Librarian at Harmarville Rehabilitation Center, provided invaluable help with references, and Pat Curran assisted with editing and typing.

CHAPTER 28

Occupational Therapy for Problems with Special Senses— Blindness and Deafness

Ann Starnes Wade

Vignettes*

Alice is a totally blind child who attends public day school with seven other blind, multiply handicapped children, ages 3 to 7. Like the others, she is developmentally delayed in adaptive and social-emotional skills, but Alice can hear, she has clear but sometimes echolalic speech, and she walks and enjoys swimming and using many items on the playground. She is moderately tactually defensive, frequently refuses to trail the wall with her hand, and she has difficulty making transitions from one situation to another. Jack, a classmate, is deaf, partially sighted, nonvocal, and delayed in all areas of development as a result of rubella syndrome. He is classified as deaf–blind, multiply handicapped, and he displays some autistic-like behaviors. Jack walks with a broad-based gait, using his residual vision to find food as well as to avoid obstacles. He knows and uses signs for drink and eat. Both children appear to crave vestibular stimulation. Occupational therapy services are included in these children's programs because their teacher has

requested them within the guidelines of federal and state special education standards. Teacher, therapist, classroom aides, and those families who can, work collaboratively with Alice, Jack, and some of their classmates. Direct occupational therapy services are provided individually on an average of three half-hour periods per week, usually in the occupational therapy department but also in halls, classrooms, and occasionally at a swimming pool. Developmental and sensorimotor integration approaches are used to attain psychosocial and cognitive-perceptual-motor goals. □

Mary is 6 years old, recently enrolled in a residential school for the deaf. Having no other physical disability, she is unlikely to be referred for occupational therapy. A volunteer recently reprimanded Mary, in sign language, when Mary kicked the volunteer apparently for not providing undivided attention. The volunteer, a skilled worker with adult deaf in another setting, later discussed with the occupational therapist the tendency of some deaf adults to interrupt, to be dependent, and to expect instant gratification; both see the need to stop this trend during childhood by (1) teaching

---

* Modified to protect confidentiality.

527

developmentally appropriate self-management, play, work-study, and social skills; (2) communicating effectively with the children as persons of worth; (3) setting reasonable limits with consistency among houseparents, teachers, volunteers, support staff, and parents; and (4) adding responsibilities and privileges as students become ready. These are areas where the occupational therapist may serve as consultant, member of a task force, as one of the providers of continuing education and sometimes as direct service provider. □

Mr. James recently lost his vision in a laboratory accident. He is wondering how he will function, declaring that he cannot do anything now that he is blind, that he must find some work other than his profession of medical technology, but what . . . and how . . . His wife and parents are upset, not sure how to help and nearly as shocked as Mr. James. Now past the medical crisis, he is due to be discharged from the hospital within a week to 10 days. Occupational therapy, social work, and nursing are involved in treatment and discharge planning, under the leadership of the ophthalmologist. □

Mrs. Turner is a blind, diabetic woman proud of her Mexican-American culture, her numerous young grandchildren, and her independence. She is receiving physical and occupational therapy in a southern rehabilitation center. Her left leg was amputated due to diabetic gangrene 6 months ago, and she wants to walk with a "wooden leg" rather than be confined to a wheelchair. She also wants to return to her two room dirt floor cottage, rather than living with one of her children. Coming from a rural area to this metropolitan one and a rehabilitation center whose mostly Anglo-American staff all seem to be under 30, she is attempting to manipulate the situation in order to cope with so much strangeness. □

Mrs. Reed is a widow with marked arthritic deformities that confined her to a geriatric chair in an intermediate care facility (nursing home) that serves many deaf residents. Because of her arthritic hands, Mrs. Reed's sign language and generally phonetic fingerspelling are difficult to receive. Her "geri-chair" tray was adapted with alphabet and a few symbols to clarify communication and to make possible some communication with nonsigning people. Until she had eye surgery to improve her vision, she needed the 1¼ inch high letters to enable her to receive others' messages too. Since surgery and new corrective lenses, she can see to receive American Sign Language, to write, and to read what others write or print at an elementary level. She also communicates by tracing words or letters with her finger when pencil, paper, and laptray are not available or when her fingers are too painful to hold a pencil. Mrs. Reed often uses her left hand to help position her right hand more correctly for certain letters of the manual alphabet. Having recently discovered that she can slowly maneuver a regular wheelchair within the building, Mrs. Reed and staff are preparing a new, narrow laptray that will permit both communication and mobility. Her improved vision enables use of smaller letters and the addition of some frequently used words including her name, address, and phone number. Nursing personnel, activities director, and occupational therapist have shared ideas and services with this spunky woman. □

Mr. Williams is an elderly bachelor who has Usher's syndrome, which rendered him deaf at birth and gradually, during middle adulthood, blind. Other family members are unable to maintain close contact, so he has resided in a residential facility for the deaf and deaf–blind. Because of a strong desire to regain his independence, Mr. Williams received and successfully completed orientation and mobility training and training in safe, independent living through state rehabilitation services for the blind. This involved the client, an orientation and mobility specialist, a rehabilitation teacher of the blind, and a certified interpreter for the deaf. Mr. Williams receives sign language and finger-spelling by placing his hands over the signer's hands, with occasional clarification by tracing numbers in the palm of his hand. He signs and fingerspells, sometimes accompanied by an approximation of speech that can give some clues or, when he is excited, can be confusing. In meetings, he sometimes needs to be reminded by contact signing not to use his voice while signing, since he cannot see or hear when the meeting formally begins nor when people try to "shush" him. He uses a timer-clock-activated vibrating pad under his pillow as an alarm. This gentleman's personal organization skills are good, but he does want and need sighted, signing help for checking cleanliness and colors of certain clothing, for shopping, for learning current news, for keeping up with sporting events, and for reducing his sense of isolation. Having been blind for about 15 years and institutionalized for 10 of these, he is relatively unfamiliar with inflated prices and with changes in technology, marketing, etc. Occupational therapy and social work services have been needed for psychological and physical reasons in the interim between completion of independent living training and actually moving into an apartment. (Independent living training had been arranged before the facility employed an OTR). Purposeful activity, which appealed to him, mainly in the nature of making salable items such as rake-knitted hats and scarves, woven rugs, and hand-rubbed wooden pieces, has helped him wait more patiently, sleep and feel better, use less chewing tobacco, and earn a little pocket money. (When sighted he had supplemented his factory wages by hand-crafting items.) Shopping, cooking, eating, and cleaning up are important for reality of prices, for personal satisfaction, and for refinement of skills. A joint effort of personnel is helping him to establish the habit of writing messages and lists, following established channels for personal assistance rather than seeking help or conversation from staff each time during the day that he thinks of something. These behaviors will enhance relationships both in his current environment and in the independent living apartment complex for elderly, deaf, and physically disabled persons. Covered by state funds, the rehabilitation teacher will review training and reorient him as soon as he has moved to the apartment. Social work and occupational therapy services will discharge him when he moves, but volunteers will assist him biweekly to shop, bank, place items for sale through a senior citizens craft outlet, attend deaf-blind club functions, etc. □

Significance of Visual and Auditory Senses

Interdependence with Other Senses

Both vision and hearing are *distance,* or *distant* senses. These are primary channels by which most individuals gather information and receive pleasure from the environment without making physical contact with it. *Near* senses of touch, movement, taste, and smell are also important; information transmitted via touch-tactile, kinesthetic-proprioceptive, gustatory, and olfactory channels requires direct contact or, in the case of olfaction, closer range. Particularly during infancy and early childhood, the individual seeks to touch, manipulate, taste, and smell himself/herself and the surroundings, as well as to look and listen. Vision and hearing become increasingly sophisticated and reliable in the course of normal development. The match between near and distant sensory data gathered and integrated during early exploration and manipulation of the world gradually enables the child to identify human and nonhuman sounds, objects, scenes, and events through visual and audi-

tory information. Contributions of visual and acoustic senses are understandably great both in the development and continuation of communication skills, perceptual-motor ability, including purposeful manipulation and mobility within one's environments, psychosocial function, and cognitive capability. This should not imply that a blind or deaf person cannot develop and use all residual and intact senses to their full extent, but it does present challenges to the individuals, their families, and the professional persons who work with them.

Nature of Visual and Auditory Problems

Deficits in Vision

The legal definition of blindness in the United States refers to visual acuity that cannot be corrected to better than 20/200 feet or 6/60 meters. That is, the legally blind person, even with maximum correction, cannot see the Snellen or similar chart with the stronger eye from a distance of 20 feet or 6 meters any better than a person with normal visual acuity can see it from 200 feet or 60 meters. An individual may also be considered legally blind if he/she has no peripheral vision, that is, the visual field is restricted to less than that of a 20-degree angle so that he or she sees no more than what a fully sighted person might see through a tube or tunnel.[1,2]

Legal definitions of blindness allow a wide range of visual problems and abilities to be classified as blind. Total blindness, the complete inability to see, accounts for about 20% of these.[3] A person may be legally blind yet have some *near visual acuity,* corrected or uncorrected, sufficient to read ordinary newsprint, large print, or something in between the two. Normal near visual acuity can be described as 14/14, achieved by accurately reading the 14th, or smallest print line on a Jaeger test type reading card at a distance of 14 inches.[4] Unless there is an eye disease that contraindicates, there is apparently no damage to the visual system even if the individual must hold a book or object only a few inches from the eyes. Each individual will vary in the manner and effectiveness with which he/she uses his/her visual acuity.

A blind person may have *no* awareness of environmental light, may have *light perception,* which is awareness of light versus dark, or may have *light projection,* which is the ability to indicate the light source.[5] The capacity of a legally blind person to perceive enough visual information to permit safe independent movement in the environment is called *travel vision.*[6]

About a half million people in the United States have been classified as legally blind, but another million visually impaired persons do not meet the criteria for legal blindness. One functional definition refers to those who cannot read ordinary newsprint, which requires a corrected visual acuity of 20/50.[7] These people, and the legally blind with some residual vision, may be called *low-vision,* visually handicapped, or partially sighted.

A person legally blind in one eye may not be classified as such if acuity in the other eye is greater than 20/200. These individuals, as well as those with scotomas, amblyopia, color blindness, and central nervous system disorders of visual perception, also warrant attention for their problems. Since a person may not qualify for additional tax deductions and other benefits unless *legally blind,* the classification can be significant for financial reasons.[8]

Primary causes of blindness are diabetic retinopathy (leading cause of adult blindness), glaucoma, cataract, retinitis pigmentosa, detached retina, macular degeneration, rubella (especially maternal), retrolental fibroplasia, and in third world countries, trachoma that is a preventable contagious disease of the eye exacerbated by malnutrition and poor hygiene. These conditions are described and discussed in terms of prognosis and implications in a useful 1979 publication of the American Foundation for the Blind.[9] Other visual problems may be due to injuries, malignancies (especially retinoblastoma), and conditions and diseases affecting the central nervous system in utero, childhood, and later life. Some visual field deficits are of psychogenic origin. Ordinarily as a person steps back from an item he/she is viewing, the visual array expands accordingly. Similarly, the person with organic tunnel vision can see more as he moves farther from the subject or scene. In contrast, persons with psychogenic field deficits characteristically do not perceive an expanded visual array at a greater distance, but they continue to identify only the original subject matter.[10]

Previously sighted persons who lose their vision are generally referred to as the *adventitiously* or *newly blind.* Those born without sight or with severely impaired vision are known as *congenitally blind.* Whenever a sensory loss occurs, it tends to be isolating and to effect a type of sensory deprivation. The impact on development must receive particular attention to avoid severe secondary handicaps.

The Blind Child's Development

As long as a blind infant can hear, smell, or feel his/her mother often enough in some meaningful way, the infant will come to recognize his/her mother. If stimuli typical of mother are absent, even though the little one is within her vision, to the infant she is absent. In fact, until the infant develops object permanence, mother ceases to exist. Ordinarily vision plays a significant role in development of object concept, but if the blind infant has sufficient opportunity and encouragement to use and refine the other senses while manipulating and responding to human and nonhuman objects, the milestone will be reached. The blind child's abilities to hear and to begin to associate words with objects and events and to move, explore, and manipulate objects become particularly important to the development of object recognition and permanence, relationship-building, and concept formation.

Fraiberg and associate psychiatrists[11] have studied the development of blind and sighted children. They found that otherwise normal, totally blind infants (1) tended to lie passively in their beds with their arms abducted to each side, elbows flexed to 90 degrees, hands at head level; (2) could distinguish parents from a stranger by the age of 6 to 8 months even when all were silent and the stranger attempted to hold the infant just as his parents did (this is within the normal range, or nearly so, of discrimination of strangers, which begins at approximately 24 weeks)[12]; (3) *did not spontaneously reach* for objects unless shown by auditory input, from tapping the toy on table or floor, that the object they had just been holding or touching was within reach; (4) could localize sound at about 10 months of age; and (5) began to creep *only after they could both localize sound and reach.* Finally, the blind children developed the apparently innate smiling response as do sighted infants, but they did not further develop or maintain true smiling in infancy, except occasionally for the mother, probably because imitation and reinforcement of the smile were hardly possible. Interpersonal relationships between parents and blind infant can be affected by this apparent lack of facial responsiveness on the part of the infant, as well as by the parents' shock at discovering their child cannot see.

More recently, Fraiberg[13] has reported that sensorimotor and emotional development are dependent upon a good mother-child relationship in the early months and years. Given that not-easily-established good relationship, some blind children are in fact able to smile spontaneously and appropriately. Fraiberg and her associates emphasize the need to work with and through the mother to assist the development of a positive relationship with her child and to stimulate crucial development throughout the sensorimotor period. Without that stimulation, Fraiberg has found that blind infants and young children may achieve static postures but may lack purposeful mobility and hand skills, and may lag in language, intellectual development, and social development.

Deficits in Hearing

Deafness has been defined as the inability to hear and understand speech through the ear alone. This definition and the following classifications have been used for the 1971 National Census of the Deaf Population and in the Model State Plan for Rehabilitation of Deaf Clients.[14] In 1971, there were approximately 13.4 million hearing-impaired persons, of whom nearly two million were deaf.[15]

The person who cannot hear and understand speech may be described according to the phase of life at which deafness occurred. An individual is said to be *prelingually deaf* if he/she did not have or lost his hearing prior to the development of speech, or *prevocationally deaf* if he/she became deaf before reaching 19 years of age. *Adult deafness* refers to loss of hearing ability at or after age 19. The earlier deafness occurs, the more severely handicapping it is likely to be; however, regardless of age of onset, loss of hearing is usually accompanied by emotional problems. Schein, editor of the Model State Rehabilitation Plan, cautions that the size of the deaf population has grown and that it shifts in regard to growth rate. He calls attention to the unusually large number of deaf persons under age 25, due to the rubella epidemics of 1964–1965 producing the "rubella bulge" and to the fact that many deaf workers currently have "jobs in declining industries or occupational categories."[16] *Hard of hearing* is the term for hearing impairments less severe than deafness. In childhood these may affect language development, with effects of later onset depending upon one's occupation and need for oral verbal communication.

Intensity or loudness, the amplitude of sound waves, is measured in decibels or dB. Ordinary conversation registers approximately 60 dB. The frequency of sound waves, known as pitch, is usually measured in cycles per second or hertz. The lower-pitched speech sounds are those such as *o* in *go, d* and *g* in *dog;* higher tones include *f* in *puff, s* in *say, school,* and *this.* Adequate auditory perception of speech requires hearing between 500 and 2000 hertz (low to high respectively), but frequencies from 16 to 16,000 hertz are audible to persons with normal hearing. Early hearing impairment may first be detected when testing for sounds at 4000 hertz. Loss is usually gradual and may go unnoticed or undiagnosed for some time. If audiometric tests reveal an average auditory loss of 16 dB for frequencies of 500, 1000, and 2000, the individual is considered to have a *beginning hearing impairment.* A person is classified as *deaf* when the average auditory loss is 82 dB or more for those frequencies.[17]

There are two major categories of deafness. In *middle ear* or *conduction deafness,* when sounds are conducted by air rather than bone, there tends to be greater difficulty in hearing lower frequencies. This type impairment may respond well to treatment. The greater problem in *perception* or *nerve deafness,* which is usually permanent though occurs less frequently, is for the higher frequencies, whether sound is conducted by air or bone. If the hearing impairment involves the cochlea, slight increases in sound intensity may, through recruitment, be perceived as much louder, even to the point of pain.[18]

Deafness may be attributed to hereditary nerve deafness, brain defects, birth trauma, congenital (maternal) rubella, maternal ingestion of certain medications during pregnancy, and early infections such as cerebrospinal meningitis and encephalitis.[19,20] Premature infants, athetoid cerebral palsied, and others whose blood type is incompatible with their mothers' Rh negative type have a higher incidence of deafness than other infants.[21] Otosclerosis, which may first be identified during adolescence, is the primary cause of deafness among active adults.[22] Continuous loud noises can damage the inner ear, but there are no conclusions regarding intermittent intense noise. Incidence of deafness increases with the age of the population. Although more women than men have otosclerosis, after age 55 there are more men than women with hearing loss.[23,24]

The Deaf Child's Development

If all other senses are intact and appropriately stimulated, the nonhearing child will develop object recognition, object permanence, and interpersonal relationships based on visual, manual, and physical exploration and the internal and external results of these experiences. Communication through smiling, other facial expressions, body language, gestures, and possibly sign language will be the basis for the young child's "labeling" of objects, events, and feelings. Later more formal manual signs, finger spelling, lip or speech reading, printed words, and symbols may supplement the infant language. If the nonhearing child's back is turned or the child is not visually attending in the parent's direction, the child's inability to respond to his/her parent's words or footsteps as one or the other approaches may affect their relationship. However, when the child does see them, their appearance may be acknowledged with a genuine smile and animation. Particularly before a definite diagnosis of deafness, the young child may be perceived and treated as stubborn, withdrawn, peculiar, or retarded as a result of apparently fluctuating attention.

There is some evidence[25,26] that if the deaf infant is reared by deaf, signing parents, he/she will likely achieve greater emotional stability and maturity than the deaf child who develops in an environment where communication and understanding are usually inadequate, often the case with hearing parents.

Most prelingually deaf persons without other physical disabilities ultimately develop keen visual and manual abilities, but receptive and expressive, oral and written language has usually fallen far behind. A small percentage may learn, laboriously, to speak and/or to speech read, but the deaf who learn these at a more adequate level usually had at least some hearing through the language development years. Some deaf never develop sign or oral language but communicate by means of gestures, signs that have meaning only among immediate family or group members, pictures, and demonstration. This is not necessarily an index of intelligence or lack of it but does greatly complicate communication with both deaf and hearing persons.

Inability to hear conversation and other environmental sounds tends to result in some fear of the unknown even among the sophisticated deaf, and often in the suspicion—sometimes well-founded—that others are talking about them or preventing their knowing all that is being said.[27] Failure to communicate in a language that *all* group members can understand *all the time* may severely retard ego development in the prelingually and prevocationally deaf, and may offend and isolate the adult deaf. Such are the observations of *deaf leaders* in the field of deaf rehabilitation.[28]

Besides the lack of self-confidence found in many deaf persons, it has been said that some deaf also have a "gimme" attitude that takes the form of overdependency on and/or exploitation of hearing and successful deaf individuals. It may be that this expectation of instant gratification is due in part to the inability to hear all the planning, problems, and preparation associated with events, services, and purchases that simply seem to appear. Overprotection and paternalism at home and in service arms of society may also erode motivation and incentive. These, then, are problems that compound the common problem of most deaf—that of a communication gap, or chasm, with hearing society, including many in medical and rehabilitation services.

Deaf–Blindness or Blind–Deafness

Both combinations of deaf-blindness and blind-deafness are included in the heading because some libraries catalog according to the second term, even though most use the first. Some professional workers in this field use the word order to designate which condition occurred first.[29] Since most persons with combined hearing and visual losses are congenitally deaf persons who become blind,[30] the term *deaf–blind* is usually employed. Often there is residual vision, as well as visual memory, on which to capitalize in rehabilitation. As suggested in the preceding sections on visual and hearing deficits, the combined loss of both distant senses may be due to hereditary or congenital causes, to infections, or to central nervous system trauma, and it may ultimately accompany or be complicated by the aging process.

Usher's syndrome is a combination of congenital deafness and *retinitis pigmentosa* that, although hereditary, results in gradual loss of vision. There is no known cure other than prevention through genetic counseling. It is found in about 50% of the deaf-blind population.[31] Many of these persons will have sign language and writing skills, and many may have some functional speech, although they cannot hear. However, the loss of vision will necessitate slower signing, received tactually in the hands or within whatever possible field (tunnel vision) of vision the person may have. Corrective and magnifying lenses may help; however, blindness may become total.

If the person was blind before becoming deaf or hard-of-hearing, he/she may continue to use Braille, good English, and voice; he/she may function with auditory memory, but will be cut off from some or all external auditory stimulation. Amplification should be explored.

The major cause of deaf–blindness in children is maternal rubella during the first trimester of pregnancy.[32] Because of the other organs affected by the rubella virus, some of the deaf-blind children suffer cardiac problems, motor and/or mental retardation, hyperactivity, and in some cases, autistic-like behaviors.[33]

The Deaf-Blind Child's Development

The world of the infant who is both deaf and blind consists only of those human and nonhuman objects that can be felt, smelled, tasted, and manipulated. Fortunately many deaf-blind individuals have some vestige of one or the other distant sense, so that residual vision or hearing, however small, can be used to aid in motivation, orientation, exploration, and satisfaction of many such children. Recalling the tendencies toward passivity of blind infants, and the attentional problems of deaf infants, one has some notion of the probable need to *bring* the world *to* the deaf-blind infant and vice versa, *and* in a manner appropriate, acceptable, and meaningful to the child. Until touched, this infant may receive no stimuli that say someone or something is near. Medical staff and parents may not initially have been aware of the profound sensory loss, and thus they may have found no reason to handle the newborn differently from any other full-term or premature infant.

Mouchka,[34] the knowing parent of a deaf-blind child, who has also had experience with other similarly handicapped youngsters, noted that these infants behave differently, within three categories: (1) they do not respond to any apparent stimuli but remain passive; (2) they consistently respond vigorously, protectively, and hypersensitively to any attempt to handle them; or (3) they cry most of the time whether they are being handled or left alone. These findings correlate with reports from parents and caretakers of other deaf-blind children and with those of Chess and associates,[35] psychiatrists who have studied children handicapped as a result of the rubella syndrome. Additional cardiac and neurological problems can compound the sensory deficits and can make homeostasis even more precarious, which may explain the extreme sympathetic nervous system responses of some multihandicapped children as well as the apparent vegetative state of others. Before object recognition can be attained there must be homeostasis and sufficient meaningful sensory information to permit the infant to sense and respond to the mother or another object. A trusting relationship is based at least in part on sufficient appropriate stimuli that the infant can somehow perceive as satisfying, predictable, and dependable. The demanding and frustrating roles of parents of such handicapped children require ongoing acknowledgment, support, and guidance by empathetic, creative, and competent health care professionals.

Object recognition and permanence, relationships, and communication can be developed slowly if the infant is neurologically and motorically able to tactually and kinesthetically experience and explore self, mother, father, crib, food, toys, and larger environment, augmented by relevant sensory information through all possible channels. Consistent tactual symbols and signs, tactile-kinesthetic rhythms, motions, and vibrations will gradually become representative of objects and events experienced, contributing to language development and the establishment of trusting relationships with others who can use the language.

Educational programs for deaf-blind children have accepted any child whose disabilities prevent his/her benefiting from programs offered the blind or the deaf child. Generally speaking, the most progress has been made by children who become adventitiously disabled, rather than congenitally deaf–blind. Legislation enacted after the 1964–1965 epidemics has helped prepare more special education teachers, habilitation programs, sheltered workshops, and centers that offer "therapeutic work" and independent living services to those too low functioning to cope with even sheltered employment.[36,37]

Occupational Therapy Services to Persons with Impaired or Absent Distant Senses

Nature of Clients Served by Occupational Therapists

Preliminary data from the American Occupational Therapy Association's 1982 member survey (about 50% response) indicates that fewer than 1% of OTRs and COTAs presently serving clients checked visual or hearing disabilities as being among their clients' three most frequently occurring health problems. (Visual disabilities—OTRs 0.3%, COTAs 0.3%; hearing disabilities—OTRs 0.1%, COTAs 0.2%.)[38] This is likely to include therapists who practice in schools, rehabilitation centers for the blind, special hospital units, and possibly some nursing homes. However, it is also probable that the majority of occupational therapists encounter among their clients with varying health problems at least a few persons who are *also* blind, partially sighted, deaf, hard of hearing, or a combination.

Nine occupational therapists from various places in the United States responded to my inquiry in "Member Hotline" of the April 1981 *Occupational Therapy Newspaper*,[39] regarding where and how occupational therapists and occupational therapy assistants are serving blind, deaf, visually and hearing impaired persons. Five OTRs work in state or local, residential or day schools or school systems serving deaf or deaf-blind or deaf-multiply handicapped children ages 0–22, with one of these schools employing a COTA to work with visually impaired students. Two of the five OTRs' roles specifically include some consultation and direct service in the areas of prevocational assessment and life adjustment. Two OTRs, from separate residential schools for mentally retarded, indicated that many residents have some type of visual handicap. An OTR employed by a society for the blind, serving adults from 17 to over 90 years of age, reported a caseload of mostly newly blind who are referred for development of self-confidence and refinement or development of remaining senses. Other services there included a deaf-blind program and treatment emphasizing sensory integration for many congenitally blind and some newly blind. A public health OTR indicated that of 12 clients at the initiation of the visting O.T. program, four were legally blind and a fifth was visually impaired. Their primary diagnoses were multiple sclerosis, CVA, quadriplegia, and cerebellar degeneration. All were homebound and confined to wheelchairs. The therapist reported close coordination with a society for the blind.

One occupational therapist's thesis delves into the need for O.T. involvement in the rehabilitation of the visually impaired (not totally blind) adult patient, who she believes is already part of the general occupational therapy caseload.[40] She found that, of the 61% of 180 Missouri occupational therapists who responded to a resource questionnaire, 89% had encountered one or more visually impaired patients in the course of practice. She further states that only 19% reported that they felt they were able to offer comprehensive services to those clients.[41] To that end she has prepared a guide for occupational therapy with the low-vision patient, including problems, aids, roles of occupational therapy, and the inexpensive equipping of an O.T. clinic to meet needs of these clients with or without additional health problems.[42]

A review of recent American Occupational Therapy Association materials indicates that some other OTRs and a COTA working with the blind and partially sighted are also finding sensory integrative treatment approaches relevant[43,44] and/or have been moved to share insights into sensory problems of the elderly[45] and treatment methods for blind and visually-impaired persons.[46,47] Public Laws 94–142 (Education of All Handicapped Children Act) and 95–602 (Rehabilitation Act Amendments of 1978) have broadened the scope of services available to handicapped children and adults, including the visually and hearing impaired, blind, deaf, and multiply involved. This has implications for occupational therapy within educational, sheltered workshops, independent living, and other rehabilitation settings. To date, the adult deaf population is the most underserved due to a communication gap.

Special Considerations for Occupational Therapists Serving Visually and Hearing Impaired Persons

Attitude and Personal Preparation

The occupational therapist and other team members must have healthy, realistic, and flexible attitudes toward blindness and deafness and must see the potential for developing or redeveloping and maintaining satisfactory functioning by persons with these problems. Positive and realistic attitudes can be facilitated through reading biographies, professional literature, and journals or newsletters published by

groups of visually or hearing-impaired persons and especially by interacting with blind and deaf persons. Besides the selected bibliography, agencies and organizations are listed at the end of this chapter so the reader may write for general or specific information, publications, or perhaps a film.

For a more personal, subjective experience, one can wear a blindfold, opaque sunglasses, or earplugs designed to reduce industrial or other noxious sound. This simulated disability can provide insights if it is maintained in a variety of situations for at least several hours, but the wearer must remember that this is only a very temporary disability and it is not conducted to win praise or instant rapport with a client. The experience can approximate some experiences of adventitiously lost sight or hearing, but it cannot provide as much understanding of the circumstances of congenitally blind or deaf persons, because the learner will not erase his visual memory or language development. Occupational therapy students who have simulated disabilities including the sensory ones have been careful to do so responsibly, either explaining the purpose to laypersons or being consistent and behaving appropriately from the time they leave class or home in the role of a disabled person until they return.

Communication and Interaction

If the deaf or deaf-blind client is known to use sign language and fingerspelling, and if he/she does not read and write understandably, the therapist should arrange in advance for a certified interpreter. Exceptions to this are if (1) the resident has understandable speech and the therapist can sign and fingerspell well enough to introduce self, state purpose of visit, and ask or answer the necessary questions; or (2) the therapist has good receptive as well as expressive skills for American Sign Language (AMESLAN, ASL) or manual English, whichever the client uses. Basic vocabulary is the same in ASL and signed English. In ASL, however, word order in short sentences may vary; articles are omitted; actual time sequence determines order of phrases or clauses; verb tense is indicated by context or by use of words like "finish, yesterday, tomorrow"; one sign concept is used to represent several English words; much facial and body language is used to show meaning; and few words are fingerspelled.[48]

A certified interpreter may be located through the Registry of Interpreters for the Deaf. Usually the interpreter will sign with the deaf person for a few minutes to determine his receptive and expressive skills so the interpreter can use the most appropriate method and vocabulary when interpreting for the therapist. I prefer to introduce myself, explain that I am learning to sign but am slow, introduce the interpreter, and then proceed with my business. The therapist asks questions and gives information to the deaf person through the interpreter who will sign to the client in the style needed, moving the lips without voice while doing so, although one may request vocalization also to understand concepts. When the client signs his/her response, the interpreter will "reverse interpret," speaking to the therapist, also converting ASL to English if necessary. Interaction between client and therapist is confidential unless otherwise agreed with client. Interpreters as well as therapists have codes of ethics.

For any ongoing program with the signing deaf and deaf–blind, it is my opinion and experience, shared with many others in the field, that the personnel must learn to sign. Most deaf and deaf-blind persons are patient with slow reception of their signs and fingerspelling (Fig. 28-1). Some enjoy teaching new signs, and nearly all receive hearing persons more readily when we are obviously trying to communicate in their language.

Although many deaf adults use combined sign language, facial and body expression, and lip reading with or without speech (referred to as total communication or simultaneous method), some deaf persons do not express or receive signs or speech well. Formal assessments of language skills are likely to be con-

ducted by other professionals, but the occupational therapist should discern what communication methods the client can use effectively for daily and emergency needs, such as transportation, job, exchanging information, and locating resources. One listens to and watches the client, communicating with him/her by voice, pencil and paper or magic slate, illustrations (pictures or on-the-spot drawings), touch, sign language, demonstration, or gesture.

Deaf and hard-of-hearing persons may read lips as well as facial expressions (speech read), but much of English is not visibly discernible to lip readers. One must be careful to articulate carefully yet not to exaggerate lip and tongue movements when speaking to a lip-reading person, and to be certain to face the person with the light on the speaker's face while keeping hands away from the mouth. Body and facial language need to be consistent with signs and/or speech.

Mindel and Vernon,[49] a psychiatrist and a psychologist accepted by the deaf community, have suggested that many deaf persons tend to use a mannerism reminiscent of the age at which it is natural and acceptable to communicate without words. The mannerism is the smile, which for the sighted but deaf infant can be reinforced and is one of the foundations for a warm relationship with parents and others. Rather than conveying a true feeling of pleasure, however, a deaf person of any age may smile (or nod) at the speaking, hearing person both to conceal the fact that he/she did not understand all of the spoken message and to avoid embarrassing the speaker. Hearing persons also may nod or smile for the same reasons, or to denote interest or acceptance, whether or not they understand or agree. Such mixed messages, however well-intended, may be the basis for grave misunderstandings and mistrust, especially when two parties use different language and cannot readily clarify.

If the person wears a hearing aid or is hard of hearing, one should modulate the voice, speak slowly and distinctly, near the better ear if this seems helpful, and project the voice without shouting. In groups, a microphone or public address system assists the hard of hearing. Persons dependent upon sign language or speech-reading must have an unobstructed view of upper body and/or head of speaker.

Two-way manual communication requires free hands and mental and visual (or tactile for the deaf-blind) attention. It is advisable to wear a garment that provides both pockets and a noncompeting but contrasting background for the hands. This is particularly important for partially sighted deaf signers, as is one's location. Persons with tunnel vision may need to be about 3 feet from the signer in order that the visual field can include the entire area where

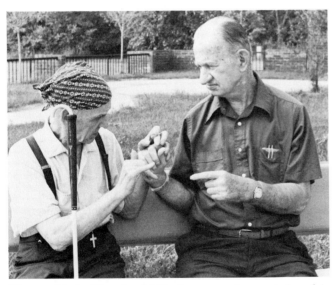

Figure 28-1. The deaf-blind person is receiving his companion's fingerspelling tactually with his left hand, while fingerspelling with his own right hand. (The individual letters visible are "y" and "x," viewed from left to right.) These gentlemen agreed to have their pictures taken in order to teach occupational therapy students some of the things that deaf and blind persons can do. (Photo by Ann Wade, with permission.)

signs are made. Fingerspelling must often be slower. If the individual must use peripheral vision, as is true for macular degeneration and pupils dilated to see around a small cataract, standing or sitting slightly to the preferred side may help prevent a stiff neck. Presbyopic individuals will prefer greater distance than myopic persons, and some will require more light on the signer than others. The principles of visual field, light, and placement of therapist and hands apply to anything the hearing or deaf low-vision client needs to see.

Unless the visually impaired or blind person is known to have a hearing loss, he/she will appreciate being spoken to in a distinct, well-modulated voice no louder than required for ordinary conversation. The speaker should identify himself or herself to the blind client when entering the room or when initiating conversation when more than two persons are in the room. Procedures or actions should be explained to the blind person before they actually begin. One must be precise but concise so the person can readily understand and remember or visualize what is described or asked. It is important to check one's facts and carefully report exact information, since the blind client cannot see to check for himself.[50] Reliable data and follow-through foster trust. Blind persons, as well as the deaf, are too frequently given reason to distrust, regardless of the motives of others.

Braille books, Twin Vision (type and Braille) children's books, and talking books in record, reel, and cassette form are available through the Library of Congress's free lending program.[51] Recorded books can be played on machines provided free by the local agency. Many persons who become blind as adults prefer not to learn Braille, so the talking book program is particularly helpful. It includes fiction and nonfiction, both general and professional. Deaf and blind persons must generally rely on Braille to read books independently, but there are some labeling and personal information systems that use raised letters or larger tactile symbols (Fishburne) so the deaf-blind person can mark containers, note and/or read short instructions, addresses, etc.[52]

For low-vision persons, magnifying glasses and monocular lenses, adequate indoor and outdoor lighting, and large print books and magazines can be of great help. Light, bright colors on oven controls and step edges may be useful. Studies[53] of the reduced visual perception of the elderly have shown that signs that consist of white or bright yellow letters and symbols against a dark background are more easily read than the reverse. Because of the yellowing of the lens, colors in the blue, green, or violet range become more difficult to distinguish, making it advisable to use bright colors of red, orange, and yellow.

Code book and separate medical and school emergency communication cards to facilitate essential messages between deaf and nonsigning persons are available through the National Association of the Deaf. Communication boards and cards can be helpful for nonsigning, possibly illiterate, or aphasic deaf. These are listed in some educational, speech and language, and general rehabilitation materials catalogs, but they can also be made by the OTR or COTA, preferably with the client. Picture/word selection should be undertaken in collaboration with client, family, and nursing personnel. To my knowledge, the deaf do not use Blissymbols, unless there is some other disabling condition that prevents signing and reading words. Blissymbols are printed symbols in various combinations designed to be an international conceptual communication system now used with some severely handicapped, nonvocal persons[54] although originally designed as an effort toward world peace.[55]

Teletypewriters (TTYs) are becoming more common and somewhat less expensive than previously. These devices enable two persons to type messages on special typewriters that convert each letter or symbol to an audible signal, transmit it by telephone (as do some other computers), and then reconvert the signals to a typed message. Typing skill and use of some keys especially for TTY need to be learned by the persons who use this equipment. Many transportation and other agencies now list a TTY number as well as the regular phone number so that the deaf may communicate directly. For the deaf-blind who use Braille, there are some TTYs with additional devices that convert Braille to signals and back.[56]

Mobility

For blind and deaf-blind individuals, development or restoration of mobility is of great importance. Independent travel skills should be taught by specially trained teachers called orientation and mobility specialists. A full course in orientation and mobility requires approximately 180 hours for the adventitiously blind person.[57] Prior to or along with the course, family, friends, workers, and the blind person should be taught the correct way for the blind to use a sighted guide. The guide walks about a half-step ahead of the blind partner, who grasps the guide's arm just above the elbow (Fig. 28-2). Both hold their upper arms close to their bodies for more effective detection of movement. It becomes less necessary for the guide to alert the partner to curbs, stairways, turns, and stops since the blind person can detect these through the guide's movements. Obstacles such as doorsills, uneven pavement, or ice should still be identified and located for the blind

Meaningful and Purposeful Activity

Selection of Activity

Certain considerations have already been described in discussions of object concept and general development, deficits in vision and hearing, and communication. Activity selection is important in assessment as well as in relation to client's goals and needs. For assessment purposes, interviews must be validated and supplemented by performance that will indicate what type of functional or potentially functional residual vision and hearing are present, under what circumstances (if any), and how the other sensations are received, perceived, and used for function. Age and stage-appropriate pursuits and natural performance should be combined with whatever specific sensory testing is needed to glean just enough information on visual, auditory, tactual, kinesthetic, proprioceptive, vestibulo-gravity, olfactory, and gustatory senses. The more severely visually and/or auditorially and multiply handicapped the person, the more careful and creative the therapist must be to find as many resources as the person has.

For treatment purposes (or consultant recommendations) those activities that have most relevance to the client's major life-tasks or occupations (*e.g.*, student, self-care, earning a living, selecting and preparing for a vocation, homemaking, adjusting to retirement, learning to get along with others) are the most appropriate. Those that have the most immediate survival value and/or that spark interest or motivation should be given priority. From that perspective, re-establishing contacts with employer, creditors, and significant others by telephone, tapes or typing, and direct contact could be most relevant for a newly blind worker with adequate verbal, tactile, and social skills. Depressed, apathetic, or dependent clients are a special challenge. Learning to problem-solve while trying familiar and adapted methods of self-care is an appropriate multifaceted activity. Pursuing a work-related activity, rather than a craft, could enhance worker-image and, if performed with one or more others in an appropriately structured situation, could also enable development or resumption of interpersonal skills. If individuals lack the ability to enjoy themselves, play, recognize, and abide by reasonable limits, and/or feel comfortable with others, then play or leisure activities including games, crafts, and hobbies in an atmosphere of fun and acceptance have much merit.

Within those major activities or pursuits, the occupational therapist now must assist the client to use residual skills to the maximum, and to compensate

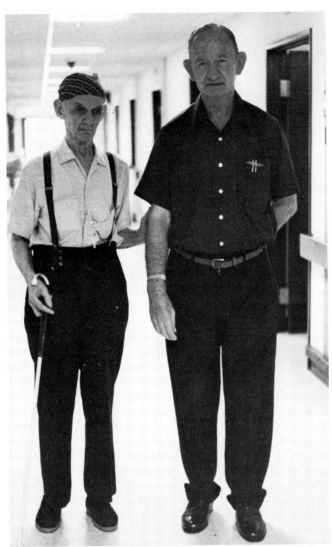

Figure 28-2. When they begin to move, the blind gentleman will drop back a half step, maintaining grasp at or just above his companion's elbow. White cane technique was adequate for navigating hall independently in spite of obstacles, but a crowded lobby and walk outdoors are more comfortably managed when his friend serves as sighted guide. (Photo by Ann Wade, with permission.)

person; sights and landmarks along the way can be described for enjoyment and enlightenment. The client should also practice detecting changes in surfaces underfoot, and localizing and identifying sounds and scents. Some blind persons may eventually use guide dogs. Special training courses are available for this.[58] Dogs can also serve to alert some deaf persons to significant sounds, and they can be trained by their owners or others to obey manual as well as spoken commands.

with other senses and with modified or adapted methods or materials. Therefore, activities should be selected that incorporate one or more of these requirements at the appropriate degree of difficulty for challenge or comfort and success. It is wise to begin with something the client has indicated is a priority, or at least an interest, and to use it to increase rapport as well as to reinforce positively the use of intact senses while working on a familiar or desired task. The tasks should lead, especially initially, to the strengths of the person, such as capitalizing on the oral/verbal and auditory abilities of the blind person; activities, such as discussing news and playing word games or crossword puzzles with the therapist can then augment tactual abilities to learn to dial or press the numbers for telephone calls, to use a tape recorder, and to identify coins. Likewise, the deaf person could demonstrate visual and manual skills by visual inspection and sorting of products, materials, or job samples relevant to him/her or by performing some mechanical or sewing task, either of which should be introduced by demonstrated, written, or illustrated directions and/or the communication method he/she uses. Hair care, shaving with an electric razor, stuffing envelopes, or pinching the dried leaves from a sturdy plant could enable the deaf-blind person to succeed with tactual-kinesthetic skills, as could tactual inspection of wood products or roller bearings for slight rough spots. Learning to use compensatory methods and aids and to evaluate their worth should occur in the context of activities important to the partially sighted, blind, hard-of-hearing, deaf, or deaf-blind person (Figs. 28-3, 28-4).

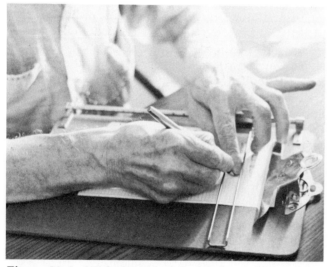

Figure 28-3. With the aid of the Marks writing guide, plus his own kinesthetic, tactile, and visual memory abilities, the blind man prepares a grocery list. (Photo by Ann Wade, with permission.)

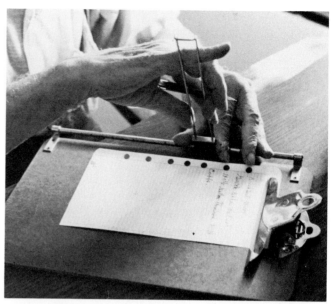

Figure 28-4. The guide bars are moved down the page at regular intervals as determined by notches in the rod on left side. A movable piece on the guide bars can be set where script stops, helpful when interrupted before completing a line or paragraph. (Photo by Ann Wade, with permission.)

Presenting and Teaching a New Activity

Careful preparation is needed before instructing any client or client group in an activity, but some aspects should be stressed. Therapists must be clear on the number and sequence of steps in the process, the most concise but precise words or sign concepts to use, the actual performance of the task according to directions with the materials and tools available, and the constraints and consequent compensatory methods required by the client. It facilitates understanding through visualization and handling to have samples of not only the finished product but also of each major step in the processes, if this is at all feasible and applicable.

In presenting the task or end-product activity, therapists should relate the process, materials, and/or product to something the individual has done previously, and they should state the goal or purpose that may or may not be the same as the final result or product. Time must then be given for the visually or hearing-impaired client to examine the examples and materials. Then each step with an example, if applicable, is introduced and taught one at a time. *Deaf* persons need time to watch the instructor and then to examine the example while communication ceases until ready for the next step. A return demonstration of that step may be the best method of determining that the client understood and can follow the directions, and it may also be the best reinforcement of learning. As with other learning situations, check to see if there are questions about that step in the process before proceeding. *Blind* persons need explicit directions in a minimum of words, before and/or while handling the example, with careful attention to left, right, over, under, and texture, because they will rely on visualization and memorization as they learn. Again, successful or corrected completion of each step as presented enables learning by experience. The *deaf-blind* client requires signed and/or fingerspelled, Braille, or other tactual instructions, with time to examine and manipulate examples and materials, with or without actual physical guidance of hands, but definitely with ongoing supervision to be certain of understanding and successful action. The process is most time-consuming for the deaf-blind; one instructor–volunteer for each of these persons in the group is initially almost essential. Patience is needed during the entire process with any sensory-impaired client and with oneself; careful advance preparation will maximize patience and effectiveness, but the therapist will still need to be flexible for various unforeseen difficulties or on-the-spot adaptations.

When the therapist becomes familiar with the client's demonstrated learning style and abilities, it may be advantageous to assist the client to continue the activity independently without the therapist being present. Key examples and cards for steps, written or Brailled in a style understood by the client, can facilitate this. Later the client may learn independently through video or audio tape-recorded, Brailled, or printed and illustrated magazines or instructions.

Organizing Materials

To compensate for little or no vision, it is essential that the partially sighted, blind, or deaf-blind person have good organizational abilities or at least the habit of maintaining consistent arrangement of belongings and appointments. Although not imperative for the deaf or hard-of-hearing, prompt and orderly management of things and affairs at home and on the job are desirable attributes of effective persons.

If materials feel the same but are different colors, each color must be kept in a separate container, or be labeled in some manner if large, like clothing. The containers may be distinguished by Braille, Fishburne, or other tactually perceived label; by an assigned number of rubberbands around the container; or by the shape or other property of the container itself. During a supervised activity it may be sufficient to designate the contents of separate and identical containers by their locations on the table.

Rather than searching through numerous containers for dissimilar items, it also is sensible to sort and label groups of like items. Labels may be affixed to rubberbands that may be placed on new cans when old are empty. Clothing may be identified by patterns of French knots sewn in a consistent location in like garments or by small abbreviated aluminum Braille labels similarly tacked, or even by safety pins or order of hanging or placing in drawers. File folders, papers, and addresses may be marked and organized using tactile and common-sense systems. Color-coded files, labels, and large print may be sufficient for partially sighted persons. It is important for safety as well as convenience that foods, cleaning products, grooming items, and medicines be unmistakenly identified, labeled, and separately organized. Work simplification principles are useful to all persons, but they may be applied according to personal need and preference.

Locating, Ordering, Purchasing and Obtaining Materials

Many deaf, blind, or low-vision clients need help initially in locating the source of a particular item or service, whether it be groceries, food, information, craft, recreation, or work needs. The client should then record the location, independently or with assistance, in a method that they may independently retrieve and pursue. He/she might travel to stores or services by bus, feet, car or cab, or write, type, or telephone an order and pay for it in the most advantageous way. There are some individuals who will need considerable help in these areas, but it is possible for many to become independent given the right location, funds, mobility, communication, and money management skills. Teachers, occupational therapists, social workers, and others have important functions, along with family members, to teach and expect the maximum amount of responsible independence.

Activity Applications

The preceding paragraphs on organization and procurement of materials and services apply particularly to Mr. Williams, Mr. James, Mrs. Reed, and Mrs. Turner, described in the vignettes. The women will need either to write for materials or to telephone, with the deaf woman using a TTY; otherwise, they will need public or private transportation by bus or van equipped with a wheelchair ramp or lift operated by someone else and with appropriate help at their destinations. The blind amputee could transfer from her wheelchair, and therefore, she could use a car with driver-helper; but arthritic deaf Mrs. Reed is unable to weight-bear for standing or sliding board transfer, so she needs to remain in a chair to avoid difficult two-person transfer into a car.

Before he was ready to function at home again, newly blind Mr. James had to regain confidence in himself, orient himself to his surroundings and belongings, and gain mobility within his immediate environment and with a sighted guide. In situations like this, personal care is particularly important, because it is comprised of familiar and repeatable skills, it influences and reflects the self-concept of the person, and it influences others' attitudes toward the individual and toward blindness. Personal care including bathing, hygiene, dressing, and care of teeth and hair are more likely to be routine, automatic, and quickly resumed. With encouragement, Mr. James began to manage these at bedside, and then in the bathroom with stand-by assistance a few times from a therapist or orderly. Mr. James was encouraged to use good posture, to look or turn directly toward the one to whom he is speaking, and to interact with sighted, blind, and partially-sighted individuals. He decided to extend his right hand when meeting others to invite their handshake. Problem solving with the client about difficulties helped his success and also set the tone for rehabilitation. Skills requiring stereognosis and kinesthesis, like eating and all related activities (*i.e.*, buttering bread, cutting meat, and managing salt, pepper, and sugar) were taught and practiced in his room or in O.T. (walking there using therapist as sighted guide), because Mr. James was sensitive about being clumsy and messy. He progressed rapidly, and he soon taught his family that visualizing the plate as a clock face assists communication about the location of food and other items, such as meat at six o'clock and water glass in line with one o'clock.

Analysis of his skills and the requirements of his job began in the hospital with the therapist. He and the social worker contacted his employer and services for the blind before discharge, so that he knew what to expect in terms of cooperation, workers' compensation, and assistance. He expressed some interest in computer programming and medical writing, either in the context of his medical technology profession or related areas. Although Mr. James' supervisor seemed hesitant, he indicated willingness to cooperate if professionals and James would tell him what to do.

Applying the section on meaningful and purposeful activity to Alice and Jack, those blind and deaf-blind developmentally delayed children (see first vignette), are presently in need of appropriate self-care and play skills and other adaptive behaviors. They require much tactile cuing. Alice requires oral preparation and instructions, whereas Jack needs to have his visual attention directed to items, actions, and simple signs; both then receive tactile and kinesthetic demonstration through the teacher's or therapist's assistance throughout the activity. Therapist and child should be in the correct position for independent dressing and other performance once the procedure is learned through corrective and positive feedback, and occasional appropriate reward (hug, treat, favorite activity). The children should also learn where clothing, soap, towels, toys, and so forth are consistently and conveniently stored so they can become able to obtain and replace materials. Sensory clues to the activities should also be emphasized, such as hearing, seeing, feeling water running, scents of soap or food, time of day (before or after certain meal, daylight or dark, chime of clock), sounds or sights of toys, and dishes. It is important to assist these children to be independent in small components of tasks, if not in the entire task, so that they can perform increasingly adequately and they can be meaningfully self-directed. Routines are helpful, if not imperative to begin with, but should be varied slightly once learned so that the child can accept some flexibility and can transfer learning to other situations. Some sensory integrative treatment strategies are also employed to influence appropriate tactile and vestibular functions and to facilitate achievement of developmental tasks and self-management.

Other Media and Methods

Occupational therapists also use games and crafts to assist a person to develop confidence and tactile, kinesthetic, and auditory skills. Braille or Fishburne labeled cards, Braille dice, Scrabble letters, Bingo cards, and games such as adapted checkers, chess, and Chinese checkers are useful. Many large dice and dominos have deep enough depressions for dots that the person can determine numbers by feeling the pattern and counting the depressions. However, Sevel and Hart[59] noted that their eye patients found a raised spot easier to distinguish than a depression. The American game "Cootie" or British "Beetle" are assembly type games that can be played tactually.

Patterns may be cut in fabric, paper, styrofoam, leather, or wood by attaching a firm cardboard or plastic pattern with paper clips, pins, or rubber cement, with the blind or partially sighted person then following the edge with one or more fingers and guiding regular or electric scissors, coping saw or safety handle knife. If the person is diabetic, incoordinated, or has peripheral neuropathy, the therapist will observe precautions and avoid sharp tools. Templates can be used successfully for tracing or for applying glue and sand, beans and gravel. Ceramics and papier-maché offer opportunities to create, and

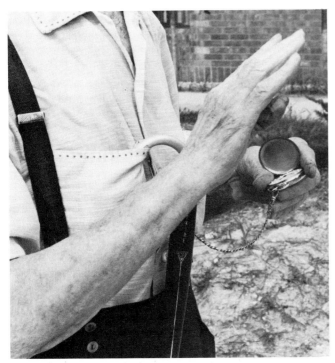

Figure 28-5. A Braille pocketwatch enables its owner to perceive tactually that the time is five after four (the four is seen here). Also note that the cane has been hooked in chest pocket to free hands, yet make retrieval certain. (Photo by Ann Wade, with permission.)

they can be glazed or painted by pouring, dipping, spraying, or brushing as the person and therapist decide, depending on ability. When working with materials that may be easily dropped, such as beads, it is helpful to work over a tray or box lid so that objects may be retrieved by the worker.

Special tools, clocks, games, and other Brailled or tactually usable items for the blind are listed in the Braille and typed catalogs of the American Foundation for the Blind. A variety of items will be carried by local vision centers or rehabilitation centers for the blind (Fig. 28-5).

The telephone company will install a special receiver on the conventional telephone so that the user may amplify the incoming message by turning a dial. Lights sensitive to audible sounds are used by some people who need an alternate means of perceiving doorbell, telephone, TTY or alarms, and infant or invalid calling. These are available through security-system retailers and some hearing aid dealers.

Vocational Considerations

Deaf and blind persons, like many disabled persons, are good and reliable workers when they have been successfully oriented, and they often have lower absenteeism than nonhandicapped persons because they value their jobs. The deaf tend to be *underemployed,* that is, employed for tasks or positions that do not use all their education and capabilities and that therefore do not pay well.[60] It is often difficult for deaf who are multiply disabled, ethnic minority group members, or low achievers to find employment; they especially need intensive and creative habilitation. Although deaf persons are usually excluded from medical professional education and subsequent qualification and employment as registered nurses, therapists, physicians, and technologists, they are beginning to be educated for paraprofessional work in these areas.[61] Communication continues to be the greatest problem, with earlier overprotection and immature attitudes complicating the situation. Deaf persons in service work need to find an appropriate way to let clients know that they do not hear and in what manner the employer and other persons can catch their attention and communicate. Technology is improving; for example, blood pressure can be read by a computerized stethoscope, which reports the results like a digital watch or clock thereby eliminating the need to listen, except to check discrepant results.

Rusalem cautions against restrictive lists of occupations suitable for the blind.[62] If lists are open-ended and allow for individual interests, abilities, and modifications of certain job methods, they may be a reasonable starting point. Technological advances are opening doors for blind workers, with computerized "voices" for output of some machines. Blind and partially-sighted persons can be found in a full range of occupations, from professions to unskilled labor, although some positions within a field are not feasible (*e.g.,* medicine). Persons already working in one field may find it possible to return to that work following loss of vision, if the employer can be convinced that it is acceptable and cost-effective. If the specific functions are not amenable to blindness, there is often some other position in the same company that the blind person can assume. Since returning to the established workplace may be faster than changing jobs, it may be psychologically as well as financially beneficial.

When developmentally blind and deaf or visually or hearing-impaired persons obtain work, their job-related personal–social skills may need more attention and improvement than do the actual tasks. Self-care, management of personal affairs, social behavior, general work habits, transportation, and communication should be assessed and improved as needed. Groups or individual adolescents and adults might benefit from using some or all of the chapters in *Career Planning for the Blind,* copyrighted by Hadley

School for the Blind,[63] and the therapist should find *Coping with the Unseen Environment*[64] useful for vocational rehabilitation. Occupational therapists and related personnel serving deaf and severely handicapped deaf will find pertinent and practical information in the *Proceedings of the National Forum VII on Careers for Deaf People* (1974)[65] and in the final report of a grant to Crossroads Rehabilitation Center on *A Program for the Severely Handicapped Deaf.*[66] Both stress the need for personal and career development and work adjustment training, with the former also emphasizing the need for deaf school children to be helped to develop the ability to think for themselves, learning to recognize and set goals, to problem solve, and to give as well as take. The Crossroads program includes objectives, methods, forms, research data, descriptions of all aspects of the program including a variety of living arrangements and representative case studies. The most current edition of the *Model State Plan for Rehabilitation of the Deaf* indicates needs and the current state of the art. Although not specifically mentioning occupational therapy, except as it can be understood under medical rehabilitation, the plan described can use occupational therapists with deaf experience to help implement.[67] For generic occupational therapy information, the reader is encouraged to refer to chapter 17 on "Prevocational Training."

Role of Occupational Therapy with Family and Agencies

Blindness and deafness are accompanied by profound isolation. Partial loss can also disrupt meaningful interaction with the human and nonhuman environments. Communication channels must be kept open, reopened, or discovered to enable the individual to give and receive understandable messages about feelings, needs, support, and information. Adventitious loss or diminution of sight or hearing will of course be mourned, with the individual passing through any or all of the stages of reaction to loss. Without family support and professional help, however, the person may plateau at early stages or may regress. The premorbid personalities of the individual and family members and their attitudes toward blindness and/or deafness will affect adjustment to the sensory loss as well as the family's treatment of the individual (*i.e.*, rejection, overprotection, ambivalence, embarrassment, and encouragement). Congenital loss will not be mourned initially by the individual, but it will certainly affect parent(s) or other primary care-givers, who may initially experience shock, denial, anger, embarrassment, and/or re-

jection of the infant. The congenitally handicapped child may begin to experience these reactions to disability when he/she begins school or when coping with many other problems during adolescence, at which time it is so important to be like one's peers. Even if peers are similarly disabled, by this age the young person is aware of things that nondisabled teenagers can do such as driving a car, conversing easily in a group or on the telephone, and being more independent generally.

Whether the occupational therapist is serving the client directly or as a consultant, it is important to ascertain that client and family/significant others' needs for emotional support and guidance are being recognized and met in the most appropriate way. This may require that a specific professional be designated; that *could* but does not have to be the occupational therapist. Interagency cooperation may be needed to assure that this is taken care of. If client and/or family are not ready to acknowledge a problem or need for help, the avenue to help should nevertheless be kept open, with the client group knowing how to contact the agency or a trusted person within the agency and with nonforcing contacts from professionals at reasonable intervals. This seems particularly important when there is a blind or deaf-blind infant involved, because initially the best stimulation can be provided through the mother who is very likely to need support, guidance, and some physical relief from other tasks. Without visual experience, early sensorimotor development can be easily retarded unless the mother or caring mother-substitute consistently provides the handling and nurturing that the baby needs.[68] Professional personnel who may visit in the homes of blind or deaf clients include public health nurses and therapists, caseworkers, family interventionists, visiting teachers, and rehabilitation teachers for the blind. Some parent organizations or groups of low-vision, blind, hearing-impaired, or deaf individuals might send representatives to offer support and socialization opportunities (Fig. 28-6). Professional personnel must be careful to protect confidentiality by asking the client and support representatives independently for permission to introduce, without giving specific information until both parties agree, and then not providing more than essential and approved information. Depending upon the individual center and state, services for the blind and deaf may be comprehensive and nonstereotyped, or less than that. For example, some states and facilities may be much more progressive in the types of prevocational and vocational exploration and rehabilitation available and in the type of job placement and follow-up. Regardless, the occupational therapist can cooperate

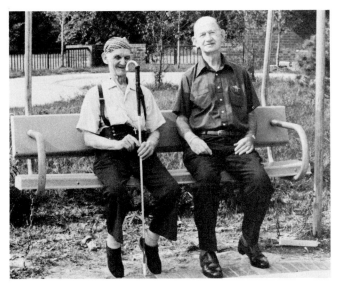

Figure 28-6. Movement in the sturdy swing, fresh air, sunshine, and companionship are enjoyed by these deaf friends, one of whom is also blind. (Photo by Ann Wade, with permission.)

with state and local agencies as needed for the client, with the ultimate goal being the realistic coping and satisfactory survival of the blind or deaf person in his/her environment.

Additional Opportunities and Responsibilities Related to Visual and Hearing Losses

Prevention of Unnecessary Sensory Losses

Along with others in the field, occupational therapists need to practice as well as to teach such preventive measures as innoculation against rubella for all females of child-bearing age; precautions against the handling of cats and litter boxes by pregnant females, because cats may transmit toxoplasmosis that may produce deaf–blindness and mental retardation in the developing infant; annual ophthalmologic examinations for diabetic individuals, and at least biannual examinations for all persons 40 years old and above for glaucoma and cataract, as well as for refractive errors and other possible eye diseases or conditions; wearing of safety goggles; careful use of cyanoacrylics; protection of the ears against prolonged industrial, traffic, and other loud sounds; and adequate vision and hearing screening and prompt eye and ear examination by medical specialists, especially for individuals with injuries, communication, and learning problems and other disabilities.

Public and Professional Education and Awareness

Through reading, viewing films, TV, and radio productions, and by becoming acquainted with many capable blind, deaf, and deaf-blind persons, occupational therapists, professional colleagues, and the general public can learn that blindness and deafness do not have to be isolating disabilities, more horrible than other handicapping conditions. Instead, they can become able to appreciate the range of characteristics and methods—some special, some ordinary—that are found among successful persons who have visual, auditory, or combined handicaps or losses. We can share knowledge of compensatory methods and materials with families and other professionals and paraprofessionals who may initially miss the potential for certain functions. By complimenting TV stations that use interpreters or captions to inform the deaf, and by acknowledging those networks and producers who participate in *closed-caption* programming (available only on sets that have a user-purchased closed-caption converter) and the newspapers and guides that indicate such programs, the deaf and those interested in them can reinforce current efforts. Similarly, public acknowledgment or information about talking book programs, radio reading services for the blind, and services available through the telephone company are educational and encouraging to the providers.

More Effective Use of Resources

The American Occupational Therapy Association has a packet of information on blindness, deafness, and deaf-blindness that therapists can request and share. Some major resources are listed at the end of this chapter and in many of the books cited in the references and bibliography. To make these and the many other resources available to visually and auditorially limited persons, their families, and therapists, each of us can maintain a file of potentially useful information and also can be willing and able to direct questions to others who may be better sources than we. Mutual sharing, rather than a defensive stance regarding what occupational therapy can do, seems to be healthier and more beneficial to clients and ultimately even to our profession. Prompt, clear requests or referrals for further assistance to the client, with a follow-up check, may make the critical difference in whether a client achieves independence and whether the family receives timely and appropriate counseling.

Summary

The principles and treatment approaches in occupational therapy as a whole definitely apply to our work with clients who are additionally or only blind, deaf, or deaf–blind. Some methods must be modified and certain materials are available to facilitate some processes. Attitudes of the client, family, and professional personnel serving the client are one significant determining factor in prognosis for rehabilitation. Preparation for working in these areas includes specific learning about visual and hearing impairments and treatment methods, examining, and if necessary, improving one's attitude toward the disability and developing sufficient skill to communicate understandably with the client. All occupational therapists need great patience, empathy, ability to know when and how to take a psychological approach different from the supportive one with some clients, and sufficient creativity and ingenuity to modify procedures to suit the needs and personality of the individual client. When the reader meets a client who has a sensory problem, with or without other problems, it is hoped that it will be a challenging and beneficial experience for both parties.

References

1. Chusid, J. G.: Correlative Neuroanatomy and Functional Neurology, ed. 15. Los Altos CA: Lange Medical Publications, 1973, p. 85.
*2. Lowenfeld, B.: Our Blind Children: Growing and Learning with Them, ed. 3. Springfield IL: Charles C. Thomas, 1971, pp. 9–10.
3. Hutchinson, E., and Wagner, E.: Occupational therapy for the blind and partially sighted. In Willard, H. S., and Spackman, C. S. (eds.): Occupational Therapy, ed. 4. Philadelphia: J.B. Lippincott, 1971, p. 491.
4. Chusid: Correlative Neuroanatomy, p. 261.
5. Lowenfeld: Our Blind Children, p. 10.
6. Bourgeault, S. E.: Blindness—a label. Ed. Visually Handicapped 6:1–5, 1974.
7. Hutchinson and Wagner: Occupational therapy for blind and partially sighted, p. 490.
*8. Yeadon, A., et al.: Living with Impaired Vision: An Introduction. New York: American Foundation for the Blind, 1979, p. 10.
9. Ibid., p. 21–29.
10. Chusid: Correlative Neuroanatomy, p. 85.
11. Fraiberg, S.: Parallel and divergent patterns in blind and sighted infants. Psychoan. Study Child 23:264–300, 1968.
12. Gesell, A., and Armatruda, C.: Developmental Diagnosis: Normal and Abnormal Child Development, ed. 2. New York: Harper & Row, 1969, p. 435.

*13. Fraiberg, S.: Insights From the Blind: Comparative Studies of Blind and Sighted Infants. New York: Basic Books, 1977. Chapters 5, 6, and p. 273.
*14. Schein, D. (ed.): Model State Plan for Rehabilitation of Deaf Clients: Second Revision. Silver Spring MD: National Association of the Deaf, 1980, p. 2.
15. Ibid.
16. Ibid., p. 3.
17. Chusid: Correlative Neuroanatomy, p. 267.
18. Ibid., p. 268.
19. Sereni, F., and Principi, N.: Clinically harmful consequences of drug administration to the pregnant woman and the infant. In Ziai, M. (ed.): Pediatrics, ed. 2. Boston: Little, Brown & Co., 1975, pp. 55–58.
*20. Mindel, E. D., and Vernon, M.: They Grow in Silence: The Deaf Child and His Family. Silver Spring MD: National Association of the Deaf, 1971, pp. 25–30.
21. Ibid., p. 27.
22. Chusid: Correlative Neuroanatomy, p. 267.
23. Atchley, R. C.: The Social Forces in Later Life: An Introduction to Social Gerontology, Belmont CA: Wadsworth Publishing Co., 1972, p. 54.
24. Chusid: Correlative Neuroanatomy.
*25. Schein, J. D.: The deaf community. In Davis, H., and Silverman, S. R. (eds.): Hearing and Deafness, ed. 4. New York: Holt, Rinehart and Winston, 1978, pp. 513, 522.
*26. Norris, C. (ed.): Letters from Deaf Students. Eureka CA: Alinda Press, 1975. (Booklet available from National Association of the Deaf).
*27. Pettingill, D. G.: Adjustments of the deaf. Printed from an address before a workshop, Understanding the Deaf Client, 1964. In Deaf Adults, collection of papers on problems of deaf people. Silver Spring MD: National Association of the Deaf.
28. Ibid.
29. Personal communication with Marguerite Moore, Certified Interpreter for the Deaf and Instructor, Columbus OH, July 1981.
30. Yeadon: Living with Impaired Vision, p. 55.
31. Ibid.
32. Ibid., p. 57.
*33. Chess, S., Korn, S., and Fernandex, P.: Psychiatric Disorders of Children with Congenital Rubella. New York: Brunner-Mazel, 1971, pp. 82–87, 120–130.
34. Mouchka, S.: The deaf-blind infant: A rationale for and an approach to early intervention. In Proceedings from the Fourth International Conference on Deaf-Blind Children, August 1971, at Perkins School for the Blind, Watertown MA, pp. 212–225.
35. Chess, Korn, and Fernandez: Psychiatric Disorders of Children.
36. Yeadon: Living with Impaired Vision, p. 29, 57, 59, 62.
37. Schein, D. (ed.): Model State Plan re: Title VII of P.L. 95-602. p. 31.
38. American Occupational Therapy Association, Operations Research Division, Rockville MD, August 1982.
39. Occupational Therapy Newspaper. The American Occupational Therapy Association. Member Hotline, Rockville MD, April, 1981.

---

* Asterisked items in reference section are also recommended for bibliography.

40. Baron, L.: The adult low vision population: An area of concern for occupational therapy. Master's thesis, Washington University, St. Louis MO, August, 1981.

41. Ibid. Personal communication with the author, October, 1981.

*42. For information on how to obtain the guide, with her permission contact Leslie Baron, M.S., OTR, 5602 Green Springs Drive, Houston TX 77066.

43. Ramm, P., Charles, S., Clark, J., and McCammon, M.: Sensory integration programming for the visually impaired, 0–22 years. Institute described in Official Program for 1981 Annual AOTA Conference, Denver, Colorado, p. 23–24.

*44. Baker-Nobles, L., and Bink, M. P.: Sensory integration in the rehabilitation of blind adults. Am. J. Occup. Ther. 33:559–564, 1979.

45. Maloney, C.: Sensory losses common to elders. General Session #121, Official Program for 1981 Annual AOTA Conference, Denver CO.

46. Schaefer, K. J., and Specht, T. R.: A light probe adapted for use in training the blind. Am. J. Occup. Ther. 33:640–643, 1979.

47. Seltser, C. G.: A COTA initiated program for visually handicapped patients. Therapeutic interaction with blind and visually impaired patients. COTA Forum topic and General Session #5, Official Program for 1981 Annual AOTA Conference, Denver CO, p. 36.

*48. Riekehof, L. L.: The Joy of Signing: The New Illustrated Guide for Mastering Sign Language and the Manual Alphabet. Springfield MO: Gospel Publishing House, 1978, pp. 11–12.

49. Mindel & Vernon: They Grow in Silence.

*50. Rouse, D. D., Gruber, K. F., and Bledsoe, C. W.: Occupational therapy for blind patients. Am. J. Occup. Ther. 10:252–53, 1956.

*51. United States Library of Congress, Division for the Blind and Physically Handicapped, Washington DC.

*52. Kates, L., and Schein, J. D.: A Complete Guide to Communication with Deaf-Blind Persons. Silver Spring MD: National Association of the Deaf, 1980.

53. Pastalan, L. A.: Lecture–demonstration at Ohio State University, Industrial Design Program, Columbus, 1976.

54. Blissymbolics Communication Institute, Toronto, Canada.

55. Bliss, C. K.: Semantography. Australia, via personal communication with Ann Banks, Blissymbolics Communication Resource Teacher, Columbus, Ohio, 1981.

56. Kates and Schein: A Complete Guide.

57. Koestler, F. A. (ed.): The Comstac Report: Standards for Strengthened Services. New York: National Accreditation Council for Agencies Serving the Blind and Visually Handicapped, 1966, p. 231. Cited in Lydon and McGraw: Concept Development for Visually Handicapped Children, rev. ed. New York: American Foundation for the Blind, 1973, p. 5.

*58. If Blindness Occurs: Practical Suggestions for Those Who Live or Work with Newly Blinded Persons. (Booklet), Morristown NJ: The Seeing Eye, Inc. (This agency also lends a film on the subject.)

*59. Sevel, D., and Hart, J. A.: Occupational therapy for the hospitalized eye patient. Am. J. Occup. Ther. 23:339–343, 1969, p. 340.

60. Schein, The Deaf Community, pp. 515–517.

61. Rawlings, Trybus, Delgado, and Stuckless (eds.): A guide to college/career programs for deaf students. Washington DC: Gallaudet College, 1978. Description of postsecondary programs, jointly prepared with National Technical Institute for the Deaf, Rochester Institute of Technology, N.Y.

*62. Rusalem H.: Coping with the Unseen Environment: An Introduction to the Vocational Rehabilitation of Blind Persons. New York: Teachers College Press, 1972, p. 97.

*63. Crawford, F. L.: Career Planning for the Blind: A Manual for Students and Teachers. New York: Farrar, Straus and Giroux, 1966 (available in regular and large print, Braille and talking book form, p. xii).

64. Rusalem: Coping with the Unseen Environment.

*65. Austin, G. F., (ed.): Careers for Deaf People. April 1974. Washington DC: U.S. Department of Health, Education and Welfare. Office of Human Development, Rehabilitation Services Administration. (Also available from National Association of the Deaf.)

*66. A Program for the Severely Handicapped Deaf: Final Report of RSA Service Grant 30-p-65000/5; a section 301(b)(1) project. Indianapolis IN: Crossroads Rehabilitation Center, 1978. (Available from National Association of the Deaf).

67. Schein. Model State Plan, 1978, pp. 25–27, 31–36.

68. Fraiberg: Insights from the Blind, pp. 40–42, 220, 273–4.

Bibliography

American Foundation for the Blind: An Introduction to working with the aging person who is visually handicapped. New York: 1977.

Asenjo, A.: A Step-by-Step Guide to Personal Management for Blind Persons, ed 2. New York: American Foundation for the Blind, 1974.

Bauman, M. K.: Guided vocational choice. New Outlook for Blind 69:354–360, 1975.

Bolton, B. (ed.): Psychology of Deafness for Rehabilitation Counselors. Baltimore: University Park Press, 1976.

Cristarella, M. C.: Visual functions of the elderly. Am. J. Occup. Ther. 31:432–440, 1977.

Drillien, A. M., and Drummond, M. B. (eds.): Neurodevelopmental Problems in Early Childhood: Assessment and Management. Oxford: Blackwell Scientific Publications, 1977. (Distributed in U.S. by J.B. Lippincott.)

Fox, J. V.: Improving tactile discrimination of the blind: A neurological approach. Am. J. Occup. Ther. 19:5–7, 1965.

Gloor, B., and Bruckner, R. (eds.): Rehabilitation of the Visually Disabled and the Blind at Different Ages. Baltimore: University Park Press, 1980.

Gregory, S.: The Deaf Child and His Family. New York: John Wiley & Sons, 1976.

Guldager, V.: Body Image and the Severely Handicapped Rubella Child. Watertown MA: Perkins School for the Blind, 1970.

Hanninen, K. A.: Teaching the Visually Handicapped. Columbus OH: Charles E. Merrill, 1975.

Harley, R. K., Henderson, F. M., and Truan, M. B.: The Teaching of Braille Reading. Springfield IL: Charles C. Thomas, 1979. (For material on prereading—tactual, auditory, physical, emotional and intellectual readiness, as well as for Braille itself.)

Harrity, R., and Martin, R. G.: The Three Lives of Helen Keller. Garden City NY: Doubleday & Co., 1962.

Haug, O., and Haug, S.: Help for the Hard-of-Hearing: A Speech Reading and Auditory Training Manual for Home and Professionally Guided Training. Springfield IL: Charles C. Thomas, 1977. (Some pointers for hearing persons and information about care of hearing aids.)

Hill, L.: Nationally speaking: Working with blind preschoolers. Am. J. Occup. Ther. 31:417–419, 1977.

Katz, L., Mathis, S., and Merrill, E.: The Deaf Child in the Public Schools: A Handbook for Parents of Deaf Children. Interstate Printers & Publishers, Inc., 1974.

Kielhofner, G., and Miyake, S.: The therapeutic use of games with mentally retarded adults. Am. J. Occup. Ther. 35:375–382. (Although not directed to the deaf or blind population, principles may be applied.)

Mikalonis, Huffman, Gaddy, Gillis, and Heater: Leisure Time Activities for Deaf-Blind Children. California State Dept. of Health. Joyce Motion Picture Co., 1974.

Moersch, M. S.: Training the deaf-blind child. Am. J. Occup. Ther. 31:425–431, 1977.

Rouse, D., Gruber, K., and Bledsoe, C.: Occupational therapy for blind patients. Am. J. Occup. Ther. 10:252–53, 1956. (As timely now as then.)

Scott, E., Jan, J., and Freeman, R.: Can't Your Child See? Baltimore MD: University Park Press, 1977.

Sloan, L. L.: Recommended Aids for the Partially Sighted. Including A Nontechnical Explanation of Basic Optical Principles. New York: National Society for the Prevention of Blindness, 1971. (Well-illustrated and informative, even though there have been new developments.)

Sperber, A.: Out of Sight: Ten Stories of Victory over Blindness. Boston: Little, Brown & Co., 1976.

Woodring, J., and Gregg, J.: Occupational therapy in the rehabilitation of the blind. Am. J. Occup. Ther. 9:136–138, 1955. (Still relevant.)

Wright, D.: Deafness. New York: Stein and Day, 1969. (Personal account followed by sections on history and treatment of deafness.)

Yoken, C.: Living with Deaf-Blindness: Nine Profiles. Washington DC: National Academy of Gallaudet College, 1979. (Available from National Association of the Deaf.)

Resources

Alexander Graham Bell Association for the Deaf, 3417 Volta Place, N.W., Washington DC 20007. Publication: *Volta Review* and others.

American Deafness and Rehabilitation Association, 814 Thayer Avenue, Silver Spring MD 20910. Publication: *J. of Rehab. of the Deaf*.

American Foundation for the Blind, 15 West 16th Street, New York NY 10011.

American Occupational Therapy Association, Developmental Disabilities Specialties Section, 1383 Piccard Drive, Rockville, Md. 20850. (Some 1981 and 1982 Newsletters feature O.T. with hearing and visually impaired children.)

American Printing House for the Blind, 1839 Frankfort Avenue, Louisville KY 40206.

Association for Education of Visually Handicapped, 919 Walnut Street, Philadelphia PA 19107.

Centers & Services for Deaf-Blind Children, Bureau of Education for Handicapped, U.S. Office of Education, 400 Maryland Avenue, S.W. (Donohoe Bldg., Rm. 3155), Washington DC 20202. Write for list of single and multistate centers for deaf-blind children.

Helen Keller National Center for Deaf-Blind Youths & Adults, 111 Middle Neck Road, Sands Point NY 11050. Publication: *Nat-Cent-News* and others.

John Tracy Clinic, 806 West Adams Boulevard, Los Angeles CA 90007. (Has correspondence courses for families of deaf and deaf-blind infants and children.)

National Association of the Deaf, 814 Thayer Avenue, Silver Spring MD 20910. Publication: *The Deaf American* and others.

National Association for Visually Handicapped, 305 East 24th Street, New York NY 10010.

Registry of Interpreters for the Deaf, P.O. Box 1339, Washington DC 20013.

Acknowledgments

To the residents, staff, volunteers, and administrator of Columbus Colony for Elderly Care, Incorporated, Westerville, Ohio—a caring, communicating facility for deaf, deaf–blind, hard of hearing, low vision, blind, and multiply disabled deaf, sponsored by the Ohio School for the Deaf Alumni Association and funded in part by HEW.

To the professional colleagues, children, and families at Colerain School, Columbus, Ohio and beyond.

To Elaine Ainsworth, OTR; Leslie Baron, OTR; Barbara Boyer, AOTA, Operations Research; Arlene C. Finocchiaro, OTR; Mike Hillis, OTR; Arlene Innman, OTR; Marguerite Moore, Interpreter and Sign Class Instructor; Cay Reilly, OTR; Suzanne Onderdonk, OTR; Crystal Overholt, OTR; Joyce Vargo, teacher; and others, for responding to my questions.

And special thanks to the gentlemen who graciously allowed me to take their pictures in order that occupational therapy students may see some of the many things that deaf and deaf–blind people can do.

CHAPTER 29

Occupational Therapy with Children— Spatiotemporal Adaptation

Elnora M. Gilfoyle and Ann P. Grady

The philosophical base of occupational therapy, as articulated by The American Occupational Therapy Association, expresses the profession's belief that individuals' can influence their own state of health through active participation in purposeful activities.[1] The Association's philosophical statement addresses relationships among development, purposeful activity, and adaptation. Mental and physical development, culminating in mental and physical health, are enhanced when an individual can purposefully control, change, or make use of the physical and social environment. Purposeful, directed use of the environment, through activities involving other persons, space and/or objects, is meaningful to the person acting. Such activity usually promotes change in the individual in the form of higher level physical and social development and more effective adaptation.

Adaptation implies change in an individual's functioning in order to meet the demands of the environment and to serve the needs of self. Such needs range from survival to self-actualization. Purposeful activities facilitate adaptation by providing challenges to functional abilities and motivation to strive for more mature levels of biological, psychological, and social adaptation.

When developmental and/or adaptation processes are interrupted by biological, psychological, or environmental insults, dysfunction in development and maladaptation may result. An occupational therapist uses purposeful activities to prevent, remediate, or help the person adjust to dysfunction or disability and/or facilitate a person's adjustment to his dysfunction. In each instance, whether the goal of therapy is directed toward prevention, (re)mediation, or adjustment, the changes that occur are primarily modifications of bodily functions used for adaptation.

For children, play is considered purposeful as it has meaning to the child by promoting development and maturation. According to Reilly,[2] play is a biosocial phenomenon in that play is a process that influences biological and sociological systems as well as a process dependent upon biological and sociological systems. Reilly includes the psychological aspects of play inherent within the social context. Others[3,4] use the term biopsychosocial to emphasize all three components. Therefore, play is a biopsychosocial phenomenon and a vital aspect of childhood.

The biological aspects of play are three fold. First, play is considered biological because it is both an event and process characteristic of living organisms.

Second, as a result of the system's biological growth, play becomes more complex over time. More complicated play activities are possible over time because the child is changing biologically (developmentally) acquiring capabilities to direct more difficult actions. As play activities increase in complexity, the nature of play directs higher level actions, because the child tends to automatically challenge the self-system by pursuing more intrinsically complex play activities. Higher levels of play stimulate and result in higher level responses from the child.[5] In a biological sense, the continuous change in the purposefulness of play for a child, based on the increasing complexity of play activities selected, challenges the child to make use of the most efficient and highly developed responses available for the task. Therefore, the nature of play changes with the child and the child changes as a result of play experiences.

The psychological and social aspects of play are gleaned from the child's organization of environmental experiences that require growth and change in the system's perceptual, cognitive and emotional functions. A child associates play activities experienced with self, other children, adults, objects and space, thus, he makes judgments about "self" in relation to the environment.[6] Through play associations the child discovers roles, rules, and relationships as they are at a given time and as they change over time. As with the biological changes in play, changes in psychosocial aspects of play are derived from maturation of the child's system and from more complex challenges from the environment. As the child is called upon to adapt to more complicated play situations, higher levels of organization are required. With higher levels of organization, integration within the system is enhanced, preparing the child to adapt to further challenges in play, as well as adapt in other functions. Therefore, the biopsychosocial purposes of play are adapted to direct more mature functions.

Reilly identifies three phases of play: exploration, competence, and achievement. During the exploration phase, new objects, persons, and routines arouse curiosity. If the novelty of the object or happening is too great, the child may withdraw or avoid the situation. If the new situation is not stimulating enough, the child will not be interested. But if the new environment feels safe, the child will explore it and learn more about objects, relationships, and trust of self and others. The competency phase is characterized by repetition of familiar activities leading to mastery of the tools of the environment and development of skills and feelings of self-confidence.

Achievement, the last phase, is built upon trust and confidence with one's skills. A child plays according to the established cultural standards and to

his expectations of self or internal standards for performance. When play experiences provide opportunities to meet externally established and internally developed standards, achievement is acquired.[7]

Relationships between play and biopsychosocial development are further elaborated by Erikson.[8] Erikson has contributed concepts relating to the developmental sequence of play. He proposes that play is "a function of the ego, an attempt to synchronize the bodily and the social processes with the self."[9] The theory of development of play begins with *autocosmic* play. According to Erikson, autocosmic play is infant's play, which is centered on the body. Autocosmic play provides experiences for the baby to learn to master his/her own body and to establish a body sense; therefore, with autocosmic play, an infant learns to influence the environment with the use of his/her body.

The next period proposed by Erikson is termed *microsphere* play, which constitutes the small world of manageable objects or toys. With microsphere play, the child learns to master "things." Ego enhancement is gained by mastering the small world of toys and objects within the environment. During the preschool age period, the social world expands for the youngster, and play reaches into a world shared with others. Play at this time is termed *macrosphere*. In macrosphere play, the child extends self and begins to acquire self-identity. During the period of macrosphere play, Erikson believes that the youngster's world of social interactions expands to include peers and adults outside the immediate family group, thus enlarging his/her scope of interactions.[10] The developmental sequence of play described by Erikson parallels the biosocial components of play as proposed by Reilly.

In addition to play, self care, pre-school and school tasks are the initial occupations of childhood that promote adaptation of the biopsychosocial environment. Normally developing children make use of their maturing system and their environment to develop functions required for play, self-care, and school tasks. Functions can be adapted to a variety of purposes. If the purpose sought exceeds the functional capacity to adapt, then functions are modified or changed to meet the need. Hence, a child's adaptation to and with his environment becomes a continuous process of function-to-purpose-to-function—and so on.

Children who are not developing normally, or children whose development is interrupted by disease or injury, experience delay or disruption in the function-to-purpose adaptation process. In a therapeutic environment, the meaningful activities related to play, self-care, and school can be used to stimulate development of the functions required to adapt. Through adaptation, functions can be modified as required to accomplish a specific goal. Purposeful activity, then, becomes the therapeutic link used by an occupational therapist to facilitate functions needed to adapt.

Play is particularly useful to the therapist since a child's natural drive to play motivates the child's engagement with activities that are known to enhance maturation and, hence, adaptation of functions. Play activity can be used to assess a child's abilities and needs, as the media for intervention, as well as a means to measure the success of intervention. Functions observed in play activities give insight into self-care and school abilities. Further evaluation and/or intervention by the therapist determines how functions are being adapted to activities in other environments. Therapeutic use of purposeful play activities ordinarily sought by children is the occupational therapist's medium. Facilitating adaptation through purposeful activities and providing opportunities to generalize adaptation of functions to many activities, situations, and environments is the therapeutic process of occupational therapy. A unique contribution of occupational therapy to pediatric health care programs is the use of purposeful activities to therapeutically facilitate adaptation.

What are the functions children develop and use for play, self-care, and school activities? How are basic functions adapted to a variety of activities, and does adaptation modify functions when activities change? What kinds of problems do some children have adapting and why? How does an occupational therapist use purposeful activities to treat the developmental problems of children? Attempts to answer these, and other questions, led to the development of a theory about the process of spatiotemporal adaptation. The theory attempts to explain associations between and causes for environmental events and processes which are adapted by the child. Through adaptation of events and processes, development of functions occur. Environmental events and experiences have both spatial and temporal dimensions that influence functions and adaptation. Thus, the theory is termed "spatiotemporal adaptation."

Theory of Spatiotemporal Adaptation

Occupational therapy values movement and activity as the means by which children find meaning in their actions and more complex movements evolve, providing the child with increased abilities to master activities and expand his environment. Higher levels of movements and activities enhance the child's sense of competence, thus encouraging the child to move about. Movement and activity are so commonplace that society takes them for granted. However, these everyday commonplace experiences are the vital aspects of development. Movement and activity provide meaning to environmental interactions by enhancing a person's investigation of his/her surroundings; by increasing his/her space; by linking self and objects; by enhancing self-satisfaction; and by promoting social relationships. Through movement and activity, a child acquires abilities to seek and obtain nutrition; to protect self; to perceive self and objects and their relationships; to pursue the world; and to acquire feelings of autonomy and competence. Movement puts the child in relationship with his/her surroundings, and through this relationship, a child can have an effect upon the environment, as well as be affected by the environment. Through this transactional relationship of child and environment, adaptation occurs.[11]

Adaptation is a dynamic process of expanding the child's repertoire of movements and activities. Through adaptation, more complex movements evolve that provide the child with increased abilities to expand his/her environment. Increased movement provides the child with a sense of competence to move about within the environment and to engage in goal-directed, purposeful experiences.

Experiences become purposeful when the active participation with behaviors and activities is meaningful to the nervous system to enhance maturation. Actions are meaningful when the feedback associated with the actions provide directions and efforts of function that are more mature or at a higher level than those previously experienced.[12] Facilitation of higher level or more complex movements and activities is inherent within the adaptation process.

The above discussion summarizes the basic concepts of the spatiotemporal adaptation theory.[13] The theory developed through the authors' quest to answer two basic questions:
1. How do children learn movement patterns?
2. If the process of learning movement patterns can be identified, would the process be applicable to therapeutic programs for handicapped children with movement disorders?

Currently, the theory provides rationale and guidance with assessment and treatment programs designed to serve children with developmental deviations. In addition, the theoretical statements specified in the theory provide directions for research and study. Through research, empirical data will be available to provide answers to the above questions. Hopefully, as a result of theory construction and research, occupational therapists will be able to achieve the mission of pediatric health care—to facilitate a developmental process by which a child can achieve his/her potential for functioning.

Idea for Theory

The basic idea of the spatiotemporal adaptation theory is that a person's developmental course is influenced by environmental experiences of movement and activity. Activity, as defined in the theory, is "action," the vital component of all change or modification.[14] Movement, as defined in the theory, is the primary means for activity, resulting in "interaction." Movement results in change, and it is basic to activity. Movement and activity are linked together in purposeful actions.

Spatiotemporal adaptation is a process by which the child discovers and absorbs the environment. Spatiotemporal adaptation is defined as the continuous, ongoing state or act of adjusting bodily processes required to function within the spatial and temporal dimensions of the environment. The process of spatiotemporal adaptation has a developmental sequence and matures with the alteration or modification of performance. Through spatiotemporal adaptation of purposeful movements and activities, growth, maturation, and developmental processes are enhanced.

Growth is defined as the biological/structural changes of the body (*i.e.*, skeletal/muscular); maturation as the change/modification within the individual's neurophysiological systems; and development as the alteration/modification of functions and processes used to adapt to the spatial and temporal dimensions of the environment. Although each term has a distinct meaning, there is a constant interrelationship among growth, maturation, and development. The interrelationship has an impact upon adaptation and contributes to the uniqueness of each child's developmental process, as well as to the uniqueness of the child's self-system.

Therefore, spatiotemporal adaptation is a process of continual interactions among growth, maturation, development, and environmental transactions. The term *environment*, as used in reference to adaptation, is all inclusive. Environment is the complete setting or surrounding, that is, the milieu, including self, other persons, objects, the earth, space, and the relationships within space. Thus, environment is everything with which an individual interacts.

The spatiotemporal adaptation process of environmental interaction has four components: assimilation, accommodation, association, and differentiation. *Assimilation* is the sensory process of taking in or receiving information that is external to or within the self-system (*e.g.*, a ball is seen as coming toward one's self; the hands are perceived as being inside one's pockets). *Accommodation* is the response or the motor process of adjusting the body to react to the incoming stimulation (*e.g.*, as the moving ball is perceived, the body posture is modified; the hands come out of the pockets and are directed in front of the body in preparation to catch the ball). *Association* is the organized process of relating the sensory information with the motor act and of relating present and past experiences with each other (*e.g.*, relating the perception of the moving ball with the accommodation of the body, the perception of the contact of body with ball in space and time, as well as the present act of catching the ball with past experiences of ball catching). *Differentiation* is the process of discriminating those essential elements of a specific behavior that are pertinent to a given situation, and distinguishing those that are not pertinent, thereby, modifying or altering the behavior in some manner (*e.g.*, discriminating the degree of the forearm supination/flexion pattern used to catch the ball, thus modifying the movement and position of the arms so that the actions of catching the ball become more accurate and efficient.)

Inherent in the spatiotemporal adaptation process is the integration of sensory input, motor output, and sensory feedback. The assimilation process can be likened to sensory input, accommodation to motor output, and association–differentiation as the vital components of sensory feedback that occur as one performs within the spatial and temporal dimensions of the environment. The sensorimotor-sensory process of adaptation is integrated by the self-system. Through integration, a child organizes sensorimotor information from environmental experiences.[15] Thus, integration is the child's "inner path" to discovery. The term sensorimotor-sensory (SMS) emphasizes the importance of sensory feedback integration with the initial sensory input and motor accommodation.

Prior to further discussion of spatiotemporal adaptation, a brief summary of related research and developmental theories contributing to its construction will be presented. The information shall be discussed according to intra-uterine, maturational, and environmental factors affecting development.

Intra-uterine Factors

Human adaptive behavior has its beginnings in early prenatal life, with reflex activity of the fetus being the foundation for movement.[16,17] Motor behavior is an expression of the functional capacities of the entire system, not just of its parts.[18,19] Motor behavior, reflexive in early life, develops as an expanding total pattern.[20–22] During intra-uterine development, generalized reactions of head and trunk develop prior to localized responses.[23,24] In addition, generalized responses of withdrawal develop and remain predominant over pursuit reactions.[25-27] The newborn is thus dominated by proprioceptive reflexes and avoidance reactions with the exception of pursuit reactions of the mouth.[28-30] Fetal reactions are characterized by total movement patterns, as the whole controls and guides its parts.[31] The more mature localized responses develop as components of primitive total patterns, which develop in an expanding total pattern, generalized to localized, cephalo to caudal, and proximal to distal.[32-34] In addition to reflexes and generalized movements, the newborn has a crude form of visual perception, indicated by preference to patterns.[35] The newborn's development of perception is indicative of intrauterine experiences providing sensory awareness of the fetal environment.

The above factors, gleaned from the literature, suggest that the reflex activity of the fetus is the foundation for learned movement patterns. Specific local responses of motor actions are components of earlier total responses. In addition, there is a crude quasi-perceptual relationship between the fetus with the intra-uterine environment.

Maturational Factors

John Hughlings Jackson[36] proposes that the central nervous system has a hierarchical functional organization that is responsible for voluntary motor actions. Generally, it is accepted that the nervous system does not function in isolation, and that all parts of the system are influenced by and influence the activities of the other parts.[37] McGraw proposes that most of the cortex is not functioning as a control for behavior at birth; therefore, movement patterns of early infancy may be under subcortical control.[38-40] Subcortical nuclei mature earlier, being prepared to influence the infant's actions.[41,42] In addition, maturation of the nervous system is not uniform; maturation of several levels occurs simultaneously in relation to different body segments and functions.[43] As a result, maturity of motor actions for specific functions may occur prior to maturity of other actions, and there will as well be divergent development of body segments until the whole is established.[44]

Penfield[45] introduced the concept of a subcortical system of integration that is responsible for the initiation of crude movements. According to Szumski, the central-cephalic system sends impulses to subcortical motor areas that activate the spinal cord and brainstem of the infant.[46] At the same time, this system sends impulses directly to the cortical motor areas of the cerebrum, facilitating pyramidal pathways.[47]

Coordinated movements are a result of various feedback mechanisms of peripheral and central nervous systems.[48-53] The influences of the vestibular mechanism upon motor activity and tone,[54,55] and the limbic-midbrain circuits that influence attention and motivation, contribute to hierarchical functional organization.[56-58] Therefore, it is "unwise to attribute specific patterns of neuronal activity to particular functions of the nervous system, since central nervous system activity is found to be essentially adaptive and does not seem to depend on any specific group of circuits."[59]

Environmental Factors

The adaptation of an organism to its environment, along with sensory integration and hierarchical maturation of the nervous system, characterize the developmental concepts of Jean Piaget.[60] Development is dependent upon the continual formation of new, higher order, intercoordinated sensorimotor systems.[61-63] Although life begins with certain neurological and anatomical structures, these structures do not determine functioning. The structures may inhibit or facilitate motor activity, but the child's interaction with the environment accounts for the development of functional performance.[64] Movement provides the means by which the child can interact with the environment.[65] During environmental interactions, purposeful movements are made by the child to increase his/her awareness of space, to manipulate the environment, and to communicate with persons and/or objects within the environment.[66] Holt proposes that sensorimotor activity is important as an integrating mechanism for linking together the components of development.[67] As the child develops, progressively more complex sensorimotor responses become a part of his/her repertoire.[68]

Theoretical Concepts

Information gleaned from the literature regarding intra-uterine, maturation, and environmental factors supports the constructs of the spatiotemporal adaptation theory. Within the theory, four major groups of theoretical concepts can be identified:

1. There is a relationship between the primitive reflex actions of an infant and his/her resulting higher level reactions; there is also a relationship between perception and sensorimotor functions.[69-71]

2. Acquired behaviors have an impact upon present actions, and present actions influence acquired behaviors by modifying the more primitive actions into higher level behaviors and activities.[72-74]

3. Phasic and tonic reflexes and movement reactions experienced during the early years of life are purposeful for sensorimotor learning and development of skilled performances.[75–78]
4. Interaction with the events of the environment provides the impetus with which one adapts; adaptation of environmental interactions is a lifelong developmental process.[79,80]

These four theoretical concepts can be illustrated by the ever-widening continuum of a spiral (Fig. 29-1). Spiraling emphasizes the process by which one adapts to the spatial and temporal dimensions of the environment in order to learn skilled performances. Three important principles of the adaptation process as emphasized by the spiraling continuum can be specified:

1. Adaptation to new experiences is dependent upon past acquired functions.
2. During the integration of past functions with the actions of new experiences, past functions are modified in some manner, resulting in higher level, more mature functions.
3. The integration of higher level functions influences and increases the maturity of lower level functions.

Spiraling, as a continuous process, provides the framework for the spatiotemporal adaptation theory.

Throughout the spiraling process, a network of spontaneous sensorimotor-sensory actions occurs.

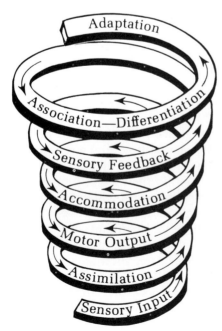

Figure 29-1. Spiraling continuum of spatiotemporal adaptation.

These observable actions are expressions of a child's functional abilities and adaptation process. In addition, the observable actions of a child serve as an expression of a child's sensorimotor-sensory integration and modification of lower level responses. For example, the foot contact reflexes that facilitate total flexion and extension of the legs of the neonate are modified throughout development to form higher level patterns of reciprocation. Observing a child's reciprocal patterns provides an expression of the spiraling process of lower level responses being integrated into the child's repertoire of functions to the extent that the lower level responses may not be identified. Although the lower level reactions may lose their original identity, their trace effects contribute to higher level functions. Thus, spiraling illustrates that a child does not acquire totally new functions; rather, functions are modifications of older lower level responses.

Spiraling also emphasizes the importance of the adaptation components of association–differentiation. Association–differentiation of old with new and new with old provides the basis for modifications of functions as well as the basis for developing perceptions. Perception is here defined as the sensory judgment and feeling given to one's experiences and environment. Perception requires thought and memory and as such cannot be separated from the cognitive processes of development. Therefore, perception and cognition are vital aspects of adaptation, and they have an important role in the process of learning skilled performances.

Sensorimotor functions provide the child with the foundation for acquiring perceptions of environmental experiences. The ability to perceive is dependent upon the process of integrating sensory input, both external and internal to the body, with the motor act and then associating and differentiating the new experience with past acquired functions. Thus, the spiraling adaptation of purposeful actions augments perception.

The importance of sensory feedback becomes more apparent when one considers that without association–differentiation, sensory input would remain at a receptive level. Through environmental experiences, a child builds a network of perceptions. As perceptions are adapted into the child's repertoire, concepts regarding the child's environmental interactions evolve. Sensorimotor functions provide the foundation by which the child interacts and acquires perceptions and concepts; perceptions–concepts are basic to spatiotemporal adaptations. Therefore, the spiraling integration of sensorimotor functions, perceptions, and concepts is inherent within the adaptation process used by a child to discover the spatiotemporal world.

As a child interacts, the challenge and demands of environmental events may exceed his repertoire of functions. When the demands or purpose of the event exceed the functions available, stress situations occur. In the stress situation, certain aspects of the more primitive or lower level functions will be utilized to adapt to the demands of the environment. For example, in patterns of early sitting and walking, shoulder retractions and elbow flexion, as aspects of the lower level prone extension posture, can be observed (Fig. 29-2). The youngster "calls up" aspects of the lower level pattern in order to facilitate the extension necessary for maintaining trunk stability in the vertical posture. As sitting and walking experiences are repeated, the lower level functions are associated and differentiated, so that the essential elements are integrated to form higher level adaptations. In this example, the essential elements of the postural extensor tone are differentiated from the shoulder-retraction and elbow flexion pattern of the prone extension posture. Through repeated experiences and the spiraling process, the self-system modifies the more primitive functions used for trunk stability into a higher level, more mature pattern for vertical postures (Fig. 29-3).

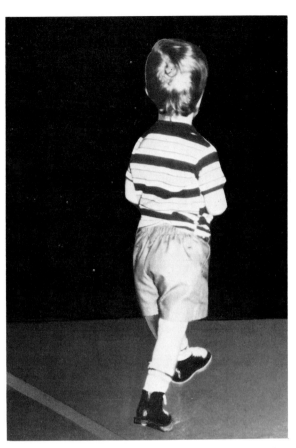

Figure 29-3. Mature postural pattern for vertical postures illustrating trunk stability.

The effects of stress upon a child's spatiotemporal adaptations are further illustrated in Figures 29-4 through 29-7. Figure 29-4 illustrates the child adapting with a beginning form of the Landau reaction. When deprived of vision, as in Figure 29-5, the sensory integration process is altered. The stress created by altering sensory integration results in the child's use of a lower level asymmetrical posture to provide stability in the suspended position. Figure 29-6 illustrates a 5-year-old boy walking on a balance beam with his eyes open. In the figure, the boy utilizes an appropriate balance reaction to adapt to the demands of the balance beam task. Compare the balance reaction in Figure 29-6 with Figure 29-7 of the boy walking on the balance beam while his eyes are closed. Note the lower level immature functions of asymmetrical positions used to adapt. The changing integration that occurs with vision occluded results in a stress-like situation with the boy adapting by "calling up" more primitive patterns to meet the challenge of the environment.

Spatiotemporal stress is a natural phenomenon that is observed throughout the developmental process.[81] Through the association–differentiation components of adaptation, the child integrates aspects of

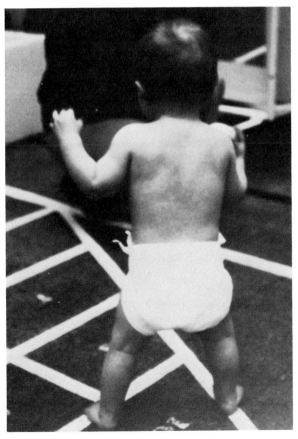

Figure 29-2. Early walking pattern illustrating shoulder retraction and elbow flexion—aspects of prone extension to facilitate trunk stability.

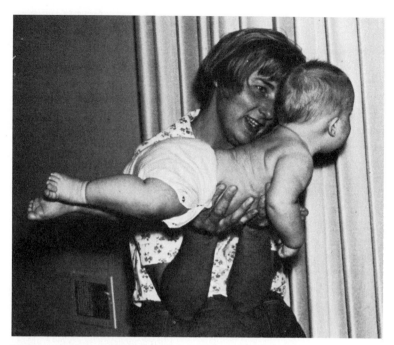

Figure 29-4. Adaptation with early development of Landau reaction. Note extension and midline orientation.

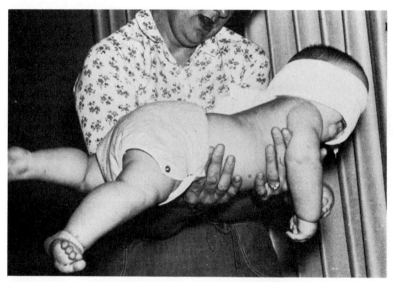

Figure 29-5. Stress condition facilitating use of lower level asymmetrical pattern to adapt.

lower level functions that are essential for performance and thus he/she modifies the more primitive response in some manner. Modification results from the spiraling integration of old with new and new with old, and higher level functions emerge. Therefore, spatiotemporal stress is a vital stimulus for development, as it becomes the motivating force that stimulates a child to adapt to the constant changes of the environment.

Environmental factors that contribute to spatiotemporal stress include the effects of gravity upon the child's position and the complexity of movement patterns required to interact, as well as the sensorimotor, perceptual, cognitive and social requirements of the activity. These factors influence the adaptation process to "call-up" previously adapted functions to adapt to the demands of the environment. Spatiotemporal stress occurs primarily in three situations:

1. when adapting to new experiences;
2. when the sensorimotor-sensory integrative process is altered;

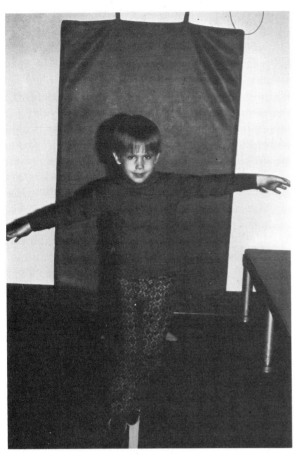

Figure 29-6. Adaptation with mature strategies with midline stability and equilibrium reactions.

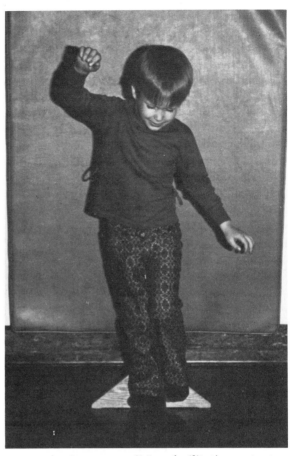

Figure 29-7. Stress condition facilitating adaptation with immature, asymmetrical pattern.

3. during the transitional phases of developmental progressions.

In summary, the theoretical concepts of the spatiotemporal adaptation theory can be illustrated by a spiraling continuum. The spiraling process emphasizes the integration of old with new and new with old, as well as the continuous, ever-expanding process of development. Inherent within spiraling are the components of association–differentiation that play a vital role in modification of older, more primitive functions to higher level patterns used to interact with the environment. The modification process evolves from the child's discoveries of the world that may be influenced by spatiotemporal stress situations. In addition, spiraling emphasizes the importance of the integration of sensorimotor experiences, perceptions of experiences, and formations of concepts.

Through the specification of the spiraling framework, additional concepts can be identified:

4. Adaptation is a sensorimotor-sensory process, dependent upon the interaction between movement and event (activity) and the interrelationship of movement, perception, and cognition.

5. Spatiotemporal adaptation is a spiraling process with increasingly more complex movement patterns gradually emerging from the lower level acquired functions as a result of continual environmental interactions.

6. Lower level functions may emerge during adaptation of events when the demands of the events exceed the functional capacities of a child, creating a stress situation.

7. Stress is a natural phenomenon as well as a vital stimulus for development. Integrating lower level functions with new experiences result in modification of functions to higher levels.

Theoretical Statements

Major developmental phases occurring within the spiraling adaptation process as well as major classifications of the process have been identified. Classifications of the process have been specified according to their proposed functions and termed (1) posture and movement strategies; (2) purposeful behaviors; (3) purposeful activities; and (4) skilled performances. These classifications have been created to further delineate the spiraling process of function-to-purpose-to-function and so on. The major developmental phases occurring with the spiraling process are termed: (a) primitive, (b) transitional, and (c) mature.[82]

The classifications of the adaptation of functions and the phases of the process have been organized into theoretical statements:

1. Sensorimotor learning results through the linkage of movement and activity functions that develop as a result of the adaptation of posture and movement strategies, intrinsic motivations, and goal-directed activities.
2. The final outcome of linking and adapting strategies, behaviors, and activities is the acquisition of skilled performances in play, self-care, and school.
3. Spatiotemporal adaptation occurs through primitive, transitional, and mature phases, with each phase having a distinct purpose.

The theoretical statements propose a process of learning how to perform. To gain comprehension regarding the proposed process, the following definitions of strategies, behaviors, activities, and skilled performance are presented. Following these definitions, there is a discussion that briefly defines the adaptation sequence according to primitive, transitional, and mature phases.

Developmental Functions

Posture and Movement Strategies

Strategies are basic processes of neuromuscular-skeletal functions used to adapt to the events of the environment. Strategies supply the system with the ability to "move" or "not move" in certain patterns. Postural strategies control movement, and movement strategies give rise to action.[83] Movement strategies promote and sequence changes in position and combine muscle actions so that one movement flows into another. Posture and movement strategies are functions of the nervous system, and they ultimately become adapted as spontaneous movement patterns available for skilled performance.

The components of strategies include the neural functions of phasic and tonic reflexes; righting, support, protective, and balance reactions; and the muscular functions of mobility and stability. In addition, the skeletal systems provide the framework for posture and movement. Strategies are patterns of movement and control that manage and coordinate the bodily functions used to adapt. Strategies are

adapted into sequences of functions used with sensorimotor behaviors and activities.[84]

Purposeful Behaviors

Purposeful behaviors link together posture and movement strategies into sequences for the innate functions used for creeping, sitting, rolling, standing/walking, and reaching/grasping. Purposeful behaviors are self-starting and self-perpetuating. They are the innate progressions of normal sensorimotor development. Behaviors are goal-directed toward the accomplishment of the behavior itself, for example, the goal to creep, to roll, to sit, to stand, to grasp, etc. Behaviors are purposeful when the actions of the behavior have meaning or purpose to the self-system resulting in maturation of functions. Through the development of behaviors, stability and mobility muscle functions and reflex/righting reactions are linked into posture and movement strategies. The linking of posture and movement strategies into movement behaviors represents the spiraling adaptation of function-to-purpose-to-function.

Purposeful Activities

Activities that are purposeful link together selected functions of posture and movement strategies adapted from movement patterns acquired through the developmental sequences of purposeful behaviors. Purposeful activities are directed toward events of the environment; thus, the goals of activities are outside of self; whereas the goals of behaviors are innate. Purposeful activity depends on the child's intrinsic motivation, attention, and accomplishment to provide meaning to the self-system for change/modification of functions. The linking of strategies, behaviors, and activities evolve into spontaneous patterns of movement.

Skilled Performances

Repeated actions of movement and activities become adapted by the self-system, and they evolve into skilled performances that can be called forth for environmental transactions. Skill is the final outcome of the adaptation process. Skill is defined as the appropriate use of posture and movement in relation to the expended effort (*i.e.,* speed, timing, exertion, space, control) for the performance of an activity. Skilled performance is characterized by freedom of movement within the spatial and temporal dimensions of the environment. There is a natural responsiveness or an automatic element to skilled actions. The natural, automatic characteristics of skill result from the regulation of flow of movement in relation to the spatiotemporal dimensions. Regulation of movement flow requires temporal sequencing of posture and movement strategies in relation to the spatial confines of the environment. Efficiency and accuracy of movement regulation underlie the blending of strategies, behaviors, and activities for skilled performance. Efficiency of actions is the relationship between the amount of work that is accomplished and the force expended to accomplish the action. Efficiency is more dependent upon the child's abilities to perceive and to adapt the spatial dimensions of the environment. Accuracy is dependent upon the perception of self in relation to the temporal dimensions. Accuracy is the perception of direction, distance, control, and timing of actions.[85] Therefore, the ability to plan and execute skilled actions is dependent upon one's efficiency and accuracy of performance requirements.

With skill, movement and activity functions are appropriate for the task or situation. When skill has been acquired, there is no need to modify functions used to adapt. Thus, skill can be identified by the consistency of movement patterns for performance.[86] When skill has been achieved, movement and activity functions are no longer purposeful.

The process of linking or blending posture and movement strategies, innate motor behaviors, and activities of the environment represents the spiraling progression by which children learn functions of performance. The spiraling progression considers primitive, transitional, and mature phases.

Developmental Phases

Primitive

The primitive phase of spiraling extends from the time of conception until several months after birth. Posture and movement strategies are influenced by neonatal generalized movements, phasic and tonic reflexes, and activation of muscle functions. During the primitive phase, the infant is supported by external sources such as a crib or floor or by being held in someone's arms. Because internal control needed to support the body has not evolved, the environment provides the necessary sources of control.

Movement strategies during primitive development tend to cause undifferentiated patterns of movement. Postural strategies cause primitive holding or fixing of postures. Primitive posture and movement experiences are primarily in body segments with the body being supported by the environment.

Primitive strategies are used to adapt primitive behaviors such as head lift, primitive support on arms, protective head turning, head lag, primary crawling, upper extremity traction, hand grasp, and avoiding.[87] Primitive strategies also underlie baby's first activities, for example, seeking the nipple for feeding, visually tracking a toy, and swiping at a toy.[88]

Primitive strategies, behaviors, and activities are adapted by means of subcortical neural mechanisms (phasic and tonic reflexes) that activate muscles for total patterns. Activation of mobility muscle functions of the primitive phase initiate co-activation of muscle groups in primitive holding patterns.[89] Actions facilitated by phasic and tonic reflexes and generalized movements provide the system with primitive patterns of movement and positions that are modified into more complex functions.

Phasic reflexes activate muscles and muscle groups through a complete range of motion for undifferentiated movement patterns. Sensory assimilations that initiate primitive mobility (activation) also provide sensory feedback from the environment, increasing the baby's awareness of self and environment. The phasic reflexive motor accommodations provide exteroceptive, interoceptive, and proprioceptive information about changing positions and movements of body segments. The baby begins to associate certain sensory input with certain predictable responses, such as moving toward a touch to obtain a nipple. As the infant links sensations with outcomes, sensory awareness of self and environment evolves. As awareness of responses develops, primitive strategies are adapted to direct actions for purposeful behaviors and activities. Organization of sensations received through feedback of actions directed toward purposeful behaviors and activities provides the system with the stimuli necessary for associations, thus perceptions develop.

Tonic reflexes are observed as postures assumed by the baby in response to head and trunk position in space. Therefore, tonic reflexes also originate from a variety of exteroceptive, interoceptive, and proprioceptive assimilations. The accommodations of tonic reflexes distribute muscle tone in primitive postural patterns. These primitive postural patterns activate muscles and muscle groups in holding contractions at a particular point within the range, frequently at the end of the range.[90] Holding strategies produced by tonic reflexes facilitate development of stability muscle functions. Holding strategies are adapted to fixation-support sets (Fig. 29-8).

As the infant moves from one primitive holding pattern to another, he receives feedback about changes in distribution of tone. The baby's awareness of changes of posture and tone prepares him/her for postural strategies to be adapted to higher levels

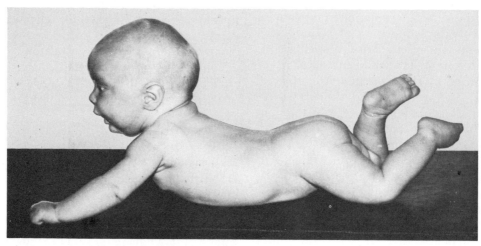

Figure 29-8. Fixation-support postural set.

of internal control, thus freeing the baby from dependency upon the environment for support. The mobility and stability functions experienced with phasic and tonic reflexes are integrated to initiate the co-activation muscle functions characteristic of the transitional phase.[91]

Transitional

The transitional phase of spiraling adaptation begins a few months after birth and culminates when the child acquires the internal posture and movement control necessary for mature functions of behaviors and activities. The major purpose of transition is the modification of primitive reflexes, muscle functions, and undifferentiated generalized movements into mature strategies, behaviors, and activities. The developmental process of transition is characterized by the adaptation of primitive reflexes to higher level vertical and righting reactions, as well as support and protective reactions. Muscle functions of the transitional phase are co-activation of muscle groups to support the joints and combined mobility and stability actions to allow movement from stabilized joints.

Reactions, like reflexes, distribute muscle tone in specific posture and movement strategies according to whether the strategies are adapted to behaviors for rolling, creeping, walking, or adapted to activities such as feeding oneself, walking to the store, drawing pictures, or writing. The terms associated with reactions are like reflex terms in that they describe specific accommodations or a series of accommodations to particular sensory stimuli. Reactions can be differentiated from reflexes by their greater complexity and inconstancy of response.[92] Whereas reflexes are simple, predictable responses to one or two sensory stimuli, reactions are complex functions that result from integration of multisensory assimilations.[93] Facilitation of the higher level reactions serves to

dampen the primitive reflexes as control mechanisms for posture and movement.

Posture and movement strategies are modified by means of combined mobility and stability functions and by the effects of chaining upon reactions. Chain reactions are neurological mechanisms observed when an initial movement of a reaction is followed by a predictable series of movements. Therefore, chain reactions help establish movement links so that one movement automatically flows into the next appropriate movement.[94] Chain reactions provide the self-system with experiences of movement links and flow of movement. The linking together of movements experienced during transition will be adapted to higher level movement sequences for mature functions.

Transitional strategies serve to provide the system with the internal control necessary to assume and maintain behaviors such as prone extension posture, on-elbows and on-hands support, propping self in sitting, being pulled to stand, and bouncing.[95] In addition, strategies and behaviors of the transitional phase are linked and adapted to activities such as reaching and grasping a toy with a palmar grasp, patting toys with hands, probing at objects with the index finger, and bringing toys to the mouth for exploration.[96] Active participation with the events of the environment provides the stimuli for the blending of strategies, behaviors and activities, thus maturation is further enhanced.

Combined mobility and stability functions are adapted to provide the baby with some degree of self-control over movements in space and movements from postures. Combined strategies are adapted in bilateral-linear sets (Fig. 29-9). Bilateral-linear sets allow body movement backward, forward, and side-to-side. Thus, the bilateral-linear functions are adapted to behaviors and the youngster acquires movement patterns for rocking, bouncing and

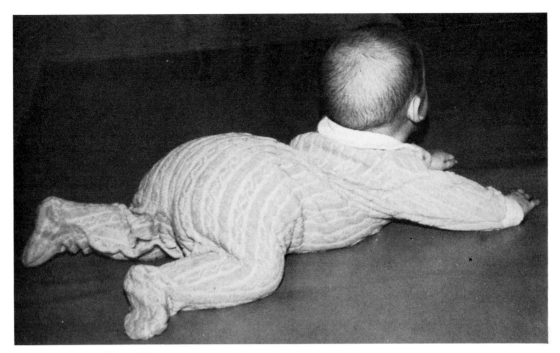

Figure 29-9. Bilateral-linear set.

pushing-pulling the body within the saptial and temporal dimensions of the environment.

Movement of the body further activates muscle groups and facilitates the development of the movement synergies needed to assume new positions in space. As the transitional phase progresses, combined mobility and stability functions from movement and posture synergies are blended. Differentiated strategies emerge that are adapted to behaviors that provide the youngster with the ability to control his position, to shift weight, and to free nonweight-bearing extremities to move out into space.[97] Free movement reflects the evolution of blended mobility and stability functions that are adapted to behaviors, such as on-hands reaching, crawling, deliberate rolling, supported walking, reach and grasp patterns, forearm supination and pronation, as well as instinctive grasp for activities.[98]

The progression of development from external to internal control requires that mobility and stability functions to be differentiated from each other. Differentiated strategies allow weight-shift sets to emerge (Fig. 29-10). Weight-shift sets are adapted for behaviors that require stabilizing for support in order to move out to interact with the environment.[99]

During transition, weight-shift behaviors are an inefficient two-step process. First weight is shifted, then movement follows. For example, forward progression is accomplished by laterally shifting weight to one side, followed by movement forward. As the two step process is repeated, stabilizing and moving become integrated into a sequence. In addition to the regulated sequence of weight-shift, during the later phase of transition, adaptations of righting, support, and protective reactions facilitate rotation between trunk and pelvis. Rotation enhances differentiation of body and body segments. With differentiated strategies, the youngster can move his extremities freely, first from the shoulder or hip. The differentiated strategies and free movement behaviors are adapted to activities such as shaking a rattle or scribbling with a crayon.[100] As blended mobility and stability functions progress to more distal movements, and differentiated strategies evolve from rotation/counter-rotation patterns, mature functions emerge.

Mature

Mature behaviors and activities are controlled by automatic balance reactions and by blended mobility-stability functions. Automatic balance reactions include midline stability and equilibrium reactions, adapted from transitional strategies.

Midline stability reactions are barely discernible postural adjustments around the midline of the trunk and proximal joints. Midline stability reactions control postural adjustments within a confined area related to the center of gravity. As soon as the body moves away from its center, equilibrium is elicited to regain balance.

Equilibrium reactions encompass several observable sequential movements:

1. Movement away from the center of gravity to the

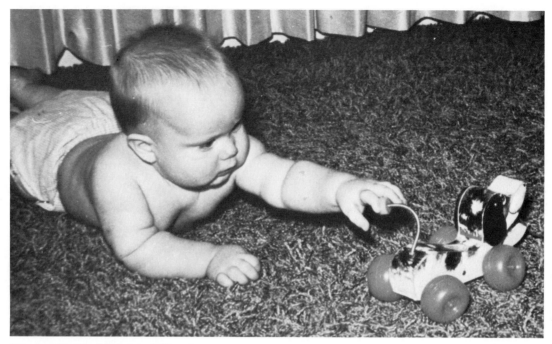

Figure 29-10. Weight-shift set.

extent that balance may be lost elicits rotation of head and upper trunk back toward the center.

2. Lower trunk segments counter-rotate to balance the rotational effect of the upper portions and control the degree of rotation. As upper portions of the body come back to midline, there is a barely observable reverse in the rotational and counter-rotation patterns of the upper and lower segments in order to stop the adjustment at midline.

3. Extremities on one side of the body may extend and abduct to assist the body back toward center alignment by pulling.

4. Opposite extremities may extend and abduct in preparation to protect and support the body if balance is lost, or if the already weight-bearing, opposite extremities experience increase in stability distribution to support the shift in weight bearing.[101]

Automatic balance reactions of the mature phase blend mobility and stability functions to achieve mature internal control by adapting movement/counter-movement postural sets (Fig. 29-11). The movement/counter-movement mature postural set provides control by stabilizing a movement with a simultaneous antagonist movement. This mature postural set is primarily executed by finely balanced rotation and counter-rotation around the central axis.[102]

Mature strategies are adapted to mature behaviors of deliberate rolling, walking, reaching, and prehending.[103] Mature functions result from control and refined blended mobility–stability. With mature functions, freely moving extremities are controlled by counter movements; that is, the shoulder moves back as the hand reaches forward, the pelvis moves back as the leg swings forward. In addition to control by counter-movements, necessary control of the distal joints of the fingers and thumb provides for mature manipulative prehension behaviors. The adaptation of mature strategies and behaviors provides a variety of movement patterns for activity. Movement/counter-movement postural sets and blended mobility-stability functions form a basis for the development of automatic movement/activity patterns that are adapted for a variety of performance skills.[104]

The above discussion of the primitive, transitional, and mature phases of spatiotemporal adaptation emphasizes the linking of strategies, behaviors, and activities. As posture and movement strategies are adapted to sequences of movement behaviors, postural sets evolve. In addition to postural sets, the spatiotemporal adaptation process contributes to the development of perceptual sets.

Perceptual Sets

During the spiraling adaptation process, the linking of movements with events/activities of the environment provides the basis for acquiring perceptual sets. Perceptual sets are formed from the organization of

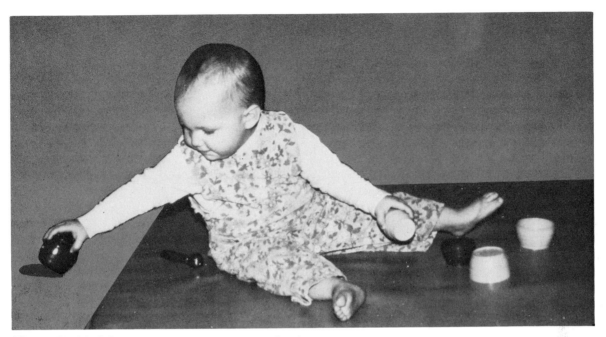

Figure 29-11. Movement-countermovement set.

sensory information external to and internal within the self-systems. Perceptions of functions used to direct efforts for interaction with the events of the environment are the basic foundation for the acquisition of sensorimotor perceptions. Sensorimotor sets are unique patterns of movements specific to each individual's acquired functions used for activity performance. As the youngster seeks out and absorbs his environment, neuromuscular functions acquired with postural sets are adapted to activities. Through the association of functions and activities, perception of actions evolve. Thus, the blending of postural sets with activities enhances sensorimotor perceptions. Sets are formed and become available as automatic sensorimotor programs that can be called forth to interact with the environment. In addition to the perceptions of movement and activity functions of sensorimotor patterns, the social and emotional perceptions of self and relationships impact the development and adaptation of perceptual sets. Social-emotional perceptions evolve from one's perceived judgments and feelings about his intrinsic abilities as well as expectations of self and/or expectation standards of one's culture. Social-emotional perceptions have a direct impact upon sensorimotor abilities, likewise perceptions about the intrinsic sensorimotor abilities impacts social-emotional perceptions. Therefore, sensorimotor and social-emotional perceptions are integrated to form perceptual sets. Perceptual sets influence interactions as the social-emotional and sensorimotor components of sets have a direct impact upon the process of adapting.[105]

The creation of perceptual sets occurs through the transactions of the child with his/her biological, psychological, and sociological environments. Perceptual sets are biopsychosocial phenomena that are acquired by the child through play. Through play, a child develops those functions required to perform within the environment and to engage in more demanding activities.

Summary of Theory

The theory of spatiotemporal adaptation has been constructed to answer questions about how children learn movement patterns. Adaptation of the spatiotemporal dimensions of the environment is described as a process of functions-to-purpose-to-functions to interact with the environment. Adaptation as defined for use within the theory is the continuous process of adjusting the bodily processes required to function within the spatial and temporal dimensions of the environment. Movements and activities are linked together for purposes of interacting with the environment so that, through movement and activity, a person's developmental course will evolve into skilled performances. Therefore, the spatiotemporal adaptation theory proposes that children acquire movement patterns through the process of adapting basic neural and muscular functions to purposes of movement and activities with self and environment. As basic functions are adapted to purposes, higher level functions emerge. The integration of functions with purpose through purposeful interactions of biopsychosocial events represents the spiraling process of the theory.

Spiraling considers not only the relationships of primitive actions with higher level, more mature actions, but also the development of skilled performances as modifications of earlier, more primitive actions. Spatiotemporal adaptation of function-to-purpose-to-function is viewed as a threefold spiraling process with higher level, more complex movement sequences emerging from the integration of lower level functions with actions being experienced as a result of the demands of the environment.

During the normal course of development, environmental situations may provide stress experiences for a child. Stress is a natural phenomenon and a vital stimulus for development as integrating lower level functions with new experiences result in higher level adaptations. In stress situations, lower level functions are called forth to adapt to the environmental demands; thus, stress enhances the spiraling integration of old with new.

Inherent within spiraling is the adaptation of posture and movement strategies to behaviors and activities. The adaptation of functions through the strategy-behavior-activity process evolves into skilled performances. Adaptation of functions occurs through the interrelationship of movement-activity experienced in a child's play. Through play experiences occurring during primitive, transitional, and mature phases, a child's self-system forms postural and perceptual sets. Blending of sets provides sensorimotor-perceptual links that are available for adaptations of environmental interactions.

The spatiotemporal adaptation theory provides an understanding of the process of adapting functions for the development of skilled performance. Application of the theoretical concepts and statements to therapeutic programs for children with movement disorders will be discussed in the following section.

Application of Theory

What types of problems do some children have adapting and why? How does an occupational therapist use purposeful activities, or spatiotemporal adaptation theory, to evaluate and treat developmental problems of childhood? According to the theory, most normal children experience difficulty adapting to their environment at different times or under certain conditions, for example, in adapting to new experiences, adapting when their sensorimotor-

sensory integrative process is temporarily altered, or adapting during transitional periods of development. Normal children experiencing stress frequently resolve the problems encountered by trying different ways to accomplish their goal. By modifying their approach to the problem, children expand their repertoire of solutions to particular types of problems, and ultimately develop more mature, or higher level, functions that serve more challenging purposes. Children with developmental problems are not so fortunate. The child's dysfunction, whether congenital, acquired, or environmental, is likely to interfer with the normal progression of spatiotemporal adaptation. For children with developmental problems, every experience can seem like a new experience. The child's sensorimotor-sensory integrative processes may be altered by a deficit rather than a temporary change in one or more sensory processes. The child may need some type of intervention to be able to develop beyond primitive or transitional ways of functioning to more mature ones.

Idea for Application

Spatiotemporal adaptation theory addresses some problems children have when otherwise normal challenges to their developmental capabilities become unmanageable and *distressful*. The idea of applying theoretical concepts about normal development to developmental disabilities came from experiences observing normal child development and adaptation, while simultaneously evaluating and treating children with known dysfunctions. Some correlations between the two groups of children became evident:

1. There is a similarity between patterns used by normal children during their primitive/transitional developmental phases and patterns continually used by children with dysfunction (Figs. 29-12 and 29-13).
2. The tendency for normal children to use previously acquired patterns to adapt under stress is also evident with dysfunctioning children, but the latter group is frequently unable to make use of stress to move to higher levels of development—the old patterns are not adapted.
3. Children with dysfunction continue to perform at primitive levels, or continue to attempt higher level activities by using lower level functions.

Although a dysfunctioning child's developmental and adaptive performance seems to reflect patterns

Figure 29-12. Comparisons of normal and abnormal patterns. (*A*) Normal prehension ▶ pattern of the 4-year-old. (*B*) Total grasp, dysfunction pattern for 4-year-old. (*C*) Total grasp, normal pattern for child 18 months old.

Comparisons of Normal and Abnormal Patterns

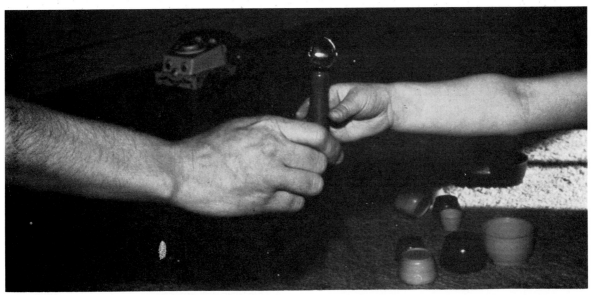

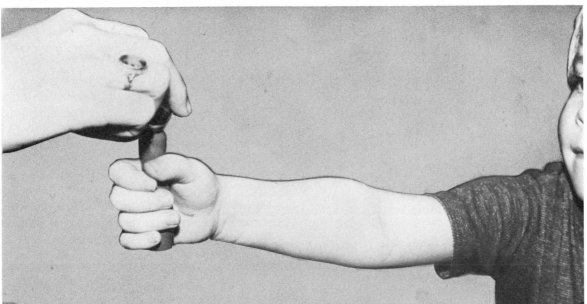

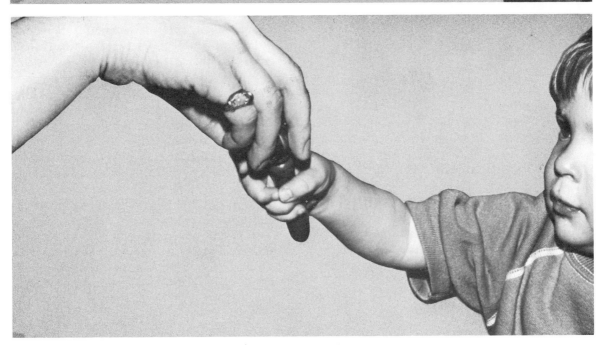

Comparisons of Normal Patterns and Patterns of Dysfunction

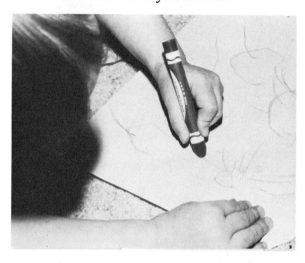

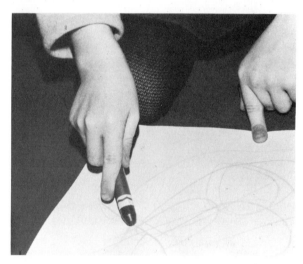

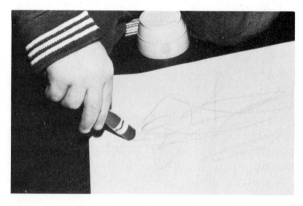

Figure 29-13. Comparisons of normal patterns and patterns of dysfunction. (A) Prehension, a mature adaptation for child of age five. (B) Modified palmar grasp, an immature adaptation for child of age five. (C) Palmar grasp, a mature adaptation for an 18-month-old child.

used by normal children at less mature stages, the child with problems is not a mirror-image of an immature normal child. There are significant differences:

1. Many conditions that interrupt normal development, such as cerebral palsy and acquired brain trauma, are accompanied by abnormal muscle tone. When primitive patterns are influenced by abnormal tone and repeated beyond their normal span of usefulness, they develop into posture and movement strategies unique to brain dysfunction. They are no longer true reflections of immature patterns. However, knowing where a particular combination of postures and movements may have originated in normal development, before the influence of abnormal tone, can help the therapist assess the level of functioning and therapeutic potential of children with developmental problems.

2. Cognitive abilities and emotional states also contribute to the differences between normal immature and truly dysfunctional patterns of posture, movement, and adaptive performance. Children with limited cognitive potential seem to possess some movement patterns unique to retardation. These patterns are often repetitive and purposeless in terms of function. Lower than normal muscle tone may also accompany retardation and certain other syndromes, greatly reducing support for higher level, more complex movement patterns. In addition, some children are not motivated cognitively or emotionally to pursue a behavior, such as rolling or walking, for its own sake. Other children may attain innate behavioral levels and move around, but may not be interested or capable of interacting with events, objects, or persons within their environment. A knowledge of the normal progression of linkages between postures, movements, behaviors, activities, and skills is useful for assessing the differences between developmental delays and uniquely abnormal patterns. It also helps in determining whether cognitive or emotional delays, rather than primarily sensorimotor involvement, are impeding development.

3. Repeated use of primitive and/or transitional functions to adapt to higher level purposes by children with sensorimotor dysfunction closely reflects the performance patterns of normal children under normal developmental stress. The cognitive ability of these dysfunctioning children ranges from moderate retardation to above normal intelligence. However, it is likely that, since the dysfunctioning child has repeated the pattern so much more frequently, often without success-

fully achieving a goal and often without any normal variation or dissociation of essential from nonessential components, the pattern will appear more stereotyped and poorly adapted, more clumsy and awkward, than when it is a normal pattern for children.

Theory and Dysfunction

The stress reactions of childhood, which are so vital to a normal child's progress, become distress reactions for children with developmental problems. The dysfunctioning child's responses to gravity, demands for complex movement, or the need to pass complicated developmental milestones add up to a disability in development. Developmental disability results from any condition, trauma, deprivation, or disease (congenital, acute, progressive, or chronic) that interrupts or delays the sequence and rate of normal growth, development, and maturation. The source of interruption or delay, such as brain trauma, environmental deprivation, or deficits in sensory processing, may cause the dysfunction initially. The resulting interference in sensorimotor-sensory processing further compromises the individual's ability to adapt.

There is a relationship between the maturation of one's nervous system, purposeful environmental stimuli, and adaptive responses. When the nervous system is deprived of meaningful stimuli, and when the nervous system cannot make a meaningful response to the stimuli, effective maturation cannot take place.

Harris[106] portrays the nervous system as "a series of interacting functional units" that are involved in a continual interplay at different structural levels. The units carry a variety of information and, if one unit works ineffectively, the other units are affected in some manner. Maturation and the resulting developmental behaviors become disorganized in proportion to the degree of involvement or impairment of the neural connections, of the interaction between the units and nuclei, and of the interaction between integrative structures. Maladaptation results from the inadequate maturation of the nervous pathways. Myelination of these pathways does not occur and synaptic connections do not develop fully nor at the proper time.[107]

Sensorimotor-sensory processing can be affected, whether the problem is primarily in receiving stimuli, in responding to stimuli, or in differentiating responses. Deficits in *sensory assimilation* may become a source of dysfunction when a child is deprived of meaningful stimuli. This can occur when a child is neglected, abused, lives in a nonstimulating or over-stimulating environment, or when the child's capacity to make use of stimuli is limited. Whenever sensory assimilations are inadequate for normal response, motor accommodations are limited and sensory feedback is diminished, further limiting sources of sensory assimilation.[108]

Difficulty with *motor accommodation* due to deficits within the nervous system results in the absence or poor execution of motor responses to stimuli. The responses are often at a lower level than needed for adaptation to occur. Feedback from abnormal movements and from immature responses provides poor assimilation for sequential responses or higher responses. This perpetuates adaptation at lower, rather than higher, levels. Children with brain trauma initially seem to have difficulty with accommodation.[109]

Even though their potential for assimilation and accommodation may be basically intact, some children have difficulty processing *sensory feedback*. They fail to *associate and differentiate* feedback, which is needed for developing efficient strategies to adapt at higher levels and for developing sensory judgment required for the development of perception. These children are often considered as children with sensory integrative dysfunctions.[110]

When distress interrupts any portion of the sensorimotor-sensory process, it affects the child's functioning as a whole entity. Its effect may be immediately observable, or it may take years to manifest itself.

Dysfunction or disability in development may be manifested as primitive or transitional pathology, or as abnormal patterns. Primitive pathology reflects adaptive patterns that have been retained beyond their normal time span. It is accompanied by a corresponding failure to develop higher level strategies to adapt to particular situations (Fig. 29-14). Primitive pathology includes the use of undifferentiated movement patterns, primitive phasic and tonic reflexes, prolonged retraction or fixation, and incomplete or absent righting reactions, as well as inadequate stability and mobility development.[111]

Transitional pathology reflects use of transitional patterns of behavior, such as undifferentiated movement synergies, prolonged stability control, bilateral-linear sets, weight-shift sets, and poor movement control.[112] Primitive and transitional pathology is usually characteristic of children diagnosed as affected by delay or disabilities of development, as well as children with sensory integrative dysfunction.

Abnormal patterns are characteristic of children with cerebral palsy and other forms of specific brain involvement (Fig. 29-15). Abnormal muscle tone is the significant factor separating primitive and transi-

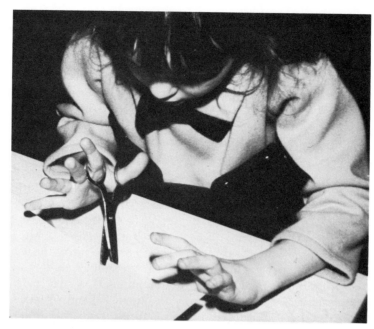

Figure 29-14. Dysfunction illustrated by primitive finger extension used to adapt.

tional pathology from abnormal patterns. The use of lower level patterns may be similar, but hypertonic, hypotonic, or fluctuating muscle status is a unique characteristic of abnormal patterns.[113]

Theories concerning normal child development,

and specifically the spatiotemporal adaptation theory, can be useful to health professionals responsible for identifying children with dysfunction, assessing the extent of dysfunction and potential for improvement, and planning and implementing

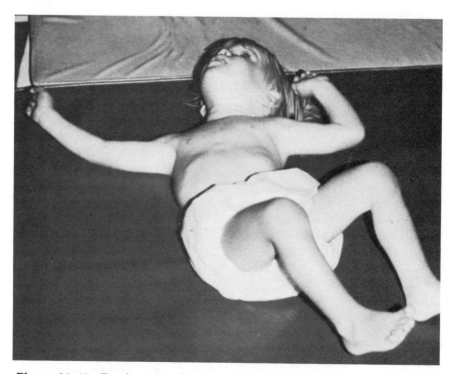

Figure 29-15. Dysfunction illustrated by pathological asymmetrical posture and tone.

treatment and evaluation progress. The theory, as discussed in the previous sections, can be expressed in the form of theoretical concepts. These concepts can be applied to evaluation, treatment planning, or assessment of progress in specific therapy programs. They can also provide a point of departure for research designed to determine the effectiveness of therapeutic intervention.

Theoretical Concepts

1. Acquired or congenital pathology, resulting in disabling conditions of development, impacts the spiraling adaptation process. Lower and higher level actions are not integrated to modify strategies, behaviors, and activities for mature performances.[114]
2. When lower level actions are not modified through the spiraling adaptation process, purposeless actions and dysfunction occur.[115]
3. Environmental situations that promote purposeless and dysfunctional actions are distressful transactions for the child, resulting in spatiotemporal maladaptation.[116]
4. Spatiotemporal maladaptation of environmental transactions is a process of repeated dysfunctional performances that are meaningless to the system and that result in developmental disabilities.[117]
5. Developmental disabilities are characterized by abnormal postural tone, abnormal patterns of movement, and/or persistant use of primitive and transitional strategies, behaviors, and activities beyond the normal or expected period of adapting those actions.[118]
6. A child with disabilities of development can benefit from a therapeutic program designed to facilitate the spiraling process of spatiotemporal adaptation.[119]

The first five theoretical concepts provide the basis for the emergence of the sixth, a concept directly related to therapeutic programs for children with developmental disabilities. The sixth concept provides the rationale or theoretical orientation on which occupational therapists can base their selection of therapeutic methods and activities. Thus, spatiotemporal adaptation theory with its spiraling framework provides an orientation and model by which therapeutic actions and reasoning can be based.

The theoretical orientation of spatiotemporal adaptation has as its core the spiraling process of modifying a child's actions by facilitating higher level functions. The orientation has the objective of linking strategies, behaviors, and activities for adaptation to skilled performances. Inherent within the development of skill is the adaptation of postural and perceptual sets that become a part of the self-system to be called forth for automatic performances.

Regardless of one's theoretical orientation to therapy, therapeutic actions and reasoning must respect the laws of development that have emerged from scientific evidence. Just as the genetico-environmental (nature-nurture) law governs developmental mechanisms, so does the law of individual differences.[120] The law of individual differences reinforces the fact that no two human beings are alike nor will they react to a given stimulus in the same exact manner. Therefore, therapeutic models for intervention must respect the genetic and environmental continuum, as well as uniqueness of each person. Thus, therapy must be adaptable for each individual and his/her assessed needs and abilities.[121] The spiraling adaptation model of therapy does not provide step by step techniques, rather, it provides a system or orientation by which a variety of treatment methods and activities can be applied to meet the needs of each unique individual. Because individuals are unique, treatment cannot be standardized nor defined as "fit" for a given population or specific handicap. Therapy must be individually formulated, just as each person is.[122]

The theory of spatiotemporal adaptation provides the underlying concepts and principles by which individual treatment programs can be formed. Central to the concepts and principles of spatiotemporal adaptation is the philosophy of the profession, that "purposeful activity facilitates the adaptive process." Therefore, therapy based upon the spatiotemporal adaptation theory includes the use of activities in such a manner that the child's active participation with the activity facilitates purposeful actions. These are adapted by the self-system through the spiraling process.

Purposeful activity is the point of departure for occupational therapy intervention programs; however, the impact of therapy depends upon the change or modification of dysfunction that children elicit within themselves through attention to and active participation in activity. Modification of dysfunction occurs in a spiraling process; thus, the principles of spiraling development and adaptation provide a framework for therapeutic programs. Spiraling adaptation of activities stresses the overlap of strategies, behaviors, and activities.

A child with disabilities can benefit from therapy that facilitates adaptation; however, therapy does not just mirror the normal adaptation process. Recapitulation of the normal process may only augment the already present dysfunction or disability. For example, facilitating the normal posture and movement patterns of primitive reflexes may only enhance the child's continued participation in undifferentiated or fixation patterns. Within normal development, a baby frequently calls forth elements of prone extension to reinforce needed trunk stability; to recapitulate this process may only enhance an abnormal pattern by increasing extension tone and repeating the undifferentiated pattern. Facilitation of neck extension or primitive kicking patterns may produce scissoring, may increase extension tone, and may prevent the development of hip flexion.[123] Also, caution must be taken regarding the speed and repetition of movement; movement that is too fast may increase tone, facilitate an excited state, or produce sensory overload. Another factor to consider is the temporal aspect of activity performance; activities requiring a quick reaction time or fast movement may elicit a less mature response and may cause distress. Another factor to consider is the level of the activity being presented. The therapist should not force activity nor present activities at too high or too low a level for the child to adapt.

Methods and activities for occupational therapy programs make use of the spiraling model. Spiraling makes its therapeutic impact through a process of "reciprocal interweaving" or reincorporation of several sequential levels of development.[124] Using the idea of spiraling for facilitation of higher levels and modification of lower level functions, guidelines for selection of therapeutic methods and activities include consideration of the following:

1. specific aspects of actions that are one level below the child's present functioning level;
2. facilitation of specific aspects of a performance that is one level above the child's present functioning level.

Using the lower, present, and higher levels of activity performance provide a method for facilitating association and differentiation of lower and higher level actions for modification of functions.

During the treatment process, a therapist observes responses and reactions, and he/she attempts to assess the child's ability to interpret feedback from the activity performances. Sensorimotor stimulation to enhance "reciprocal interweaving" of levels of functions is therapeutic only when the feedback is appropriate. The child's involvement with and interest in his or her actions provide valuable clues to the child's awareness and use of feedback, as does the child's progress. During treatment, a child must guide and direct his or her own actions. The child is the best judge of the appropriateness of an activity. Therefore, throughout the adaptation program, the child is the best indicator of the impact of activity, as the child's performance is a functional expression of the self-system.

The Therapeutic Process

Preparation

Preparation, facilitation, and adaptation are viewed as a threefold process for occupational therapy intervention programs.[125] *Preparation* is both the preliminary and ongoing process of enhancing readiness and use of the neural and muscular functions in posture and movement strategies. The purpose of preparing strategies for use is to attempt to achieve a state of homeostasis within the self-system. Preparation in a therapy session attempts to do for the child what strategy development accomplishes in the normal adaptation process. Preparation includes normalizing postural tone (by increasing, decreasing, or stabilizing tone); increasing the range of motion and strength; promoting subcortical attention; securing a balance of the inhibitory-facilitory state; and controlling sensory input to prevent deprivation and overload. In addition to preparation of the child's internal environment, the process also uses the external environment to assist in bringing strategies forth for purposeful use.

Facilitation

Facilitation is the continued successive application of the necessary stimulus to elicit an adaptive response. The facilitory process includes the use of external means applied during therapy for enhancement of an appropriate reaction. The stimulus may be the position, activity, and/or what the therapist may provide directly to the child in order to enhance both stability and mobility components. The major purpose of facilitation is to provide needed and appropriate input for association and differentiation. With distress/dysfunction, the system cannot associate and differentiate the pertinent elements of one action for adaptation to another. Thus, stimuli are used to provide opportunities for the association and differentiation components to occur. These vital components of adaptation are best facilitated through therapeutic control over "reciprocal interweaving," the reincorporation of several levels of actions through the spiraling process.

Adaptation

Adaptation as a therapeutic mode gives purpose to performance. Adaptation is the process of promoting a child's ability to differentiate those aspects of a behavior sequence pertinent for purposeful activity. Adaptation involves the connection of movements and events or actions to goals outside the body.

Therapeutic linking promotes association and differentiation by structuring and guiding the child's active participation. The therapist must have knowledge of those components, patterns, or sets from a behavior that a child needs to "call forth" for adapting to the demands of the environment. Therapeutic adaptation promotes the positive use of spatiotemporal stress and prevents distress.

The concepts and principles inherent in the therapeutic model of spiraling adaptation are next presented as theoretical statements regarding pediatric occupational therapy.

Theoretical Statements

1. Activities for and methods of therapeutic intervention involve the process of structuring events so that the person's transactions with those events will provide experiences that are purposeful and directed toward a goal.
2. Purposeful, goal-directed activities are selected to facilitate adaptation. The purposefulness of these activities are dependent upon the person's attention to and active participation with the events of the environment.
3. Purposeful, goal-directed activities are meaningful for the self-system when participation in the activity enhances maturation of the system by directing an adaptive response that is at a higher level than acquired functions.
4. Higher level adaptive responses result from the spiraling process of integrating lower level and present functions with higher level activities; thus, lower level acquired functions are modified.
5. The spiraling adaptation process of modifying lower level functions is dependent upon a certain degree of association and differentiation of specific components of the lower level functions with the activities being experienced.
6. Methods and activities are selected with the knowledge that adaptation spirals through primitive, transitional, and mature phases of strategies, behaviors, and activities that occur at the same time within different body segments.
7. Methods and activities of therapy are selected to facilitate "reciprocal interweaving" of strategies, behaviors, and activities for adaptation and the development of skill.

Identification of theoretical statements related to therapeutic methods and activities provides insight. It is an essential aspect of therapeutic reasoning. These statements provide specifications for an intervention program designed to facilitate adaptation through active participation in goal-directed, purposeful behaviors and activities.

Summary

Application of spatiotemporal adaptation theory provides the underlying concepts and principles from which treatment programs emerge. Concepts of theory and principles for treatment have been organized into a spiraling model involving the "reciprocal interweaving" of strategies, behaviors, and activities for adaptation to skilled performances. Inherent within the therapeutic model is the sensorimotor-sensory approach for enhancement of spatiotemporal adaptation. The use of goal-directed activities that are purposeful for the self-system is also central to this model.

The theory of normal and abnormal spiraling adaptation is expressed in this chapter in terms of theoretical concepts and statements. The identification of concepts and statements inherent to the theory may be useful for clinicians planning intervention, for educators teaching occupational therapy students, and for researchers investigating adaptation.

References

1. The Philosophical Base of Occupational Therapy. Resolution #531-79 Representative Assembly Minutes—59th Annual Conference. Am. J. Occup. Ther. 33:785, 1979.
2. Reilly, M. (ed.): Play as Exploratory Learning. Beverly Hills: Sage Pub. Co., 1974, p. 122.
3. Mosey, A. C.: Three Frames of Reference for Mental Health. Thorofare NJ: Charles B. Slack, 1970.
4. Takata, N.: The play milieu. Am. J. Occup. Ther. 25:281–284, 1971.
5. Florey, L.: Studies of play: Implications for growth, development, and for clinical practice. Am. J. Occup. Ther. 35:519–524, 1981.
6. Reilly, M.: Play as Exploratory Learning, Chapter 3.
7. Ibid., p. 145–148.
8. Erikson, E. H.: Childhood and Society. New York: WW Norton & Co., 1963, p. 259.
9. Ibid., p. 263.
10. Ibid., p. 211.
11. Gilfoyle, E., Grady, A., and Moore, J.: Children Adapt. Thorofare NJ: Charles B. Slack, 1981, p. 48.
12. Ayres, A. J.: Sensory Integration and Learning Disorders. Los Angeles: Western Psychological Services, 1972, p. 276.
13. Gilfoyle, Grady, and Moore: Children Adapt, Chapter 3.
14. Erikson, J.: Activity, Recovery, Growth. New York: WW Norton & Co, 1976, p. xi.
15. Ayres, A. J.: Sensory Integration and The Child. Los Angeles: Western Psychological Services, 1979, p. 184.
16. Holt, K.: Movement and child development. In Clinics in Developmental Medicine, no. 55. Philadelphia: J.B. Lippincott, 1975, pp. 10–15.

17. Flavel, J.: The Developmental Psychology of Jean Piaget. Princeton: Von Nostrand, 1963, pp. 85–90.
18. Twitchell, T. E.: Attitudinal reflexes. The Child with Central Nervous System Deficit. U.S. Printing Office, Children's Bureau Pub., No. 432, 1965, pp. 77–84.
19. Jacobs, M. J.: Development of normal motor behavior. Am. J. Phy. Med. 46:41–50, 1967.
20. Ibid., pp. 41–50.
21. Barr, M. L.: The Human Nervous System, ed. 2. New York: Harper & Row, 1974.
22. Eccles, J. C.: The Understanding of the Brain. New York: McGraw-Hill, 1973.
23. Crelin, E. S.: Functional Anatomy of the Newborn. New Haven: Yale University Press, 1973.
24. Gilfoyle, Grady, and Moore: Children Adapt, pp. 7–36.
25. Moore, J.: Concepts from the Neurobehavioral Sciences. Dubuque IA, Kendall Hunt, 1973, pp. 33–38.
26. Szumski, A. J.: Mechanisms underlying normal motor behavior. Am. J. Phys. Med. 46:52–68, 1967.
27. Twitchell, T. E.: Normal motor development. The Child with Central Nervous System Deficit. Children's Bureau Pub. no 432, US Dept of H.E.W., Washington DC, US Gov. Printing Office, 1965, pp. 85–89.
28. Moore: Concepts from the Neurobehavioral Sciences, pp. 34–35.
29. Szumski: Mechanisms underlying normal motor behavior, pp. 52–68.
30. Twitchell: Normal motor development, pp. 85–89.
31. McGraw, M. G.: The Neuromuscular Maturation of the Human Infant. New York: Hafner, 1966.
32. Gilfoyle, Grady, and Moore: Children Adapt, Chapter 2.
33. Hunt, J. McV.: Intelligence and Experience. New York: Ronald Press, 1961.
34. Jacobs, M. J.: Development of normal motor behavior.
35. Fantz, R., Fagan, J., and Miranda, S.: Early visual selectivity. In Cohen, L., and Salapatek, P. (eds.): Infant Perception: From Sensation to Cognition, Vol. 1. New York: Academic Press, 1975, pp. 249–343.
36. Taylor, E. (ed.): Selected Writings of John Hughlings Jackson. London: Hodder and Stoughton, 1932, p. 64.
37. Ibid., p. 64.
38. McGraw, M. G.: The Neuromuscular Maturation of the Human Infant.
39. Gilfoyle, Grady, and Moore: Children Adapt, Chapter 2.
40. Beintema, J. D.: A neurological study of newborn infants. Clinics in Developmental Medicine, no 28. Philadelphia: J. B. Lippincott, 1968.
41. André-Thomas: The neurological examination of the infant. In Clinics in Developmental Medicine, No. 1. Philadelphia: J. B. Lippincott, 1964, p. 1.
42. Beintema, A neurological study of newborn infants.
43. Penfield, W.: Mechanisms of voluntary movements. Brain 77:1–17, 1954.
44. McGraw, M. G.: The Neuromuscular Maturation of the Human Infant.
45. Penfield. Mechanisms of voluntary movements, pp. 1–17.
46. Szumski. Mechanisms underlying normal motor behavior.
47. Ibid., pp. 52–68.
48. Luria, A. R.: The functional organization of the brain. Sci. Am. 222:66–72, 78, 1970.
49. Eldred, E.: Peripheral receptors: Their excitation and relation to reflex patterns. Am. J. Phy. Med. 46:69–87, 1967.
50. Buchwald, J. S.: Exteroceptive reflexes and movement. Am. J. Phys. Med. 46:121–128, 1967.
51. Stelmach, G., and Larish, D.: A new perspective on motor skill automation. Research Quart. Exercise Sport 51:144–157, 1980.
52. Ewert, J. P.: The neural basis of visually guided behavior. Sci. Am. 230:34–42, 1974.
53. Gernandt, B. E.: Vestibular influence upon spinal reflex activity in myotatic, kinesthetic and vestibular mechanisms. Ciba Foundation Symposium. Boston: Little, Brown & Co. 1967.
54. Ibid.
55. Gillingham, K.: A Primer of Vestibular Function, Spatial Disorientation and Motion Sickness. Brooks Air Force Base, Texas, USAF School of Aerospace Medicine, 1966.
56. Fisher, E.: Factors affecting motor learning. Am J. Phys. Med. 46:511–516, 1967.
57. Penfield: Mechanisms of voluntary movements, pp. 1–77.
58. Szumski: Mechanisms underlying normal motor behavior, pp. 52–68.
59. Ibid., p. 64.
60. Flavel: The Developmental Psychology of Jean Piaget, p. 44.
61. Ibid., pp. 16–19.
62. Gilfoyle, Grady, and Moore: Children Adapt, pp. 4–5.
63. Buchwald, J. W.: General features of nervous system organization. Am. J. Phys. Med. 46:88–113, 1967.
64. Flavel: The Developmental Psychology of Jean Piaget, pp. 16–19.
65. Gilfoyle, Grady, and Moore: Children Adapt, p. 1.
66. Ibid., p. 79, 135–137.
67. Holt: Movement and child development, p. 12.
68. Gilfoyle, Grady, and Moore: Children Adapt, p. 47.
69. Ibid., p. 4.
70. Holt: Movement and child development, p. 10.
71. Jacobs: Development of normal motor behavior, pp. 41–50.
72. Flavel: The Developmental Psychology of Jean Piaget, pp. 16–19.
73. Gilfoyle, Grady, and Moore: Children Adapt, pp. 47–50.
74. McGraw: The Neuromuscular Maturation of the Human Infant.
75. Peiper, A.: Cerebral function in infancy and childhood. New York: Consultants Bureau, 1963.
76. Gilfoyle, Grady, and Moore: Children Adapt, pp. 58–62.
77. Beintema, D. J.: A neurological study of newborn infants.
78. Bobath, K.: The motor deficit in patients with cerebral

palsy. Clinics in Developmental Medicine, no. 23. Philadelphia: J. B. Lippincott, 1966, pp. 2–5.

79. Gilfoyle, Grady, and Moore: Children Adapt, pp. 135–137.
80. Turvey, M. T.: Preliminaries to a theory of action with reference to vision. In Perceiving, action and knowing, Toward an Ecologicalpsychological Theory. Hillsdale: Skew/Bransford, 1979, pp. 211–259.
81. Gilfoyle, Grady, and Moore: Children Adapt, pp. 51–54, 174–175.
82. Gilfoyle, Grady and Moore: Children Adapt, p. 65.
83. Ibid., p. 57.
84. Ibid., pp. 58, 79, 136–137.
85. Ibid., p. 137.
86. Ibid., p. 137.
87. Ibid., pp. 122–123.
88. Ibid., pp. 138–142.
89. Ibid., pp. 64–66.
90. Ibid., p. 66.
91. Ibid., p. 69.
92. Ibid., p. 58.
93. Ibid., pp. 58–62.
94. André-Thomas: The neurological examination of the infant, p. 11.
95. Gilfoyle, Grady, and Moore: pp. 122–123.
96. Ibid., pp. 143–144.
97. Ibid., pp. 66–73.
98. Ibid., pp. 146–149.
99. Ibid., p. 66.
100. Ibid., p. 149.
101. Ibid., p. 75.
102. Ibid., pp. 66, 76.
103. Ibid., pp. 122–123.
104. Ibid., p. 76.
105. Ibid., p. 137.
106. Harris, F. A.: Multiple-loop modulation of motor outflow: A physiological basis for facilitation techniques. Phys. Ther. 51:391–396, 1971.
107. Harris, F. A.: The brain is a distributed information processor. Am. J. Occup. Ther. 24:264–268, 1970.
108. Gilfoyle, Grady, and Moore: Children Adapt, p. 178.
109. Ibid., p. 178.
110. Ibid., p. 179.
111. Ibid., pp. 184–187.
112. Ibid., pp. 188–192.
113. Ibid., pp. 193–194.
114. Ibid., p. 177.
115. Ibid., pp. 178–179.
116. Ibid., p. 210.
117. Ibid., p. 210.
118. Ibid., pp. 183–194.
119. Ibid., pp. 207–216.
120. Ibid., p. 220.
121. Ibid., p. 220.
122. Ibid., p. 207.
123. Bobath, K., Bobath, B.: Cerebral palsy. In Pearson, P., Williams, C. (eds.): Physical Therapy Services in the Developmental Disabilities. Springfield IL, Charles C. Thomas, 1972, pp. 31–185.
124. Ames, L. B., Lig, F. S.: The developmental point of view with special reference to its principle of reciprocal neuromotor interweaving. J. Genet. Psychol. 105:195–209, 1964.
125. Gilfoyle, Grady, and Moore: Children Adapt, pp. 215–216.

CHAPTER 30

Pediatric Occupational Therapy *Patricia Ann Ramm*

Therapists share with parents a mutual fascination blended with an ongoing curiosity about the nature of children's behavior and development. As ever increasing numbers of occupational therapists enter the field of pediatric occupational therapy, there is a need for comprehensive material on this subject. But to provide such requires that a wide range of considerations be addressed.

Basic to the topic of pediatric occupational therapy is the need for understanding human functional systems and their interrelationships. The blending of this understanding with knowledge about the variety and types of pathologic or disabling conditions that make an impact upon young children form a foundation for understanding the effect of these conditions on children's functional abilities and behavior.

Functional disorders or differences, stemming from disease or other causes, have an intimate relationship with the child's dynamic developmental process, and they further expand the complexity of this topic.

Gilfoyle and Grady's theoretical framework of spatiotemporal adaptation has provided a major contribution to pediatric occupational therapy. The continuum of acquiring integrated sequences of move-

ment as a means of gaining skilled performance is fundamental to the subject of this section.

This broad yet intricate subject would nevertheless suffer, unless thought is given to the influence and interrelationship that parenting and care giving has on the child's state of health and function. Bonding, parenting skills, cultural values, health practices, and health knowledge are but a few of the more crucial factors that need equal consideration.

Basic professional preparation of occupational therapists is an important factor as well. There is professional agreement that the basic premise of occupational therapy necessitates therapists' first level of preparation should be as a generalist. Further, at the present time, the field of occupational therapy has no professionally identified specialization. Despite this, the practice of pediatric occupational therapy presents an immediate challenge to the entering or inexperienced therapist to respond swiftly and effectively to children's needs for services requiring highly specialized skills. Admittedly, this is not unique to occupational therapy pediatric practice alone, but it is a growing and expanding factor in this area of practice.

For example, in the area of pediatric occupational therapy assessment alone, the number, type, and complexity of examinations that therapists are providing is greater than in any other specific area of occupational therapy practice. A number of valuable occupational therapy pediatric screening and assessment mechanisms are now being readied by trial testing and standardization. Use of advanced occupational therapy assessment and diagnostic procedures has and will continue to result in exciting advances and expansion of occupational therapy pediatric services. Yet the present status of pediatric occupational therapy practice is that many unusually demanding and specialized skills are required of the entering therapist if quality care is to be assured.

In most areas of occupational therapy, changes are occurring in settings where services are being provided. This is especially so in pediatrics. The reasons for such changes are the major advances in medical science and litigated human rights guarantees.

Though pediatric occupational therapy services primarily address the human condition, such services often face impositions based on the condition of the service setting. It would be true to say that the parameters of the professional services are closely tied to the delivery system or type of health service system available to the therapist. Though the traditional role of pediatric practice continues to exist in acute and convalescent care hospitals, large numbers of therapists are extending pediatric occupational therapy services to advance functional performance of children in community and educational programs. Viewing pediatric occupational therapy on a developmental continuum relating to the model depicted by Johnson expands the subject's perspective to include prevention, early detection, remediation, treatment, restoration, referral, and health maintenance as components of that practice.[1] This perspective underscores the variety of facilities and service settings that therapists are encountering in this field of practice. Home settings, neonatal intensive care units, well-child clinics, infant-parent centers, private or public school programs, regional educational service centers, specialized pediatric intermediate care units, and state sponsored schools for the deaf and blind are appropriately utilizing occupational therapy services. Experienced pediatric occupational therapists are developing their own private clinics specializing in services for children with learning disabilities, and they are finding their services well utilized.

Each of these examples, including hospital-based programs, offer uniquely important, though differing, opportunities for practice. Settings vary in structure from informal to highly technical and complex systems. It is the ethical responsibility of each therapist to offer occupational therapy knowledge and skill appropriate to the client's needs, despite the constraints of settings and service systems. It is an equally important responsibility of each therapist to use the occupational therapy knowledge base to work collaboratively in attaining the overall constructive mission of each particular health delivery system.

Expanded examples of indirect but valuable pediatric occupational therapy services include the following:

1. screening of populations to identify the children who need services;
2. consulting with other related professionals or agencies who need services;
3. educating parents, teachers, and care-givers to influence children's development.

In this chapter, children are viewed in a variety of dimensions—as unique human beings living with different kinds of parents, families, and living in different kinds of conditions—the whole of which is affected by physical, emotional, and/or social insult. To avoid any tendency to oversimplify or fragment the topic, a schematically based model (Fig. 30-1) is presented to depict the relationship of occupational therapy to children, their family, or care-giver, when the children are experiencing a human system dysfunction. The model indicates broad types of insults and emphasizes consideration of the key functional systems therapists most frequently address. Included in this diagram are initiating points for occupational therapy services and linking of restorative analysis or outcome determination for termination, referral, or continued services with or without change.

Insult

In this model, the human organism under consideration is the young child. Basic consideration of insult factors has been categorized into three major components that are biological, psychological, or social in nature. But children and adults alike rarely experience an insult that is isolated and that does not have related consequences to the human being overall. Biological insults under consideration often relate to physical dysfunction stemming from disease, injury, genetic, structural, or chemical factors. Psychological and sociological factors are entwined and are frequently indigenous to the pediatric occupational therapy process. Psychologically, harm may occur to any child regardless of economic condition and opportunity. Social disadvantages have a complex effect on children both negatively and in some cases

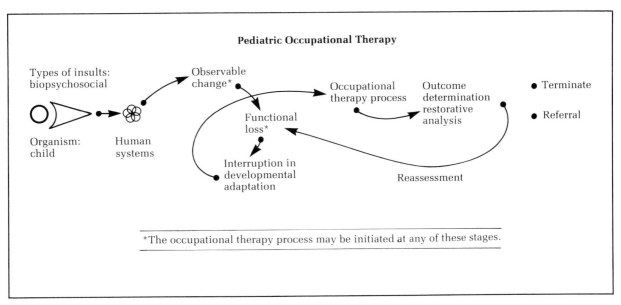

Figure 30-1. A model depicting the interrelationship of the occupational therapy process to biopsychosocial insult to human (child) function.

paradoxically, because of the human support mechanisms that may be available. These support mechanisms may provide an impetus for advantageous change whether psychological or social or both through health providing services.

Human Functional Systems

A simplification of key human systems used in the conceptual models are listed together with the function of each system in Table 30-1. Included are observable change outcomes when such systems are insulted. This list of changes is representative but they should not be considered all inclusive.

The Pediatric Occupational Therapy Process

The occupational therapy process is a complex system that must be ordered in terms of achieving improved functional and behavioral goals if the therapist is to achieve beneficial outcomes for pediatric clients and their families. Figure 30-2 depicts the various stages of the process.

A subsequent discussion of these stages are present in general terms. Chapter 31, entitled "Occupa-

tional Therapy Process in Specific Pediatric Conditions" provides the following:
- case discussion
- schematic drawing of the individualized child-oriented problems and treatment or intervention program
- narrative or graphic information illustrating and describing an appropriate occupational therapy evaluation, plans, and goal setting/objectives
- procedures for accomplishing these identified goals
- readjustments that are further discussed and diagrammed in some cases.

Evaluation

The key to the occupational therapy process is evaluation. A diagram that identifies key factors that influence children's health and developmental potential is presented in Figure 30-3. In the broadest sense, this diagram is a reminder that while on one hand the occupational therapy evaluation addresses a great number of these factors (see items in Fig. 30-3); on the other hand, the information this process yields closely relates to information being processed by other involved professionals or persons. The effectiveness of the evaluation process will be augmented

Table 30-1

Human System	Function	Observable Changes
Circulatory Cardio	Oxygenation	1. Dyspnea (difficulty with breathing, especially during feeding) 2. Edema (fluid retention) 3. Cyanosis (bluing of nailbeds, lips, or fat) 4. Fatigue 5. Underweight and/or poor weight gain 6. Pallor 7. Unexplained vomiting 8. Shallow, grunting, or rapid respiration 9. Cough 10. Clubbing of fingers 11. Wheezing 12. Periodic apnea 13. Gagging 14. Flaring of nostrils
Gastrointestinal/Urinary	Digestive/Absorption/ Filtration/Elimination process	1. Obesity or poor weight gain 2. Milk tolerance 3. Edema 4. Nausea/vomiting 5. Anorexia (poor appetite) 6. Diarrhea/constipation 7. Fever 8. Abdominal/flank/pubic tenderness 9. Lethargy/weakness 10. Abnormal skin texture
Endocrine/Metabolic	Maintenance of Homeostasis	1. Poor weight gain 2. Abnormal growth patterns 3. Excessive thirst/urination 4. Abnormal skin texture 5. Sweating 6. Abnormal activity (state) levels (*i.e.,* hypo-hyper) 7. Alterations in attention/attention behavior
Musculoskeletal	Structural Framework	1. Joint abnormality 2. Asymmetrical posture 3. Stiff/difficult movement 4. Pain in joints on movement or handling 5. Swelling of joints 6. Inability to feed effectively (poor suck ability) 7. Lack of smooth, coordinated movement 8. Congenital abnormalities
Neurological	Regulation of Behavior/ Physiological Function	1. Seizures 2. Tremor 3. Alterations in sensation 4. Hypotonia (ragdoll) 5. Hypertonia (stiff) 6. Sudden "startle-like" movements 7. Jerky random movement 8. Attention alerting disturbances 9. Sleep pattern disturbances 10. Lack of smooth coordinated movement 11. Congenital abnormalities 12. Visual, hearing deficiency, muteness 13. Poor feeding

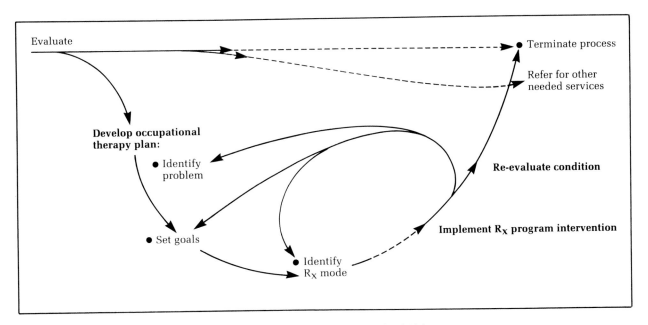

Figure 30-2. Model of the occupational therapy process with children.

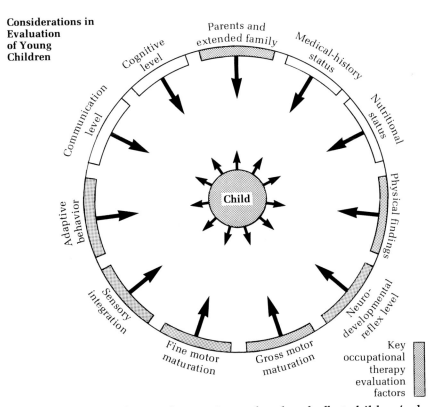

Figure 30-3. A diagram of key factors that are interrelated and affect children's development and behavior.

if a true climate of collaboration and coordination is present.

Fundamentally, the evaluation process in any endeavor is the foundation for any change effectiveness. In pediatric occupational therapy, the emergence of great numbers of useful evaluation instruments or tools that have differing types of focus demand therapists' careful attention. In the past, it has been suggested by Lewke[2] that therapists and other related health providers often err in the appropriate selection of evaluation measures. An error of this nature will diminish the effectiveness of the occupational therapy process. Therefore, it is essential that therapists correctly administer the test measures that are standardized with proven validity and reliability, and that they clearly understand the population studied and the intended use for such tests, and that proven measurements of error be considered. Figure 30-4 presents useful tests and measures and the categories that each test measures or addresses. A description of features and sources of many of these tests is included in Chapter 11.

Often a therapist finds that decisions about the treatment plan for the child will need to take into account less tangible influences identified through observation and judgment of the child, the family, and the child's environment. Sample questions that guide the therapist's investigative thinking into these less tangible but fruitful avenues of consideration are listed below:

- What is the child's state (excitation) level primarily? Is there a lack of or marked increase in the alteration of the child's state level?
- Are there significant alterations in the child's level of comfort?
- Are the child's coping patterns maladaptive?
- Is the family coping pattern effective?
- Is the family structure supportive?
- Is there a grieving process present with the family or possibly with the child? Is it acute, anticipatory, or delayed?
- Is there a potential for injury, trauma, or further complication?
- Is there a need for or a lack of knowledge about the child's condition?
- Is there noncompliance with the helping process? If so, why?
- What is the level of parenting skills?
- Are there nutritional alterations?
- Is there dysrhythm in the sleep-rest cycle of the child, mother, or care giver?
- Is there sensory or social isolation?
- Are thought processes impaired?
- Is there a communication impairment?

Again, these questions are presented as samples to encourage and direct therapists to fully address less tangible but related and important factors that often clarify the occupational therapy plan and the ordering of therapists' goals.

To complete the evaluative stages of the occupational therapy process, the therapist must address and synthesize a multiplicity of data collected relating to the child's status:
1. physical
2. neurodevelopmental
3. motor performance
4. sensory integration
5. adaptive behavior

Figure 30-5 is an example of a comprehensive evaluation tool useful in the identification of a young child's developmental abilities. This type of assessment enables therapists to pinpoint levels of reflex maturation, sensory integration, gross and fine motor skill attainments in daily living skills as a basis for planning the occupational therapy program. This data must be viewed and interrelated with information about the child's social, cultural, and familial condition. From this synthesis a tentative plan of treatment should be followed by problem identification objectives and R$_x$ procedures. This synthesizing process is frequently the most complicated stage of work for therapists. If this stage of work is well executed, the ordering of occupational therapy processes, goals, objectives, and procedures will advance the child's functional ability to the highest level of expectation.

The Occupational Therapy Plan

The occupational therapy plan evolves from the occupational therapy evaluation process identifying strengths and weaknesses that the child is experiencing and that may influence the child's world. The beginning of the occupational therapy plan evolves from these identified factors. Problems should be clarified as stated goals. Many times broad goal statements will be needed as a guide in the overall occupational therapy plan. To achieve these major goals, therapists must delineate more specific short-range goals or objectives that can be clearly stated as measurable objectives. From such objectives, treatment procedures and modes can be planned to implement the objectives and to adjust procedures in an orderly system.

Adjustment of therapeutic goals, objectives, and methods for attaining such are based on the success or lack of success in reaching these treatment objectives. Objectives achieved or not achieved require careful examination by occupational therapists providing direct services, as well as by supervisors and administrator-managers of occupational therapy ser-

(*text continues on page 587*)

	Develop-mental	Motor function or reflex	Sensory integra-tion	Neuro-physio-logical	Other (specify)
Barraga-Diagnostic Assessment Procedure (of Efficiency of Visual Function)	X				X(use of vision & visually impaired children)
Bayley Scale of Infant De-velopment	X				
Callier-Azusa Scale	X				X(assessment of multi-handicapped children.)
Denver Developmental Screening Test—Revised	X				
Developmental Assessment for the Newborn or High Risk Infant	X	X	X	X	
Beery's Developmental Test of Visual Motor Integration			X		
Gesell Developmental Tests	X				
Gestational Age Assessment	X				X(cutaneous musculo-skeletal)
Goodenough-Harris: Drawing Test			X		X(cognitive maturation)
Illinois Test of Psycholinguistic Abilities			X		X(cognitive)
Joint Mobility		X			X(musculo-skeletal)
Miller Assessment for Pre-schoolers	X	X	X	X	X(learning potential)
Neonatal Behavioral Assessment Scale (Brazelton)	X	X	X		
Neurological Assessment during the First Year of Life (Amile-Tison)	X	X	X	X	
Ordinal Scales of Infant Psycho-logical Development (Uzgaris-Hunt)	X	X	X		
Parent Denver Questionnaire	X				X(parent stimulation)
Pre-Term Behavioral Assessment Scale (Als-Brazelton)	X		X	X	
Reflexes in Motor Development (Crutchfield, Barnes, Heriza)		X			
Southern California Sensory Inte-gration Tests	X	X	X	X	
Southern California Postrotary Nystagmus Test			X		

Figure 30-4. Frequently used tests and measures by categories.

Infant-Parent Training Program
Sensory Motor Integration Assessment

Code: 1 + 5 = Present in increasing strength

A = Absent

(#) = Abnormally present

(A) = Abnormally absent

Child's name _____
Birthdate _____
Diagnosis _____
Referral source _____
Examiners _____

	Date	C.A.	M.A.	M.Q.
Test 1				
Test 2				
Test 3				
Test 4				

Comments

I. Neuromuscular Reflex and Gross Motor Development

Position	Reflex				
1. sup	Rooting				1.
2. sup	Sucking				2.
3. sup	Traction				3.
4. sup	Moro				4.
5. sup	Crossed extension				5.
6. sup	Flexor withdrawal				6.
7. sup	Plantar grasp				7.
8. pr	Galant				8.
9. sup	Neonatal neck righting				9.
10. vert	Plantar placing legs				10.
11. vert	Neonatal positive support				11.
12. vert	Spontaneous stepping				12.
13.	Tonic labyrinthine prone				13.
14.	Supine				14.
15. vert	Plantar placing arms				15.
16.	ATNR				16.
17. sup	Palmar grasp				17.
18. sup	Avoidance reaction				18.
19.	Labyrinthine righting prone				19.
20.	Supine				20.
21.	Tilting				21.
22.	Optical righting prone				22.
23.	Supine				23.
24.	Tilting				24.
25. pr	Landau				25.
26. vert	Visual placing arms				26.
27. vert	Visual placing legs				27.
28.	STNR				28.
29. sup	Neck righting				29.
30. sup	Body righting				30.
31.	Instinctual grasp				31.
32.	Equilibrium prone				32.
33. vert	Positive support				33.
34. vert	Protective extension forward				34.
35. sit	Protective extension sideways				35.
36.	Equilibrium supine				36.
37.	Equilibrium sitting				37.
38. sit	Protective extension backwards				38.
39.	Equilibrium Quadriped				39.
40.	Equilibrium standing				40.
41. std	Staggering reaction (protective)				41.

Grading: 1 2 3 4

Gestational age/wks: 28 32 34 35 36 37

Age in months: 0 1 2 3 4 5 6 7 8 9 10 11 12 13 15 18 21 24 30 36 48 60

Figure 30-5. Infant-Parent Training Program.

	Voluntary activity**	
1. pr	Lifts head slightly	1.
2. sup	Rolls part way to side	2.
3. sit	Head bobs erect	3.
4. pr	Suspension, lifts head	4.
5. sup	Symmetrical posture	5.
6. pr	Weight on forearms	6.
7. sit	Head steady	7.
8. pr	Lifts head 90 degrees, turns	8.
9. sup	Pulled to sit, no head lag	9.
10. sup	Rolls to side	10.
11. pr	Arms extended, chest raised	11.
12. sup pr	Rolls both ways	12.
13. sup	Lifts legs high in extension	13.
14. sup	Pulled to sit, assists	14.
15. sup	Lifts head	15.
16. sit	Sits erect momentarily	16.
17. std	Bears large part of weight	17.
18. sit	Leans on hands briefly	18.
19. std	Stands briefly, hands held	19.
20. pr	Pivots	20.
21. sit	Sits steadily	21.
22. std	Stands holding rail	22.
23. sit	To hands and knees	23.
24. sit	Leans forward, re-erects	24.
25. pr	Crawling	25.
26. std	Pulls to feet at rail	26.
27. pr	Raises and lowers from sit	27.
28. pr sit	Creeps and hitches	28.
29. std	At rail lifts foot	29.
30. sit	Pivots in sitting	30.
31. std	Cruises	31.
32. std	Walks hand held	32.
33. std	Lowers to floor from stand	33.
34. std	Walks, one hand held	34.
35. kn	Assumes, maintains kneeling	35.
36. std	Walks few steps alone	36.
37. std	Stands momentarily alone	37.
38. std	Walks, starts, stops	38.
39. std	Stands independently	39.
40. pr	Creeps upstairs	40.
41. std	Runs stiffly	41.
42. std	Squats in play	42.
43. std	Upstairs, one hand held	43.
44. std	Small chair, seats self	44.
45. std	Downstairs, one hand held	45.
46. std	Upstairs, holds rail	46.
47. std	Walks and runs	47.
48. std	Up, down stairs, marks time	48.
49. std	Kicks large ball	49.
50. std	Jumps with both feet	50.
51. std	Walks backwards	51.
52. std	Walks on tiptoe	52.
53. std	Rides tricycle	53.
54. std	One foot, momentarily	54.
55. std	Jumps high	55.
56. std	Upstairs, alternate feet	56.
57. std	Jumps distance	57.
58. std	Stands on one foot	58.
59. std	Downstairs, alternate feet	59.
60. std	Hops on one foot	60.

**Criteria based on Hoskins, T.A., Squires, J.E., Dev. assessment, Phys. Ther., 53:117-126, 1973.

Figure 30-5. (*continued*)

II. Physical Findings

A. Posture
1. _____
2. _____
3. _____
4. _____

B. Muscle tone
1. _____
2. _____
3. _____
4. _____

C. Range of motion
1. _____
2. _____
3. _____
4. _____

	Date	C.A.	F.M.A.	F.M.Q.
Test 1				
Test 2				
Test 3				
Test 4				

D. Adaptive appliances
1. _____
2. _____
3. _____
4. _____

E. Other findings or comments
1. _____
2. _____
3. _____
4. _____

III. Activities of Daily Living

A. Feeding

Method
1. _____
2. _____
3. _____
4. _____

Quantity
1. _____
2. _____
3. _____
4. _____

Texture
1. _____
2. _____
3. _____
4. _____

Sensitivity
1. _____
2. _____
3. _____
4. _____

Assistance devices indicated _____

Reflexive feeding

	Grading			
	1	2	3	4

0–life
1. Gag reflex
2. Rooting
3. Suckling

1–5 mos.
1. Tongue protrusion
2. Bite reflex
3. Suck–swallow

Figure 30-5. (*continued*)

Voluntary feeding

	1	2	3	4
4 mos. 1. Lip closure				
2. Sucking				
3. Anticipates food on sight				
6–9 mos. 1. Vertical chewing				
2. Holds own bottle				
9 mos. 1. Rotary chewing				
2. Lateral tongue movement				
3. Tongue protraction				
4. Tongue retraction				
5. Tongue to palate				
6. Finger feeding				
12 mos. 1. Grasps spoon (picks up)				
2. Drooling controlled except at meals				
3. Drinks from cup (if held)				
15 mos. 1. Holds cup; quickly tips				
2. Inserts spoon in dish; poor filling				
3. Spoon to mouth; may turn over				
18 mos. 1. Fills spoon with food				
2. Drinks from cup, 2-handed				
3. Diff. inserting spoon				
4. Considerable spilling				
2 yr. 1. Drinks cup, 1-hd. repl. cup				
2. Feeds self from spoon				
3. Automatic swallowing				
3 yr. 1. Feeds self c̄ spoon; may spill some				
4 yr. 1. Feeds self with fork				

B. Dressing

	1	2	3	4
1 yr. 1. Cooperates in dressing				
2. Removes socks (from toe)				
2 yr. 1. Removes shoe (untied)				
2. Pushes down pants and removes				

C. Grooming

	1	2	3	4
2 yr. 1. Washes, dries hands (partl.)				
2. Wipes face				

D. Written communication

	1	2	3	4
1 yr. 1. Discr. use of crayon				
18 mos. 1. Spontaneous scribbling				
2 yr. 1. Vert.-horiz. patterns				
3 yr. 1. Copies circles				
2. Copies vertical				
3. Copies horizontal				
4. Imitates X				

Comments

1. _____
2. _____
3. _____
4. _____

Figure 30-5. (*continued*)

IV. Upper Extremity Functional Activities

A. Prehension and bilateral hand usage

			Grading			
			1	2	3	4
1–4 mos.	1. Both hands fisted	R				
		L				
	2. Mass motor activity reac.	R				
		L				
	3. Hands open	R				
		L				
	4. Plays regarding hands	R				
		L				
	5. Brings hands to mouth	R				
		L				
4–8 mos. Voluntary grasp pronation	1. Palmar	R				
		L				
	2. Ulnar	R				
		L				
6 mos. Eye-hand coordination	1. Arms used, shoulder cont.	R				
		L				
	2. Raking grasp	R				
		L				
	3. Transfers object	R				
		L				
7 mos.	1. Radial palmar grasp	R				
		L				
8 mos.	1. Lateral pinch	R				
		L				
9 mos.	1. Crude pincer grasp	R				
		L				
10 mos.	1. Pikes finger in hole	R				
		L				
12 mos.	1. Precise pincer	R				
		L				
	2. Bangs 2 obj. together	R				
		L				
	3. Supinated grasp develop.	R				
		L				
12 mos. con't.	4. Reaches for large object, both arms	R				
		L				
	5. Brings 1" cube over another					

		Grading			
		1	2	3	4
15 mos.	1. Places objects in and out of container				
18 mos.	1. Builds 3-blk. tower				
	2. Tosses ball undir.				
	3. Puts peg in 1" hole				
	4. Turns pg. 2-3 at time				
2 yr.	1. Turns pg. 1 at time				
	2. Strings beads (1")				
	3. Builds 6-blk. tower				
	4. Throws				
	5. Hand pref. R L				
3 yr.	1. Builds 9-blk. tower				
	2. Assists with 1 hand				
	3. Screws lid on jar				
	4. 10 pellets in bottle (30 sec.)				
	5. Grasps w/extended wrist and good thumb opposition				
	6. Turns door knob with forearm rotation				
	7. Imitates cube bridge				

Comments:

1. _____

2. _____

3. _____

4. _____

Figure 30-5. (continued)

V. Sensory Integration

A. Tactile processing

Comments   1. _____   2. _____   3. _____   4. _____

Seeking   1. _____   2. _____   3. _____   4. _____

Avoids/withdraws   1. _____   2. _____   3. _____   4. _____

B. Postural adaptation

Comments   1. _____   2. _____   3. _____   4. _____

Seeking reinforcements   1. _____   2. _____   3. _____   4. _____

Withdraws/insecure   1. _____   2. _____   3. _____   4. _____

Phasic/lacks midline
stability   1. _____   2. _____   3. _____   4. _____

C. Bilateral motor integration

Comments   1. _____   2. _____   3. _____   4. _____

Midline   1. R-L _____ L-R _____   2. R-L _____ L-R _____   3. R-L _____ L-R _____   4. R-L _____ L-R _____

Head rotation   1. _____   2. _____   3. _____   4. _____

Trunk rotation   1. _____   2. _____   3. _____   4. _____

D. Motor planning

Comments   1. _____   2. _____   3. _____   4. _____

Moves to pursue object
efficiently   1. _____   2. _____   3. _____   4. _____

Mounts efficiently   1. _____   2. _____   3. _____   4. _____

Reproduces imitative   1. _____   2. _____   3. _____   4. _____

E. Visual processing

Comments   1. _____   2. _____   3. _____   4. _____

Eye preference   R _____ L _____   R _____ L _____   R _____ L _____   R _____ L _____

Fixates on light   1. _____   2. _____   3. _____   4. _____

Uses neck rot. to pur.   1. _____   2. _____   3. _____   4. _____

Isol. eye move. to pur.   1. _____   2. _____   3. _____   4. _____

Eyes follow past 90°   1. _____   2. _____   3. _____   4. _____

Converges   1. _____   2. _____   3. _____   4. _____

Midline disturbance   1. _____   2. _____   3. _____   4. _____

Quality of ex. ocular
pursuit   1. _____   2. _____   3. _____   4. _____

Postrotary nystagmus   1. _____   2. _____   3. _____   4. _____

   1. L _____   2. L _____   3. L _____   4. L _____

   1. R _____   2. R _____   3. R _____   4. R _____

Figure 30-5. (*continued*)

F. Auditory-language processing

Comments _____

		Grading		
	1	2	3	4

1 mo.   Responds to sound

3 mos.   Vocal noise, resembles speech

4 mos.   Turns to noise and voice

6 mos.   Distinguishes angry/friendly voice

9 mos.   Comprehends a few gestures

10 mos. Comprehends and waves "bye-bye"

24 mos. Attains 50 word vocabulary or 2-word sentences;
         Im. absent models; pretends; reconstructs memories

30 mos. 3-word sentences

36 mos. Adult grammatical structure

G. Comments:

1. _____

   _____

2. _____

   _____

3. _____

   _____

4. _____

   _____

Figure 30-5. (*continued*)

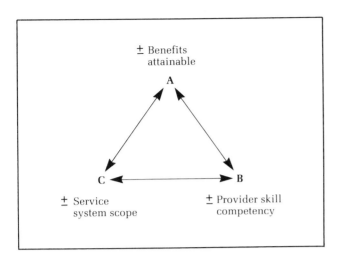

± Benefits
attainable

A

C ⟷ B

± Service
system scope

± Provider skill
competency

Figure 30-6. (*A*) Problems in attainment of benefits often relate to realistic goal setting. Competent evaluation, and ability to synthesize information and to prioritize client needs are a primary consideration.

(*B*) Problems in the actual skills of providers once identified often can be addressed through staff education whether group or individual, and when possible through hands on experience.

Above and beyond actual therapeutic competency, therapists need to consider less tangible factors of performance. Competent skills and sensitivity in touching, handling, communicating, and initiating voluntary movement with young children supersede all other treatment procedures in importance. Some therapists possess these abilities innately. Others are conscious of the importance of such skills and may find the greatest help in acquiring such is facilitated through experience with therapists who demonstrate or provide models of such skills.

(*C*) The reality of present pediatric occupational therapy practice in enlarging areas of the service delivery system was previously discussed in the introduction of this section. The lack of attainment of therapeutic goals because of service delivery limitations should be analyzed on the following basic factors: (1) Can the system be modified so that treatment objectives and procedures can be implemented? (2) If the system cannot be modified, and direct R_x measures based on sound objectives and goals are unrealistic, further considerations should be made of the value of consultative or educational process. Refer to the chapter on Health Systems in this text for further information.

vice programs. Therapeutic goal achievement may be directly related to the actual quality of the service provided, or may be complicated by other factors inherent in the service system.

Alterations in the therapeutic plan, because of the lack or partial attainment of objectives, should address the following questions:

- Within the goal or objective-setting process were the benefits (or objectives) realistically attainable?
- Within the skill level of the service provider, were the goals–objectives achievable?
- Within the structure and scope of the service delivery system, was the attainment of the goals–objectives possible?

Figure 30-6 is presented to assist and encourage this type of feasibility analysis as a means of refining and improving therapeutic planning for more effective treatment results.

References

1. Johnson, J. A.: Delegate assembly address—April 19, 1976. In Hopkins, H. L. and Smith, H. D. (eds.): Willard and Spackman's Occupational Therapy, ed. 5 Philadelphia: J. B. Lippincott Co., 1978, pp. 111.
2. Lewke, J. H.: Current practices in evaluating motor behavior of disabled children. Am. J. Occup. Ther. 30:7, 403–419, 1976.

CHAPTER 31

The Occupational Therapy Process —In Specific Pediatric Conditions

Patricia Ann Ramm

The following chapter presents specific pediatric conditions that occupational therapists often address. These specific diagnostic topics are presented by means of the conceptual model, in most cases, so that equal emphasis is placed on the causative nature of the condition, the characteristics of the condition, and the manner in which an individual child within his or her living condition is affected. Preliminary, history, background, and evaluation information is blended in the evaluation stage to advance the actual implementation of the therapeutic intervention or treatment process. In most conditions, an illustration of the appropriate treatment processes is presented in relation to the therapeutic goals and objectives. Frequently, further evaluation and adjustments to the plan, goals, and methods are also presented to clarify the therapeutic process as an ongoing basis.

Occupational Therapy with Neonates or Infant Services

With the expanding, complex service delivery model available to the neonate today, it is imperative that occupational therapy services be established as a vital part of this health service in nurturing the frail infant and in promoting interaction of the family. The role of the occupational therapist in this highly specialized service delivery model can be as multifaceted as the practice itself. The skills needed by the occupational therapist in this field are directly related to the entry point of occupational therapy services in this service continuum. There are three major areas of neonatal involvement that occupational therapists may be asked to provide:

1. Direct services to the infant in the special care unit.
2. Consultation services to house staff and discharge planning.
3. Follow-up services—posthospital discharge.

Each occupational therapy service model will be presented through discussion and case study illustration.

Figure 31-1, Neonatal Community Follow-up Services, depicts by flow chart the range and order of services needed by neonates, depending on the degree of physical involvement or impairment. Before any level of intervention can be initiated, there are basic considerations that must be addressed by the occupational therapist. They include, but are not limited to, the following:

1. Physical Plant (in hospital)
   - Nursery structure—policies and procedures

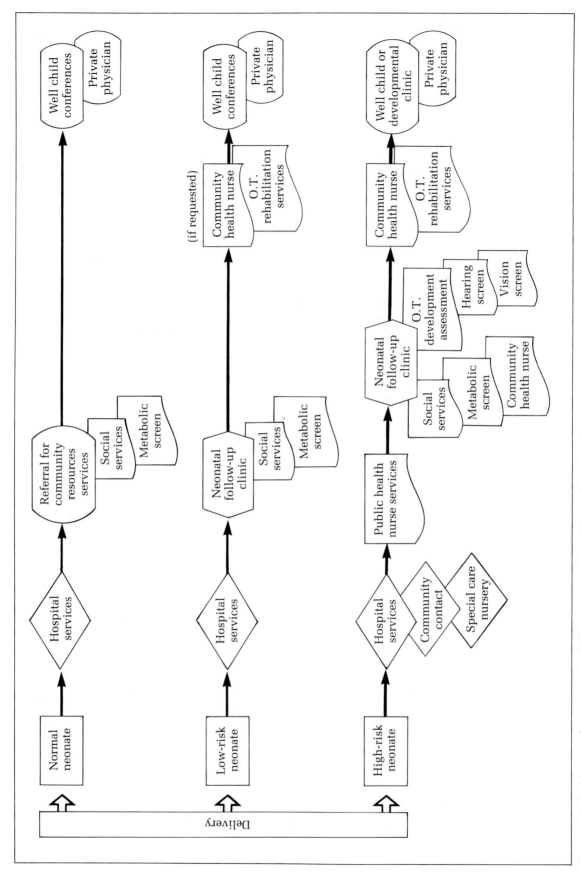

Figure 31-1. Neonatal community follow-up services (flow of services).

- Hospital policies governing service delivery
- Responsible agent for the unit management
- Responsible agent for the medical care of the child
2. Family and Care Givers
   - Who are they?
   - Do they visit?
   - What is their understanding of the infant's condition?
   - What is their level of acceptance and/or grief?
   - Who is responsible for primary care (hour by hour) to the infant? In hospital? At home or community?
   - Goals or expectations for the infant.
3. Medical/Health
   - Develop a knowledge base regarding conditions commonly treated in special care unit.
   - Become skilled in determining developmental expectations based on current medical status.
   - Become skilled in predicting developmental outcomes based on hard assessment data.
   - Be aware of *medical* priorities. An occupational therapist's intervention may need to be delayed.
   - Remember that the therapist is only one part of a very specialized team—all team members provide valuable knowledge and skill in assisting the neonate's survival.
   - Develop an understanding of the neonatal systems as a means of advancing each infant's development through a system of continued care.
4. Assessment
   A comprehensive developmental assessment in the nursery should include the eight areas presented in the Developmental Assessment for the Newborn or High-Risk Infant, Figure 31-2, which are:
   - Tonus and postural behavior
   - Reflex-response behaviors
   - Orthopedic considerations
   - Asymmetry items
   - Adaptive responses
   - Sensory motor/sensory integration
   - Nasal-oral/feeding functions
   - Social-medical history

Occupational Therapy in Direct Special Care Nursery Services

Case Study A

Greg was born prematurely at 30 weeks of gestation. He was the first child of a 31-year-old white female. The mother had received limited prenatal care, and she had planned a home delivery for her child because she was opposed to "modern medicine" and hospital care in general.

At birth Greg weighed 1310 gm (2 lb,14.2 oz) and was border-line appropriate size for his gestational age. His admitting diagnosis to the special care unit was respiratory distress syndrome secondary to prematurity. Greg's first week in the unit was filled with life-threatening episodes. He continued to have spells of apnea, and he exhibited minor seizure activity for the first 4 weeks of life. Once he was medically stable, an occupational therapy assessment and intervention program was requested. See Figure 31-3 for detailed findings.

At the time of evaluation, Greg's chronological age was 4 weeks compared to his minus 8 week gestational age. Nevertheless, his reflexive behavior was found to be within normal limits, but postural responses and tone appeared asymmetrical and slightly increased on the right. He continued to be difficult to handle and to hold at times. On occasion he would appear to become "hyperalert." The slightest additional stimuli would increase his activity level and the subsequent amount of intervention required to calm him.

Greg's mother appeared to have great difficulty in dealing with the nursery environment and her child's fragile condition. The act of touching her child seemed to require great effort. Greg usually cried when his mother did touch him, but he would calm for nursery personnel. This reinforced his mother's sense of inadequacy and insecurity in the situation.

The mother required considerable support and assistance in understanding her son's current environment. A systematic approach to the mother's growing process had to be undertaken as well as assisting her move through her grieving process. During this early phase, the mother continued to exhibit anger and bargaining as part of her grief. Although she gradually accepted the occupational therapist as her resource, and began to relax around the therapist, she remained skeptical of the other nursery personnel and fearful of the physician. The occupational therapist was able to share positive aspects about Greg's condition with her, as a means of reducing her anxiety relating to her child's pathological problems. Occupational therapy recommendations included the following:
1. Hold a conference with the mother regarding positive interactions she can have with her son.
2. Provide a framework for mother to interact with her son.
3. Normalize environment with inhibition activities.
4. Continue to monitor the occupational therapy

(*text continues on page 594*)

<table>
<tr><td colspan="2" align="center">

Developmental Assessment for the Newborn or High-risk Infant
Nursery and Follow-up

</td></tr>
</table>

Social History

Name: _____   Parent's Name:_____

MR#:_____   APGAR:_____   Address _____

DOB:_____G.A.:_____Adjust:_____   _____

B.W._____ B.L.:_____B.H.C.:_____   Phone_____

Hospital: _____   _____

Referring Physician:_____   Area_____WCC_____PHN_____

Attending Physician: _____   Medical Hx. 1°D$_x$ _____

Subs. Pediatrician: _____   2°D$_x$ _____

Address: _____   _____

_____   _____

Scoring Key

+ = Present   UE = Upper extremity   Sym = Symmetrical
0 = Absent   LE = Lower extremity   Asym = Asymmetrical
< = Decreased/diminished   R = Right   NT = Not tested
> = Increased/emerging   L = Left   # = Screening
WNL = Within Normal limits

Assessment

	1	2	3	4
C.A.				
G.A.				
Date				
Exam.				

I. Tonus and Pastural Behavior

	+ present	0 absent
Hypertonia Elv. Palpe. Sup.		
Setting Sun Sign		
Marked Strabismus		
Sustained Nystagmus		
Hypertonicity—Neck Ext.		
Opisthotomus		
Asym Posture of Limbs $\frac{R}{L}$		
Facial Sasym. $\frac{R}{L}$		
Ankle Clonus $\frac{R}{L}$		
Postural Tone: Hyper.		
(static) Hypo-		
Fluc.		
Postural Tone: Hyper.		
(dynamic) Hypo.		
Fluc.		
Other: _____		

State (describe)

1. Deep sleep   2. Light sleep   3. Drowsy
4. Quiet alert   5. Active alert   6. Crying

Initial		
Intermediate		
Ending		
Assess. Time		

II. Reflex/Response Behavior

Rooting G28→3m				
Sucking G28→7m				
Moro G28→7m				
Cros. Ext. G28→1–2m				
Galant G32→2m				
Neo Nck Rtg. G34→4–5m				
Placing G34→1–3m				
Neo Posit. Supp.				
Auto Walking G37→2m				
ATNR (post) B→3m				
ATNR (evoke) B→4–6m				
TLR (prone) B→4m				
TLR (supine) B→4m				
Palmar Gsp. B→4m				
Planter Gsp. B→10m				
Landau 1–4→12–18m				
Neck Rtg. 4–6m→5y				
Body Rtg. 4–6m→5y				
Pos. Supp. 3→8m				
Optical Rtg. (pr) 2m→				
(supine) 6m→				
(lateral) 8m→				
Lateral Prop. 7–8m→				
Parachute 8–9m→				

(C) CGJ-MAN '80
Adapted from CGJ-CFR '78/80

Figure 31-2. Developmental assessment for the newborn or high-risk infant: Nursery and follow-up.

III. Orthopedic Conditions				
ROM—UE				
LE				
Neck				
Ventral Flexion of Neck				
Ventral Flexion of Trunk				
Extension of Trunk				
Contractures (rept)				
Dislocations (rept)				
Fractures (rept)				
Adductor <: ☦				
40–80 (1–3m)				
70–110 (4–6m)				
100–140 (7–9m)				
130–150 (10–12m)				
Heel to ear				
80–100 (1–3m)				
90–130 (1–6m)				
120–150 (7–9m)				
140–170 (10–12m)				
Popliteal <				
80–100 (1–3m)				
90–120 (4–6m)				
110–160 (7–9m)				
150–170 (10–12m)				
Dorsiflexion of Ft.				
60–70 (slow)				
10 (fast)				
Scarf sign:				
(1–3m)				
(4–6m)				
(7–9m)				
(10–12m)				

IV. Asymmetry Items (note side)				
Flapping Foot (↑)				
Sq. Window (↓<)				
Flapping Hand (↑)				
Lat. Rot. Head (↑ to)				
Lat. Rot. Trunk (↑ to)				
Other				

V. Adaptive Responses				
Self-consolability:				
readily				
attempts				
unable				
Spontaneous Behavior:				
active				
average				
listless				

VI. Sensory Motor/Sensory Integration				
Tactile: hypersensitive				
hyposensitive				
acceptant				
Position in space to Chg.				
Visual—eyes open				
pursuit of image				
localization				
tracks to midline				
tracks past midline				
Auditory—alerts to noise				
activates to voice				
localizes voice				

VII. Nasal/Oral Feeding Function				
Breathing/Nasal/Oral				
Palate—elevated				
cleft				
Tongue—midline				
deviated				
Suck—spontaneous				
closure				
burst/sequence				
Swallowing—seq. with suck				
tongue thrust				
Feeding—Type				
Position				
Tolerance to feed				
Choking spells				
Feeding History:				

Additional Comments (please date)

Voluntary Activities—see attached:
(Yes) (No)

Figure 31-2. (*continued*)

VIII.

A. Voluntary Activity—Gross Motor			
sit—Head bobs erect 1m			
pr—Wt. on forearm 3m→			
sit—Head steady 3m→			
pr—Head-90° 4m			
sup—Pulled to sit—no lag 4m			
sup/pr—Rolls both ways 5m			
sit—sits erect momen. 6m			
stdg—Bears weight 6m			
sit—Sits steadily 7m			
sit—To hands & knees 8m			
pr—Crawling 8m			
pr—Raise & lower fr. sit 9m			
stdg—Cruises 11m			
stdg—Walks hand-in-hand 11m			
stdg—Walks few steps—I 13m			
stdg—Runs stiffly 15m			
stdg—Squats in plan 15m→			

B. Voluntary—Fine Motor			
Reflex Grasp 0→4m			
Palmar Graps 4→8m			
Ulnar Graps 4→8m			
Control from Shldr 6m→			
Lateral Pinch 8m→			
Deliberate Release 9m→			
Precise Pincer/rel. 11m→			
Opposition 12m→			
2-cube tower 12→25m			

C. Voluntary—Self-care			
Finger Feeding 9m→			
Drinks from cup 12m→			
Grasps spoon 12m→			
Cooperates Drsg. 1y→			
Pushes down pants 2y→			
Toilet Trained 2½y→			

D. Voluntary—Communication				
Prespeech—Laughs 6wk–3m				
Recept—anticipates care				
Food 4m→				
Responds to own name 7m→				
Gestures				
Shake head "no" 4m				
Wave bye-bye 7m				
Shake head "yes" 12m				
Vocalizations				
Throaty sounds 9m				
Strong cry 1m				
"Talks" back when				
talked to 8m				
"Mama-Dada" unspec. 8m→				
"Mama-Dada" spec. 10→				
Unintelligible jabbering 10–14m				
Combines 2 wds 14m→24m				
Names 1 picture 20m→30m				

IX. Parental Concerns:

X. Other comments: (dysmorphic features)

Figure 31-2. (*continued*)

intervention program to adapt to medical changes.

Initial interaction between mother and child were highly structured. The occupational therapist began by encouraging the mother to scrub and gown, enter the unit, and sit by her child. The process of touching the child was more involved because of his hypersensitivity to light touch. The mother had to be willing to use a firm touch pressure with a child she viewed as extremely fragile. Progressive touch and consolability techniques were discussed and demonstrations were shared with the mother.

Direct service to Greg provided by the therapist included activities that would decrease the external stimuli he received 24 hours a day, as well as provided for short periods of structured activity or inactivity. Specific approaches included swaddling for proximal joint pressure and warmth to calm him, as well as slow stroking to increase tactile acceptance. Other inhibition techniques included draping the respirator head gear to reduce visual stimuli during nine feedings to decrease reflux. While being fed, Greg was not rocked or moved because he seemed to convert all stimuli into increased excitatory state, therefore diminishing his feed response. Since a major goal with a preterm

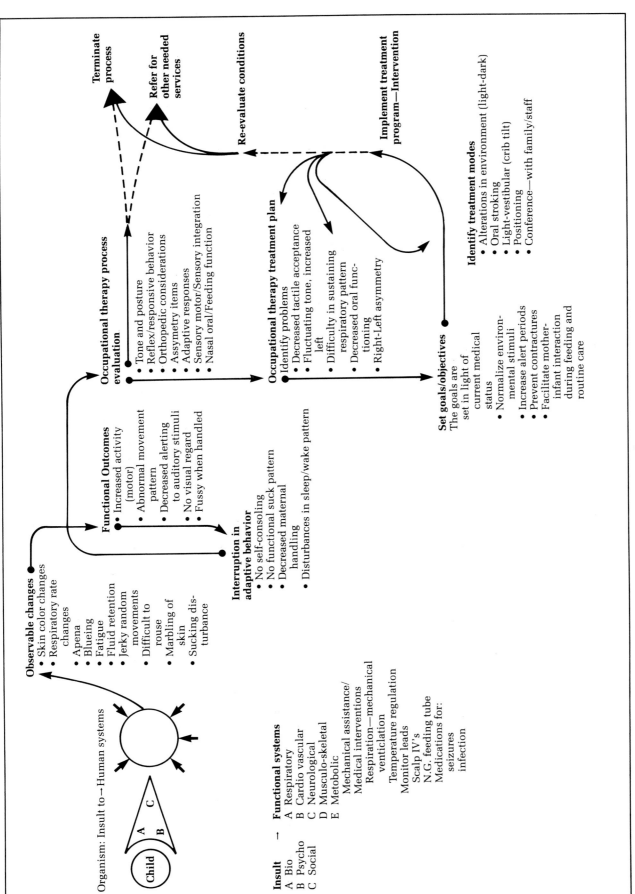

Figure 31-3. Occupational therapy program with a neonate (direct special care nursery service). Case study: Greg.

infant is weight gain, the acceptance of the feeding is all important. To increase usable alert periods, highly structured and controlled periods of gentle rocking were used while Greg was on the respirator.

Although Greg continued to exhibit specific postural tone defiency and asymmetry, his increased registration of touch, handling and other external stimuli reduced markedly as the previously described therapeutic measures were implemented by the occupational therapist, medical staff and Greg's mother. The major goal of Greg developing an acceptance of feeding was gradually attained. This improvement in his nutritional status laid the groundwork for improving Greg's overall developmental potential. □

Occupational Therapy Consultation Service to House Staff and Discharge Planning

Case Study B

Kelly was a 34-week-old (SGA) female, small for her gestational age, born of a 20-year-old mother. Kelly's primary referral to special care nursery was because of amnionic bands resulting in a congenital lack of the development of distal segments of the left foot (four toes) and right thumb. Additional work-up showed microcephaly, abnormal spike waves on EEG tracings, and a normal CAT scan.

Kelly's mother was a single parent living with her mother, a younger brother, and a 4-year-old son (Kelly's brother) in a city-sponsored housing project. Kelly's mother worked the 3 to 11 shift in a local plant. The grandmother planned to be the primary care-giver for the infant.

In response to a request for consultation by the neonatologist, the occupational therapist made an initial chart review, determined an appropriate time to visit in accordance with the nursery schedule, and advised the charge nurse of intent.

Reports from the unit nurse were that even with intense stimulation, such as undressing, sponge bathing, and redressing, Kelly did not rouse. She was also unresponsive to the insertion and removal of nasogastric tubes for feedings.

When the occupational therapist visited, Kelly was at midfeed (approximately 40 minutes before her next feeding). Assessment was done and clinical observations were made. See Figure 31-4 for system review and findings. In summary, no functional alerting to auditory, visual, vestibular, or tactile stimuli was noted. Kelly demonstrated severely decreased muscle tone in her upper extremities and,

proximally, at her hips. A positive stretch reflex was present bilaterally at the ankles. Oral motor assessment showed no reflexive suck or rooting present in this 38-week-old infant (adjusted gestational age by assessment). She appeared extremely small and globally nonresponsive.

Goals were outlined for the nursery staff since the occupational therapist would not be the primary provider, and plans to re-evaluate were made. Recommendations included:
1. Intensive alerting activities eight times per day, per feed.
2. Positioning recommendations to realign proximal joints.
3. One nipple feeding per day.
4. Re-evaluation by occupational therapist in one week. Consider formal occupational therapy program.
5. Conference with mother regarding expected delay in discharge.

Occupational Therapy Consultation Service Program

Occupational therapy consultation service for Kelly included recommendations for the nursery staff and key considerations in discharge planning. Recommendations and demonstrations were given to the nursery staff in the following:
• feeding
• positioning
• behavioral observations

Brief feedings were suggested, with 1 to 3 minute alerting periods, prior to the eight daily feeds. The alerting activities for the baby included tactile and vestibular stimulation. (Note: intercranial hemorrhage and major cardiac concern had been ruled out.)

Often a neonate is very sensitive to movement. To a newborn, the act of being picked up from a supine position or turned from prone to supine may be an overwhelming vestibular input. The recommendations for Kelly included moving her from prone to supine, picking her up, and lateral rocking. Once these maneuvers were completed a series of light tactile alerting actions to encourage rooting and sucking responses were initiated. Swaddling during the feed as well as continuation of alerting responses was encouraged. In an attempt to facilitate the development of a suck response, it was also recommended that a nasogastric tube feeding be replaced with a nipple feed. During the first 5 to 7 minutes of the nipple feed, an infant should be allowed to pace the rate of the feed. The nurse was shown basic oral facilitation, involving stroking and

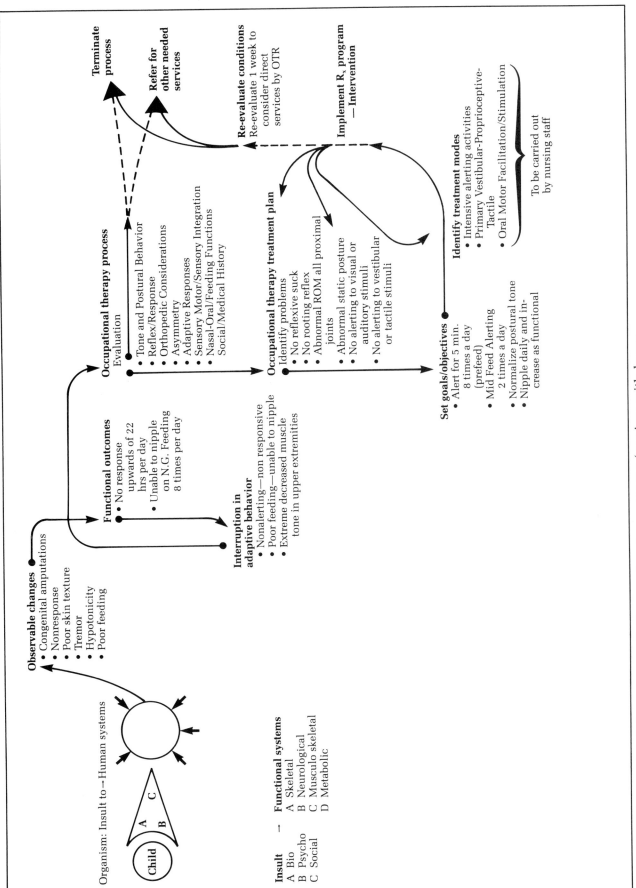

Figure 31-4. Occupational therapy consultation services to a neonate (services with house staff and discharge planning). Case study: Kelly.

positioning. Because of staffing limitation, the feedings were conducted every 3 hours for no more than 30 minutes per feed.

Basic positioning was suggested to realign the child's proximal joints, including towel rolls at the lateral hip border with a flexion assist at knees while supine. Prone positioning was unassisted with the exception of head rotation. Alternating side lying with full support to encourage proximal input was utilized approximately 15 minutes out of every 2 hours.

A conference of Kelly's medical care-givers regarding early discharge planning focused on the child's lack of response and failure to nipple. Discharge was contingent on weight gain, increased periods of alertness, and ability to feed without the nasogastric tube. Lengthy conferences with the mother and grandmother to assist them in understanding the complexity of the feeding and responsiveness of the infant were conducted.

Following these conferences, a request for direct occupational therapy services was issued by the neonatologist in an attempt to facilitate the child's attaining discharge status. □

Occupational Therapy Services Postdischarge (Follow-up)
Case Study C

Patrick was referred for developmental assessment at the chronological age of 6 months. Born in a small hospital of a rural community about 50 miles from the regional neonatal center, he was the second child of an upper middle-class family. The pregnancy and delivery had been uneventful. He was an appropriate size and weight for his estimated 36–38 weeks gestational age. However, he had demonstrated early neonatal distress. He remained in his local hospital for 10 days because of reported "minor difficulties in maintaining body temperature" and "brief periods of apnea." After his condition appeared to be stabilized, he was sent home.

At 14 days of age he was admitted this time to the regional neonatal center in respiratory distress. Febrile seizures were observed within the first 24 hours, although no infectious agents were isolated. The child initially required mechanical ventilation, progressed to enriched air, and was weaned to room air. During a 12-week hospitalization, Patrick's mother stayed with a friend in the city and was able to visit daily. His father visited on weekends but remained at the family home to oversee his business.

One month after discharge Patrick, at age 6 months, returned to the Regional Center for a routine medical follow-up visit. It was at this point he was referred to the occupational therapist for development assessment. Both parents and a 4-year-old sibling were present during this assessment. The father did not stay in the room for the full assessment. Patrick appeared quiet and alert. Mother was motionless while holding the child; she did not rock or stroke him. Upon movement or light touch he became fussy and cried. When placed prone on a mat on the floor, he strongly objected to the positioning. He held a toy in each hand but did not transfer a toy from one hand to the other or engage the toy at midline. No mouthing of the objects occurred during the assessment. Detailed findings can be seen on the schematic Figure 31-5. Recommendations included the following:

1. Weekly home visits for one month by the occupational therapist.
2. Formal re-evaluation in 30 days.
3. Pending re-evaluation findings, consider referral to an outpatient center with an infant-parent program near child's home.

The occupational therapy follow-up goals included increasing Patrick's acceptance of tactile stimuli as a means of facilitating child-parental interaction and attempting to increase the parents' understanding of Patrick's medical-health status in relation to his current behaviors. The approach included an awareness of appropriate motoric and reflexive developmental progression and facilitation methods.

Suggested activities were incorporated into daily activities, and pleasurable transactions between parent and child were encouraged. This was especially important because of the parents' level of acceptance of any concerns about their child. The father actively denied any problems with his son and assured the therapist any special exercises or programming were unnecessary. The mother, however, welcomed suggestions on ways to make her son easier to handle and less fussy. The specific program consisted of organized full body rubs once a day and a series of stroking activities at bath time in water, progressing to a brisk dry-off period. Mother was also taught care-giver consoling techniques and was instructed in methods to encourage Patrick to console himself. During the course of service delivery she was instructed in the developmental continuum of motor, social, and language skills. This process allowed the mother to view her son as a whole being within the family environment and to develop more appropriate expectations for him.

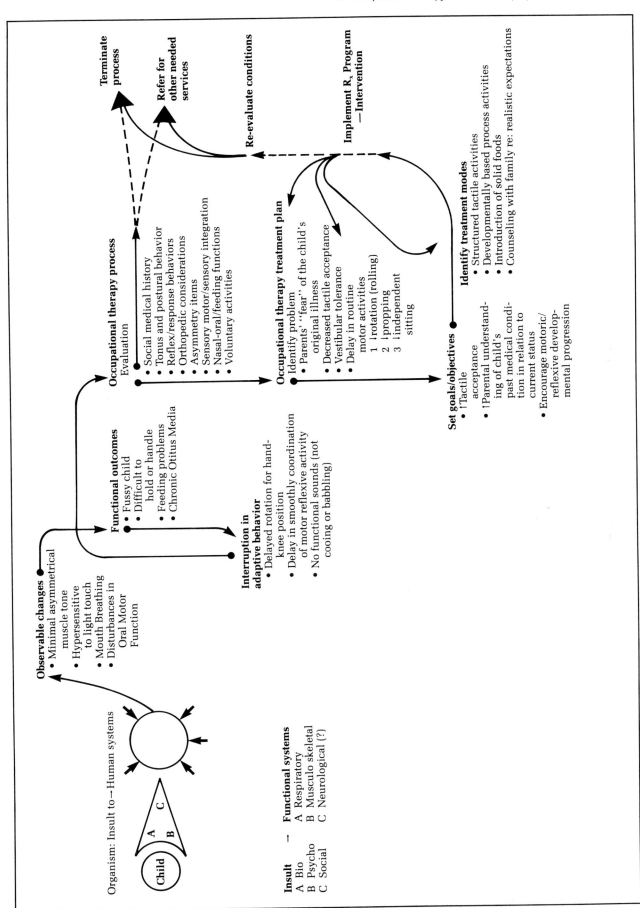

Figure 31-5. Occupational therapy program for a neonate (postdischarge follow up). Case study: Patrick.

By the end of the first month noticeable changes occurred in Patrick's sleep–wake cycle, ease of handling, and general behavior. His father was beginning to move from his active denial to admitting that his son was less than perfect. He began to question the rationale behind therapeutic intervention and agreed to accompany his wife to the formal re-evaluation scheduled in a week. □

The role of the occupational therapist in neonatal services is extremely complex—but no more or less complex than the young client to be served. The concepts offered are simple and can become the foundation for the multiplicity of skills and expertise the occupational therapist must possess in serving the neonate. The primary concept is that the neonate must be considered as a unique being with certain unique life qualities, and that he or she is a member of a particular family unit and community. This, plus his genetic endowment and experiences, is the key to his development. The second concept is that the occupational therapist is one of many providers and care-givers involved with the infant. While many of these providers are appropriately concerned with sustaining the child's life, the occupational therapist's concern and services should address the quality of that child's life—today and in the future.

Congenitally Blind or Visually Impaired Child

Occupational therapists involved in the evaluation and treatment of young children with suspected developmental disabilities will in all probability encounter within their referral population a significant number of children who exhibit visual impairment or, in fact, who may be congenitally blind. In some cases, children who were birthed prematurely and who are less than 12 months of age may have a visual deficiency status and prognosis that is clouded or incomplete. In some cases, therapists may encounter a baby who seems visually handicapped, but who has not been so identified. Because of the advances in survival of high-risk neonates, (in which birthing may occur as nearly as 24 weeks gestation, with a birth weight of 16 oz or less) and because of the increased incidence of visual impairment in these cases, the previous discussion of neonates is directly applicable to the early experiences of the child and family. Survival of the baby is the overwhelming goal and desire for parents. Preoccupation with the child's circulation, respiration, and nourishment status preclude consideration of the consequences of impaired vision on the child's development.

As the child reaches physical and medical stability, parents then can address their concerns about the child's development and to what degree visual impairment will hamper their child's developmental potential. The occupational therapist serving a blind or visually impaired child and family has an important opportunity. Careful developmental assessment and critical interpretation are needed. Many contenitally blind or visual impaired children exhibit multisensory integrative problems, and their neurophysiological development varies from the sighted child in certain predictable patterns. Helping the child to achieve developmental gains directly, and also helping parents to recognize and enhance their vital contributions to the young child's development, is the thrust of occupational therapy in this field of endeavor.

General physical sensory variations of young congenitally blind children include the following:

- diminished muscle tone accompanied by poor joint stability in some cases
- irregularity in neurodevelopmental reflex presence and maturation
- delayed or partial acquisition of gross and fine motor skill
- irregularity in somatosensory and vestibular processing
- sensitivity to or misunderstanding of sensory stimuli.
- means—ends (motor output)
- gestoral—imitation
- cause—effect (inductive reasoning)
- spatial relationships

Sensitivity to or misinterpretation of sensory stimuli by the child can be determined by the therapist during the assessment process and by information provided by the parents and by observation. Those senses under suspicion are listed with observable behaviors as an outcome:

Olfactory—Poor appetite or adversive behavior to certain foods on the basis of odor

Oral Tactile—Difficulty in accepting variations of food texture or feeding instruments

Tactile—Discomfort with touch contact, especially to certain clothing, dressing process, bathing, cuddling, and comforting

Tactile Proprioceptive—Voluntarily withdraws from support of self with upper and lower extremities to surface

Tactile Proprioceptive–Vestibular—Responds negatively to unfamiliar handler, especially to imposed movement in space, or generally is earthbound by strong preference

Auditory—Frightened frequently by unfamiliar voices and environmental sounds

A lack of early mutual visual attention of the infant and parents may disrupt early bonding communication links between the child and parent.

Through neurodevelopmental reflex testing, a therapist gains much needed information. Therapists frequently need to review the basis of reflex testing. Through this understanding the therapist is assisted in determining the child's response to:

- light and firm tactile stimuli
- proprioceptive stimuli
- spatial organization
- reaction to surface
- optical organization of space (when some vision is present)

Reflex testing, combined with vestibular testing, allows the therapists to understand the child's processing and organization in a definitive way. Some of the discrete variations in reflex maturation most frequently seen in the first years of life are:

- prolonged moro reflex to loss of position
- prolonged avoidance reflex
- deficient labyrinthine head righting reflex, especially prone
- delayed or absent landau
- poor or disordered proprioceptive placing reflexes, both legs and arms
- delayed support mechanisms

As a consequence, equilibrium reactions in all planes and protective extension reactions are delayed. The gross motor milestones attainment frequently varies in a particular order. The delays are observed in:

- diminished oral/facial weakness
- diminished head/neck performance against gravity, especially in prone extension with neck rotation to left or right
- diminished prone extension performance on forearms and hands
- delay in prone progression; creeping and hitching
- deficiency in active transitions of coming and lowering to both sit and, later, stand
- delays in squatting in play
- delays in walking freely and running
- delays in all gross motor tasks requiring discrete midline stability

See Figure 31-6, which illustrates contrasts in motor performance of congenitally blind children and sighted children.

The attaining of fine motor skill is strongly dependent on somatosensory processing efficiency. If efficiency is present, many fine skills occur in an orderly fashion; however, even in these cases the use of instruments for eating is characteristically delayed, though cup use is not.

When sensory motor integration deficiency is present, and especially in the case of somatosensory deficiency, the early developmental understanding basic to skill attainment may occur or not occur in disorder. Problem area domains include:

- Object permanence
- A lack of visual feedback regarding socially appropriate behavior needs consideration. Efforts to provide alternate methods of gaining such understanding are needed on an ongoing basis.
- A lack of visual feedback of nonverbal communication influences overall appropriate behavior and assumes pragmatical ideation. As verbal communication develops, literal approaches and interventions may promote more appropriate development behavior.
- Auditory motor transactions can be stress producing and may have a negative influence on behavior and adaptation.

The better the therapist's ability to understand and communicate to the parent the unique nature of the development of their congenitally blind or visually impaired child, the greater the possibility of correctly developing a plan of treatment that incorporates the parent in the process. This joint effort enables the child to have an improved prognosis for success in the development of skills.

Case Study

History

Beth was born prematurely at a gestational age of 22 weeks, weighing 1 lb, 11 oz. After birth her weight dropped to 1 lb, 6 oz. Along with prematurity, she was medically diagnosed as having Respiratory Distress Syndrome (RDS), complicated by marked cardiac dysfunction, and there was little hope for her survival. However, treatment and nurturing offered through the services of a hospital neonatal intensive care and nursery program advanced her physical-medical status over a 5-month period so that she was stabilized for discharge to her parents.

Parental Information

Beth's parents were reared and lived in a rural setting, which was 60 miles from Beth's medical support system. Her parents were in their late 30s. The family also included two boys aged 14 years and 7 years. The oldest had a mild hearing impairment. Both parents had long wished for a baby girl, and

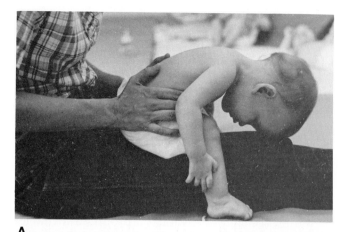

A

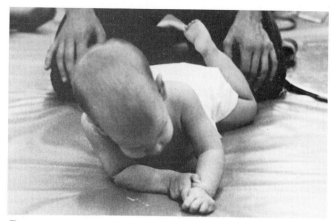

B

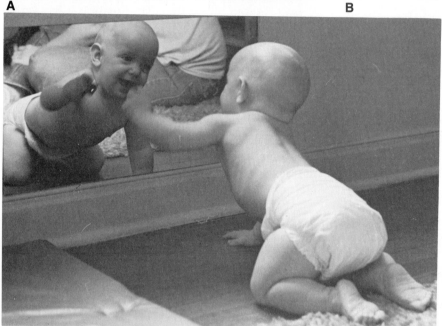

C

Figure 31-6. A contrast of motor performance of congenitally blind children and sighted children. (*A*) Poor extensor ability of trunk and neck seen in a congenitally blind child. (*B*) Lack of prone stability of a blind child in attempted prone progressions. (*C*) A sighted child demonstrates the automatic development of trunk stability. Note the importance of vision and searching in encouraging extensor development.

Beth's mother had experienced several miscarriages in this attempt prior to her pregnancy with Beth. In general, Beth's parents were experienced and comfortable in their parenting role and responsibility. They were obviously solicitous in their attitude toward their children. In general their management expectation of their children was to encourage useful orderly behavior. The family attended church regularly, and church values were a part of the family's daily life. It is important to know that Beth's mother was an efficient manager of the household and that she carried the chief responsibility for that and the children's care.

Beth's mother was quick to note and question Beth's visual attention when Beth was discharged home. Within two weeks of discharge Beth had a complete visual examination that revealed her to be cortically blind due to Retrolental Fibroplasia. The mother's grief over her daughter's blindness was

and continued to be a major factor of concern in infant–parent treatment programming.

Figure 31-7 depicts the initial occupational therapy program.

Occupational Therapy Program

An initial occupational therapy evaluation was conducted when Beth was physically stable and her neonatologist felt her resistance to infection was satisfactory. Her chronological age was 13 months (gestational age 9½ months). Beth required considerable restriction from contact with others outside the home in order to prevent her exposure to respiratory diseases for 8 months after discharge from the hospital. As a consequence, her mother experienced limited social contact during this period. Her examination was conducted at a community infant–parent program and was the first

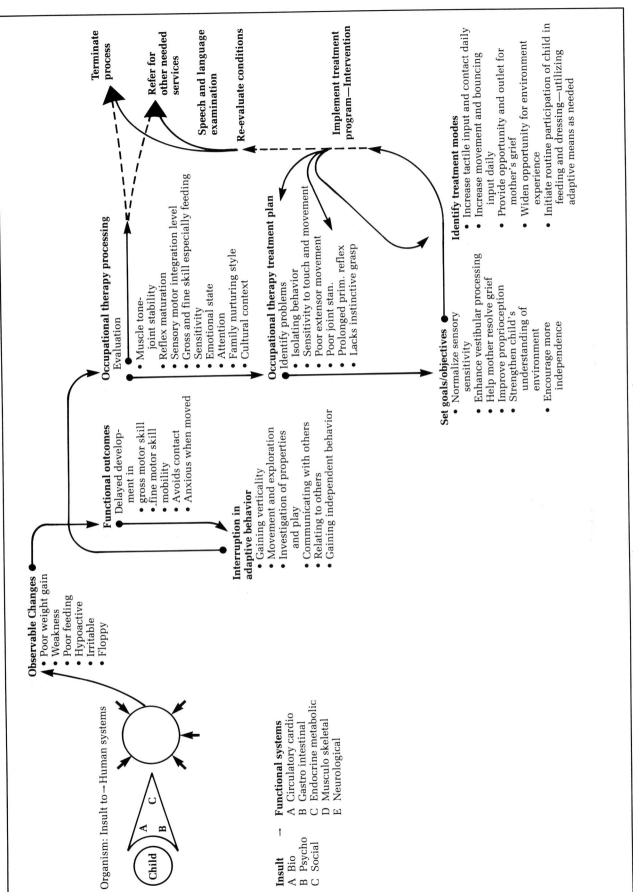

Figure 31-7. Occupational therapy with a congenitally blind child. Case study: Beth.

real opportunity for the parents to express their needs and concerns about their child's development.

Examination of Beth revealed the following. She appeared pale, small and her skull was elongated due to positioning during her hospitalization. She was quiet when unattended. She alerted to sound, but did not orient. The mother felt Beth could distinguish between low and high sounds. But she was fearful of low voices, and was afraid of being picked up by male family members including her father. During testing she displayed fussiness when handled, and she withdrew from light touch stimuli. She strongly objected to being placed in prone position.

Physically she was weak and floppy. All reflex responses were underactive; no pathological tone condition was noted. Primitive tonic neck reflexes prevailed, though her tonic labyrinthine prone reflex was absent. Labyrinthine righting was demonstrated in supine but was absent in prone and tilting responses. There was no landau. Proprioceptive reflex testing such as plantar and palmar placing was weakly present. Neck and body righting was stronger. Tactile related reflex testing produced an avoidance of limbs, but some slight evidence of instinctive searching with her hands was noted. The most dynamic response in testing was her moro response of complete embrace to loud sound and loss of position (backwards 45 degrees). Some slight incurvature of the spine was seen in prone equilibrium testing, which was her only advanced reaction. Her reflex profile was that of a 5-month-old child, with certain exceptions often seen in congenitally blind children as described earlier in the discussion.

Gross motor skills were displayed to a 5-month level, except for raising chest on extended arms and head lag in pull to sit. She rolled both ways and lifted her legs in extension, but could not sit independently, momentarily. Her gross motor quotient compared to her gestational age was 55%.

Her fine motor skills were quite depressed. She had no palmar grasping reflex, tending to not grasp generally, though she could bring her hands to her mouth and was scheming to use the thenar emmenances of both her hands plus her two feet to prop her bottle while her mother fed her the bottle. No swiping behavior was present, and instinctive hand use was limited to feeding time where she reached briefly for bits of food and occasionally for her spoon. The mother was encouraging Beth to search for parts of her body, particularly her feet. She was teaching Beth to assist in pulling off her socks.

Optokinetic testing produced no response, but blinking occurred to testing. No resting nystagmus was present, and there was no response to postrotary nystagmus testing. The mother felt that Beth might have some light perception. Beth's alerting to odors was minimal. She registered little interest in toys other than musical or chiming ones. She disliked fuzzy and furry toys.

The mother was quite open in expressing her concerns about her daughter, including:
1. A frustrating hope that Beth might see someday. She cried as she said, "Oh if she could only see her pretty dresses."
2. Worry over Beth's poor appetite and slow weight gain. She also found feeding time frustrating because of Beth's picky appetite.
3. A fear of Beth's delicate health.
4. Fear that when Beth cried or fussed, she was experiencing pain due to eye pressure, despite the lack of medical support to this belief.

Following the evaluation, the parents and staff held a planning conference to jointly determine goals and objectives that would assist Beth's development. Because the family lived a distance of 60 miles from the infant–parent center, and considering Beth's somewhat fragile condition, the decision was made to arrange a home treatment program. A home therapist would provide both treatment to Beth and train the family in appropriate therapeutic interventions. Weekly visits were provided, and an occupational therapy program was implemented (see Beth's Occupational Therapy Program—13 months).

Re-evaluation

At the next regularly scheduled 3-month evaluation, Beth, now 16 months old (gestational age 13 months), demonstrated some substantial gains in development. She showed marked improvement in behavior including less fussiness and crying. The mother felt the remaining crying episodes were occurring when Beth was hungry. The entire family were now enjoying Beth because she was happier and responsive to them when handled or touched. Beth now had a good appetite and was accepting a variety of foods. Reflex maturation was seen in inhibition of moro reflex and avoidance. Tonic neck reflex presence was diminishing, while improved labyrinthine righting, and emergence of equilibrium response in prone, supine, and sitting were emerging. Good positive support of lower extremities and instinctive grasp were noted. She was placing and protecting with upper extremities forward and to the side. Reflexively, Beth was now programmed for gains in gross motor patterns and improved mobility.

Beth's Occupational Therapy Program: Chronological Age—13 Months; Gestational Age—9 Months, 15 Days		
Therapeutic Goals	Objectives	Examples • Methods • Modes • Procedures
I. Normalize tactile sensitivity as a means to reduce isolating behavior.	IA. Increase child's contact with family members, objects of significance in the home.	IA. 1. Swaddle the child before child is handled by family other than mother. Play soothing music while handling. 2. Give firm rubdowns daily, especially before handling or tactile contact play. Emphasize palms of hands. 3. Encourage child to explore family members' facial features and hands. Encourage self touch. Use bells on ankles and wrists. Use appropriate labels as child contacts. 4. Encourage child to touch and hold objects common to child's daily experience. Name first then offer touch experience. Ex.: food, clothing, toys, mother's things, father's things, and brother's items. 5. Encourage Beth's exploration of hands/arms, feet/legs, face and skull with a manual vibrator. 6. Explore Beth's response to vibrating surface, especially when child demonstrates prolonged crying with cause.
II. Enhance vestibular processing as a means to improve adaptive behavior.	IIA. Child will increase tolerance to movement.	IIA. 1. Jigglers will be added to child's crib legs. 2. Mother will manually turn child slowly 10 x's to right and left; mother will tilt child in all directions 5 x's; mother will lower child 10 x's while holding the child erect. (Use swaddling if poorly tolerated). 3. Mother will gently swing child in a hammock on a basinette mattress. Child should be in prone or supine position. In prone chest wedge should be used.
III. Help mother resolve grief.	IIIA. Channel mother's grief. B. Reduce the mother's anxiety about her child.	IIIA. 1. Provide time to listen to mother's feelings about Beth. 2. Give mother emotional support as needed. B. 1. Encourage mother to share home therapy program with other family members.

Therapeutic Goals	Objectives	Examples • Methods • Modes • Procedures
		2. Encourage mother to share feeding responsibilities with father and older brother.
		3. Encourage family to resume previous socialization and leisure activities.
		4. Encourage mother to have ½ day/week away from care duty.
	C. Increase mother's knowledge about blind children's development.	C. 1. Encourage mother to communicate with other parents of blind children.
		2. Provide information and sources of information on blind children's development.
IV. Improve proprioception as a means to increase mobility.	IVA. A child will achieve raising chest on extended arms during playtime on own initiative.	IVA. 1. Bounce child in crib in prone, supine supported sitting and puppy with elbow support in extension. Add quadriped over bolster as stabilizer is achieved in puppy.
		2. Move bouncing activity to suspended hammock with spring as child's tolerance increases.
	B. Encourage rolling as a means to an end.	B. 1. Encourage rolling on a padded surface 3-5 x's to right and left. Use bottle as a lure, or a musical toy.
V. Strengthen child's understanding of her environment.	VA. Identify rooms of household by means of distinctive sounds.	VA. 1. Have mother examine each room in household and add noise factor to each room. Ex.: wind chimes at backdoor, radio in bedroom, TV in den, in backyard, etc.
	B. Plan a daily routine in which Beth is exposed to all areas of household.	B. 1. Child will spend time in kitchen, laundry room and bathroom, bedroom, garage-backyard and front porch.
VI. Encourage more independence.	VIA. Child will eat with more independence.	VIA. 1. Child will hold bottle during feeding.
		2. Child will have opportunity to finger feed a portion of every meal.
		3. Child will drink from a cup with lid and will place hands on cup to steady.
		4. Child will hold spoon and take tastes from spoon with help.
	B. Child will cooperate in dressing and assist.	B. 1. Child will remove socks.
		2. Child will reach and co-contract during dressing process.

Her neck strength and organization were improved. She no longer demonstrated head lag; she could sit steadily and lean forward, and re-erect. Her performance on the floor was markedly improved. She not only raised her chest in prone on extended arms, but she could also pivot 90 degrees to right and left. As Beth became more comfortable in her world, she used rolling to explore her world. Gross motor skills were at a 7-month level.

All goals in feeding and dressing were accomplished. She was finger feeding, holding her bottle, accepting cup use, and assisting a little with spoon feeding. She quite automatically removed her shoes and socks and was far easier to dress. Her upper extremity skill included swiping, reaching, transfer, and she had crude pincer skill, voluntary release. She did not bang two objects together, but she did bang on surface and demonstrated crossing midline ability.

Her response on the postrotary nystagmus test was hyporeactive. There was no change in her visual status. The mother and father discussed their continued hope for eye surgery to help Beth see.

Changes and upgrading of Beth's home program were discussed with the family. A treatment plan was implemented during the next 4-month period of treatment (see Beth's Occupational Therapy Program—16 months).

At the next regularly scheduled 4-month evaluation, Beth at age 20 months old (gestational age 17 months) again demonstrated continued developmental gains in most parameters; her gross motor age was 12 months and her fine motor skills were in a range of 12–18 months level. Other advances were as follows:

1. Improved overall communication and minimal crying behavior overall. More use of gestures to make her needs known. No expressive speech.
2. Reflexive maturation with good equilibrium in prone, supine, sitting, and quadriped.
3. Improved mobility by means of prone progression, with emerging creeping and hitching, able to mount and lower from couch.
4. Improved searching ability within her own bedroom, living area, and kitchen. Family and staff were elated with her increased evidence of orientation as her mobility advanced.
5. Though all self-help skills were continuing to advance, she tended to cling to manual searching of foods in self-feeding with a slow acceptance of the use of utensils for feeding.
6. Improved prehension and instinctive grasping, good opposition. More abilities to place objects, stack objects. Recognizing familiar objects by touch.

Both staff and family felt Beth's gains in sensory integration were fundamental to her major increases in function and improved adaptive behavior. The family expressed more confidence in Beth's future, but at the same time they were pursuing eye surgery for Beth in the next several months. The surgery was to attempt to reattach the retina of the right eye. If the operation was successful, the ultimate that could be achieved would be an increase in Beth's light perception. (Note: The surgical process was subsequently carried out as planned, but it lacked success in improving Beth's visual status.) Beth's family continued to work conscientiously with their therapist in advancing Beth's development.

Over the following year and a half Beth made great strides in gaining gross motor and fine motor skills. Though she was a happy child who learned to sing songs and imitate what she heard, language development, especially expressive speech, was slow. Her enrollment in a nearby special class for visually handicapped children at age 36 months was a turning point for Beth. Subsequently Beth's ability to communicate markedly improved, which greatly enhanced Beth's potential for learning and functioning. □

Brachial Plexus Injury

Discussion

A brachial plexus injury to a child at birth will result in damage to the peripheral nerves from injury to their roots at the site of the injury. The most common type of brachial plexus injury is of the upper arm, or Erb's Palsy, which involves the upper trunks of C5–6. A less common type of brachial plexus injury is of the lower arm and hand, or Klumpke's type, which involves the trunks of the C8—T1 level. The child with these injuries has deficits in the musculo-skeletal and neurological systems of a lower motor neuron lesion type, involving both the motor and sensory nerves to the involved arm.

The child with an Erb's type of palsy will characteristically keep the arm in an adducted and internally rotated position, with little to no elbow flexion and little shoulder motion. Hand muscles are usually active, but the child has little opportunity to experience the normal adaptations to the developing use of the hand due to the limited arm motion. There are varying degrees of injury, with different amounts of residual muscle strength and potential for return in the first year or two of life. Often the child has little opportunity in those early years to experience inherently normal patterns of arm and hand movement and, as a result, learns to make little use of both

Beth's Occupational Therapy Program:
Chronological Age—13 Months; Gestational Age—9 Months, 15 Days

Therapeutic Goals	Objectives	Examples • Methods • Modes • Procedures
I. Continued normalization of tactile sensitivity as a means of encouraging improved adaptive behavior and socialization.	IA. Child will initiate touching and tolerate being touched. B. Encourage improved tactile discrimination and localization.	IA. 1. Continue firm rubdowns daily. 2. Continue vibratory play. 3. Continue use of vibrator board as a calming means. B. 1. Play sticky tape game; place sticky tape on varying body locations, have child pull off tape. 2. Continue to have child contact self and others. Name first then have child touch these body parts. 3. Continue and expand contact with objects common to household and child's experience. 4. Encourage tactile searching for objects using sound clues.
II. Enhance vestibular processing as a means of improving mobility, function and adaptive behavior.	IIA. Child will tolerate swinging. B. Child will tolerate tilting and respond. C. Child will tolerate sliding and initiate movement in sliding. D. Child will demonstrate improved response to angular vest stimulation.	IIA. 1. Child will swing in a suspended hammock in all directions for 5-10 minutes (3 sec. arcs). Positioned in prone, supine and sitting. B. 1. Child will tilt on a moderately firm surface in prone, supine, puppy and supported quadriped. (Use well inflated rectangular air cushion on 2 inch mat.) Use slow rate, wait for response. C. 1. Child will slide down an incline plane on stomach on back and seated. C. 2. Child will use prone progression down incline plane. To be done 2 x's each or more feet if desired. D. 1. Child will turn slowly in hammock seated, side-lying and supine 12 x's in one direction followed by ½ turns in the reverse direction.

Therapeutic Goals	Objectives	Examples • Methods • Modes • Procedures
III. Improve proprioception as a means to increase child's mobility.	IIIA. Child will move in prone progression automatically during play time and as a means to end.	IIIA. 1. Child will wear weighted vest and cuff weights during proprioception ties. Weighted pockets Weighted cuff
	B. Child will maintain supported quadriped independently.	
	C. Child will initiate creeping and hitching for 2 feet before lowering into prone progression for means to end.	A,B,C. 1. Child will bounce in a suspended hammock with spring on a firm surface in sitting puppy position, and quadriped with limited support.
	D. Child will stand supported by rail, 2 hands, child will raise one foot at rail and take initial side steps.	D. 1. Add supported kneeling and standing, bounding as skill emerges.
IV. Strengthen child's understanding and orientation to home setting as a means of gaining increased function, mobility and independence.	IVA. A child will move and search for centers of interest in each of the principal rooms in the home setting.	IVA-B-C. Orientation Process This orientation process is appropriate for child who has reflex organization for movement, either by prone progress or creeping and hitching. (Skull sensitive children may prefer to move backwards creeping. Because this is detrimental to orientation, it should be inhibited.) Reciprocal prone progression Creeping and hitching Backward (discouraged) A. 1. As tactile sensitivity subsides and child is exploring objects and toys, particularly objects with sound should be kept in a box. The box should initially be stationed under or near the child's bed. Noise from jigglers on bed will help the child locate the box and facilitate search. The box should be kept without variation is the same location until child is automatic in locating the box.

Therapeutic Goals	Objectives	Examples • Methods • Modes • Procedures
	B. Child will move and search the parameters of each room she frequents.	B. 1. Then the box should be used to orient the child to the entrance(s) to the room and the parameter (walls) of the room. Once the child can trace the room in on direction, the pattern can then be reversed.
		As the child accomplishes this in one area, a similar process is used in other principal areas.
	C. Child will move and search out pathways leading from one room to another.	C. 1. Box of interest should be placed to encourage child to search and move through spaces requiring change of direction to right and left, and reversed patterns. Varying floor surfaces aid the child to distinguish areas. Scooter board movement may be used to facilitate this progress.
V. Encourage development of more independent funcion in daily living skills.	VA. Child will eat independently with supervision.	VA. 1. Child will hold cup with lid and drink without assistance.
		2. Child will spoon feed as a principal means of feeding with some spilling with adapted spoon and bowl.
		3. Child may use fingers to discriminate foods and eat with fingers foods that are appropriate.
	B. Child will initiate undressing skills and assist in dressing.	B. 1. Child will remove shirt overhead, and push off pants from hips, at bath or bed time.
VI. Continue to encourage resolution of mother's grief over time.	VIA. Continue to channel mother's grief into useful pursuits.	VIA. 1. Continue the processes described in initial program Goal III A, B and C.

hands in play. It is often easier for the child to develop use of one hand to the neglect of the other than to try to use a hand that neither moves nor feels normally. This works to the detriment of strengthening returning muscle power and developing use of residual muscles in bilateral play, self-care, and other functions.

Occupational Therapy

Occupational therapy intervention at an early age can contribute to potential for improved muscle function by careful positioning of the arm for optimum muscle protection and strengthening. Equally important is the contribution of the occupational therapy program to help the child develop functional use of the arm in play by positioning the arm to permit the child to see and use the arm and hand in early infant play. It is also important to help the parents work with the child for optimum gains, to learn to handle the child correctly to foster good arm use, and to learn to accept the residual deficits that do remain. Accepting the fact that the child will generally have some permanent deficits is not easy for the parents, but the occupational therapist may enhance parents' acceptance as they become involved with the child in the treatment program.

Case Study

Pat was medically diagnosed as having a brachial plexus injury at birth. She was referred to the occupational therapy service at 6 weeks of age. She maintained her right arm in an adducted and internally rotated position with elbow extension. Wrist and finger motion was present but limited. Her primary hand position was fisted, a normal position for a baby of her age. There was no marked passive limitation of motion in her arm, and she tolerated her mother handling and ranging her arm. Her lack of response to handling the right arm indicated a possible deficit in sensation of the right arm. Normal infant patterns of motion at this age generally include some elbow flexion, arm abducted slightly away from the side, and some external rotation particularly in startle and crying reactions. In her case these patterns were lacking. Tone and motion patterns in the left arm and hand were normal, as were her head, neck, and leg reactions. Figure 31-8 depicts the occupational therapy process as planned for this child and her family.

This was the first child of a young mother. The father did not take an active role in the child's program, and the young mother at first seemed

unable to comprehend the need for a treatment program for her child. Fortunately for this child, a grandmother was part of the extended family and took over the major responsibility for guiding the child's program at home. By the third and fourth visits, the young mother had grown in her ability to comprehend and work with the therapy program and with the child.

Problems noted in this child were as follows:
1. Limited active shoulder and elbow flexion musculature in right arm.
2. Possible lack of sensation and no ability to place her arm where she visually compensated for lack of sensation.
3. No ability to use her right arm in normal random waving motions.

Goals and objectives for the occupational therapy program were established as follows:

GOAL 1: Increased Muscle Strength in Right Arm
  Objective: Develop sufficient muscle strength in shoulder and elbow to enable Pat to place her arm in a position for hand use by the time she is 8 months old.

GOAL 2: Increase Sensory Awareness in Right Arm
  Objective: Pat will be aware enough of her right arm to turn when someone touches her right hand by the time she is 8 months old.

GOAL 3: Increase Functional Use and Awareness of Right Arm in Total Body Scheme
  Objective: Achieve a position for her right arm that would place her hand so Pat will be able to engage in some hand play between her hands.

The mother was instructed in a home program of 1) passive ranging of the right arm, 2) positioning of the right elbow in flexion by pinning an Ace bandage loop sling to the child's clothing and placing her right arm in the sling with elbow flexed for one-half of the day, 3) positioning of arm in abduction and slight external rotation by use of pillows when child was lying on her back in bed, 4) sensory stimulation to the right arm by means of rubbing and stroking many times a day, and 5) maintenance of equal play by the mother with the child's right and left arms. The mother was also encouraged to prop Pat's right arm under the child's chest when she was on her stomach and to encourage Pat to lift up her head and push up with her left arm.

The child was re-evaluated 6 weeks later, when she was 3 months old. She had developed better use of her shoulder in that she was swinging her arm through about one-fourth of the range of motion of the left arm. Her elbow was kept in a slightly more

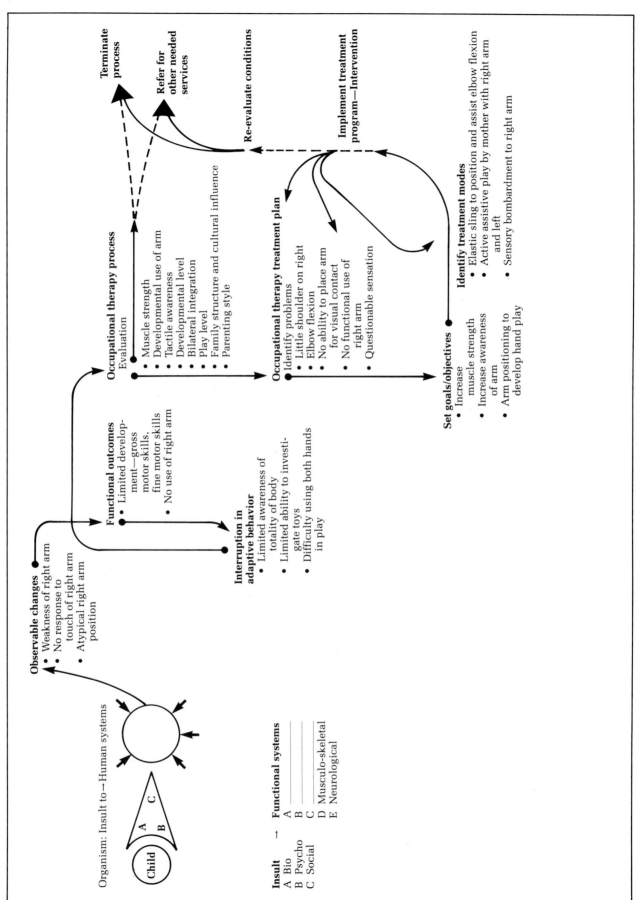

Figure 31-8. Occupational therapy program with an infant with a brachial plexus injury. Case study: Pat.

flexed position, but no elbow flexion was seen actively. More finger flexion and extension was seen, but she had increased in her tendency to keep a tightly clenched fist rather than losing this reflexive posture as she had done in the left hand. She also maintained her wrist in a sharply extended posture that is not normal for this age. She had continued to move through other developmental milestones, such as lifting her head well when on stomach, slight tension of her neck when pulled to sitting, relaxed hand on left, and momentary grasp on rattle.

Additional problems noted since the initial evaluation included an increased wrist hyperextension tendency and a clenched fist hand. Because of these additional problems the following objective was added:
GOAL 1:

Objective 2: Develop a hand that is relaxed and slightly open at rest and one that Pat is able to open and close around toys.

Treatment instituted was the wearing of a special cock-up orthosis that prevented wrist hyperextension. The orthosis positioned her fingers in extension at the metacarpal phalangeal joints to encourage active finger extension. The mother was advised to have Pat wear this orthosis 1½ hours, three times a day. She was also advised to continue with the previous home program with special emphasis on helping Pat move her right arm along with her left arm in play activities.

Pat was re-evaluated again at 6 months of age. At that time she was making excellent use of her right arm in reaching activities. Arm and shoulder motion was not normal, but her efficiency in reaching for toys was almost equalized between right and left. Her right hand was relaxed most of the time, with tension noted primarily in the thumb and index finger. She demonstrated palmar grasp with the right and used the right hand together with the left for holding larger objects. Elbow flexion still lagged behind, and all bilateral arm motions were accomplished with the extended right elbow. In supine with her right elbow propped in a slightly flexed position, she was able to flex her elbow slightly using the biceps occasionally. In all other positions she was unable to activate the right biceps. When on her stomach she supported herself with the right and left arm equally. She had not started to creep or crawl, so use of her right arm in this pattern was not evaluated. Problems still noted were:

1. lack of right elbow flexion unless maximally assisted;
2. lack of full arm raising on the right;
3. slight difficulty in opening thumb and index finger on the right.

Additional objectives were developed as follows:
GOAL 1:

Objective 3: Develop elbow flexion sufficiently for her to bring objects toward her.

Objective 4: Continue to develop free opening and closing of her right hand, especially thumb and index finger, sufficiently to allow her to handle toys.

GOAL 3:

Objective 2: Monitor use of right arm in developmental activities so that, as growth and development causes the need for more complex hand activities that require two hands, Pat is able to make sufficient use of the right hand to accomplish the developmental task.

The mother was again instructed in a home program, with the focus of the program now being on propping the right elbow in a bent position and helping Pat make use of the slight biceps that is present. The child was not ready for a walker at that time; however, an overhead sling with spring assist were to be added to encourage elbow flexion. Developmental activities of propping on both elbows; reaching out with both hands; and handling, dropping, and picking up toys were to be encouraged. Ongoing re-evaluations at regular 2 to 4-month intervals were scheduled until maximum benefits are achieved. □

Spina Bifida

Discussion

The child born with spina bifida starts life with a limited number of opportunities to experience the full spectrum of sensorimotor experiences that contribute to normal growth and development. The child has no bowel or bladder control and varying degrees of sensory and motor loss to the lower extremities and trunk. The child may also have some degree of hydrocephalus and may or may not have a shunt to drain the cerebrospinal fluid to another part of the body.

The implications of this disability include a variety of losses of normal developmental experiences and the opportunity to experience normal developmental adaptation. The spina bifida child has limited mobility and, therefore, misses out on many of the normal experiences of movement, such as rolling over, rocking on his or her stomach, creeping, crawling, running, and jumping. The child may frequently be sick, and parents are necessarily more cautious and careful in handling the child. This will further limit the child's opportunities for movement, such as being bounced and swung around, and for normal social interactions with parents and peers. Sensation is also deficient in a portion of the body, so the child is receiving less than normal sensation from which to learn about his or her body and the world around.

These basic deficiencies in normal experiences, if not treated, will have a delaying effect upon development, especially in those areas that are strongly dependent upon normal tactile and vestibular input, such as eye control, integration of both sides of the body, and good motor planning. When these are coupled with an untreated hydrocephalus that results in neurological deficits, the child's delays can result in marked learning deficits. Occupational therapy intervention at a young age can provide the child with an opportunity to experience some normal tactile and vestibular responses that will enhance the child's normal growth and development and will prevent developmental delays that would result in learning problems in later years.

Case Study

Mary, diagnosed as having spina bifida at birth, was first seen by the occupational therapist when she was 4 years old. See Figure 31-9, which depicts the occupational therapy program plan. The human systems involved were circulatory, intestinal–urinary, musculoskeletal, and neurological. Mary presented no hydrocephalus condition. The observable changes in Mary were:

1. No active foot and ankle muscles, poor knee muscle strength, good hip muscle strength. She walked with bilateral long leg orthosis and a walker.
2. No sensation from the knees down.
3. No bowel and bladder control.
4. Frequent infections of the urinary tract and respiratory system.

The occupational therapy initial evaluation revealed the following functional losses and interruption in developmental adaptation.

1. No response to postrotary nystagmus test after 10 seconds of spinning nor any response after a repeat test of 20 seconds' duration.
2. No ability to achieve a correct prone extension-holding pattern to overcome the dominance of the tonic labyrinthine reflex when prone. This deficit would be expected in her legs due to lower extremity weakness, but she also could not lift her head and shoulders and was very frightened of the position.
3. No protective extension or parachuting reaction.

4. Poor attention to task. She frequently talked rather than attending to assigned play activities.
5. Limited experience on normal playground equipment. She was still frightened of most new play activities that involved total body motion.
6. Eye tracking was nonexistent. She did not even attempt to pursue the object by moving her head as many 4-year-olds will do.

Fine motor skills were at age level, as were self-care skills. She even attempted the difficult task of putting on her long leg orthosis. The family was very supportive and had attempted to seek medical advice at an early age. As a result, urinary tract infections had been kept at a minimum. She had been referred to a physical therapist by 10 months of age, but this was her first referral to an occupational therapist. There was a younger brother in the family, and play between Mary and her younger brother was quite normal for the ages of the two children in spite of the fact that Mary was more confined and limited in her activities.

Occupational Therapy Program

Occupational therapy intervention was necessary to achieve the following goals and objectives:

GOAL 1: Child Will Be Able to Develop Improved Vestibular Responses to Movement.
  Objective: Mary will show slight nystagmus (after 6 months of treatment).
GOAL 2: Child Will Be Able to Integrate Primitive Reflexes As a Means to Achieving Normal Adult Reflex and Movement Patterns.
  Objective: She will be able to lift her shoulders, arms, and head when on her stomach for 10 seconds, and will be able to play in this position with moving activities for 10 minutes without fatigue.
  Objective: She will be able to throw her arms out protectively four out of five times when turned upside down.
GOAL 3: Child Will Be Able to Develop Improved Eye Tracking Ability.
  Objective: She will be able to eye track smoothly horizontally three times and vertically three times, after 3 months of treatment.
  Objective: She will be able to eye track diagonally smoothly two out of three times after 6 months of treatment.
GOAL 4: Child Will Be Able to Develop Attention to Performance Tasks at Her Age Level.
  Objective: She will be able to follow therapist's oral directions in the treatment

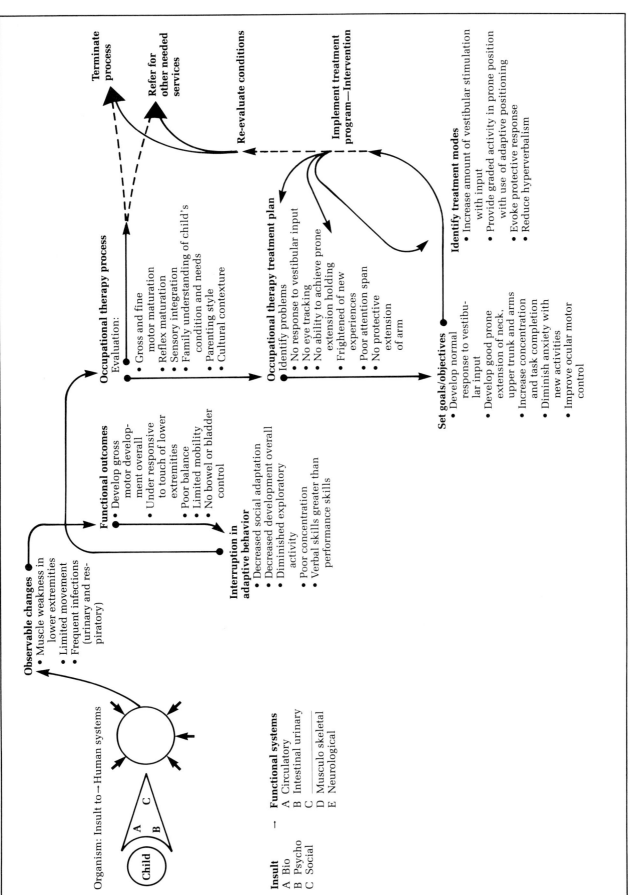

Figure 31-9. Occupational therapy program with a spina-bifida child. Case study: Mary.

sessions three out of four times without extraneous conversation.

Objective: She will be able to play appropriately with a toy of her own choice for 15 minutes.

She was treated weekly in an outpatient treatment center, and a home program was designed for the parents to use between treatment sessions. Her therapy program consisted of a variety of vestibular activities including spinning in a hammock, riding a scooterboard, swinging in an infant swing that supported her unstable legs, rocking in a "Play All" toy, and being bounced on a spring horse. Due to the weakness in her legs, she could not bounce herself on the horse.

She was also started in a program that would encourage the development of a good prone extension-holding pattern by positioning her on a scooterboard which was adapted to accommodate for some of her structural deformities. Her hips were tight in flexion, and her lower back was lordodic. This caused her to be angled in an uncomfortable position downward when on her stomach contributing to her dislike of this position. By wedging at her hips and upper trunk, she was placed in an optimum position to foster good upper trunk and head extension. By propelling herself on the scooterboard very rapidly, she was able to stimulate more automatic head lift. This treatment procedure was also designed to encourage better eye tracking.

Her parents were shown how to design a similar scooterboard for home use. They were supportive of the need to build this equipment and used it at home as a supplement to the weekly occupational therapy session. After the parents watched and helped with the child's treatment program for several treatment sessions, the family was provided with a home program to be carried out daily with Mary. The child's younger brother also enjoyed the same activities, so peer play time was used to provide the optimum activities to enhance this child's development. By using the peer play time for the exercise program, less attention was drawn to the special treatment. This avoided the conflicts frequently arising in family situations when one child receives special treatment.

After 3 months in the program Mary was able to:
1. Lift shoulders, arms, and head when on her stomach for 10 seconds and play in this position for 20 minutes without fatigue.
2. Consistently throw both arms out to protect herself when turned upside down.
3. Attend to assigned performance tasks for 20 minutes.
4. Eye track horizontally five times smoothly.

She had not made any gains in correct nystagmus following spinning nor had she gained any vertical or diagonal eye tracking. Her treatment program was revised to increase emphasis on the activities for these two areas, and she continued in the outpatient program for 6 more months. She was referred to the school-based therapist when she entered school at age 5. After a year in school, the school-based therapist reported that Mary had continued to make gains in eye tracking and attention span, and was having no trouble in the regular classroom. At 6 years of age she still did not show any nystagmus response to spinning for 10 seconds. She continued on a home program of stimulation to her vestibular system. The school-based therapist re-evaluated her progress frequently and made suggestions to the family, but Mary was not provided direct occupational services because her classroom performance was excellent.

Although at 6 years of age this child still shows a neurological deficit in motor and sensory control of her lower extremities and a significant lag in her vestibular processing, the occupational therapy intervention enabled her to reach a more balanced level of growth and development allowing her to function in the regular classroom. Attention span and eye tracking deficits seen at age 4 could have hampered classroom performance without the intervention and remediation provided through the occupational therapy program. □

Down's Syndrome

Discussion

Basic and general understanding of children with Down's Syndrome is clouded by a history of long-standing misinformation. Despite more advanced methods, both lay persons and professionals often lack sufficient or current information about this condition, characteristics of development, and specific developmental potential. Advances in cytogenetic studies do enable physicians to provide a more timely and accurate diagnosis. Accurate type of Down's syndrome identification does clarify whether the genetic insult is hereditary or an accidental mutation. These advances are of great importance to Down's Syndrome children and the parents. Nevertheless, for parents of newborn or young Down's Syndrome children, the paucity of help in learning to parent their child and in understanding the development of their child is a major problem. Occupational therapists have an important early and long-range role in assisting both the parents of and Down's Syndrome children to attain their individual development potential.

Physical Characteristics

Certain physical characteristics of Down's Syndrome children are classic and familiar:

- shortened limbs and fingers
- slanted eyes with skin fold over eyelid
- small mouth with enlarged protruding tongue
- simian line
- speckled iris
- high incidence of congenital heart defects
- increased incidence of leukemia
- mental retardation

Other physical characteristics of importance to the child's development, though less well known, are:

- floppiness at birth and generalized low muscle tone prevalence in early years. Note: Special weakness of trunk flexors and, in general, poor muscle co-contractibility
- hyperextensibility joints system, especially the hips, limbs, and digits
- poor muscle tone of oral facial mechanism
- increased and prolonged tactile sensitivity with diffuse tactile discrimination deficiency
- increased sensitivity to gravitational adjustment
- hyporeactive postrotary nystagmus
- poor bilateral motor coordination

Because of the altered sensory integration, the following variations often occur in neurodevelopmental reflex maturation:

- diminished suck reflex
- accentuated gag reflex
- diminished palmar reflex
- prolonged exaggerated moro reflex
- prolonged flexor withdrawal and avoidance reactions of hands and feet
- delayed proprioceptive placing of limbs and "air sitting" response to positive support testing
- poor optical righting, especially supine reactions
- poor body on body righting
- delayed equilibrium responses, especially quadripedal and standing

Some of the motor problems that are outcomes of the previous stated conditions are:

- a general delay in gross motor milestone attainment based on body instability, weakness, and often fear of imposed handling or imposed touch sensation
- skull sensitivity, also feet and hands sensitivity
- prolonged head lag in coming to sit
- child avoids weight bearing on feet—air sits or retracts lower extremities
- child often incorporates creeping with knee extension pattern

- child may have hyperextended knees, pronated feet in walking pattern

Some examples of characteristics are shown in Figure 31-10.

Other predictable outcomes based on these Down's Syndrome variations in development are as follows:

- difficulty in early nurturing ability with later selectivity in foods basically tied to gag reflex influences and poor chewing ability
- delays in prehension overall
- delays in finger feeding due to sensitivity of hands to messiness
- splintered hand skill development with some compensation because of delayed or organized mobility

In general, Down's Syndrome children are usually classically dyspraxic based on vestibular somotasensory dysfunction.

Case Study

History and Background

Jane, a 20-month-old Down's Syndrome child, had a history of delayed development, recurrent respiratory infection, and allergies, despite general good health. Jane had received comprehensive developmental services prior to initial evaluation.

Jane's parents were newly located following the completion of their graduate studies in applied sciences. Both parents' ages were in their late 20s. Each had secured promising positions in the field of their study. They had little experience in handling or caring for young children, Jane being their first and only child. Both were equally committed to their careers and their child. Communication between the parents seemed good. Household responsibilities were shared equally by the parents. The father demonstrated innate nurturing skills while the mother, an assertive person, seemed less at ease. The father assumed equal or more responsibility for Jane's care. Both held high anticipation for their child's individual development and high expectations for those providing services directed toward such goals. They demonstrated good coping skills relating to Jane's high-strung behavior and frequent temper outbursts. They initiated a request for developmental services, including occupational therapy services from a community infant–parent training program. Figure 31-11 depicts that process.

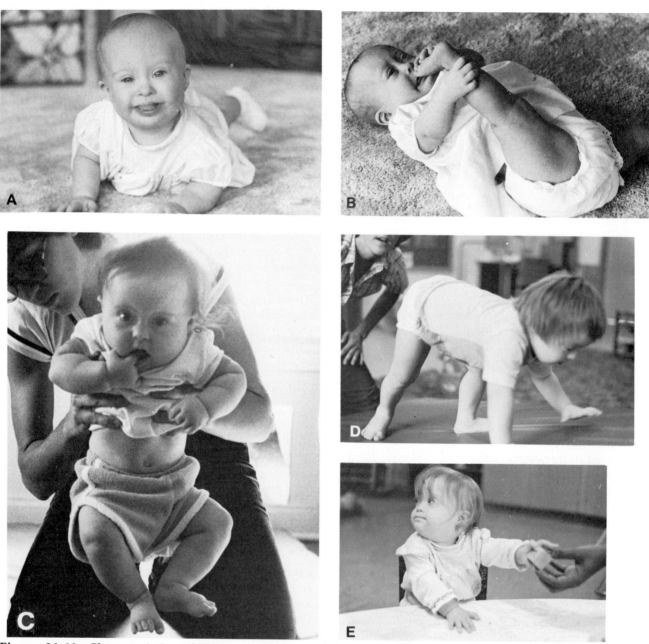

Figure 31-10. Characteristics of Down's-syndrome children's motor development or performance. (*A*) Oral–facial weakness. (*B*) Hyperextensible joints, especially hips. (*C*) Diminished proprioception and tactile sensitivity seen in delayed positive support of lower extremities. (*D*) Extended knee creeping compensating for diminished proprioception and joint stability. (*E*) Poor attention and concentration in fine skill performance.

Occupational Therapy Program–Initial Evaluation

During the initial evaluation on Jane at 20 months, she was noted to have moderately low muscle tone with a presence of hyperextensible joints of the limbs and digits. A key problem area was identified in the markedly limited mobility of the child. The child could sit with a fairly straight back when placed, and could roll to right and left, but was delayed in independent coming to and lowering from sit. When pulled to sit, she assisted but still demonstrated head lag during the first 45 degrees of movement. Delay was also noted in lower extremity weight bearing and support. The child avoided surface contact by air sitting more than 50% of the

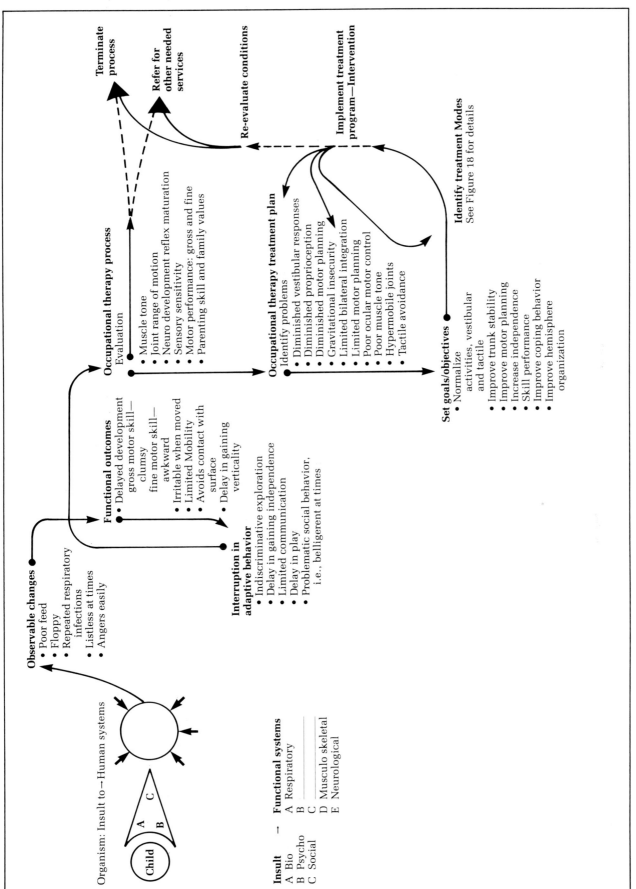

Figure 31-11. Occupational therapy with a Down's syndrome child. Case study: Jane.

time. She had recently gained pivoting in prone and had emerging skills in reciprocal progression in the prone position. Reflexively, she continued to show some hand and foot avoidance, though instinctive grasping was moderately present. She had poor placing of hands and absent visual placing of legs. The overall gross motor level was 6–7 months with a motor quotient of 35% indicating significant deficiency.

In contrast, fine motor performance was in advance of gross motor. In feeding, she had a good appetite and was eating a wide variety of foods, chewing fairly well, independent in cup use and finger feeding, and was able to help with spoon feeding. In dressing she was generally cooperative, and was able to take off her socks and shoes when untied. In general manipulation she banged blocks together, reached for large objects, approximated a 1-inch cube over another, and threw a ball undirected. She was beginning to discriminate a crayon and used it appropriately. She was using both the right and left hand equally well, and was just beginning to automatically cross midline with the right. In general, her fine motor skills clustered at 12–15 months or roughly at 60%–75% of chronological age expectancy.

Sensory factors of significance were as follows:

- tactile avoidance, with diffused and poor discrimination; oral sucking behavior; irritability to light touch on the back of the neck, abdomen, hands, and feet
- proprioception—under registered—seeking such on her own limits
- vestibular processing—poor postural organization with diminished response to postrotary nystagmus testing; alarmed and irritated by linear vestibular input when imposed
- visual processing—visually attentive, but lacked smooth ocular motor performance depending on neck rotation primarily; convergence limited, with midline interruptions
- visual search relating to object permanence judged to be at 8 months, and in obtaining objects she could push away an obstruction to obtain a wanted object
- motor planning—limited gross motor planning in evidence, though fine motor planning included imitation of repetitive simple gestures and in some cases she was examining, letting go, and initiating some "give me" transactions

A treatment and educational planning meeting was held with the parents following completion of the child's evaluation. Evaluation results were explained along with the identified problems, goals, and objectives.

Proposed treatment and educational modes or procedures to assist in achieving short-range goals were explained, including suggested home program activities. Though the parents agreed to the plan that focused on improving Jane's sensory motor integration and adaptive behavior, they questioned whether or not more emphasis should be placed on cognitive activities for Jane. Staff provided further explanation of the need for sensory motor organization for their child as a basis for cognitive development, explaining that in Jane's case, improved sensory integration would reduce her sensitivity and would lead to improved mobility, understanding, and function. There was agreement that Jane would attend daily classes at the Center, that would provide sensory motor integration intervention, along with speech–language, educational, and social developmental activities. Home programming with parent training was agreed to as well. Formal re-evaluation was tentatively scheduled for 3 months following initiation of programming activities.

The outline of the treatment plan (see Jane's Occupational Therapy Program—20 months) includes major therapeutic goals, with specific objectives and suggested modes or procedures. Ongoing adaptation or adjustment of these procedures is required as objectives are achieved or when methods appear to be inappropriate. Jane's attendance for programming at the Center was regular. Home programming visitation by the Center therapist was highly irregular due to parent cancellation. The reason given for the numerous cancellations of home visit appointments was work-related conflicts.

Re-evaluation

Jane was 24 months old at the time of re-evaluation. She continued to have hyperextensible joints and moderately low muscle tone, but she had made major gains in mobility. Improved motor planning for movement transitions were seen in new skills in raising and lowering from sit, and from sit to hands and knees. The ability to creep and hitch were demonstrated with some instability. Because of this instability, she continued to use reciprocal prone progression as her chief mode, which was at that time a very efficient skill. Though she continued to air sit 25% of the time, when handled she showed emerging lower extremity positive support, and was standing at a rail and beginning to lower to sit. She could pivot in sitting and no longer showed head lag

Jane's Occupational Therapy Program: Chronological Age—20 Months

Therapeutic Goals	Objectives	Examples • Methods • Modes • Procedures
I. Normalize tactile sensitivity as a means to increase gross and fine motor function/mobility.	IA. Child will air sit infrequently (1 out of 10 x's) when lowered in handling.	IA. 1. Apply firm tactile stimulation generally to child 2 x D. 2. Provide manual otolithic stimulation in all positions including supported standing to tolerance. 2 x D.
	B. Child will weight bear in standing hold to rail.	B. 1. Using external motivator, child will be assisted in transitional movement to achieve standing during purposeful play. 5x during a 30 minute period.
	C. Child will explore familiar objects using both instinctive and voluntary grasp with avoidance interference.	C. 1. As in A.1 plus moisten body with water generalized especially extremities. 2. Child will search for objects partially hidden in a box containing styrofoam stuffing, crumbled foam or pan of water for 10 minutes.
II. Improve proprioception especially trunk stability, as a means to increase gross motor function/ mobility.	IIA. Child will maintain static quadriped position during activity.	IIA,B,C. 1. Using a weighted vest and cuff weight child will bounce on a flexible surface such as an air mattress with assist, 5-10 minutes. Other means of bouncing, firm padded board in hammock on springs when in quadriped be sure palms are flattened. Weighted/vest Cuff weights Firm surface suspended/by hammock & spring
III. Normalize gravitational insecurity and improve vestibular processing to enhance adaptive behavior.	IIIA. Child will tolerate swinging.	IIIA. 1. Child will swing on suspended pendulum swing with spring seated for 5 minutes (3 second arcs)
	B. Child will tolerate tilting.	B. 1. Child will tilt on firm surface in prone, supine, sitting and puppy position.

Therapeutic Goals	Objectives	Examples • Methods • Modes • Procedures
	C. Child will initiate and tolerate sliding.	C. 1. Child will slide down an incline plane on stomach and in seated position 2 times minimal or more frequently to desire.
IV. Improve motor planning as a means to increase gross and fine motor function.	IVA. Child will attempt to imitate complex gestures. B. Child will raise and lower from sitting. C. Child will move to hands and knees.	A. 1. Child will attend to task demonstration and initiate movement grossly. B&C. 1. Using external motivator, child will perform these transitional movements during play activities 5 times during a 30 minute period.
V. Improve bilateral integration.	VA. Child will cross midline right and left in seated activities. B. Child will cross midline in prone activities.	VA. 1. Child will place objects in a receptical to right of midline with left hand and vice versa 10 times. B. 1. Child will turn, while prone, using alternating hands, to right and left in hammock.
VI. Improve ocular motor control.	VIA. Child will track object using eye muscles with minimal rotation.	VIA. 1. While lying supine child will follow a slowly swinging 3″ ball of contrasting color.
VII. Improve the level of independence in activities of daily living.	VIIA. Child will eat with minimal assistance. B. Child will partially remove shirt and pants.	VIIA. 1. Child will be fitted with scoop dish, non slide and spoon with handle of ⅝″ diameter. Spoon should be bent slightly to compensate for poor supination stability. 2. Child should use feeding equipment at school and home daily. Assistance may be needed in practice of filling spoon. B. 1. Child will practice removing button shirt or loose T-shirt over head in 1 minute D, at school and home with encouragement. 2. Child will practice removing pants from knees when seated, in 2 minutes with encouragement D, at school and home.

coming to sit. The key changes in reflex status were seen in lessening plantar grasping; less avoidance of hands and feet; improved visual-labyrinthine righting in supine; improved placing of limbs, especially her hands and arms; improved equilibrium in prone supine and sitting; and emergence of protective reactions sideways. Gross motor skill level had reached 11 months, with a gross motor quotient of 42%.

Improved fine motor skill was also apparent. Jane now demonstrated independent spoon and two-handed cup use, though she was quite messy and needed a watchful eye at mealtimes to prevent chaos. She was beginning to wipe her mouth. In dressing she was able to partially remove upper and lower garments. She was beginning to scribble with a stubby crayon. Her pincer grasp was precise as was opposition, and she could now release a block carefully, place a peg in a hole, and on occasion leaf pages one at a time. She was continuing to use some oral exploration, but she tended to rotate and examine objects more often.

Sensory integration factors of significance were:

- tactile avoidance—now less pervasive but continued to be noted, especially with lower extremities and feet; continued oral seeking behavior, at times, poor tactile discrimination now noted in two-point discrimination.
- proprioception continued to be under registered—continued to be sought by herself; changes were noted in her improved willingness to allow others to control her excessive drive. Poor concentration seemed to be linked to poor proprioception and cocontractability
- vestibular processing-improving postural organization with continued hyporesponsiveness to postrotary nystagmus testing; no longer alarmed by linear vestibular input when imposed—but now sometimes angered; now seeking angular vestibular stimulation
- motor planning—improved gross motor planning as reflected in gross motor milestone attainments; able to get off chair; fine motor planning and imitation level include clapping, waving bye bye, imitating two gestures in twinkle–twinkle, making faces spontaneously and on occasion in imitation.

Resetting Goals, Objectives, and Methods

A joint parent-staff meeting was held following Jane's reassessment at 24 months. The parents were encouraged by Jane's advances in mobility and skill gains. They were concerned about Jane's behavior because of her continued temper outbursts that sometimes occurred in handling, often when the child was unable to get her needs met, and in some cases when expectations required Jane to "be still" for any length of time. Jane's parents were worried about her short concentration. The staff explained the related nature of sensory integration dysfunction to irritable behavior and anger, to poor organization, and hence, to poor concentration. The staff urged that they be given more opportunity to assist the parents in home management techniques and sensory integration opportunities. The parents agreed to make a more concerted effort to organize a supportive home program and to meet regularly with a home program therapist. The adjustments in goals, objectives, and methods are presented in Jane's Occupational Therapy Program—24 months.

Subsequent re-evaluations of Jane at age 29 months and 34 months, and conferences with parents, confirmed the successful achievement of motor skills to 85% of age expectancy in fine and gross function. She was moving freely in space at home and outdoors, was running stiffly, squatting in play, mounting stairs, and descending while using a rail. On occasion her parents did carry Jane, but principally for their own convenience or when Jane was tired. Jane could self-feed fairly well, undress with ease, and she was learning to unfasten. She was partially toilet trained. She was concentrating for longer periods; working simple puzzles; stacking blocks to seven high; and imitating vertical, horizontal, and circular patterns with chalk and crayon on a vertical and horizontal surface. Jane's skill performance was not splintered but generalized. She was playing with dolls symbolically and demonstrated many skills in her use of objects in symbolic play. Her construction of objects in space, such as arranging chairs at a table, ordering large plastic boxes, and using objects for intended purposes, was expanding daily. Parents and staff noted with satisfaction that as tactile, proprioception, and vestibular processing normalized, Jane had not only gained skills, but her stormy behavior had subsided and she was far easier to manage. An extra bonus was Jane's markedly improved ability to follow oral instructions for motor output. Overall communication was advancing as well.

Staff and parents agreed to continue Jane's program with an upgrading of sensorimotor integration objectives until age 36 months. They also agreed that Jane could profit from a combination of early childhood programming (to continue needed therapeutic measures) with normal 2+-year-old nursery experiences. The transition to this was a fairly smooth one for Jane and her family. At age 48 months a follow-up indicated continued sensorimotor integration, good mastery of skills

Jane's Occupational Therapy Program: Chronological Age—24 Months

Therapeutic Goals	Objectives	Examples • Methods • Modes • Procedures
I. Improve the continuity of the treatment program.	IA. Train parents in skills necessary to provide sensory motor integration programming as a part of their daily life pattern.	IA. 1. Hold planning meeting at child's home, review the new therapeutic objectives and procedures and how they will promote development. 2. Determine those procedures the parents will be able to incorporate over time. 3. Help parents obtain, construct or install equipment or supplies needed for program. 4. Teach by demonstration and example those techniques judged to be of greatest value to parent and child. 5. Have parents assist in procedures, then demonstrate the procedure independently. 6. Give genuine praise for effort, be lert to caution about procedures. 7. Give particular consultation, and demonstration method for controlling behavior during therapeutic procedures and in general daily living encounters.
II. Continue to normalize tactile sensitivity to improve gross/fine motor function/mobility.	IIA. Child will not exhibit air sitting when lowered in handling. B. Child will cruise independently and walk with hands held. C. Child will explore unfamiliar objects instinctively or voluntarily without avoidance.	IIA. 1. Continue to apply firm tactile stimulation generally. 2. Continue otolith stimulation especially in kneeling and supported standing (5 min. 00) B. 1. Using external motivator child will move independently in biped using furniture for support or hands of therapist during purposeful play. C. 1. As in A1 plus misting to body generalized. Child will search for objects that are varied in texture and use, that are placed on shelves that require child to kneel or standing to obtain for (10 minutes D).

Therapeutic Goals	Objectives	Examples • Methods • Modes • Procedures
III. Normalize gravitational insecurity and improve vestibular processing to enhance adaptive behavior.	IIIA. Child will increase tolerance to swinging.	IIIA. 1. Child will swing on platform in prone—supine, seated and puppy position for 5 minutes (4 sec. acrs).
	B. Child will increase tolerance to tilting.	B. 1. Child will tilt on a firm surface in the quadriped, kneeling and in supported standing 5 minutes D.
	C. Child will increase tolerance to sliding.	C. 1. Child will slide down inclined plane on a metal disc seat facing forward, backward and sideways; also in puppy position forward and backward to tolerance D.
IV. Improve proprioception, especially trunk, shoulder girdle and hands.	IVA. Child will propel himself with use of upper extremities.	IVA. 1. Positioned in seat or prone position in hammock, child will pull himself/herself through space by means of suspended dental dam strip 10x's 2x D.
	B. Child will place hands more effective and initiate backwards protective extension.	B.*1. Child will use protective extension when moved while seated on carpeted barrel. 10x's D. *Continue use of cuff weights and weighted vest.
V. Improve motor planning as a means to increase gross and fine motor function	VA. Child will attempt to copy therapist's demonstrated gestures in goal directed task.	VA. 1. Child will pull bead on string, stack beads 3-6 high, turn crank on toy, spin large top.

Therapeutic Goals	Objectives	Examples • Methods • Modes • Procedures
VI. Improve bilateral integration.	VIA. Child will demonstrate use of assisting hand. B. Child will cross midline in 2 step activities.	VIA. 1. Child will remove cap from pen, hold jar while unscrewing lid, hold bead while stringing same with dominant hand. B. 1. Child will move forward on scooter in prone position through a simple maze requiring turns of 180° to right and left using alternating hands. 10 feet trip 2x's.
VII. Improve ocular motor control.	VIIA. Child will track and converge as a part of a purposeful task.	VIIA. 1. Child will push and catch a 6″ ball while seated 10 x's D.
VIII. Improve the level of independence in activities of daily life.	VIIIA. Child will eat independently without supervision. B. Child will completely removal of shirt and partial removal of pants.	VIIIA. 1. Using adaptive feed equipment, child will feed all meals routinely with less spilling. B. 1. Child will remove button shirt or loose T-shirt at nap time and bath time. B. 2. Child will take off pants when below hips.

overall, and, in particular, good visual motor integration. This marked gain in ability to copy symbols was only one of a number of evidences that gave support to a hopeful future of Jane's academic potential and overall development. □

Autism

Discussion

Autistic children demonstrate a marked deviation in development, exhibiting classic characteristics that pediatric occupational therapists need to be aware of. Autism was first identified as a distinct syndrome by Kanner[1]. Through Kanner's work, other researchers intensified efforts to identify etiological factors and characteristics of the condition and to determine which treatment or methods of treatment were effective. To date research has yet to identify the exact physical cause of autism.

Autistic children display unusual social developmental characteristics. Often they are unable to relate appropriately to their parents, siblings, peers, and others they encounter in their environment. They often display an indifferent or detached behavior. Their language may be delayed or absent. Often a deficiency is noted in reception or registration. In many cases symbolic representation in expression is lacking, and the child's expressions are limited to echolalic production. In other cases expressive language organization is disordered, and characteristically, pronoun references are poor. Because of the late-ness, absence or peculiarity of their child's ability to communicate, initially parents often seek professional help from physicians, psychologists, social workers, and speech pathologists. In other cases, parents seek help for their child because they recognize that their child is not relating to themselves (the parents) and that he or she has unusual behaviors—in some cases very obsessive—that prevent the child's ability to advance in acquiring generalized function.

More recent investigators of autism (Ornitz and Ritvo)[2] have identified neurophysiological disorders as a major factor in autism, focusing on sensorimotor and perceptual motor processing as contributing factors. Ornitz[3,4] raises pertinent questions about the relationship of vestibular processing efficiency to autism. Recent researchers in the field of autism have recognized the inadequate ability of autistic children to process, organize, interpret, and respond to sensory information. Pediatric occupational therapy skills/services are specifically related to the improvement of such processing deficiencies as a means of promoting improved functional and behavioral/adaptive outcomes. As such, autism evaluation and treatment should include occupational therapy services. The treatment of this disorder should include the services of occupational therapists because of their therapeutic skills in developing such sensorimotor organization for functional behavioral advancement.

Specific characteristics identified in autism[5,6] include the following:
- onset prior to 30 months
- perceptual and sensory processing disturbances, as a possible result of distorted sensation, faulty modulation of sensory input, and impaired discriminative ability
- deviations in rate of development marked by periods of rapid growth, followed by plateaus
- inability to relate to others noted in such behaviors as aversion to physical contact, delay or absence of social smile, and lack of anticipation of being picked up
- unusual relating to objects with a need to "maintain sameness" (Kanner) in the environment, leading to rigid, inflexible, and controlling personality traits; frequently, manipulation of toys is inappropriate and maladaptive where spinning, twirling, rubbing, and feeling of them is common
- speech and language disorders marked not only by delayed development but also abnormal features, including echolalia, pronoun reversal, and monotonous and atonal quality expressing little emotion; language-related functions in general are seriously impaired, including symbolic play, abstraction, understanding of gestures and writ-

ten language, sequential tasks (primarily temporal in nature) and meaning in memory processes
- unusual motility or spontaneous motion patterns, either intermittent or continuous, repeated in serial fashion; includes hand-flapping, finger-flicking, and toe-walking
- mental retardation is diagnosed in a high percentage of autistic children, as most cannot perform adequately on IQ tests and generally perform throughout life as mentally impaired individuals
- seizure disorders likely to become manifested with increasing age, even in those with normal EEGs and neurological examinations early in life
- "soft" neurological signs often found, including low muscle tone, poor coordination, drooling, short attention span, hyperactivity, hypoactivity, and hyperreflexia

Efforts to identify possible explanations for this complex, behaviorally and clinically defined syndrome have led to inconclusive findings. Some authors have investigated parental traits and socioeconomic conditions,[7,8] noting a preponderance of highly intellectual, obsessive professional parents, lacking in emotional warmth.

Most investigators now agree that central nervous system dysfunction is the basis for autism. Consideration given to prenatal and perinatal causes, association with viral diseases, genetic factors, and biochemical and metabolic elements has not produced a significant explanation of etiology. These parameters continue to be studied in hopes of finding not only the reasons for the occurrence of autism, but additional modes of intervention to increase the functional capacity of individuals involved.

Prognosis for future outcome with autistics in developing functions necessary for independent living is more hopeful for the mildly involved and those with fewer complicating and associated disorders, such as mental impairment and other development delays. Higher IQ, earlier language development, and earlier demonstration of appropriate play seem to be indicators of a more hopeful outcome.[9,10] However, the number who can live and work unaided is small, with most requiring assistance and supervision throughout life.

Intervention strategies are as varied as the possible causes and include behavioral approaches, milieu therapy, play therapy, neurodevelopmental treatment approaches, and pharmacotherapy provided in medical and educational settings.

Of particular interest to the occupational therapist who applies neurological and developmental principles in treatment is the disordered sensorimotor integration often displayed by autistic children. Responses to stimulation can be elevated or reduced, in various instances, in the same child. Autistic children may be noted to lack response to painful stimuli; to lack or have delayed startle response; to lack visual attention to new events within the environment; or to be unaware of auditory input. In contrast, the therapist may note exaggerated responses to sensory stimuli that create observable stress in the child, who attempts to avoid or block out the sensation. The child who seeks to whirl and rock himself in one instance may display fear of vestibular activity in another. Oral-tactile sensitivities are noted by the child's aversion to foods of thick consistency and/or rough texture. Avoidance of certain odors may occur, yet the child may smell objects in his hand prior to mouthing them in exploration.

Seeking of stimulation is a commonly observed trait, especially of apparent input to the tactile, proprioceptive, and vestibular systems. Rubbing and twirling of objects in the fingers, probably to produce tactile stimulation, is noted in some autistic children. One adult[11] reports a great need for heavy pressure, finding comfort and relief from stress when receiving significant amounts of such pressure input. Rocking, head-rolling and head-banging, twirling, and hand-flapping may be methods of stimulation through proprioceptive and vestibular channels. Becker[12] reports Ayres' observations that autistic children seek joint traction to a degree that most individuals would find painful.

Auditory and visual input may also be sought in unusual, yet persistent and obsessive ways. Generally, it appears that there is preference for input through the proximal senses (somatosensory, vestibular, gustatory, and olfactory) over the distal senses (auditory and visual) for environmental exploration. If sensory modulation is inadequate, even information through the early-evolving tactile, proprioceptive, and vestibular systems may be of little value if the child cannot make sense of those inputs in forming the basis for advancing social, movement, and learning strategies. These sensory channels are the primary focus in applying the theoretical principles of sensory integration, as occupational therapists attempt to enhance the foundation for increasingly sophisticated adaptive functions.

In investigating responses to sensory input as predictors of outcome in sensory integrative therapy, Ayres and Tickle[13] found that those autistic children who were hyperresponsive or oriented to certain types of stimuli showed greater gains in treatment than those who were hyporesponsive. It is suggested that children whose nervous systems are receiving some sensory input, but who fail to organize that information, have an advantage over those who do not register the information because of an inability or failure to orient to stimuli. It seems easier in therapy, through controlled sensory input, to help modify information that is entering the child's brain than to activate new or nonfunctioning neural circuits.

Children typically learn through movement and play, gaining information about themselves, about objects in the environment, and about themselves in relation to objects and others. Movement is basic to learning, laying the foundation for percepts, concepts, and abstract reasoning in addition to establishing the child's self-identity. Black, et al,[14] found that within a confined area, equipped for gross motor activities, autistic children engage in more imitative play and display more appropriate play behaviors than in spaces where no objects or other smaller toys are presented. In the latter situations more repetitive and solitary behaviors are noted.

Planned and controlled sensory input used in active play helps to facilitate more appropriate and adaptive behaviors in children, and it offers the occupational therapist an important and vital mechanism by which to impact on a child's total growth and development.

Case Study

Raymond, age 5 and diagnosed as autistic to a moderate degree, was born prematurely at 6 months gestation. He remained on a respirator for 2 months before he was physically stable enough to be held by his parents. His mother reported that toxemia occurred during her pregnancy. Both parents are teachers and concerned about their child's needs, although they lack understanding about the implications of his handicap as they expect him to eventually be like other children his age. They have become more aware of the severity of his disorder since the birth of their second son, now 10 months old. The younger child is developing at a typical rate and appears to be free of any dysfunction. There is no reported history of familial disorders such as autism.

Raymond attends a special education program for severely emotionally impaired students five afternoons a week. He has used repetitive echolalic speech for approximately 2 years, and he lacks ability to make his needs known appropriately through verbal means. Raymond seldom makes eye contact and prefers to work in isolation at any task in which he becomes engrossed. He does not spin objects nor does he exhibit hand-flapping or body-rocking, but he is an occasional toe walker.

Raymond's behavior, noted as hyperactive, distractible, compulsive, and sometimes aggressive, prevents him from being a candidate for standardized sensory integration and intelligence tests. Although Raymond's sensitivity hampers such testing, clinical behavior indicates an obvious presence of ability for performing simple tasks.

Obsessiveness in play is a noted characteristic as Raymond places objects adjacent to one another in a continuous line and becomes markedly disturbed if their order is disrupted. He usually puts toys and objects in his mouth upon picking them up before manipulating them to any extent with his hands. Other than these behaviors, play is disorganized and inappropriate for most tasks.

Observation and interpretation of his activities reveal a decided craving for tactile stimulation, as he is often noted to rub objects on his arms, legs, stomach, face, and hair as he handles them; however, he is extremely aversive to touching by other people. When overly aroused, he chooses to wrap himself in a blanket and hide in a confined space while sucking his thumb. Low muscle tone and poor cocontraction are noted with hyperextensibility of fingers and elbows, scapular winging, and lordotic trunk. Raymond lacks adequate tonus of the flexor muscles preventing him from ever holding on to a person who is carrying him. This problem has also been noted when he has been carried in piggyback fashion. Slight head lag is observed when he is pulled to sit. He refuses to play in a prone-lying position for any period of time, probably as a result of inadequate extensor tone that would allow him to perform against gravity. He is unable to maintain the quadruped (all-fours) position for creeping; instead, he rests on his heels and scoots along the floor to maneuver. He prefers to move while upright and generally runs rather than walks. He occasionally performs activities such as swinging, rocking, or jumping, which may enhance input through the vestibular system, but this does not seem to appeal to him as much as tactile input through self-stimulation.

Raymond eats most foods and can adequately handle a spoon, fork, or cup, but often stuffs large quantities in his mouth at one time. He likes to smear food on his face and head while eating. Except for feeding, toileting, and some undressing, he is dependent in self-care.

Treatment Goals and Objectives

Children with dysfunction who are motivated usually have an inner drive that can be tapped for increasing self-direction. Occupational therapists should provide the opportunity for the child to achieve success while being appropriately challenged. This process leads to increased adaptive capacity and enhances the child's confidence and self-concept. Ayres[15] emphasizes that therapists

follow the child's cues, offering in treatment the type and amount of sensory input that he or she seeks and needs in tasks geared to his or her developmental level.

Children like Raymond, who are not well-directed by internal sources and who demonstrate poor orientation and sensory modulation, require particular sensitivity to their behavior as indicators of their sensorimotor needs. The ability of the therapist to interpret their activity as an outward expression of a disorganized and dysfunctioning central nervous system is the key to the therapeutic process. Therapists may be required to impose cautiously more external control and direction on the autistic child who lacks the innate ability to direct himself. Therapists should observe developmental principles, working in early developmental positions (prone, supine, and quadruped) and initiating activities with the child in a gradual sequential order. Changes from one task to another should be at a pace that respects the level of the child's needs and ability to learn and benefit from an activity.

An occupational therapy summary interpreting Raymond's behaviors indicated the following key problems:

1. Decreased attention span includes limited eye contact, distractibility, and hyperactivity
2. Inadequate modulation of tactile input as evidenced by his craving for stimulation yet aversion to touch and stimulation by others
3. Signs of poor neuromuscular status, including:
   a. low muscle tone in flexors and extensors
   b. poor co-contraction
   c. instability in early developmental positions
4. Inappropriate play due to lack of adequate sensorimotor foundation and as seen in immature manipulation and use of objects and obsessive behaviors
5. Inadequate social skills resulting from all problems as noted

Major Occupational Therapy Goals (in order of priority/progression)

1. Decrease arousal, including hyperactivity, distractibility, and aversion to touch
2. Increase attention span
3. Increase physical stability through facilitation of muscle tone and cocontraction, especially of midline trunk and proximal joints
4. Improve visual attending and eye contact
5. Enhance tactile discrimination
6. Facilitate play behavior through appropriate use and manipulation of objects

Treatment Methods with Suggested Procedures for Achieving Goals

1. Decrease arousal through inhibitory methods which calm the CNS, including:
   a. decreased environmental auditory and visual stimuli
   b. slow, rhythmical movements provided by manual rocking
   c. proprioceptive input through resisted activities, joint compression and traction, working against firm object or gravity
   d. pressure–touch on body as tolerated, given manually, such as swaddling child, rolling child in a blanket, or sandwiching child between mats
2. Facilitate total body flexion. The flexed position is one of the first total body patterns to occur in infancy. It is seen as an important element in development for organizing the child through symmetrical bilateral movement. Hand and/or feet may be engaged at midline and provide the experience of self-exploration through touch and movement. Awareness of self and understanding of body movements are further enhanced and guided through vision, leading eventually to coordinated action of eyes and hands together.[16] The flexor pattern then is critical to the development of midline behavior and organization, beginning with the eyes and including symmetrical extremity movements, especially with the integration of the ATNR at 12–16 weeks. Example: move child on bolster using prone position; encourage improved holding while riding piggyback.
3. Enhance physical stability by increasing muscle tone and cocontraction especially of midline trunk, and proximal muscles, through:
   a. Linear vestibular input (provides input to the spinal tract supplying extensors). Example: prone forward motion in hammock or on inflated ball
   b. Proprioceptive input as applied through resistance, compression, and traction. Example: quadriped position on firm surface pushing forward against moderately firm surface
   c. Reinforcement with above, through prone play where resistance of the extensors to gravity is maximally enhanced
   d. Resisted sucking activity (the first cocontraction pattern in infancy). Example: vary the resistance of child's suck effort by lengthening straw or thickening the liquid used

4. Provide appropriate tactile stimulation to enhance discrimination. Avoid light tactile input that is arousing and that could lead to aversive reactions. Emphasize firm touch–pressure and proprioceptive input as tolerated. Ayres[17] has also found that vestibular stimulation can help to organize and modulate tactile functions, depending on the responses of the child, through common connections within the central nervous system. Example: linear vestibular input—up and down, back and forth, and side to side movements seem to be more organizing

Summary

Progress over a 3–6 month period of therapy was seen in Raymond's decreasing destructive behavior toward himself and others. He improved in tolerance to prone position and activity while in that position. Some reduced tactile self-stimulation was noted on a gradual basis. Further, an increase in overall stability was noted leading to improvement in his organization base and his potential for function. □

Sensory Integrative Dysfunction: Developmental Dyspraxia

Discussion

Certain categories of sensory integrative dysfunction have been identified[18–21] in which disorders of the tactile, proprioceptive, and/or vestibular systems are suspected to contribute to disruption in typical development processes. Such system disorders are manifest in deviations in movement, behavior, and learning.

Developmental dyspraxia seems to be the most frequently observed sensory integration disorder. This dysfunction is seen in an inability to plan and to execute movement patterns of a skilled or nonhabitual nature. Praxis, or motor planning, is a uniquely human function that relies on an understanding of one's own body and how it operates within and relates to the external world. This type of understanding is formed internally and is based on appropriate and adequate input and processing through the channels of the tactile, proprioceptive, and vestibular systems. These systems are the first to mature and function in infancy and continue as movement feedback mechanism. The focus of this discussion of dyspraxia relates to problems beginning early in life, stemming from a disorder in the developmental processes rather than that of an individual whose dyspraxia is the result of a traumatic injury later in life.

Several aspects of human movements are basic to understanding the concept of motor planning,[22] including:

- those that are automatic and reflexive in nature
- those that are an inherent part of the human repertoire of movement strategies
- those that require motor planning

The latter leads to the acquisition of specific skills and the ability to learn new, unfamiliar, and complex tasks. Postural reactions fall within the first category, where processing of sensory input produces automatic responses without conscious effort to changes in position. These reactions, directed primarily by the brainstem, may be inefficient in the child with sensory integrative dysfunction, because they are based upon assimilation of sensory information.

Certain movement patterns, such as creeping and walking, are an inherent part of human development. The human nervous system is programmed in such a way that these actions occur during the normal course of development as maturation allows. The child may need stimulus to execute motor planning strategies when first demonstrating these acts, but generally most children acquire these abilities without having to be shown how to do them. The child with minor nervous system disorders, such as sensory integrative dysfunction, may show few problems in achieving these motor milestones.

As a child learns to master certain skilled tasks, there is a need to concentrate and direct energy toward the specific movement sequences that are necessary to complete these tasks. This involves the complex assimilation and integration of sensory input at several levels of the CNS in order to organize an appropriate motor response for the task. With repeated effort, the child eventually develops skills that become familiar and that can then be repeated in rapid manner as needed without great concentration. These skills comprise a certain motor skill "library." For example, most dressing tasks require children to initially direct great attention to the task. Eventually the ability to initiate and complete these acts rapidly and without much thought is gained. The dyspraxic child often experiences a paucity of skills, although once the child has learned a skill, he can usually perform it well under familiar conditions.

Motor planning demands attention that enables the brain to direct movements in a specific manner. This is a highly complex function in childhood because it depends upon processing and organization throughout the central nervous system, from the brainstem to the cerebral hemisphere. When a new or unfamiliar aspect of a learned skill is presented, motor planning is generally required in order to deal effectively with that aspect and to complete the task. For example, the child may learn to skip a rope with practice and become quite efficient at it. Introducing some change, such as skipping rope backward, requires the programming of some different actions and demands attention and concentration in order to learn the task. Eventually, with practice, most children learn to become efficient at this altered activity. The dyspraxic child may need more practice or may fail to learn the task because he or she cannot put all of the components together.

Performance of skilled tasks, even those that have been learned and are slightly altered, present the greatest problem to the dyspraxic child. Where motor planning problems are a result of sensory integrative dysfunction, the child often lacks the input needed to develop an understanding of his body, his movements, and his ability to impact effectively upon the environment through movement; this presents the occupational therapist with a complicated therapeutic picture.

Because the child with developmental dyspraxia experiences a decreased capacity to impact upon the environment, he may feel overwhelmed and powerless, failing to recognize himself as an animated being. Emotional lability is common. The child often cannot figure out how to get into or out of unfamiliar motor situations. He may avoid competitive activities where inadequacy would be obvious. The child may lack imagination and may fail to initiate active play. One may note a stubborn or uncooperative attitude resulting from a need to avoid change.

In summary, the following are identifying characteristics of developmental dyspraxia:

1. Difficulty in performing skills not previously mastered, where motor planning is required.
2. Sensory processing deficits, often in the tactile system, and occasionally in the vestibular and proprioceptive systems.
3. Low muscle tone, generally poorer in flexors than extensors. Flexor muscles are used primarily for phasic and skilled movements while extensors serve tonic and postural functions.
4. Generally poor coordination, accident-prone tendency, and disorganized movement. The child exhibits excessive concentration when approaching a new skill. Inefficiency and awkwardness of movements are noted.
5. Emotional instability, easily frustrated; appears to have an unwillingness to change.
6. Generally normal onset of developmental motor milestones but delay in acquisition of skills such as dressing and appropriate manipulation of toys

(blocks, puzzles, etc.). Deficient skills are noted overall, with the child relying on a few learned skills that have been acquired through considerable effort and practice.

Case Study

Michael is 6 years old, the third child in a family of four children, and the only boy. The mother indicated that there were no problems during pregnancy and delivery, but she felt there was something different about Michael as compared to her other children. She reported that he seemed to maintain a distance from other people and preferred remaining in his crib to being held and rocked. He was a very quiet baby and, though only moderately active, he achieved most motor milestones within the age-expected ranges. He was breast-fed for 8 months, and solid foods were introduced at 6 months. He indicated particular food preferences and tended to avoid eating meats and vegetables. He disliked bathing, hair-washing, combing, and brushing his teeth. The father noted that Michael was found crying several times as a baby when caught in corners or on furniture, and when Michael could not independently get himself moved out of these situations. He was resistant to any boisterous play compared to his siblings, and he was severely distressed if jostled or swung in the air. As a toddler and preschooler he was happier looking at books or being read to, and he is now beginning to read. His parents are interested in helping Michael but find him a confusing and frustrating child. They have sought family counseling because they feel responsible for his unhappy disposition.

Michael was referred to occupational therapy by his kindergarten teacher. She reported that Michael seemed to be a bright child, but he hesitated to become involved in activities with his peers. He had difficulty holding and using tools, such as crayons, pencil, or scissors, and often destroyed his papers or threw them away. On the playground he made use of most of the available equipment, but he refused to participate in group games. Crying and pouting were commonly observed, with occasional temper tantrums when a situation became too frustrating. Michael has been referred to the school social worker for evaluation and has received speech therapy services for severe articulation problems.

An attempt was made in occupational therapy to evaluate Michael's sensory integrative abilities via the Southern California Sensory Integration Tests, but he could not maintain his attention long enough nor adequately follow directions to obtain reliable results via this assessment. The therapist found that clinical observation of performance in exploratory play and assessment of neuromuscular status and reflex integration was necessary to determine his strengths and weaknesses, while additionally trying to establish rapport with him. A developmental history was also obtained from his parents.

Clinical observation revealed several problems. Michael refused to remove his clothing, would not lie prone on any surface, and balked at new experiences of a variety of types. Slight hypotonicity was noted upon palpatation in combination with hyperextensible fingers and elbow joints. His ability to track visually moving objects was poor. Movement on uneven surfaces evoked fearful reactions, and he would not allow himself to be picked up. In nonstructured exploratory play Michael was cautious, but curious, about the toys and equipment, and he manipulated many of them. When concentrating intently on a task that he was trying to learn, he appeared to be thinking through each step and often drooled or squinted in the effort. His awkward movements suggested poor body awareness that was further evidenced by his inability to change position quickly or efficiently move around objects. He often collided with equipment and tripped over toys. When he attempted to retrieve a ball that rolled under a table, Michael, in unplanned and slow sequence, turned himself around, climbed on the table, then got down and crept sideways on the floor before he could accomplish his goal. It was obvious that he had no idea what maneuvers his body should follow toward successful completion of the intended act.

Treatment Goals and Objectives

In spite of Michael's resistance to standardized test conditions, his performance and behaviors were evidence of disordered sensory and motor abilities. The following problem areas were addressed through occupational therapy programming:
1. Impaired sensory processing functions:
   a. Tactile system problems as evidenced by aversion to handling and grooming, possible avoidance of textured foods, and sensitivity to uncovering his body.
   b. Poor proprioceptive mechanisms as shown in low muscle tone and inability to make use of and learn from his movements. Speech articulation problems may reflect both tactile and proprioceptive problems leading to poor awareness of oral movements.
   c. Inadequate vestibular activity as seen in his fear of displacement from the earth, poor visual tracking, low muscle tone, and inefficient righting and equilibrium reactions.
2. Impaired neuromuscular status and reflex

integration noted with low muscle tone and deficient postural reactions.

3. Severe motor planning problems as evidenced by his inability to move efficiently and skillfully through even simple motor tasks, and the need to direct intense concentration on performance. Tool manipulation difficulties were a reflection of this condition.
4. Behavior problems and inadequate social skills.

Major Goals in Occupational Therapy

1. Decrease aversion to touch, handling, and movement.
2. Enhance functions of the tactile, proprioceptive, and vestibular systems.
3. Improve postural reactions.
4. Enhance motor planning ability.
5. Decrease inappropriate behaviors. (Although this was the reason for referral, this goal is related to 1 to 4 major goals.)
6. Improve self-concept.

Treatment Methods and Suggested Procedures for Achieving Goals

1. Decrease aversive reactions through:
   a. Proprioceptive input in resisted activities. Example: In quadriped position child pushes or pulls weighted objects.
   b. Pressure–touch as tolerated; avoid light tactile stimuli that is interpreted as uncomfortable. Example: A large inflated ball is rolled over child in prone or supine position.
   c. Movement in slow, gradual ranges using calm, rhythmical input. Example: Child is rocked over ball, or rides pendelum swing while his feet touch the floor.
2. Enhance sensory system function as aversion decreases emphasizing the following:
   a. Proprioceptive input. Example: Give manual joint approximation or traction to child or encourage push-off wall activity in different positions on scooter board.
   b. Discriminative tactile activities. Example: Taking clue from child noted to exhibit improved tolerance to varying floor surfaces while walking barefoot, increase other opportunity for tactile exploration (environmental) by feet and hands.
   c. Carefully graded (gradual) movement. Example: encourage movement on a variety of objects to the point that the child initiates climbing activity.

3. Build midline stability as the basis for postural reactions. Trunk stability must be achieved first and is facilitated through increased muscle tone via vestibular input, especially linear stimulation, and tactile and proprioceptive stimulation. Example: tapping and vibration (myotendenous junction). Resistance to and movement against gravity is advanced through proprioceptive and vestibular mechanisms. Example: linear stimulation in the following directions (*i.e.*, up and down, back and forth, and side to side movement). All activity should encourage an automatic unconscious control of body. These procedures lead to enhanced movement around and away from the body axis.
4. Enhance motor planning built upon somatosensory and vestibular processing and adequate postural reactions. Use simple movement activities and increase complexity as child can complete with success while being appropriately challenged. Add skills to the child's repertoire. Follow the child's cues and present tasks appropriate for his abilities. Do not force him to perform.[23] Example: Encourage child to go under a table, or go under table and chair, crawling. Have child build a simple bridge-like structure or large blocks and then maneuver through the structure by crawling or by means of a scooter board.
5. In reducing demands made upon the child and allowing him success in his play, self-concept is enhanced and frustration is reduced. As ability to successfully impact upon and interact with the environment increases through sensorimotor and cognitive channels, the child's behavior can be more appropriately and productively directed without the need to act out.

Summary

Although certain substantial changes in Michael's sensory integration process and behavior were achieved in a 3 to 6 month period, the identification of his problems had an even greater impact on his parents and family. Their ability finally to understand the underlying reasons for their child's performance difficulties and behavioral reactions markedly improved their ability to help Michael. As the result of improved parenting, Michael demonstrated improved coping skills (less crying and sulking) and better ability to verbalize his feelings of frustration. Teachers, therapist, and family could observe the outcome of improved motor planning seen in his ability to engage in more creative and imaginary play, in general, and use of tools and materials. He still avoided most children's games because of a lack of ability to organize game procedures and to predict outcomes at such a level. □

Child Abuse and Neglect

Discussion

For centuries child abuse or neglect has been known to exist in varying degrees (and to have had certain endurance by society). Herod's destruction of males, the degradation and forced use of children as laborers during the Industrial Revolution, and more notably the descriptive work of Dickens are reminders of the exploitation of children over time. During the last two decades, child abuse has become a major concern in the United States, with most states adopting laws that require the reporting of medical incidents of child abuse while providing immunity for those reporting abuse in good faith. Once the reporting of child abuse was required by law, the extent of the problem began to reach both public and professional attention. By record, child abuse is the second most common cause of death of young children in the United States. Two thirds of the child abuse or neglect incidents occur with children 3 years or younger. Permanent brain damage or other handicaps result in approximately 25% of the cases reported.[24]

Child abuse occurs by physical abuse or neglect, sexual abuse, and emotional abuse or neglect, and though they may occur in combination, physical abuse has the clearest diagnostic base and is the most frequently reported incidence. Incidence of physical neglect, whether deliberate or willful neglect, is more difficult to determine because of the influence of poverty or lack of means to provide adequate child sustenance. Incidence of sexual abuse is the least reported, whether assaultive or nonassaultive. Defining and managing abuse that is emotionally based is by far the more difficult because of the limited reportable physical evidence. The variation of cultural and social expectations of children further complicates what is truly emotional abuse or neglect. Failure to thrive and various learning disabilities have definitely been linked to emotional abuse and neglect—an important consideration for occupational therapists.

Physical abuse occurs most frequently to children at 0 to 3 years of age. Sexual abuse, whether male or female, may occur at any age, but is more frequently seen in the school-age or adolescent girls. Emotional neglect or abuse is nonrestrictive to age.[25]

In general occupational therapists considering this particular problem area may find more than one area of potential useful service. Because the characteristics of adults involved in child abuse have been iden-

tified, therapists' services may need to be directed toward identifying individuals with high risk for abusing, or assisting in determining whether abuse has occurred, or even more importantly, developing interventions to benefit families involved in abuse. The occupational therapist's evaluation of young children with known or suspected history of abuse or neglect is strongly recommended because of the child's potential for short or long-range problems in learning and adapting.

Characteristics of Abusive or Neglectful Parents

Parents are the most frequent abusers of children, though relatives, stepparents, or guardians may also be involved.[26] Basically, abuse is an outcome of past or present problems or stresses that the abusive parent has little control or ability to deal with, such as:

1. Lack of maturity—young parents with unmet needs often lack understanding of their children's behavior or needs.
2. Unrealistic parental expectations of the child, or the child may have *special needs* that prevents the child from meeting parents' expectations.
3. Unmet emotional needs of parents—parents may have problems relating to adults and may expect the child to satisfy their need for love, protection, or self-esteem.
4. Frequent family crises—incidental or ongoing, financial, emotional, or physical problems can explain abusive behavior in parents.
5. Lack of parenting knowledge or skill—many abusive parents know little about the various stages of child development, and often they have no model of successful family patterns to draw from.
6. Poor parental childhood experiences—often abusive parents were reared in a physically or emotionally traumatic pattern.
7. Family social isolation—abusive families often lack any support network of friends or family to help with simple or complex problems encountered in rearing small children.
8. Alcohol or drug abuse related activity limits parents' ability to rear children effectively.

Signs of Physical Abuse or Neglect

Therapists may have an opportunity to assist in the acute identification process of abused children. Key factors are listed:

• Evidence of repeated, multiple, or significant injuries.

- Parental delay in seeking medical care.
- Child has a vacant stare, lies very still when approached.

It is important to note that physicians have the key role in determining physical abuse. Medical diagnosis of physical abuse to children has been greatly refined. Radiologic laboratory studies of blood coagulation help establish a profile of present or past abuse patterns. But it is the responsibility of therapists to be alert to evidence of abuse and neglect and to have an understanding of the laws governing abuse in their particular state.

In general, therapists need to become familiar with the types of skin and subcutaneous tissue changes, whether bruises, burns, scalds, or wasting, that are typical of abused or neglected children. Injuries to ears, nose, mouth, and head follow unusual and identifiable patterns that differ from usual accidental patterns. An excellent reference for obtaining such information is *Clinical Symposia: The Abused Child.*

Other visible signs of abused or neglected children should include children who are undernourished, inadequately clothed, or left unattended. Sometimes these children will exhibit aggressive negative behavior on a constant and repetitive basis. Other children may exhibit excessive withdrawal behavior and may be unable to relate to others, especially other children.

Occupational Therapy with Abused or Neglected Children and Their Families

Occupational therapists have an important role with parents who are abusive/neglectful or who have potential for such. Therapists' goals with such parents should:

- Establish and maintain regular, not threatening, contact with the family.
- Promote a sense of parental adequacy.
- Support strengths of the parent-child relationship.
- Strengthen parents' understanding of their child and capability in child handling and nurturing; children's motor developmental process; nursing, feeding, and nutritional skills.
- Encourage improved child-rearing skills.
- Be alert to signs indicating continued abuse and, in such a situation, take appropriate action.

Often, a therapist can appropriately use her skills in handling, feeding, promoting gross and fine motor development, and demonstrating alternate approaches to behavior control as a model for parents.

Occupational therapy skills are even more directly related to services for children who have experienced abuse or neglect. Children, especially those 3 years or younger, who fail to thrive or grow in size, who have developmental disability, or whose behavior is withdrawn or maladaptive, are high risk for abuse or neglect or may be the result of neglect. Often mental retardation is a factor in cause or result in abused and neglected children.

The occupational therapist's evaluation of abused/neglected children should be comprehensive and complete. Frequently therapists are asked to determine motor developmental status of the child as base line information when the question of abuse is being investigated. Sometimes the therapists may be asked to develop an intervention program that would augment the child's motor development or improve behavior regardless of the domicile determination. In many cases the therapist may have the opportunity to provide services to the child and parent or caseworker. When the abusing parents are judged to be temporarily or in fact incapable of controlling their abusive behavior, the occupational therapist's role may be more as an evaluator and guide to agency personnel who will sponsor the care and service to the abused or neglected child.

In any event, the occupational therapy assessment of abused and neglected children under 4 years of age should address:

1. Neuro-developmental reflex maturation levels.
2. Gross motor developmental skill levels.
3. Fine motor developmental skill levels.
4. ADL skill developmental level.
5. Sensory integration to include tactile, proprioceptive, kinesthetic, vestibular, and ocular organization.

The referral of a child with a history of abuse or neglect to an occupational therapist suggests that the child is exhibiting significant or observable behaviors of concern. In young children these observable behaviors may include:

- overly compliant behavior
- social withdrawal, may not make eye contact
- lack of autonomy, with little exploring behavior or asserting behavior
- acting-out aggressive episodes, leading to alienation—isolated state
- apathy—helplessness
- retarded growth

Other concerning factors leading to referral are listed:

- hyperactivity—tendency to become overstimulated easily
- poor concentration and attention

- suspected mental retardation
- delay in developing daily living skills, especially irregularity in feeding habits
- delay in developing gross and fine motor skills

The occupational therapist examiner should review the referral of an abused or neglected child carefully in light of the person, professional, institutional/agency referral service, or case manager. The purpose of the referral must be addressed during the child's evaluation. But it is the ethical responsibility of the therapist to determine primarily the child's developmental, functional, and adaptive behavior levels and status as a means of identifying the child's individual needs. A summary or report of the evaluative process should include recommendations for improving the child's status as appropriate, while addressing directly the purpose of the referral. In some cases the therapist may be asked to address the question of parent ability or effectiveness in caring for the child.

It is important to note that the opportunity and feasibility for direct occupational therapy services may, in some cases, be limited or unnecessary. Often recommendations and advice to the referring service about the child's strengths and weakness, how to encourage improved functional ability in motor performance, adaptive behavior, concentration, or other areas of concern may be the major contribution of the occupational therapist. When treatment is strongly recommended, the therapist needs to state that opinion clearly and to work assertively to eliminate barriers to the provision of needed services.

Case Study

History and Background

Gabriel, a child of Hispanic extraction, experienced severe infantile abuse from both his natural mother and stepfather. The identification of four separate incidents of untreated bone fractures inflicted during his first year of life led to the removal of Gabriel from his parents by the State Human Resource Department. Subsequently he became a ward of the State. Gabriel then had six different foster home placements during the following 18 months. These placements were, in some cases, in homes where Spanish was spoken and, in other cases, where English was spoken.

By the time Gabriel was 2½ years old his behavior and limited communication skills were recognized as a problem. Specifically, he was hyperactive, hard to control, and had a speaking vocabulary of 3 to 5 words. At that age he underwent psychiatric, otological/audiological, and speech/language examinations. He was labeled mentally retarded due to environmental deprivation, functioning at an overall 18-month level.

By the time he was 35 months old, the State Human Resources Department referred Gabriel for occupational therapy evaluation. His then current foster parents were considering adopting him. Both the state agency and the foster parents were seeking definitive information about the child's development. The couple was in their early thirties; the foster mother was a certified kindergarten teacher who was not employed at that time. The father was a state agency employee. The foster parents reported specific concerns about Gabriel's communication, poor concentration, and behavior at meal time. Whenever food was presented Gabriel responded by gorging himself; this was a special concern of the foster parents. The occupational therapy process is depicted in Figure 31-12.

Occupational Therapy Program

Gabriel's occupational therapy assessment consisted of an evaluation of:
- general physical findings, including muscle tone
- reflex maturation
- gross and fine motor skill attainment
- daily living skill performance
- sensory integration and sensitivity
- visual motor integration
- adaptive behavior

The findings of the assessments were as follows:
1. Historically the child was adequately nourished and small in stature. His normal muscle tone was low, but joint stability was adequate. No observable deformity was noted.
2. Child demonstrated delays in higher level reflex maturation, exhibited certain primitive reflex patterns of a nonobligatory nature. Midline stability was diminished, and balancing was poor.
3. Gross and fine motor skills had advanced to 24 months. A gain of approximately 6-months motor maturation since his examinations at chronological age 30 months.
4. Despite poor concentration, the child performed certain daily living skills fairly adequately to a 30-month-old level, such as removal of garments. He was clumsy in performance and awkward in those skills requiring dexterity. The foster parents reported the child had difficulty remaining seated during mealtime, and they were dismayed over the child's continued

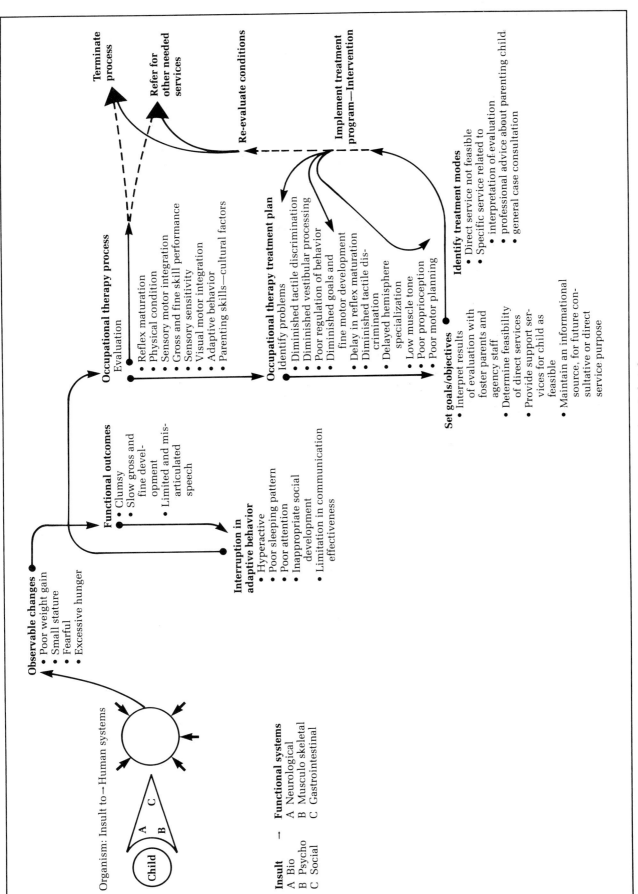

Figure 31-12. Occupational therapy program with an abused child. Case study: Gabriel.

gorging of foods despite their efforts to discourage these behaviors.

5. Sensory integration testing indicated tactile processing was deficient in discrimination and localization. Diminished vestibular responses were noted in postrotary nystagmus testing. Proprioception and motor planning ability were deficient. On the K. E. Beery Developmental Test of Visual Motor Integration,[27] he scored an age equivalence of 30 months. He was noted to be significantly tactilely defensive and underreceptive to movement and spatial organization.

Additional factors relating to hemispheric specialization included:

• lack of specialization for preferred hand or eye usage
• poor contralateral use of right or left hand

Six adaptive behaviors during testing were significant:

• the child was overstimulated, became disruptive if confined for fine skill performance activity
• child overresponded to gravitational testing and demonstrated increased falling behavior apparently on a sensoral need basis
• auditory motor organization was poor (*i.e.*, poor response to verbal directions for action)
• once overstimulated or angered, the child seemed to sustain this intensified state level for a fairly prolonged time, lacking ability to calm himself or to respond to efforts to help him calm

Parents reported difficulty in scheduling the child's rest patterns. It was difficult for the child to take afternoon naps, and bedtime was a nightly battle with erratic early morning waking, also a part of the problem. The foster parents did feel that Gabriel was showing some improvement in understanding them on a verbal basis and by other more subtle factors. They also felt that Gabriel was showing signs of settling into a less frantic pattern of behavior, but they expressed concerns about the prognosis for improved behavior.

Following the completion of the child's evaluation, an interagency family conference was held. Results of communication and occupational therapy evaluations were shared with the parents. Information about overall developmental level and potentials were discussed, along with the speech pathologist's findings. The occupational therapist encouraged both agency and foster parents to consider the child's developmental delay as one that could be altered by structuring the child, continuing improved nutrition, and giving sensory

integration treatment enhanced with language and educational therapy. The conference recommendations were favorable, indicating a general expectation for the child's increased ability to function in a nearly normal capacity if the child had the opportunity for bonding with caring parents who could provide a structured nurturing environment. The opportunity and need for occupational therapy to enhance motor functional, sensory integration, and improved adaptive behavior was strongly encouraged, as was continued speech/language training.

Both agency personnel and foster parents appeared to view Gabriel's developmental future constructively. However, before adoption was concluded, the foster mother became pregnant. At this point, the couple elected not to proceed with the adoption of Gabriel, principally because of the welcomed pregnancy, but also because of Gabriel's behavior problems and hyperactivity.

Although Gabriel benefited from this foster-living arrangement for the next 7 months, no specific therapeutic interventions were provided. Slow advancement in development and communication continued, and some gradual improvement in the child's behavior was evident. However, no further occupational therapy case contact opportunity occurred until Gabriel was adopted at 43 months by a single woman in her early 30s. She had a rich background in education of young children in normal and special nursery programs. At the request of the agency and adoptive parent, a special occupational therapy consultative conference was held to assist the new parent in organizing a program that would structure the child's daily activities and guide management of the child's behavior. The child qualified for early childhood educational programming (4 hrs/daily) that included occupational therapy and speech therapy services. The mother was advised to explore this opportunity once the child made an adjustment to his new home setting. Specific recommendations were also made for updated sensorimotor integration testing following early childhood admission. Although this case conference concluded the official service, informal contacts were made by the adoptive mother during the following 6 months, considered as the transition period. All progress was favorable, including Gabriel's adjustment to his new home and mother and ultimately to the early childhood program. Of interest to the occupational therapist were the sensory integration evaluation findings conducted by the early childhood therapist. Gabriel was diagnosed as mildly dyspraxic on a vestibular basis. The program provided daily therapy and aided the mother with a home program. Prognosis for advancement within the normal range in speech development and behavior was considered good. □

Summary

This chapter has been prepared in light of the expanding opportunity for occupational therapists to practice in the field of pediatrics and because of the expanding needs, both for knowledge and performance, of therapists who choose to work in this area.

This chapter provides both general and specific considerations underlying effective pediatric occupational therapy practice. Pediatric therapists are urged to view the child in the context of his world and the influence of biopsychosocial insult to the child's overall development and functional potential. Constraints or opportunities for occupational therapy effectiveness are addressed in relation to differing service-delivery systems. The importance of evaluation, treatment planning, goal setting, and adjustment is related to occupational therapy effectiveness as well.

A conceptual model for considering the occupational therapy process is presented to clarify and unify this process, and is applicable to a wide range of pediatric conditions. Certain conditions are presented in this way, along with narrative case studies that describe treatment program planning, including the actual treatment procedures or intervention used to achieve identified occupational therapy goals.

The quest for clinical competence in pediatric practice is unending. As therapists gain one level of accomplishment, they often find this knowledge leads to the recognition of the need for further study and understanding if quality of occupational therapy services are to be provided to children.

Acknowledgments

To the staff of the Austin Travis County Infant Parent Program of Austin, Texas; to Esther Bell, MA, OTR, FAOTA; Cynthia Jones, MS, OTR; and Gretchen Reeves, MA, OTR, for their assistance and contribution to the preparation of this chapter.

References

1. Kanner, L.: Autistic disturbances of affective contact. Nervous Child 2:217–250, 1943.
2. Ornitz, E. M., and Ritvo, E. R.: The syndrome of autism: A critical review. *Am. J. Psych.* 133:609–621, 1976.
3. Ornitz, E. M.: Vestibular dysfunction in schizophrenia and childhood autism. *Comp. Psychiatry* 11:159–173, 1970.
4. Ornitz, E. M.: Neurophysiologic studies. In Rutter, M. (ed.): Autism: A Reappraisal of Concepts and Treatments, pp. 117–139. New York: Plenum Press, 1978.
5. Rutter, M.: Diagnosis and definition. In Rutter, M. (ed.): Autism: A Reappraisal of Concepts and Treatment. New York: Plenum Press, 1978.
6. Ornitz, Ritvo: The syndrome of autism: A critical review.
7. Bettelheim, B.: The Empty Fortress. New York: Free Press, 1967.
8. Lotter, V.: Epidemiology of autistic conditions in young children—II. Some characteristics of the parents and children. *Soc. Psych.* 1:163–73, 1967.
9. Lotter, V.: Factors related to outcome in autistic children. J. Autism Child. Schizophr. 4:263–277, 1974.
10. Lotter, V. Follow-up studies. In Rutter, M. (ed.): Autism: A Reappraisal of Concepts and Treatment, pp. 475–495. New York: Plenum Press, 1978.
11. Grandin, T.: What is being autistic like? CSSID Newsletter 8:6–7, 1980.
12. Becker, M.: In unpublished notes from Conference on Sensory Integrative Dysfunction. Cincinnati, June, 1979.
13. Ayres, A. J., and Tickle, L. S.: Hyper-responsivity to touch and vestibular stimuli as a predictor of positive response to sensory integration procedures by autistic children. Am. J. Occup. Ther. 34:375–381, 1980.
14. Black, M., Freeman, B. J., and Montgomery, J.: Systematic observation of play behavior in autistic children. J. Autism Child. Schizophr. 5:363–371, 1975.
15. Ayres, A. J.: Sensory Integration and Learning Disorders. Los Angeles: Western Psychological Services, 1972.
16. Sherick, I., Greeman, G., and Legg, C.: Some comments on the significance and development of midline behavior during infancy. Child Psychiatry Hum. Dev. 6:170–183, 1976.
17. Ayres, A. J.: From comments at CSSID Faculty Meeting. Cincinnati, June, 1981.
18. Ayres: Sensory Integration and Learning Disorders.
19. Ayres, A. J.: Interpreting the Southern California Sensory Integration Tests. Los Angeles: Western Psychological Services, 1976.
20. Ayres, A. J.: Sensory Integration and the Child. Los Angeles: Western Psychological Services, 1979.
21. Silberzahn, M. A.: Sensory integrative theory. In Hopkins, H. L., and Smith, H. D. (eds): Willard and Spackman's Occupational Therapy, ed. 5. Philadelphia: J. B. Lippincott, 1978, pp. 134–140.
22. Ayres: Sensory Integration and the Child, pp. 91–95.
23. Ayres: Sensory Integration and Learning Disorders, pp. 256–266.
24. United States Department of Health, Education and Welfare: The Diagnostic Process and Treatment Programs in Child Abuse and Neglect, Publication No. (OHD)-76-30069, Washington, D.C., 1976.
25. Ibid.
26. McNeese, M. C., and Hebeler, J. R.: The abused child: A clinical approach to identification and management. CIBA Clinical Symposia 29:5, 1977.

27. Beery, K. E.: Developmental Test of Visual Motor Integration. Chicago: Follett Publishing Co, 1967.

Bibliography

American Occupational Therapy Association. Principles and Guidelines of Occupational Therapy Ethics, 1977.

American Occupational Therapy Association. The Role of Occupational Therapy in Early Childhood Intervention, 1981.

American Occupational Therapy Association. Standards of Practice for Occupational Therapy Services for the Developmentally Disabled Client. Developmental Disabilities, 1976.

American Occupational Therapy Association. Standards of Practice in Schools, 1980.

Amiel-Tison, C: A method for neurologic evaluation within the first year of life. Curr. Probl. Pediatr. 7:1, 1976.

Angelucci, A., et al.: Early visual stimulation. Austin TX: Texas Education Agency Special Education Service, 1979.

Apgar, V.: Perinatal problems and the central nervous system. The Child with a Central Nervous System Deficit. Children's Bureau Publication, No. 432, 1965.

Ayres, A. J.: The Effect of Sensory Integrative Therapy on Learning Disabled Children. Los Angeles: Center for the Study of Sensory Integrative Dysfunction, 1976.

Ayres, A. J.: Interpreting the Southern California Sensory Integration Tests. Los Angeles: Western Psychological Services, 1976.

Ayres, A. J.: Sensory Integration and the Child. Los Angeles: Western Psychological Services, 1979.

Ayres, A. J.: Sensory Integration and Learning Disorders. Los Angeles: Western Psychological Services, 1973.

Ayres, A. J.: From comments at CSSID Faculty Meeting. Cincinnati, June, 1981.

Ayres, A. J., and Tickle, L. S.: Hyper-responsivity to touch and vestibular stimuli as a predictor of positive response to sensory integration procedures by autistic children. Am. J. Occup. Ther. 34:375–381, 1980.

Barnes, M. R., Crutchfield, C. A., and Heriza, C. B.: The Neurophysiological Basis of Patient Treatment, Vol. 2. West Virginia: Stokesville Publishing Company, 1978.

Barraga, N.: Increased Visual Behavior in Low Vision Children. American Foundation for the Blind, 1964.

Becker, M.: In unpublished notes from Conference on Sensory Integrative Dysfunction. Cincinnati, June, 1979.

Bennett, F. C., Sells, C. J., and Brand, C.: Influences on measured intelligence in Down's Syndrome. Am. J. Dis. Child. 365:700–703, 1979.

Bettelheim, B.: The Empty Fortress. New York: Free Press, 1967.

Black, M., Freeman, B. J., and Montgomery, J.: Systematic observation of play behavior in autistic children. J. Autism Child. Schizophr. 5:363–371, 1975.

Brazelton, T. B.: Neonatal Behavioral Assessment Scale. Clinics in Developmental Medicine, No. 50. London: William Heinemann Medical Books, Ltd., 1973.

Brown, C. C. (ed.): Infants At Risk. Pediatric Round Table Series No. 5. New York: Johnson and Johnson Baby Products Company, 1981.

Brown, R. J. K., and Valman, H. B.: Practical Neonatal Pediatrics, ed. 3 Oxford: Blackwell Scientific Publications, 1975.

Campbell, S.: Facilitation of cognitive and motor development in infants with central nervous system dysfunction. Phys. Ther. 54:346–353, 1974.

Carter, R., and Campbell, S.: Early neuromuscular development of the premature infant. Phys. Ther. 55:346–353, 1974.

Chance, P. (ed.): Learning Through Play. Pediatric Round Table Series No. 3. New York: Johnson and Johnson Baby Products Company, 1979.

Clark, D. L., et al.: Effects of vestibular stimulation on nystagmus responses and motor performance in the developmentally delayed infant. Phys. Ther. 56:414–420, 1976.

Clark, D. L., et al.: Effects of vestibular stimulation on nystagmus responses and motor performance in Down's Syndrome children. Phys. Ther. 57:524–527, 1977.

Clark, D. L., et al.: Vestibular stimulation influence on motor development on infants. Science 196:1228–9, 1977.

Dargassies, S. S.: Neurological Development in Full-Term and Premature Neonates. Amsterdam: Excerpta Medica, 1977.

Dubowitz, L., et al.: Clinical assessment of gestational age in the newborn. J. Pediatr. 77:1, 1970.

Farber, S.: Sensorimotor Evaluation and Treatment Procedures for Allied Health Personnel. Indianapolis: Indiana University School of Medicine, 1974.

Frailberg, S.: The Magic Years. New York: Scribners, 1959.

Frailberg, S.: Parallel and divergent patterns in blind and sighted infants. Psychoanal. Study Child 22:264–300, 1968.

Frailberg, S., Siegel, B. L., et al.: The role of sound in the search behavior of a blind infant. Psychoanal. Study Child 21:327–357, 1966.

Franz, R. L.: Visual perception from birth as shown by pattern selectivity. In Stone, L. J., Smith, H., and Murphy, L. B. (eds.): The Competent Infant: Research and Commentary. New York: Basic Books, 1975.

Gilfoyle, E. M., and Grady, A. P.: A developmental theory of somato-sensory perception. In Henderson, A., and Coryell, J. (eds.): The Body Senses and Perceptual Deficit. Boston: Boston University, 1973.

Gilfoyle, E. M., Grady, A. P., and Moore, J. C.: Children Adapt. New Jersey: Charles B. Slack, Inc., 1981.

Grandin, T.: What is being autistic like? CSSID Newsletter 8:6–7, 1980.

Gregory, R. L.: Eye and Brain, The Psychology of Seeing, ed 2. New York, Toronto: McGraw-Hill Book Co., 1973.

Harper, R., and Yoon, J.: Handbook of Neonatology. Chicago: Year Book Medical Publishers, 1979.

Hebb, D. O.: The Organization of Behavior: A Neurophysiological Theory. New York: John Wiley & Sons, 1949.

Hoskins, T. A., and Squires, J. E.: Developmental assessment: A test for gross motor and reflex development. Phys. Ther. 53:117–125, 1973.

Jabbour, J. T., Duenas, D. A., Gilmartin, R. C., and Gottlieb, M. I.: Pediatric Neurology Handbook, ed 2.

Flushing: Medical Examination Publishing Company, Inc., 1978.

Jastrzembska, Z. S. (ed.): Effects of Blindness and Other Impairments for Early Development. American Foundation for the Blind. New York: McGraw-Hill, 1973.

Johnson and Johnson Round Table. Maternal Attachment and Mothering Disorders. New York: Sausalito, California, Johnson and Johnson Baby Prod. Co., 1974.

Jones, C. G., and Monkhouse, M. A. Developmental assessment for the newborn or high risk infant—nursery and follow-up. Austin-Travis County Health Department, 1980.

Kanner, L.: Autistic disturbances of affective contact. Nervous Child 2:217–250, 1943.

Klaus, M. H., and Fanaroff, A. A.: Care of the High Risk Neonate. Philadelphia: W. B. Saunders, 1973.

Komich, M. P., et al.: The sequential development of infants of low birthweight. Am. J. Occup. Ther. 27:398–402, 1977.

Koroners, S. B.: High Risk Newborn Infants. St. Louis: C. V. Mosby Co., 1976.

Langley, B., and DuBose, R.: Functional Screening for Severely Handicapped Children. Distributed by special permission, 1979.

Lewke, J. H.: Current practices in evaluating motor behavior of disabled children. Am. J. Occup. Ther. 30:403–19, 1976.

Lotter, V.: Epidemiology of autistic conditions in young children—II. Some characteristics of the parents and children. Soc. Psychiatry. 1:163–73, 1967.

Lotter, V.: Factors related to outcome in autistic children. J. Autism Child. Schizophr. 4:263–277, 1974.

Lotter, V.: Follow-up studies. In Rutter, M. (ed.): Autism: A Reappraisal of Concepts and Treatment. New York: Plenum Press, 1978.

Ludlow, J. R., and Allen, L. M.: The effect of early intervention and pre-school stimulus on the development of the Down's Syndrome child. J. Ment. Defic. 23:29–44, 1974.

McGraw, M. B.: The Neuromuscular Maturation of the Human Infant. New York: Hafner Publishing Co., 1963.

McNeese, M. C. and Hebeler, J. R.: The abused child: A clinical approach to identification and management. CIBA Clinical Symposia 29:77, 1977.

Milani, C. A., and Gidon, E. A.: Pattern analysis of motor development and its disorders. Dev. Med. Child Neurol. 9:631–638, 1967.

Money, J.: The syndrome of abuse dwarfism: Psychosocial dwarfism or reversible hyposomatotropism. Am. J. Disabled Child. 131:508–513, 1977.

Montague, A.: Touching: The Human Significance of Skin. New York: Harper & Row, 1978.

Moore, J. C.: Neuroanatomy Simplified. Dubuque: Kendall-Hunt, 1969.

Morgan, S. B.: Development and distribution of intellectual and adaptive skills in Down's Syndrome children: Implications for early intervention. Ment. Retard. 17:247–9, 1979.

Ornitz, E. M.: Neurophysiologic studies. In Rutter, M. (ed.): Autism: A Reappraisal of Concepts and Treatments. New York: Plenum Press, 1978.

Ornitz, E. M.: Vestibular dysfunction in schizophrenia and childhood autism. Compr. Psychiatry 11:159–173, 1970.

Ornitz, E. M., and Ritvo, E. R.: The syndrome of autism: A critical review. Am. J. Psychiatry 133:609–621, 1976.

Powell, L.: The effect of extra stimulation and maternal involvement on the development of low-birth-weight infants and on maternal behavior. Child Dev. 44:106–113, 1974.

Reilly, A. P. (ed.): The Communication Game. Pediatric Round Table Series No. 4. New York: Johnson and Johnson Baby Products Company, 1980.

Rutter, M.: Diagnosis and definition. In Rutter, M. (ed.): Autism: A Reappraisal of Concepts and Treatment. New York: Plenum Press, 1978.

Sherick, I., Greeman, G., and Legg, C.: Some comments on the significance and development of midline behavior during infancy. Child Psychiatry Hum. Devel. 6:170–183, 1976.

Smith, D. W.: Recognizable Patterns of Human Malformation, ed 2. Philadelphia: W. B. Saunders, 1976.

Trotter, S., and Thoman, E. B. (eds.): Social Responsiveness of Infants. Pediatric Round Table Series No. 2. New York: Johnson and Johnson Baby Products Company, 1978.

United States Department of Health, Education and Welfare. The diagnostic process and treatment programs in child abuse and neglect. Publication No. (OHD) 76-30069. Washington, D.C., 1976.

Uzgaris, L. D., and Hunt, J. M.: Assessment in Infancy. Chicago: University of Illinois Press, 1975.

Williamson, J. W.: Formulating priorities for quality assurance. J.A.M.A. 236:631–637, 1978.

CHAPTER 32

Occupational Therapy with Children— Cerebral Palsy *Margaret V. Howison*

The occupational therapist who works with cerebral palsied children must focus attention on the integration of the many aspects of a child's development. These include the physical, sensory, perceptual, emotional, cognitive, cultural, and social aspects. It is necessary for the occupational therapist to understand normal developmental sequences before evaluating and treating the individual with cerebral palsy. This chapter presents a problem-solving rationale for occupational therapy intervention for individuals with cerebral palsy. It is based on a neurodevelopmental approach to human development and treatment. The emphasis is on infants and children. However, some basic concepts apply to working with adult cerebral palsy patients.

Historical Perspective

Cases of cerebral palsy have been mentioned throughout recorded history. Perhaps biblical references to a man who was "a cripple from his mother's womb, who never had walked" (Acts 14:8) or "the man who was sick of the palsy" (Matthew 9:2), describe individuals with cerebral palsy.

It was not until 1843 that William John Little of England (1810–1894) first discussed what he called "infantile spastic paralysis." This became known as "Little's disease." In 1862 Little presented an accurate paper on the etiological factors of cerebral palsy. This described the problem as one resulting from prenatal, natal, and immediate postnatal influences.[1]

For many years cerebral palsy was treated from a surgical perspective that was based upon surgeons' experiences in treating poliomyelitis.[2] The enthusiasm for surgical intervention to correct deformities, to provide stability, and to improve motor control waned as assessment showed that deformities recurred or new ones developed.

In 1932, Winthrop M. Phelps (1894–1971) began developing a new approach. Phelps had been influenced by Bronson Crothers' work in the field of pediatric neurology. Phelps became aware of the necessity for including exercise, muscle training, and bracing in the treatment of cerebral palsy.[3] He gradually moved away from the use of surgical intervention, except in cases of bone deformities in older children. Phelps eventually coined the term cerebral palsy (C.P.) to distinguish the condition from mental retardation.

Since Phelps' era, various nonsurgical approaches have evolved, emphasizing neuromuscular training. They include neuromuscular reflex therapy, developed by Fay and Doman-Delacato; neurodevelopmental treatment, developed by Bobath; the neurophysiological approach, developed by Rood; and proprioceptive neuromuscular facilitation, developed by Kabat, Knott, and Voss. (See Chapter 7, section 2).

Persons involved in the fields of neurology and psychology have studied early disorders more carefully. This has led to a closer study of the early stages of development. At the same time, people working in the area of pediatrics have enhanced knowledge regarding the newborn and the newborn's neurological status. These changes and increased interest have led to both earlier diagnosis and more successful treatment of cerebral palsy.[4]

Modern sophisticated obstetrical and neonatal care, together with the practice of referring at-risk infants for treatment before they are 1-year-old, may lessen the number of severe disorders.[5] The children who may be less severely involved as a result will hopefully be able to lead relatively normal and productive lives.

Definition, Incidence, and Etiology

Cerebral palsy is defined as a nonprogressive lesion of the brain occurring before, at, or soon after birth that interferes with the normal development of the immature brain. The resulting impairment of the coordination of muscle action with an inability to maintain postures and balance and to perform normal movements and skills is common to all cases.[6] Because the parts of the brain are interrelated, there may be many associated neurological abnormalities, such as sensory deficits, speech problems, sensory integration deficits, intellectual impairment, seizure disorders, and emotional problems.

Cerebral palsy occurs in approximately two per one thousand live births.[7] Thirty percent of incidences of cerebral palsy seem to be caused by prenatal complications, 60% by perinatal complications, and 10% by postnatal complications.[8]

Cerebral palsy may be inherited. Other *prenatal* causes are infection such as toxoplasmosis, rubella, and cytomegalic inclusion disease; prenatal anoxia (lack of oxygen) caused, for example, by an umbilical cord around the neck; prenatal cerebral hemorrhage (abnormal bleeding) caused by maternal toxemia or direct trauma; Rh factor such as kernicterus resulting from Rh complications; metabolic disturbances such as diabetes; harmful exposure to x-rays; bleeding in the first trimester; drug toxicity such as vitamins A and D; or multiple conceptions.[9]

Perinatal causes include anoxia from respiratory obstruction, placental abnormalities, maternal anoxia, hypotension, or breech delivery; trauma or hemorrhage from disproportions and malpositions, forceps application, induced labor, sudden pressure changes in a precipitate delivery, prolonged labor, or cesarean delivery; and prematurity.[10]

Postnatal causes include trauma from skull fractures, wounds, and contusions of the brain or from subdural hematomas; infections such as meningitis, encephalitis, and brain abscesses; toxicity from lead, arsenic, and coal tar derivatives; vascular accidents such as congenital aneurysms or hypertensive disorders; anoxia from CO_2 poisoning, strangulation, or hypoglycemia; and neoplasms or the developmental effects of tumors, cysts, or hydrocephalus.[11,12]

Normal and Abnormal Development

Basic Components of Normal Development

Before the occupational therapist can successfully treat an individual with cerebral palsy, knowledge of normal development is essential. The therapist should be able to differentiate between what is 1) *normal* at a given age, 2) *primitive* or normal at one age but abnormal at another age, and 3) *abnormal* or not seen in the normal child at any period of development.

Normal movement is built upon the development of righting, equilibrium, and protective extension responses or reactions. A righting reaction brings one up in space, an equilibrium or balance reaction keeps one in space, and a protective extension response occurs when one goes beyond the point of balance. The occupational therapist must be familiar with the normal components of movement that make up these three reactions in order to evaluate and treat patients in a functional, creative way.

An infant's first movements are primitive and gross. They are not purposeful nor are they cortically controlled.[13] These motions help to establish a range of motion in joints so that the muscles around the joint can develop control. In time, random movements develop into symmetrical, bilateral movements of the arms and legs; both arms or both legs move together. This symmetrical activity then breaks down to dissociate one extremity from the other; one extremity is able to move independently of the other. All development progresses from head to foot as the extensor and flexor components of movement develop. The proximal muscles develop first to give midline and trunk control with the distal muscles developing later. A combination of head to foot and proximal to distal development brings in the diagonal components of movement essential for righting and balancing responses.

Lois Bly, a physical therapist, has made an in-depth study of the development of normal components of movement. She describes four general characteristics of movement: there must be 1) *a point of stability,* 2) *a point of mobility,* 3) *weight shift,* 4) *a reaction to weight shift.*[14]

A point of stability refers to the base of support or what is maintaining a child in a given position. The hips are the point of stability in sitting; the feet support the standing child; the hands and knees maintain the creeping child. Stability may be either external or internal. External, or positional, stability is found when the child uses his or her anatomical structures to broaden the base of support. Two examples of this are when the child "circle sits" with hips abducted and externally rotated with knees flexed and feet touching each other, and when the child sits with hips in wide abduction with knees extended. Internal stability is when the child develops both muscle and joint control.[15] This is the mature stability necessary for functional movement.

The second characteristic of movement is *a point of mobility.* This identifies the place where movement is required, for example the joints involved in a motion. When one lifts an arm, the point of mobility is in the shoulder and the point of stability is in the hips.[16]

The third characteristic of movement is *weight shift.* Every movement causes a weight shift. It may be an anterior, posterior, lateral, or diagonal shift. A sitting child reaches forward; this necessitates an anterior weight shift. An infant shifts his weight backwards to lift his head and chest off the surface; this is a posterior weight shift. He moves his weight from one elbow to the other; this is a lateral weight shift. He transfers his weight to one side in order to reach out with the opposite arm; this is a diagonal weight shift. It is necessary to know the direction of weight shift in order to elicit a righting reaction. Weight shift may be initiated by muscle action, visual stimulation, and head turning. If a child has steadied himself with a positional point of external stability, he will not be able to shift his weight effectively.[17] Internal stability is important for this component of movement.

The fourth characteristic of movement is *reaction to weight shift.* One child may react by falling, demonstrating lack of control. Another may use a righting reaction in which her head and trunk come into alignment. She may use protective extension by stretching out her arms. Another may use a balance or equilibrium response to keep himself in space.[18]

While the infant's development progresses from head to foot and from proximal to distal control; he or she acquires the extensor, flexor, lateral flexor, and rotational components of movement necessary for righting, equilibrium, and protective extensor responses. Before an infant can gain control of a joint, full range of motion and muscle elongation must occur. Developing full range of motion and elongation of muscles are two key points in treatment planning. When an infant is born, he or she comes from the compact environment of the womb where the neck and back extensor muscles have been elongated. For this reason, the infant's first controlled movements are of extensor muscles.[19] An infant's extensor development will normally stay several months ahead of its flexor development.

When prone, the neonate uses neck retraction to lift and turn the head. The side to which the head is turned is the side that is weight bearing. The infant's arms are flexed, adducted, and internally rotated; the elbows are behind the shoulders. He or she has posterior pelvic tilt; the legs are adducted, flexed, and externally rotated with the feet in dorsiflexion. The newborn has a traction and grasp reflex response.[20]

When supine, the neonate does not have the flexion needed for controlled movements. The hips, ankles, knees, and elbows spring back when passively extended;[21] this is called *physiological flexion.* The neonate's head is not in the midline, but it is also not fully rotated to the side. When eating and/or crying, the infant's head tends to be in the midline. The head is turned toward the side bearing more weight. When pulled to sit, a newborn has total head lag. When held in a sitting position, the head flops forward. The neonate's shoulders are forward with the arms flexed, adducted, and internally rotated with the hands clenched into fists. He or she is able to bring the back of the hand to the mouth but not in the midline. He or she still has posterior pelvic tilt, legs are flexed and adducted with slight outward rotation. Because of the neonate's posterior pelvic tilt, he or she kicks in the air.[22]

Within 3 months, the infant has developed sufficient prone extension to lift his or her head up to 90°, and is able to rotate it freely. The infant now has early proximal control of horizontal abduction and horizontal adduction that allows forearm weight bearing with proprioception into the shoulders. The elbows have come forward and are in line with the shoulders. This allows the infant to have upper extremity external rotation. The 3-month-old infant has lumbar extension with the pelvis down. Hip extension has decreased, but the infant's hips continue to be flexed, abducted, and externally rotated.[23]

When supine, the 3-month-old assumes more

symmetrical positions. Neck flexors have developed, so the head is held near the midline. The infant's eyes converge. He or she brings the arms together on the chest, but does not reach out in space. The infant pulls at his or her clothing. There is controlled internal rotation of the arms and forward flexion. The infant's legs tend to assume the "frog-legged" position, in which there is increased external hip rotation and abduction and the feet are together. When kicking, more of the foot hits the surface.[24]

When sitting, the 3-month-old infant holds his or her head up. Increased back extension has developed that is reinforced with scapular adduction and humeral extension. The infant tends to lean forward because of low muscle tone in the lower back and hips.[25]

At 6 months of age, the infant has well-developed neck extension when prone. He or she pushes up on extended arms. The narrower base of support and neutral shoulder rotation allows the infant's hands to point straight ahead. The 6-month-old maintains an extended arm position to shift weight to one side while reaching out with the opposite arm. The infant may be able to push backwards on the stomach. A child of this age extends both legs vigorously to "play" in this newly developed extension pattern.[26]

When supine, the 6-month-old infant demonstrates increased flexor control by touching the feet with his or her hands. The baby reaches out in space with extended arms. He or she transfers objects from one hand to the other. He or she can roll from supine to prone.[27] When pulled to a sitting position, a 6-month-old infant lifts his or her head independently and pulls with the arms. Increased flexor control lets the child flex the legs at the hips and counterbalance with knee extension.[28]

This overview of gross motor development in newborn, 3-month-old, and 6-month-old infants illustrates some components of movement and their relationship to the next level of development. In summary, extension is normally well developed in the neck at 0 to 4 months, the midback by 3 to 4 months, the hips by 5 to 6 months, the knees by 6 months, and the feet by 6 to 8 months. As stated earlier, flexors usually lag behind extensors. Flexion is normally present in the neck by 5 months, abdominals by 6 to 7 months, and hips by 7 to 8 months. Lateral flexion is controlled in the neck by 4 months and in the trunk by 5 to 6 months. Rotational components are usually developed in the upper trunk by 4 to 5 months, lower trunk by 6 to 7 months, and sitting position by 10 months.[29] The components of movement guide the therapist in preparing treatment plans for assisting the cerebral palsied child to attain the appropriate developmental milestones.

Normal and Abnormal Blocks in Development

There are four major areas where the normal infant may have a temporary block in development: the neck, shoulders, pelvis, and hips. If the infant has not developed sufficient control of an area, the development may be blocked distal and/or proximal to that point.[30] As mentioned previously, persons with cerebral palsy may maintain some primitive movement patterns. A block in development which was normal at 3 months of age may be seen in the older child and adult and be a part of primitive and/or abnormal motor development pattern. Awareness of these blocks can guide the therapist in evaluating and planning treatment.

There are two types of neck blocks: *neck hyperextension* and *neck asymmetry*. *Neck hyperextension* is extension of the occiput on the atlas. It is normally seen in the 1- to 3-month-old infant. Hyperextension is normally counterbalanced by the development of the neck flexors and leads to elongation of the neck. Head extension is balanced by head and cervical flexion. The child with cerebral palsy may show primitive and abnormal development when flexor control does not develop sufficiently to counterbalance extension. This may result in the neck's never becoming elongated. Also, head extension is never balanced by head flexion (chin tuck) although cervical flexion develops.

Neck asymmetry causes the head to be turned to one side. It may occur in combination with neck hyperextension. There is a lack of symmetrical development of the flexors necessary to bring the head to the midline and to suppress the stimulation of the asymmetrical tonic neck reflex. Neck asymmetry is normally seen in the infant until the age of 3 to 4 months when flexors develop and bring the head to the midline, allowing symmetry to develop, the eyes to converge, and the hands to come together. Children with cerebral palsy may show primitive and abnormal development when they do not have symmetrical development of their flexors. They may have poor midline control of their heads. Their eyes may have difficulty converging, and their hands often do not come together. Also, cerebral palsied children may have difficulty bringing their hands to their mouths and faces, which decreases the tactile stimulation they experience.

Because shoulder development is directly related to neck development, the presence of a neck block may cause a shoulder block to occur. There are two types of shoulder blocks: *scapulohumeral tightness* and *scapular adduction*.

Scapulohumeral tightness is normal in infants from

1 to 3 months of age when the elbow is normally held behind the shoulder in prone. As the upper trunk flexors and scapular stabilizers develop, the infant's arms move forward so that the elbow is in front of the shoulder. This causes elongation of the muscles between the scapula and humerus. This is only possible after the scapula has become proximally stabilized on the chest wall. This allows scapulohumeral dissociation that permits upper extremity external rotation, forearm supination and pronation, and that allows for the fine motor development of the wrists and fingers. When this does not take place in the child with cerebral palsy, the arms cannot move forward because of poor development of flexor control that causes tightness of the muscles between the scapula and humerus. The upper extremities are kept internally rotated. No dissociation occurs between the scapula and humerus, causing them to move as a unit. This inhibits the development of fine motor control in the upper extremity.

In the normal developmental sequence, *scapular adduction* reinforces back extension and stability. It is normal in infants aged 4 to 5 months when they are placed in prone suspension. This is seen in the Landau response. It is later seen in the initial stages of sitting, standing, and walking independently. It is always counterbalanced by equal trunk flexor control. If this normal balance does not occur, primitive and abnormal development may result. Because of poor scapulohumeral dissociation, scapular adduction causes the arms to retract. The scapula muscles do not become stabilized on the trunk, preventing dissociated upper extremity function. Lack of dissociation prevents the arms from coming forward for forearm support, prevents upper extremity function in unsupported sitting and upper extremity function in standing and walking.

A child with neck and shoulder blocks often compensates for these limitations in ways that lead to abnormal development. These compensations are usually seen in sitting. A child with poor head control elevates the shoulders to provide head stability that further limits the possibility of lateral head righting and head rotation. The shoulders will become tighter and their mobility more limited when they are elevated. This increases neck hyperextension, humeral adduction, and humeral hyperextension. Neck hyperextension limits downward gaze, which leads to a forward jaw thrust, and makes lip closure more difficult.

There are two types of pelvic blocks: *anterior pelvic tilt* and *posterior pelvic tilt*. Anterior pelvic tilt or lordosis can be seen in a prone four-month-old infant. When the infant reaches 4 to 5 months of age, anterior pelvic tilt is balanced by the abdominal muscles. Later the abdominals and hip extensors work

together. This elongates the iliopsoas muscles. When supine, anterior pelvic tilt can be balanced when the infant puts his or her hands on knees, feet in the mouth, and hands on feet in the air. It is muscular control of the hips that provides stability for prone forearm weight shifting. In a cerebral palsied child, anterior pelvic tilt stays strong because it is not opposed. This may cause primitive and abnormal development. Abdominal muscles may not develop; the iliopsoas muscles are never elongated. The lower extremities stay abducted, flexed, and externally rotated in a frog-like position with no hip stability. Supine balancing activities may never occur. Low extensor tone in the hip muscles may cause the child to flop forward when placed in a sitting position. A cerebral palsied child may "circle sit," using legs for positional stability. This causes the child to use neck and trunk hyperextension to lift the head and trunk. The child may also compensate by "W" sitting in which the hips are internally rotated and knees flexed, allowing child to sit between his or her legs. This provides a broad base of support but may lead to dislocated hips. He or she uses anterior pelvic tilt to lock the lower extremities into a position that stabilizes the pelvis. This may cause the child to hyperextend the trunk. The child's legs may remain abducted when standing. Because there is insufficient hip control to shift weight, the child compensates by abnormally adducting the hips and keeping the feet wide apart. Adducted thighs rather than trunk control give the child external stability. He or she shifts weight by using lateral trunk flexion to the weight-bearing side instead of elongating the weight-bearing side of the normal balance reaction.

Posterior pelvic tilt results from normal co-contraction of the abdominals and hip extensors. If this co-contraction does not develop, the child with cerebral palsy will lack hip joint mobility. Spastic hip extensors may become shortened and may lack mobility. This, in turn, limits the hip flexion; when a child tries to flex the hips, the pelvis is pulled back during sitting, which increases extensor tone in the trunk. This may throw the child backwards. The child compensates by pulling the trunk forward into abnormal flexion. This leads to abnormal hip adduction and eventually to strong internal rotation of the hips. Long sitting (sitting with the legs extended forward) is difficult and nonfunctional for the child with a posterior pelvic tilt. He or she may resort to "W" sitting, which gives a more functional stable position. He or she keeps the pelvis back, thighs together, and feet apart for a wide base of positional support.

There are two types of hip blocks: *pelvic femoral tightness* and *hip extension adduction. Pelvic femoral tightness* is normal for infants from 3 to 4 months of age. Their legs are abducted, flexed, and externally rotated in a frog-legged position. This position changes when the iliopsoas becomes elongated and the development of normal hip extension, adduction, and internal rotation on a stable trunk allows the legs to come together. Lower extremity dissociation develops through a weight shift and elongation of muscles on the weight-bearing side. If the child with cerebral palsy continues to experience a pelvic femoral tightness hip block, his or her legs will not come together and will remain in a frog-like position. There is no lower extremity dissociation or weight shifting capability.

Normal *hip extension and adduction* occur as a result of the development of hip extensors with good abdominals, and hip adductors with good extensors. These are balanced by hip flexors and abductors. All of these are working together on a stable, integrated trunk. The child who has cerebral palsy may have an unstable trunk because he or she does not have good abdominals. Without a stable trunk, normal hip extension and adduction cannot occur. The legs may extend and adduct instead as a result of abnormal trunk flexion.

Classification of Cerebral Palsy by Muscle Tone

There are four types of cerebral palsy: spasticity, athetosis, ataxia, and flaccidity. The presence of abnormal muscle tone is common to all types. Most cases, however, are mixed and do not fit into a clearcut diagnostic classification. Often it is more meaningful to the therapist to refer to the type of muscle tone rather than a concrete classification. It is interesting to note that the superficial muscle tone is often not the same as the underlying tone. When the superficial muscle tone is inhibited, the underlying tone is often low.

Spasticity

Spasticity refers to extreme and above normal muscle tone. Spastic individuals usually have quadriplegic, diplegic, hemiplegic, or sometimes paraplegic involvement.

The *severely spastic* person has high muscle tone with little change in the degree of tone. There is constant co-contraction of muscles that inhibits relaxation while awake or asleep. Because they tend to assume a few abnormal postures, these individuals are more vulnerable to developing deformities including scoliosis; kyphosis; flexion deformities of the hips,

knees, and fingers; forearm pronation contracture; subluxation of the hip; and shortening of the heel cords with inward or outward turning of the foot (equinovarus and equinovalgus respectively). Movement occurs only when strongly stimulated. This movement is labored and remains within a limited range of motion. Primitive spinal patterns are often completely inhibited by tonic reactions. Startle reactions are common in many cases. Tonic patterns are seen in the tonic neck and tonic labyrinthine reflexes and also in a positive supporting reaction. Associated reactions can be felt, but little movement is observed. Righting reactions, protective extension, and equilibrium reactions are often absent. Neck righting, however, may be present.

The individual with *moderate spasticity* may have normal to high muscle tone, is usually able to move around, and may be able to walk. The degree of high tone is negatively influenced by the amount of stimulation received from effort, emotion, speech, and sudden stretch. More spasticity is seen in the agonist than in the antagonist muscles and more occurs distally than proximally. Deformities may develop from the maintenance of abnormal postures, the use of stereotyped abnormal patterns, and the associated reactions in lesser involved parts. These deformities may include kyphosis; lordosis; hip subluxations or dislocations; flexion contractures of hips and knees; tight hip inward rotators; tight hip adductors; and heel cord shortening with foot rotation.

Although the moderate spastic possesses a greater range of motion, it is usually not complete throughout every range. Learned skills are performed in primitive and abnormal patterns without selectivity of movement. Total movements may be in synergies or patterns. There may be voluntary use of spinal and tonic reflex patterns for purposive movements. Primitive spinal patterns of total flexion or extension are common. A strong startle response is usually present. The tonic neck and tonic labyrinthine reflexes and positive supporting reactions are often present. Reactions in the form of associated movements are strong. Some righting reactions may be present. Equilibrium reactions are often developed in sitting and kneeling positions, but not in standing and walking positions. An individual's size and weight may eventually necessitate the use of a wheelchair. As a child grows bigger, he or she may become more spastic because of the increasing effort needed to move around.

The *mildly involved spastic* individual often is able to stand up despite having incomplete righting and equilibrium responses. Because of his or her level of movement, deforming factors are minimal. This child seems motor driven and is often difficult to treat. As the child's speed builds up, muscle tone and tension increase. Mildly spastic children may have more diplegic and hemiplegic involvement. They learn to compensate for their problems effectively while still young.

Athetosis

Athetosis refers to muscle tone that fluctuates from low to normal and, in some cases, to high. Usually there is quadriplegic involvement, but sometimes there is only hemiplegic involvement. It is rare for an individual to have pure athetosis. It is often combined with spasticity, tonic spasms, or chorea movements.

Individuals with athetosis like to move. They often maintain abnormal and persistent primitive patterns of movement. One compensation they may make involves the use of an asymmetrical tonic neck reflex to attain stability. The reflex pattern often involves the right side with the right arm extended and the left arm flexed. They will use the left hand for functional activities. Individuals with athetosis cannot hold their heads in the midline because of this primitive reflex. The head is used to control gross motor movements. If the head is turned, the rest of the body will assume the appropriate asymmetrical tonic neck reflex position. Because athetoid individuals have no gross motor midline, they have difficulty developing a visual midline involving head, hands, and eyes. This negatively influences perceptual skills.

Because an athetoid child has better control of the feet than of proximal muscles, he or she will start to develop extensor tone from the feet up rather than from the head down. The neck and shoulders may be locked into neck and shoulder blocks to assist in stabilization.

Low fluctuating muscle tone allows a broad range of motion in all joints. Joint dislocation may result from this hyperextension. The shoulders especially may dislocate easily and painlessly. When this occurs, it is difficult to attain joint stabilization.

ATHETOSIS WITH SPASTICITY. The athetoid with spasticity seems to have moderate spasticity in proximal areas and athetosis in distal areas. Muscle tone fluctuates between normal and high. Deformities are less frequent than in the spastic type but may occur as flexor deformities in the hips, elbows, and knees. There may be some co-contraction in proximal joints. Such individuals often lack selective movement and grading of muscle action. There is some control throughout the midranges. Postural patterns are similar to those with moderate spasticity. Primitive spinal patterns are present but modified by involuntary movements. There are strong influences of the tonic neck reflexes (symmetrical and asymmetrical) and the tonic labyrinthine reflexes. Although usually present, righting reactions are unreliable because of the intermittent influence of tonic reflexes.

ATHETOSIS WITH TONIC SPASMS. In the athetoid individual with tonic spasms, muscle tone changes from low to high. Lack of co-contraction causes excessive extension or flexion. Strong postural asymmetry influenced by tonic neck reflexes that are more exaggerated on one side may cause deformities to develop. These may include scoliosis; kyphoscoliosis; dislocation of the hip on the skull side; and flexor contractures of the hips and knees if the individual has been sitting for long periods. Occasionally the hips, fingers, or lower jaw sublux. There is hardly any voluntary control of movements because of strong, intermittent tonic spasms. Extreme postures of flexion or extension are assumed. There seems to be more involuntary movement in distal areas than in proximal parts. Because the individual either is in tonic spasm or has low muscle tone and is unable to move, primitive spinal patterns are usually not present. Strong tonic patterns are seen in the asymmetrical and symmetrical tonic neck reflexes and the tonic labyrinthine reflexes. Righting, equilibrium, and protective extension reactions are absent.

CHOREOATHETOSIS. The individual with choreoathetosis has muscle tone that fluctuates from low to normal and from low to high. There is no co-contraction. Deformities are rare, but there is a tendency for subluxation of the shoulder and finger joints to occur. There are extreme ranges of motion with no grading of midranges. The large jerky involuntary movements seem to be more proximal than distal. Hands and fingers are weak, but often coordination is good in free movement. There is a lack of selective movement and fixation of movement. Primitive spinal patterns are present but modified by the athetosis. There are intermittent tonic reflex patterns. Righting and equilibrium reactions are present to some extent, but coordination is abnormal. Protective extension of the arms is abnormal and often absent.

PURE ATHETOSIS. The individual with pure athetosis has muscle tone that fluctuates from low to normal. There are rarely any deformities. There may be some transient subluxations of the shoulder and finger joints, and there is lack of co-contraction. Twitches and jerks of individual muscles or even muscle fibers are seen. Slow, writhing involuntary movements that are more distal than proximal and lack of fixation are characteristic. Primitive spinal patterns are present but modified by athetosis. These patterns are less primitive and more selective than in choreoathetosis. There is rarely any tonic reflex influence. Righting, equilibrium, and protective extension reactions are present but involuntary movements interfere with them.

Ataxia

Ataxia refers to muscle tone that fluctuates from below normal to normal. Usually there is quadriplegic involvement. It is rare to see a case of pure ataxia, as they are usually mixed. Children with ataxia may look normal at rest, but, in severe cases, they experience tremors when awake. Intension tremors and nystagmus are common.

Because ataxic individuals lack a point of stability, muscular co-activation is difficult for them. They do not like to move. They use primitive rather than abnormal patterns with little reflex influence. This causes gross, total patterns of movement. They have difficulty grading movements within a small range, and they will often overshoot targets. They use "fixing" or will stabilize themselves against any point of contact to gain stability. They use their eyes to keep their heads in the midline. If they look to the side, they may lose their balance.

These children may have developed righting responses, but these are uncoordinated, exaggerated, and poorly utilized. Equilibrium responses may be developed, but they are not coordinated. Ataxic children may be slow to move to regain their balance, and their movements are poorly timed and not smooth. They use protective responses to "fix" and lock themselves into stable positions. They walk on the medial border of their feet with their legs abducted to provide a wide base of support. They may reach out with their toes to feel their way and then bring their legs over their feet. Ataxic children use a flexor component to help stabilize themselves. If thrown off balance, they pull into flexion to protect themselves.

They may "fix" or stabilize with their mouths, which causes slow, thick speech. They may "fix" or stabilize their tongues between or against their teeth to know where it is. The tongue, like the head, is held in the midline with little lateralization or interplay. During feeding, ataxic children may hold their lips against their gums to keep track of where they are. They may have difficulty coordinating suck–swallowing and breathing.

Flaccidity

Flaccidity is characterized by fluctuating low muscle tone. This may be seen in either an infant or a toddler. Initially, the child is flaccid but later, with maturation, he or she may be classified as spastic, athetoid, or ataxic. Involvement is usually quadriplegic.

These children have little to no sensory or stretch feedback to stimulate movement and therefore stay passive. Because they may not be able to move, they may only respond with their eyes. Because they have no head control, eye movements may not be smooth unless they are supine. It is important to check for eye brightness. These babies do not cry much. When they do cry, it is shallow and low. They are considered "good" babies and therefore often will get less attention and will experience less interaction with adults during their crucial first 6 months of life.

The physiological flexion seen in the normal neonate does not occur. Infants of this type may look like premature infants. However, they do not build up muscle tone as "premies" do; they may stay flaccid until 2 years of age. The longer the child is flaccid, the greater the probability of mental retardation. As this infant matures, it is important to watch for signs of spasticity and/or athetosis. The infant who "fixes" or stabilizes his or her shoulders and lower back may become a spastic. The infant who "fixes" or stabilizes in trunk extension may become an athetoid.

The child may first attempt to move when in extension. If the flaccid child does not become a spastic or an athetoid, he or she will learn to "fix" using extension to come up against gravity. This occurs most frequently when the child is propped in a semireclining position and pushes back into the surface using extension. When supine, the child will play in extension. The child's hips go into outward rotation, attaining a frog-like position. Because this child spends much time supine, tonic labrynthine reflexes become strong and pull him or her further into the surface. When prone, the flaccid child may not lift the head. As extensor tone develops, the child seems stronger; however, flexion does not develop at the appropriate rate. The flaccid child has a flat, narrow chest and a poor, shallow breathing pattern. Any respiratory infection may be life threatening.

Some infants may stay flaccid until 6 months of age. Then the process is reversed and by 18 months they may have passed the appropriate developmental milestones. These infants are usually more responsive to their environment and seem more visually alert.

Associated Neurological Abnormalities and Problems

Occupational therapists must be aware not only of the motor implications of cerebral palsy but also of other problems and neurological abnormalities that may be associated with it. Studies have shown that most children with cerebral palsy have anywhere from two to seven additional disorders.[31]

It is estimated that 50% of children with cerebral palsy have *disturbances of vision*. This may result from a lack of eye coordination that occurs especially when there is quadriplegic involvement. There may be internal or external squints or strabismus. This may be alternating or fixed and may cause lack of accommodation. Lack of conjugate movement may cause an impairment of stereoscopic vision. The child may not be able to move his or her eyes and thus must move the head. Strong neck retraction may limit the athetoid child's ability to look down. A strong asymmetrical tonic neck reflex may fix the eyes or may prevent the eyes from moving over the midline. Total blindness may be caused by the increasingly rare retrolental fibroplasia and by optic atrophy. It is likely that the cerebral palsied child who may also be hemiplegic will have visual field deficits from optic radiation.[32]

An estimated 25% of children with cerebral palsy have some type of *auditory disturbance*. The most common auditory problem is high frequency deafness. This is most likely to occur as a result of neonatal jaundice suffered by the athetoid child, but it is also common in the spastic child. There may be auditory imperception or agnosia.[33]

Speech disturbances are seen in approximately 25% of cerebral palsy cases.[34] The most common problem is dysarthria, which is pseudobulbar palsy seen in the spastic, athetoid, and mixed types. Aphasia is rare. Apraxia of the mouth, throat, and larynx may cause an inability to speak.[35]

Impairment of stereognosis is common in the individual with hemiplegic involvement. There may be a more subtle global problem with the spastic quadriplegic child.

Sensory integrative disorders are seen in approximately 14% of individuals with cerebral palsy.[36] Apparently, incidence is higher among spastic children. This may be the result of a brain lesion, of the child's inability to explore the environment, or of learning disorders.

An estimated 50% to 75% of children with cerebral palsy have *below average intelligence*.[37,38]

Seizure disorders are seen in approximately 25% of cerebral palsy cases.[39] Any type of seizure may occur, but seizures are usually generalized. Seizures are more common with hemiplegia of postnatal origin. They are rare among athetoid children.[40]

Emotional problems are common among children with cerebral palsy. They are often compounded by emotional immaturity, since these children tend to be dependent upon their families. This may result from physical dependency or because of isolation from normal children. The degree of acceptance of and adjustment to disability is primarily the result of both the problem itself and the reactions of the child with the immediate environment of parents and family.[41]

Some individuals with cerebral palsy exhibit a *weak self-image*; their ability to feel a sense of self-worth and/or responsibility may be minimal. They may experience difficulties in group situations and in interpersonal relationships. They may withdraw from social interactions.

A few studies have been done on the *personality traits* that may accompany cerebral palsy. It seems that athetoid children tend to have less emotional stability and to be "explosive." Spastic children seem to have "obsessive compulsive" personality traits and may find it difficult to adapt to new situations.

In some cases the associated problems are more limiting than the motor abnormalities.

Assessment

Accurate assessment of the individual with cerebral palsy is essential for functional treatment planning. Thorough evaluation should be done to determine the child's developmental levels. The physical, sensory, perceptual, emotional, cognitive, cultural, and social components of development should all be considered.

The occupational therapist should be aware that there is no single evaluative tool that defines the many abnormalities seen in the cerebral palsied child. Instead there are many tools that can be used in conjunction with each other. A correctly selected combination results in a more accurate evaluation. The following are a variety of evaluative tools that the occupational therapist should be acquainted with and should be able to utilize in the assessment process. Many of the evaluation tools that may be used with the cerebral palsied child are the same as those in the chapter on assessment. A few especially useful tests have been singled out and are listed below.

1. *Developmental Programming for Infants and Young Children—Early Intervention Developmental Profile*[42] and *Pre-school Developmental Profile* by Rogers and D'Eugenio[43] is one of the more comprehensive evaluation tools. It assesses children from birth to 6 years of age in the areas of gross motor development, self-care, perceptual and fine motor development, and language and cognition.
2. *Denver Developmental Screening Test* by Frankenburg and Dodds[44] screens children for developmental delays. It assesses children from birth to 6 years of age in the areas of gross motor development, language, fine motor development, adaptive behaviors, and personal-social behaviors (Figs. 32-1 and 32-2).

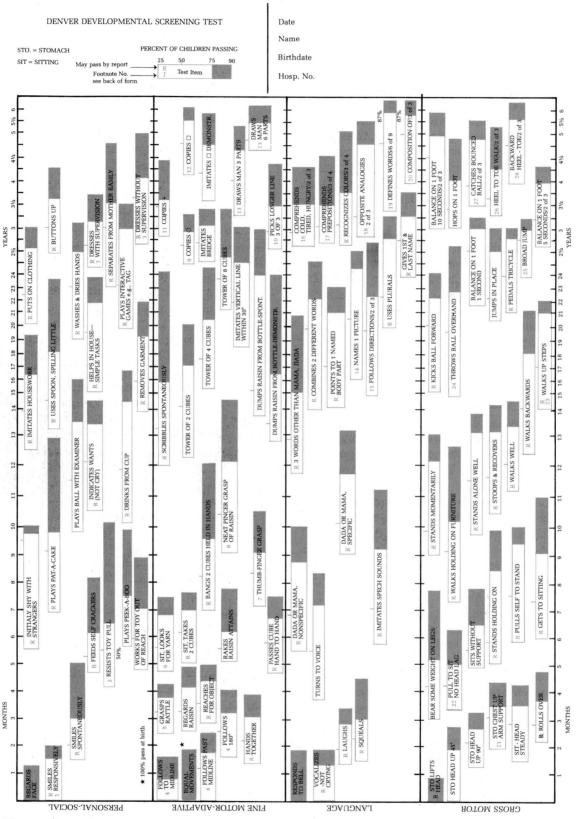

Figure 32-1. The Denver Developmental Screening Test. © 1969 by W. K. Frankenburg, MD, and J. B. Dodds, PhD, John F. Kennedy Child Development Center, University of Colorado Health Sciences Center, Denver. Printed with permission.

DATE
NAME
DIRECTIONS
BIRTHDATE
HOSP. NO.

1. Try to get child to smile by smiling, talking or waving to him. Do not touch him.
2. When child is playing with toy, pull it away from him. Pass if he resists.
3. Child does not have to be able to tie shoes or button in the back.
4. Move yarn slowly in an arc from one side to the other, about 6″ above child's face. Pass if eyes follow 90° to midline. (Past midline; 180°)
5. Pass if child grasps rattle when it is touched to the backs or tips of fingers.
6. Pass if child continues to look where yarn disappeared or tries to see where it went. Yarn should be dropped quickly from sight from tester's hand without arm movement.
7. Pass if child picks up raisin with any part of thumb and a finger.
8. Pass if child picks up raisin with the ends of thumb and index finger using an overhand approach.

9. Pass any enclosed form. Fail continuous round motions.
10. Which line is longer? (Not bigger.) Turn paper upside down and repeat. (3/3 or 5/6)
11. Pass any crossing lines.
12. Have child copy first. If failed, demonstrate.

When giving items 9, 11 and 12, do not name the forms. Do not demonstrate 9 and 11.
13. When scoring, each pair (2 arms, 2 legs, etc.) counts as one part.
14. Point to picture and have child name it. (No credit is given for sounds only.)

 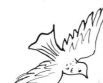 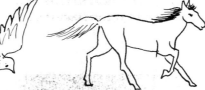 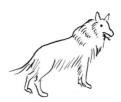 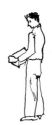

15. Tell child to: Give block to Mommie; put block on table; put block on floor. Pass 2 of 3. (Do not help child by pointing, moving head or eyes.)
16. Ask child: What do you do when you are cold? ..hungry? ..tired? Pass 2 of 3.
17. Tell child to: Put block *on* table; *under* table; *in front* of chair, *behind* chair. Pass 3 of 4. (Do not help child by pointing, moving head or eyes.)
18. Ask child: If fire is hot, ice is ?; Mother is a woman, Dad is a ?; a horse is big, a mouse is ?. Pass 2 of 3.
19. Ask chilkd: What is a ball? ..lake? ..desk? ..house? ..banana? ..curtain? ..ceiling? ..hedge? ..pavement? Pass if defined in terms of use, shape, what it is made of or general category (such as banana is fruit, not just yellow). Pass 6 of 9.
20. Ask child: What is a spoon made of? ..a shoe made of? ..a door made of? (No other objects may be substituted.) Pass 3 of 3.
21. When placed on stomach, child lifts chest off table with support of forearms and/or hands.
22. When child is on back, grasp his hands and pull him to sitting. Pass if head does not hang back.
23. Child may use wall or rail only, not person. May not crawl.
24. Child must throw ball overhad 3 feet to within arm's reach of tester.
25. Child must perform standing broad jump over width of test sheet. (8½ inches)
26. Tell child to walk forward, ⬤⬤ ⬤⬤ ⬤⬤ ⬤⬤ → heel within 1 inch of toe. Tester may demonstrate. Child must walk 4 consecutive steps, 2 out of 3 trials.
27. Bounce ball to child who should stand 3 feet away from tester. Child must catch ball with hands, not arms, 2 out of 3 trials.
28. Tell child to walk backward, ← ⬤⬤ ⬤⬤ ⬤⬤ ⬤⬤ toe within 1 inch of heel. Tester may demonstrate. Child must walk 4 consecutive steps, 2 out of 3 trials.

DATE AND BEHAVIORAL OBSERVATIONS (how child feels at time of test, relation to tester, attention span, verbal behavior, self-confidence, etc.):

Figure 32-1. (*continued*)

3. *Bayley Scale of Infant Development* by Bayley evaluates the young child in motor development, language, and cognitive skills.[45]
4. *Pre-Speech Assessment Scale: A Rating Scale for the Measurement of Pre-Speech Behaviors from Birth through Two years* by Morris[46] evaluates the normal and abnormal characteristics of feeding and pre-speech behaviors.
5. *American Academy of Mental Deficiency Adaptive Behavior Scale* by Nihira, Foster, Shellhaas, and Leland[47] serves as a guideline for development of a life tasks program for the young adult and adult.

Intervention

The treatment of the individual with cerebral palsy is a 24-hour-a-day process. The treatment team may consist of the occupational, physical, and speech therapists, the physician, psychologist, and nurse. The family is also an integral, active part of the treatment team. In addition, the child often sees a pediatrician, neurologist, developmental pediatrician, orthopedist, physiatrist, and psychiatrist. To this team the occupational therapist brings his or her skills in developmental assessment and individual problem solving. The child is viewed as a total being.

Before any evaluation or treatment can be effective, a mutual respect and acceptance needs to grow between the individual and the therapist. Children need to know that they are cared about, that they are important, and that they are unique.

The occupational therapist identifies the physical needs, emotional or maturational level, intellectual level, and specific interests of each person. The therapist in conjunction with the family and, if possible, the child, then plans a highly individualized program and presents a choice of several appropriate activities. In choosing activities, the therapist considers the cultural background, age level, physical ability, interests, and the functional level of the child.

Home programs are an essential part of the total treatment process. The goals and activities that make up these programs must meet the needs of not only the children but also of their families. One family may be able to follow an elaborate treatment program whereas another family may be able to do only one small activity. If the activities are too complicated or too time consuming for their capacity, family members may feel overwhelmed and do nothing.

Many remediation techniques may be combined with age-appropriate activities. Besides toys, games, books, and crafts, everyday practical activities may be suggested. These activities may include helping to mix cookies, knead bread, fold laundry, hang up clothes, dry unbreakable dishes, or dust. The activity may simply be playing near and/or in a cabinet of pots and pans. All of these are normal developmental experiences that an individual with cerebral palsy may miss. The occupational therapist, in his or her unique professional role, plans a therapeutic environment that includes these activities in conjunction with treatment.

The family of a child with cerebral palsy may experience many emotional strains and practical problems. Occupational therapists must be sensitive to this and should help families cope with these difficulties. Parent support groups are an important part of the entire treatment process. These groups bring together families who have gone through or are going through similar problems and feelings. Group members may be able to help each other through difficult times and to new adjustment levels.

Occupational Therapy Treatment

General Occupational Therapy Treatment Principles and Remediation Techniques

The treatment principles and processes that will be presented here are based on the Neurodevelopmental Treatment (N.D.T.) method that is based on the works of Dr. and Mrs. Karl Bobath. Mrs. Bobath, whose background was in gymnastics and movement and who had studied both normal and abnormal development in-depth, used these principles in the treatment of both the hemiplegic and cerebral palsied individual. She relied heavily on Dr. Bobath's neurophysiological knowledge to validate her findings.[48] Many others have pursued the N.D.T. approach and have continued to build upon the Bobaths' work.

The basis of the N.D.T. approach is to establish the balance necessary to be upright in space. This balance is built on the development of normal righting, equilibrium, and protective reactions.[49] It is necessary to look at the components of the righting, equilibrium, and balance responses needed for functional movement. By definition, the cerebral palsied child has high, low, or fluctuating muscle tone. When abnormal muscle tone is inhibited, the righting responses inherent in most children may be able to develop. The child is a motor-sensory-motor being. In moving, the child gains the proprioceptive feedback that prompts him or her to move again. Initially, the therapist should provide the components of movement the child needs. Later, as the child begins to develop inner control, the therapist decreases external control. The extent to which the individual with cerebral palsy responds to treatment is directly related to the amount of brain damage sustained. For this reason, some may show more progress than others. Most will respond to some degree based on their innate ability.

The N.D.T. program does not emphasize primitive and abnormal reflexes. Rather, it seeks to facilitate the normal components of movement that provide a solid basis for motor development and integration. When such components are missing, primitive patterns persist and abnormal reflexes are dominant.

The occupational therapist's goal is to inhibit abnormal and/or primitive movement patterns and to facilitate normal righting and balance responses. The concepts of normal development on which a treatment program is based have been presented throughout this chapter. They include the following:

1. A muscle must be elongated before it can work.
2. A joint must have full range of motion before internal control can be developed.
3. Weight bearing throughout a joint for proprioceptive feedback is necessary to develop weight shift.
4. Weight shift and a reaction to weight shift are essential for development to occur.
5. The capability of movement normally develops from head to foot and from proximal areas to distal areas.
6. Normal components of movement are the foundation of a treatment program.
7. Treatment must be symmetrical, that is, both sides of the body are treated regardless of the degree of involvement.

If the occupational therapist applies these basic concepts, he or she should be able to problem solve and to provide a functional treatment program for a child with cerebral palsy regardless of the type of muscle tone.

The therapist may want to use various pieces of therapeutic equipment to assist in moving and manipulating the child. These may include therapy balls that vary in size from 1 to 4 feet in diameter. Rolls or bolsters may vary in size from 3 inches to 24 inches in diameter and may be several feet long. Wedges, large stuffed animals, and many other devices may be used. The best equipment the therapist has available is his or her own body. For example, the therapist's legs may be used as bolsters or inclined planes. A child will sometimes accept the warmth of the therapist's body when he or she will not accept a ball or bolster.

Although treatment concepts in this chapter refer to the "child," the same concepts are used with the adult. However, the child has a developing motor system and usually will show more progress than the young adult and adult. The infant under 1 year old will show the most progress.

Application of Basic Concepts

High Tone or Spasticity

The basis for treatment of the child with high muscle tone is the use of *movement to reduce tone*.[50] Initially, movement is passive to elongate muscles in the trunk and extremities. This allows greater mobility, active movement, and decreased muscle tone. A ball or roll may be used. The child is picked up in the desired position and placed on the ball; he or she is not placed on the ball and then positioned. To position and pick up a child who is prone, the therapist places one arm under the child's thighs and one arm under the extended arms. This puts the child in an extended, elongated position. (It is easy to lose control of a wiggly child, nonetheless.) To reduce tone, the child is slowly rocked on the ball. The more proximally the child is held, the less trunk work he or she must do. As muscle tone is reduced, the child may be held further down on the legs.

If the child's trunk is asymmetrical or if the child pulls his or her arms down from the extended position, it may be necessary to further elongate the side. To passively move an arm, grasp it above the elbow and then move it. If the arm is grasped below the elbow, there is a tendency for the child to pull into flexion. (This should also be remembered when dressing and bathing a child.) With the arm on the shortened or tight side held over the head, the child may be rolled to that side to elongate the muscles. Gentle rocking may continue forwards, backwards, sideways, and diagonally. Care should be taken that the hip on the elongated side is in line with the body. If it is flexed, it will not allow for a good stretch. A flexed hip may be a compensation to avoid stretching and using that side. This type of elongation is especially beneficial for children with hemiplegic involvement. Additional elongation may be done by having the child prop up on an elbow when in a sidelying position. It is necessary to do all activities to both sides of the child's body. The child should be assisted to move in the appropriate sequential manner needed to assume elongation on the opposite side. This gives the child much needed sensorimotor feedback. He or she should not be bodily lifted off a surface and "plopped" into another position.

The child with high muscle tone needs *mobility with stability in larger ranges and movements*. This can be exercised and developed using the basic concepts of weight shift and elongation. For example, a child is placed on the elbows when prone. He or she initially maintains the prone position with no weight

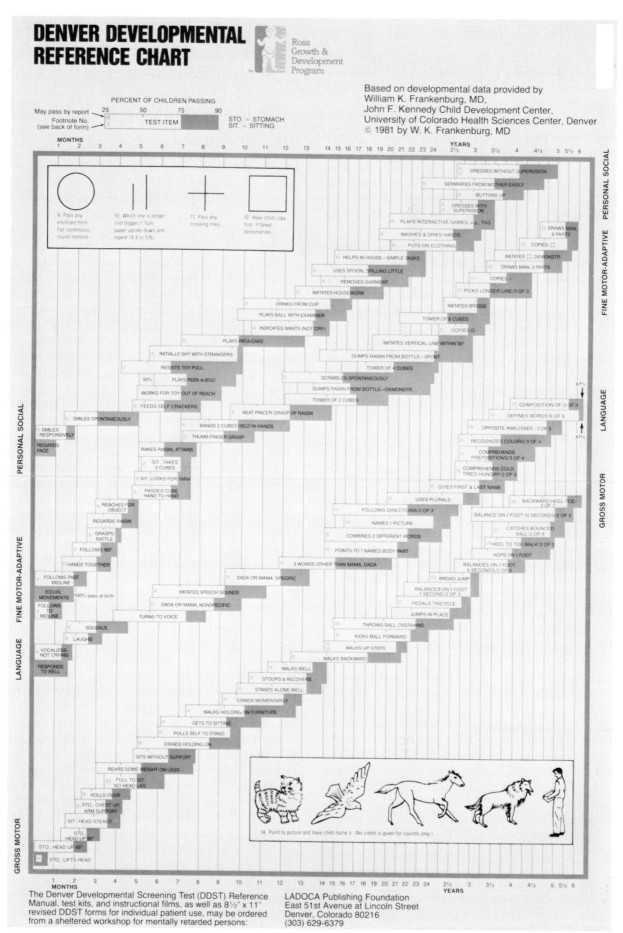

Figure 32-2. The Denver Developmental Reference Chart. © 1981 by W. K. Frankenburg, MD, John F. Kennedy Child Development Center, University of Colorado Health Sciences Center, Denver. Printed with permission.

DIRECTIONS

This Denver Developmental Reference Chart has been developed as a parent counseling aid to parallel a smaller version of the Denver Developmental Screening Test, which helps to determine whether or not a given child's developmental status falls within established norms. Health professionals need to administer and interpret each item on the Screening Test according to standardized procedures and then plot the development of each child in their practice on a separate form. They then may use this Reference Chart, which has been designed in size and format for this purpose, as an office aid to discuss a child's development with the parents.

1. Try to get child to smile by smiling, talking or waving to him or her. Do not touch him or her.
2. When child is playing with toy, gently pull it away from him or her. Pass if he or she resists.
3. Child does not have to be able to tie shoes or button in the back.
4. Move yarn slowly in an arc from one side to the other, about 6″ above child's face. Pass if eyes follow 90° to midline. (Past midline; 180°)
5. Pass if child grasps rattle when it is touched to the backs or tips of fingers.
6. Pass if child continues to look where yarn disappeared or tries to see where it went. Yarn should be dropped quickly from sight from tester's hand without arm movement.
7. Pass if child picks up raisin with any part of thumb and a finger.
8. Pass if child picks up raisin with the ends of thumb and index finger using an overhand approach.
9. , 10., 11., 12. (See directions on face of chart. When giving items 9., 11., and 12., do not name the forms. Do not demonstrate 9. and 11.)
13. When scoring, each pair (2 arms, 2 legs, etc.) counts as one part.
14. (See directions on face of chart.)
15. Tell child to: Give block to Mommie; put block on table; put block on floor. Pass 2 of 3. (Do not help child by pointing, moving head or eyes.)
16. Ask child: What do you do when you are cold? . . . hungry? . . . tired? Pass 2 of 3.
17. Tell child to: Put block *on* table; *under* table; *in front of* chair; *behind* chair. Pass 3 of 4. (Do not help child by pointing, moving head or eyes.)
18. Ask child: If fire is hot, ice is ____? Mother is a woman, Dad is a ____(man)? A horse is big, a mouse is ____? Pass 2 of 3.
19. Ask child: What is a ball? . . . lake? . . . desk? . . . house? . . . banana? . . . curtain? . . . ceiling? . . . hedge? . . . pavement? Pass if defined in terms of use, shape, what it is made of, or general category (such as banana is fruit, not just yellow). Pass 6 of 9.
20. Ask child: What is a spoon made of? . . . a shoe made of? . . . a door made of? . . . (No other objects may be substituted.) Pass 3 of 3.
21. When placed on stomach, child lifts chest off table with support of forearms and/or hands.
22. When child is on back, grasp his or her hands and gently pull him or her to sitting. Pass if head does not hang back.
23. Child may use wall or rail only, not person. May not crawl.
24. Child must throw ball overhand 3 feet to within arm's reach of tester.
25. Child must perform standing broad jump over width of test sheet (8½ inches).
26. Tell child to walk forward, ∞∞∞∞→ heel within 1 inch of toe. Tester may demonstrate. Child must walk 4 consecutive steps, 2 out of 3 trials.
27. Bounce ball to child who should stand 3 feet away from tester. Child must catch ball with hands, not arms, 2 out of 3 trials.
28. Tell child to walk backward, ←∞∞∞∞ toe within 1 inch of heel. Tester may demonstrate. Child must walk 4 consecutive steps, 2 out of 3 trials.

Figure 32-2. (*continued*)

shift. The child then either weight shifts to one elbow or is assisted to shift by the movement of the therapy ball. The weight-bearing side is elongated, an early component of a balance response. The opposite and non-weight-bearing side becomes free to move in space. Depending upon the placement of a toy or other stimulus, the child will reach out and develop larger ranges of movement. Mobility is increased through weight shift and elongation. Trunk mobility is increased through the prone-on-elbows position and later by the prone-on-extended-arms position. This will be discussed in more detail under gross motor development.

Verbal commands often make the child with high muscle tone tense. It is important to use other methods of communication such as touch, movement, and appropriate play to communicate.

Fluctuating Tone or Athetosis

The key to working with a child who has fluctuating tone or athetosis is to work on *steadying the tone and achieving midline orientation.* This may be done by giving the child firm, steady pressure through the joints with symmetrical positioning. For example, a therapist can lay a child supine on a pillow so that the neck is slightly flexed, shoulders are forward, and arms are across chest. The therapist sits in front of the child with his or her legs on either side of the child to help cradle the trunk and shoulders and to control movements. The child's hips and pelvis are positioned against the therapist's body. Steady, controlled pressure is given through the shoulders to steady muscle tone. The therapist grasps the child's pelvis and gives a downward stretch while flexing the child's trunk. This will elongate the child's neck and back and give him or her the feeling of steady, stable movement as the knees come into close reaching range of the already midline-oriented arms. The child with fluctuating muscle tone works well within small ranges and small movements. If midline control of head or arms is lost when attempting to touch knees, the therapist may use his or her feet and/or legs to bring the shoulders and arms symmetrically forward. This should also reorient the head. The therapist will usually be able to control arm use from the shoulders without actually moving the arms. The older child may not be interested in touching the knees and feet and will need an appropriate stimulus such as a toy or piece of food placed on the knees or feet. In the above activity, the therapist has given the child stability in conjunction with movement, increased trunk control, and practice of small movements within small ranges.

When a child is moved into more upright positions, more inner control is needed. From the curled-up position just described, the child is brought to a sitting position. The therapist lies back on an inclined plane and brings the child forward to sit with the child's legs either straddling the therapist's trunk, to put weight on his or her feet, or extending in a long sit. The therapist's legs are used as a back support. Side-to-side and forward-to-backward movements facilitate weight shift in the trunk. Another sequential movement from the curled-up position is to bring the child into a sitting position in front of the therapist. Weight shift may be done through the trunk and compression down from the shoulders to increase muscle stability. Midline orientation of head and arms is necessary. The further down on the trunk, hips, or legs the child is held, the more trunk control he or she needs to use. If the child seems fearful and appears to be holding on tightly or "fixing," it may be necessary to move up the trunk for support and to go back to some preparation activities such as elongation.

It is important to work on balance responses while in an upright position. An upright position may be sitting, standing, or half-standing with the support of a piece of equipment. Balance responses develop through weight shift to a weight-bearing side that allows the other side and/or trunk to be free to move and react.

The more stability the therapist gives the child with fluctuating muscle tone, the more the child uses and depends on it. The child should be given support only as needed. For this reason, the treatment must be active, with the therapist removing and replacing his or her hands often to encourage the child to develop inner control.

Verbal commands work nicely with this child. The therapist states his or her intention before touching and moving the child. However, the child with fluctuating muscle tone is difficult to treat because he or she is always changing.

Low to Normal Muscle Tone or Ataxia

The ataxic child needs to have *movement with stability* (as opposed to the athetoid child who needs stability with movement). Because the ataxic individual wants to stay still, therapy involves increased trunk movement and assistance in developing righting and balance or equilibrium reactions. These are incorporated into small, slow movements. For example, the child can sit on a large ball without feet touching the floor. At first, the therapist gives the child proximal hip support by either holding the child on either hip or holding him or her with one hand on the lower abdomen and one hand on the lower back. When the child is in this stable, supported position, the ball is moved in slow, small movements to encourage weight-shift reactions in the child's trunk. The child should feel comfortable and not have the need to stabilize by pulling into flexion or into any convenient surface. If this occurs, the treatment may be on too high a level, and it may be better to return to prone activities or to find a more supported position. If the sitting position is tolerated and functional, the child can be held further down on the thighs. To help stabilize low to normal tone, the therapist gives compression down through the shoulders while controlling the legs with his or her elbows. This is done intermittently. The ataxic child uses the eyes to "fix" or stabilize by cuing in on a stable visual target.

During treatment he or she needs constantly changing intermittent support from the therapist. Any consistent pressure or weight provides an opportunity for "fixing." The child needs the opportunity to react to the movement that is imposed on him or her. For example, the moving surface of a roll or ball may be used. It is necessary to increase muscle tone but not to the point of making the child spastic. Careful monitoring of muscle tone can prevent this.

Low Muscle Tone or Floppy

The child with low muscle tone (the "floppy" child) needs *weight-bearing with movement* to stimulate tactile and proprioceptive input. Muscle tone must be increased. This is done through compression activities such as bouncing up and down, and compressing head into shoulders or shoulders into trunk, arm into shoulder and leg into hip. For example, the child can be placed over a roll and passive compression can be applied to the joints. While the trunk is supported on the roll, the child is positioned to experience weight-bearing on one arm. By assisting and maintaining the child's arm in alignment with the body, the trunk is moved over the arm to give joint compression and weight bearing with movement. This is done with each extremity working from elbow and knee weight-bearing to extended arm and leg weight-bearing. Bouncing and compression can also be done while the child is sitting on the therapist's lap. When the child is sitting, the more the arms are used for support, the less the trunk is used. Positional stability of wide hip abduction and external rotation is often used to increase the base of support rather than active use of the trunk muscles. For this reason, it is important to keep the child's hips and legs in a more neutral and adducted position.

Specific Remediation Techniques

Preparation

The child needs to be prepared before treatment can be done successfully. Preparation refers to the steadying of muscle tone. Suggestions for reducing or increasing muscle tone in each diagnostic area were given under "Application of Basic Concepts." Preparation also includes elongation of muscles and full passive range of motion in a joint.

After the child has been prepared, the therapist uses the normal developmental continuum as a basis for treatment planning. The type of preparation is specific to the abnormal muscle tone. It may be necessary to incorporate preparation activities into many parts of each treatment session as the child may become tight and unstable and may need to have preparation activities repeated. The therapist's flexibility is essential to meet the specific needs of each child.

Gross Motor

The treatment program follows the normal developmental sequence. Components of movement necessary for higher level functions are facilitated first.

One of the first gross motor tasks for the infant is lifting and turning the head. The same applies for the child with cerebral palsy. Normal positions must be studied and used. Because less gravitational pressure is exerted on an upright head, it is easier to raise the head from a vertical position. If a child is prone on a large ball, the ball may be rolled backwards to place the child upright. Pressure down through the shoulders and on the large proximal trunk muscles of the back will help to facilitate neck extension and to give a posterior weight shift. The heel of the therapist's hand is used for pressure or facilitation as fingers could pinch the child's skin. If the child's elbows are adducted and behind the shoulders, trunk stabilizing of the proximal back muscles will be used to lift the head. This elongates the anterior trunk muscles and facilitates bringing the arms forward. If the child is placed on the ball with the elbows forward or under the shoulders, this serves to mechanically elongate the trunk. This will help the child use neck extensors but may not facilitate stabilizing the scapula on the chest wall for later development of upper extremity dissociation and independent use. While the child remains prone, the ball may be moved forward for more gravitational pressure and sideways or diagonally to bring in lateral head righting responses. If the child holds his or her head in an asymmetrical position, pressure over the pectoralis muscles in front of the shoulder will facilitate turning of the head toward the side facilitated. Pressure on either the flexor (front) and/or extensor (back) surface of the trunk will facilitate head and neck flexor or extensor movements. The therapist may need to maintain backward, downward pressure on the child's shoulders and trunk to assist in holding up the head. As voluntary control begins to develop, facilitated or stabilized control should be lessened. To voluntarily lift the head, the child needs a stable pelvis that is lower than the head. The therapist may need to place his or her hand on the child's buttocks to stabilize the pelvis. A toy, bright mobile, interesting book, or person may encourage visual attention and may interest the child in lifting the head. Midline placement of the head while the child is on the elbows will allow midline orientation for symmetrical bilateral upper extremity activities.

Head control may also be facilitated while the child is in a sitting position, because there is less of a gravitational pull. If the child has little or no neck control, the therapist needs to use his or her hands to support the head while also supporting the rest of the body. Firm co-contraction of the neck and trunk muscles and bouncing the child also builds up muscle tone. While fully supported and receiving intermittent facilitation, the child is moved forward, backward, and side to side to stimulate head and neck righting responses.

The therapist helps the child to lie prone on elbows by facilitating the pectoralis muscles in front of the shoulder. His or her hands are placed under the child's chest, and pressure is applied in front of the shoulder. This also allows the therapist to shift the child's trunk to one side for weight shift. It is important to let the child experience the movement needed to achieve a position rather than to be placed in a static position. For this reason, the sequential transition from one activity to another is an integral part of treatment.

While the child is in a prone position and raised up on the elbows, the sideways movement of a ball facilitates lateral weight shift. The weight-bearing elbow is brought under the shoulder to provide increased proprioceptive and kinesthetic feedback. When the child is able to turn his or her head from side to side without looking to the weight-bearing or face side, an important milestone has been reached. Head movements are becoming dissociated from trunk movements. He or she is able to turn the head to either side while maintaining weight on one side. Side-to-side weight shift frees the nonweight-bearing side for other actions. The higher the child reaches, the more weight shift, weight bearing, and elongation on the opposite side. The child also experiences the upper-trunk rotation necessary for higher-level activities. Reaching higher helps the child push up on extended arms, which elongates the lower back and mobilizes the pelvis.

Developing an ability to shift weight from side to side when prone on elbows helps the child to roll over. The child falls off balance and initiates a turn to the side by using the neck or shoulders. Pressure down through the shoulder and side facilitates a lateral righting response necessary for rolling. The child's legs must not be "frogged" or they will block the rolling pattern.

The child may be facilitated in moving from a prone position to a sitting position and back after having shown some early trunk rotation, such as reaching out in prone. Any piece of equipment may be used that will assist both therapist and child. With the child lying prone on elbows, the therapist facilitates weight shifting by holding the child under the shoulder. The therapist facilitates a lateral righting response on the opposite side by pressing down through the side with his or her other hand. If the child has some hip stability, he or she is turned and brought into a sitting position with guidance only from the shoulder. The nonweight-bearing side leads. The child goes back into a prone position by reversing the process, in which case the weight-bearing side leads. A slow transition from one position to another facilitates the trunk muscles more. A fast movement uses momentum rather than muscle power.

The child may be brought to a sitting position from a sidelying position. The therapist places his or her right arm under the right shoulder and arm of the child and his or her left hand on the child's left hip. While leading with the hip or the nonweight-bearing side, the hip is rotated backwards, and the child is encouraged to push up on extended arms to rotate to a sitting position. Initial assistance at the weight-bearing shoulder may be necessary. This pattern of movement is easier when the child faces away from the therapist. The child is brought down to a sidelying position using the same basic pattern, except that the shoulders lead. When the child comes up to a sitting position, the hips or nonweight-bearing side lead. When going down to a sidelying or prone position the shoulders or weight-bearing side leads. It is important to do the same activity on both sides of the body.

The child must use his or her muscles the most in the transition stage from flexion to extension and from extension to flexion. He or she should be encouraged to "play" or move slowly within this transition to strengthen abdominal muscles, which are essential for a stable trunk. The oblique abdominal muscles need to be facilitated in order to develop both lower trunk rotation and stability. To facilitate the oblique abdominals, the therapist places the heel of his or her hand on the lower part of the abdomen just above the pubic bone. Pressure on the muscle and the pull of the therapist's hand guides the child in the desired direction. Depending upon the child's diagnostic classification, the child is facilitated in using small or large movements.

When moving from the sitting position, placement of the child's arms and knee and the type of weight shift dictates whether he or she ends up side sitting, prone, or on hands and knees. Placement of toys can encourage rotation into a side sitting position. Facilitation of the oblique abdominals on the weight-bearing side increases trunk rotation. The more abduction of the weight-bearing arm, the easier it is for the child to go into a sidelying and prone position. With the weight-bearing arm under the shoulder and the hip flexed, the child rotates to hands and knees by reaching out with the non-weight-bearing arm. The child may need elongation of the nonweight-bearing shoulder and side, and diagonal pressure on the abdominals of the weight-bearing side. When the child is on hands and knees, side to side weight shift of the upper or lower trunk brings the extremities into weight bearing in line with the body. The normal baby mobilizes the pelvis and increases balance by rocking on hands and knees. The child with cerebral palsy must do the same thing.

It is more important for the child to move in and out of the hands-and-knees and sitting positions than it is for him or her to move forward or to creep on hands and knees. The transition between these positions builds up the muscles needed to creep and to develop more upright skills. It also helps the child increase balance reactions. The transition phases may be facilitated on balls and bolsters that move with the child.

When the child moves from hands and knees to a half-kneel position, weight is shifted to one side. The opposite-side abdominals are facilitated to externally rotate and flex the nonweight-bearing leg. The weight-bearing leg is in line with the body. The child may stay on extended arms with weight on one knee and the opposite foot. Some children creep in this position. Side-to-side and forward-to-backward weight shift increases balance responses. Rotation of the nonweight-bearing side to further shift the weight over the weight-bearing knee will bring the child into a half-kneel position. Elongation of the nonweight-bearing side assists in standing up. Moving in and out of the different stages of movement builds and reinforces the components necessary for balance reactions to develop.

Fine Motor Movement

Fine motor movement (the basic hand skills of reaching, grasping, releasing, and fine prehension) is developed through weight bearing on the upper extremities. As this is incorporated into the treatment program, the child will show an increasing refinement of hand skills.

The basic concepts of establishing a treatment plan should be followed. The child needs full range of motion and elongation of the proximal areas before the distal areas can be free to function. The child may be placed over a bolster on his or her side with the arm over the bolster and the hip on the same side as extended as possible. Movement of the roll will give additional stretch to the side to decrease muscle tone and to increase range of motion. At the same time, the child may be encouraged to reach out to pop bubbles or bat a balloon for more extensor and rotational activities. He or she may play a game or read a book in front of the roll. When the therapist feels that the tone on the stretched side is reduced, the child may be rotated to sit while the elongated and extended side is maintained. The shoulder may then be given full range of motion, after which the child may go back into an upper extremity weight-bearing position. This may be done by having the child prop up on an extended arm in long or side sitting, push up on elbows or extended arms in a prone position, or side lie raised on an elbow or extended arm. Instead of coming to a sitting position after being stretched and elongated over the roll, the child may go into a prone position and onto the opposite side for elongation.

If the therapist and child choose to stay in the sitting position, the child sits on the floor or on a movable object such as a bolster or smaller ball. To encourage bilateral shoulder movements, the child and therapist may place large necklaces and hats on each other. The child may reach to touch a light object such as a mobile or a bubble. The child may put his or her hands on the therapist's shoulders or head while being moved on the ball or bolster. These activities also reinforce trunk stability and balance.

While the child is prone and raised on the elbows, he or she receives the proprioceptive and kinesthetic feedback necessary to dissociate the elbow from the shoulder. Elbow movement is a necessary part of self-feeding and dressing.

As control develops in the shoulders, a change from internal to external rotation occurs. Corresponding to shoulder control, weight bearing on the heel of the hand progresses from the ulnar side to the radial, or thumb, side of the hand. Weight bearing facilitates an open hand. The weight-bearing side of the hand corresponds to the finer hand skills. Initially, there is an ulnar–palmar grasp. The fingers on the ulnar side of the hand flex to make contact with the palm of the hand. When the weight shifts to the radial side of the hand, a radial palmar grasp develops. The fingers on the radial side flex to make contact with the palm of the hand. When the weight shifts to the thenar eminence, the thumb rotates into contact with the fingers in lateral prehension. As the thumb becomes more active, the finer prehensile skills of inferior and superior pinch develop.

A stable trunk, elongation and range of motion of the shoulders, and the facilitation of weight shift and weight bearing through the shoulders help the finer skills to develop. Following weight-bearing activities, the child may be given small objects to pick up and play with. These include raisins, Cheerios, and small, safe toys. A game may be made up using small wads of paper, cotton, or styrofoam chips.

It is important for the therapist to remember that fine motor skills can only develop on a stable gross motor base.

Handling

Good handling techniques are basic to a treatment program. A child who receives appropriate and consistent physical handling will more than likely do better than a child who receives poor, inconsistent handling and has a "good" treatment program. Good handling includes the way a child is picked up, carried, and positioned into sitting, prone, supine, and sidelying. Handling is an important part of the child's everyday world. When handling the child, it is important to inhibit primitive and abnormal patterns. For many children, a flexed position is the most functional.

To pick a child up from a supine position, the therapist should gather him or her into flexion. To do this, the lifter slides one arm under the child's shoulders and upper back, making sure that the neck is supported in flexion on the lifter's arm and the child's arms are forward. At the same time, the lifter slides the other arm under the child's knees and flexes both the hips and knees. In this gathered-up position, the child is lifted comfortably. It is important to keep the child's head and arms forward and the knees higher than the hips.

If the lifter needs to have a free arm, the initial lifting process is started. Then the child is shifted to the side of the lifter that controls the child's legs. The child faces forward and the upper trunk is controlled against the lifter's chest and arm. The child's legs may be held at one or both knees. This allows the lifter to use one arm in interacting with the child. Older children and adults are lifted the same way, but two lifters may be needed.

If the child is carried facing out, it allows him or her to look at and interact with the world. To increase trunk rotation, one knee can be pulled up toward the opposite shoulder. If a child is prone, sidelying, or sitting, he or she is turned and lifted in the same gathered-up position.

When supine, the child with cerebral palsy usually needs a pillow under the head and shoulders to increase upper trunk flexion and to decrease muscle tone. Care is taken to ensure that the child brings the

arms together at the midline. If he or she cannot do this voluntarily, small rolled-up towels are placed next to the trunk and under the shoulders. If the child has increased stiffness in the legs, a roll is placed under the buttocks to increase trunk flexion. The knees should be positioned higher than the hips.

Sidelying places the child in a position where primitive and abnormal patterns have the least effect. The head, hips, and knees are flexed. The arms are free to come together at the midline. The trunk is slightly flexed. If the top leg is flexed forward over the bottom leg, it is easier to maintain the position. A pillow may be placed at the back and/or under the upper trunk and head. A "side lier" is commercially available. It simulates a corner and provides both support and straps that help maintain the child's position.

Feeding (Oral-Motor)

Normal Reflexes

Normal oral-motor behavior begins in prenatal development at approximately 7½ weeks, menstrual age. (Menstrual age refers to age of the fetus as measured by the time from the onset of the mother's last normal menstrual cycle.)[51] Tactile stimulation applied to the perioral area facilitates the first fetal oral reflex activity.[52]

Table 32-1 indicates fetal reflex activity of the face as a result of tactile stimulation applied to the area innervated by the trigeminal nerve, the fifth cranial nerve.[53] During the normal postnatal development, primitive oral reflexes can be observed in the newborn.

Table 32-1 *Fetal reflex activity of the face*

Response	Area stimulated	Menstrual age
Mouth opening	Lower lip	9½ weeks
Swallowing	Lips	10½ weeks
Momentary lip closure and, with repeated stimulation, swallowing	Lips (and/or tongue)	12½ weeks
Maintained lip closure	Lips	13 weeks
Protrusion of upper lip	Upper lip	17 weeks
Protrusion of lower lip	Lower lip	20 weeks
Protrusion and pursing of both lips simultaneously	Lips	22 weeks
Audible sucking	Lips	29 weeks

Based on data from papers of Hooker, cited in Jacobs, M. J.: Development of Normal Motor Behavior. Am. J. Phys. Med. 46:41–42, 1967.

ROOTING REFLEX. This reflexive response persists from birth to 3 to 4 months of age and can be seen in sleeping infants up to 7 months of age.[54] The turning of the head in the direction of tactile stimulation that is applied in a light stroking manner at the corner of the infant's mouth is characteristic of this reaction. Touching the upper lip elicits lip and tongue elevation accompanied by mouth opening and head extension. The opposite reaction occurs when the lower lip is stimulated. The lip and tongue depress, the mouth opens, and the head flexes.[55] These reactions are thought to be associated with the infant's search for the nipple of the mother's breast.[56] The reflexive response may diminish immediately after feeding; therefore, it is observed best when elicited in a hungry infant.[57] In the newborn, most responses to direct tactile input take the form of avoidance or protective withdrawal reactions (*i.e.*, the infant moves as far away from the input as possible). The rooting response is one of the first reactions of the neonate that enables him or her to pursue tactile input, thus allowing the infant to make contact with the external environment.

SUCK SWALLOW REFLEX. The normal duration of this primitive response is from the first or second day of life to 2 to 5 months of age.[58] Tactile stimulation applied to the infant's lips by the nipple of the mother's breast or bottle results in lip closure followed by a rhythmical movement of the tongue and jaw enabling the infant to obtain food. Usually three repetitive sucks followed by swallowing make up the rhythmical pattern.[59] Sucking action is performed by the elevation and applied pressure of the anterior aspect of the tongue against the nipple. This movement elicits the release of the liquid. Swallowing and transferring of the liquid to the back of the oral cavity is the function of the posterior aspect of the tongue.[60] Nonnutritive sucking can also be observed in the neonate. This is sucking action in the absence of food.

PROTECTIVE GAG REFLEX. This is an oral reflex normally present from birth that gradually becomes weaker when chewing occurs but does persist throughout life. Tactile input to the posterior aspect of tongue or soft palate will normally elicit a gag response. The gag response is thought to be hyperactive if it is facilitated in any other area of the oral cavity.[61]

BITE REFLEX. This reaction can normally be seen from birth. It gradually diminishes around 5 to 6 months when rotary chewing develops. A rhythmic opening and closing of the mouth is elicited by direct application of a tactile input to gums, teeth, or tongue.[62]

Normally, the infant's response to tactile stimulation in the oral area is very sensitive. From birth, the infant engages in hand-to-mouth activity.[63] By 6 months of age the total patterns of either complete flexion or extension are modified by combined patterns of flexion and extension enabling the infant to bring the feet to the mouth. Oral exploration of body parts is not only important for the development of body image but also helps to desensitize the low threshold to tactile input. Another important developmental milestone is the object to mouth exploration particularly dominant in children 6 to 7 months of age.[64] This not only teaches the child about the external environment, but it also decreases oral sensitivity. When finger feeding begins and various consistencies of food are introduced, the infant will be able to accept food and spoons without facilitating the primitive oral reflexes, particularly gagging.[65]

BABKIN REFLEX. This reflex is a normal neonatal response characterized by the opening of the infant's mouth when pressure is applied to the palm of the hand.[66]

MENTAL PALMAR REFLEX. This normal reflexive response is characterized by observable movements of the infant's chin, elicited by the light touching of the infant's palm.[67]

Normal and Abnormal Development

The feeding process includes all the components that are part of a normal feeding pattern, such as sucking, swallowing, biting, chewing, self-feeding, accepting food texture, and the many complicated and interrelated movements necessary to accomplish each one of these.

The individual with cerebral palsy may not be able to take food and/or liquids in the normal way or may not be able to feed himself or herself. He or she may have primitive and/or abnormal oral patterns resulting from high, low, or fluctuating muscle tone causing a lack of balance between the extensor and flexor muscles. Such a balance is needed to produce normal stable head, shoulder, and trunk control and it provides the basis for the development of the fine motor oral control necessary for eating. Many oral motor problems may be the result of or compensations for blocks in development causing abnormal oral characteristics.[68] Neck blocks may result in abnormal oral characteristics. There may be jaw thrust in which there is a strong downward extension of the lower jaw. The jaw may appear to be stuck open, and the child may have difficulty closing his or her mouth.[69] Jaw thrust may occur during any phase of the feeding process.

The individual who maintains a neck block may exhibit lip and cheek retraction in which there is a drawing back of the lips and cheeks so that they form a tight horizontal line over the mouth. This limits lip closure. The teeth usually show, and there is often a constant smile. The child may compensate by having a purse-string action of the lips and may try to counteract the basic tendency toward retraction by pursing or pulling the lips forward.[70]

Neck hyperextension and the pull of gravity may cause tongue retraction in which there is a strong pulling back of the tongue into the pharyngeal space. The tip of the tongue is not even with the gums or in approximation with the lower lip as it should be. It is often pulled back toward the middle of the hard palate and may be in firm approximation with the hard or soft palate. This makes it difficult to place a nipple, cup, or spoon in the child's mouth or to initiate a swallowing response. The airway may also be cut off by the tongue.

A tongue thrust may be a compensation for a neck block.[71] It may be defined as a forceful protrusion of the tongue from the mouth. It is frequently arrhythmic; its intermittent occurrence breaks a previously sustained rhythm.[72] The thrusting of the tongue may interfere with any phase of the feeding process. The individual may compensate for a neck block by having abnormally strong jaw closure. Such tight, involuntary closure of the jaw often makes opening the jaws difficult. This is related to excessive flexor tone throughout the body or to self-stimulation of a tonic bite reflex.[73]

A bite reflex is the rhythmic closing and opening of the jaws when the gums or teeth are stimulated. This may be in the form of an easy phasic bite with slight chewing motion during stimulation, or a strong tonic bite. In the tonic bite reflex, the jaw closes strongly and often does not open easily.

The cerebral palsied child may lack the ability to produce his or her own tactile stimulation. This may cause oral tactile hypersensitivity, which results in the child's resisting textured foods. It may also lead to a jaw thrust, tonic bite, lip and cheek retraction, lip purse, tongue thrust, and tongue retraction.

An individual with a neck block may further compensate by using strong shoulder elevation to help stabilize his or her head during oral activity. This may increase tightness throughout the chest, inhibiting the respiratory and feeding process.

Shoulder blocks may result in other abnormal oral characteristics and compensations. Scapulohumeral tightness may cause the use of elevated, internally rotated shoulders to stabilize the head. Shoulder elevation increases neck hyperextension, which may cause the many problems associated with a neck block. Tightness in the upper chest limits both res-

piration and the feeding process. Scapular adduction does not allow the hands to come together at the midline. This prevents the child from providing his or her own tactile oral desensitizing. Tension across the chest may limit respiration and the feeding process. Neck hyperextension may be increased, which may cause related oral problems.

The therapist may simulate each of the blocks and their oral consequences in order to experience personally a little of what the individual with cerebral palsy feels:

1. *Neck hyperextension:* Is it easy or hard to close the mouth? If the jaw opens too wide, is a jaw thrust possible? Is there tightness across the mouth that could cause lip retraction and a purse-string compensation? What has happened to the tongue? Is it retracted? What if food is placed in the mouth? Does it cause a tongue thrust? Is there a tendency to use tongue retraction and elevation to the hard palate to keep food out of the air passage? Does an attempt to bite cause an abnormally strong response? Have the shoulders elevated to maintain stability?

2. *Neck asymmetry:* How does it feel to swallow? Try to close the mouth. Is there jaw deviation? Does the jaw want to snap shut, retract, or thrust?

3. *Scapulohumeral tightness:* With the shoulders elevated, how does it feel to swallow and breathe? Is there a tendency for the neck to hyperextend?

4. *Scapular adduction:* With the shoulders adducted and externally rotated, how does it feel to swallow and breathe? Is there a tendency for the neck to hyperextend?

The therapist may further experience oral motor problems by having someone else feed him or her while in these primitive abnormal positions.

Using a problem-solving model based on the abnormal oral characteristics as compensations for blocks in development, the components essential for a successful remediation program are *stability* and *symmetry*.

Stability may be both internal and external as discussed under "Basic Components of Movement." Internal stability develops along a developmental continuum. An infant has a suckle pattern because of no jaw stability and a small oral cavity. A 2-year-old will bite on the rim of the cup because he or she does not have enough internal stability to hold the jaw steady as he or she drinks. A 3-year-old should have the internal jaw stability needed to hold the cup between the lips.

External stability is the additional control needed by, and/or given to, individuals who have not developed their own internal control. The child does this when biting on the cup rim. The therapist provides external stability until the child develops internal stability in oral as well as other motor skills.

There are two types of external stability that will be discussed. These are *positioning* and *jaw control*. To position a child for feeding, stability and symmetry are essential. There are different ways to position a child. Common to all are the following components:

1. head forward with the chin tucked or down,
2. head in the midline,
3. shoulders forward,
4. arms internally rotated,
5. hands in the lap,
6. trunk straight,
7. hips and knees flexed to at least 90°.

The infant or baby may be cradled in the feeder's arms in the above position. This encourages eye contact and communication with the feeder. If the feeder needs both hands free to assist the baby, he or she may sit tailor or Indian fashion and cradle the baby in his or her lap. The baby's head is at the feeder's knee. The shoulders may be brought forward and internally rotated by the feeder's legs. The baby's hips may be flexed at a 90° angle in the center of the lap.

A young child may sit on the feeder's lap. One of the feeder's arms may be used to control the child's neck and upper trunk while feeding with the other arm.

The baby may be placed in an infant or car seat that has been adapted. A "Feeder Seat" by Tumbleforms may be used for a child who needs the support of a larger infant seat. This may be placed in a beanbag chair, regular chair, or against the wall. It may be reclined or positioned vertically depending upon the needs of the child. A beanbag chair may be arranged to position a child functionally. It may need to be over corrected to allow for settling of the Styrofoam "beans." An inflatable infant bathtub called a "Tubby" may be used as a back support for the larger child in the beanbag chair. It centers the head and brings the arms forward. An adapted seating device such as a wheelchair or "care chair" may also be used for feeding. A high chair may be adapted to meet the above criteria.

The child may be placed supine on a firm inclined wedge placed on the feeder's lap and resting against a table edge. A very firm pillow may be used. The child faces the feeder. The hips and knees may be flexed and adducted with the feet resting on the feeder's abdomen, or else the hips may be abducted, with the legs straddling the feeder's hips.

Because mealtime is a time of direct communication, it is better to feed the child from the front. If this is not feasible, the therapist may feed the child from the side. The food should always enter the child's mouth at the midline. The side position may be necessary for certain types of jaw control. A child with excessive flexor tone may be fed in prone either on a wedge or bolster. He or she should be encouraged to lift his or her head to get the food. A severely involved child, who cannot be positioned in a seating device, may be fed in a sidelying position. A "Side Lier" by Tumbleforms may be used. The same basic criteria must be met.

It is often necessary to position the child functionally by adapting the child. To bring the head forward in a chin tuck in the midline, a rolled-up towel or small roll may be placed at the base of the skull. This must be high enough to elicit a chin tuck in which the neck is flexed. The chin must not jut forward and the neck must not hyperextend over the top of the roll. A conveniently shaped stuffed animal such as a stuffed snake may be used. This acts as a neck roll but also may go behind the shoulders to bring them forward. The neck may be brought forward by appropriate placement of the head against the feeder's elbow or knee. A small wedge or molded head piece may be placed on a wheelchair or "care chair." The occipital area of the skull should be avoided as pressure on this area causes hyperextension of the neck.

To position the shoulders forward with the arms internally rotated and the trunk straight, a rolled up towel may be placed on either side of the trunk and behind the shoulders. The thickness of the roll depends on the amount of internal rotation the child needs.

Before a child's hips and knees can be flexed to a 90° angle, the child must be positioned to sit on the buttocks or ischial tuberosities and not on the tailbone or sacrum. To do this, stand behind the child, grasp under the upper thigh, and roll the child's pelvis under and pull him or her back. A small roll may be placed under the knees to maintain the desired flexion.

The angle of feeding is important. The child should be as upright as possible but reclined enough to allow the child to keep the food in the mouth, chew it, and swallow it.

The very hypotonic child who will not stay positioned long enough to eat may need some additional help. If the arms are elevated, spinal extension will increase. This will help him or her stay in position and will also facilitate the entire feeding process by increasing general muscle tone. A towel or roll across the child's chest and under the arms will help to maintain the position. The child's arms may be placed over the edge of a high table. The feeder's arms may go across the chest to elevate the trunk. A child who seems to get "stuck" or who stops eating in the middle of a meal (and is not full) may be helped to resume the feeding process by elongating the trunk. He or she may be so tight that eating is no longer possible.

When functional positioning does not provide enough stability, jaw control may be necessary. The child may not have enough internal stability to control the jaw because of high or low muscle tone and/or persistent primitive, and/or abnormal, oral patterns. He or she may have jaw thrust, jaw retraction, jaw asymmetry, exaggerated opening or closing, poor lip closure, and/or tongue thrust.

There are two types of jaw control. One type uses two fingers and a front approach (see Fig. 32-3). The distal phalanx of the feeder's thumb is placed in the center of the child's chin at the base of the lower lip. Inward and upward pressure is applied to control jaw opening and closing. The feeder's index finger is placed under the child's chin at the base of the tongue to control jaw movement. The feeder's wrist may be placed on the upper chest to facilitate upper trunk flexion and chin tuck.

The second type of jaw control uses three fingers and a side approach. The feeder stands to the side or behind the child (see Fig. 32-4). The therapist's thumb is placed on the child's jaw line to control lateral jaw movements. The index finger is positioned on the child's chin. Inward and upward pressure is applied to control jaw and lip movements. The middle finger is placed under the chin to control jaw opening. This method allows for more external con-trol of chin tuck and neck elongation. The feeder's body against the child can be used for additional control.

Jaw control is not needed with every child. When it is used, the feeder must not get so caught up in controlling the jaw that he or she inadvertently puts a finger in the child's eye or ear. The child should not be held so tight that there is no independent jaw movement. He or she needs to move the jaw during the feeding process but at the same time to have enough stability to experience a more functional feeding pattern. This is especially important with infants who normally have an unstable jaw. The feeder should only give the child the amount of external stability necessary. Perhaps there is enough internal jaw control for the developmental level and only lip control is needed. The program must be geared to the individual's needs.

Some children may be too sensitive in the oral area to accept jaw control. Compromise between the feeder and child may be necessary. In the meantime, an oral desensitizing program may be initiated. With the hypersensitive child, it may be possible to gradually "sneak in" and give light jaw control at an important feeding phase. Jaw control is increased as tolerance develops.

Treatment

When planning a feeding program, the therapist should be aware of the difference between a feeding management program and a therapeutic feeding program. A management program involves getting food into the child and includes optimum positioning. A therapeutic feeding program emphasizes righting and balance responses as the basis for feeding development; the child has a more active role. A treatment program seeks to increase oral motor development, whereas a management program seeks to solve an immediate need. Both are important. The infant and young child may initially need both a management program and a therapeutic feeding program for development. The older child or adult may need a management program.

Using the developmental framework to analyze feeding activities is important. The anatomic size of the infant's oral area and the lack of stability greatly influence the ability to take foods. As the oral area grows, more tongue movement is possible. This necessitates more stability of the head, neck, and upper trunk for the finer oral skills of sucking, swallowing, biting, and chewing to develop. As textured foods are introduced, the child must use more refined feeding abilities.

SUCKING. Sucking is the rhythmic method of drawing soft food or drink into the mouth with a

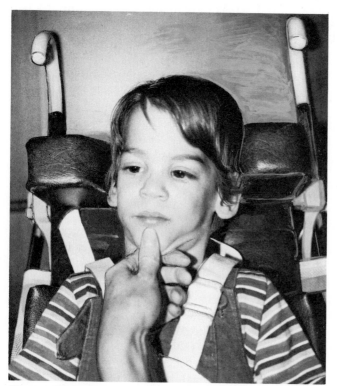

Figure 32-3. Jaw control: two fingers from the front.

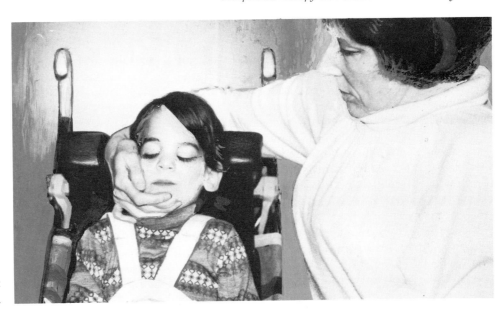

Figure 32-4. Jaw control: three fingers from the side.

negative pressure component. Tongue action is primarily up and down. Negative pressure builds up within the oral cavity because of firm approximation of the lips. This helps to pull soft food and liquid into the mouth.[74]

The early infantile method of sucking is called *suckling*. This involves a definite extension/retraction movement of the tongue. Liquid or soft food is obtained through a rhythmic licking action of the tongue combined with strong jaw opening and closing. There is frequently a rather loose approximation of the lips. The tongue does not protrude beyond the borders of the lips.[75] Tongue action in suckling should not be confused with the hard forceful protrusion of the tongue thrust.

An infant or child may have a weak or absent suck. It may be a medical necessity to tube-feed the infant to provide nourishment. A nasogastric (N/G) tube goes in one nostril and down to the stomach. The N/G tube may negate the child's gag response. This type of tube may be used for a temporary feeding problem.

Another type of feeding tube is the gastric tube, which goes through the abdominal wall directly into the stomach. This requires a surgical procedure called a gastrostomy. This is used with a child who has a long-standing feeding problem and who cannot take foods by mouth. A positive aspect of the gastric tube is that the child does not experience the negative oral input that he or she receives when an N/G tube is inserted or removed. An oral stimulation program may be used. The child is given some food by mouth, but the rest goes directly into the tube.

It is important for an individual to receive oral stimulation at the same time as he or she is tube-fed. The filling of the stomach should be associated with oral activity. If possible, he or she should be held while fed, to communicate with the feeder. This early communication is essential for bonding with the feeder and for later communication skills.

The normal infant increases the suckle pattern by moving the tongue within the small oral cavity. The only way that the tongue can move is in an extension/retraction pattern as it rubs against the hard palate. Since all treatment is based on normal development, the therapist facilitates a suckle by rhythmically stroking the hard palate with his or her finger pad. It is important to find the individual's own rhythm for all phases of sucking. This includes sucking from the bottle, cup, and spoon. Rhythmic stroking of the spoon on the lower lip may increase the strength of the suck. The faster the food moves from the front of the mouth in a controlled pattern, the less likely the child is to choke. Slow transit time may cause choking.

A child with poor oral control may aspirate food into the lungs. This may cause aspiration pneumonia. A child who gurgles in his or her throat may aspirate. Using the chin-tuck-head position should decrease this possibility. Feeding the child with the neck extended should be avoided, as this allows direct access from the oral cavity to the lungs. Giving oily liquids to children who may aspirate is not recommended. The body can absorb a water-based liquid, such as juices, more easily.

The infant or child with a poor suck needs many oral experiences. Because of blocks in development, the child may not have been able to put the hands in his or her mouth. The normal infant will first put the dorsum of his or her hand in the mouth. Later he or she will turn the wrist to put a fist in the mouth. A child with a poor suck needs to experience the same sequence. This also helps to desensitize the mouth. The therapist may put his or her hand in the child's mouth. The child should be introduced to a pacifier and small, textured toys to chew and suck on. A weak suck may be facilitated by helping the child move his or her lips and cheeks in a rhythmic pattern. This may be done with toys as well as with a bottle.

When working with a bottle-fed infant, the therapist may want to experiment with different types of nipples. A "preemie" nipple with a cross-cut hole often works well. This is a soft rubber nipple used with premature infants. Some come with a small cross-cut hole, which may be enlarged with small scissors. (Small suture or nail scissors work well.) The "x" cut lets the child control the flow of liquid. As he or she sucks or bites on the nipple, the liquid flows into the mouth. When he or she releases the nipple, the liquid stops flowing. This allows time for the child to process what is in the mouth. It may be necessary to assist the infant with jaw control and/or cheek facilitation. A nipple with an enlarged hole is not good. It will allow too much liquid to flow into the child's mouth. He or she may not be able to swallow so much, and could aspirate some of it.

If the child will suck on a pacifier but cannot or will not suck from a bottle or spoon, a pacifier may be used to elicit a suck and then be quickly exchanged for a bottle or spoon. When high muscle tone is present, a child may have a hard, nonproductive suck. The child's position should be evaluated. The neck may be hyperextended. Repositioning the child in flexion will facilitate a functional suck. Jaw control may be needed to control ungraded jaw movements and to provide stability.

SWALLOWING. Initially, swallowing is part of the suck–swallow or suckle–swallow pattern. The infant is dependent upon the suckle or suck to trigger a swallow. He or she gradually dissociates swallowing and can swallow whenever food is in the mouth. This necessitates movements of the tongue, lips, and cheeks that help to form a bolus from the food and to send it to the back of the mouth for the final swallow.[76]

A child may hold liquid or food in the mouth and may have a slow swallow. A quick, light touch between the child's upper lip and nose may facilitate a swallow. Some children will both suck and swallow slowly but automatically if they are given the time to do it. A feeder who is in too much of a hurry might not give a child enough time to suck and swallow. Gentle bouncing and rocking may provide vestibular stimulation, which might help the child to swallow. There are times when a child may need the help of gravity to swallow. He or she may need to be in a semireclined position with the chin tucked. As the child gains control of swallowing, he or she may be brought into a more upright position. Children should not be fed in a fully supine position.

It is easier to form a bolus for swallowing if the food is finely ground and a little dry. For this reason, textured foods should be used. Some children may scatter the food in their mouth and need liquids to either form a bolus from the food or wash it down.

A child with low muscle tone may keep the mouth open. This makes swallowing difficut. This individual responds well to a therapeutic feeding program that builds up muscle tone. He or she needs oral play. Quick stretching of the lips and cheek may increase muscle tone. Jaw control during feeding, with emphasis on lip closure, is important. Light, quick tapping of the lips will facilitate lip closure. The therapist must be cognizant that some children have to breathe through their mouths and will need to keep them open.

A child with lip retraction may not be able to close his or her lips to suck and/or swallow. The upper lip may appear to be very thin. The teeth and upper gums may be visible. Stretching the lip muscles may lower muscle tone and decrease lip retraction. While controlling the child's jaw and lips, the therapist places an index finger under the lip with the back of the finger to the teeth or gum. Then the finger is rolled out of the mouth, stretching the lip forward. This should be done to each quarter of the lip. Enough time should be allowed for the child to swallow after each stretch. This exercise may be done in preparation for feeding. An individual with lip retraction may also have a tonic bite reflex. The therapist needs to be cautious when placing a finger in the child's mouth. If the therapist is not quick enough and a child bites down on his or her finger, the child's jaws may be opened by flexing the child's head forward and opening the jaws with pressure on the outside, back part of the cheeks between the teeth.

BITING AND CHEWING. Biting and chewing are more voluntary aspects of feeding. Although they have their origins in early reflexive movement patterns that are triggered by stimulation of the gums and/or tooth receptors, they remain at a reflexive level for only a brief period. Munching is the earliest form of chewing. Munching seems to evolve from a combination of the tongue pattern seen in a true suck and the jaw pattern seen in a phasic bite reflex. It involves a flattening and spreading of the tongue combined with an up-and-down movement of the jaw. The jaws make a definite biting or chewing rhythm. The tongue does not move in a lateral direction, which would be necessary to transfer food to the teeth for real chewing. Munching remains a part of the adult chewing pattern and is observed when food is not being transferred.[77] The untrained person may confuse a primitive phasic bite reflex with munching and/or chewing.

Chewing is the process of using the teeth and/or tongue to break up and pulverize solid pieces of food in preparation for swallowing. The chewing pattern progresses from the primitive phasic bite-and-release pattern, to a nonstereotyped vertical movement, and then to the diagonal rotary jaw movements that occur as food is transferred to the side or middle of the mouth by the tongue. These movements continue to be refined until they become smooth and well-coordinated. They finally develop into the circular, rotary, jaw movements that occur as the child transfers food across the midline from one side of the mouth to another.[78] The development of gross motor extension and flexion, diagonal trunk patterns, and rotational trunk patterns needs to be well-established before fine oral movements occur. Placement of food between the child's teeth facilitates chewing.

The phasic bite-and-release pattern is the first, primitive form of biting to occur. Next, the child learns to quiet the jaw and develops a holding posture. Later, the child will be able to bite a soft object, like a soft cookie, in a sustained, controlled manner. Still later, the child will be able to bite a hard object, like a hard cookie, in a sustained manner but with excessive movement.[79] Finally the child develops a sustained, controlled bite with head in midline and appropriate grading of jaw movements. Using food with different textures facilitates biting. The child progresses from a soft cookie, to crisp food such as pretzels, to hard cookies. Lunch meat, hot dogs, and other soft meats may be introduced.

Oral hypersensitivity negatively influences the feeding process. The child may not accept anything into the mouth. He or she may refuse all lumps of food. There may be a history of not putting the hands or toys in the mouth. He or she may take objects to the lips without mouthing them. This child may have a very active gag reflex. The infant normally has a large gag-sensitive area. This may not yet have been integrated. The child may refuse to allow anyone to brush his or her teeth or wash his or her face. He or she may turn away when touched on the face. (There may be a difference between light and firm touch. Light touch is less acceptable than firm touch.) A dislike of being held and/or rocked may go with the whole syndrome.

The therapist should give the child firm tactile input to the trunk and then progress up to the arms and mouth. When this is tolerated, the child needs oral play around and inside the mouth similar to that discussed under *Sucking*. The firm tactile input provided by swaddling and close-fitting knitted clothing may be helpful. After a bath, a brisk rubdown with a towel will provide input. The child needs to feel and experience many different textures and sensations on the body. The same progression of hands in his or her mouth working up to toys discussed under *Sucking* may be done. Flavors may be added to hands or toys.

Oral digital stimulation may be done after the child tolerates having his or her face touched. At first, the lips are touched and rubbed. Then he or she is touched and rubbed between the lips. When the child allows the therapist to put his or her finger in the child's mouth, the gums may be rubbed. One quarter of the mouth is done at a time. Starting at the back of the mouth, the finger makes small, firm circular movements. It is brought forward and out of the mouth at the midline. While maintaining external jaw and lip control, the therapist must wait for the child to swallow. Each quadrant is done in the same way. The inside of the gum ridge and cheeks may also be rubbed. The child should not be forced to accept the stimulation. If he or she resists, the child is saying that it is aversive. It is necessary to find compromise between the child's immediate needs and the therapeutic program.

A child who will not accept textured foods may gag and/or spit out the smallest lump. It is best to process table foods in a blender and gradually add thickening such as instant potato, baby cereal, or bran. Work up to fork-mashed foods. The child may find softer foods such as pasta more acceptable.

Some children may be hyporesponsive to oral stimulation. They may lack sensory awareness in the oral area. They need a sensory program similar to that needed by the hypersensitive child. The therapist should be aware that a child may have been so sensitive in the mouth that he or she needed to "shut down" his or her sensory system to survive. This defense mechanism may make him or her appear unresponsive.

Some children may gag and/or vomit frequently. Physical problems must first be ruled out. A common cause of vomiting is called esophageal reflux. The esophagus does not close off sufficiently to hold food in the stomach. Food or gastric juices flow back into the esophagus and may be vomited. Reflux is common in the infant who "spits" or vomits small amounts of food. Reflux can be surgically corrected. If the child might have this condition, he or she should be kept sitting for at least 3 minutes after he or she is fed to allow gravity to help keep the food down. The child who vomits may be a "ruminator." Ruminators stimulate themselves by bringing up partially digested food that they may spit out or reswallow. A developmental psychologist is needed to help formulate a behavior-oriented program.

There are several ways to interrupt gagging. The

child's head needs to be flexed forward. Rapid tapping under the chin at the base of the tongue and lips may reduce the muscle tone that has built up. The therapist must move quickly, cover the child's mouth, and move out of the "line of fire."

Drooling often occurs in individuals with cerebral palsy. Drooling may be mild to severe. Remediation is directly related to the development of upper trunk and head control. This is the foundation on which to build the sucking and swallowing components of oral movements. Lip and jaw closure are especially important.

Food Intake

Until the child develops sufficient oral control, he or she should be fed. Self-feeding may cause associated abnormal reflexive movements in the oral area and in other areas of the body. Before one feeds a child, it is best to prepare the child as one does before a treatment session. Hopefully this will help him or her to use innate abilities optimally. Symmetrical, stable, functional positioning is necessary.

A small, flat spoon is often easier for the child to accept. A small amount of food is placed on the end of the spoon. The spoon is presented to encourage chin tuck and midline orientation of the head. It should be placed about one third of the way back on the tongue with slight downward pressure. Time should be allowed for the lips to close on the spoon and for the sucking process to begin. Jaw and lip control may be needed. The child should use his or her lips to clean the spoon. The food should not be scraped on the upper teeth as this may cause a tongue thrust and/or extension–retraction suckle pattern. To facilitate the use of both lips, the spoon may be withdrawn from the child's mouth using a slightly upward diagonal pattern. Sufficient time must be allowed for swallowing.

If chewing or increased lateral tongue movements are treatment goals, the food should be placed on the side of the child's tongue or between the teeth. Placement should facilitate the forming of a bolus for swallowing.

If more lip closure is needed, more food may be placed in the child's mouth. He or she may continue to chew with the mouth open but might close it to swallow so as to keep the food in the mouth.

Spoon-feeding may require compromises between the child and the feeder. A child with a tonic bite may need quick movement of the spoon in and out of the mouth to prevent a bite reflex. The child's teeth and gums should be avoided, as touching them could stimulate the reflex.

Most children are able to drink from a cup, even when they cannot drink from a bottle. It is essential

that the child controls the amount of liquid that flows into the mouth. A cut-out cup works well. This is a soft plastic or paper cup that has been cut out on one side to accommodate the nose and to allow the feeder to closely monitor the child's drinking. Place the uncut edge of the cup on the child's lower lip and allow some liquid to flow to the lip. Wait for him or her to initiate a suck. Although he or she may be slow to start the process, the child may have the ability to do it. Liquids should not be poured into the child's mouth as this makes it harder for the child to suck and swallow. If the child does not have the ability to initiate a suck, it may be necessary to pour a small amount of liquid into his or her mouth. Jaw and lip control may be necessary throughout the drinking sequence. It should be maintained until swallowing is completed. He or she may need to swallow several times for every mouthful. If the child swallows immediately, the feeder may leave the cup in place for several suck-swallow sequences before giving the child a short break to breathe. Symmetrical, stable, and functional positioning is necessary. The feeder must not let the child's head tip back because this increases the possibility of aspiration. Downward pressure on the sternum or breastbone will help induce chin tuck.

If the feeding program is not working the way the therapist wishes, he or she should re-evaluate all areas of it. More preparation may be needed. The key areas of positioning should be reassessed. Is the child compensating with poor patterns? Are there too many distractions? Does he or she dislike the food?

The type of food used influences the feeding process. Thin liquids can be difficult to handle. Fruit nectars and juices thickened with fruit sauce might be easier to suck and swallow. Powdered instant breakfasts, powdered milk, and baby cereal may be used to thicken liquids and to add nourishment to the diet.

Commercial baby foods are not recommended. It is cheaper and usually more appetizing to puree, grind, mash, or chop table food. This also lets the child acquire the taste preferences of the rest of the family. Pureed foods are often more difficult to handle than finely ground foods, which tend to become liquid and may be drooled back.

Milk may increase the thickness of mucus. A nondairy formula may be better for a baby who has difficulty handling secretions. Oily fluids such as beef and chicken broth may help to thin mucus, but they should be used with caution with children who aspirate. As was previously mentioned, oily liquids are slower to be absorbed into the system if they get into a child's lungs.

Beef and pork may be difficult to chew. Softer meats, such as hot dogs, lunch meats, veal, lamb, and chicken, are easier. Chicken and turkey roll are especially good. They are soft and easy to finger-feed. Cheese and boneless fish are usually even softer. Foods combining several textures may be difficult for a child to process. These include soups with vegetables and noodles and vegetables with skins, such as corn, lima beans, and peas. They are soft inside but have a firm outer covering. Finger foods include the softer meats that have been cubed, rolled, or stripped. Vegetables, such as carrots, beets, potatoes, and green beans, may be cut and cooked in a shape that is easily finger-fed.

If the child is having difficulty forming a bolus to swallow, gummy, cakey foods should be kept to a minimum. Tepid foods are more readily accepted than hot or cold foods. This is especially true of the child with hypersensitivity in the oral area.

Self-Feeding

When the child has integrated primitive oral patterns and/or developed sufficient oral control, self-feeding may be initiated. A child may be motivated but may continue to have oral motor problems. It may be necessary to make a compromise between the child's goal of self-feeding and the therapist's goal of developing better oral control.

Self-feeding may be started at snack time with the introduction of finger foods. The child must be in a symmetrical, stable, functional position at a table or in a high chair. The child's feet should also be supported. The same principles apply to self-feeding that apply to feeding in general.

A preparation period before feeding will increase the child's ability to eat. Self-feeding skills may develop parallel to fine motor skills. The foods offered should be appropriate for the child's type of grasp. If a child has a palmar grasp, rolled lunch meat or a slivered hot dog might be good. If he or she has a fine pincer grasp, raisins or Cheerios might be good. He or she may need to compensate and/or stabilize himself or herself by leaning on the elbows. A higher table can help stabilize the child's upper trunk.

Spoon-feeding will progress as with the normal child. A regular spoon should be tried first. If the child lacks the supination needed to place the spoon in the mouth, a spoon can be bent to accommodate his or her needs by twisting the bowl down. A few children may need a built-up spoon handle. The use of a swivel spoon, in which the bowl moves to remain level, is less common. A drawback of a swivel spoon is the fact that it may continue to move as it nears the mouth. This makes it difficult for the child to place the spoon in the mouth. If the child cannot scoop with a spoon, stabbing the food with a fork may be more functional.

The less special equipment used, the better. A lip on the child's plate may keep the food from slipping off. Scoop dishes that have a built-up side to assist with filling a utensil are available. They usually have a nonskid bottom that stabilizes them. A commercial product called "Dycem" is an excellent nonskid material to place under a plate. A flat, wet washcloth placed under a dish will provide some resistance to sliding. A small plastic cup without handles is the most functional for a child's use because it provides a larger surface to hold on to. Handled cups tend to reinforce scapular adduction and to increase muscle tone. Covered cups are often just a step up from a bottle. Straw-drinking seems to reinforce neck hypertension; as the liquid is sucked up a straw, the individual tends to go into hyperextension. Straw-drinking should be used with caution and carefully evaluated.

Dressing

The acquisition of dressing and undressing skills by the child with cerebral palsy should follow the same sequence as for the normal child (Table 32-2).

Initially it is necessary to encourage a child to develop an interest in dressing and undressing. But as the child's abilities increase and he or she becomes developmentally ready, cooperation should increase.

A normal child is most commonly dressed while in the supine position. This position may make a cerebral palsied child more rigid and will unecessarily complicate the dressing process. Laying the small

Table 32-2 *Acquisition of Dressing and Undressing Skills*

Age	Skill
12 mo.	cooperates with dressing, i.e., extends arms to put in sleeve
18 mo.	purposefully removes socks
2 yr.	removes unlaced shoes
	removes pants with assistance over hips
3 yr.	removes clothes completely except for small buttons and back fastenings
	unfastens medium-sized buttons
	puts on underpants, socks, and shoes
4 yr.	fastens large buttons
	laces shoes
5 yr.	fastens medium-sized buttons
	dresses self except for bows and small buttons
6 yr.	ties bows

Adapted from Finnie, N.: Handling the Young Cerebral Palsied Child at Home, ed. 2. New York, E. P. Dutton & Co., 1975.

child across the therapist's knees or lap, prone with arms and legs extended, makes dressing much easier. The child's extremities can easily be manipulated into clothing, and the whole child is in a therapeutically functional position.

The best way of dressing a child is to sit the child between the therapist's legs with the child leaning forward at the hips, with legs abducted and knees flexed. This decreases extensor tone. One should describe and name each article of clothing as it is used and each part of the body as it is moved. At first it may help to work in front of a mirror so that the child can see what is happening. When the child begins to assist the therapist, the mirror should be removed as the reversed mirror image may be confusing.

For the child, adolescent, and adult dominated by flexor or extensor tone, the sidelying position seems to neutralize excess tone and facilitates the dressing process. When rolling an individual from side to side, the knees and hips should remain flexed to inhibit extensor tone.

If the person must be supine, a hard pillow should be placed under the head and shoulders to break up the extensor tonus. Knees and hips should be flexed and abducted.

Whichever position is used for dressing the child, it should be symmetrical. Note the following suggestions:
1. Put the more affected limb in clothing first.
2. Straighten the arm before putting it in a sleeve.
3. Hold the arm at the elbow or above to move it. If resistance is felt, do not attempt to pull the arm through a sleeve by pulling on the hand. This causes the whole arm to flex and the shoulder to retract.
4. Before putting on shoes or socks, the leg should be flexed.

If the child wears braces, remove them by unfastening them at the most proximal point and work distally toward the feet. When putting braces on, be sure that the child's heel is placed firmly down into the shoe before lacing and securely tying the bow. Continue to work from distal to proximal. Two adult fingers should fit under each closure for a comfortable fit.

According to Finnie,[80] a child should be ready to undress when he or she knows body parts, is aware of self in space, and can name or recognize clothes.

Some children can dress while sitting in a sturdy low chair. If the child does not have enough balance to lean forward when sitting, several alternatives may be used. The child may sit between the therapist's legs for support. A triangular chair may be used either on the floor (Fig. 32-5) or raised on a platform

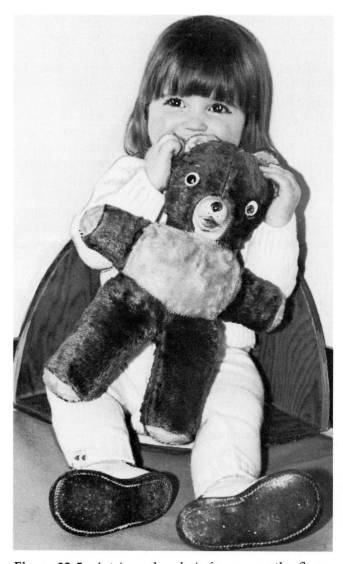

Figure 32-5. A triangular chair for use on the floor.

A corner or wall may provide additional support (Fig. 32-6).

An older and more severely involved child may not be able to sit. If head control has been attained, he or she may be able to dress and undress from a side lying, prone, or supine position. A simple pants pusher or pants puller is often needed.

While sitting with hips and knees bent, the child may remove socks by pulling on the toe end of the sock or by sliding a thumb down the back of the leg and over the heel. The sock may also be rubbed off the toes either by using the other foot or against the floor. It is helpful to avoid stretch and elastic socks. Tube socks are easier to put on than those with a heel.

In order to put on socks the child should have knees and hips bent. The sock is opened with two hands and the child is encouraged to make a "big

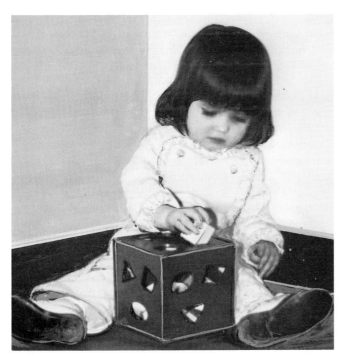

Figure 32-6. A corner may provide additional sitting support.

mouth with the opening" in order to put all toes in at one time. Some children will try to put the sock on the big toe first and will try to stretch it across to the little toe. This often leaves the little toes out of the sock or pops the sock off the foot. In this case it helps to start with the little toe and stretch the sock over the big toe.

Removing underpants or trousers may be done while sitting or lying down. The child shifts his or her weight to push them over the hips and down the legs. To put underpants or trousers on, the child is flexed at knees and hips. After feet are in the correct holes, the child may stand up, kneel stand, or roll from side to side to pull them up.

Unlaced shoes may be kicked or rubbed off. Two colored laces may be used to encourage unlacing. When first putting shoes on the feet, the laces should be very loose. A flexed and abducted leg is necessary. High-top shoes are easier to put on if loops are sewn on at the tops. These keep the back of the shoe from being crushed. Tying bows can be a difficult process to learn. When the child is ready for tying, the same words of instruction should be employed during each teaching session.

Many children seem to benefit from the "backward-chaining" method of instruction. The therapist ties the bow up to the last step and then asks the child to complete the process. As each step is mastered, the child continues working backwards

until the entire process has been completed. It is important to follow the same process with each article of clothing.

Taking off pullover and front-opening shirts can be done in several ways. The usual way is to cross one's arms, grasp either side of the bottom, and pull the shirt up and over the head. One or both hands can be used to grasp the collar. Children usually pull their nondominant arm out of the sleeve first. The dominant side sleeve is either shaken or pulled off by the other hand. Some children prefer to remove both arms from the sleeves, then pull the shirt off and over their heads. Another way to take off a shirt is to remove the nondominant arm from the sleeve and to pull the shirt over the head and off the opposite arm. Most methods can be used while lying supine or prone.

The process is reversed when a child puts a shirt on. The child's arms are put in first and then the shirt is pulled over the head, or vice versa. The more involved side goes in first, and the dominant arm in last. The "duck-the-head" method is helpful in putting on a front opening shirt or coat. The garment is positioned with the collar near the child, label side up. The arms are placed in the sleeves and the whole shirt is tossed over the head.

Buttoning and unbuttoning should be learned on the child's own clothing or on a button vest (Fig. 32-7). (Buttonboards are nonfunctional since they put the buttons in a position not related to the child's body.)

Few clothing adaptations are necessary for individuals with cerebral palsy. Clothing should be loose fitting to facilitate putting on and removing. Velcro closures can be used if an individual's coordination is too poor for handling buttons, zippers, or snaps. Sometimes a buttonhook is helpful, and the addition of a large loop to a zipper may prove advantageous. Adolescents may need pants pushers or pullers. Trousers with elastic tops alleviate waist closure problems.

When older children are referred to occupational

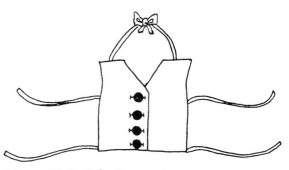

Figure 32-7. A button vest.

therapy for treatment, the area of dressing is often something they need to learn. It often seems easier for a parent to dress a child than to take the time to teach the child how to do it. This may happen because parents have not been included in their children's treatment programs and do not know how to help. This exemplifies how essential it is for the occupational therapist to work with the parents in the early stages of treatment and to continue to do so throughout the entire treatment process. Occupational therapists may find that they have "itchy" hands, and that it is hard not to assist children as they slowly struggle to dress themselves. However, it is worthwhile to be patient. Children feel a special pride when they master a task. The first time a severely involved adolescent can say, "I don't have to wait for someone to dress me. I can do it myself" is an especially proud moment.

Chair Adaptations

The basic principles of positioning and handling also apply to chair positioning. The child sits with the trunk straight, hips and knees flexed to beyond 90°, with the legs abducted. The ankles are at 90°, and the feet are supported. The child's elbows rest comfortably on arm rests or lapboard.

Adapting chairs is a highly individualized process. The occupational therapist should be aware of the many aspects of the individual's needs in order to problem solve with the child and family to determine which adaptations are most suitable.

There are many seating devices available. A sturdy infant seat or car seat may be appropriate for a baby. A small child may use a regular stroller with or without adaptations. Specially designed inserts for strollers are available if needed (Fig. 32-8). An older child or small adult may need a large stroller called a "Pogon buggy" with a specially designed insert. A "care chair" or "travel chair" may meet the needs of the child and his or her family. It has several positions that range from reclined to upright at table height. It folds to attach to a car seat and is used for safe transportation.

A wheelchair may be appropriate for some individuals. The same adaptations used in the stroller insert (Fig. 32-8) may apply to provide proper fit in a wheelchair. Solid seat and back inserts keep the trunk straight and the shoulders forward. To increase trunk symmetry and midline orientation, long, foam-padded wedges are added to the solid back. They are placed laterally and extend from under the arm to the waist or hip, fitting closely against the trunk.

The depth of the seat should come to an inch or two behind the child's knees to provide normal flexion. A pillow may be placed behind the child to push

him or her forward to achieve this position. The seat upholstery may be removed and a specially made insert put in its place. This insert should be made to the child's dimensions and be of the proper depth to provide flexion for the knees. A firm wedge-shaped seat that is higher in the front than in the back may be used to increase hip flexion.

To inhibit adduction of the legs, a molded seat insert may be made to fit the child. This insert places the pelvis in a neutral position, the hips in flexion, and the legs in abduction. It may have a built-in wedge shape. The back may incorporate lateral support wedges for the trunk. An individual with low muscle tone and excessive abduction may use a molded seat insert to provide more adduction of the hips and trunk control. A foot rest can be positioned so that the knees are slightly higher than the hips to decrease extensor tone. The entire sole of the foot should be supported to prevent extension (see Fig. 32-8).

A "U" shaped head support is used for the child unable to hold his head up and in the midline. It is angled so that the center of the "U" is at the base of the skull. This elongates the neck extensor muscles. The side projections of the "U" are angled under the child's ears. This facilitates chin tuck as well as midline orientation.

A lapboard may be used to provide the individual with a stable surface on which to eat, play, and work (Fig. 32-9). It is positioned at elbow height for comfort and to assist external stability. For the baby and young child, a toy bar may be added. Objects may be hung directly in front of the child at a height which is easily accessible. The toys are always available to encourage reaching into space at the appropriate level for shoulder and back extension and eye–hand coordination. The visually handicapped child will always have toys near him.

High chairs, commode or potty chairs, and other devices may be adapted using the same basic ideas.

A triangular chair provides good support for the individual with cerebral palsy. It rests on the floor, giving the child support while allowing him or her to experience the normal developmental activity of playing on the floor (Fig. 32-5). The back of the chair comes to the child's shoulders to provide lateral and back support. The child's knees come to the edge of the seat to allow slight flexion while long sitting. The child is also able to circle sit in a triangular chair. Abductor wedges may be placed on the seat to inhibit adduction. A triangular chair may also be raised on a platform and fitted with a small table. This gives back, side, and frontal support. The child's elbows rest comfortably on the table. One can sit in the chair to eat, play, or even complete schoolwork.

Seating adaptions and devices are used to aug-

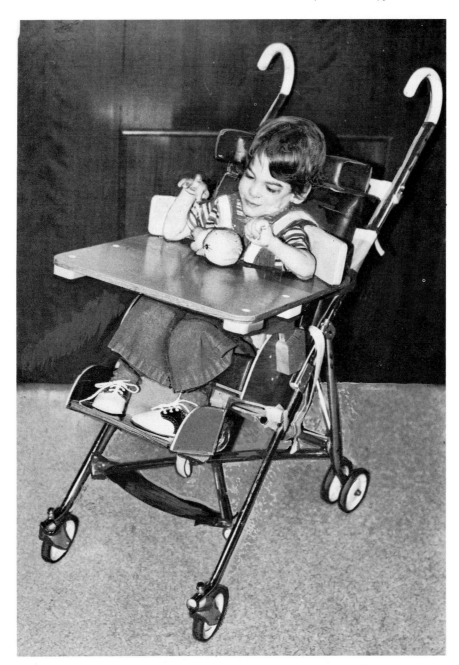

Figure 32-8. A stroller adapted with a specially designed inset.

ment development and treatment. They are modified to meet the needs of a changing child. The low-tone child may easily conform to the shape of a seat.

Some occupational therapists build all the adaptions for their patients. Others may be part of a seating team in which someone else constructs the equipment. The decision-making process involved in selecting seating adaptations requires a team effort.

Communication

The basic human need to communicate one's joys, sorrows, needs, ideas, frustrations, anxieties, and sense of belonging may be thwarted in the cerebral palsied individual because he or she is unable to express himself or herself through the spoken word. The individual may be intelligent but too severely involved physically to talk or to control the head, trunk, and upper extremities. Oral control may be insufficient for speech. The occupational therapist, together with the speech therapist, can provide a means of nonverbal communication.

In the early stages of treating and handling the young infant, communication between mother and infant is stressed just as it is with the normal child. Because of the added special needs of the infant with

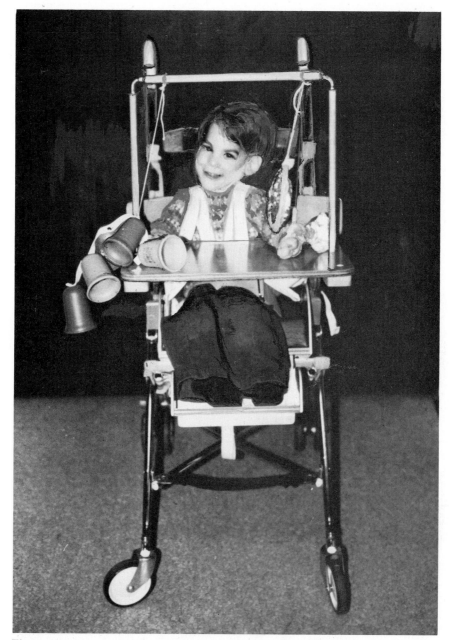

Figure 32-9. A lapboard and toy bar with suspended toys for ready access.

cerebral palsy, early communication skills are often overlooked. These skills usually begin with face-to-face contact between mother and infant. In order to gain and hold the infant's attention, good external control of the child's head and shoulders is necessary.

The occupational therapist should be sensitive to the subtle nonverbal messages that a child may give. Increased muscle tone may mean the child is upset, excited, hurt, needs the bathroom, or wants attention. Darkness under the eyes may mean the child has a headache. Excessive drooling may mean the child is under emotional stress. Closing the eyes may mean the child is retreating from the environment.

For older children who still have not developed

speech, alternate means of language expression are utilized. The simplest form of communication is indicating "yes" or "no" or by moving a body part. This may be done by blinking the eyes, looking up, moving an arm or leg, or turning the head. Some intelligent children have learned to blink the Morse code in order to communicate.

The next level of communication for the nonverbal child may be the use of a language board or book. This may be a lapboard secured to a wheelchair or a book or card that is carried. A language board is covered with either plexiglass or a clear plastic material to protect it from drooling and everyday wear and tear. The child points to the board using fist, finger, elbow, eyes, paper straw, or headstick. A headstick may be fastened to a headband that is attached to the child's forehead.

Several types of boards are possible. A ring board has plexiglass rings ⅝ inch to ½ inch thick. These are glued to the top of a plexiglass board. Used to reduce involuntary movements, the rings can be large in diameter and spaced far apart or they can be small in diameter and spaced close together. The written insert is attached under the board. The writing shows through the rings.

A ring board adapted for a headstick has smaller rings about ¾ inch in diameter. These may be arranged like a typewriter keyboard or in a list form with phrases. The child points to the message with a headstick.

Flat boards may list important words and phrases. The child points to the words or phrases in the appropriate column to convey the message.

A more sophisticated form of language board utilizes number and color coding of the words. Colors and numbers are spaced along the edges of the board. In the center, a color- and number-coded grid has many words or phrases on it. The nonverbal child uses his or her eyes to point to an appropriate color first and then to a number. This locates a word on the grid to relay a message. Either whole sentences, phrases, or individual words may be placed on the grid.

It is important that the material is positioned within the child's functional area of movement. Correct positioning maintains body symmetry and will not facilitate abnormal postural reflexes.

The language board changes as the child's abilities develop. The first board may have objects on it such as a toy toilet and small cup. The next board may have pictures on it. These may come from magazines, familiar photographs, or simple drawings. Pictures may depict needs such as the toilet, drink, food, bed, television, Mother, Father, places to go. As the child's reading skills develop, words replace pictures. Eventually, words may be arranged by parts of speech and increase in complexity. For some nonverbal individuals, an alphabet card and pointer may be sufficient to meet their communication needs. The letters may be arranged alphabetically or as on a typewriter keyboard.

Electronic aids are now available for the nonverbal individual. Three basic approaches with these aids are scanning, encoding, and direct selection. Scanning generally refers to the placing of appropriate phrases, letters, or symbols in a line or a grid configuration. The individual then controls a system that goes through each step until the desired message is completed. Encoding refers to a more complex system of controls in which a particular pattern of numbers or letters is used to relay a message. Usually

there is a series of activating switches. Direct selection refers to communication by direct input. An example would be a small calculator type device that allows the individual to spell a word or message on the keyboard. This is then displayed on the device.

Communication aids can be controlled using many different switches. A rocking lever may be activated by gross hand or arm movement or by a mouth- or headstick. A tongue switch may be activated by the tongue or lips. A pneumatic switch is activated by either blowing or sucking. A rocking level may be adapted to a chin switch. An arm slot control holds the arm on a desired switch without activating other ones. Some devices are activated by a beam of light.

References

1. Samilson, R. L. (ed.): Orthopaedic Aspects of Cerebral Palsy. Clin. Develop. Med., Nos. 52/53. London: William Heinemann, 1975, p. 1.
2. Ibid., p. 3.
3. Ibid.
4. Bobath, K.: The Motor Deficit in Patients with Cerebral Palsy. Clin. Develop. Med., No. 23. London: William Heinemann, 1975, preface.
5. Ibid.
6. Bobath, K., and Bobath, B.: Cerebral palsy. In Pearson, P. H. (ed.): Physical Therapy Services in the Developmental Disabilities. Springfield, IL: Charles C. Thomas, 1972, p. 31.
7. Gordon, N.: Pediatric Neurology for the Clinician. Clin. Develop. Med., Nos. 59/60. London: William Heinemann, 1976, p. 134.
8. Bobath and Bobath: Cerebral palsy, p. 33.
9. Berzins, G. F.: Causes of cerebral palsy. Mimeographed handout, 1972.
10. Ibid.
11. Ibid.
12. Gordon: Pediatric Neurology.
13. Mohr, J.: Basic neurodevelopmental treatment course. Unpublished class notes, 1978.
14. Bly, L.: Neurodevelopmental treatment baby course. Unpublished class notes, 1980.
15. Ibid.
16. Ibid.
17. Ibid.
18. Ibid.
19. Ibid.
20. Mohr: Unpublished class notes.
21. Bly, L.: Normal motor development: The first twelve months. Mimeo. 1980.
22. Mohr: Unpublished class notes.
23. Bly: Normal motor development: The first twelve months.
24. Ibid.
25. Ibid.
26. Mohr: Unpublished class notes.

27. Bly: Normal motor development: The first twelve months.
28. Ibid.
29. Mohr: Unpublished class notes.
30. Bly, L.: Abnormal motor development: Blocks. Mimeo., 1980. All references in this section are to this source.
31. Samilson: Orthopaedic Aspects, p. 7.
32. Bobath and Bobath: Cerebral palsy, p. 35.
33. Bobath and Bobath: Cerebral palsy, p. 36.
34. Samilson: Orthopaedic Aspects, p. 8.
35. Bobath and Bobath: Cerebral palsy, p. 37.
36. Samilson: Orthopaedic Aspects, p. 8.
37. Ibid.
38. Gordon: Pediatric Neurology, p. 145.
39. Ibid., p. 8.
40. Ibid., p. 145.
41. Bobath and Bobath: Cerebral palsy, p. 36.
42. Rogers, S., D'Eugenio D.: Developmental Programming for Infants and Young Children: Assessment and Application, ed 2. Ann Arbor: University of Michigan Press, 1981, vol. 2.
43. Ibid., vol. 5.
44. Frankenburg, W. K., and Dodds, J. B.: Denver Developmental Screening Test, rev. ed. Denver: La Doca Foundation, 1981.
45. Bayley, N.: Bayley Scales of Infant Development. New York: Psychological Corp., 1969.
46. Morris, S. E.: Pre-Speech Assessment Scale: A Rating Scale for the Measurement of Prespeech Behaviors from Birth through Two Years, experimental ed. Milwaukee: Curative Rehab. Center, 1980.
47. Nihira, K., Foster, R., Shellhaas, M., and Leland, H. American Academy of Mental Deficiency Adaptive Behavior Scale, rev. ed. Washington: Am. Acad. of Mental Def., 1974.
48. Mohr: Unpublished class notes.
49. Ibid.
50. Ibid.
51. Shepard, T., and Smith, D.: Prenatal life. In Smith, D., and Marshal, R. (eds.): Introduction to Clinical Pediatrics. Philadelphia: W. B. Saunders, 1972.
52. Jacobs, M. J.: Development of Normal Motor Behavior. Am. J. Phys. Med. 46: 41–42, 1967.
53. Ibid.
54. Fiorentino, M. R.: Normal and Abnormal Development. The Influences of Primitive Reflexes on Motor Development, p. 10. Springfield, IL: Charles C Thomas, 1972.
55. Jacobs: Development of Normal Motor Behavior, p. 47.
56. Colangelo, C., Bergen, A., and Gottlieb, L.: A Normal Baby: The Sensory-Motor Processes of the First Year. Valhalla NY: Blythedale Children's Hospital, 1976, p. 5.
57. Ibid.
58. Mueller, H.: Facilitating feeding and pre-speech. In Pearson, P. H. (ed.): Springfield IL: Charles C. Thomas, 1972, p. 287.
59. Davis, L.: Pre-speech development. In Connor, F., Williamson, G., and Siepp, J. (eds.): A Program Guide for Infants and Toddlers with Neuromotor and Other Developmental Disabilities. New York: Teachers' College Press, 1976, p. 211.
60. Colangelo, Bergen, and Gottlieb: A Normal Baby, p. 5.
61. Mueller: Facilitating feeding and pre-speech, p. 287.
62. Davis: Pre-speech development, pp. 211–212.
63. Brazelton, T. B.: Neonatal Behavior Assessment Scale. Clin. Develop. Med., No. 50. Philadelphia: J. B. Lippincott, 1976, p. 41.
64. Gesell, A., et al.: The First Five Years of Life. New York: Harper & Row, 1940, p. 23.
65. Davis: Pre-speech development, pp. 211–212.
66. Jacobs: Development of Normal Motor Behavior, p. 47.
67. Colangelo, Bergen, and Gottlieb: A Normal Baby, p. 7.
68. Alexander, R.: Neurodevelopmental Treatment Baby Course. Unpublished class notes, 1980.
69. Morris: PreSpeech Assessment Scale.
70. Ibid.
71. Alexander: Unpublished class notes.
72. Morris: Pre-Speech Assessment Scale.
73. Ibid.
74. Ibid.
75. Ibid.
76. Ibid.
77. Ibid.
78. Ibid.
79. Ibid.
80. Finnie, N.: Handling the Young Cerebral Palsied Child at Home, ed 2. New York, E. P. Dutton & Co., 1975.

Bibliography

Ackerman, N.: Early Identification and Intervention Programs for Infants with Developmental Delay and Their Families: A Summary and Directory. National Easter Seal Society for Crippled Children and Adults, Chicago, 1973.

Ambrose, J. A. (ed.): Stimulation in Early Infancy. London: Academic Press, 1969.

Andrews, B., et al.: Cerebral palsy: My baby is slow. Patient Care 21 (1972).

Ayres, A. J.: Sensory Integration and Learning Disorders. Los Angeles: Western Psychological Services, 1972.

Banus, B.: The Developmental Therapist, ed 2. Thorofare NJ: Charles B. Slack, 1979.

Battle, C. U.: Disruptions in the socialization of the handicapped child. Rehabil. Lit. 35 (1974).

Beintema, D. J.: A Neurological Study of Newborn Infants. Clin. Develop. Med., No. 28. London: William Heinemann, 1968.

Bergen, A.: Selected Equipment for Pediatric Rehabilitation. Valhalla NY: Blythedale Children's Hospital, 1974.

Bobath, B.: Abnormal Postural Reflex Activity Caused by Brain Lesions, ed. 2. Clin. Develop. Med. London: William Heinemann, 1971.

Bobath, B.: Motor development, its effect on general development, and application to the treatment of cerebral palsy. Physiotherapy 57:526–531, 1971.

Bobath, B.: The very early treatment of cerebral palsy. Develop. Med. Child Neurol 9:373–390, 1967.

Bobath, B., and Bobath, K.: Motor Development in the Different Types of Cerebral Palsy. London: William Heinemann, 1975.

Bobath, K., and Bobath, B.: An analysis of the development of standing and walking patterns in patients with cerebral palsy. Physiotherapy 48:144, 1962.

Bosley, E.: Development of sucking and swallowing. Cerebral Palsy J., 26, no. 6 (1965).

Bosma, J.: Fourth Symposium on Oral Sensation and Perception. National Institutes of Health, Bethesda MD, 1973.

Bosma, J. (ed.): Symposium on Oral Sensation and Perception. Springfield IL: Charles C Thomas, 1967.

Bower, T. G. R.: Development in Infancy. San Francisco: W. H. Freeman, 1974.

Bower, T. G. R.: A Primer of Infant Development. San Francisco: W. H. Freeman, 1977.

Brazelton, T. B.: Infants and Mothers. New York: Delcorte Press, 1969.

Brazelton, T. B.: Psychophysiologic Reactions in the Neonate. J. Pediatr., 58, no. 4 (1961).

Brazelton, T. B., Koslowski, B., and Main, M.: The origins of reciprocity: The early mother-infant interaction. In Lewis, N., Rosenblum, L. (eds.): The Effect of the Infant on Its Caregiver. New York: John Wiley & Sons, 1974.

Breakey, A., Wilson, B., Wilson, J.: Sensory and Perceptual Functions in Cerebral Palsied. J. Nerv. Ment. Dis. 158:70–77, 1974.

Bullock, Dalrymple, Danca: Communication and the nonverbal. Am. J. Occup. Ther. 28:150–152, 1975.

Burton, White: Human Infants. Englewood Cliffs NJ: Prentice Hall, 1971. Summary in Kopp, C.: Reading in Early Development. Springfield IL: Charles C. Thomas.

Campbell, S. K.: Facilitation of cognitive and motor development in infants with central nervous system dysfunction. Physiotherapy 54:346–353, 1974.

Caplan, F. (ed.): The First Twelve Months of Life: Your Baby's Growth Month by Month. Princeton NJ: Edcom Systems, 1973.

Carlsen, P.: Comparison of two occupational therapy approaches for treating the young cerebral palsied child. Am. J. Occup. Ther. 29:267, 1975.

Carter, R., and Campbell, S.: Early neuromuscular development of the premature infant. Physiotherapy 55:1332–1341, 1975.

Cliff, G., and Nymann, C.: Mothers Can Help. A Therapist's Guide for Formulating a Developmental Text for Parents of Special Children. El Paso TX: The El Paso Rehabilitation Center, 1974.

Connor, F. P., Williamson, G. G., and Siepp, J. M. (eds.): Program Guide for Infants and Toddlers with Neuromotor and Other Developmental Disabilities. New York: Teachers College Press, 1978.

Crickmay, M. C.: Speech Therapy and the Bobath Approach to Cerebral Palsy. Springfield IL: Charles C Thomas, 1970.

Cristarella, M.: Comparison of straddling and sitting apparatus for the spastic cerebral palsied child. Am. J. Occup. Ther. 29:273–276, 1975.

Crothers, B., and Paine, R. S.: The Natural History of Cerebral Palsy. London: Oxford University Press, 1959.

Danella, E.: A study of tactile preference in the multiply handicapped child. Am. J. Occup. Ther. 27:457, 1973.

Developmental disabilities: Current problems of early detection and management (Clinical Conference). Brain Dev. 2:149–70, 1980.

Dubowitz, V.: The Floppy Infant. Clin. Develop. Med. No. 31. London: William Heinemann, 1969.

Egan, D. F., Illingsworth, R. S., and MacKeith, R. C.: Developmental Screening 0–5 Years. Clin. Develop. Med. No. 30. London: William Heinemann, 1969.

Enright, D.: Cognition—An Introductory Guide to Theory of Jean Piaget for Teachers of Multiply Handicapped Child. Watertown MA: Northeast Regional Center for Services to Deaf-Blind Children, 1977.

Erhardt, R.: Sequential levels in development of prehension. Am. J. Occup. Ther. 28:592–596, 1974.

Farber, S.: Sensorimotor Evaluation and Treatment Procedures for Allied Health Personnel, ed. 2. Purdue University at Indianapolis Medical Center, 1974.

Fiorentino, M. R.: A Basis for Sensorimotor Development: Normal and Abnormal. The Influence of Primitive Postural Reflexes on the Development and Distribution of Tone. Springfield IL: Charles C. Thomas, 1981.

Fiorentino, M. R.: Normal and Abnormal Development. The Influences of Primitive Reflexes on Motor Development. Springfield IL: Charles C. Thomas, 1972.

Fiorentino, M. R.: Reflex Testing Methods for Evaluating C.N.S. Development. Springfield IL: Charles C. Thomas, 1979.

Frailberg, S.: The Magic Years. New York: Scribners, 1959.

Fulford, F. E., and Brown, J. K.: Position as a cause of deformity in children with cerebral palsy. Dev. Med. Child Neurol. 18:305–14, 1976.

Gesell, A.: The ontogenesis of infant behavior. In Mussen, P. H. (ed.): Carmichael's Manual of Child Psychology, ed. 3. New York: John Wiley & Sons, 1970.

Gibson, J. J.: The mouth as an organ for laying hold on the environment. In Bosma, J. F. (ed.): Symposium on Oral Sensation and Perception. Springfield IL: Charles C Thomas, 1967.

Gilfoyle, E., and Grady, A.: A developmental theory of somatosensory perception. In Coryll, J., and Henderson, A. (eds.): The Body Senses and Perceptual Deficit. Boston University Symposium, March 1972.

Ginsberg, H., and Opper, S.: Piaget's Theory of Intellectual Development: An Introduction. Englewood Cliffs NJ: Prentice-Hall, 1969.

Golden, G. S.: The effect of developmental disabilities on mental health. J. Sch. Health 49:260–262, 1979.

Gralewicz, A.: Play deprivation in multihandicapped children. Am. J. Occup. Ther. 27:70, 1973.

Haberfellner, H., and Rossiwall, B.: Treatment of oral sensorimotor disorders in cerebal palsied children. Preliminary report. Dev. Med. Child Neurol. 19:350–352, 1977.

Hemiplegic Cerebral Palsy in Childhood and Adults. Report of an International Study Group. Cin. in Develop. Med., No. 4. London: William Heinemann, 1961.

Holser-Buehler, P.: The Blanchard method of feeding the cerebral palsied. Am. J. Occup. Ther. 20:1, 1966.

Holser-Buehler, P.: Correction of infantile feeding habits. Am. J. Occup. Ther. 27:6, 1973.

Ilg, F., and Ames, L. B.: Child Behavior. New York: Harper & Row, 1955.

Illingsworth, R. S.: The Development of the Infant and Young Child: Normal and Abnormal, ed. 4. Baltimore: Williams & Wilkins, 1970.

Illingsworth, R. S.: An Introduction to Developmental Assessment in the First Year. London: National Spastics Society. William Heinemann, 1962.

Ingram, T. T. S.: Clinical significance of the infantile feeding reflexes. Develop. Med. Child Neurol. 4:159–169, 1962.

Johnson, and Mogarb: Developmental Disorders: Assessment, Treatment, Education. Baltimore: University Park Press, 1976.

Kessler, J. W.: Parenting the handicapped child. Pediatric. Ann. 6:654–661, 1977.

Knott, G. P.: Attitudes and needs of parents of cerebral palsied children. Rehabil. Lit. 40:190–195, 206, 1979.

Komich, P., and Tearney, A.: The sequential development of infants of low birth weight. Am. J. Occup. Ther. 27:396, 1973.

Kong, E.: Very early treatment of cerebral palsy. Develop. Med. Child Neurol. 8:198–202, 1966.

Kubler-Ross, E.: On Death and Dying. New York: Macmillan Publishing Co., 1969.

Largent, and Waylett: Follow-up study on upper extremity bracing of children with severe athetosis. Am. J. Occup. Ther. 28:341–347, 1975.

Leiper, C. I., Miller, A., Lang, J., and Herman, R.: Sensory feedback for head control in cerebral palsy. Physiotherapy 61:512–518, 1981.

Levine, and Billie: An Approach to the Treatment of the Cerebral Palsy Child. Long Island NY: Suffolk Rehabilitation Center, 1973.

Levitt, S.: Treatment of Cerebral Palsy and Motor Delay. Philadelphia, J. B. Lippincott, 1977.

Lewis, M., and Rosenblum, L. (eds.): The Effect of the Infant on the Caregiver. New York: John Wiley & Sons, 1974.

Manning, J.: Facilitation of movement—the Bobath approach. Physiotherapy 58:403–408, 1972.

Minde, K. K.: Coping styles of 34 adolescents with cerebral palsy. Am. J. Psychiatry 135:1344–1349, 1978.

Montgomery, P., and Richter, E.: Sensorimotor Integration for Developmentally Disabled Children: A Handbook. Los Angeles, CA: Western Psychological Services 1977.

Morris, S.: Program Guidelines for Children with Feeding Problems, 1974. Illinois State Pediatric Institute (1640 W. Roosevelt Road, Chicago IL 60608).

Norton, Y.: Neurodevelopment and sensory integration for the profoundly retarded multiply handicapped child. Am. J. Occup. Ther. 29:93, 1975.

Paine, R. S., et al.: Evolution of postural reflexes in normal infants and in the presence of chronic brain disorders. Neurology 14:1036, 1964.

Paine, R. S., and Oppé, T.: Neurological Examination of Children. Philadelphia: J. B. Lippincott, 1966.

Pearson, P. and Williams, C. (eds.): Physical Therapy Services in Developmental Disabilities. Springfield IL: Charles C. Thomas, 1972.

Peiper, A.: Cerebral Function in Infancy and Childhood. New York: Consultants Bureau, 1963.

Phillpot, R.: Headstick helmet for cerebral palsied children. Am. J. Occup. Ther. 28:291–292, 1975.

Piaget, J.: Play, Dreams and Imitation in Childhood. New York: W. W. Norton & Co., 1963.

Piaget, J., and Inhelder, B.: The Psychology of the Child. New York: Basic Books, 1969.

Prechtl, H., and Beintema, D.: The Neurological Examination of the Full Term Infant. Clin. Develop. Med., No. 12. London: William Heinemann, 1964.

Provence, S., and Lipton, R. C.: Infants in Institutions: A Comparison of Their Development with Family Reared Infants During the First Year of Life. New York: International Universities Press, 1962.

Rosenbloom, L.: The consequences of impaired movement: A hypothesis and review. In Holt, K. (ed.): Movement and Child Development. London: William Heinemann, 1975.

Rosenbloom, L., and Horton, M. E.: The maturation of fine prehension in young children. Dev. Med. Child Neurol. 13:3–8, 1971.

Rugel, R., et al.: The use of operant conditioning in a physically disabled child. Am. J. Occup. Ther. 25:247, 1971.

Saint-Anne Daregassies, S.: Neurodevelopmental symptoms during the first year of life. Develop. Med. Child Neurol. 14, 1972.

Scarr-Salapatek, S., and Williams. M.: The effects of early stimulation on low-birth-weight infants. Child Devel. 44 (1973).

Schaffer, H. R., and Callender, W. M.: Psychologic effects of hospitalization in infancy. Pediatrics 24 (1959).

Stern, F.: A review of the reflex development of the infant. Am. J. Occup. Ther. 25:155–158, 1971.

Stone, L. J., Smith, H., and Murphy, L. B. (eds.): The Competent Infant: Research and Commentary. New York: Basic Books, 1975.

Tyler, W., et al.: Interpersonal components of therapy with young cerebral palsied. Am. J. Occup. Ther. 28:395, 1974.

Tyler, and Kahn: A home-treatment program for the cerebral palsied child. Am. J. Occup. Ther. August: 437–440, 1976.

Vanderheiden, G. C. (ed.): Non-Vocal Communication Techniques and Aids for the Severely Physically Handicapped. Baltimore: University Park Press, 1976.

Walsh, G.: Cerebellum, Posture and Cerebral Palsy. Clin. Develop. Med. No. 8. London: William Heinemann, 1963.

Walsh, G.: Measuring ocular motor performance of cerebral palsied children. Am. J. Occup. Ther. 28:265, 1974.

Wolff, P. H.: The serial organization of sucking in the young infant. Pediatrics 42:943–956, 1968.

Wyke, B.: The neurological basis of movement: A developmental review. In Holt, K. (ed.): Movement and Child Development. London: William Heinemann, 1975.

Acknowledgment

To Joyce Perella, who contributed the section on oral reflexes.

CHAPTER 33

Occupational Therapy with Children— The School Setting *Nancy Allen Kauffman*

The child's role as a student dominates a large percentage of time in the developmental years. The occupational therapist's task in this setting is clearly not to provide academic instruction but to facilitate competencies that will help the child benefit from the total educational experience.

Private schools for the handicapped were the first educational programs to hire occupational therapists. By the early 1970s, therapists were being hired by public as well as private schools to evaluate and treat not only the physically handicapped, but also the severely mentally retarded, some of whom had previously been at home because they had been excluded from public education. Therapy for many other handicapping conditions followed.

The number of occupational therapists employed in schools increased from 4% of the total American Occupational Therapy Association (AOTA) membership in 1973 to 10% in 1978. This rapid expansion was accompanied by a lack of uniformity of policy, problems of communications, and blurring of roles between educational, medical, and therapeutic personnel at state as well as local levels. In the 1970s, with funding assistance from federal agencies, AOTA established research programs to investigate existing and potential roles of occupational therapists in

schools. These programs culminated in a comprehensive training program conducted in 1981 in every state to train occupational therapists for the specific role of providing services in an educational setting.[1]

Papers presented through the World Federation of Occupational Therapists in 1980 documented occupational therapists' growing involvement in educational settings not only in the United States but also in Ireland and New Zealand.[2] In 1980 the AOTA Representative Assembly passed Standards of Practice for Occupational Therapy in Schools (see Appendix C), and in 1981, a Position Paper, The Role of Occupational Therapy as an Education-Related Service.*

With the passage of new federal legislation, the need for appropriate personnel in every school district had been mandated to take place by 1978. Pressure on school boards and administrative personnel by parent advocate groups became an effective method of creating positions in many states. However, budget cuts associated with the early months of President Reagan's administration threatened therapy positions in schools as well as other child care facilities in 1981.

---

* Published in the American Journal of Occupational Therapy. Vol. 35, No. 12, p 811, 1981.

Legislation

In the early 1970s there was a legislative trend at the state level initiating educational rights for the retarded and other handicapped persons. Section 504 of the Federal Rehabilitation Act of 1973 was intended to eliminate discrimination against handicapped citizens.

PL94–142

In 1975 the federal government responded further to state legislative changes, and President Gerald Ford signed into law the Education of the Handicapped Act, PL94–142. It required free and "appropriate" public education for all handicapped children including the learning disabled; speech, language, hearing, and vision impaired; or physically, mentally, or emotionally impaired. Education in it's broadest sense was intended,[3] and some states had to include handicapped from age 3 to 21 by 1980. The new law gave schools several years to comply because of the wide ranging changes it required. The changes had a dramatic effect on occupational therapy that was specifically included as a "related service."

One emphasis of the law was the mainstreaming of as many handicapped children as possible into regular education classes, a concept commensurate with the normalization concept developed during the preceeding decades. Normalization recommends conditions for the handicapped as close as feasible to the mainstream of society. The Cascade System (Fig. 33-1) is a theoretical prototype used in many states as a conceptual framework for providing educational services from the handicapped. Children are placed in "the least restrictive alternative," or in other words, the class that best fits their needs and is as close as possible to the everyday classroom. Also called the inverted pyramid, this system assumes the greatest number of handicapped children can be absorbed into mainstream education, thus allowing financial resources to be directed to the most handicapped. Ideally, support from counseling, educational, and therapeutic services is provided as needed to facilitate each transition, which is made as soon as educationally feasible.[4]

Due Process

Parents or guardians now have the legal right to examine all school records. They also participate with professionals in making educational placement decisions and in developing the diagnostic-prescriptive Individualized Educational Program (IEP) that must

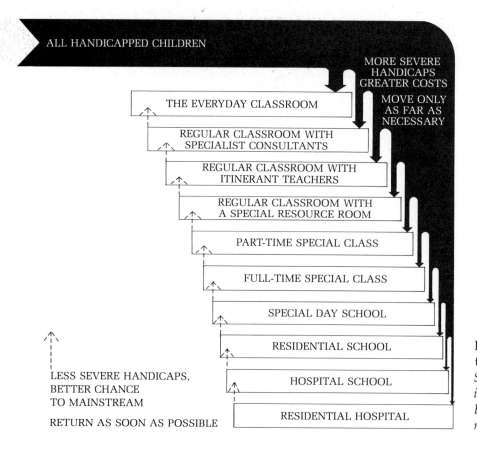

Figure 33-1. The Cascade System. (*From One Out of Ten: School Planning for the Handicapped, p. 7, 1974. Courtesy of Educational Facilities Laboratories, New York.*)

be written annually for each child. They may bring trained advocates to help them understand and protect the rights of their child at these meetings. Parents are entitled to "due process" of the law in safeguarding their child's rights in these matters. They may bring legal counsel and other professionals of their choice before an impartial Fair Hearing Officer of the state in order to question school decisions. Therapists must be prepared to present testimony at such a hearing, and to be cross-examined by lawyers representing the parent and the school district.

TIPS TO HELP REDUCE ANXIETY IN PREPARING TESTIMONY FOR A DUE PROCESS HEARING

Rely on the high standards of documentation you have maintained. They will help "prove" your testimony.

Organize testimony carefully. Include treatment goals, objectives, and progress measured by pre- and post-testing.

Informally review your testimony with a co-professional who has testified or a due process lawyer.

Read Bateman[5] or other introductory Due Process information.

Have in hand records that might help you document answers to questions posed during cross-examination.

Project confidence and self-assurance but not presumptuousness.

Use clear communication without therapy jargon. State observations and behaviors, not hypotheses (about causes of deficits).

Answer questions as asked by the lawyers. Do not say more than you are asked.

The law requires public participation in the development of educational policies, and occupational therapists have presented testimony at state public hearings and federal level House and Senate subcommittee hearings. They also participate in state task forces within departments of Health and of Education for determining the role of occupational therapists within school systems.

Additional Legislative and Judicial Changes

By 1981 many states had adopted statutes requiring an excess of the usual 180 school days if regression in skills following an extended vacation would be ex-

pected to be excessive, and recoupment or regaining of the lost abilities would be unduly slow, especially in self-care skills. Simultaneously, a movement was astir at the federal level to consider reducing the mandate for provision of related services to an optional status. Block grants were being considered, a policy in which large sums of federal money with few restrictions would be provided to state and/or more local educational administration. Since priorities would be established at state or local levels, some occupational therapists were apprehensive.

On June 29, 1982, the Supreme Court ruled local school districts were not obliged to provide all services that handicapped children need in order to reach their full academic potential. While they must provide free appropriate public education that "benefits" the handicapped child, no particular level of education was required.*

The case on which the Supreme Court ruled involved only one deaf student's education and was not a class action lawsuit. However, its potential impact for the 4.4 million handicapped students in the country was much broader, and therapists were relieved that the written decision reiterated that handicapped children were entitled to both "specialized instruction and related services"† (which include occupational therapy).

Team Approach

It is important to understand the role of the occupational therapist within the particular local school system by first studying the state and local hierarchy of administration and service delivery. Does the therapist fit into the health chain of command or that of education? How are therapy services provided locally and statewide? Are local parents strong advocates in favor of occupational therapy for their children?

The occupational therapist functions often as a member of the local school system interdisciplinary committee, which makes decisions about placement of children in programs at various levels of the Cascade. These decisions are based on such things as developmental level, adaptive ability, academic performance, social maturity and behavior, in addition to Intelligence Quotient (IQ). The committee recommends placement based on the primary cause of the child's learning problem. If a secondary problem, such as emotional overlay, has developed, appropri-

---

* Greenhouse, L.: Schools Backed on Limiting Aid to Handicapped. New York Times, June 29, 1982. p. 1.

† Rehnquist, W. H.: Excerpts from Justices' Opinions in Case of a Deaf Girl and School District. New York Times, June 29, 1982. p. B4.

ate education emphasizing treatment of the primary problem often eliminates it.

Gilfoyle[6] emphasizes the importance of knowing how to participate effectively in the group decision-making process. In addition she points out the need for communication skills that enhance understanding by other members of the team. Jargon specific to occupational therapy should by avoided unless it has been carefully adapted to the school environment, so the team members receiving the information can process it.[7] Hypotheses regarding causes of deficits in observable behavior should be clearly stated as such.[8] It is important for therapists to become familiar with tests frequently used by each team member in order to better interpret results. A task analysis, after observing pertinent tests being administered, is one effective method.

The role of members who usually serve on the interdisciplinary committee within school systems will be described later. Others who may serve as interdisciplinary committee members or who may provide consultation are medical, neurological, psychiatric, and optometric personnel. Important team members who do not serve on interdisciplinary committees are teachers of art, music, and physical education. These teachers may have been specially trained to work with handicapped children. The child, classroom aide, and volunteer also play important roles in the team effort of teaching the handicapped child.

Interdisciplinary Team Members

Members of the interdisciplinary committee assist in formulating decisions on appropriate placement and educational programming for children:

School Principal or Program Director: These committee members interpret local administrative policies in special education.

Counselor: The counselor brings to the interdisciplinary committee awareness of both the child's family milieu and a variety of placement services within the community and the school system.

Parent: The parent, as the primary care-giver of the child, helps set goals commensurate with family expectations. Parents, with the help of their trained advocate or lawyer, may initiate suggestions regarding educational placement and programming or, through team meetings, may be better prepared to give informed consent.

Psychologist: The psychologist reports mental age or I.Q. scores, cognitive and adaptive functioning, and sometimes social and emotional information resulting from projective tests. Consideration of scores and quality of performance on tests and

subtests given by the psychologist may give diagnostic information that can reduce the amount of time spent in evaluation by the therapist. Figures 33-2 and 33-3 suggest interpretation of subtest scores from two psychological tests. A breakdown of subtest scores may have to be specifically requested.

Educational Evaluator: This specially trained teacher reports results of standardized tests of academic and readiness achievement levels in number concepts and in the developmental sequence of listening, speaking, reading, and then writing. The evaluator also makes observations about the child's learning style that may differ widely from the child's strengths and weaknesses in tactile, kinesthetic, visual, or auditory modalities. For example, the child may score low in tests of auditory processing but may learn to read better through listening than looking tasks.[9] The diagnostician may report on perceptual, language, and motor performance if they are not tested by other services.

Special Education Teacher: Teachers sometimes have responsibility for making reports to the interdisciplinary committee as well as teaching. The classroom teacher is the most significant person in the educational program because of having the most consistent contact with the handicapped child. This teacher makes recommendations about

THE TASKS	Verbal	Perceptual-Performance	Quantitative	General Cognitive	Memory	Motor
1. Block Building		P		GC		
2. Puzzle Solving		P		GC		
3. Pictorial Memory	V			GC	Mem	
4. Word Knowledge	V			GC		
5. Number Questions			Q	GC		
6. Tapping Sequence		P		GC	Mem	
7. Verbal Memory	V			GC	Mem	
8. Right-Left Orientation		P		GC		
9. Leg Coordination						Mot
10. Arm Coordination						Mot
11. Initiative Action						Mot
12. Draw-A-Design		P		GC		Mot
13. Draw-A-Child		P		GC		Mot
14. Numerical Memory			Q	GC	Mem	
15. Verbal Fluency	V			GC		
16. Counting and Sorting			Q	GC		
17. Opposite Analogies	V			GC		
18. Conceptual Grouping		P		GC		

Chart showing the contribution of the eighteen tasks to the six scales

Figure 33-2. Plan of the McCarthy Scales. (*From McCarthy, D: McCarthy Scales of Children's Abilities, 1972. Courtesy of the Psychological Corporation, New York.*)

Figure 33-3. Content of test items of the Wechsler Intelligence Scale for Children (WISC-R). (*Modified from Waugh, KW, and Bush, WJ: Diagnosing Learning Disorders. Columbus, Charles Merrill, 1971.*)

THE TESTS	Spatial	Quantitative	Sequencing	Perceptual organization	Conceptualization and verbal comprehension	Ability to concentrate: Distractibility	Visual motor integration: Fine motor	Verbal expression
● VERBAL SCALE Information					✓			✓
Similarities					✓			✓
Arithmetic		✓			✓	✓		
Vocabulary					✓			✓
Comprehension					✓			✓
Digit Span	✓	✓				✓		
● PERFORMANCE SCALE Picture Completion	✓					✓		
Picture Arrangement			✓		✓			
Block Design	✓			✓				
Object Assembly	✓			✓			✓	
Coding	✓		✓				✓	
Mazes	✓						✓	

the everyday social maturity and behavior as well as academic, perceptual, and language performance of children in the classroom. The resource room teacher sees mildly handicapped children for a portion of each day to work on specific deficit areas. The itinerant special education teacher travels to schools or homes for the purpose of either screening and teaching children or suggesting to regular teachers academic intervention methods for mildly impaired children.

Physical Therapist: The physical therapist reports on quality of movement, reflex development, equilibrium reaction, gait, and gross motor development.

Speech and Language Clinician: This member of the interdisciplinary committee reports test results of the child's receptive language (comprehension or decoding of what is heard) and expressive language (encoding through the use of linguistic symbols). For both expressive and receptive language, consideration is given to the child's use of sounds (phonology), meaning (semantics or vocabulary and concepts), and grammar (syntax and morphology). Integration (inner associative language processing such as categorization and understanding of analogies) is also considered as well as retention (memory) and such perceptual problems as auditory discrimination and speed of verbal response.

Occupational Therapist: The occupational therapist reports the quality and level of functioning of the child in the areas evaluated (see Assessment and Program Planning sections of this chapter). Service delivery may be provided through direct, hands-on intervention. However, an evaluation and treatment model that can be integrated right into the home and classroom environments (rather than the isolated once a week model in the artificial therapy environment) is recommended by Sternat *et al*, particularly for the severely handicapped student.[10] On the other hand, the role of the therapist may include writing programs or making suggestions to be carried out by teachers, aides, parents, or volunteers. In that case the therapist monitors progress through occasional re-evaluation and updating of program suggestions. The therapist may also supervise or manage others and must provide and receive training to enhance professional skills and quality of service delivery to children.

In carrying out the role of school system therapist, every effort should be made to maintain close professional involvement with parents through telephone or personal contact as well as written test results and progress reports. Team meetings that include parents provide a useful forum for exchange of information, and parents should be urged to attend. Parents may appreciate guidance toward reading publications such as "The Exceptional Parent" magazine[11] and books written for parents, or joining such national organizations as the Association for Children with Learning Disabilities (A.C.L.D.), Association of Retarded Citizens (A.R.C.), and Council of Exceptional Children (C.E.C.) (see Glossary).

Assessment

Evaluation of handicapped school children provides the basis for planning treatment and, in some cases, identifies which children need special help. Children with severe handicaps tend to be placed in appropriate programs at an early age. But for others, the need for special education is not readily apparent.

The goal of screening is to identify children who need help without interfering in the lives of those who have only a mild and temporary developmental delay. Screening during the preschool or kindergarten years allows early detection of children with learning disabilities, minimal brain dysfunction, mild mental retardation, or mild emotional disturbances. Early special class placement or special help within the mainstream classroom helps prevent development of secondary emotional overlay resulting from learning failure in later grades. It also provides intervention procedures at a critical time in the child's life when they will be most helpful. Keeping the child in the mainstream classroom or returning the child there at the earliest opportunity is currently considered most desirable.

In many school districts, preschool children are screened and tested as early as age 3 based on referrals from parents, physicians, and community agencies. Thorough reviews of screening methods and tests for this age group are presented by Stangler, et al,[12] Lerner, et al,[13] and the Educational Staff of Chapel Hill.[14] The beginning therapist may wish to screen children with mild handicaps using the *Pre-School Screening System*[15] or the *Learning Accomplishment Profile*.[16] The *Developmental Test of Visual-Motor Integration*[17] by Beery and Buktenica is standardized down to age 2 and also includes guidelines for informal assessment of earliest form copying skills.

Mildly impaired children having only subtle problems often are not identified until kindergarten or first grade. Occupational therapists, along with educators, language specialists, and medical personnel, may play a key role in district-wide and local school methods for finding such children and planning suitable programs for them. Several examples of group screening procedures will be discussed.

In one school district, teachers identified children with suspected problems by color coded name tags as occupational therapists led the whole class through informal screening tasks. The therapists observed especially carefully the children whose colored tag suggested the likelihood and severity of subtle problems in motor skills, perception, or sensory-based poor behavior. Classroom recommendations for training of problem children were made, and a small percentage of children was recommended for further standardized testing.

Another school district sent a team of medical and educational personnel to individually observe and screen a few problem children identified by each teacher. Recommendations were made to the teacher and parents for managing the specific educational and behavioral problems. Later the team returned and used additional test measures for the one or two children who, in spite of several months of maturation and special teaching techniques, still had the greatest problems.

Volunteers were used in Forth Worth Public Schools to assist professionals in testing children using a locally developed screening instrument.[18]

The School District of Philadelphia developed a learning disabilities checklist to be marked by classroom teachers for each of their kindergarten or first grade students.[19] It eliminated the need for screening by specialists. Although the attempt was made to write items observable during normal classroom activities, many teachers resisted the extra burden of evaluation. Such a checklist could be used for parent observation or for school use where teachers have been trained and motivated. The checklist, typical of many developed around the country, did serve one of its purposes: to familiarize teachers with behavioral and performance characteristics of young children with subtle learning problems. Easily understood phrases were checked as occurring frequently or seldom, and cover the topics listed below:

Behavior. Items in this section cover hyperactivity; distractibility and impulsiveness; overreaction to change, excitement or unexpected touch, sounds or smells; hypoactivity; focusing on irrelevant details; difficulty completing tasks; perseveration; inconsistent academic performance; and difficulty with peer relations.

Motor Coordination. These items test for placing 2 feet per tread when climbing or descending stairs;

clumsiness or awkwardness in moving or catching a ball; inability to hop three times or skip; difficulty copying pantomimed body positions especially when crossing the midline; difficulty touching the tip of the nose with the little finger with eyes closed; inability or awkwardness in bead stringing, coloring, pasting, buttoning, cutting, or holding a pencil.

Orientation. Items tested are body image; drawing a person; under- or overreaching for objects or colliding with people or things; environmental disorientation; confusion of directional words such as up and before; inappropriate placement or size of drawings or writing on paper; and difficulty understanding schedules and elementary time concepts.

Visual Motor Integration. These include difficulty matching symbols or pictures and recognizing a figure when only fragments are presented; difficulty with puzzles or connecting dot patterns; switching of hand use while cutting, throwing, drawing, or eating; and inability to copy correctly a circle, cross, square, or X.

Language. These items test for poor auditory figure ground and discrimination; inability to categorize or classify objects ("mistakenly groups large with small, round with flat, toys with clothing, etc."); inability to reproduce simple sound rhythms; poor auditory sequencing of three spoken simple directions; inability to repeat the sequence of three words or numbers and to easily and rapidly recall words or names of familiar items (note: a combination of poor rote auditory memory plus difficulty with word calling in a child often means the child will need long-term special education services); avoidance of spoken language; inability to rhyme; difficulty communicating events sequentially or in complete sentences.

Using the Child Development Chart, Table 33-1, a therapist can quickly determine the normal age at which children acquire commonly tested abilities. The chart reads developmentally down from the top to the bottom. It also reads across from left to right, as some developmental sequences on the right side of the chart may be interrupted because of deficits in developmental sequences on the left side. For example, equilibrium (in the fourth column) may not be developing properly because of poorly inhibited reflexes (first column). Body scheme and eye-hand coordination (columns three and seven) may be negatively affected by poor sensory development, which appears in an earlier column. Inadequate development of language (the last column) in some cases may be a reflection of poorly integrated visual percepts or sensory information. The use of the chart

is intended to promote continual awareness in the mind of the therapist of all the goals established for each child, and their interrelationship. Also, the chart can be helpful in talking with parents, recommending developmental activities, or making general judgments about children's performance levels.

Following the use of such screening methods as those described above, or on the direct referral of educational or medical personnel, therapists will further evaluate children showing evidence of dysfunction. They may use informal functional assessments based largely on clinical impressions; or they may use standardized tests, which compare a child's performance with that of many other children. Standardized test administration methods must be followed exactly and may require special training, as for example the Southern California Sensory Integration Tests.[20]

In addition to clinical impressions and standardized tests, the therapist may use criterion referenced tests, some of which have instructional activities suggested to remediate each test item or section in which the child needs additional help. Criterion reference tests, now widely used to establish goals and objectives, evaluate performance on specifically described skills or knowledge without comparisons between individuals as in standardized testing. Skills are arranged in a sequence at the discretion of the test author, and an attempt is usually made to list skills in the order in which they are normally acquired. Specific skills on the test that have not yet been acquired are trained, and the criterion of the test is 100% mastery.[21] One example of a criterion referenced test is *The Learning Accomplishment Profile.*[22]

The beginning therapist wishing to evaluate the subtle problems of the young mildly impaired child is advised to use the Developmental Test of Visual-Motor Integration,[23] The Motor-Free Visual Perception Test,[24] and the Bruininks-Oseretsky Test of Motor Proficiency.[25] Southern California Sensory Integration Test administration must be learned through a certification course.

Other chapters in this textbook suggest appropriate assessment tools for various types of handicaps found in the school-age population. Part four: Evaluation Process and Procedures describes methods of testing range of motion, muscle strength, sensation, motor skills, sensory integration, cognition, developmental reflexes and reactions, eating, writing, activities of daily living, and prevocational and vocational skills. In addition, assessments are included for cerebral palsy (Chapter 32) and hand rehabilitation (Chapter 25). In addition, Lerner, et al,[26] and Gilfoyle[27] give thorough annotated bibliographies of published screening and evaluation tools for children.

Table 33-1* *Child Development Chart

	Items closer to top of each column suggest remedial sequences for problems observed closer to bottom of column. Items in left hand columns suggest possible causes of problems in certain columns further to the right.			
	General reflex development	*Sensory development*	*Body scheme*	*Equilibrium*
0–3 mo.	• 0–2 mo. Phasic/movement spinal cord reflexes predominate. Limbs coordinated in total flexion or extension. • 0–6 mo. Static, brainstem mediated reflexes are present. Stimulation of labyrinths or neck muscle feedback changes distribution of muscle tone throughout body.	• 1–4 wk. Infant differentiates: Tactile (touch, pressure) Temp. (hot, cold) Taste (sweet, sour, salty, bitter) Vision (see vis. percept. column) • Infant also experiences vestibular input, internal chemical changes, audition.	• 1 mo. Mass motor activity reaction to stimuli. • 3 mo. Plays regarding hands.	• 2 mo. prone, head and chest up to 45° recurrently • Head bobs when sitting, back rounded.
3 mo. to 1 yr.	• 4–15 mo. Midbrain mediated reactions in all-fours position help child right self, turn over, assume crawl & sit positions. Maximum concerted effort 10–12 mo. • 6 mo. Equilibrium reactions under cortical control begin to gradually modify, inhibit & dominate righting reactions if muscle tone is normal. Results in standing, walking, well-coordinated person.	• 3 mo. Tickle reaction.	• 4–6 mo. Plays with hands and feet in supine. Hands come together in play. • 5–6 mo. Pats mirror image • 7–8 mo. Plays peek-a-boo	• 3 mo. Prone, supports weight on forearms. • 5 mo. Pull to sit. No head lag. • 6–8 mo. Sit, head erect. • 7–9 mo. 4-point kneel; rocks back and forth.
1–2 yr.			• 12–18 mo. Points to 2 of own body parts.	• 12–13 mo. Kneel/stands. • 14 mo. Stands. • 14–18 mo. Walks; feet wide apart, arms in primary balance role

Developed from Ayres, Banus, Beery, Berry, Bobath, Cattell, Colarusso & Hammill, Cratty, Dale, Denhoff, Erhardt, Fantz, Fiorentino, Frostig, Gardner, Gesell & Armatruda, Gilfoyle & Grady, Gibson, Hull & Hull, Kephart, Llorens, Miller, Moore, Norton, Oseretsky, Pearlson, Piaget, Wiig & Semel.

Age norms are approximate. Authors vary. Children vary. Development does not really occur in separate rows and columns. All parts of the nervous system influence each other.

Bilateral integration	*Visual perception*	*Eye-hand coordination*	*Language*
• 1–4 wk. Assymetrical postures predominate. • 2 mo. supine, child can hold head in midline & extremities symmetrical. • 2 mo. Eyes begin to follow past midline.	• 3–4 wk. At 10″ discriminates ⅛″ stripes from plain surface. • 1–2 mo. Discriminates stylized face from oval pattern. Also color. • 2 mo. Visual size & near distance constancy developing. Unable to apply them simultaneously. • 2 mo. Recognize visual cliff.	• 0–4 wk. Reflexive grasp. No eye-hand coordination. Touch tells when to grasp. • 1–4½ mo. Fixates on light monocularly. • 2 mo. Prone, head and chest up for forward vision. • 3 mo. Eye follows across midline and past 90°. • 3 mo. Plays regarding hands.	• 1 mo. Responds to sound. Undifferentiated crying. • 2 mo. Single vowel sounds, coos. • 3 mo. Vocalizes pleasure in response to social stimuli. Vocal noises resemble speech. • 2 mo. Discriminates intonations and 2 voices.
• 4–6 mo. Hands together in play. • 6 mo. Symmetrical arm use & postures predominate. • 7 mo. Transfers toy 1 hand to the other. Hands cross midline. • 7–8 mo. Creeps amphibian; tactile stim. to stomach. • 7–8 mo. Bunny hops. • 7–9 mo. 4-point crawl; homo then hetero-lateral.	• 6–7 mo. Discriminates + ○ □ △. 3-dimensional discrim. easier than 2-dimensional. • 8–24 mo. Convergence to 2″ from nose. Divergence to 20″. Primitive depth perception. • 9 mo. Recognizes danger of visual cliff.	• 4 mo. Rotates head to inspect surroundings. • 4–6 mo. Visually pursues lost toy. • 6 mo. Eye-hand coord. begins. • 6 mo. Palmar grasp. • 10 mo. Crude release. Pokes finger in holes.	• 3 mo. Chuckles. • 4 mo. Turns to noise & voice. • 6 mo. Distinguishes angry-friendly voice. • 6 mo. Intonational jargon. • 9 mo. Comprehends a few gestures, intonations, "no-no," "hot." Echolalia. • 10 mo. Word-like syllables: ma-ma-ma, da-da-da. Comprehends & waves bye-bye.
• 11–12 mo. Cruises sideways, holding furniture. • Creeps up stairs. • 15 mo. Creeps down stairs.	• 15 mo. Looks selectively at pictures in book. • 21 mo. Aligns 3 blocks for train. • Object permanence	• Imitates scribble. • 12 mo. Neat pincer grasp. Supinated grasp developing, wrist extended. • 13 mo. Good release. • Tower of 2 cubes. • 15 mo. Places objects into & out of containers. • Spontaneous scribble.	• 12 mo. First word, usually noun. • Action response to commands. • 1–5 word vocabulary.

Table 33-1 (continued)

	General reflex development	Sensory development	Body scheme	Equilibrium
1–2 yr. (Cont.)				usually at or above shoulder height. • 17 mo. Stoops to pick up toy without losing balance.
2-yr. old			• Identifies 2 body parts from picture. • Touches tummy, cheek, arm, leg, mouth, hair.	• Up & down stairs independently, 2 steps per tread holding on. • 2½ yr. Jumps, 2-foot take off. Tiptoes briefly. • Runs. Walks sideways & backwards. • Kicks ball on request.
3-yr. old		• Vision occluded, matches grossly different textures, e.g., sandpaper & satin.	• Knows front, back, side of self. Also chin, neck, forearm.	• Jumps from 12″ height, feet together or 1 ft. lead. • Up stairs 1 foot per tread, no support. Down 2 steps per tread, no support. • Hops 1 foot 2, 3 times. • Climbs 3 rungs. • Squats. • 3½ yr. Tandem walks 10 ft.

Bilateral integration	Visual perception	Eye-hand coordination	Language
		• 18 mo. Turns pages, 2 or 3 at a time. • Uses spoon, cup well. • 21 mo. Puts large pegs in pegboard.	• 1-word sentences. • Can mentally perform behavior before physically perform. • Produces all vowel sounds. • 1½ yr. Extension of word meanings; over-generalizations. • 50-word vocabulary, mostly nouns.
• Rhythmical bounce, sway, nod, swings arms.	• Enjoys watching moving objects. • Simultaneous visual size & distance constancy developing. • 20/70 visual acuity. • Points to pictures of familiar objects. • 2½ yr. Adds chimney to 3-cube train • Begins matching colors.	• Hand preference beginning. • Tower of 6–7 cubes. • Strings large beads. • Throws. • Imitates / • 2½ yr. Imitates —, ○ • Copies / • Pours well, glass to glass.	• 2-word sentences that are functionally complete. • Imitates absent models; pretends; reconstructs memories. • Knows "in" and "under." • Knows "I," "you," "me," "mine." • 2½ yr. Telegraphic speech. • 3-word sentences.
• Walks swinging arm with opposite leg, arms free of shoulder ht. balance position. • Pedals tricycle. • Weight shift in throwing. No step into.	• Tends to react to entire stimulus rather than label separate parts, especially if unfamiliar. • Picks longer line 3 of 3 times. • Imitates cube bridge • 3½ yr. Recognizes 2 colors named.	• 10 pellets into bottle in 30 sec. • Tower of 9–10 cubes. • Copies —, ○ • Simian pencil grasp (fist clenched). • Turns doorknob, forearm rotation. • Unbuttons accessible buttons. • May shift handedness. • Catches large ball, arms extended. • 3½ yr. Imitates X.	• Has adult grammatical structure. Complete simple-active sentences. • Uses sentences to tell understandable stories. • 3½ yr. Speech disfluency. • "Why" questions. • Names 1 color.

Table 33-1 *(continued)*

	General reflex development	Sensory development	Body scheme	Equilibrium
4-yr. old		• Names heavier of 2 weights. • Discriminates different scents. • Compares different textures, e.g., soft, smooth.	• Draws man with head and legs.	• Stands 1 foot 4 sec. Broad jumps . . . • standing—8–10″ • running—23–33″
5-yr. old	• Primitive reflexes inhibited or dominated. In supine & all-fours child can turn head side-to-side, up, down without elbows, shoulders, or knees changing angle. • Can flex in supine & extend in prone positions for 10 sec. • Sits and stands symmetrically from supine with only slight body rotation.	Vision occluded . . . • discriminates ○□☆ blocks (stereognosis). • points to touched finger 1/2 times. • points to within 3″ of stimulus spot on arm. • points to hand &/or cheek touched singly or simultaneously.	• Copies Simon Says postures. • Draws 6-part unmistakable man with body. • Points front, back, near, up, down, with eyes closed. • Can clench and bare teeth. • Aware of, but confuses left and right. • In pictures identifies object that is beside, between, in middle, in front of.	• Down stairs, alternating feet, no support. • Stands 1 foot 6–8 sec. • Balances on tiptoe, 1/3 trials. • Running broad jump 28–35.″ • Jumps 10″ high hurdle. • Begins balance beam backwards. • Tries roller skates, jump rope, stilts.
6-yr. old				• Jumps over rope 20 cm. high. • Standing broad jump 3 ft.

Bilateral integration	*Visual perception*	*Eye-hand coordination*	*Language*
• Runs with good arm-leg coordination. • Up and down stairs 1 foot per tread. • Gallops. • 4½ yr. Skips, 1 foot only (lame duck skip).	• With increasing age child tends to differentiate stimuli in environment, esp. when specific language labels applied to them. • Slow down of rapid visual acuity development since birth. • Matches shapes (same color and size). • Can find simple familiar overlapping outline figures. • Builds 6-block pyramid. • 4½ yr. Copies gate ⌂	• Follows moving object smoothly with eyes ↔ ↕ ↘ ↗ ↻ • Copies + • Imitates □ • 10 pellets into bottle in 25 sec. • Bounces ball awkwardly. • Tries to cut on straight line.	• Transforms kernel sentences. • 4-word sentences, some complex or compound. • Intuitive thought begins, less concreteness. • Little word analysis; deals with whole sentences. • Counts 3 objects, though imperfectly. • Uses slang. • Understands syntax, grammatical contrasts beyond production ability. • Repeats 3 digits. • 4½ Names primary colors. • 4½ yr. Perceives differences in concrete events.
• Mimics pointing to ipsi- or contralateral ear or eye. 2/3 trials. • Can reproduce simple rhythmic clapping. • Marches in time to music.	• 20/30 visual acuity. • Difficulty with orientation. Can detect ↕ reversals easier than ↔ reversals after instruction. • Difficulty performing closure necessary to distinguish incomplete ○ □ ▢ • Simultaneous size constancy & form discrim. developing. • Imitates 10-block pyramid. • 5½ yr. Begins to mentally rotate simple shapes for solving puzzles.	• Tripod pencil grip. Begins flex I.P. joint. • Copies ╱ □ ╲ ✕ • Imitates △ • Sequential finger opposition (1, 2, 3, 4) with visual regard and minor associative movements. Slow. • Throws 16" playground ball 10–11 feet. Catches bounced large playground ball.	• Embeds phrases, clauses in sentences. • Develops percepts of number, speed, time, space. • Inner logic & imaginative thinking. • Categorizes by likeness & difference. • Marked increase in vocab. comprehension (not use). • Repeats 4 digits • 5½ yr. Mean length of response = 4.9 words.
• Skips alternately. • Throws stepping with foot opposite throwing arm.	• Begins to identify imbedded familiar outline figures. • Recalls 3½ of the 9 Bender Gestalt figures.	• Copies △ ✳ • Ties shoelaces. • 6½ yr. Hand dominance established.	• Command of every form of sentence structure. • Mean sentence length rapidly increasing. Now 6.5 words.

Table 33-1 *(continued)*

	General reflex development	Sensory development	Body scheme	Equilibrium
6-yr. old (Cont.)				
7-yr. old	• Arises from supine to standing in 1–1.5 sec.	• Vision occluded, can reproduce - × ○ drawn on back of hand 1/2 trials.	• Good jumping jacks. • Can knit eyebrows. • 7½ yr. Stabilizes arms and trunk against much resistance. • Knows left and right on self.	• Stands on 1 foot, eyes closed, 3 seconds. • Can hop and jump accurately into small squares. • Walks 2″ wide balance beam.
8-yr. old			• Eyes closed, points right & left. • Can wrinkle forehead.	• Crouches on tiptoes without falling 1/3 trials.
9-yr. old			• 9½ yr. Discriminates left & right on facing person.	• Runs 16–17 ft./sec. • Jumps over rope 15″ high 2/3 trials. • Jump, clapping hands 3 times, 1/3 trials.
10–12 yr.				• 10 yr. Hops 50 ft. on 1 foot in 5–6 sec. • 11 yr. Standing broad jump 4½–5 ft. • 12 yr. Standing high jump 3 ft.

Bilateral integration	Visual perception	Eye-hand coordination	Language
	• May still reverse some letters or numbers.		• Asks for and attempts to verbalize explanations, causal relationships.
• Can tap floor alternately with feet.	• 20/20 visual acuity. • b-d, p-q confusions resolved. • Builds 6-block pyramid from memory.	• Grips pencil tightly, often close to tip. Pressure may be heavy. • Good sequential finger opposition (1, 2, 3, 4). • Drops 20 coins, one at a time, into open box in 16 sec. • Accurately taps swinging suspended ball 2/5 tries. • 7½ yr. Copies ◇◇	• Good speech melody & facial/hand gestures. • Good inner language. • True communication; shares ideas. • Mean length of response 7.2 words. • Repeats 5 digits • 80% know comparative relationships (e.g. bigger than)
• Good 2-2, 2-1, 1-2 hop. • Can run into moving jump rope but cannot alter step.	• Identifies heavily embedded familiar figures. • Notices and labels component parts of stimulus more than does younger child. • Capable of attending to both whole and part.	• Laces 8 beads in 20 sec. • Places 10 pairs of matchsticks in box in 16 sec.	• Skilled use of grammatical rules. • Acceptable articulation.
	• Closure figure recognized and seen as incomplete. • Notices wholes & parts simultaneously in figures composed of familiar objects.		• 80% know passive relationships (e.g. person was hit by). • 75% know familial relationships (e.g. "your mother's father").
	• 11 yr. & above. Recalls 5½–6 of the 9 Bender Gestalt figures.	• 10 yr. Draws 3-dimensional geometric figures. • 10 yr. Judges & intercepts pathways of small balls thrown from a distance. • 12 yr. Linear perspective seen in drawings. • Anticipates locomotor & manual responses to rapidly moving objects, e.g., where to catch ball whose complete trajectory is not observable.	

Lists of tests for screening and evaluating learning impaired children are available from federally funded Area Learning Resource Centers and local centers, sometimes called Special Educational Instructional Materials Centers (SEIMC). These centers, in many locations around the country, also have samples and lists of educational curriculum materials. *The Mental Measurements Yearbook,* edited by Oscar K. Buros[28] and published every several years, is an important reference book that groups tests by topic and that includes several critiques of each one by authorities in the field.

When screening and testing children, constellations in results of all testing must be considered rather than single low scores. Even normal children may fail in some aspect of motor, sensory, or psychosocial functioning. Plan goals and make recommendations that are relevant to the presenting educational problem,[29] for providing therapy to improve an irrelevant area that happens to score low is not the goal. All the testing methods described are only as valuable as the program planning that results from them.

Program Planning and Documentation

Following the use of assessment procedures such as those just described, the occupational therapist documents test results in writing, including all the areas outlined in the AOTA "Uniform Occupational Therapy Evaluation Checklist" (see Appendix F). Information related to the client's personal data and history as well as the referral are included. The checklist also urges therapists to include skill/performance in independent living, sensorimotor areas, cognition, psychosocial areas, therapeutic adaptation, and prevention (see Uniform Occupational Therapy Evaluation Checklist[30] for details of subcategories). In addition to this initial evaluation report, the therapist also keeps daily progress records of treatment programs and of recommendations made to teachers, administrators, parents, or volunteers. Once or twice a year, therapists who treat children send descriptive reports home and write formal progress notes that are added to the child's school records.

When planning a program, the occupational therapist considers all areas assessed that might have pertinence to quality of performance in the educational environment. Specific documentation of planned treatment is now required by law, although school personnel are not held accountable for children's progress.

Often the therapist is required to write a portion of the student's Individualized Educational Program

(IEP). The IEP includes a statement of present educational levels, annual long-term goals (a general statement of treatment intent), and short-term objectives. The latter are written in behaviorally observable (not theoretical) terms and include conditions under which they will take place, terminal behavior, a measurable criterion level, and anticipated completion date[31] (see IEP Plan, Fig. 33-4).

Figures 33-5 and 33-6, adapted from Llorens and Seig,[32] show a method of organizing treatment goals for whole classes or small groups of young children. Such an evaluation record provides a visual chart of assets and deficits. The therapist administers only those tests most suitable to the age and capability levels of the child. While one inadequate score within a particular heading is usually insignificant, clusters of low scores indicate treatment goals. Individual subtests cannot be considered as separate entities, and caution should be used in determining the importance of any one subtest score, but listing them on such an evaluation record helps point out clusters of low scores.

Test results of 5½-year-old Richard, a learning disabled student, are recorded in Figure 33-5 as an example of the use of this evaluation record. A diagnostic-prescriptive program for improving motor and perceptual functioning might be correlated as follows: through sensory integrative techniques the therapist would use vestibular and tactile stimulation, and developmental activities to enhance motor planning, body scheme, reflex development, ocular control, and visual perception. Following three auditory sequential directions, using the scooter board, could frequently be included in the activities. The physical education teacher could emphasize prone extension and supine flexion along with games involving moving specific body parts. The classroom aide, volunteer, or resource room teacher could supervise Richard's copying of specifically selected inch cube and pegboard designs to help fine motor and prereading perceptual skills. Independent desk work could include worksheets emphasizing imbedded geometric shapes and alphabet letters for visual figure-ground discrimination. The parents could be providing daily tactile stimulation and discrimination at home. Such a complete program could be organized by the therapist or might be planned and agreed upon by all the professionals at a team meeting. The language therapist would be emphasizing Richard's associative language processing and the speed with which he makes oral responses. Awareness of the language problems helps all members of the team understand his learning style better.

The columns listed in Figure 33-5 are only examples of test results or developmental activities that could be listed. Other standardized or observational

Individualized Educational Program Plan (I.E.P.)
(abbreviated version)

Name___Richard (R.)_____   Date of Birth_____

Address _____   Today's Date _____

School_____ Grade/Program_____   I.E.P. Review Date _____

	Date started	Frequency or % of time	Expected duration of services
Primary assignment Integration into regular education (Opportunities for child to participate with mainstream children during school hours.) Related Services (e.g. transportation, O.T., P.T., speech, audiology, psychology, counseling, social work, etc.)		(e.g. 20% of each school day) (e.g. 30 minutes 2 times per week)	

Reason for assignment _____

Administrative person responsible for program _____

I.E.P. Planning Meeting Participants_____   _____

_____   _____

Present Educational Levels	Curricular Area	Assessment Procedure	Date	Program Planner
(Results of testing: clinical impressions, standardized tests, criterian referenced measures, etc.)		(tests used)		

Curricular Area (e.g. gross motor)   Annual Goal (e.g. improve balance)

(e.g. fine motor)   (e.g. improve eye-hand coordination)

Short Term Objectives	Criteria for Successful Performance
(e.g. With eyes closed (R.) will correctly touch one body part to another on command	. . . . . 3 times in sequence on 3 successive days.)
(e.g. With a ½ inch diameter pencil (R.) will maintain correct pencil grip while coping ◯, □, & △	. . . . with shapes clearly discernible.)

Figure 33-4. Individualized Educational Program Plan (IEP)

TABLE 24–2. Evaluation Record For the Mildly Neurologically Impaired.

Headings	Column items	Test scores (Richard)			
	Classroom #				
	Age	8½			
	I.Q.	83			
	Behavior	α			
Reflex development	ATNR	α			
	Prone Ext. (Kep)	↑			
	Supine Flex.	↑			
	Cocontract'n	→			
	Postrot. Nystag. (SC)	+?			
	Sitt'g Blance	α			
	Forw'd Bal. Beam (Kep)	α α			
	Sideway Bl. Bm. (Kep)	α			
	Backw'd Bl. Bm. (Kep)				
	Stand'g Bal. (SC)	+! −?			
	Static Bal. (Dev)	α			
Bilateral integration	STNR creep (Bndr)	α			
	Midline Xing (SC)	→			
	Bilat. Mot. Cord. (SC)				
	Dbl. Circles (Kep)				
	Skip (Kep)				
	2-2, 2-1 hop (Kep)				
	Hand Dominance / Eye Foot	R / R ℓ			
Body scheme and tactile discrim.	Imitate Post. (SC)	2d			
	Imitate Post. (Kep)				
	Perc. Mot. (Dev)				
	Sequ. Mot. (Dev)				
	Point Body Parts (Kep)	4			
	Angls in Snow (Kep)	+!			
	Kinesthesia (SC)				
	Man. Form. (SC)	+1.2			
	Fing. Identif. (SC)	−.9			
	Graphesthesia (SC)				
	Loclz'n Tac. Stim. (SC)	−1.7			
	Dbl. Tact. Stim. (SC)	−1.2 α			
	Tactile Dfsivenes (SC)	α			

CLASS DAYS: ____ TO ____
TIME: ____

Figure 33-5. Evaluation Record for the Mildly Neurologically Impaired.

Evaluation Record for the Mildly Neurologically Impaired—(Continued)

Code for standardized tests indicated in parenthesis:

Kep — Kephart's Purdue Perceptual Motor Survey

SC — Southern Calif. Sensory Integration Tests

Dev — Devereux Test of Extremity Coordination

Beery — Beery-Buktenica Test of Visual Motor Integration

MVPT — Motor Free Test of Visual Perception

Blank score indicates item not tested because (a) it was not age appropriate, or (b) new insight into deficit areas would not result.

			Richard			
Fine motor	Mot. Acc. (domin.)	(SC)	-24			
	(non-domin.)	(SC)				
	Vis. Mot. Integr.	(Beery)				
	Design Copy	(SC)				
	Pencil Grip		→			
	Handwriting		→			
	Sequent. Fing. Tip Touch		→			
	Fine Motor	(Dev)				
	Ocular Fixation		∝			
	Ocular Pursuit	(Kep)	→			
	Ocular Converg.	(Kep)	→			
Spatial orientatn	Environmntal Disorientation		∝:9			
	Posit. in Space	(SC)	∝:9-7			
	Space Visualiz.	(SC)	7-7			
	Reversals: letter—word					
	Reading L. to R. direct.					
	R-L Discrim.	(SC)				
Vis. discrim. & fig. grnd.	Perceptual Quotnt	(MVPT)	→			
	Figure Ground	(SC)	→			
	Letter Recogn'tn		→			
	Recogn'tn of error	(Beery)	→			
Memory — Vis'l	Sequence of 4 color beads		∝			
	Sequ. of 3 vis. instrctns		∝			
	Memory test items	(MVPT)				
	Posit. in Space mem.	(SC)	∝			
Aud	Repeat 3 wrds or #'s		→			
	Sequ. of 3 audit. directns		→			
Language	Receptive		∝			
	Expressive		∝			
	Integrative (Associative)		→			
	Auditory Discrim.		∝			
	Word finding (naming)		→			
	Sound-symbol assoc.					
	Speed of Auditry Process'g		→			

After testing use soft pencil to fill in scores on pages 1 and 2 for only those items tested. Then with soft red pencil make hachures in boxes of pertinent low scores indicating current treatment objectives. Use the Evaluation Record to see goals common to the whole group, to zero in on particular children's deficits when part of the group is suddenly absent, and for ready reference when talking with parents and teachers. Erase and change scores often as children show progress.

Figure 33-5. (*continued*)

Class	Gross motor and reflexes		Equilibrium		Bilateral integration	Domin: Hand	Body scheme	Tactile and sensory	Self help	Social emotional
		PRNT	Dynamic	Static		Eye				
Names ↓		L				Foot				
		R								

	Eye/hand coordination			Perception		Memory and speed of processing	Language	Cognitive adaptive		
	VMI	Dexterity	Ocular motility	Spatial orientation	Visual discrimination and figure ground				I.Q.

Figure 33-6. Evaluation Record for Young or Moderately to Severely Handicapped Children.

score columns could be substituted, for example pertinent subtests of the WISC-R or McCarthy tests.

Figure 33-6 shows a similar group evaluation record designed for younger or more handicapped children. Rather than listing standardized tests, space is left under each heading for listing particular skills or clinical observations indicating strengths or deficits for the particular age group. Red pencil hachures can be used to mark columns indicating current treatment objectives as they do in Figure 33-5.

Interpreting Performance

Testing and treatment of the youngster in the special education setting may be complicated by undetected deficits in visual, auditory, or tactile acuity. On the other hand, a child may hear well and express himself well verbally but may have a severe impairment in auditory reception. In that case automatic or learned reliance on visual cues may cause misinterpretation of such instructions as "I'm drawing a line on top of the black line. If I go off the black line by accident [like this] I come back on the black line again [like this]."[33] One bright language impaired child with excellent auditory acuity proceeded half way around the 1972 version of the Southern California Motor Accuracy Test with regularly spaced pencilled projections off the tracing line in spite of many verbal efforts by the examiner to halt the practice! On the other hand "Do this, this, and this after you roll to the ladder," may be an impossible activity for the child who cannot remember the sequence of three visual stimuli or who does not understand the temporal concept "after." It is important to know a child's sensory, language processing and cognitive deficits as well as to task analyze testing and treatment requirements in order to understand the full impact of a child's performance.

Implementing the Program

The value of occupational therapy treatment techniques in educational settings is a controversial issue among some educators and doctors. Strongly worded adverse opinions have appeared in print.[34-36] Therapists must be prepared to counter with research results and carefully compiled articles supporting the importance of sensory integration,[37-40] motor programs,[41] and other occupational therapy techniques.[42] While special education classes and medication have consistently been shown to produce academic gains in learning disabled children,[43] training visual perception[44] and motor performance have not. School therapists should be alert to relevant new scientific reporting in their own and other professional literature, and they should continually investigate and scientifically evaluate their own testing and treatment data.

The therapist is encouraged to seek advanced training in sensory integration, neurodevelopmental treatment, and other specific forms of treatment. However, it is important to avoid the tendency to apply one treatment method exclusively or to follow a bandwagon approach to solving children's problems. Drilling in splinter skills should be avoided, and a broad developmental program should be emphasized.

Occupational therapy treatment is intended to allow the child to be able to direct cognitive skills toward the academic task at hand rather than toward execution of balance, motor planning, fine manipulation, and so forth. Therapy prepares the child to learn; however, it does not result in increased academic performance unless accompanied by an appropriate academic program. The therapist should avoid removing a child from the classroom unless therapy is clearly warranted and ongoing assessment indicates progress is being made.

Improved quality of life is the goal in occupational therapy. Emotional and social factors as well as physical needs should be considered. Play, the primary occupation of the child, is an important consideration in program planning. Activities should be fun and should foster in the child a positive self-image. As one therapist put it, every pediatric occupational therapy treatment program should include Play, Pleasure, and Success. Clark, et al,[45] point out that play is intrinsically motivating, and self-direction by the child should play a major role in therapy, accompanied by artful vigilance by the observant therapist. They point out that therapy is an art that is best carried out within a healthy helping relationship that values the child as an important contributor to the process. On the other hand, the child must not be permitted to misbehave or misuse activities to the detriment of his own progress or that of his classmates.

Management of Behavior

Hyperactivity often causes behavior management problems and inaccurate interpretation of performance capability, particularly in a large group of developmentally impaired children. Helping a child learn to manage his own behavior may be one goal of therapy. In addition, it is important for children to leave therapy quietly controlled and ready to resume desk work without disrupting the academic classroom.

Medicine prescribed by the child's doctor is likely to be helpful if the cause of the hyperactivity is organic, particularly if the child consistently demonstrates hyperactivity, poor impulse control, and short attention span. The central nervous system stimulant Ritalin is most often effective, while the amphetamine Dexedrine is a good second choice. It is thought that possibly the stimulants may act on the reticular activating system, a part of the brainstem that receives and sorts out stimuli. In a few cases the tranquilizers Thorazine and Mellaril may help reduce anxiety.[46,47] The use of medication should be accompanied by special education, environmental control, and, sometimes, counseling.

Hyperactivity may also be psychogenic. It may be caused by emotional overlay secondary to a learning problem, or it may reflect an inconsistent child-rearing approach. In this case the child is physically able to control his behavior but is preconditioned not to do so.[48]

Management of hyperactive behavior, particularly if it is of psychogenic origin, requires firmness, structure, and environmental controls. Such controls might include reducing distractions, defining performance expectations clearly, and giving clear warnings of impending minor changes. Keeping an accurate daily record of types and forerunners of inappropriate behavior in the classroom helps determine the cause of hyperactivity and effectiveness of intervention procedures.[49]

Behavior modification, currently widely used in the field of education, is a particularly useful method of managing hyperactive behavior of psychogenic origin and of bringing about improvement in specific performance goals. Performance is assessed first, and terminal goals or "behavioral objectives" are established. Positive rewards or reinforcements that are important to the child are determined so that they may be given upon successful completion of each small step approaching the goal. Negative or incorrect behavior or performance are usually ignored and are not negatively reinforced by scolding or criticising. Primitive rewards are often edible. Interim rewards, such as paper tokens that can be traded in for treats or privileges, are more therapeutically desirable, and social rewards such as a handshake or a smile are the highest level. Frequency of rewarding is decreased as the child's performance improves.[50,51]

Mildly impaired children, even the very hyperactive, learn to sit quietly on their special spots waiting for treatment to begin when they know the star they then receive can later be exchanged for free play time. They understand when newly performed activities are listed on an "I can do" sheet to take home. On individually written self-paced activity sheets each step leading to correct skipping can be checked off as it is mastered.

Consistency of expectations and rewards is impor-

tant, especially when working with a group. Motivating and allowing a child to make the decision to cooperate has more positive results than trying to force conforming behavior. Having a child help establish his own goals often fosters cooperative behavior.

In a difficult to control class, it may be necessary to plan the same activities for the whole class. In that case formal structure or calming activities, at least at the beginning and end of the session, may be necessary to establish control.

This finely delineated sequence of steps might be helpful when working with more than one or two students simultaneously:

1. have equipment ready and highly motivating activities planned (some will have been selected by the students);
2. position children with enough space between to perform task;
3. gain undivided attention of the group;
4. introduce equipment and wait until reaction subsides;
5. briefly and clearly explain the task using three or fewer sequential directions;
6. demonstrate;
7. gain undivided attention;
8. have one or all children demonstrate verbally or physically that they understood directions;
9. gain undivided attention;
10. signal start of task;
11. continually reward appropriate performance verbally or with a pat, handshake, star, privilege, or other reward;
12. conclude task specifically by change in positioning of children or equipment or by some other specific means. Avoid the temptation of rushing into a new activity before the children have had time to "change gears."

The experienced therapist may wish to make efficient use of time with a well-controlled group of mildly impaired children by using "learning stations" or "circuit training." At several positions around the room, equipment or activities are placed for use by one or two children. It is important for each unsupervised activity to provide its own feedback so the child knows whether he performed correctly. (Did the beanbags go in the can? Did you catch the ball?) Children change stations at their own volition, or as "the gong sounds," or as the therapist directs. With this method all children are therapeutically engaged with activities or equipment that can be used by only one child at a time. The therapist stays with the station that is least safe or that needs to have feedback provided. Also each child could be directed only to those particular stations within his treatment program. Classroom and physical education teachers are often experts in using this method, and they would be helpful models.

Expanding the Therapist's Role

Occupational therapists must be prepared to provide programs for a wide variety of handicapping conditions (see appropriate treatment sections of this textbook). The age of students served runs the gamut from infant stimulation and preschool programs in some school districts through the grade school years and on into secondary education programs and vocational high schools. For the mainstreamed population, the therapist must be able to suggest classroom or home activities to help the nonspecial education student who manifests mild motor or perceptual difficulties.

In addition to seeking expertise in treating or consulting for the varied handicapping conditions, the well-prepared therapist acquires information regarding the organizational and legal idiosyncrasies of educational systems (for example, through the training program "Occupational Therapy Educational Management in Schools" offered by the American Occupational Therapy Association). Various consultancy and supervisory roles are explored—even telephone monitoring of programs being carried out under the therapist's supervision in distant schools. Membership on school curriculum development committees is encouraged, particularly for motor or preacademic programs.

Organizations such as A.C.L.D., A.A.M.D., A.R.C., and C.E.C. (see Glossary) offer opportunities for reciprocal sharing between educators, parents, and therapists. Increasing involvement and professional contributions by therapists in local chapters, national conventions, and journal or newsletter publications of these organizations help highlight the expanding role of the school therapist. Other new publications[52,53] and well-established journals[54,55] also indicate the increasing interest in therapy services for children.

Therapists point out to others the unique contributions they are qualified to make within the total educational program while remaining open to opportunities for role release exchange with other educational professionals. Role release for the therapist involves encouraging classroom faculty members to carry out therapeutic activities, sometimes in conjunction with achieving IEP objectives, and helps the therapy become an integral rather than peripheral part of the learning process.[56] A guide for helping other members of the educational team establish developmental sequences for training gross and fine motor development in the mildly impaired follows.

Providing Developmental Program Planning Guidelines

The developmental sequences in the Child Development Chart on pages 690 to 697 provide a basis for creating nonacademic school curriculum ideas to share with teachers, physical educators, parents, and aides. The following ideas, based on that chart, stress gross and fine motor development. They may be adapted for many types of handicapping conditions, but are particularly suitable for the early grade school-aged mildly impaired child. The ideas are written in language intended to be clearly understandable to educators and parents. They are divided into four sections:
1. Body Scheme (which includes sequenced items listed under Sensory Development on the Child Development Chart);
2. a combined section of Reflex Development and Balance Skills (the latter from the Equilibrium section);
3. Coordination of the Two Body Sites (from the Bilateral Integration section of the chart);
4. Eye-Hand Coordination (which also includes some developmentally sequenced items under Visual Perception).

Behaviors in the left column of each of the four sections are arranged approximately developmentally, and some include approximate age norms. Therefore they can be used by educational personnel for informal evaluation/data gathering to determine *general* areas that need remedial help, for developmental program planning, and for re-evaluation. This would not, of course, replace the standardized and developmental testing to be done by the therapist. Early "Behaviors" are generally, though not absolutely, prerequisite to later behaviors, and they may have to be mastered before progress in later behaviors can be expected. Adjacent behaviors may be interchangeable.

The behaviors in the left column may also be stated in positive terms by therapists or educators for writing behavioral objectives as a part of diagnostic-prescriptive Individual Educational Programs (IEPs).

Body Scheme

Body Scheme is the unconscious awareness of the physical and sensory components of one's self. It includes awareness of the physical structure, movement/functions, and positions of the body and its parts in relation to each other and to objects in the environment. As used here it also includes the ability to recognize and interpret touch and pressure to the skin. Children with good body scheme accurately imitate new body postures or movements; have smoothly coordinated movements on the playground, particularly when trying new actions; adequately point to or name body parts (assuming that language comprehension and memory are adequate); usually draw human figures' age appropriately; and interpret touch/pressure to the skin comfortably and accurately.

If these behaviors are observed

Cannot comfortably accept ordinary new or unexpected touch/pressure to skin. Has aversion to haircuts, new clothes, sand play, mudpies, love-pat on shoulder, injections, bare feet in grass, wind through hair.

Try these activities, strategies, or materials

- Apply firm, well-modulated pressure in rapid rhythm. Teacher rubs back/arms during rest time.
- "Time out" four times daily for child's *self-rubbing* of arms, tummy, legs, neck, and face. With rapid back and forth motions use *child's* choice of soft or rough fabric, carpet piece, baby oil, hairbrush, or paint brush.
- Present a variety of textures/sensations in calm, well-structured atmosphere: ice cubes, warm water, textured fingerpaints, sand play, rotary electric shoe polish brush, vibrator, tug of war on tummy in grass, electric hair dryer, inchworm race on back on grass or thick carpet.
- Avoid unexpected touch by teacher/students. Encourage "thinking space" between children in line; position desk to avoid accidental touch; praise verbally rather than with love-pats unless child sees the "pat" approaching.
- Slowly encourage physical contact within child's toleration level—lapsitting, arm around shoulders, hand pat on hair.

Is unable to imitate simple body postures/movements accurately.

- Give visual, verbal, *and* tactile clues. Manually move child to appropriate position so movement/position can be felt and learned through experiencing it.
- Encourage movement/contact of all body parts with different textures and surfaces: mat, shredded paper, blankets, floor, grass, brick wall, and smooth wall.
- Mimetics, pantomime, obstacle courses, animal walks, Simon Says "do this," "See a Lassie."
- Trampoline, cheerleader yells, signal flags, mat stunts.
- Child wiggles through rungs of leaning, suspended, or sidelying ladder with predetermined movements or climbs in and out of holes cut into refrigerator shipping cartons.
- Action songs: I'm a Little Teapot, Inky Dinky Spider, Two Little Ducks, Little Cottage in the Woods, My Hat It Has Three Corners.
- Child performs familiar movements in slow motion: walking, especially against resistance, walking backwards, crawling, skipping.

If these behaviors are observed

Try these activities, strategies, or materials

- Child reproduces silhouette of partner's body positions (use film projector light), then verifies by measuring/feeling silhouette against wall.

Inaccurately uses and points to own body parts as directed.

- Beginning with easiest to learn (facial features, arm, side, leg), teach body-part awareness, being alert to child whose problem is not poor body image but poor language comprehension or poor auditory-motor match (can understand words but can't carry out appropriate movement response without visual clue).
- Then work on identification of more difficult body parts (wrist, knee, shoulder, elbow, ankle, neck, waist, etc.)
- One sequence of teaching body parts (achieved over a long period of time) is to have child:
    touch and move part while repeating the name of the part
    touch and move part, eyes shut
    touch part to object (from standing, sitting, lying down positions) while repeating the name of the part
    touch part to object, eyes shut
    touch part to part ("put your ankle on your knee")
    touch part to part, eyes shut
    name part independently
    "place ankle higher than shoulder," or "back higher than head," or "ear lower than knee"
- Refer to body image instructional sequences recommended in *Developmental Sequences of Perceptual Motor Tasks.*[57]
- Child rapidly and firmly rubs body parts while naming:
    "paint" with wet or dry brush
    rub off "mud" or "ice cream" with hand-sized towel/carpet
    wrap body part with yarn or bandage
    at goal line rub powder off "hurt" ankle or wrist held in air during lame puppy race.
- Point out body parts and movements during doll play or on pop-singer posters.
- Sing "Dem Bones," "Head and Shoulders—Knees and Toes," "Looby Loo," "Hokey Pokey."
- Play Busy Bee (partners touch back-to-back, ankle-to-ankle, etc.) or Simon Says (naming one body part while teacher demonstrates the wrong one—for advanced players).
- Be alert to the idea that pointing to or naming body parts is only one step in "knowing" body image.

With eyes closed, cannot point to location of one or two touches on body parts (approximately age 5).

- Emphasize identification of and tactile stimulation to body parts.
- Emphasize activities suggested for imitation of simple body postures/movements.

If these behaviors are observed	*Try these activities, strategies, or materials*
Does not know meaning of in front, back, beside, in, up, above, out, by age 5. Has difficulty negotiating obstacles and judging distances, especially if blindfolded.	• Eyes closed, child points to objects in familiar room, then verifies by looking, approaching, and *touching* with specified body parts. • Place three to five 8-inch numbers around room. Eyes closed, children point to numerical answer to simple verbal math problem, then verify. • Eyes closed, child touches one body part to another; touches body part to object in environment; goes through obstacle course; follows thick-rope path; touches environmental objects to front, side, top of body planes. • Child applies verbal directional labels to gross body movements and fine manipulative placement of small objects. • Child uses beanbags, plastic or playground balls for target or goal throws or dodge ball. Increase spatial awareness through eye-body, eye-hand, and foot-eye coordination activities.
Is unable to draw six-part recognizable person with body (approximately age 5).	• Look for other indications of delayed eye-hand coordination. • Emphasize awareness of body parts and imitation of postures (above).
Cannot discriminate simple shapes traced on skin with eyes closed.	• Help child identify large simple shapes traced on back, hand, or tummy using "point to the answer" method instead of "draw the answer" (eye-hand coordination may be poor) or naming answer (language deficits may be present). Advance to more complex shapes and to naming shapes. • Seat teams facing forward. Trace shape or letter on back of last child on each team. Each child traces on back of person in front. Child in front of each team traces that team's shape on chalkboard. • Identify hand-sized objects felt in bag but not seen. • Child identifies finger touched by partner when eyes closed or points to spot(s) touched by partner or by "it" in circle game.
Cannot name heavier of two weights (approximately age 4); with eyes closed cannot tell whether one finger has been moved to up or down position by partner/teacher by age 7½; cannot stabilize arms and trunk against much resistance.	• Children do tug of war while standing, sitting, and lying down. • Encourage pressure on joints through resistance: walrus, crab, seal walk, wheelbarrow race, crawling with partner facing child and pushing against shoulders, stretching inner tubes, partners trying to force wrists together or apart. • Compression of joints through jumping, leaping, trampoline, and bouncing board.
Has poorly developed sense of rhythm. Awkwardly performs rapid alternating motions using opposite muscle groups.	• Rhythm band, marching, dancing, musical activities, and Lummi sticks.

<table>
<tr><td>*If these behaviors are observed*</td><td>*Try these activities, strategies, or materials*</td></tr>
</table>

If these behaviors are observed	*Try these activities, strategies, or materials*
	• Provide definite, clear auditory rhythm signal (drum or triangle beat) with each separate motion response. This may need to be accompanied by touch-pressure clue. Example: angels in snow movements slowly to beat of metal triangle, with touch by teacher to appropriate limb for those children who need this extra clue.
	• Child performs rapid opposing motions on signal or to beat of music: palms down, palms up index finger touch tip of nose, tip of finger held at arm's length tongue protrudes straight forward, retracts into mouth protruding tongue touches one side of open mouth, then opposite side child repeatedly says sound "puh, puh, puh" or "buh, buh, buh" or "tuh, tuh, tuh" heel-toe, heel-toe tap while sitting, standing.
Does not know right/left on self with eyes closed (approximately age 8); right/left on facing person (approximately age 9½).	• Point out freckle or tiny scar on child's right or left hand to help in discrimination. • Child identifies randomly distributed right and left hand/foot cutouts. • Footsie Game. Advance player on game board number of spaces written on correctly identified foot "playing card" drawn from pack. • Zip Zap. (Circle Game. "Zip" means name, right neighbor, "Zap" means name left neighbor. Encourage speed.) • Blindfold one child. Others give verbal directions to lead child to target, (*e.g.*, three steps to right, two steps backwards, two steps to left).
(if these advanced Body Scheme tasks are difficult for a child, return to "behaviors" and "activities" for younger children.)	• Use facing pairs of objects such as trucks, TV sets, chairs, to demonstrate and quiz diagonal aspect of right and left before applying labels to right or left of facing object. *Later* teach right and left on facing person.

Reflex Development and Balance Skills

As early primitive postural reflexes decrease in importance, the normally developing child acquires more advanced balance skills which allow automatic equilibrium responses. These responses first develop with the infant in a lying down position, then in sitting and kneeling on hands and knees, and finally in standing and walking positions. Training for delayed balance skills should proceed in the same developmental sequence. Early "behaviors" are generally, though not absolutely, prerequisite to later behaviors and should be mastered first. Grade school children with good balance skills have good head and trunk stability while sitting and/or standing, walk with feet close together and with hands swinging reciprocally at sides, and walk a balance beam, hop, jump and leap comfortably.

If these behaviors are observed	*Try these activities, strategies, or materials*
Has very inadequate sitting balance and difficulty "leading with the head" when rolling.	• Log and egg rolls, somersaults on mats or down inclines. (Make more difficult up incline, against

If these behaviors are observed

Try these activities, strategies, or materials

resistance, or holding beanbag between knees.)
- Move head separate from stable body in backlying position to look in various directions on cue, including looking at toes without lifting back.

Is unable to lie on stomach on small pillow and hold head, shoulders, arms, knees and toes off floor (for 10 seconds, by age 5½).

- Back raises with feet held; leg raises with trunk held. Kraus Weber position. Push ups.
- Scooter board activities on stomach.

Is unable to curl up in a ball while lying on back and hold head, arms, feet off floor (for 10 seconds, by age 5½).

- With chin on chest and arms bent and folded, child kicks ball across floor with sole of foot, kicks balloon over short "net," rides bicycle motion with legs while hips off floor, blows tissue off chest.
- Child rides gym scooter on back, with head and feet up, using hands to pull forward on suspended rope or ladder rungs.
- On monkey bars and jungle gyms, child attains and then holds upside down, curled up position while looking forward.

Cannot stand from back-lying position almost symmetrically by age 5½ or 6. Must turn nearly onto stomach or hands-knees position before reaching standing.

- From back-lying, child quickly jumps up and runs or moves to goal or target with minimal trunk rotation.
- From standing position, child stoops, reaches for object across midline, picks it up from floor, and returns to standing position.

Squirms or readjusts posture often in sitting position. Has difficulty sitting on unsteady or tipsy equipment, especially if not holding on.

- Child seat-walks on buttocks—race or stunt.
- Play musical chairs on tipsy seats, no hands.
- Partners sit back to back, lock elbows, then try to stand. Partners face each other, hold hands, and touch soles of feet while rocking far forward and backward.
- Child sits on and rides swing, seesaw, sliding board, barrel lying on its side, board with hubcap screwed under it so curve touches floor, scooterboard, one-rope swing.

Has difficulty balancing in hands and knees position on unsteady surface or in three-point position (one hand or foot raised), especially if head is turned toward one side.

- In hands-and-knees position, child rocks forward and backward, head facing forward. With forehead, child taps suspended ball so it hits target on wall or knocks over bowling pins on chair.
- Vary head position during hands-and-knees balance activities so eyes look at targets forward and at either side.
- In hands-and-knees position, child rocks side to side or uses one hand or knee to push ball or beanbag to goal.
- Place color card (or vocabulary word, letter or number) under each hand and knee. Instruct child to "lift yellow (or #7) hand (knee) and hold for 5 seconds." Advance to lifting two limbs, and later three.

If these behaviors are observed	*Try these activities, strategies, or materials*
Is unable to jump in place, climb stairs one foot per tread without holding on, squat or briefly tiptoe (approximately age 4).	• Child jumps off of short, then taller, objects, then jumps over flat, then taller, obstacles. • Child runs up incline and jumps off in various directions and postures. • All teachers and parents cooperate to remind child about one foot per stair tread. • Stunts or musical games encourage squatting (ducklike), walking on tiptoes (fairies and tall people), and jumping (over imaginary brooks, obstacles).
Cannot heel-toe walk, broad jump, hop on one foot briefly, descend stairs one foot per tread without holding on (approximately age 5).	• Play potato-on-a-spoon race, dodgeball with plastic beach ball, hopscotch with two feet and later one foot, potato sack race, hopping tag, and trampoline. • Child heel-toe walks on tape, fat rope, balance beam, and side of ladder.
Does not try roller skates, stilts, jump rope (approximately age 6). Cannot high jump 8 inches, broad jump 3 feet.	• Introduce skates, coffee-can stilts, wooden-pole stilts, jump rope (first teacher turns, later self-turning occurs).
Is unable to crouch on tiptoes (approximately age 8), jump clapping hands three times (approximately age 9), hop 50 feet in 5 seconds by age 12.	• Advanced balance beam activities. • Simple track and field events.
(If these advanced tasks are difficult for a child, return to "behaviors" and "activities" for younger children.)	

Coordination of the Two Body Sides

This skill indicates the body's motoric ability to function as a whole. Developing children first initiate purposeful movement with both arms/legs similarly, and later reciprocally (*i.e.*, with one limb after another in steady rhythm). Children also first perform movements without crossing the body's midline (a theoretical plane or line drawn from the center of the forehead straight down to a point between the feet), and later with midline crossing. It is recommended that training of motorically delayed children proceed in the same sequence. Children having good coordination of the two body sides have adequately established hand dominance with adequate assist by the nondominant hand; spontaneous crossing of the midline when appropriate; and smooth, coordinated patterns of walking, running, and skipping (within age expectancy).

If these behaviors are observed	*Try these activities, strategies, or materials*
Is unable to creep, tummy off floor, with opposing hand and knee moving almost simultaneously before the age of 12 months.	• Bunny hopping with two knees moving ahead simultaneously is an immature pattern that should be discouraged in the school-aged youngster. • Child creeps facing target at eye level, hands and tops of feet flat on floor, and pointing straight (not away from or toward midline of body). See *The Bender-Purdue Reflex Test and Training Manual*.[58]

If these behaviors are observed	*Try these activities, strategies, or materials*
	• As correct reciprocal pattern of arm/leg movement develops, add resistance to forward movement at the shoulders and ankles. Resist backward creeping at the buttocks. • Introduce puppy, kitty, and wild animal walks and races, and obstacle courses.
Walks and runs without opposing reciprocal arm and leg movements at age 4.	• If hands are held at shoulder level during walking/running, train balance skills. • Invert tricycle. Child rotates wheel with reciprocal hand motion on pedals. • Child pulls rope, hand-over-hand, to move gym scooter seat toward goal, to lift weighted pulley rope. "Pedal" gym scooter with hands moving reciprocally. • Introduce tricycles, pedal cars, Big Wheels, Sit 'n' Spin, Irishmail cart.
Cannot gallop, sashay, slide-step well, or skip with one foot only (lame duck skip) (approximately age 5).	• Encourage reciprocal hand and foot rhythms: xylophone, bongo drums, Ali Babba and the Forty Thieves, wheelbarrow walk, step-together-step sideways to music. • New skills may have to be taught and learned with two hands moving together first, later hands moving reciprocally. • Teach component skill parts of gallop, sashay, slide-step, lame duck skip, and crab walk.
Inaccurately imitates pantomimed midline crossing postures (approximately age 5). Avoids spontaneous midline crossing.	• Play Simon Says with midline crossing, Lummi sticks, crepe paper humming, lasso motions, target throws across midline (also during scooter rides), partner hand-clap games (Peas porridge, Miss Mary Mack, Oh Little Playmate, Pretty Little Dutch Girl), folk dancing steps (Heel-toe cross over; grapevine). • Hurry-Hurry Relay (team game: pass each of many items, two hands together, sideways to team mates until all items reach winning bucket). • Child taps suspended ball sideways with palms. Advance to backs of hands, then palms when arms crossed. • Child creeps along rope or line with knees straddling, hands crossed to opposite side. If necessary, give touch clue to indicate next hand movement.
Cannot skip alternately and exhibits much difficulty learning to throw a ball with proper weight shift onto foot opposite the throwing arm (approximately age 6½).	• Skipping: teach slow step-hop pattern on each foot. Place straight rope between feet, or place one foot on board, one foot on floor. Thus child can see and feel difference between the two feet and can begin to predict the feel of the slow step-hop rhythm. (If the board on which one foot practices step-hop is unsteady and clatters on the floor with each step-hop, it gives an additional auditory

If these behaviors are observed	*Try these activities, strategies, or materials*
	clue.) Teach reciprocal arm rhythm simultaneous to step-hop by moving arms correctly for the child.
	• Introduce component skills of throwing, pitching, and catching.
Has not established good hand dominance (approximately age 6½ or 7).	• Check for assymmetry of discrimination in identifying small objects by touch; in recognizing shapes drawn on hand; in recognizing which finger is touched. Train accordingly. (Hand that doesn't feel things adequately may "refuse" to accept dominant role.)
	• Check again for midline crossing. If each hand works independently only on its own side of the body, neither accepts dominant role.
Cannot perform good jumping jacks or tap floor alternately with feet (approximately age 7). Cannot hop alternately 2 right–2 left or 3 right–1 left foot patterns (approximately age 8). Cannot throw small ball 40 to 60 feet (approximately age 9).	• Child performs angels in snow, jumping jacks, and commando crawl (tummy touching floor) with variety of specified arm/leg movements.
	• Introduce advanced reciprocal hand/foot rhythms, slowly advancing up to need for balance while performing. Sample sequence: 2 right, 2 left rhythm on xylophone 2-2 stamp of feet while sitting 2-2 stamp of feet while standing 2-2 hop *once* while holding teacher's two hands 2-2 hop *once* without holding hands 2-2 hop several times, holding hands 2-2 hop several times, not holding hands
(If these advanced tasks are difficult for a child, return to "behaviors" and "activities" for younger children.)	• Child bounces ball in pattern or 2 right–2 left or 3 right–1 left.

Eye-Hand Coordination

Good eye-hand coordination is seen in the child who cuts, writes, works puzzles, manipulates small materials, and performs motor self-care activities age appropriately and with a good dominant/assistive hand use pattern. Behaviors are listed approximately by degree of difficulty (*i.e.*, in the sequence in which they are normally acquired). Success in more difficult classroom behaviors can be expected only if earlier levels have been mastered.

If these behaviors are observed	*Try these activities, strategies, or materials*
Is unable to focus on object with both eyes as it moves nearer to and farther from face (convergence).	• Teacher or other child slowly moves straw as child tries to put toothpick inside.
	• Child tries Forward Pass ball-on-rope toy by Developmental Learning Materials.[59]
Is unable to follow moving object (with eyes only, head not moving) thru 160° arc vertically, horizontally, diagonally, and in a circle. Eyes do not move smoothly and together. (Be sure visual acuity has	• Child tries ball activities using first balloons, large plastic beach balls, whiffle balls, and later large playground balls, then firmer balls, then smaller balls.

If these behaviors are observed	*Try these activities, strategies, or materials*
been examined. Persistent or exceptional ocular problems should be referred to a vision specialist.)	• Coat-hanger bats for balloons can be made by stretching nylon stockings over hanger pulled to square shape.
Does not poke finger into small hole. Is clumsy in picking up small items between thumb and index finger.	• Child places small objects into and "fishes" them out of small necked container. This can be timed. • Child tears—tissue (easiest), paper, manila folder, rag (hardest)—while holding between thumb and index finger. • Pinch and squeeze seeds or small discs (toward target), clothespins, and metal clips.
Has difficulty using wrist in side-to-side movements and palms-up/palms-down rotation. Grasps without wrist slightly extended.	• Child rings handbells, turns doorknobs, and unlocks with keys. • Child unscrews nuts and bolts, bicycle spokes from their end-casings or lids from small photo-film can containers.
Balances poorly on floor and chair so hands and forearms are not free to develop manipulative skills.	• Train sitting balance.

Has difficulty rolling clay into snake shape, later ball shape. Is clumsy when pasting, gluing, using even large paint brush, throwing ball with voluntary release. Displays generally inadequate eye-hand coordination in spite of adequacy in previously mentioned eye-hand behaviors.	• Child practices spreading fingers apart and squeezing them together while they are *straight*.*
	    squeeze tiny sponges, eye droppers between fingers
	    squeeze cardboard between straight fingers or finger and thumb so it cannot easily be pulled away
	    spread rubberband wide with straight fingers
	    suddenly spread apart straight fingers without moving wrist, and knock beads or blocks off desk.
	• Finger plays: Inky Dinky Spider; church and steeple.*
	• Child walks balloon up and down wall with fingertips. Advance to small plastic ball, Ping-Pong, golf, and playground balls.*
	• Look for body scheme difficulty and train accordingly.*
	• Introduce coloring accurately, dot-to-dot, tracing, mazes, lacing cards, pipe cleaners, beads, jacks, chalkboard road (trace on, wet fingers on, wet paintbrush on).†
	• Child glues outline of letters, then sprinkles on glitter.†
	• Squirts out lit candle with water pistol.†
	• Pastes tiny things accurately (*e.g.*, holes punched) using toothpicks.†
	• Try commercial games such as Perfection, Numbers Up, Drop in the Bucket, Pick Up Sticks, Operation, Etch a Sketch, Cross Fire.†

---

* Fine motor dexterity activities.
† Eye-hand coordination activities. (Can be adapted to all later age activities.)

If these behaviors are observed	*Try these activities, strategies, or materials*
	• Child traces on graph paper through empty squares as directed (right, left, up, down); guesses letter reproduced.† (Can be adapted to all later ages.)
Has not established use of one dominant hand at a time with other hand helping, for example, in stringing large beads, later small beads; folding paper with definite crease (although inaccurately).	• All of the above activities plus Origami paper folding. • Look for and train problems in coordination of two body sides.
Does not reach across midline of body spontaneously to pick up and put down objects.	• Look for and train problems in coordination of two body sides.
Has difficulty making tower of 9- or 10-inch-cubes or 3-cube bridge before age 4 or placing small pegs in pegboard holes.	• Child practices block building, pegboards, and copying simple models. • Look for and train visual perception problems.
Cannot copy │, –, or ○ holding crayon/pencil with appropriate grip and using good assistance of non-drawing hand before age 4.	• Use plastic, three-sided pencil grippers for correct and comfortable pencil position (from Developmental Learning Materials).[60] • Encourage correct grip in all pencil, crayon, and painting activities. • Move arm, later hand, through correct motion on chalkboard, paper, and fingerpaint.
Cannot unbutton accessible buttons before age 4.	• Emphasize self-help skills, breaking each into component parts.
Does not use hands reciprocally.	• Look for and train coordination of two body sides difficulty. • Child winds thread on spool evenly, sharpens pencil, uses manual egg beater.

Is unable to cut paper fringe before age 4. (All cutting activities are listed developmentally here. Actually more advanced cutting skills develop in conjunction with more advanced eye-hand coordination skills.)	• Use four-holed scissors that can be held by both child and teacher.
	• Introduce cutting tasks in sequence listed under Behaviors.
	• Encourage:
	  elbow near waist, not away from body
	  wrist slightly extended, not slightly flexed
	  palm facing midline or face, not floor
	  all fingers flexed while cutting, not extended and wide apart
	  scissors held comfortably and consistently in thumb-finger position, preferably near knuckle of thumb but near middle of middle finger
	  assisting hand adjusting paper position to scissors, not cutting hand adjusting position to paper.

Is unable to cut across paper, generally following straight, later curved line.	• Prevent jagged edges by placing paper against center of X of scissors.

† Eye-hand coordination activities. (Can be adapted to all later age activities.)

If these behaviors are observed	*Try these activities, strategies, or materials*
Is unable to cut out simple shapes having very wide outlines and no sharp angles.	• Child cuts *slowly,* down center of "road" (outline) while rotating paper *slowly* with nondominant hand. Success measured by half of "road" (outline) appearing on each side of cut.
Is unable to cut out small ○, △, ▭, ☐.	• Encourage accuracy.
Is unable to cut cloth.	• Grade up from thin to heavier cloth. Also try manila folder paper for heavy resistance.
Is unable to cut out complex pictures following outlines.	• Look for and train visual figure-ground problems.
Has great difficulty bouncing and catching large playground ball (approximately age 5); accurately tapping swinging suspended ball two out of five tries (approximately age 7).	• Teach handball skills in sequence of throw, catch, bounce and catch, toss and catch, and strike. • Teach foot-eye skills in sequence of kick nonmoving ball, kick moving ball, run and kick, and catch with feet.
Cannot put 10 pellets into bottle in 25 seconds before age 5; 20 coins into open box, one at a time, in 16 seconds (approximately age 7).	• Encourage speed of fine motor response.
Is unable to copy +, ╱, ╲, ▭, × (approximately age 7).	• Walk outlined shapes on floor. Then use templates of straight line plus simple geometric forms. Begin with chalkboard size; advance to desk size.
Cannot draw unmistakable six-part man including body (approximately age 5).	• Look for and train other indications of body image difficulties.
Cannot oppose thumb and each finger tip sequentially while looking at fingers, even slowly and with similar but incomplete movements of opposite hand (approximately age 5); is unable to do this competently—eyes open or closed with no overflow movements in the other hand (approximately age 7).	• Encourage competency, later speed in this skill.
With inch cubes, is unable to reproduce six-block pyramid and gate (approximately age 4½); copy △, ✶ (approximately age 6).	• Look for and train other indications of visual perception problems.
Hand dominance has not been established (approximately age 6½ or 7).	• Look for and train problems in coordination of two body sides.
Is unable to copy many letters and numbers (approximately age 6).	• Encourage correct position of pencil and child's body. Paper position may vary with child's hand preference, but should be consistent. Elbow should be abducted from body sufficiently to allow slight wrist extension (not flexion) while writing. • For most learning disabled children, cursive handwriting is easier to master than manuscript. • If child forms letters consistently better with eyes

If these behaviors are observed	*Try these activities, strategies, or materials*
	closed, allow child initially to learn feel of making each letter without the need for placing it on lines or tracing letter shapes. Later child can learn to visually direct hand. • Use salt tray, heavy crayon tracing, VAKT (Visual Auditory, Kinesthetic Tactile System developed by Fernald[61]). • Use Dubnoff School Programs 1, 2, and 3 by Teaching Resources Company.[62] • Read pages 107–122 in *Teaching Children with Learning and Behavior Problems.*[63]
Is unable to reproduce letters and numbers from memory.	• Encourage visual memory and imagery as well as adequate visual perception. • Read pages 191–247 in *Aids to Psycholinguistic Teaching.*[64] • Encourage right-left body part discrimination.
Has not resolved letter and number inversions (approximately age 6) or b-d, p-q reversals (approximately age 7). Tries to write or read in right to left direction. (If these advanced tasks are difficult for a child, return to "behaviors" and "activities" for younger children.)	• Mark frequently confused letters for easier discrimination, for example, put a "stinger" (ʮ) on all b's to represent buzzing bee. • Use nondominant index finger to point out direction of pencil movement, for example, left index finger points toward round movement for right hander's b (↦), 6 (◯), 3 (⌒). • Put arrow pointing to right in upper left-hand page corner indicating left-right progression.

References

1. Gilfoyle, E. M.: Training: Occupational Therapy Educational Management in Schools. OSERS Grant #G007801499. Rockville MD: American Occupational Therapy Association, Inc., 1980, Module 1, p. 3.
2. Flynn, S.: Pediatric care in occupational therapy in Ireland. And Davidson, J. E.: Ways in which occupational therapy involves the community in treatment. World Federation of Occupational Therapists Bulletin, 1980, vol. 5, pp. 9–13, 18–20.
3. Public Law 94-142 Education for All Handicapped Children Act. As reviewed in Legislative Alert. Rockville MD: American Occupational Therapy Association, Inc., 1975.
4. One Out of Ten: School Planning for the Handicapped. New York: Educational Facilities Laboratories, 850 Third Avenue, 1974.
5. Bateman, B.: So You're Going to a Hearing: Preparing for a Public Law 94-142 Due Process Hearing. Champaign IL: Research Press, 1981.
6. Gilfoyle, E. M.: Training: Occupational Therapy Educational Management in Schools. OSERS Grant #G007801499. Rockville MD: American Occupational Therapy Association, Inc., 1980, Module 1.
7. Gilfoyle, E. M.: Training: Occupational Therapy Educational Management in Schools. OSERS Grant #G007801499. Rockville MD: American Occupational Therapy Association, Inc., 1980, Module 6.
8. Clark, F.: Advanced Interpretation Course: Moving Beyond Preliminaries. Pasadena CA: Center for the Study of Sensory Integrative Dysfunction, 1980.
9. Newcomer, P., and Hammill, D.: ITPA and academic achievement: A survey. The Reading Teacher, May: 739, 1975.
10. Sternat, J., Nietupski, J., Lyon, J., Messina, R., and Brown, L.: Occupational and Physical Therapy Services for Severely Handicapped Students: Integrated vs Isolated Therapy Models. Federal Contract No. CEC-0-74-7993. Madison WI: Madison Public Schools, 1980.
11. Schleifer, M. (ed): The Exceptional Parent. 296 Boylston Street, Boston MA.
12. Stangler, S. R., Huber, C. J., and Routh, D. K.: Screening Growth and Development of Preschool Children: A Guide for Test Selection. New York: McGraw-Hill, 1980.
13. Lerner, J., Mardell-Czudnowski, C., and Goldenberg,

D.: Special Education for the Early Childhood Years. Englewood Cliffs NJ: Prentice-Hall, 1981, pp. 302–331.

14. Educational Staff of Chapel Hill: Critical Review of Commonly Used Preschool Assessment Intruments: Resource Guide for Health Care Coordinators. Chapel Hill NC: Resource Access Project, 1977.

15. Hainsworth, P., and Hainsworth, M.: Pre-School Screening System. 1974. Pre-School Screening, Box 1635, Pawtucket RI 02862.

16. Sanford, A. R.: Learning Accomplishment Profile and Manual. 600 Jonestown Road, Winston-Salem, North Carolina: Kaplan School Supply Corporation, 1974.

17. Beery, K. E., and Buktenica, N. A.: Developmental Test of Visual-Motor Integration. Chicago: Follett, 1967.

18. Kurko, V., Crane, L. L., and Willemin, H.: Preschool Screening Instrument, Forth Worth TX: Forth Worth Public Schools, 1973.

19. The Cornman Diagnostic Center Learning Disabilities Checklist for Kindergarten and 1st Grade, ed 2. Philadelphia: The School District of Philadelphia, 1975. Out of print; available from the author of this chapter.

20. Ayres, A. J.: Southern California Sensory Integration Tests. Los Angeles CA: Western Psychological Services, 1972.

21. Gillespie, P. H., and Johnson, L.: Teaching Reading to the Mildly Retarded Child. Columbus OH: Charles Merrill, 1974.

22. Sanford, E. M.: Learning Accomplishment Profile and Manual. 600 Jonestown Road, Winston-Salem NC: Kaplan School Supply Corporation, 1974.

23. Beery, K. E., and Buktenica, N. A.: Developmental Test of Visual-Motor Integration. Chicago: Follett Publishing Co., 1967.

24. Colarusso, R., and Hammill, D.: Motor-Free Visual Perception Test. San Rafael CA: Academic Therapy, 1972.

25. Bruininks, R.: Bruininks-Oseretsky Test of Motor Profiency. Circle Pines MN: American Guidance Service, 1978.

26. Lerner, J., Mardel-Czudnowski, C., and Goldenberg, D.: Special Education for the Early Childhood Years. Englewood Cliffs NJ: Prentice-Hall, 1981, pp. 302–331.

27. Gilfoyle, E. M.: Training: Occupational Therapy Educational Management in Schools. OSERS Grant No. G007801499. Rockville MD: American Occupational Therapy Association, 1980, Module 3, pp. 18–26.

28. Buros, O. K. (ed.): Mental Measurements Yearbook, Ed 1 to 7. Highland Park NJ: Gryphon Press.

29. Clark, F.: Advanced Interpretation Course: Moving Beyond Preliminaries. Pasadena CA: Center for the Study of Sensory Integrative Dysfunction, 1980.

30. American Occupational Therapy Association: Uniform Occupational Therapy Evaluation Checklist. Rockville MD: American Occupational Therapy Association, 1981.

31. Wilder, J. M., and Wall, C.: Pennsylvania's Preschool Pilot Individualized Educational Program. Harrisburg PA: CONNECT Division of Special Education, 1976.

32. Llorens, L. A., and Seig, K. W.: A Profile for Managing Sensory Integrative Test Data. Am. J. Occup. Ther. 29:205, 1975.

33. Ayres, A. J.: Southern California Sensory Integration Tests. Los Angeles: Western Psychological Services, 1972, p. 27.

34. Accardo, P. J.: A Neurodevelopmental Perspective on Specific Learning Disabilities. Baltimore MD: University Park Press, 1980.

35. Sieben, R. L.: Controversial Medical Treatments of Learning Disabilities. Academic Therapy 13:133–147, 1977.

36. Lehrer, R. J.: An open letter to an occupational therapist. J. Learn. Disabilities 14:3–4, 1981.

37. Ayres, A. J.: A response to defensive medicine. Academic Therapy 13:149–152, 1977.

38. Ayres, A. J.: Improving academic scores through sensory integration. J. Learn. Disabilities 5:24–28, 1972.

39. Ayres, A. J.: The Effect of Sensory Integrative Therapy on Learning Disabled Children. Pasadena CA: Center for the Study of Sensory Integrative Dysfunction, 1976.

40. White, M.: A first-grade intervention program for children at risk for reading failure. J. Learn. Disabilities 12:231–237, 1979.

41. Cratty, B. J.: Motor development for special populations: Issues, problems, and operations. Focus on Exceptional Children 13:1–11, 1980.

42. Kauffman, N. A., Kinnealey, M. S., and Gressang, J. D.: The Role of Occupational Therapy in the Education of the Learning Disabled Student. Philadelphia PA: Cornman Diagnostic Center, 1980. Out of print; available from the author of this chapter.

43. Silver, L. B.: Acceptable and controversial approaches to treating the child with learning disabilities. Pediatrics 55:406, 1975.

44. Hammill, D. D.: Thoughts to consider before beginning a visual perception program. In Hammill, D. D., and Bartel, N. R.: Teaching Children with Learning and Behavior Problems. Boston: Allyn and Bacon, Inc., 1975.

45. Clark, F., Mailloux, Z., and Parham, D.: The Art of Therapy. Pasadena CA: The Center for the Study of Sensory Integrative Dysfunction, 1981.

46. Haslam, H. A., and Valletutti, P. J. (eds.): Medical Problems in the Classroom. Baltimore: University Park Press, 1975, pp. 294–297.

47. Lecky, P.: Drug Management and Survival Techniques for Parents and Teachers. Lecture during Programming for Learning Disabilities Conference. Philadelphia: St. Joseph's College, 1974.

48. Murray, J. M.: Is there a role for the teacher in the use of medication for hyperkinetics. J. Learn. Disabilities 9:30, 1976.

49. Ibid.

50. O'Leary, K. D., and O'Leary, S. G.: Classroom Management: The Successful Use of Behavior Modification. Elmsford NY: Pergamon Press, 1972.

51. Stephens, T. M.: Directive Teaching of Children with Learning and Behavioral Handicaps. Columbus OH: Charles Merrill, 1970.
52. A Newsletter for the School-Based Therapist, P.O. Box 3772, Amity Station, New Haven CN 06525, Synops Publishing Co.
53. Campbell, S. K. (ed.): Physical and Occupational Therapy in Pediatrics. 149 Fifth Avenue, NY, NY 10010, The Haworth Press.
54. Kratoville, B. L. (ed.): Academic Therapy. 20 Commercial Boulevard, Novato CA, Academic Therapy Publications, Inc.
55. Senf, G. M. (ed.): Journal of Learning Disabilities. 101 East Ontario Street, Chicago IL 60611, The Professional Press, Inc,
56. Lyon, S., and Lyon, G.: Team functioning and staff development: A role release approach to providing integrated educational services for severely handicapped students. J. Assoc. Severely Handicapped 5:250–263, 1980.
57. Cratty, B.: Developmental Sequences of Perceptual-Motor Tasks. Freeport NY: Educational Activities, 1967.
58. Bender, M.: The Bender-Purdue Reflex Test and Training Manual. PO Box 899, San Rafael CA, Academic Therapy Publications, 1975.
59. Developmental Learning Materials. 7440 Natchez Avenue, Niles IL 60648.
60. Ibid.
61. Fernald, G.: Remedial Techniques in Basic School Subjects. New York: McGraw-Hill, 1943.
62. Dubnoff School Programs 1, 2, and 3. 100 Boylston Street, Boston, Teaching Resources Corporation, 1975.
63. Hammill, D., and Bartel, N.: Teaching Children with Learning and Behavior Problems. Boston: Allyn and Bacon, 1975.
64. Bush, W. I., and Giles, M.: Aids to Psycholinguistic Teaching. Columbus OH: Charles E. Merrill Co., 1969.

Acknowledgments

The author wishes to acknowledge the support and assistance of Cheryl Elizabeth, Richard and Philip, and to thank Thomas DiRenzo, physical education teacher, for his contributions to the game and activity suggestions.

CHAPTER 34

Gerontology   *Linda A. Johnson*

Defining Practice Area

Scientific investigations of the aging process and study of the social consequences of aging populations are to a great extent phenomena of the post-World War II era. The definition of gerontology is literally the study of later maturity and old age in its biological, psychological, and sociological aspects. The term gerontologist is applied to those educators and researchers who study problems of aging as they are currently manifested.

Those who deal primarily with the elderly in their practice are usually called gerontologists only when they also conduct research on problems of aging encountered with their clients. The term geriatrics, which specifically refers to the physiology and pathology of old age, has traditionally been used to describe this field of occupational therapy. With the research of Lorna Jean King, Mary Reilly, and others, which has expanded the boundaries of our practice, there is considerable evidence to support the use of the broader term gerontology.

Occupational therapists utilize a medical model of practice but expand its parameters to include the concept of normalization. This implies an abililty to enable a client to grow, adapt, change, and move toward self-directed behavior and independence of function. Within this process, accepting necessary limitations of chronic disability, the therapist's role is that of a facilitator who enables the individual to make his or her own decisions on goals, assures an awareness of realistic alternatives, and assists him or her in achievement of goals. The therapist does not impose values but assists the individual to function as independently as possible within his or her own cultural system and physical limitations. Each elderly person has his or her own readiness to capitulate to disability. Given the same degree of disability, some choose independence, to whatever degree it is possible, while others prefer the security of a protective environment.

Therapists in this field work within the framework established by current gerontological theories and the public policies that they determine. The philosophical bases of occupational therapy enable the occupational therapist to make a unique contribution to this field. Unlike other disciplines, which develop theories describing society, occupational therapy seeks individualized and client-oriented solutions to problems.[1] There is a real question as to whether the former approach does not, by its very nature, predetermine the outcome of intervention, resulting in a self-fulfilling prophecy; whereas the latter approach allows intervention to be flexible, based on individual needs, choices, and possible solutions to problems. Publicizing the results of this therapeutic approach can influence both the theories and the public policies toward realistic and constructive change. Within the past five years, legislators in many states have introduced legislation to broaden the application of publicly provided services for the elderly to permit true alternatives to nursing home admission, enabling the frail elderly to live independently for longer periods with supportive services in the home. Oregon's Senator Packwood has introduced a bill in the Senate (1981) to establish, under the Social Security Act, a ten-state, six-year, demonstration program to test implementation of an organized system of noninstitutional, long-term care services.

Attitudes Toward Aging

Our youth-oriented, technological society has, by its very nature, created some of the problems of aging. Rapid technological advances have made obsolete many of the skills accumulated by our elders in their lifetime. The young tend to ignore their counsel. A transient population has been destructive to the three-generation family concept, so that young people often have no intimate contact with old people.

The mass media projection of the "young is beautiful" concept implies, when it is not stated overtly, that "old is ugly." We are told to get rid of that gray in our hair, prevent wrinkles in our skin, use the toothpaste, deodorant, or soap that will keep us sexually attractive. Even Geritol is advertised by the young and beautiful. Old people are often pictured as cranky, demanding, incompetent, and ill.

Current attitudes still closely resemble those reflected in the 1952 study done by Tuckman and Lorge.[2] They asked one group of young people and another of old people to describe old age. *Both groups* characterized old people as economically insecure, in poor health, lonely, resistant to change, and failing in physical and mental powers. When these attitudes are coupled with the concrete facts of our inflationary economy with high unemployment, it is not surprising to note some antagonism in the controversy over retirement age or opposition to increasing benefits for the aged. Alex Comfort wrote that "Unique to our culture is its rejection of the old, their exclusion from work and their accustomed social space, their premature burial by society as 'unpeople', and a rich and erroneous folklore of mental decline, infirmity, asexuality, ineducability, and the normality of causeless mental disorder in the old. Shared, unfortunately by the old themselves and by physicians, both mental and physical ill health are seen as requiring no explanation provided the subject is 'old.'"[3]

Theories of Aging

Sociologists, psychologists, and biologists have produced theories to explain what they see as phenomena of later adulthood and old age. An understanding of these theories is helpful in understanding both the basis of public policy and the rationale behind much research in gerontology. Some of the major theories are touched on in this section.

Sociology

The *disengagement theory of aging* was one of the first theories developed by sociologists and has been a center of controversy ever since.[4] It states that there is a gradual, mutual withdrawal or disengagement of the individual and society from each other, and that this is a natural and inevitable process which continues until the final withdrawal into death. This theory has been repeatedly questioned and challenged by gerontologists.

The *continuity theory* is based on the assumption that identity is a function of relations and interactions with other people.[5] Individuals who are most successful continue to maintain interaction with society after retirement, involving themselves in appropriate community, family, and interpersonal relationships. They continue to maintain both identity and ego strength.

The *activity theory* is closely related to the continuity theory, and, with that theory, is accepted increasingly as research supplies more supporting evidence.[6] It suggests that the majority of aging persons maintain fairly constant levels of activity and engagement with society and that the amount of engagement or disengagement is more influenced by past lifestyle and socioeconomic forces than by any inevitable biologic or psychologic force within either society or the individual. It proposes that maintaining or developing substantial levels of physical, mental, and social activity contributes to successful aging.

Psychology

The *psychoanalytic view* states that the sense of identity established in early life produces consistent behavior throughout life, that character structure becomes relatively fixed in early adulthood, and that, even though the ego becomes an increasingly strong change agent, the essential nature of the personality remains stable.[7] Jung and Erikson took exception to this theory. Jung described the increase in introversion in middle and late life, and the reorganization of value systems. Erikson outlined eight stages of ego development in life, each representing a crisis or choice for ego development. Erikson's eight stages of development are the following:[8]

1. Development in the infant of a sense of trust versus distrust
2. Development in later infancy of a growing sense of autonomy versus a sense of shame and doubt
3. Development in early childhood of a sense of initiative versus a sense of guilt
4. Development in middle childhood of a sense of industry versus a sense of inferiority
5. Development in adolescence of a sense of ego identity versus role confusion
6. Development in early adulthood of intimacy versus ego isolation
7. Development in middle adulthood of generativity (expanding ego interests and a sense of contributing to the future) versus ego stagnation
8. Development in late adulthood of a sense of ego integrity (a basic acceptance of one's life as having been inevitable, appropriate, and meaningful) versus a sense of despair, equated with a fear of death

Peck felt that Erikson's eight stages should be expanded, that his sixth and seventh stages cannot successfully be deferred beyond the age of 30, leaving the eighth stage to represent in a "global, nonspecific way all the psychological crises and crisis–solutions of the last 40 or 50 years of life.[9] He suggests four stages that occur in middle age and three in old age. Peck's stages in middle age are the following:[10]

1. Valuing wisdom versus valuing physical powers, using the wisdom gained through the lifetime's experience to accomplish a good deal more than younger people in a different way to compensate for waning physical powers
2. Socializing versus sexualizing in human relationships, redefining men and women as individuals and companions, the sexual element becoming decreasingly significant
3. Cathectic flexibility versus cathectic impoverishment or the ability to shift emotional investments from one person to another or from one activity to another
4. Mental flexibility versus mental rigidity. This critical issue may arise in middle age when individuals have reached peak status, have worked out the answers to life, and may be tempted to avoid further effort to devise new or different solutions

Peck's stages in old age are the following:[11]

5. Ego differentiation versus work–role preoccupation, frequently precipitated by retirement,

necessitating development of alternatives that can produce a sense of satisfaction and worth.
6. Body transcendence versus body preoccupation, or the ability to create satisfying relationships and develop creative activity of an intellectual nature to combat the tendency to preoccupation with bodily ills.
7. Ego transcendence versus ego preoccupation, the development of an awareness of the enduring significance of one's achievements as contributions to the future to overcome an inward preoccupation and withdrawal

Social psychologists have other theories such as that of Brim, who argued that there are no personality dispositions that are persistent across situations, that personality can be defined as the sum of social experiences and social roles.[12] Another approach, represented by Schaie, suggests that we should look to social and historical contexts more than to developmental processes for explaining differences between age groups.[13]

Biology

Biological theories of aging deal largely with attempts to discover causes for cellular deterioration resulting in the various aspects of biological aging.[14] Scientific knowledge has become so extensive that simple explanations no longer suffice. One theory considers the question of whether the aging process constitutes deliberate biological programming or if the present life span of an individual is all that can be expected, considering the chemical complexities of the human being. Another is that of the accumulation of copying errors, which holds that the individual eventually dies because cells develop copying errors, and those errors in copying, in turn, reduce metabolic efficiency and interfere with the capacity for repair.

Normal Aging and Development in Late Life

Social and Economic Status

In spite of negative societal images of aging, social losses, and economic constraints that are sometimes severe, the majority of our aging population are coping more or less adequately with the numerous crises of late life. Ninety-five percent of individuals over the age of 65 are living outside of institutions. In 1974, 30% of individuals over 65 were employed.[15] Brickfield reported that in 1978 only 14% of the elderly population were living below the poverty level, compared with 25% in 1970. He divided the over-65 population into the 'enjoyers,' the 'survivors,' and the 'casualties.' The 'enjoyers' had incomes over $8,000 with assets of $26,000 or more. Twenty-seven percent fit into this category, 46% of them women. 'Survivors,' 61% of this population, are "balancing between longevity and resources." Only 12% were termed 'casualties,' the group described as crushed by the difficulties of old age.

Personal adjustment for the aged requires finding self-fulfillment through socially accepted means. Tibbitts lists the needs of the aged as follows:[16]
1. To render some socially useful service
2. To be considered a part of the community
3. To occupy increased leisure time in satisfying ways
4. To enjoy normal companionships
5. To achieve recognition as an individual
6. To have opportunities for self-expression and a sense of achievement
7. To receive health protection and care
8. To experience suitable mental stimulation
9. To have suitable living arrangements and family relationships
10. To find spiritual satisfaction

To satisfy these needs, which he also describes as rights, Tibbitts identifies certain obligations which must be fulfilled earlier in life:[17]
1. To become and resolve to remain active, alert, capable, self-supporting, and useful as long as circumstances permit, and to plan for retirement
2. To learn and apply sound principles of physical and mental health
3. To develop potential avenues of service after retirement
4. To share with others the benefits of one's experience and knowledge
5. To adapt to changes that age will bring
6. To maintain constructive and pleasant relationships with family, neighbors, and friends

Dr. Richard Besdine stated in a 1981 lecture that of all the old people ever born who lived to 65 years the majority are living now.[18] The number of people aged 85 or older has increased 209% in the past 25 years and will increase 84% in the next 25 years. By the year 2000, 70% of a physician's time will be spent treating patients over the age of 65.

Development in Late Life

Closely related to the psychoanalytic view of development represented here by Erikson and Peck are the contributions of a group, largely psychologists, developed in a series of West Virginia University Life-Span Development Conferences.[19] The fourth conference, held in 1975, represented an attempt to bridge the gap between theorist and practitioner, and included contributors from many related fields. They defined human development as the process that occurs between conception and death, reflecting the efforts of the individual to reconcile himself or herself to the two poles of his or her existence.[20] The study of life–span development is limited by the breadth of its scope, including as it does, social, economic, political, and historical influences, as well as by time constraints, acknowledging that "in the long run, we are all short term." Indication of change and growth in individuals past middle age is of particular significance for therapists working with the elderly. Riegel feels that crises, conflicts, and contradictions throughout the life span ought to be regarded as constructive confrontations and the basis for development rather than in a negative manner as causes for disruption.[21]

Lieberman describes intact survival as the ability to maintain the same level of competence and behavior after a crisis as before.[22] He points out that this is survival, not necessarily bliss. Those elderly who were able to maintain a consistent and coherent self–image remained intact. Survival techniques and characteristics in old age differ from those of other stages. They include possessing an adequate level of cognitive and physical resources to bring to bear on crisis management. The degree of environmental change is directly related to the adaptive demands required for change, and consequently, to the degree of stress. Growing old gracefully, he says, is an invention of the poets, rather than an adequate guide to survival. The older person relies less on social strengths learned earlier and is forced to use his own introspective resources. The individual who is aggressive, irritating, narcissistic, and demanding is more likely to survive than the passive, accepting "good guy." Survivors may have a pugnacious, even suspicious stance toward the world, perceive themselves as the center of the universe, but maintain crucial skills for appraising their environment. Dylan Thomas might have been describing survival when he wrote the lines: "Do not go gentle into that good night; Rage, rage against the dying of the light."

Sexuality in Aging

This subject rates a separate section, not because it is really different from sexuality at any other age, but because our society thinks it is. Actions considered normal in a 35 or 40-year-old are considered deviant in a person in his or her 70s. "A dirty old man" is usually an elderly man expressing normal sexual interest in a woman, be she young or his own age.

Kinsey and Masters and Johnson all report sexual activity continuing into the 70s, and less frequently, into the 80s, despite the general metabolic decline and lowered thyroid function that diminish production of sex hormones as aging progresses. Sexuality, in its more general sense of sexual identity, has implications in interpersonal relations. It continues as a vital force as long as an individual maintains contact with reality, and to some degree as long as life persists. An attractive appearance, and its recognition by others, is important to sustain this sexual identity in the frail elderly, as it is for everyone. With progressive diminution of sight, hearing, and touch sensitivity, the person's intimate and social spaces shrink. For example, at the normal distance for social interaction, a hearing impaired person cannot hear; a visually impaired person may not perceive facial features. As a result of these deficits, the individual often is hypersensitive, and feels he or she is a bother to others with nothing interesting to offer to a relationship. Response to the frail elderly requires tact, respect, awareness, and a belief in the innate value of human beings regardless of age.

Inappropriate sexual behavior, particularly within institutions, can arise in response to a number of causes, from boredom to a cry for attention and recognition as a person. It can usually be eliminated by appropriate recognition of its cause and acceptance by staff of the normal sexual needs of residents. Complaints are frequently heard of masturbating in public areas, which may be solved by permitting masturbation in the resident's room in private. "Pawing" of female staff members by male residents can be handled by a calm, nonjudgmental statement of expectations, with the recognition that touch is as natural to the aged man as to his younger counterpart. It is important that the staff of the institution be aware of the socially deprived nature of the residents' environment.

The aging homosexual person is becoming a more visible consideration in this field, about whom little has been written to date. Social attitudes may create special problems for the homosexual, not only in adjustment, but in accessibility of services.

Aging and Disease
Vulnerability to Disease

Old age should not be equated with disability and disease. Loss of function is caused by disease, not old age.[23] Over three quarters of the elderly population describe themselves as well in spite of one or more chronic conditions they have learned to live with. There are normal decrements in body tissues with increased age, but these occur within the individual's

reserve capacity rather than in the *front line critical functions*.[24] Vulnerability to illness is increased. Reduced function of liver, kidneys, and other organs, including resting cardiac output, lowered maximum breathing capacity, and reduced metabolism, slowing of reflexes (including righting reflexes), and gradual sensory losses increase the susceptibility of the elderly to the effects of disease and reduce their tolerance to drugs, including alcohol. They are especially vulnerable to drug intoxication, dizziness, and falling, the dangerous consequences of stimulus deprivation and depression. In addition, the symptoms of disease in the aged are often blurred and nonspecific, and consequently make diagnosis difficult and very easy to ignore. The term *senility* is defined as the gradual loss of physical or mental function and well-being of an elderly person.[25] It describes a condition that in infants is called *failure to thrive*, and is cause for active intervention. Unlike the case of infants, in the aged, diagnostic efforts are often neglected because "at that age what else can you expect?" Adequate recognition of what is now considered the normal physiology of aging can prevent or cure many of the disabilities commonly considered inevitable to the aging process. It is especially important for physicians and health care practitioners to use this knowledge.

Physiological Impairment

Physiological decrements of the normal aging process predispose the elderly to specific diseases that are considered "diseases of the aged." Among these are minor cerebral infarction, stroke, hypothermia, which often masquerades as stroke, hypertension, hypothyroidism, osteoporosis, arthritis, Parkinsonism, myocardial infarction, mild, late-onset diabetes, pneumonia, drug intoxication, depression, and dementia. In addition, tuberculosis is now considered a disease of old age, usually occurring as reactivation of old disease.[26] Glaucoma, untreated in younger years, is a leading cause of blindness in the elderly. Malnutrition is also a frequent problem due to a multitude of factors.

The aged, of course, are also subject to the same diseases that occur at any age. With this group of diseases as well as with those listed previously, diagnosis is often complicated by the presentation of nonspecific symptoms and the likelihood of multiple pathologies.[27] Nonspecific symptoms may include any or all of the following: refusal to eat, headache, dizziness and falling, loss of mobility, new incontinence, withdrawal, acute confusion, worsening dementia, and failure to thrive (senility). Besdine mentioned, in a series of studies done in England and the United States, that 80% of patients over 70 with myocardial infarction had no chest pain. Thirty percent presented only the symptom of confusion or dementia. Dementia has been present before blood tests revealed the diagnosis of anemia, and may be the only symptom of drug intoxication, depression, metabolic disorders, hypothyroidism, and a host of other pathologies. Other reversible causes of dementia are congestive heart failure, infections with fever (especially urinary infections, tuberculosis, and bacterial endocarditis), subdural or epidural hematomas, chronic pain, sensory deprivation (especially poor hearing), and hypoglycemia.[27] Alex Comfort notes that "old people who 'become crazy' do so because they have always been crazy, because they are sick, or because we drive them crazy."[28] Palmore warns, "The belief that mental illness in old age is inevitable, untreatable, disabling, and irreversible becomes a self-fulfilling prophecy."[29] It leads to lack of prevention and treatment, which in turn confirms the belief.

Intellectual Impairments

Recent research into the causes of dementia was prompted by recognition that up to 80% of nursing home residents are diagnosed as having chronic brain syndrome, organic brain syndrome, dementia, senility, senile dementia, or confusion, in varying degrees. Researchers identified a similarly large population in the community. They project a rapid increase of the problem in the future, based on statistical projections of the rising percentage of aged in the population and their increased longevity. Jarvik estimates that dementia will reach epidemic proportions by the year 2000 unless means are discovered to reverse the disease processes.[30] Results of that research have clarified terminology and emphasized the importance of recognizing those dementias that are reversible.

The terms *chronic brain syndrome* and *organic brain syndrome* are equivalent to dementia and describe the irreversible, organic brain damage which is characterized by a slowly progressive loss of mental capacity including memory, orientation, and ability to do serial tasks. Reversible dementias have the same characteristic symptoms, but are caused by a variety of conditions that timely treatment may relieve or cure. Confusion is a minor delerium usually induced by disease or a traumatic change in living conditions. This clears fairly rapidly with treatment. Senile dementia is usually synonymous with dementia, but is occasionally used interchangeably with senility. Senility is probably the most misused term applied to the elderly, often signalling lack of proper diagnosis and treatment.

Dementia

Dementia occurs in 10% of the elderly population and is seriously disabling in 5%.[31] Of the 10% of dementia cases, from 10% to 30% would be reversible if treated in time. The major cause of reversible dementia is drug intoxication. Tolerance to drugs is reduced in the elderly. Their proneness to multiple pathologies results in 12% of the population taking from 25% to 30% of the prescription drugs in this country. In addition, they take 40% of all over-the-counter drugs, and borrow some from neighbors.[32] Krupka refers to studies that show the greatest danger is in self-administration of drugs at home. Investigators found that three drugs are the most that an elderly person can manage correctly.[32] Besdine recommends that normal drug dosage should be reduced by 10% for every decade over 40 to allow for the normal aging body's decreasing tolerance to drugs.[33] Drugs particularly likely to cause dementia include barbiturates, antihypertensive drugs, diuretics, and tranquilizers, especially Valium.[34] All of these drugs are commonly used by the elderly. Krupka emphasizes that adverse drug reactions accelerate with increased drug exposure as in the use of long-term prescriptions for chronic conditions.[35] Of hospital patients he studied, receiving at least six different drugs, 81.4% had adverse drug reactions. These are caused by age-related differences in absorption, distribution, metabolism, excretion, and in alterations of drug action at receptor sites. Drug intoxication, disease processes, pseudodementia (which is a manifestation of depression), "nursing home disease," and occasionally misdiagnosed psychiatric illness, account for the 10% to 30% of dementias that are reversible.

"Nursing home disease" is a type of pseudodementia.[36] This may result from a combination of boredom, lack of demand, social deprivation, and chemical restraint by overdose of tranquilizers given for the convenience of untrained staff and to prevent complaints. It is reversible by withdrawal of medication and restitution of social responsibilities. Untreated, it rapidly becomes a true dementia. As a manifestation of depression, pseudodementia has a characteristic difference from true dementia. The patient may complain of severe cognitive loss, but when pressed to perform, improves considerably. In true dementia, the patient attempts to gloss over deficits and, when pushed to perform, deteriorates in performance.

Differential diagnosis of dementia includes a large battery of tests to identify disease processes and drug intoxication, including computed tomography (CT scan) to identify brain pathology.[37] Brain atrophy that may show up is not necessarily symptomatic. Some brain atrophy is normal in aging and does not affect brain function. Tests should also include a mental status exam. Besdine feels the mental status exam is an essential part of the yearly physical exam for early recognition of cognitive changes. The exam includes items to test orientation, memory (both recent and remote), simple arithmetic calculations, language usage, and any recent change in social functioning, judgment, and abstract thinking.[38] Of these, judgment may be the critical factor in determining whether or not an individual can continue to live alone.

The Diagnostic and Statistical Manual of the American Psychiatric Association, Third Edition (DSM III), lists two major causes of the organic, irreversible dementias.[39] They are primary degenerative dementia or senile dementia, Alzheimer type (SDAT), and multi-infarct dementia. Post mortem study has shown that brain pathology of primary degenerative dementia is identical with Alzheimer's presenile dementia, though its onset occurs later in life. Researchers are working on the theory that it may be caused by a virus or a deficit in brain chemistry, so that in the future it may be treatable. It has an insidious onset and a uniformly progressive, deteriorating course. Multi-infarct dementia, in contrast, is caused by strokes, which cause deterioration of personality and intellect, and causes stepwise deterioration in intellectual function rather than a uniformly progressive one, with some intellectual functions relatively intact early in its course. Focal neurological signs and symptoms are present. There are other minor causes of irreversible dementia such as alcoholic dementia, which remains stable if the patient stops drinking, dementia following head trauma, dementia following anoxia, and dementias concurrent with specific neurological diseases including Huntington's chorea and Parkinson's disease.

Depression

Depression is the commonest disease in old age, being clinically present in 20% to 45% of people over 65. "Age in our culture is depressing," to quote Comfort, and the aged also have an endogenous predisposition to depression.[40] It may be confined to somatic complaints of backache, fatigue, or cancer phobia, or may be visible as pseudodementia. It is the most likely underlying cause of otherwise unexplained sudden or gradual downhill changes. It is a medical emergency for two reasons: (1) because of the high risk of suicide or death from "giving up," and (2) because it is treatable, often with spectacular results. The highest suicide rate in the world is for male

Caucasions over the age of 80. Women attempt suicide oftener but are not as likely to succeed. Suicide threats from this age group must always be taken seriously. Depression may be accompanied by acute anxiety, confusion, or fear of losing one's mind. These manifestations are especially associated with a move to unfamiliar surroundings. Unexplained withdrawal and apathy, loss of appetite, unusual hypochondria, increased irritability, early waking, and other sleep disturbances may all be symptomatic of depression. Psychiatrists say that one way to identify depressed people is that they are depressing. Because of its tremendous influence on the quality of life, if for no other reason, depression should always be treated.

Other Affective Disorders

Paranoia is a frequent diagnosis that may accompany mania or depression, or may stand alone.[41] It should be distinguished from well-founded anger, frustration, and suspicion of relatives as well as from symptoms of sensory deprivation, especially poor hearing. Paranoid ideas also serve to fill in gaps caused by sensory or cortical defects to "make sense of the senseless." Carefully monitored medication may relieve symptoms.

Abnormal behavior of many varieties may increase under pressure of societal rejection. Self-neglect may result in a gradual increase of weakness and confusion. Loss of morale is inherent in the concept of senility. At all other ages, society tends to support the attempts of the patient to cope. In old age, society promotes the propriety and naturalness of decline. A hardy individual can resist this pressure, but any symptoms of impairment increase the anxiety that society may be right after all. In old age, we see the syndrome of self-willed death, which otherwise is confined to believers in sorcery.

The Occupational Therapist in Gerontology

Wiemer's chart on Traditional and Nontraditional Practice Arenas (1978) lists the roles of Occupational Therapist, Registered (OTR) and Certified Occupational Therapy, Assistant (COTA) as follows: OTR— professional clinician, educator, administrator, researcher, academician, consultant; COTA—technical clinician, administrator, consultant, educator.[42] The role of the COTA is expanding rapidly in the profession, and this is certainly true in gerontology practice. The term "occupational therapist" refers to both OTR and COTA, the difference being in the professional and technical level of application of occupational therapy techniques.*

The occupational therapist is concerned with three aspects of health care for the aged: preventive care, acute care, and chronic or long-term care. There are an increasing number of job opportunities for therapists in all three areas, although not all are specifically designated as occupational therapy positions, and some require additional training.

Preventive Care

Multiservice centers offer social and recreational opportunities for elders and are usually housed with a variety of other services such as legal aid, nursing clinics, Housing and Urban Development offices, income tax consultants, and other appropriate services. They serve as community centers for senior citizens. Directors of these centers could appropriately be occupational therapists. The centers provide an excellent opportunity for community education on health, nutrition, and safety measures to aid in prevention of illness and accidents as well as promote physical and mental health.

Hospital discharge planners act as liaison with the community when a patient is discharged from the hospital, contacting community agencies that provide appropriate follow-up care in the patient's community. Such agencies as senior citizens' centers, hot lunch programs, Meals on Wheels, Visiting Nurse Association, home health agencies, and homemaker services can assist in completing the patient's rehabilitation and aid in maintenance of independence. Planners frequently make home visits to determine the adequacy of the home environment. An occupational therapist is well qualified for this role.

Home health aide training is done in Oregon for the State Department of Health by occupational therapists. The therapists provide the same type of training given to restorative aides in nursing homes: range of motion, ADL techniques, transfer and gait-training techniques, basic nutritional principles, and safety measures.

Preretirement planning is another area occupational therapists are entering. In increasing numbers, corporations, unions, businesses, and continuing education centers are offering courses for individuals to

begin planning for the economic, social, and leisure changes after retirement.

Planning housing for older people is an area with great potential for occupational therapists. Elimination of architectural barriers, planning work areas suitable for the disabled (particularly kitchen and laundry areas), providing protective devices such as appropriate doorknobs for the arthritic or feeble, and compensating for poor eyesight with well-lighted stairs, handrails, and well-marked top and bottom steps are considerations unknown or overlooked by most architects and builders. While initially these devices are no more expensive than ordinary construction, they can be quite costly later. There is a desperate need for appropriate housing for the partially disabled within the community.

Public education opportunities are exemplified by the Seattle therapist who worked with a video tape expert from a local public broadcasting station. They investigated the possibility of using video tapes to involve tenants of a high rise residence for the elderly in discussion of the change of pace and lifestyle that benefit the arthritic and to demonstrate protective devices to prevent deformities.

Acute Care

Hospitals and stroke care units are a familiar site in which occupational therapists treat the aged. These roles are discussed elsewhere in this text.

Home health agencies, and Visiting Nurse Associations are established under Medicare to meet federal guidelines, though they are not limited to Medicare patients. They provide at least two services, nursing plus one or more of the following: occupational therapy, physical therapy, speech–language pathology therapy, and social work. Some are associated with county or state health departments or local hospitals. They are limited to the treatment of the homebound patient, providing essentially the same services as those available in rehabilitation centers, and can also provide any special equipment needed for the patient. In addition to filling a therapist's regular role, the occupational therapist with some administrative training could initiate and direct a home health agency. (See Chapters 36 and 37 on Home Health).

Arthritis treatment centers, found in hospitals, clinics, outpatient centers, or doctors' offices, should include occupational therapy. The therapist's interpretation, in concrete terms in a living situation, of the doctor's prescription for a balanced regime of rest and exercise is often critical to success for the client. Ability to teach human energy-saving methods of performing everyday living and housekeeping tasks and to point out simple adaptations that can be

---

* Project to Delineate the Roles and Functions of Occupational Therapy Personnel in the Detail Needed to Serve as a Basis for the Construction of Proficiency Examinations. Department of Health, Education and Welfare, Public Health Services, National Institute of Health, Bureau of Health Manpower Education, Division of Allied Health Manpower, Contract No. NO 1 AH 24172. Washington, D.C.: American Occupational Therapy Association, 1973.

made in the household and new ways of performing familiar tasks can be the means of preventing otherwise inevitable deformities.

State receiving hospitals and crisis care units for the treatment of acute psychiatric problems are also familiar to occupational therapists. Their role in these settings is discussed elsewhere and is virtually the same as for other age groups.

Detoxification centers are growing in number in urban areas to treat the acute stages of alcoholism. Many of their patients are aged. There is an increasing recognition of the role occupational therapists can play in the evaluation and treatment of the alcoholic.

Chronic Care

Rehabilitation institutes and skilled care facilities, formerly called extended care facilities, actually fall between the areas of acute and chronic care. Occupational therapists are well recognized as part of the rehabilitation team. The aged form a large part of their patient population. Therapists should assume responsibility for ensuring good follow-up care for these patients when they are discharged.

Nursing homes providing skilled and intermediate care are required to have a full-time activity director. Few nursing homes have an OTR on their staff, although many have recognized the advantages of hiring certified occupational therapy assistants. OTR's often act as consultants to the COTA or activity director, provide inservice training for staff members, and sometimes also provide direct service for individuals. The consultant's objective is to integrate concepts of restorative care into the overall plan of patient care in the skilled nursing facility. To accomplish these goals, the consultant works with the administrator, the director of nurses, and the activity director.

Day care centers and day health care centers are being developed in many urban areas. They are designed to provide an additional alternative to institutional care for individuals with varying degrees of physical or mental disability. Ideally, they provide structured activity within a therapeutic environment, offering group process to the outpatient as well as one-to-one therapy when needed. The focus is on health care, physical and occupational therapy for rehabilitation and maintenance, social services, and nutrition. Occupational therapists usually are participants in the treatment team but too seldom assume administrative and developmental responsibilities for the programs.

State mental hospitals are familiar sites for occupational therapists and have many aged patients. Notable among contributions by occupational therapists in evaluation and treatment of chronic schizophrenics is that of Lorna Jean King.[43]

Homes for the aged, boarding homes for the aged, retirement homes, retirement villages, and public housing units for the aged must be mentioned separately for, at present, there is little or no involvement by occupational therapists in most of these sites. The contributions that could be made at administrative as well as planning and evaluation levels are as numerous as in the other areas mentioned. They require a combination of the requisite skills and the ability to prove the need for their qualifications to those who are financially accountable for the operation of such facilities.

Need for Research

Occupational therapy's unique frame of reference can be applied to many research areas. Critical research, which applies a survey of current literature to specific provision of services, is rare in the field at present. Neugarten points out the need to delineate processes that underlie adult change and especially to find operational definitions.[44] She also complains that the phenomena that preoccupy the experimentalist are seldom those that concern the professional dealing with real life problems of clients. There is need to point out factors of environment, experience, and social roles that are primary in understanding stability and change in adult personality. Establishment of objective measures to define the categories of "frisky, frail, and fragile" would enable more appropriate assistance to be offered to those individuals involved than does the present use of actuarial tables of probability.

Care must be taken to pose initial questions in research projects so as to ensure valid results.[45] In developing the methodology, the researcher must remain objective and should carefully review related studies, assessing their validity in the context of the current study. The final step, which must not be overlooked, is ensuring availability of the research to those professionals who may profit from it. Occupational therapists often fail to publish their studies in appropriate journals outside their own field and, hence, are scarcely recognized in the broad field of gerontology.

Philosophical Base of Treatment

"The uniqueness of occupational therapy lies in its use of goal directed activity by the patient in a structured environment to trigger the unfolding of a need for adaptation."[46] The meaning of the activity, its choice, and the degree of satisfaction provided are determined by the *patient's* needs, interests, and motivations, and are directed toward his or her meaningful involvement in problem-solving tasks or creative performance. To quote Yerxa, "We need to reaffirm to ourselves and society the significance of the mundane stuff of daily living. . . For what we value is what existence is all about, finding meaning in all that we do, from cooking a meal to rocking a child to sleep, to tending roses or building sand castles. Our service depends upon the person acting in some new and uniquely meaningful way that moves him or her to a new state of healthfulness."[47]

Other disciplines operate from theories derived from observations of group manifestations in society. From these theories, they serve and advise their clients, anticipating results predicted by statistical data. There is always the possibility that the client's reactions may be the result of the professional's expectations. Public policy is determined by the existing norms as interpreted by researchers and theoreticians and, hence, reinforces those norms. The occupational therapist, with the basic premises from which he or she operates, can provide a new dimension to this process.

Implied in these premises are critical factors too often forgotten or ignored by professionals from many disciplines in working with elderly clients. The inherent decision-making ability of human beings does not magically disappear at age 65, as our youth-oriented society often implies. Options for lifestyle should refer to the individual's choices within the limits of real possibility, not those of a professional plan of what would be good for that individual. *There is no formula for "understanding old people"*—old people are as different and as complex as human beings at any age.

The therapist must see himself or herself as a facilitator whose professional qualifications can enable a client to make the best possible use of remaining capabilities to achieve his or her own goals. It is in the realm of goal setting that particular care must be exercised to listen to the individual, to identify sufficiently with that person, to help the person realize what he or she can realistically achieve, and to assist the individual in setting goals that are not only possible but important and affirming.

There is a great temptation to assume that old people are sick people and assign them what Parsons calls a sick role.[48] The assumption is made that the sick person is unable to fulfill social responsibilities and, furthermore, should not do so; the sick person cannot make himself or herself well and therefore, must be cared for; being ill is undesirable, so the individual has an obligation to cooperate with those who care for him or her in order to become well. With this concept as an almost subliminal assumption, it is easy to see how providers of services to the aged might fall into a caretaker role rather than that of a

facilitator towards independence. A very human tendency to exercise power over fellow human beings can lead to an even more insidious leaning toward the role of benevolent dictator. The therapist must be both objective and concerned—objective enough to make a realistic evaluation and concerned enough to discern patient-oriented goals.

Treatment in Gerontology

The elderly clients seen by the occupational therapist for treatment, whether in an institution or in the community through Visiting Nurse Associations, home health agencies, or day treatment centers, are remarkably similar. The term frail elderly is descriptive of their delicate balance between illness and health. For a variety of reasons, the elderly people in the community do not usually seek medical help until a crisis occurs. Both groups average three chronic conditions each, such as arthritis, arteriosclerosis, glaucoma, and osteoporosis, so it is rare to see a patient with only one problem.

The nursing home patient has an additional problem of adjustment to an unfamiliar environment. Many new residents suffer a period of mild to severe confusion, which abates once adjustment has been made. This process of adjustment requires the skillful support offered by staff members. Without it, sometimes even with it, many old people die rather quickly after such a radical change. Moving to the nursing home may be the most radical change of the individual's lifetime, and occurs when he or she is both mentally and physically least able to cope with such a transition. For most individuals, this move is viewed as "the beginning of the end." They must part with most of their personal possessions; few are fortunate enough to have the privacy of their own room. Ability to continue making personal decisions varies with the degree of physical or mental infirmity but is, at best, considerably restricted. There is a heightened awareness of impending death. Institutional management, in spite of recent improvements in many areas, is still geared more toward the convenience of staff than toward the individual needs of residents and tends to be dehumanizing.

Lieberman, commenting on the quality of institutional environments, stated that "maladaptive reactions to institutionalization are reduced considerably if the new environment is able to support an individual's previous life style."[49] He describes a good environment as one which encourages expression of individuality, is emotionally supportive, and is tolerant of deviant behavior. In contrast, a bad environment provides a high level of care and a great deal of supervision, catering to dependencies and treating residents as children. This, in support of previous lifestyle in essence, is the philosophy of occupational therapy in an institution. It is a tall order, requiring some compromises because of the number of individuals involved. A few nursing homes are taking tentative first steps away from the hospital model and are beginning to adopt a more resident-oriented model. Occupational therapists, utilizing basic principles of professional practice, should be prime movers in this trend.

Evaluation

Patient evaluation is a complex process. Part of it can be completed quickly, but part will be done in conjunction with the first phases of treatment. The skills of that therapist are put to a real test, especially the ability to "evaluate the individual's capacity to relate to and master his environment," and then provide a program design which speaks to his task mastery needs.[50] The therapist's attitude and the relationship developed with the patient are critically important to success. A sincere belief in the patient's ability to progress is as important as professional competence. Rapport must be developed based on mutual respect and trust. Liking the patient is not essential, though it is desirable. Respect, optimism, hope, and the ability to project these feelings to the patient are important. A patient who is so depressed he or she is unable to project hope for anything pleasant in the future is likely to die, as Comfort says, from "giving up." It is often necessary to overcome a patient's deep distrust and suspicion of nosy, interfering strangers, or at the other extreme, his or her total helplessness and dependence. Both extremes require professional objectivity, patience, respect, and optimism in the form of realistic expectations.

Evaluations should include the following:

1. Medical history—This may be sketchy or nonexistent. It can be supplemented by information from patient, family, physician, or friends.
2. Current diagnoses and medications (including over-the-counter medicines)
3. Referral information—who referred the patient, date, and purpose of the referral
4. Physical evaluation—active and passive range of motion, sitting balance and righting reflexes, sensory deficits (hearing, vision, sensation, kinesthesis, stereognosis), communication problems (language, speech, receptive or expressive aphasia, for instance), coordination, level of physical tolerance
5. Activities of Daily Living (ADL) dressing, grooming (combing hair, make-up, shaving), mouth care (including dentures), washing hair, bathing (both bowl and tub bath), eating (including socially acceptable manners), ambulation and, if patient is wheelchair bound, transfers, competence in planning and carrying out leisure activities (where applicable), any adaptive equipment required
6. Social history—when and where patient was born, family members, relationship, whether employed, patient's occupation, educational level, religion or other significant values, present and former hobbies and interests, any recent change in quality or quantity of relationships and social activity
7. Mental status—a mental status evaluation can be done in a nonthreatening, informal manner as part of a getting-acquainted process and need not be done all at the same time. It includes the following:
   orientation to time (at least season and year), place, and person,
   abstract reasoning (such as explaining the meaning of a proverb),
   memory, both recent and past (recent memory is most often defective in dementia),
   ability to solve simple arithmetic problems,
   judgment (a complex function often critical to determining ability to live alone),
   emotional state (anxiety, depression, or paranoia almost always accompany the onset of dementia)
8. Reliability of patient's information—assessment sometimes requires considerable skill, and it is wise to check information with at least one other reliable source. Social skills persist intact and often cover up considerable cognitive deficits. Depression, euphoria, dementia, or something as simple as fear of failure or wishing to please (or discourage) the therapist may distort facts.

For further detail, see Part 4, Evaluation Process and Procedures.

Program Development

Occupational therapy is based on meaningful, goal-directed activity. Therapeutic success depends on the degree to which the therapist is able to ascertain the patient's goals and tailor a program to ensure visible success at each step on the way toward that goal. Depression, despair, feelings of helplessness and uselessness are the major obstacles to motivating a patient to participate in a treatment program. Occupational therapy is done not to, but with the patient. The occupational therapist may be the only person within the patient's support system who is able to see the importance of something as simple as a midmorning cup of coffee with a friend to provide motivation for rehabilitation. The mundane things of life *are* important, particularly for the frail elderly. Also, it must be remembered that we are gregarious animals requiring interpersonal relationships. Feedback from another human being is essential to retaining a coherent self–image, which in turn is critical to survival. The first simple goals may have to be set by the therapist to prove that progress is possible, and often include physical abilities observed by the therapist that the patient has not yet recognized he or she has.

Positive feedback on the smallest improvement is important. It must be sincere and honest because these patients are hypersensitive to condescension and insincerity. A positive attitude and realistic expectations from the therapist usually prompt a positive response.

The program should include, in conjunction with the skills for dressing, grooming, eating, bathing, toileting, and ambulation, a degree of competence in attaining a balance of work, play, and leisure activities. These could be as simple and basic as putting away clothes, knitting, and picking out a favorite television program to watch.

Dementia is a common problem among frail elderly patients. The therapist should encourage physicians to check for possible causes of reversible dementia. He or she can certainly alleviate some of the symptoms.

Sensory deprivation is one factor that can cause brain damage when associated with isolation. A variety of stimuli are required to maintain a consistent personal image and to retain contact with the external world. Stimulation inhibits as well as excites. Violent, emotional storms may result from stimulus deprivation. Deterioration of sensory receptors (sight, hearing, touch, balance, kinesthesis, stereognosis) results in loss of information from the external world, making that world a lonely, frightening place. Sights, sounds, and even words lose their meaning as fantasy replaces environmental stimulation and increases isolation. Absence of stimulation leads to deterioration of physical activity, social participation, intellectual status, and overall personality integration—in short, symptoms of dementia.

Program goals include the following:

1. Reduce sensory deficits, where possible, with properly fitted eyeglasses and properly functioning hearing aid that is best suited to the type of hearing loss.
2. Maximize physical condition by minimum medications properly administered, treatment of de-

pression or illness, physical exercise, and good nutrition.
3. Reduce isolation by increasing social interaction.
4. Simplify the environment and develop a consistent, repetitive routine with calendar and written reminders (for instance, directions for dressing, preparing a simple breakfast, and taking a walk, making certain the territory is familiar).
5. Use remaining skills, requiring acute observation.
6. Emphasize sensory input with exercises that focus on body image, body parts, and their location in space, awareness of movement through use of rhythmic music, an auditory stimulus, and activities that stress tactile and olfactory stimulation.

For further detail, see Part 5, General Treatment Process and Procedures; and Part 6, Chapter 21, Functional Restoration Theory, Principles, and Techniques and Chapter 22, Functional Restoration: Specific Diagnosis for specific disabilities.

Death and Dying

This subject merits study and a thoughtful self-evaluation of feelings and attitudes by occupational therapists and other professionals working with the aged population. Certainly with the frail elderly population most of us serve, almost any illness could be terminal, though most of them are not. On the positive side, Lieberman, in writing of death as a "life crisis," feels that the crisis proportions of the issue are the invention of the young rather than the old.[51] His experience has been that most old people are quite willing to discuss their thoughts and feelings about death at great length. It is as if they are dealing with another developmental task and are coping adequately with it. Crises, he feels, occur primarily with unsolved problems of life—unresolved problems in relationships with family, for example—rather than with death.

Kastenbaum suggests that there are some things we do not want to know about old men and women.[52] We may resist the prospect of becoming intimately involved in the old person's world including vulnerability and anxieties about death. "Why let ourselves in for vicarious suffering? Why borrow misery from the future? Aversion from intimate contact with the aged is common." Kastenbaum feels that a self-discovery component should be added to the training of those preparing for a career with the aged.

The aged person must either make some type of adjustment to the thought of impending death or build up defenses as shields against the prospect.[53] A realistic acceptance of death is a part of emotional maturity.

It is commonly held that one's life passes in review when facing death. The theory of the life review, developed by Butler, suggests one such mechanism.[54] Life review is defined as a process of looking backward that has been set in motion by the imminent prospect of death. Butler feels that it accounts for the increase of reminiscence in the elderly, that it contributes to the occurrence of certain disorders in later life, particularly depression, and that from it also evolve such characteristics as candor, serenity, and wisdom among certain old people. It occurs not only in old people but in younger people who expect death, such as those who are fatally ill or condemned to death.

Contemplation of early experiences from the perspective of age often results in expanded understanding and may give new and significant meaning to life. It is tragic when the insight leads to a sense of total waste. One group that seems prone to depression and despair is made up of those who avoided living in the present, expecting the future to bring the rewards they sought. This philosophy brings great disillusionment in old age. Those who have consciously injured others, whose guilt is all too real, suffer terribly in this process. Butler feels that, possibly as a result of the life review, personality can change in old age. He has noticed positive, affirmative changes reported by the aged themselves.

Feifel, as well as other investigators, confirmed that, for many old people, a belief in a life after death is a great comfort, going a long way to reduce the element of fear.[55] For a few individuals, a strong belief in retribution for sins in the afterlife is very threatening. It is a great comfort for many to have children and grandchildren in whom they see a continuity of their own life.

Some residents in nursing homes, for the most part, see death as preferable to continuing illness or chronic disability. According to Kalish's concept, these persons may already have become "socially dead" in their own eyes as well as in the eyes of others, and thus view their impending death as timely and welcome.[56]

What causes the fear and anxiety that often prompt hospital or nursing home staff, from the aide to the doctor, to avoid unnecessary contact with dying patients? As Kastenbaum suggests, there should be a conscious analysis of one's attitudes and training to prepare one to assume a constructive role with individuals who are anticipating death.[57] The occupational therapist may be able to stimulate interest in enabling the staff members to become more aware of the needs of dying patients. The staff should be alert to the need of some elderly individuals to discuss and resolve old conflicts and to assure themselves that their lives have indeed had some meaning. A therapist can let the old person know, in an appropriate manner, that it is all right to talk about death, if he or she wishes to do so, now or at some future time. The person who is threatened by impending death often has a great need to discuss it. The dying person should be enabled to put his or her affairs in order, to make a will, to discuss funeral arrangements, and to ascertain any other matters that should be resolved. Family members are often too emotionally involved to be able to listen comfortably. Even the doctor, committed to the saving of lives, may be unable to respond appropriately. Health–care personnel who have come to terms with their own anxieties may provide the necessary empathy and support. These procedures, appropriate to occupational therapy, are important to the dying person to achieve "closure," enabling him or her to be at peace with self and family, to create a feeling of fulfillment and a sense of worth as an individual.[58] See also section on "Role of the Occupational Therapist in Death and Dying" in chapter 35, General Medicine and Surgery.

References

1. Butler, R. N.: The life review: An interpretation of reminiscence in the aged. In Neugarten, B. (ed.): Middle Age and Aging. Chicago: University of Chicago Press, 1968, pp. 18–30.
2. Tuckman, J., and Lorge, I.: The best years of life: A study in ranking. J. Psychol. 34:137–149, 1952.
3. Comfort, A.: The Practice of Geriatric Psychiatry. New York: Elsevier, 1980, p. 2.
4. Palmore, E.: Sociological aspects of aging. In Busse, E. W., and Pfeiffer, E. (eds.): Behavior and Adaptation in Late Life. Boston: Little, Brown & Co., 1969, pp. 58–59.
5. Neugarten, B.: Personality change in late life: A developmental perspective. In Eisdorfer, C., and Lawton, P. (eds.): Psychology of Adult Development and Aging. Washington, DC: American Psychological Association, 1973, p. 324.
6. Palmore: Sociological aspects, pp. 57–59.
7. Neugarten: Personality change, pp. 314–316.
8. Erikson, E. H.: Childhood and Society, ed. 2. New York: W. W. Norton, 1950, p. 85.
9. Peck, R. C.: Psychological developments in the second half of life. In Neugarten, B. (ed.): Middle Age and Aging. Chicago: University of Chicago Press, 1968, p. 88.
10. Ibid., pp. 88–92.
11. Ibid., pp. 90–92.
12. Brim, O. G.: Socialization through the life cycle. In Brim, O. G., and Wheeler, S. (eds.): Socialization after Childhood. New York: John Wiley & Sons, 1966, p. 316.
13. Ibid., p. 317.
14. Busse, E. W.: Theories of aging. In Busse, E. W. and

Pfeiffer, E. (eds.): Behavior and Adaptation in Late Life. Boston: Little, Brown & Co., 1969, pp. 18–27.

15. Brickford, C.: Myths that distort the plight of the elderly. Modern Maturity, October-November, 1980, p. 10–11.

16. Tibbits, C.: The evolving work-life pattern. In Tibbits, C. (ed.): Handbook of Social Gerontology. Chicago: University of Chicago Press, 1960, pp. 123–125.

17. Ibid. p. 124.

18. Besdine, Richard: Lecture, American College of Nursing Home Administrators Seminar, Good Samaritan Hospital, Portland, Oregon, April, 1981.

19. Datan, N., and Ginsberg, L. H. (eds.): Life Span Developmental Psychology: Normative Life Crises. New York: Academic Press, 1975.

20. Ibid., p. 6.

21. Riegel, K. F.: Adult life crises: A dialectic interpretation of development. In Datan, N., and Ginsberg, L. H. (eds.): Life-Span Developmental Psychology: Normative Life Crises. New York: Academic Press, 1975, p. 100.

22. Lieberman, M. A.: Adaptive processes in late life. In Datan, N. and Ginsberg, L. H. (eds.): Life-Span Developmental Psychology: Normative Life Crises. New York: Academic Press, 1975, pp. 154–157.

23. Besdine, R.: Lecture.

24. Comfort, A.: The Practice of Geriatric Psychiatry, p. 8.

25. Ibid., p. 10.

26. Besdine, R.: Lecture.

27. Ibid.

28. Comfort, A.: The Practice of Geriatric Psychiatry, p. 3.

29. Palmore, E. B., Ernst, P., Beran, B., Safford, F., and Kleinhanz, M.: Isolation and symptoms of chronic brain syndrome. Gerontologist 18:468–474, 1978.

30. Jarvik, L. F.: Alzheimer's disease. Newsweek, November 5, 1979.

31. Barnes, R. F., and Raskind, M. A.: DSM-III criteria and the clinical diagnosis of dementia: A nursing home study. J. of Gerontology 36: 20–27, 1981.

32. Krupka, L. R., and Vener, A.: Hazards of drug use among the elderly. Gerontologist 19:90–95, 1979.

33. Besdine, R.: Lecture.

34. Comfort, A.: The Practice of Geriatric Psychiatry, pp. 14, 15.

35. Krupka, L. R., and Venner, A.: Hazards of drug use, pp. 90, 91.

36. Comfort, A.: The Practice of Geriatric Psychiatry, p. 8.

37. Besdine, R.: Lecture.

38. Barnes, R. F., and Raskind, M. A.: DSM-III, p. 21.

39. Ibid.: p. 20.

40. Comfort, A.: The Practice of Geriatric Psychiatry, pp. 3, 4.

41. Ibid., pp. 14, 15.

42. Wiemer, R. B.: Traditional and Nontraditional Practice Arenas. In Occupational Therapy: 2001. American Occupational Therapy Association, 1979. p. 49.

43. King, L. J.: A sensory-integrative approach to schizophrenia. Am. J. Occup. Ther. 28:529–536, 1974.

44. Neugarten, B.: Personality change, p. 318.

45. Birren, J.: Principles of research on aging. In Neurgarten, B. (ed.): Middle Age and Aging. Chicago: University of Chicago Press, 1968.

46. King, L. J.: Toward a science of adaptive responses. Am. J. Occup. Ther. 32:429–437, 1978.

47. Yerxa, E.: The philosophical base of occupational therapy. In Occupational Therapy: 2001. American Occupational Therapy Association, 1979. p. 27.

48. Parsons, T.: The Social System. Glencoe IL: Free Press, 1951, p. 436.

49. Lieberman, M. A.: Institutional Environment. University of Chicago Magazine, July-August 1973.

50. Johnson, J.: Report of 1974 Task Force on Target Populations, Part I. Am. J. Occup. Ther. 28:160–161, 1974.

51. Lieberman, M. A.: Death as a life crisis. University of Chicago Magazine, July-August, 1973.

52. Kastenbaum, R.: Epilogue: Loving and dying and other gerontological addende. In Eisdorfer, C., and Lawton, P. (eds.): The Psychology of Adult Development and Aging. Washington, DC: American Psychological Association, 1973, p. 701.

53. Jeffers, E., and Verwoerdt, A.: How the old face death. In Busse, E. W., and Pfeiffer, E. (eds.): Behavior and Adaptation in Late Life. Boston: Little, Brown & Co., 1969, p. 163.

54. Butler: The life review, pp. 486–496.

55. Feifel, H.: Attitudes toward death. In Feifel, H. (ed.): The Meaning of Death. New York: McGraw-Hill, 1965, p. 172.

56. Kalish, R. A.: A continuum of subjectively perceived death. Gerontologist 6:73–76, 1966.

57. Kastenbaum, R.: Epilogue: Loving and dying, pp. 700–702.

58. Gammage, P. S., McMahon, P., and Shanahan, P.: The occupational therapist and terminal illness: Learning to cope with death. Am. J. Occup. Ther. 30:5, 1976.

Bibliography

Normal Aging/Adjustment

Cone, J. W.: Formal models of ego development: A practitioner's response. In Datan, N., and Ginsberg, L. H.: Life-Span Developmental Psychology: Normative Life Crises. New York: Academic Press, 1975.

Costa, P. T., McCrae, R. R., and Norris, A. H.: Personal adjustment to aging: Longitudinal prediction from neuroticism and extroversion. J. Gerontology 36:78–85, 1981.

Guttmann, D.: Live events and decision making by older adults. Gerontologist 18:462–467, 1978.

Kline, C.: The socialization process of women: Implications for a theory of successful aging. Gerontologist 15:486–492, 1975.

Lawton, P.: The Philadelphia Geriatric Center morale scale: A revision. J. Gerontology 30:85–89, 1975.

Leon, G. R., Kamp, J., Gillum, R., and Gillum, B.: Life stress and dimensions of functioning. J. Gerontology 36:66–69, 1981.

Lopata, H. Z.: Widowhood: Societal factors in life-span disruptions and alternatives. In Datan, N., and Ginsberg, L. H.: Life-Span Developmental Psychology: Normative Life Crises. New York: Academic Press, 1975.

Lozier, J.: Accommodating old people in society: Examples from Appalachia and New Orleans. In Datan, N., and Ginsberg, L. H.: Life–Span Developmental Psychology: Normative Life Crises. New York: Academic Press, 1975.

Miller, M.: Geriatric suicide: The Arizona study. Gerontologist 18:488–495, 1978.

Neugarten, B., et al.: Kansas City studies of adult life. In Neugarten, B., et al.: Personality in Middle and Late Life. New York: Atherton, 1964.

Payne, E. C.: Depression and suicide. In Howells, J. G. (ed.): Modern Perspective in the Psychiatry of Old Age, Vol. 6. New York: Brunner-Mazel, 1975.

Sheppard, H. L.: Work and retirement. In Binstock, R., and Shanas, E. (eds.): Handbook of Aging and the Social Sciences. New York: Van Nostrand Reinhold, 1976.

Long-Term Care Environment

Hardiman, C. J., Holbrook, A., and Hedrick, D. L.: Nonverbal communication systems for the severely handicapped geriatric patients. Gerontologist 19:96–101, 1979.

Moos, R. H., Gauvain, M., Lemke, S., Max, W., and Mehren, B.: Assessing the social environments of sheltered care settings. Gerontologist 19:74–82, 1979.

Treatment Factors

Adams, J. E., and Lindeman, E.: Coping with long term disability. In Goelho, G., Hamburg, D., and Adams, J. (eds.): Coping and Adaptation. New York: Basic Books, 1974.

Arenberg, A.: Cognition and aging: Verbal learning, memory, and problem solving. In Eisdorfer, C., and Lawton, P. (eds.): Psychology of Adult Development and Aging. Washington, DC: American Psychological Association, 1973.

Blackman, D. K., Howe, M., and Pinkston, E. M.: Increasing participation in social interaction of the institutionalized elderly. Gerontologist 16:1, Part I, 69–76, 1976.

Butler, R. N., and Lewis, M. I.: Aging and Mental Health: Positive Psychosocial Approaches. St. Louis: C. V. Mosby, 1973.

Davis, J. W., and Blumenthal, S.: A model of risk of failing for psychogeriatric patients. Arch. of General Psychiatry 38:463–467, 1981.

Ernst, P., Beran, B., Stafford, F., and Kleinhanz, M.: Isolation and symptoms of chronic brain syndrome. Gerontologist 18:468–474, 1978.

Frankel, L. J., and Richard, B. B.: Be Alive As Long As You Live: The Older Person's Complete Guide to Exercise for Joyful Living. New York: Harper & Row, 1980.

Graney, M. J.: Happiness and social participation in aging. J. Gerontology 30:701–706, 1975.

Kaplan, J., and Ford, C. S.: Rehabilitation for the elderly: An eleven year assessment. Gerontologist 15:393–403, 1975.

Kleban, M. H., Lawton, P., Brody, E. M., and Moss, M.: Characteristics of mentally impaired aged profiting from individualized treatment. J. Gerontology 30:90–96, 1975.

Lewis, S.: A patient determined approach to geriatric activity programming within a state hospital. Gerontologist 15:146–149, 1975.

Veterans Administration Hospital: Guide for Reality Orientation. Nursing Service, Tuscaloosa AL., 1970 (revised, mimeographed).

Ward, R.: Review of research related to work activities for aged residents of long term care facilities. Am. J. Occup. Ther. 25:348–351, 1971.

Zepelin, H., Wolfe, C. S., and Kleinplatz, F.: Evaluation of a year-long reality orientation program. J. Gerontology 36:70–77, 1981.

Geriatric Medical Care

Brickner, P. W.: Home Health Care for the Aged: How to Help Older People Stay In Their Own Homes and Out of Institutions. New York: Appleton-Century Crofts, 1978.

Comfort, A.: The Practice of Geriatric Psychiatry. New York: Elsevier, 1980.

Cape, R. D. T.: Aging: Its Complex Management. Hagerstown, MD: Harper & Row, 1978.

Reichel, W. (ed.): Clinical Aspects of Aging: A Comprehensive Text. Prepared under the direction of the American Geriatrics Society. Baltimore: Williams & Wilkins, 1978.

Reichel, W. (ed.): The Geriatric Patient. New York: HP Publishing Co., 1978.

Rossman, I. (ed.): Clinical Geriatrics, ed 2. Philadelphia: Lippincott, 1979.

Philosophical Base of Treatment

Baum, C. M.: Occupational therapists put care in the health system. (1980 Eleanor Clarke Slagle Lecture) Am. J. Occup. Ther. 34:505–516, 1980.

Gilfoyle, E. M.: Caring: A philosophy for practice. Am. J. Occup. Ther. 34:517–521, 1980.

King, L. J.: Creative caring. Am. J. Occup. Ther. 34:522–528, 1980.

King, L. J.: Toward a science of adaptive responses. Am. J. Occup. Ther. 32:429–437, 1978.

Reilly, M.: Occupational therapy can be one of the great ideas of twentieth century medicine. Am. J. Occup. Ther. 16:1–9, 1962.

Yerxa, E.: The philosophical base of occupational therapy. In Occupational Therapy: 2001 AD. Am. Occup. Ther. Assn., 1979.

Sexuality and Aging

Butler, R. N., and Lewis, M.: Sex After Sixty. New York: Harper & Row, 1976.

Comfort, A.: Sexual Consequences of Disability. Philadelphia: Geo. F. Stickley, 1978.

Pompeo, M. J.: Human Sexuality and the Aging. Center for Studies in Aging, Denton, TX, 1979.

Solnick, R. (ed.): Sexuality and Aging. Ethel Percy Andrus Gerontology Center, University of Southern California, 1979.

Laner, M. R.: Growing older male: Heterosexual and Homosexual. Gerontologist 18:496–502, 1978.

Resources

Gerontological Society of America
1835 K St., NW
Washington, DC 20006

NE Gerontology Center
15 Garrison Ave.
Durham, NH 03824

Institute of Gerontology
University of Michigan—Wayne State University
520 E. Liberty
Ann Arbor, Michigan 48108

Ethyl Percy Andrus Gerontology Center
University of Southern California
Los Angeles, CA 90007

Gerontology Specialty Section Newsletter
1383 Piccard Drive
Rockville, MD 20850

Gerontology Society for your region

Gerontology centers in nearby universities

CHAPTER 35

General Medicine and Surgery

Carole Hays

Occupational therapists working in a general hospital setting have the responsibility to be knowledgeable about a variety of diagnoses, occupational therapy assessments, treatment approaches, and community resources. The individuals in this setting are acutely ill, many have more than one problem, their diagnoses are in the process of being identified, and their adjustment to problems is just beginning. Many of the clients with medical and surgical diagnoses found on the case load of an occupational therapist in a general hospital are those clients covered in other sections of this book, such as cerebral vascular accident, arthritis, and spinal cord injuries. In a general hospital the occupational therapist's approach toward individuals with such diagnoses, and others to be covered in this chapter, is somewhat different because they are treated in the acute stage of the disease. The therapist must see each client as a human being with a unique set of problems who must be viewed with sensitivity and creativity.

There are many facilities, agencies, and institutions where an individual may receive health care, but in the United States the general hospital is second only to the private doctor's office in the delivery of health care services. General hospitals serve all ages from birth to death. They are most frequently the entry point for all types of diagnostic, medical, and surgical problems such as birth defects, depression, and traumatic quadriplegia. In some areas of the country, general hospitals provide all of the acute rehabilitation and chronic care programs for both physical and mental disorders; in other areas they serve as a primary care provider for acute problems and as a referring agent to rehabilitation centers, home care programs, mental health facilities, chronic care institutions, and other health care systems.

It is important to recognize that a general hospital exists for acute care problems or for episodic care. With this philosophy and the enforcement of it by utilization review committees, the patients have very short-term hospitalizations that nationally range anywhere from 5.4 to 11 days. Therefore, it is essential that occupational therapists assess the potential benefit of treatment to referred patients so that recommendations can be made regarding whether the patient should be discharged, kept in the hospital for a longer period of time, or sent to another facility. Short-term hospitalization means that often the therapist has time to complete only the assessments and program planning, and the implementation is done by a therapist in another center, in the patient's home, or through home health care agencies. Discharge planning is vital in assuring that all patients receive quality care.

The procedures that the occupational therapist uses in a general medical and surgical setting are based upon problem solving. The process of providing occupational therapy services includes gathering data, analyzing available information and evaluations, program planning, program implementation, documenting on the medical record all the services rendered, continual reassessment, home visits, discharge planning, after-care programs as appropriate, and follow-up by the occupational therapist until the patient has reached a maximum level of functioning.

The process of initiating an occupational therapy program is essentially the same in general medicine and surgery facilities regardless of the specific diagnostic categories. With this in mind, the next section will contain an overview of occupational therapy assessment followed by examples of specific approaches to selected diagnoses and problems.

Assessment

The assessment of the patient should include a maximum amount of information gathered in a short period of time. The Uniform Occupational Therapy Evaluation Checklist (see Appendix F) or an interview form based on the Checklist is essential. In many instances it is not practical to do a complete and specific evaluation of the patient's physical status at the time of the initial interview. However, facts pertaining to whether the individual functions within normal limits and whether deficits exist should be recorded, and a complete evaluation can then be accomplished as part of the overall treatment plan.

Demographic Information

This section should include personal information: name, address, telephone number, date of birth, age and sex, referral information; date of admission to the facility, date of referral to occupational therapy, who referred the patient to occupational therapy (whether a physician or another health–care professional), and the date the patient was first seen by the occupational therapist. It should also include the diagnoses that are being addressed in occupational therapy treatment and additional diagnoses that are affecting the patient's life. The date of onset, present problems and symptoms, medications, precautions, complications, the reason for the referral, date of evaluation, and the name of the evaluation should be documented, as should personal, developmental, educational, vocational, socioeconomic, and medical histories. The

family situation, including marital status, family members at or near the home, people who are with the patient during the day and night, the family members who are employed need documentation. There should be a brief description of the home accessibility including whether it is in an urban or rural setting, the type of structure, whether it is a house, apartment, or upstairs flat, number of levels, number of steps between levels, number of stairs the patient uses in daily living, and the number of rooms. The patient's mode of transportation outside the home also needs to be assessed. Is he or she a licensed driver? Does he or she use a bus or other forms of public transportation? Does he or she assist with driving, or do others have to drive?

Independent Living and Daily Living Skills

During the initial assessment the present self-care status should be documented. Independence requires that the patient perform every aspect of that task without assistance. The areas that should be considered are grooming and hygiene, eating, dressing, functional mobility, and object manipulation. The interviewer should listen carefully to the patient's speech and determine whether impairment is present. If possible, a sample of the individual's writing should also be obtained. Accessibility of and ability to use a telephone at home and in the hospital should be determined as well as the type of telephone used by the patient. Information regarding the patient's self-concept and self-identity, situational coping, and community involvement needs to be obtained.

Work

Data should be gathered regarding former, present, and proposed occupations. Periods of employment, education or training, and job requirements and responsibilities should also be documented.

Daily Responsibilities and Activities

This should include home and/or job responsibilities, leisure-time activities, amount of time the patient is active, daily routine, who are the people presently carrying out the patient's responsibilities, and whether they can be depended on to continue during the recovery of the individual.

Sensorimotor Skills and Performance Components

If applicable, reflex integration, range of motion, gross and fine coordination, strength and endurance, sensory awareness, visual and spatial awareness, and body integration should be assessed.

Cognitive Skills and Performance Components

This review includes orientation, conceptualization, and cognitive integration.

Psychosocial Skills and Performance Components

Data gathered on self-management, didactic integration, and group interaction should be documented.

Therapeutic Adaptation

The use of prosthetic or orthotic devices should be recorded. The occupational therapist should ask and record whether the patient does or does not use adaptive equipment.

Patient's Goals

The individual's long-term and short-term goals need to be documented. Included should be the patient's understanding of the disability or disease, response to a brief description of the occupational therapy program, and attitude toward the occupational therapy program.

Therapist's Impression

The potential benefit of treatment, presumed reliability of patient responses, and interpretation of those responses, should be recorded.

Occupational Therapy Program Plan

This section should state plans for specific evaluations, treatment objectives, treatment modalities, follow-up or referral considerations, and estimated duration of occupational therapy treatment.

Examples of Treatment Programs

The assessment process is essentially the same for each referral received, but individual treatment plans are developed for each patient based on the information gathered. Certain aspects, however, are common within specific diagnostic categories.

A complete example of a treatment program is presented for myocardial infarction. Cardiac disease is the most common cause of death in the United States, and patients with this diagnosis are frequently treated in general hospitals. Some other examples of treatment plans and special services for patients with other problems are presented in less detail.

Myocardial Infarction

Myocardial infarction (M.I.) is an event that causes permanent heart damage. Tissue anoxia from occlusion of the arterial blood supply results in necrosis of muscle fibers in an area of myocardium. Eventually this shrinks and scars. The extent of functional impairment varies with the amount of damage, area of damage, length of time after the event, and patient cooperation during the acute and convalescent stages. Arrhythmia, valvular damage, thromboembolism, shock, pump failure, and anxiety states may contribute to prolonged recovery times.

The primary goal of the rehabilitation program for individuals with the diagnosis of recent acute myocardial infarction is the return to maximum functional abilities by creating a therapeutic environment that not only promotes a healing of the damaged myocardium, but also helps prevent any further insult to the heart. The objectives to be achieved in helping the individual reach this goal are (1) provision of a systematic approach to the advancement of activities throughout convalescence, (2) active participation by the patient and family in the cardiac rehabilitation program, (3) provision of an explanation to the patient of the disease process and its consequence for lifestyle, and (4) provision of emotional and psychological support for the patient and family by all members of the team.

When dealing with an acute medical problem such as myocardial infarction, it is essential that the occupational therapist consult with the nursing staff and review the medical records daily to keep current on the patient's status. The occupational therapist must also consult with the physician to determine from a medical standpoint when the patient's activity level should be reduced, sustained, or upgraded.

After receiving a referral from a physician, reviewing the medical records, and consulting with the nursing staff on the patient's condition that day, the occupational therapist should start the program by completing an initial assessment. With the data gathered from the physician, the nurse, the medical record, and the interview form, the therapist will be ready to begin planning a treatment program.

Stages of the Treatment Process

Each stage of the treatment process involves four basic areas of daily living—self-care, mobility/

CARDIAC REHABILITATION PROGRAM
ACTIVITY CHART

Name:_____   Room:_____

Admission:_____   Date program started: _____

Doctor: _____

Occupational Therapist:_____

○ Supervision needed
○ Can do without supervision
○ Activity no longer applies

	1–1.5 Mets. Stage II		1.6–2.0 Mets. + U.E. Tension (Static) Stage III		2.1–3.0 Mets. Stage IV	

Self-care	Wash hands and face	○	Bathe body in bed
			  except back and legs
				○	Eat in dining room in
					  w/c.
						○

	Feed self in bed	○	Shave self (seated, elec-
			  tric razor)
				○	Dress/undress in street
					  clothes
						○

	Fingernail care	○	Comb hair (short)	○	Go to beauty parlor in w/c.	○
	Brush teeth	○	Bathe body except back, seated at sink	○	May take shower	○

	Feed self in chair with
	  feet elevated
		○	Dress/undress in bed-
			  clothes
				○		

Mobility	Bedside commode with
	  assisted transfer
		○	Walk to bathroom for
			  toileting
				○	Walk in hall—slow pace
					  44 ft.
						○

	Chair rest with feet
	  elevated:
			Progress to walking in
			  room tid
				○	Walk in hall 44 ft. in
					  15 secs. (2 mph.)
						○

	bid. 20 min.	○	Walk in room ad lib	○	Walk in hall 55 ft. in
					  15 sec. (2.5 mets.)
					  (2.5 mph.)	

	bid. 30 min.		Sit in chair ad lib	○		

	tid. 20 min.				Walk in hall 66 ft. in
					  15 secs. (3.0 mets.)
					  (3 mph.)
						○

	*As tolerated . . .					
	tid. 30 min.	○				
	tid. 45 min.	○				
	tid. 60 min.	○				
Exercise	Deep breathing every hour—5 deep breaths	○	Quad setting	○	Straight leg raising	○
	Shoulders—1 arm at a time	○	Hips and knees	○	Trunk side bending	○

	Quad. setting—
	  1 leg at a time
		○	Straight leg raising—
			  1 leg at a time
				○	Trunk twisting	○

	Hips and knees— 1 leg at a time	○				
	Ankles and toes— 1 leg at a time	○				
Other activities	Listen to radio	○	Watch T.V. in bed sitting	○	Get items out of drawers, closet. . . .	○

	Read light weight book
	  with bookstand or
	  otherwise supported
		○	Read newspaper	○	Observe, participate in
					  recreation programs
					  in w/c talking, singing,
					  table games
						○

	Use of telephone 3–5 mins., 2–3 calls/day	○	Yarn activities	○		

	Crossword puzzles	○	Table games and
			  activities
				○	Sit outside in warm
					  weather, not in hot
					  sun
						○

	Write short letters	○	Light craft activities	○	Stair climbing	○

ambulation, exercise, and other activities of daily living or recreation. The occupational therapist usually does not see the patient during the period of complete bedrest, which is considered stage one. Stages two, three, and four are defined by energy expenditure, and the patient is progressed from one stage to the next after consultation with the primary physician.

STAGE ONE. An activity chart should be given to the individual during the first contact (see Activity Chart). The purpose and stages of the program are explained and appropriate initial activities are filled in by the therapist. The purpose of an activity chart is to demonstrate visually to the patient, family, and other staff the level of physical activity permitted. The activity program serves to maintain and increase physical tolerance, to prevent loss of muscle tone, to promote means of relaxation, to develop interests to replace previous more strenuous activities, and to aid in long-term rehabilitation and adjustment to convalescence.

STAGE TWO. At stage two, some of the self-care activities allowed are washing hands and face, feeding self in bed, fingernail care, brushing teeth, and feeding self in a chair with feet elevated. In the mobility/ambulation area the patient should be able to use a bedside commode with the cardiac method of transfer and start sitting with feet elevated in a chair twice a day for 20 minutes. After the therapist has ascertained that the condition is stable, sitting time can gradually be lengthened to 60 minutes, three times a day. Other activities allowed include listening to the radio, reading a book placed in a bookstand or otherwise supported, reading a newspaper or magazine, using the telephone for 3 to 5 minutes at a time, making two or three calls a day, doing crossword puzzles, or writing short letters. When the patient can tolerate this level of activity, the therapist consults with the physician about advancing to stage three.

STAGE THREE. During stage three, in the area of self-care, the individual should be able to bathe (except for the back and legs) in bed or seated near a sink, to shave with an electric razor, to comb short hair, and to dress and undress in bedclothes. Regarding mobility/ambulation, a patient should first be able to walk to the bathroom for toileting, progress to walking about the room three times a day, and then progress to walking about the room as desired. Other activities that can be incorporated during stage three are watching television while in bed and reading a newspaper. Light activities such as yarnwork, table games, or light crafts can also be initiated. When able to tolerate all stage three activities, the patient can

progress to stage four, in consultation with the physician.

STAGE FOUR. During stage four, in the area of self-care, the individual should be independent in eating when seated in a chair and in dressing and undressing in street clothes. The patient may take a shower. The individual should be able to do some activities such as going to an occupational therapy clinic, a hospital beauty parlor or barber shop, or a coffee shop. At this stage, ambulation includes walking in the hall at a slow pace of approximately 2 miles per hour, or 44 feet in 15 seconds. This should be progressive until the patient is able to walk in the hall at 3 miles per hour, or 66 feet in 15 seconds. Other acceptable activities would include taking items out of drawers and the closet, observing and participating in activity programs such as talking, singing, and light crafts, and sitting outside in warm weather. The individual should also be able to begin some stair climbing.

Among the indications for stopping an activity are signs of ischemia or undue fatigue, chest pain, shortness of breath, dizziness, diaphoresis, pallor, cyanosis, and nausea. Another sign for caution is incomplete recovery, indicated by fatigue one hour after an activity has been completed. All changes need to be analyzed within the context of the situation or activity. In all cases of distress, consultation with the attending physician is required before either initiating or resuming activities. Observations and actions taken are to be noted on the medical record.

It is not in the purview of this section to go into telemetry and electrocardiogram monitoring in great detail. Therapists who work in facilities that now have telemetry as a part of cardiac monitoring during the treatment program have further guidelines and methods of evaluating when to stop an activity. Comparisons between a resting, baseline tracing, and the most recent electrocardiogram strip on the medical chart may reveal significant differences, such as recently developed arrhythmias. A therapist who is employed in a work situation that has these tools available will need further inservice training and continuing education in the use of the telemetry, treadmill, electrocardiogram monitoring, and physical exercise programs. They are now being provided across the country by cardiologists, occupational therapists, physical therapists, physical educators, exercise physiologists, and others.

Environmental Evaluation

In addition to the activity program, the therapist and the cardiac patient will need to evaluate the environment. If the patient is to be discharged, some information is needed about the physical structure of the home, including accessibility of rooms and utilities, accessibility from the outdoors, levels and locations of bathrooms, the bedroom, kitchen, and work–area locations and structures. The individual's primary home–management responsibilities, child–care responsibilities, and the availability of outside help should also be assessed.

Further information on job requirements and duties needs to be obtained, including the hours of work required, the physical demands of the job such as sitting, walking, climbing, and lifting, the mental demands or stress of the job, production rate and output on the job, and the patient's responsibility for others. Free time available from work also needs to be determined. This would include lunch time, coffee breaks, and whether the patient can take extra time if needed during the day. The therapist should discuss what kinds of facilities are available at the place of employment including elevators, restrooms, health facilities, and areas available for resting. The usual method of getting to and from work, the distance and travel time, and the availability of a bus from the parking lot to the building entrance are additional considerations.

Other aspects about returning to work that need to be evaluated include the company's attitude toward part-time employment increments until an employee is able to resume full-time employment, the feasibility of a change of job within the company, and the policies of the company regarding sick leave, vacation, and retirement. All possible income such as sick pay, disability insurance, social security, other family members' salaries, and public assistance should be considered. Planning must take into account the attitude of the patient about returning to the same job, consideration of a job change, and willingness to work. Based on the information gathered, the therapist supplies the physician and the patient with recommendations about returning to work, vocational evaluation, retirement, employment opportunities that may be open to the individual, or referral to a vocational rehabilitation service. Many people are able to resume employment, but usually they are not ready for two to three months after the myocardial infarction. It is usually recommended that they return to work on a part-time basis.

Another treatment objective is a review of work simplification. This should relate to the individual's situation including home and vocational responsibilities and avocational interests.

Psychosocial Aspects

Consideration of the psychosocial problems is essential when dealing with a patient with myocardial in-

farction. The individual with myocardial infarction goes through the common stages of coping with illness, including disbelief, shock, denial, anxiety, anger, depression, and, finally, acceptance and adaptation. The patient's mood may reflect boredom, restlessness, anger, depression, anxiety, and/or loneliness. Some of the goals of the cardiac rehabilitation program should be to decrease the patient's and family's fears through the process of education and to facilitate understanding of the disease and what can be expected. The therapist should encourage the view that successful recovery from injury leads to a relatively normal and productive life. The patient and the family are able to observe concrete evidence of progress through the use of the activity chart, which documents increased activity levels and increased strength and endurance without discomfort. It is important that the therapist maintain daily contacts to establish rapport and allow maximum opportunity for discussion of the risk factors of myocardial infarction, the roles of activity, stress, limitation of activities, relationships, return to work, signs and symptoms of fatigue, and ischemia. By the time of discharge, the patient and family should have a clear understanding of these factors and should be reassured about a safe return home.

Before discharge, a home program should be developed in collaboration with the physician and the other team members. Included here is an example of a basic home program developed by the occupational therapist and the clinical nurse specialist in cardiology and reviewed by the physician. In some facilities a dietician, social worker, and other professionals may be part of the home care team. Although there are some basic premises for preparing home programs, each program must be developed for an individual on a personal basis and must be reviewed with the patient and family before discharge. Telephone contact with the patient one to two weeks after discharge is useful to check on his or her functional status and answer any questions that have arisen.

Ronald, A Case Study

Ronald, a 49-year-old male, was admitted to the emergency room with sudden onset of gripping chest pain radiating to the medial aspect of his left arm and the left side of his jaw. The pain lasted for 45 minutes. He had no history of angina,

He is an automotive engineer with a large automobile company. He is married with four children—two are married, one is away at college and his 14-year-old son, Joe, is living at home. At the onset, he was very upset, did not believe he had

had a heart attack, and could see no real purpose for a cardiac rehabilitation program.

At the end of his fourth week in the hospital he is prepared for his discharge. Passing the initial stage of denial after his heart attack, he was cooperative with the cardiac rehabilitation program, with staff and family support. An occupational therapy session was set with Ronald and his family and he was given the following home program:

Ronald's Home Program

I. First week at home (approximately fourth week after M.I.)
  A. Self-care
    1. Eating—May eat three meals at the kitchen table, with family members present.
    2. Bathing—May use shower or bathtub. Use luke-warm water and have all necessary articles nearby.
    3. Dressing—May dress self; wear comfortable, loose-fitting clothes.
    4. Grooming—All activities allowed.
    5. Hair care—Have wife or son wash your hair while you are seated in a chair.
  B. Ambulation
    1. Walking—Walk indoors for the first week at home. May walk on main level and between rooms as desired. In addition, you should walk 75 to 100 feet this week.
    2. Sitting in chair—As tolerated.
      a. Never sit for more than one hour without getting up for a short walk.
      b. When possible, elevate your legs while sitting but do not cross legs.
  C. Rest
    1. Rest at least 1 hour after each meal. This may be done in a chair with your legs elevated.
    2. Rest quietly or nap for at least 1 hour in the late afternoon.
  D. Activities
    1. Visiting—Limit visitors to family and close friends. Do not allow visitors to interfere with scheduled rest periods.
    2. Car rides—Do not take trips in the car for the first week.
    3. Meal preparation—Once cooking utensils are placed on stove, counter, or table, you can prepare one meal a day. Do not move, lift, or carry pots and pans or food to the table.
    4. Housework—Do not participate in general household tasks or yardwork for this week.

5. Sexual activity—Not generally permitted until the sixth week.
6. Other activities
  a. May continue any projects begun in the hospital.
  b. May do table-top activities for 1 hour three times a day, such as cards, puzzles, models, drafting, or painting.

II. Second week at home (fifth week after M.I.)
  A. Self-care—unrestricted
  B. Ambulation
    1. Walking
      a. May walk 100 to 200 feet daily, gradually increasing amount during the week. If symptoms of fatigue, chest pain, shortness of breath, or dizziness occur, cut back to first week's level.
      b. Avoid stairs and any steep inclines in walking.
      c. May sit on porch if outside temperature is 40°F (near 5°C) or warmer.
  C. Rest
    1. Continue resting after meals for 1 hour.
  D. Other activities
    1. Rides in car—May go for rides in car as a passenger three times this week. Rides cannot exceed 1 hour.
    2. Visting—Same as first week.
    3. Meal preparation—May prepare two meals a day this week. Must not lift or carry food, pots, or pans. Sit at table to work when possible.
    4. Household—May wash dishes, if already placed in sink. Do not wash pots and pans. This should not be done until after resting 1 hour after eating. May put dishes and silverware away if not more than two plates are lifted at a time. May dust. May assist in cutting and preparing vegetables if seated. May assist in household plant care if seated.
    5. Other activities—Can work a total of 4 hours daily, spread throughout the day. Continue previous activities. May also begin assembling light wood projects (no sawing). Allowed essential business conferences, provided they are not too numerous (one per day), protracted, or associated with tension.

After completion of these two weeks, a routine visit to your physician is indicated. Based on the physician's findings concerning your general progress, additions to your rehabilitation program will be made. □

Swallowing Program for Adults with Dysphagia

A swallowing program is conducted in close cooperation with the medical, nursing, and dietary staffs, the patient, and the patient's family. The occupational therapist, before involvement in a dysphagia program, must review the anatomy and physiology of the complex swallowing mechanism, including the specific volitional and reflexive components. The occupational therapist must understand the nerves that affect swallowing, muscle action, and what signs and symptoms may be present. Many of the treatment techniques used with the individual with cerebral palsy are applicable to the adult with dysphagia.

Swallowing impairment often results from acoustic neuroma, brain stem tumors, radical neck surgery, laryngectomy, long-term tracheostomy, multiple sclerosis, myasthenia gravis or other progressive neurological diseases, cerebrovascular accidents, and Guillain-Barré syndrome. In developing a program for a person with swallowing problems, the therapist should complete an initial assessment as presented earlier, obtaining a general history of the patient, including specific facts related to the swallowing problems. There needs to be an evaluation of the peripheral speech and swallowing mechanisms, including resistance to mouth opening, jaw deviation, tongue deviation, strength of the tongue on protrusion and retraction, soft palate function, and laryngeal closure.

Prerequisites for Treatment

Before implementing a swallowing program, there are several prerequisites. First, the patient must be mentally alert and able to follow instructions, carry them over from day to day, and concentrate on the task well enough to support a reflex behavior. Second, the physiological potential to swallow must be ascertained from the evaluation. Last, a gag reflex must be present.

If a patient has little or no gag reflex unilaterally or bilaterally, a stimulation program needs to be attempted before food is introduced. In addition, tongue mobility and good laryngeal closure should then be established through tongue exercises and stimulation to ensure propulsion of food through the mouth to the esophageal opening.

Treatment Program

Exercises to strengthen the mechanical swallowing abilities include exercises for tongue lateralization, tongue elevation, tongue retraction, strengthening the cheeks and lips, chewing, swallowing, and gag reflex. Facilitation with pressure and ice might be used together with the exercises.

The precautions in implementing a swallowing program include an awareness of aspiration, as well as choking and gagging on foods and liquids, observation for food coming out of the mouth, tracheostomy, or nose, and daily checking of the patient's weight, hydration, and intake and output to make certain the patient is receiving enough nourishment.

When the patient is ready to attempt oral feeding, several factors must be considered in the diet selection, including other methods by which the patient may be receiving nutrition or hydration (I.V., nasogastric, or other tube feedings), the therapist's evaluation results, and the patient's food preference. Specific foods are selected to provide the most sensory feedback possible to enhance the volitional and reflexive components. Considerations are that (1) food with low specific gravity, such as liquids or purees, does not excite pressor receptors in the mouth or, more importantly, the soft palate and has the tendency to leak into the trachea; (2) casein in milk products thickens mucous secretions thereby decreasing sensation; (3) pureed food may not have an aroma and often tastes bitter; (4) sweet food decreases saliva; and, (5) sour food facilitates swallowing.

The patient must trust the therapist in order to comply with the program. There are numerous emotional ramifications resulting from the inability to eat and the necessity for relearning the process; it is usually an unpleasant experience; it is uncomfortable, and can be painful. The patient is often embarrassed because he or she may be sloppy. The emotional support provided by having a confident therapist present during meals can be the most important treatment offered.

When oral food swallowing is initiated, if possible, the nasogastric tube should be removed since it depresses the gag reflex, irritates the mucous membranes, and increases secretions. It also prevents tight closure of the nasopharynx passages. Intravenous fluids are usually continued to prevent dehydration. The patient should sit in a chair at 90 degrees; the neck should be slightly flexed and the body tilted forward during the meal and for 1 hour afterwards. The food should be placed in the mouth at the point where the patient will get the most sensory feedback for the taste, pressure, and temperature of the food. The patient should begin with small amounts of food and proceed slowly.

Preferably, small portions are given five times a day, rather than large portions three times a day. Initially, the patient needs to be supervised by the occupational therapist during each meal, followed by the nursing staff, if they are instructed properly by the therapist. The ultimate goal is for the therapist to instruct the patient and family in the swallowing program so as to allow them to continue the program until independence is reached.

By following a program of evaluation, therapeutic exercises, and treatment, the majority of patients note improvement, and some completely resolve their swallowing problems.

Role of the Occupational Therapist in Death and Dying

The occupational therapist has a unique background in physical, psychosocial, and occupational performance needs. Integration of this knowledge gives the therapist the ability to see a person as a human being rather than as a disease process. Therefore, an occupational therapy service program for individuals who are dying can provide psychological support and active participation within the patient's capabilities. The activity provided should be in concert with the patient's goals and physical and mental capabilities and should provide a feeling of self-worth and productivity.

The therapist must be secure in his or her own attitude toward death and dying. The therapist must be able to listen, hear, understand, be sensitive to, and be able to respond verbally or nonverbally to spoken and unspoken requests. The ability to recognize when a patient needs you, and the willingness to give the time, regardless of personal or professional schedules, are essential. It is usually recognized that the sicker and closer to death the patient is, the less personal attention he or she receives from the hospital staff. The patient continues to receive good medical and nursing care but less love. It is an occupational therapist's responsibility to be sensitive, to be aware, to provide meaningful activities, and to care.

Case Summary—Death and Dying

Ada was a 36-year-old mother of eight children with a diagnosis of acute leukemia. Her family could visit only on weekends, because she lived 100 miles from the hospital. She was referred to occupational therapy with the problem of a reduced energy level and was instructed in work–simplification and home–management techniques. The therapist also worked with Ada and her family to set up a household routine that provided built-in rest periods so she could continue to be independent and function as a wife and mother. Because of her

husband's request, Ada was not told about her diagnosis. Two weeks after discharge, the therapist called Ada to find out how the home–management plan was functioning. Ada and her husband were satisfied with the program, and the household was running smoothly. Follow-up contacts after six months and one year were made, and the family was still managing well.

At the age of 38, Ada was readmitted to the hospital because the disease process had progressed rapidly. It was then determined that she only had a few weeks to live. She was again referred to occupational therapy for supportive care. One of Ada's goals was to make individual items of similar quality for each of her eight children, which would last as a remembrance and a reminder that she loved them. The therapist helped Ada select items that were within her capabilities and that Ada would enjoy making. They were graded from the first project, which was the most difficult, to the last item, which required less strength and was less complicated. The grading of the activities was necessary because she was expected to decline in awareness and physical capability.

The last item Ada was making was a ceramic piggy bank that required several coats of one-color glaze. On the final day she was in bed with intravenous fluids running and was alert for only 1 or 2 minutes at a time. During these intervals she still wanted to complete the project. The therapist had to help hold the brush in Ada's hand in order to finish. She and the therapist completed the glazing at 2 p.m. The therapist returned at 4:30 the same afternoon and told Ada that the piggy bank would be fired and ready the next day. No one else was in Ada's room. Her family had been notified of the severity of her condition and was on the way to see her.

Ada asked the therapist to stay with her and hold her hand. During the remaining few hours Ada was awake and alert only a few minutes at a time. She talked about her family and was told by the therapist that they were coming. She was concerned and was reassured by the therapist that she had completed all the projects and that each child would receive the present she had made. What Ada wanted most was contact with a caring human being who would be with her at the end. Ada's respiration ceased at 6:30. □

Cancer

The term *cancer* is used by the public to refer to a myriad of separate diseases with a common bond. They all begin with a disorderly growth of cells in a malignant neoplasm. The autonomous growth of abnormal tissue invades or replaces normal tissue. It can also spread to distant sites, and this is termed *metastasis*.

The location, rate of growth, spread of growth, and amount of interference with function determine the pathological effects of the disease. It often strikes in middle age, although no age group is unaffected. Causative factors have been identified, but the process remains incompletely understood. The means of slowing, arresting, or curing the disease include surgery, chemotherapy, and radiation. These can result in amputation, seriously altered ways of functioning, change in self-image, adjustment of lifestyle, and varying states of well being.

Patients with Radical Mastectomy

A referral to occupational therapy should be obtained from the physician as soon as possible after admission or after surgery. Occupational therapy services for the woman having a radical mastectomy are designed to help prevent problems of decreased shoulder range of motion and edema, to provide education through discussion, to demonstrate available adaptive equipment such as bras, prostheses, clothing, including bathing suits, and cosmetics to obscure scars. The therapist should provide activities that are therapeutic, explain which activities are contraindicated postoperatively, and facilitate the patient's psychological acceptance of her amputation and her return to the family. Physical activity usually does not begin until 4 to 10 days after surgery, in consultation with the patient's physician. The specific objectives are based on the problems the patient presents, with due consideration given to other complicating factors such as decreased strength, obesity, and hemiplegia. There should be a review of household work simplification, work simplification, and beneficial activities.

In coordination with the social service department, psychological support for the individual and the family should be offered. There are some community agencies that can be very helpful to the woman with a mastectomy, such as the Reach for Recovery Program of the American Cancer Society. The patient should be referred, if appropriate. Following discharge from the hospital, there should be a review and reinforcement of material presented during hospitalization and outpatient treatment, if needed.

Diabetes Mellitus

In diabetes mellitus, blood sugar becomes elevated as a result of a deficiency of insulin. There are other associated metabolic variations and vascular changes. The disease is controlled by stimulation of insulin production with oral medication, lessening insulin requirements by diet or weight loss, or by the administration of insulin. Balance must be achieved between available insulin, intake of food, and consumption of energy in activities. Long-standing diabetes may lead to decreased vision from retinal vessel disease, kidney lesions with failure, neuropathies, arteriosclerosis, and peripheral vascular disease causing gangrene and perhaps damage severe enough to require amputation.

There are four primary objectives for occupational therapists when working with a person admitted to the hospital with diabetes: (1) providing regulated activity to assist in insulin regulation, coordinating normal home activity with hospital routines; (2) providing an environment to allow the individual to demonstrate knowledge of diet regulation; (3) evaluating and teaching compensatory skills when the patient has associated complications that result in visual loss, sensory loss, or amputation; and (4) providing psychological support.

Following the initial interview with the patient, the therapist needs to evaluate the home and work routine and to calculate the calories expended by the individual on a normal day. The treatment program then focuses on providing activities to simulate home calorie expenditure during the hospitalization. Specifically, these may include self-care, activities of daily living, recreation, avocational interests, walking, climbing stairs, exercises, or work experiences such as collating, typing, filing, or woodworking. By providing the regulated activity program, the physician and dietician will have a better basis for insulin and diet regulation.

The role of the occupational therapist in diet regulation is to evaluate the previous dietary regime and the patient's level of responsibility for it by talking to the dietician, patient, and patient's family. The therapist would then provide the patient with an opportunity to apply dietary knowledge by planning and preparing a snack or a meal. The treatment plan may provide for therapeutic trips to stores or restaurants, which would help determine the individual's ability to maintain the diet independently.

The patient also needs a supportive milieu in which to express feelings about diabetes mellitus and to achieve realistic acceptance of it. The therapist should be able to help minimize malingering by provision of an activity program and simulated home—management responsibilities. Close coordination and a team approach with the physician, nurse, dietician, patient, family, and occupational therapist are essential.

A program for an individual with complications

or decreased function focuses on necessary compensatory skills. The program could include additional goals in ADL skills, communication, amputee training, or work simplification. Referral to appropriate community agencies, rehabilitation centers, or other health care systems may be needed.

Chronic Obstructive Pulmonary Disease

People with chronic obstructive pulmonary disease (C.O.P.D.) have difficulty moving air in and out of their lungs because airways are narrowed by spasms, secretions, or loss of elasticity of lung tissue, which allows air to be trapped in the lungs. Chronic obstructive pulmonary disease results from emphysema, chronic bronchitis, bronchiectasis, or diseases that cause pulmonary fibrosis or cardiac disease. Symptoms include decreased physical tolerance, shortness of breath, cough with production of sputum, chest pain, hemoptysis, and noisy respiration.

Four primary objectives for occupational therapists when treating patients admitted to the hospital for chronic obstructive pulmonary disease are (1) evaluating and teaching compensatory skills for loss of physical tolerance, including work simplification and energy conservation, (2) exploration of job responsibilities and vocational evaluation to decrease occupational exposure to dust and toxins, (3) provision of graded activity programs, and (4) psychological support.

The initial interview should provide the occupational therapist with information for development of treatment plans. The plans must be individualized to facilitate function as normal as is physically possible. By providing a regulated activity program, the occupational therapist provides the physician with a better baseline for the regulation of medicines. The occupational therapist may work in conjunction with the physical therapist and the respiratory therapist in the development of a breathing exercise program.

Special Treatment Procedures

Therapeutic Trip

The therapeutic trip is a community outing in which the occupational therapist and patient go outside the confines of the hospital. The purpose of a therapeutic trip is to provide the patient with practical experi-

ence, while the therapist evaluates and instructs the individual on the following concerns:
1. Architectural barriers
2. Application of previously learned skills such as transfers or handling of money
3. Ability to assume responsibility, such as obtaining a "leave on pass" order from the physician, gathering any necessary equipment, and donning appropriate clothing
4. Ability to organize and plan, such as allowing adequate time for the event, making transportation arrangements, and obtaining equipment needed
5. Ability to problem solve and be flexible
6. Ability to interact practically and comfortably with the public
7. Ability to manage a wheelchair, crutches, walker, or cane
8. Judgment about safety factors and when to seek help
9. Dependence or independence in all areas, including initiating and carrying through plans.

Before a therapeutic trip, the above objectives and methods of achieving them are discussed with the patient. Prior to, during, and following the trip, the patient is expected to assume as much responsibility as possible. Following the trip the patient and staff member should assess the patient's functioning and problem areas. Follow-up treatment programs and services are based on the outcome of the therapeutic trip as assessed by the therapist and patient.

Home Assessment

If the patient or therapist foresees problems in the return to the home from the general hospital, the therapist should arrange to do a home assessment before the planned discharge. Ideally, the therapist should arrange for the patient and the other members of the household to be present in the home during the assessment.

If possible, treatment and evaluation of performance should be completed before the home visit. The purpose of the home assessment is to determine whether barriers in the home environment will conflict with performance. By doing the home assessment before discharge, the therapist can make realistic recommendations to the patient and implement further treatment goals to ease the transition from the hospital to the home. The therapist can also determine whether further services are needed on an inpatient or outpatient basis, whether a referral to a home care program is necessary, or whether discharge to another type of facility is indicated.

The home assessment can be fairly standardized,

OCCUPATIONAL THERAPY HOME ASSESSMENT REPORT   Patient's Name
                                                 Address
                                                 Telephone Number

Date:

People who participated:
Number of levels:
Which rooms on each level:

	ACCESSIBLE ADEQUATE	NON-ACCESSIBLE INADEQUATE	RECOMMENDATIONS AND/OR CORRECTIONS NEEDED
OUTDOORS			
1. Terrain			inclines, mobility on varying surfaces
2. Porch/Patio/Balcony			
a. Stairs			railing; size; number; height
b. Doors/Doorways			threshold; direction of opening; operate knobs and locks; width
c. Maneuverability			furniture; carpeting; mobility on surfaces; adequate turning radius; throw rugs
d. Furniture			location; height; transfers
e. Plugs/Switches			location; height; ease of operation
3. Parking/Garage			distance to entrance; incline
4. Compliance with City Ordinances			ramping; exits; fire codes; building permits
5. Entrances—Front			steps; railings; surfaces; direction of opening threshold; operate knobs and locks; width
Side/Back			
HALLWAYS			
1. Maneuverability			as above
2. Plugs/Switches			as above
LIVING ROOM/DINING ROOM			
1. Doors/Doorways			as above
2. Maneuverability			as above
3. Furniture			as above
4. Plugs/Switches			as above
5. Lighting			amount location
KITCHEN			
1. Doors/Doorways			as above
2. Maneuverability			as above
3. Stove/Burners			operation and visibility of controls; location; gas/electric
4. Oven			operation and visibility of controls; open/close door; operate broiler; height; pull out/in oven rack
5. Refrigerator/Freezer			height of handle and shelves; depth; open/close doors
6. Dishwasher			loading/unloading; operate controls; portable/built in; detergent
7. Sink			garbage disposal; direction of approach; manage faucets; height; depth; countertop space; stopper
8. Plugs/Switches			as above
9. Storage			ability to reach; handles; organization; adequate amount
10. Working Surfaces			countertop heights; depth; direction of approach
11. Transportation of Items			distances; continuous surfaces for sliding objects; wheeled cart; lapboard; walker apron
12. Small Appliances			location; operation; work saving
13. Furniture			as above

OCCUPATIONAL THERAPY HOME ASSESSMENT REPORT (*Continued*)

	ACCESSIBLE ADEQUATE	NON-ACCESSIBLE INADEQUATE	RECOMMENDATIONS AND/OR CORRECTIONS NEEDED
BATHROOM			
1. Doors/Doorways			as above
2. Stairs			as above
3. Maneuverability			as above
4. Sink/Countertop Space			as above
5. Tub/Shower			manage faucets; nonskid surfaces; height; transfer; need for grab bar and/or chair
6. Toilet			need for grab bars; location of toilet paper; height; operate lever; direction of approach; transfers
7. Plugs/Switches			as above
8. Mirror			height; location
9. Medicine Cabinet			height; location; open/close door
BEDROOM			
1. Stairs			as above
2. Doors/Doorways			as above
3. Maneuverability			as above
4. Closets			direction of approach; height of rod and shelves; open/close door
5. Dresser			height; location; open/close drawers
6. Furniture (Bed/Chair)			location; heights, transfers
7. Plugs/Switches			as above
8. Lighting			as above
BASEMENT/REC. ROOM			(evaluate if use is necessary or desired)
1. Stairs/Lighting/Railing			as above
2. Doors/Doorways			as above
3. Maneuverability			as above
4. Plugs/Switches			as above
5. Furniture			as above
COMMUNICATION SYSTEMS			
1. To contact others outside home			telephone (emergency numbers easily visible, location, type, operation); signal in window; warning light
2. To contact those within home			intercom; buzzer system; bell
CLEANING			
1. Laundry Facilities			washer/dryer; location; load/unload; operate controls; detergent
2. Supply Storage			ability to reach; handles; organization; adequate amount
3. Use of Equipment			open/close containers of cleaning equipment; vacuum; mop; dustpan; broom
4. Garbage Removal			location; city ordinances; secure and tie bag; transport; use of other person
USE OF COMMUNITY RESOURCES			
1. Transportation			public (cab, bus, train); personal
2. Shopping Facilities			distance; type (mall, street); restroom facilities; use of other persons; phoning orders; architectural barriers
3. Social and Recreational Facilities			distance; architectural barriers; restroom facilities (church, parks, clubs, theaters)
4. Medical Facilities			distance; architectural barriers; restroom facilities; emergency arrangements; transportation

OCCUPATIONAL THERAPY HOME ASSESSMENT REPORT (*Continued*)

	ACCESSIBLE ADEQUATE	NON-ACCESSIBLE INADEQUATE	RECOMMENDATIONS AND/OR CORRECTIONS NEEDED
ADDITIONAL CONSIDERATIONS			
1. Other Rooms			frequency of use; accessibility; need for cleaning
2. Windows			height; location; open/close; lock; shades/curtains
3. Thermostat			location; height; operation and visibility of controls
4. Precautions when patient is alone			communication system; adequate food, water, medi- cation bowel/bladder care
5. Pursuit of Avocational interests			location of supplies; adequate space
6. Yardwork and Repairs			use of other persons; storage; use of equipment
SUMMARY AND RECOMMENDATIONS:			Briefly summarize; include persons responsible for carrying out recommendations, if possible; suggested follow-up

Date of Visit: _____

Length of Visit: _____

Signature: _____

and often a form or questionnaire is helpful. All rooms and hallways the patient will use need to be evaluated in terms of maneuverability, including carpeting, surface mobility, adequate turning radius, furniture placement, and the presence of throw rugs. The location, height, and ease of operating plugs and switches need to be noted as well as the presence of adequate lighting. Threshold, direction of door opening, ability to operate knobs and locks, and door width need to be considered. The location, heights, and possibilities of moving furniture must be recorded. In regard to stairs, the height, number of flights, presence of rails (including sturdiness and whether they are on one side of the stairs or both), and frequency of use need to be documented. Specific observations necessary for various areas of the home are listed in the Home Assessment Report (see sample Home Assessment Report).

Summary

The variety of problems that an occupational therapist encounters through referrals, evaluation, and treatment in a general hospital is limited only by the therapist's skills, knowledge, and ability to problem solve. Some additional diagnoses that might be encountered and guidelines for approaching patients suffering from them are listed in Table 35-1. The functional goal for each patient is to be as independent as possible.

The patient's problems can be as simple as an inability to open jars or as complex as adjusting to life in a wheelchair, learning about adaptive equipment, and discovering new methods of accomplishing daily life tasks. This chapter is just a beginning. To be a good occupational therapist one must continue to acquire and apply new knowledge and skills throughout one's career.

Table 35-1. *Problems encountered and guidelines for solving.*

Diagnosis	Common problems encountered	Occupational therapy services rendered
Parkinson's disease	Muscular weakness Tremors Extreme rigidity	Activities of daily living Therapeutic activities to increase coordination, range of motion, and muscle strength Work simplification
Rheumatic heart disease	Decreased physical tolerance Poor cardiac reserve	Work simplification Energy conservation Graded activity program
Scleroderma and other collagen diseases	Excessive fatigue Limited range of motion Decreased muscle strength	Therapeutic activities to maintain or increase range of motion and muscle strength Physical tolerance programs Activities of daily living Splinting Psychological support
Blood dyscrasias	Excessive fatigue	Work simplification Energy conservation Graded physical tolerance program
Renal insufficiency	Dependency on artificial dialysis Limited energy Variety of neurological manifestations Limited work potential	Hospital and home program to help maintain a balance of fluids and body chemistry by medication, activity, and diet Graded physical tolerance program Vocational (work) evaluation Avocational pursuits Activities of daily living
Hip fracture	Self-care problems, especially reaching, transfers, and lower extremity dressing Household management Nonoperative fracture treated by bed-rest or traction	Self-care evaluation and treatment Avocational program Work simplification Physical tolerance program
Hemophilia	Hemorrhage into joints causing limited range of motion	Activities to maintain or increase range of motion Vocational (work) evaluation Static splinting to prevent contracture or deformity Self-care evaluation and treatment
Obesity	Limited reach Poor cardiac reserve Poor self-concept Lack of appropriate work skills	Graded physical activity program Self-care evaluation and treatment Activity assimilation program Vocational (work) evaluation Behavior modification
Low back pain	Pain–medication cycle Inability to carry out life tasks	Work simplification with emphasis on proper methods for lifting and carrying Activity assimilation program Psychological support Behavior modification Vocational (work) evaluation

(Continued)

TABLE 35-1. *(Continued)*

Diagnosis	Common problems encountered	Occupational therapy services rendered
Thoracic surgery—cardiac	Decreased physical tolerance	Work simplification
	Unable to carry out home management tasks	Energy conservation
		Graded activity program
	Employment concerns	Psychological support
	Fear of surgery	Vocational (work) evaluation
Psychosomatic illness	Inability to function in daily life tasks	Behavior modification program
		Psychological intervention
		Avocational pursuits
		Energy expenditure programs

Bibliography

Assessment

Cautela, J. R.: Organic Dysfunction Survey Schedules. Champaign, IL: Research Press, 1981.

Hays, C., Kassimir, J., and Parkin, J.: Sample Forms for Occupational Therapy. Rockville, MD, American Occupational Therapy Association, 1980.

Krusen, F. H., et al.: Handbook of Physical Medicine and Rehabilitation, ed. 2. Philadelphia: W.B. Saunders Co., 1971.

Wittmeyer, M. B., and Stolov, W. C.: Educating wheelchair patients on home architectural barriers. Am. J. Occup. Ther. 32:557–564, 1978.

Cancer

Dudgeon, B. J., DeLisa, J. A., and Miller, R. M.: Head and neck cancer, a rehabilitation approach. Am. J. Occup. Ther. 34:243–251, 1980.

May, H. J.: Psychosexual sequelae to mastectomy: Implications for therapeutic & rehabilitative intervention. Journal of Rehabilitation. Jan. Feb. Mar. 1980, pp. 29–31.

McCorkle, M. R.: Coping with Physical Symptoms in Metastatic Breast Cancer. (Distributed by American Cancer Society, Inc.) American Journal of Nursing Vol. 73, No. 6, June 1973.

Psychosocial Rehabilitation of Cancer Patients, Rehab. Brief, Vol. III, #10, July 14, 1980. Prepared by Rehabilitation Research Institute, College of Health Related Professions, University of Florida, Gainesville, FL 32610.

Rosenbaum, E. H., et al.: Rehabilitation Exercises for Cancer Patients (Revised ed.) Palo Alto, CA: Bell Publishing, 1980.

Rosenbaum, E. H., Rosenbaum, I. R., et al.: A Comprehensive Guide for Cancer Patients and Their Families. Palo Alto, CA: Bell Publishing, 1980.

Villanueva, R.: Rehabilitation needs of the cancer patient. Southern Medical Journal, Vol. 68, No. 2, February 1975, pp 169–172.

Whitley, S. B., Branscomb, B. U., and Moreno, H.: Identification and management of psychosocial and environmental problems of children with cancer. Am. J. of Occup. Ther. 33:194–195, 1979.

Cardiac

Alpert, J. S.: The Heart Attack Handbook. A Common Sense Guide to Treatment, Recovery, and Prevention. Boston: Little, Brown and Company, 1978.

Cohn, K., Duke, D., and Madrid, J. A.: Coming Back—A Guide to Recovery from Heart Attack and Living Confidently with Coronary Disease. Addison-Wesley Publishing, 1979.

Exercise Testing and Training of Apparently Healthy Individuals: A Handbook for Physicians. New York: American Heart Association, 1972.

Fardy, P. S., Bennett, J. L., Reitz, N. L., and Williams, M. A.: Cardiac Rehabilitation: Implications for the Nurse and Other Health Professionals. St. Louis, MO: C.V. Mosby, 1980.

Gentry, W. D., and Williams, R. B.: Psychological Aspects of Myocardial Infarction and Coronary Care. St. Louis, MO: C.V. Mosby, 1975, 162 pp.

Huntley, N., (ed.): Basics of Cardiac Rehabilitation. Minnesota Occupational Therapy Association, 1978.

Meltzer, L. E., Pinneo, R., and Kitchell, J. R.: Intensive Coronary Care. A Manual for Nurses. 3rd ed., Bowie, MD: Charles Press, 1977.

Morse, R. L.: Exercise and the Heart. Springfield IL: Charles C. Thomas, 1972.

Ogden, L. D.: Activity guidelines for early subacute and high risk cardiac patients. Am. J. Occup. Ther. 33:291–298, 1979.

Pollack, M., and Schmidt, D.: Heart Disease and Rehabilitation. Boston: Houghton-Mifflin, 1979.

Semple, T., et al. (eds): Myocardial Infarction, How to Prevent, How to Rehabilitate. International Society of Cardiology, 1973.

Strickland, A.: Cardiac rehabilitation: An occupational therapist's approach. Can. J. Occup. Ther. (Canada) University of Toronto, 44:3, pp. 127–130, 1977.

The American Heart Association Cookbook. New York: David McKay, 1973.

Wendland, L.: The psychodynamics of coronary heart rehabilitation: Some basic understandings for allied health professionals. Journal of Allied Health, February 1981.

Wenger, N. K.: Coronary Care: Rehabilitation after Myocardial Infarction. New York: American Heart Association, 1973.

Wright, I. S., and Fredrickson, D. T.: Cardiovascular Diseases—Guidelines for Prevention and Care. The Inter-Society Commission for Heart Resources, Bethesda, MD, 1973.

Chronic Obstructive Pulmonary Disease

An Occupational Therapy Program for the Patient with Chronic Obstructive Pulmonary Disease: A Teaching Package for Therapists from Moss Rehabilitation Hospital. Department of Occupational Therapy, Moss Rehabilitation Hospital, 12th Street and Tabor Road, Philadelphia, PA 19141.

Berzins, G. F.: Occupational therapy program for the chronic obstructive pulmonary disease patient. Am. J. Occup. Ther. 24:181, 1970.

Haas, A., Pineda, H., Haas, F., and Ayen, K.: Pulmonary Therapy And Rehabilitation: Principles and Practice. Baltimore, MD: William and Wilkins, 1979.

Moser, et al.: Better Living and Breathing: A Manual for Patients 2nd ed. St. Louis, MO: C.V. Mosby, August, 1980.

Pomerantz, et al.: Occupational Therapy for Chronic Obstructive Lung Disease. Am. J. Occup. Ther. 29:407, 1975.

Death and Dying

Burnside, I. M.: Touching is talking. Am. J. Nurs. 73:2060–2063, 1973.

DuBois, P. M.: The Hospice Way of Death. New York: Human Sciences Press, 1980.

Kubler-Ross, E.: On Death and Dying. New York: Macmillan, 1971.

McCorkle, R.: Effects of touch on seriously ill patients. Nurs. Research 23:125–132, 1974.

Preston, T.: When words fail. Am. J. Nurs. 73:2064, 1973.

Diabetes

Creighton, C. A., et al.: Who helps the diabetic? New Physician, April 1973.

Holliman, K.: Another device for one-handed insulin management. Am. J. Occup. Ther. 33:393, 1979.

Dysphagia

Bockus, H. L.: Dysphagia. In Gastroenterology, ed. 2. Vol. I, Chapter 3, pp. 54–59. Philadelphia: W.B. Saunders, 1963.

Doty, R. W.: Neural organization of deglutition. In Code, C. F. (ed.): Handbook of Physiology, Vol. IV, pp. 1861–1902. American Physiological Society, Washington, DC, 1968.

Hendrix, T. R., and Bayless, T. M.: Dysphagia and heartburn. In Harvey, A. M. (ed.): The Principles and Practice of Medicine, ed. 18. Chapter 65, pp. 687–694. New York: Appleton-Century-Crofts, 1972.

Ellis, H.: Dysphagia. In Hart, F. D. (ed.): French's Index of Differential Diagnosis, ed. 10, pp. 217–221. Baltimore: Williams & Wilkins, 1973.

Farber, S. D.: Sensorimotor Evaluation and Treatment Procedures for Allied Health Personnel, ed. 2, Chapter IV, pp. 53–67. Indianapolis: Indiana University Press, 1974.

Gallender, D.: Eating Handicaps: Illustrated Techniques for Feeding Disorders. Springfield, IL: Charles C Thomas, 1979.

Gambescia, R. A., and Rogers, A. I.: Gastroenterology, dysphagia, diagnosis by history. Postgrad. Med. 59:211–216, 1976.

Griffin, K. M.: Swallowing training for dysphagic patients. Arch. Phys. Med. Rehabil. 55:467–470, 1974.

Huffman, A.: Biofeedback treatment of orofacial dysfunction: A preliminary study. Amer. J. Occup. Ther. 32(3):149–154, March, 1978.

Larsen, G. L.: Conservative management for incomplete dysphagia paralytica. Arch. Phys. Med. Rehabil. 54:180–185, 1973.

Larsen, G. L.: Rehabilitating dysphagia mechanica, paralytica, pseudobulbar. J. Neurosurg. Nurs. 8:14–17, 1976.

Ogg, H. L.: Oral-pharyngeal development and evaluation. Phys. Ther. 55:235–241, 1975.

Phillips, M. M., and Hendrix, T. R.: Dysphagia. Postgrad. Med. 50:81–86, 1971.

Silverman, E. H., and Elfant, I. L.: Dysphagia: An evaluation and treatment program for the adult. Amer. J. Occup. Ther. 33:6:382–392, June, 1979.

General Medicine

Beeson, P. B., and McDermott, W. (eds.): Testbook of Medicine, ed. 14. Philadelphia: W. B. Saunders, 1975.

Steinberg, F. U.: The Immobilized Patient, Functional Pathology and Management. New York: Plenum Medical Book, 1980.

Warfel, J. H. and Schlagenhauff, R. E.: Understanding Neurologic Disease: The Text Book for Therapists. Baltimore, MD: Urban and Schwarzenberg, Inc., 1980.

General Practice

Banus, B. S.: The Developmental Therapist. Thorofare NJ: Charles C. Slack, 1971.

Baum, C. M.: Occupational therapists put care in the health system. Amer. J. Occup. Ther. 34:505–516, 1980.

Goldenson, R. M. (ed.): Disability and Rehabilitation Handbook, New York: McGraw-Hill, 1978.

Handbook on Third-Party Reimbursement for Occupational Therapy Services. American Occupational Therapy Association, Inc., Rockville, MD, October 1976.

Hays, et al.: Guidelines for Interpretation of Occupational Therapy in General Practice and Rehabilitiation. Michigan Occupational Therapy Association, January 1970.

Hays, C.: Sample Job Descriptions for Occupational Therapy. Rockville, MD, American Occupational Therapy Association, 1981.

Huss, A. J.: Touch with care or a caring touch? 1976 Eleanor Clarke Slagle Lectures. Am. J. Occup. Ther. 31:11–18, 1977.

Kirchman, M. M.: The quality of care in occupational therapy: An assessment of selected Michigan hospitals. Am. J. Occup. Ther. 33:425–431, 1979.

Obesity

Humphrey, R.: A practical approach to exercise in the treatment of obesity. Obesity & Bariatric Med. 10:6, 1981.

Wise, J. F. and Wise, S. K.: The Overeaters: Eating Styles and Personality. New York, Human Sciences Press. 1979.

Parkinson's Disease

Lavigne, J.: Home Exercises for Patients with Parkinson's Disease. New York, The American Parkinson Disease Association, 1978.

Sweet, R., and McDowell, F.: A Manual for Patients with Parkinson's Disease, New York, The American Parkinson Disease Association, 1978.

Scleroderma

Rodan, G. P.: Progressive Systemic Sclerosis, Arthritis and Allied Conditions, 9th ed. Philadelphia: Lea & Febiger, 1979.

Swezey, R. L.: Arthritis: Rational Therapy and Rehabilitation. Philadelphia: W.B. Saunders, 1978.

Resources—Agencies

American Cancer Society
777 Third Ave.
New York, NY 10020

American Diabetes Association
600 Fifth Ave.
New York, NY 10020

American Heart Association
7320 Greenville Ave.
Dallas, TX 75231

American Hospital Association
840 North Lake Shore Drive
Chicago, IL 60611

American Lung Association
1740 Broadway
New York, NY 10019

American Occupational Therapy Association
1383 Piccard Drive, Suite 300
Rockville, MD 20850

The American Parkinson Disease Association
116 John Street
New York, NY 10038

Arthritis Foundation
3400 Peachtree Dr., N.E.
Atlanta, GA 30326

Arthritis Information Clearinghouse
P.O. Box 34227
Bethesda, MD 20034

Leukemia Society of America, Inc.
800 Second Ave.
New York, NY 10017

Acknowledgments

With special acknowledgments to Barbara Bly, OTR, Betty Cox, COTA, ROH, Carolyn Creighton, M.D., Linda DiJoseph, OTR, Sue Graalman, B.S., Frances R. Richardson, and the entire occupational therapy staff at the University of Michigan Hospital.

CHAPTER 36

Community Home Health Care—The Home-Bound Patient

Ruth Levine

WANTED: Experienced O.T.R. with knowledge of physical and psychosocial dysfunction. Well-organized person who is able to work without direct supervision. Flexible personality—able to adjust to a variety of social and environmental situations.

O.T.R. must be able to teach activities of daily living and motor skill retraining to both professional and nonprofessional team members as well as patients.

Job requires above-average written and verbal communication abilities.

Applicants must be able to drive in all weather conditions.

Salary and benefits are excellent. Working hours can be scheduled by applicant.

Is this job description appealing to you? If so, you might be interested in home care. If not, you might read on anyway to learn more about a growing area of occupational therapy practice. This chapter will explore the boundaries of home care practice, describe the delivery process, and comment on issues that affect the present and future of home care.

Description of Home Care

Home care can best be described as a holistic context for providing therapeutic services in the patient's home. A home care agency offers skilled professional services, such as nursing, physical, occupational, and speech therapies, medical social service, laboratory testing, and other services, including light housekeeping, shopping, and personal care. Also available are counseling services, specialized testing procedures, and visits from other health specialists such as podiatrists, dentists, and respiratory therapists.

The medically stable patient is eligible for home services. Acute medical conditions requiring complex equipment, emergency intervention, and constant monitoring are best treated in an institutional setting.

Overview of Home Rehabilitation

The occupational therapist delivers services to home-bound patients who have been referred by their physicians. The occupational therapist works in conjunction with the family and other members of the home care team to maximize the patient's functional abilities. Emotional and motivational factors are part of the recovery process. Thus, the therapist must manage both the physical and psychological aspects of delivery. Programs initiated in the hospital or rehabilitation center can be reinforced by home care teams. Other appropriate uses of home care include the rehabilitation of patients who were never hospitalized, the rehabilitation of patients who did not cooperate with institution staff, care for patients who are too ill to withstand a full-time rehabilitation program, and care for those who are terminally ill.

Case Study

Mr. Smith, a 67-year-old former truck driver, suffered a cerebrovascular accident in March of 1982. He was rushed to the hospital where his medical condition was stabilized by medication, rest, remedial diet, and bed exercises. After two weeks, he was transferred to a rehabilitation center.

The rehabilitation center staff taught Mr. Smith to bathe from a basin while in bed, dress if supervised and assisted, eat using adapted equipment, transfer with supervision and assistance, and to perform selected joint range of motion exercises with his affected upper extremity. Mrs. Smith was involved in the rehabilitation program.

Mr. Smith was fitted for a resting hand splint and arm sling. He was sent home with a tub transfer seat, wheelchair, walker, and raised toilet seat.

The rehabilitation center team felt that Mr. Smith could benefit from additional training, therefore the physiatrist ordered a home program. Three days prior to discharge, a hospital social worker referred Mr. Smith to a home care agency. The social worker described Mr. Smith's rehabilitation program and discussed his progress.

A home health agency nurse visited the day that Mr. Smith came home. The nurse evaluated Mr. Smith's condition, checked on the available medical equipment, and verified the need for other skilled services. She found that Mrs. Smith seemed anxious and threatened by her new responsibilities.

The nursing supervisor referred the case to physical and occupational therapies. The patient's diagnosis, history and address were given.

The occupational therapist visited the patient three days after he came home. The therapist found that Mr. Smith could eat pre-cut food, but was dependent on Mrs. Smith for all other aspects of his daily care. Mr. Smith's impulsive behavior, short attention span, and left visual field-cut all limited his performance in daily self-care. The home visiting team continued services for the next six months.

The occupational therapist upgraded the therapeutic exercises initiated in the rehabilitation center. Mr. Smith could use his affected arm to stabilize objects. A complete review of dressing techniques was necessary because Mrs. Smith initially found it easier to dress her husband. The occupational therapist also taught Mr. Smith to compensate for his left field-cut by using familiar cues from his environment.

After six months of training in occupational and physical therapy, Mr. Smith could dress, eat, and do light housekeeping. He could ambulate to the front door and go down the front steps if assisted. He could bathe upstairs in his bathroom, sleep in his own bed, and prepare a light meal. □

In the case of Mr. Smith, the home care team completed the patient's rehabilitation program. Much therapy was initiated by the rehabilitation hospital staff; however, much additional treatment was required to make the patient independent. The home visiting team could adjust Mr. Smith's program to the needs of his family by using the familiar setting of his home.

Definition of Terms

The following definitions will be used throughout this chapter:

Home care is an organized health service that is delivered in a patient's home. Frequently, patients with stable medical conditions can be appropriately treated at home. Home visiting team members consider the patient's problems from a holistic vantage point. Home services include nursing, home health aid, physical, occupational, and speech therapy, medical social work, EKG and other laboratory tests, and nutritional guidance. Each service is described below.

The *nurse* carries out skilled duties that include supervising medication, giving injections and nutritional advice, caring for wounds and dressings, monitoring vital signs, and teaching and supervising the patient and caretakers regarding daily care. The nurse is usually the coordinator of the patient's care; he or she supervises other nursing personnel such as home health aides.

The *home health aide* carries out the nursing care plan. Duties include bathing, dressing, and feeding the patient; carrying out and/or reinforcing therapeutic activities and exercise regimes; maintaining the environment; assisting in the preparation of meals; and providing assistance with ambulation and self-administered medications. The home health aide also offers psychological support.

The *physical therapist* employs physical agents such as heat, light, water, electricity, massage, radiation, and exercise to restore patients to their maximum level of physical function.

The *speech therapist* uses knowledge about speech, hearing, and language to plan and implement a realistic program to increase the patient's communication skills. The patient's emotions affect speech; thus psychological aspects are an important consideration in speech therapy.

The *occupational therapist* uses specified therapeutic, self-care, homemaking, and creative activities to facilitate and/or maximize the patient's level of function. Both the psychosocial and the physical aspects of the patient's condition are assessed in terms of the total context for treatment.

The *social worker* uses a problem solving approach to help patients help themselves. Options and resources are presented to the patient and caretakers in an attempt to maximize the patient's level of adjustment.

Not all of the possible home care professionals were presented in this section. Others may include a podiatrist, optometrist, dentist, homemaker, dietician, and home-visiting physician.

Home-bound patients cannot leave their homes without assistance. This is an important classification for third party carriers (insurance coverage). Ambulatory patients may be asked to travel to outpatient therapy. Some carriers refuse to cover services if patients can walk out of their house without maximum assistance.

Resources are the patient's available human and physical assets. Assets can help to balance the debilitating effects of health problems. Resources can be categorized into human and material classes.

Human resources are caretakers—people who assist with the patient's daily care. Caretaker duties include such tasks as preparing meals, caring for the patient's wounds and dressings, offering medication at the appropriate times, bathing the patient, cleaning the surrounding environment, and offering support, encouragement, and entertainment. At times, the caretaker assumes responsibility for the patient's financial obligations.

The patient's skills determine the scope of the caretaker's responsibilities and the time required to complete the daily tasks. Human resources are so important that they frequently influence the overall course of the patient's progress. There are three kinds of human resources. *Primary caretakers* assume full responsibility for all of the patient's needs. The amount of effort involved is determined by the extent of the patient's independence. If the patient is dependent in all aspects of self-care, primary care may be equivalent to a full-time job. In many cases, the burdens of patient care are added to the normal responsibilities of the caretaker. This means that the caretaker has two jobs. The work load can become emotionally and physically draining.

Secondary caretakers do not assume total responsibility for the patient's care. The secondary caretaker, however, will frequently perform routine patient care tasks, thereby offering respite to the primary caretaker.

Tertiary caretakers offer infrequent but welcome assistance. They visit the patient and provide emotional support and social contact. Also important is the periodic help given to the primary and secondary caretakers. Although tertiary caretakers are not available for daily rehabilitation training and personal care, they may perform duties such as shopping for food and medicine, transporting the patient to the doctor, and staying with the patient while the primary caretaker attends to other business.

Material resources consist of the patient's financial assets. Furniture, equipment, supplies, clothing, medication, safety equipment, and aide services can all be purchased.

Boundaries of Home Care

There are five factors that make home care delivery different from the care offered in an institution. These factors include the patient's medical condition, the resources necessary for good care, the emotional and motivational needs of the patient, the need for effective teaching in the home setting, and the shift in social roles.

Medical Condition

Elderly adults who are recovering from fractures, heart or pulmonary diseases, cerebrovascular accidents, neurological disorders, decubitus ulcers, surgical wounds, and arthritis are frequently referred to a home care agency. Younger adults and children with similar medical conditions are also eligible for care. Patients with acute medical problems should have their medical conditions stabilized before they can be offered home care services. Terminally ill patients can often remain at home if the family is able to cooperate in providing the necessary care.

Resources

Because the home care patient requires supervision and direct care, the available human and material resources become important considerations. A network of supportive friends, relatives, or neighbors may provide meals, supervision, and assistance with the patient's care. Without adequate help, the patient will find home convalescence difficult and awkward.

The home environment is also important. Temporary changes such as placing a hospital bed, commode, and wheelchair in the dining room of a two-story house may make home placement realistic.

Motivational and Emotional Factors

Patients can gain positive reinforcement from the nonhuman objects in their own home. Some patients find little comfort in the institutional environment and long for their own home, bed, food, and pets. Searles' work on the nonhuman environment substantiates the importance of the objects, smells, and sights that are present in a person's environment.[1] In many instances, a person can progress rapidly if treated at home, although this may not be true for everyone.

Importance of Teaching

Since home care practitioners commonly visit the patient only two or three times a week, with each visit averaging about 35–45 minutes, effective teaching is especially important.

Direct "hands-on" techniques are required for home care practice. Of equal importance, however, is the therapist's ability to promote patient and family independence. Effective communication by home care practitioners encourages carry-over of skills taught during visits. Home care practitioners realize that teaching skills either make or break the rehabilitation program. Thus, the practitioner must tailor each program to meet the unique needs of a particular family.

Therapists provide direct service and explain how and why a technique or activity is used. As soon as the patient and the caretaker become comfortable with it, the responsibility for the exercise or activity is turned over to the family. The patient can receive a therapeutic regime seven days a week if the patient and caretakers cooperate.

Home health aides may visit five times a week until the family caretaker network operates well. Aide visits usually decrease in frequency as the patient improves.

Shift in Social Roles

The last factor that makes home care unique is the shift in social roles. The health care practitioner enters the social hierarchy of the patient's family and friends. The therapist is a guest in the patient's house, a visitor in his or her lifespace. The reverse is true with services offered in an institution. The patient enters the institution as a temporary member of the formal social hierarchy.

As a visitor in the patient's world, the practitioner must adjust to values, traditions, communication patterns, and environmental factors. The patient's lifestyle might be unfamiliar, but the practitioner must use verbal, nonverbal, and environmental cues to promote effective interaction. Successful home care practitioners have the ability to interact in a variety of social systems. Communication skills must promote caretaker and patient cooperation.

Theoretical Overview

Delivery Model

There are several stages in the delivery of home services. After initial intervention, there is a period of gradual building during which relationships and treatment regimes are established. After this period, a plateau frequently occurs, and fewer gains take place. During this time, learning and therapeutic patterns are reinforced. Finally, the patient and the caretakers return to their former lives, and the case is discharged. The stages of this process are depicted in Figure 36-1.

Each of the five divisions in the diagram represents a phase in the treatment cycle. The umbrella of prevention arches over the entire model; this is a fundamental consideration throughout the delivery process. The five stages of this process are intervention, building a therapeutic relationship, carrying out the treatment program, discharge planning, and after-care. Each of the stages, as well as some of the issues that arise during the stage, will be discussed in detail later. In brief, characteristics of each stage include the following:

1. *Intervention.* This includes the referral, initial visit, and process of data collection.

2. *Building a Therapeutic Relationship.* In this period, the initial assessment is completed. Long- and short-term goals are established defining the focus of the occupational therapy care plan. The initial foundations for a trusting relationship are being built.

3. *Carrying Out the Treatment Program.* This is a time to teach the patient and the caretakers how to maximize the patient's level of function. Therapeutic exercises and modalities are introduced. The thrust of the team effort is to integrate the skills that the patient gains into the daily lifestyle.

4. *Discharge Planning.* During discharge planning goals are reassessed and new resources are sought out. Preparation is made for the termination of direct services. The full responsibility for care shifts back to the patient and the caretakers.

5. *After-Care.* This is a time when contact with the patient is maintained by telephone conversa-

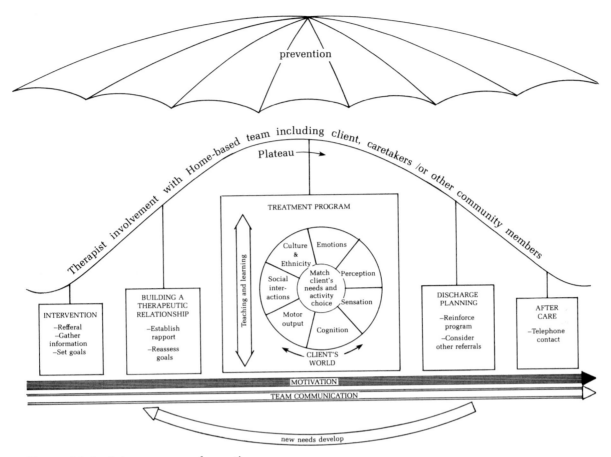

Figure 36-1. A home care schematic.

tions. If new needs arise, the process begins again with a referral.

Social Roles

No section that purports to offer background information for home care can overlook the importance of social roles. Research in sociology provides a foundation for differentiating the practical roles of the therapist in an institution and of the home-based therapist. Stated simply, the difference lies in the power they hold. "Power refers to the ability to secure one's ends in life, even against oppression."[2] In the institution, the patient has only a minimal amount of power over other team members and within the treatment process. The reverse is true in home-based therapy, where the practitioner becomes a guest in the patient's world.

Each person has a role in the social system. This social system is composed of numerous subsocieties which reflect parts of the total society. The social system is stratified; it reflects a hierarchy. The social group or society is arranged ". . . into a hierarchy of positions that are unequal with regard to power, property, social evaluation, or psychic gratification."[3]

The roles at the top of the social structure have more authority and status than those at the bottom. This ordered hierarchy of roles creates an arrangement of society that facilitates function.

Medical practitioners rarely consider the sociological aspects of the health care delivery system. Whether it is acknowledged or not, the practice of any aspect of medicine is a social act. Each practitioner has a place in the social system. The professional's role is shaped by the social system as well as by individual skills, knowledge, and attitudes. Any role, regardless of the individual who occupies the role, has certain values and functions that transcend individual differences. Professional education, liaisons, job descriptions, and status in the social hierarchy all shape individual behavior. Individuals express their roles in unique fashions while societal pressures determine the outer boundaries.

In general, the larger the social unit, the more numerous, specialized, and rigid are the roles of the participants. Communication among professionals becomes difficult. People organize around different specialty areas; those who are outside of this area do not tend to socialize or meet informally on a frequent basis. Territory becomes an important issue. The overall goals of the institution become abstract and less than obvious to members of the broader society. Individuals at the bottom of the social system do not interact with those at the top.

In an institution the patient is at the bottom of the social system and not a permanent member of the institution's social system, and thus has little power. The patient role can become depersonalized in a world of experts. Yet the goals of the institution are said to be based on serving the patient. While staff members are sensitive to individual patients, they often neglect the powerless state of this role. The recent popularity of a discussion regarding Patient Rights in the institution merely exaggerates their lack of real power.

This situation is reversed in the home setting. The therapist is a guest in the patient's house. The practitioner is a temporary addition to the family social system. The patient and the caretakers determine the therapist's role as much as do the therapist's job description and training. If the therapist does not meet the patient's needs, suggestions will be ignored or services cancelled. The patient has more control over the practitioner; therefore, the patient has more control over the treatment.

Philosophical Base

It is useful to orient oneself to specialty practice by categorizing and identifying personal values. Values become a belief system, establishing a predilection for certain objects, perceptions, people, and emotions. A refined belief system is a practitioner's philosophical base.

There are values shared by most occupational therapists. Basically, these values maintain that people have the potential to adapt, to grow, to change, and to engage in purposeful activity.[4] Occupational therapists believe that people learn by doing. The patient is considered a whole being and not merely a collection of anatomical parts. Finally, the activity process is focused on the patient's rather than the therapist's needs.

Home care therapists agree with the above values. There is, however, a difference in the manner in which the values are integrated into daily practice. The home setting requires a unique approach to patient care.

There are three values that are central to home care:

1. *Home care practice must be functional.* The O.T.R. enters the patient's world. Activity choices are limited by the family's resources and perceived needs. Communication is not done only on the verbal level. The nonhuman environment can be used to focus the occupational therapy program on activities that have meaning to the patient. Activity choices may be rejected if the family does not understand the purpose and expected outcome of the therapy program.

2. *The importance of teaching.* Interaction is a component in many occupational therapy programs, but it is essential in home care delivery. Since the patient and the caretakers are responsible for the continuity of the daily program, the occupational therapist must present the treatment in a manner that is understood by them. The professional's ability to teach is the core of home care. Necessary also is an understanding of human motivation. Motivation has a direct effect on the ability to learn.[5,6,7,8]

3. *Adapting to a variety of life-styles and values systems.* Home therapists enter a different social system every time they enter a patient's house. The therapist finds that every family operates with different values, traditions, and habits. At times, the occupational therapist does not understand the patient's hierarchy of needs. If a practitioner appreciates the complexity of a family's belief system, he or she can maintain objectivity and avoid a clash of values. The therapist must work within this belief system and respect, as well as utilize, the patient's values when making treatment decisions.

The test of an effective home program is the degree to which the treatment is carried over in the therapist's absence. A good home program is pragmatic and useful to the patient in the tasks of everyday living.

Home Delivery Process

The conceptual material presented earlier has been offered as a foundation for understanding the delivery of home-bound services. At this point, you may wish to consider some direct service issues. How does the occupational therapist obtain cases, and how is the occupational therapy program carried out?

This section can be compared to an orientation handbook. The information is useful as an introduction to home care delivery. The material is divided into the five stages of the Home Care Delivery Model (Fig. 36-1), as follows:

Intervention—referral, preparation, initial visit, and evaluation
Building a Therapeutic Relationship—establishing rapport, reassessing goals, and initiating programs
Treatment Program—activity choices, teaching and learning, coordination, architectural barriers, body mechanics, transfer techniques, and home modalities

Discharge Planning—Reinforcing program
After-care

Intervention

Intervention includes the therapist's preparation for and entry into a new case. The agency personnel intervene and offer direct patient services. The process begins with a telephoned referral to the home health agency. Patients must be under the care of a physician, who may refer the case to the agency. Social workers, nurse coordinators, rehabilitation teams, family members, and friends may also make a home care referral.

The first agency contact is usually made by a nurse. If there is no need for skilled nursing services, a physical therapist or a speech pathologist may open the case. (Occupational therapists may not open cases because they are not classified as primary providers.) Referrals to occupational therapy may be included in the physician's original orders. If not, and the patient could benefit from occupational therapy, the nurse, physical therapist, or speech pathologist may initiate a referral. The coordinating nurse will contact the patient's physician, verify the request, and obtain written occupational therapy orders.

Information commonly given in the *referral* includes the patient's: (1) location—name, address, telephone number and zip code, (2) date of birth, (3) primary and secondary diagnoses and treatment precautions, (4) recent hospitalization dates, if applicable, (5) physician and the physician's address and telephone number, and (6) name, address, and telephone number of the primary caretaker. Also listed are the date that the agency started care, the name of the person who opened the case, the other services that the physician ordered, the frequency of visits, if specified, and physician's orders.

If the patient was treated in a hospital or rehabilitation facility, the former therapist may be contacted to ensure continuity of the occupational therapy program. The referral must be answered within 72 hours of receipt. (See sample referral.)

Preparation

Preparation for the initial visit involves three steps: locating the patient's house, scheduling the visit, and selecting appropriate modalities for the evaluation. Planning maximizes the time spent with the patient as one minimizes the time wasted on nonproductive concerns. It is best to make the shortest trips between patient houses. Using a detailed map will make routing easier.

The new patient must next be contacted by telephone. Offer an introduction and ask for permission to visit. Emphasize the time and day of the visit; verify the address and discuss directions to the house that will help in avoiding traffic obstacles.

Most therapists carry a bag filled with evaluation tools and common modalities. The bag may contain a stereognosis testing kit (box filled with familiar objects), perceptual test materials (may be formal or informal tests), goniometer, watch with a second hand (pulse rate measurement), safety pin (test for neurological deficits), a blindfold (testing for proprioception), and household items (paper towels, soap, crayons, scissors, pens, pencils, and masking tape). Some therapists also carry exercise putty, rubber bands, theraplast, stacking cones, foam rubber, surgical tubing, and equipment catalogs. Splinting materials, crafts, weights, pulleys, and other equipment may be required at a later date.

Initial Visit

The initial visit is crucial to the entire treatment process. The therapist evaluates the patient's abilities, establishes a baseline for treatment progress, and determines the goals of the program. Also important is the assessment of the entire environment including caretakers and resources. Finally, the therapist must determine how to interact effectively within the patient's social system. The therapist takes in as much information as possible.

There are five tasks that must be completed during the initial session:
1. Evaluation of the patient's motor, sensory, perceptual, and cognitive abilities
2. Exploration of the patient's ability to perform life tasks
3. Assessment and integration of cues offered in the environment
4. Establishment of long- and short-term goals for the occupational therapy program
5. Projection of the time it will take to achieve the goals

Other objectives of the initial visit are to verify information about the patient's medical history, diagnoses, and treatment precautions, to meet the caretakers, and to examine the available resources.

The therapist must determine the treatment goals and the duration of services during the initial visit. Goals must include independence in self-care and upper extremity retraining. Most funding sources require evidence of *measurable, practical* progress in a reasonable period of time.

Long-term goals establish the desired outcome of the therapy regime. The success of the patient's progress will be measured in terms of the expected therapy outcome.

Short-term goals are the graded steps to attainment of long-term goals. Short-term goals are part of the mastery process.

Evaluation

The evaluation form must be completed. A case study and sample evaluation (see Occupational Therapy Evaluation and Care Plan) are included. Read the narrative and see if you agree with the therapist's evaluation.

Case Study No. 1

Mrs. Helen Rowlings is a 72-year-old former domestic worker who suffered a cerebrovascular accident four weeks ago. She has a residual right hemiplegia with severe expressive aphasia. She was treated at a teaching hospital and transferred to a Rehabilitation Center.

In the Rehabilitation Center, Mrs. Rowlings became anxious and uncooperative. The Rehabilitation Center team tried to find out why Mrs. Rowlings was so troubled. The social worker discovered that Mrs. Rowlings wanted to go home. She feared that her prolonged absence might encourage burglars and vandals. Since two boarders reside in her house, it was unclear whether she really feared for her possessions or whether she just wanted to be home.

Mrs. Rowlings had worked for the same family for 30 years, and her employer was anxious to help. Two neighbors were willing to feed and care for Mrs. Rowlings until she could assume responsibility for herself. Mrs. Rowlings was discharged to her own house and her network of caretakers. Her case was referred to a home health care agency as well.

She was visited by a nurse who ordered a home health aide for five days a week. Physical therapy, occupational therapy, and speech therapy were also required. The occupational therapist scheduled her first visit and found the patient's house on a busy urban street. Scattered throughout the block of victorian row houses were newly renovated houses.

As the therapist parked her car, she noticed that the street bustled with foot traffic. Neighbors greeted each other and children played on the pavement. Water ice was sold in front of a house in the middle of the block. The patient was seated by an open window. People stopped to greet her, and some children were coming out of her house as the therapist entered.

The therapist found a neat, but shabby interior. There were six unrailed steps to the entry. The parlor had been converted to the patient's room. Available were a hospital bed, a commode, and a four-point cane. A bathroom was situated in a corner of the breakfast room.

Mrs. Rowlings was seated in a straight-backed chair. There were three packages of cupcakes on the window sill. Next to her chair was a coffee can. Mrs. Hughes, the neighbor, explained that Mrs. Rowlings loved to chew tobacco. She used the can for the remains of her "wad."

The occupational therapist assessed the patient's skills. (Please refer to the Evaluation Form.) Mrs. Rowlings' arm was flaccid and painful. She could bathe if set-up. She could not prepare her own meals. □

Consider the complexity of the patient's situation. What factors are most significant? Note how the environment and available resources influence treatment planning. How would you plan the treatment process? What activities would be relevant to Mrs. Rowlings?

Building a Therapeutic Relationship

In the second stage of the Home Care Delivery Model, the therapist must establish a good rapport, refine treatment planning, and initiate the treatment program. Communication must be effective. The human and nonhuman environment provide information. The Case Study offered here demonstrates the importance of using cues from the environment to enhance communication.

Case Study No. 2

The occupational therapist walked up a flight of freshly scrubbed, marble steps and rang the doorbell of a twin house. Peering through the double glass doors of the glass-enclosed porch, he noted an orderly, modestly furnished porch and living room. Starched, white, ruffled curtains stood out from the window sills. Crocheted doilies adorned the dated, overstuffed sofa and arm chairs. Tiny, delicate china *objets d'art* were displayed on the sofa endtables. The focal point of the living room was a religious statue situated on an altar. The front windowsill was lined with large, potted plants. The potting soil in several pots was decorated with china figurines and large, satin bows.

A neatly attired, elderly woman hobbled to the door; she seemed hesitant and fearful. The therapist displayed his arm patch and loudly mentioned his name and their earlier telephone call. The woman

OCCUPATIONAL THERAPY EVALUATION AND CARE PLAN

Name _____ H.I.C. No. _____

Date of Evaluation_____ Age _____ Medical Record No. _____

_____ Date of Onset _____

Diagnosis _____

_____

Communication Ability _____

_____

HOME SITUATION

Architectural

Consideration _____

_____

Family Members _____

Daily Routine _____

PHYSICAL CAPACITY

	Right	Left	COMMENTS
RANGE OF MOTION/UE			
Active	___	___	
Passive	___	___	
MUSCLE TONE	___	___	
STRENGTH	___	___	
HAND CAPACITY			
Appearance	___	___	
Hook Grasp	___	___	
Lateral Pinch	___	___	
Palmer Grasp	___	___	
3-Jaw Pinch	___	___	
Opposition	___	___	
COORDINATION			
Gross	___	___	
Fine	___	___	
Bilateral	___	___	
PRONATION/SUPINATION	___	___	
SENSORY			
Sharp/Dull	___	___	
Stereognosis	___	___	
Proprioception	___	___	

Physical Endurance _____

Visual Deficits/Aids _____

Present Use of Same _____

Hearing Deficits/Aids _____

Visual Motor Perception _____

Hand Dominance _____ Change Required? _____

Comments from Perceptual Evaluation: _____

This plan was developed by Ruth E. Levine, Lynn Marcus, Jane Roda, and Carmella Strano, Community Occupational Therapy Consultants Group, and is printed with permission.

Name _____   Medical Record No. _____

ACTIVITIES OF DAILY LIVING

I - Independent   M - Maximum Assistance
A - Minimal Assistance   D - Dependent

Feeding: Dressing:

   Eat with Fork _____   UE Dressing _____
   Cut Meat _____   UE Undressing _____
   Butter Bread _____   LE Dressing _____
   Drink from Glass _____   LE Undressing _____

Hygiene: Buttons _____

   Comb Hair _____   Fasteners _____
   Brush Teeth _____   Shoes/Braces _____
   Cosmetics/shave _____   Ties/Laces _____
   Wash Upper Body _____   Sling _____
   Wash Lower Body _____

   Shower/Tub _____   General Abilities:

   Nails _____   Phone _____
   Urinal/Toilet _____   Turn Pages of Book _____

Transfers: Wristwatch _____

   Chair _____   Doorknob/Key _____
   Bed _____   Writing _____
   Toilet _____   Open/Close Drawers _____
   Tub/Shower _____   Operate TV _____
   Car _____   Lights _____
                                                 Faucets _____
                                                 Flush Toilet _____
                                                 Pick Up Articles From Floor _____

Ambulation Ability _____

Patient's Homemaker Skills (Meals prepared by) _____

Medical Equipment Available _____
Additional Equipment Needed _____
Comments _____
_____
_____
_____

Short Term Goals _____
_____

Long Term Plans _____
Treatment Frequency
and Duration _____

_____
OCCUPATIONAL THERAPIST

OCCUPATIONAL THERAPY EVALUATION AND CARE PLAN

Name _HELEN ROWLINGS_
Date of Evaluation _9/5/8–_ Age _72_

H.I.C. No. _____
Medical Record No. _4561A3_
Date of Onset _____

Diagnosis _CVA → (R) HEMI, MI. DM._

Communication Ability _PATIENT SEEMS TO UNDERSTAND BUT HAS NO FUNCTIONAL SPEECH. SHE CAN MUMBLE SYLLABLES_

HOME SITUATION

Architectural
Consideration _TWO STORY ROW HOUSE: 6 STEPS UNRAILED, 1 STEP UP TO VESTIBULE, LR (PATIENT'S BED & COMMODE) KITCHEN & PANTRY, BATHROOM ON 1st FL. IN KITCHEN, 15 STEPS RAILED (R) GOING UP TO 2nd FLOOR_
Family Members _LIVES WITH 2 BOARDERS WHO WORK DAY SHIFT_
Daily Routine _UP & DRESSED c̄ ASST. WATCHES T.V. VISITS c̄ NEIGHBORS_

PHYSICAL CAPACITY

	Right	Left	COMMENTS
RANGE OF MOTION/UE			
Active	①	NORMAL	① FLACCID
Passive	②	LIMITS	② PROM
MUSCLE TONE	FLACCID		
STRENGTH	"		SHOULDER – FORWARD REFLEX 80°—PAIN
HAND CAPACITY			ABDUCTION TO 90° – PAIN
Appearance	EDEMA		
Hook Grasp	FLACCID		ELBOW – FLEXION COMPLETE BUT
Lateral Pinch	NONE		PAINFUL, EXT. COMPLETE
Palmer Grasp	NONE		
3-Jaw Pinch	NONE		WRIST – LOOSE, FULL RANGE
Opposition	NONE		
COORDINATION			FINGERS – EDEMATOUS. TIGHT & PAINFUL
Gross	NONE		PATIENT REFUSES TO KEEP ARM
Fine	NONE		ELEVATED
Bilateral	NONE		
PRONATION/SUPINATION	FULL PROM		③ NOT TESTED – CONFUSED ANSWERS
SENSORY			
Sharp/Dull	③	③	
Stereognosis	③	③	
Proprioception	③	③	

Physical Endurance _LIMITED – GETS SOB³ (SHORT OF BREATH)_
Visual Deficits/Aids _NONE_
Present Use of Same _NONE_
Hearing Deficits/Aids _NONE_
Visual Motor Perception _③_
Hand Dominance _(R)_ Change Required? _YES_
Comments from Perceptual Evaluation: _SEE ③_

This plan was developed by Ruth E. Levine, Lynn Marcus, Jane Roda, and Carmella Strano, Community Occupational Therapy Consultants Group, and is printed with permission.

Name _HELEN ROWLINGS_   Medical Record No. _4561A3_

ACTIVITIES OF DAILY LIVING

I - Independent   M - Maximum Assistance
A - Minimal Assistance   D - Dependent

Feeding:

Eat with Fork	I
Cut Meat	D
Butter Bread	D
Drink from Glass	I

Hygiene:

Comb Hair	I - UNILATEAL
Brush Teeth	DENTURES Ⓓ
Cosmetics/shave	DID NOT USE
Wash Upper Body	I
Wash Lower Body	I
Shower/Tub	D
Nails	D
Urinal/Toilet	A

Transfers:

Chair	I
Bed	I
Toilet	I - COMMODE IN L.R.
Tub/Shower	D
Car	M

Dressing:

UE Dressing	I
UE Undressing	I
LE Dressing	M
LE Undressing	M
Buttons	I
Fasteners	A
Shoes/Braces	D - NO BRACE
Ties/Laces	D
Sling	D - REFUSES TO WEAR

General Abilities:

Phone	D - APHASIA
Turn Pages of Book	I
Wristwatch	NOT USED
Doorknob/Key	I
Writing	D
Open/Close Drawers	I
Operate TV	I
Lights	I
Faucets	M
Flush Toilet	M
Pick Up Articles From Floor	ASSISTENCE

Ambulation Ability _CLOSE SUPERVISION_

Patient's Homemaker Skills (Meals prepared by) _NEIGHBOR — MRS. HUGHES & MRS. COLEMAN. BOARDERS WILL HELP OCCASIONALLY_

Medical Equipment Available _HOSPITAL BED, COMMODE_

Additional Equipment Needed _—_

Comments _MRS. HUGHES & MRS. COLEMAN ARE PAID FOR THEIR ASSISTENCE BY MRS. ROWLINGS' FORMER EMPLOYER (MR. & MRS. JOHNSON). MRS. HUGHES IS RESPONSIBLE FOR DAY MEALS & DAY CARE; MRS. COLEMAN FOR NIGHT MEAL (5-11 PM). PATIENT HAS NO OTHER FAMILY. SEEMS AS IF MRS. ROWLINGS HAS ABUNDANCE OF VISITORS._

Short Term Goals _Ⓘ DRESSING   THERAPEUTIC EXERCIZE TO Ⓡ UE   ACTIVITIES TO INC. ACTIVITY TOLERENCE_

Long Term Plans _↑ Ⓘ ADL   ↑ FUNCTION Ⓡ UE_

Treatment Frequency and Duration _2 X WEEK ⑱_

Kelwene — OTR
OCCUPATIONAL THERAPIST

Community Home Health Care—The Home-Bound Patient **767**

HOME CARE DEPARTMENT

HOSP. NO. _____

REFERRAL FORM

H.C.
CASE NO. _____

H.I. CLAIM NO. _164 - 53 - 4173 A_

PATIENT _HELEN ROWLINGS_

SOURCE OF REFERRAL _REHAB CENTER_

ADDRESS _6622 N. 75TH ST._

ADM. DATE _3/4_   DISCH. DATE _3/10_

CITY _____ ZIP _19135_ TEL. NO. _783-2043_

PARTY RESPONSIBLE FOR CHARGES TO PATIENT _____

DATE OF BIRTH _2/17/05_ AGE _78_ SEX _F_

B.C. OR INS. CERT. NO. _____ GR. NO. _____

MARITAL STATUS S M (W) SEP. DIV.   HOSP. ACCOM. P S/P W OPD

IS ILLNESS EMPLOYMENT RELATED?   YES ☐   NO ☒

RESPONSIBLE PERSON IN HOME _NEIGHBOR: MRS. HUGHES_

PATIENT'S EMPLOYER _FORMER EMPLOYER — MR. & MRS. JOHNSON_

ADDRESS _6623 N. 75 ST., PHILA. PA. 19135_
_783-1230_ ZIP

ADDRESS _6612 OAKDALE TERRACE, WYNMOOR, PA._
_635-0782_ ZIP

PLAN OF TREATMENT—TO BE COMPLETED BY PHYSICIAN

DIAGNOSIS (PRIMARY AND SECONDARY—IN ORDER) _MI CVA (R) Hemiplegia, Diabetes_
Mellites, HT

SURGICAL PROCEDURE _____ DATE _____

PROGNOSIS _Fair_

PATIENT INFORMED: DIAGNOSIS YES ☒ NO ☐ PROGNOSIS YES ☒ NO ☐
FAMILY INFORMED: DIAGNOSIS YES ☒ NO ☐ PROGNOSIS YES ☒ NO ☐

THERAPEUTIC GOALS _Increase Independence in Self-Care & Ambulation_

MEDICAL SUPERVISION IN HOME BY _Dr. Jay Zaller_ TEL. NO. _234-5000 (page)_

ADDRESS _64 Wingdale Ave._ CITY _____ ZIP _____

HOME HEALTH SERVICES ORDERED: NURSING ☒ PHYSICAL THERAPY ☒ MEDICAL SOC. SER. ☐ SPEECH THERAPY ☐ OCC. THERAPY ☒ HOME HEALTH AID ☒

MEDICATIONS _Digoxin 0.25 mg. O.D._
Lasix 40 mg. O.D.
Aldomet 250 mg. B.I.D.
Diabenese 250 mg. A.M.

LABORATORY TESTS _Electrolyte 1X Mon   Digoxin level 1 q.o. mon._
Blood Sugar 1X mon.

DIET _Low Salt 1500 Cal. A.D.A._

ACTIVITIES ALLOWED _No Stairs graded program_

TREATMENT AND SPECIAL EQUIPMENT _Hospital bed, commode, 4 point cane_

SPECIAL INSTRUCTIONS, REACTIONS TO BE REPORTED TO PHYSICIAN _____

PATIENT TO BE SEEN BY PHYSICIAN: DATE _5/4/81_ HOME ☒ OFFICE ☐ OPD ☐

HOME HEALTH SERVICES TO BE PROVIDED ARE NEEDED TO TREAT THE CONDITION(S) FOR WHICH THE PATIENT RECEIVED SERVICES DURING THE RELATED STAY IN A HOSPITAL OR SKILLED NURSING FACILITY. YES ☐ NO ☐

I CERTIFY THAT THE PATIENT IS (1) HOMEBOUND, (2) REQUIRES THE HOME HEALTH SERVICES INDICATED ABOVE ON AN INTERMITTENT BASIS, (3) THE PATIENT IS UNDER THE CARE OF A PHYSICIAN WHO WILL REVIEW THIS PLAN OF TREATMENT PERIODICALLY.

_____
DATE

Jay Zaller M.D.
PHYSICIAN'S SIGNATURE

_____
REG. NO.

JAY ZALLER
PHYSICIAN'S NAME—PLEASE PRINT

(371-HC-1)

**HOSPITAL COPY
HOME CARE DEPARTMENT**

REFERRAL FORM

PATIENT   *HELEN ROWLINGS*   HOME CARE
                                                   CASE NO.   *3143 A*

TO BE COMPLETED BY HOME CARE NURSE

REVIEW OF PATIENT'S ILLNESS (INCL. PREVIOUS HOSPITALIZATION, LAB. FINDINGS AND SOCIAL DATA SIGNIFICANT TO PATIENT'S CARE)

PT. FOUND LYING ON FLOOR. RUSHED TO HOSP. 1X FOR CVA Ⓡ HEMI.
TRANS. TO REHAB CENTER. PATIENT INSISTS ON HOME MANAGEMENT.

BP 150/90   T. 98°   R. 70 WEAK & IRREGULAR

SERVICES ORDERED:	NURSING	P.T.	S.T.	O.T.	M.S.S.	H.H.A.
DATE OF FIRST VISIT:	*9/21*					
FREQUENCY OF VISITS:	*2-3*	*2X*	*2-3X*	*2 X*		*5X WK.*

PERTINENT INFORMATION REGARDING CARE TO BE GIVEN ___ *3X WK.*

MONITOR B/P & MEDS.   NOTE:
MAX LEVEL Ⓘ A.D.L.   *MAX. LEVEL OF FUNCTION*
MAX STRENGTH Ⓑ UE & Ⓑ LE-S   *W/IN BOUNDARIES OF*
↑ COMMUNICATION SKILLS   *CARDIAC STATUS*

MEDICAL SUPPLIES AND EQUIPMENT PROVIDED   *HOSPITAL BED, COMMODE*

_____   *Dee Jackson M. S. W.*   _____
DATE   SIGNATURE   TITLE
(371-HC-2)

Printed with the permission of Helen L. Rawlinson, Director, Home Care Department, Blue Cross of Greater Philadelphia. The form is used by all hospitals participating in the Blue Cross of Greater Philadelphia Home Care Program and Demonstration Study. (The patient on pages 645 and 646 is fictitious.)

could see the agency insignia on the therapist's car door. She smiled and opened the door.

The therapist analyzed his observations. Signs indicated that the family might have little contact with young men. If he made enthusiastic gestures, for example, they might be unfamiliar and arouse suspicion. The orderly rooms implied a formal, respectful demeanor; a boisterous person might not be well-received in this home. One might also speculate that changes should be introduced gradually; abrupt decisions should be avoided. The therapist used these cues from the nonhuman environment to enhance the effect of his communication. □

A home-based therapist needs to develop the ability to establish a rapport with people in various social systems. Developing this kind of skill depends on making good observations and evaluating what is observed. The therapist must also be aware of his or her own value systems and how they affect the perception of others.

Once communication patterns are established, the therapist may discover information that will affect the outcome of therapy. The therapist addresses the altered goals and changes the treatment plan accordingly.

The treatment regime can now be given full attention. The program is introduced to the patient and the caretaker. Once the treatment program is underway, the program moves to the third stage in the Home Care Delivery Model.

Treatment Program

The majority of patient learning takes place during the third stage of the treatment model. There are six concerns that one must address during this stage: the activity choice, the teaching and learning process, coordination among team members, architectural barriers, body mechanics and transfer techniques, and home modalities. Each topic will be discussed below.

Activity Choice

Curiosity about the activity base of occupational therapy has increased in the last two years.[9,10] The home setting offers an excellent example of the positive effects that can be derived from goal-directed activities. Few individuals will work at a task that they neither understand nor find pleasurable. On the other hand, a meaningful match between patient needs and an activity can stimulate and motivate the patient.

An easy way to begin the search for a relevant activity choice is to ask patients about their former life. What tasks did they perform in their house? How did they manage their daily life? Were they interested in any particular activities? A formal "Activity History" might help to organize your thoughts. Another strategy is to ask the patient to describe a "typical" day.

The occupational therapist tries to find an activity that will motivate the patient. Motivation is self-directed behavior that an individual pursues for internal or external reinforcement. The individual moves toward a goal. Occupational therapy relies on both extrinsic and intrinsic motivation.

Goal-directed behavior, stimulated by rewards outside of an organism can be called extrinsic motivation. Intrinsic motivation, on the other hand, is dependent on an internal reward system. The individual will pursue an idea or task to fulfill an inner need. This need is not based on the satisfaction of basic drives, such as hunger, thirst, or libido. "Intrinsic motivation builds toward self-reward in independent action that underlies competent behavior."[11] Crucial factors in the environment determine the extent that an individual is motivated by intrinsic rewards.

Successful home care programs are carried over when the occupational therapist is not present. The choice of activity promotes the patient's goals hopefully generating some intrinsic rewards.

Teaching and Learning

If you are a student, you are engaged in the teaching and learning process. Although the complexity of teaching and learning is seldom acknowledged, every person has unique learning needs. Thus, there are no definitive rules that can be used as a guide to success.

There are some basic tenets that might serve the home care practitioner. Center the learning on the patient's goals and expectations. Modalities should promote goal attainment. Activity selection must have a moderate degree of difficulty, but the choice should not foster anxiety. The occupational therapist slowly increases the patient's level of participation. The responsibility for a daily program will ultimately rest with the patient and the caretakers. Finally, feedback is offered to help the patient learn how to self-monitor.[12]

Programs should be written out so that other caretakers and team members can follow the instructions. Teaching aides—pictures, samples, demonstrations, and cues—help to facilitate the teaching and learning process.

Coordination

Coordination determines the degree to which the home care team is able to work together. The home care team has two parts: the patient and caretakers, and the professional staff. This diverse group is most effective when it functions as a unit. Although the patient is the focal point of the delivery process, each individual views the patient's condition from a different perspective. All views must be respected. Diverse opinions must be organized into a unified effort (Fig. 36-2).

It is difficult to create a home care team. However, if several professionals assume the responsibility for coordination, the communication channels can begin to open. The patient, who is the focus for care, should be informed of and included in all communication. No decision can be made with out his or her participation. If the patient is unable to take part in decision making, a family member or caretaker should be included in the discussions. In keeping with this spirit of family participation, conferences can be held in the patient's house.

A healthy team should have conflicts and problems. Issues should be identified and aired. Skilled group members are able to separate subjective issues from objective goals. This is why the home care practitioner needs to understand group dynamics. Such knowledge can be gleaned from a balance of practical experience and a theoretical base.

The patient and the caretakers, who are together for most of the day, form the hub of the wheel of effort. The wheel cannot roll forward unless all of the team members that operate around it move in the same direction. Figure 36-2 illustrates this concept. The team must work toward similar goals.

It will be remembered that primary, secondary and tertiary caretakers constitute the caretaker network. The caretaker network, or the hub of the wheel of effort, is the bedrock of effective home care. Cooperative participants reduce the stress of caring for the ill family member. On the other hand, the stress of illness taxes the family's resources. If some of the family members are uncooperative, the wheel of team effort cannot move forward.

Patient care requires time and effort. Eventually, stress may tax communication among the closest family members and friends. Specialists should assist the family and help members with any interaction problems. This assistance should be offered before the situation deteriorates and family members have no energy left to invest in cooperation.

It is helpful to discuss the patient's assets and strengths as well as liabilities and weaknesses. The patient's premorbid lifestyle should be explored in an effort to understand the present situation. New information may alter the thrust of care and reorder treatment priorities. Professionals may also encourage increased use of secondary and tertiary caretakers. No caretaker should feel overburdened. Family members may be reluctant to admit that they need help.

Case Study No. 3 is an example of a functional caretaker network.

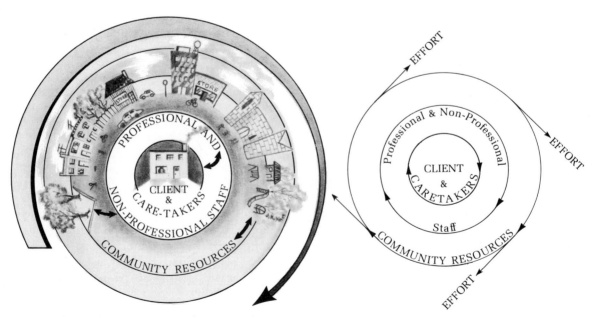

Figure 36-2. The wheel of team effort. All of the unique goals and skills of all the team members must be organized into a unified effort. All members must move in one direction so that the treatment can move forward.

Case Study No. 3

The Stylowski family has a network of caretakers. Mr. Stylowski suffered a fracture of his right humerus and hip one month ago. He was treated in the hospital and discharged to his own home. Mrs. Stylowski is the primary caretaker. She oversees the exercise regime, dressing, and bathing activities. All this is done at the same time that she continues her "normal" household and shopping chores.

Mr. Stylowski's brother, Stephen, and his wife Maria are the secondary caretakers. They live five miles from the patient. They visit Mr. Stylowski almost every night on their way home from work. They assist with shopping, heavy cleaning, and occasionally with the exercise programs.

The patient's daughter, Lydia Holmes, lives 30 miles away. She is a working mother with house, work, and family responsibilities. Lydia stops to see her parents every other week. Her uncle asks her to complete selected errands—shopping for special equipment, drycleaning, and staying with her father when her mother goes out to Bingo once a month. □

Communication

In the home setting there are three basic forms of communication—face-to-face interaction, telephone communication and written communication.

Face-to-face communication takes place in the patient's home or in the agency. This type of interaction may be difficult to arrange for a team because each team member has a different schedule and visits the patient at a different time. Team goals and roles must be resolved early in the treatment process because they could block communication and progress.

Written communication may be used in lieu of a face-to-face interaction. On an informal level, notes may be left in the patient's house for other team members. Telephone discussions may prove to be a more effective method of exploring issues and potential areas of confusion.

Another form of written communication takes place after each patient visit—the progress note. The importance of documentation cannot be avoided in the home situation. Many fiscal intermediaries have stringent requirements for documentation that must be followed to qualify for reimbursement.

Communication creates a sense of teamwork that is satisfying to all of the members. The following quote underscores the effort that one must invest to develop a team.

"It is naive to bring together a highly diverse group of people and expect that, by calling them a team, they will in fact behave as a team. It is ironic indeed to realize that a football team spends 40 hours per week practicing teamwork for those two hours on Sunday afternoon when their teamwork really counts. Teams in organizations seldom spend two hours per year practicing when their ability to function as a team counts 40 hours per week."[13]

Architectural Barriers

One factor that affects the outcome of a home care program is physical in nature. Architectural barriers can impede patient progress. Economic factors limit large-scale changes in many homes. Few people have access to the resources that would be needed to renovate basic structures such as the bathroom and kitchen fixtures. The therapist must assess the type of changes that would be helpful and possible. Little is gained from an exploration of changes that can never come about.

Another less obvious factor is cultural in nature. While some people enjoy change that will facilitate their daily performance, others regard adjustment with new discomfort. The total expenditure of energy needed for change is not considered possible. The daily, smaller energy expenditure attached to the current inconvenience seems more acceptable. Sometimes the only stable part of the patient's world is the unchanging nonhuman environment. The illness may have upset and altered everything else, including roles and relationships. Investment in the secure and unchanging environment may be more reasonable to some people.

The therapist who blindly suggests extensive change in this type of situation may encounter a brittle and resistant audience. It seems logical to suggest minor changes like moving a bookcase one foot to the left to free a passage for wheelchair accessibility. However, the patient may not wish to crowd the picture that hangs next to the bookcase. The nonhuman world may be the last place that remains unscathed by illness.

The best approach for the therapist to use cannot be precisely outlined. Patients must be assessed in the context of their nonhuman environment and social interaction patterns. There is no need for the therapist to invest energy in attempting to foster change when the patient or caretaker do not think that any benefit can be gained from the alterations. Some ideas may be accepted at a later date.

Change was precluded in the next example because of cultural and economic factors. This family was limited in income and provincial in outlook. The family could not value the suggestions of an "outsider." The therapist could raise questions but could never expect to see immediate results. The therapist's role regarding changes to the environment was, at best, that of a catalyst. The only change that was considered was the addition of a snack table to the right side of the refrigerator. Any others would have been too costly. The family seemed to accept the idea, but the item was never purchased. Possibly after the case was discharged, the family was able to develop its own solution to the problem.

Case Study No. 4

The Hagers have resided in their small row house for 30 years. The brick house is over 150 years old; it is situated in a blue-collar residential district in a large metropolitan area.

Mrs. Hager is 54 years old. She has a residual left hemiparesis. Her recovery is complete except for a decrease in shoulder function. A Winter-Haven perceptual test revealed a possible deficit in visual memory and spatial relations. She can dress independently although her performance is slow. The occupational therapist has been actively involved with Mrs. Hager's training for 2 months. The long-term goal is to "maximize independent

functioning." The short-term goal is to help Mrs. Hager be independent in the kitchen.

The therapist found that Mrs. Hager used her disability. She could now garner the sympathy and support of her two teenaged children. She agreed to try to work in the kitchen only because her children could not cook very well. The biggest problem that hindered progress was the layout of the kitchen and the breakfast room. (See floor plan in Fig. 36-3.)

Whenever Mrs. Hager wished to take things out of the refrigerator, she had to walk back several feet to place the objects on the table. The food then had to be transferred into the pantry. Mrs. Hager refused to consider carry-all baskets. She felt that they "looked funny." The therapist suggested that a snack table be placed next to the refrigerator. The client agreed but never was able to procure the item. The stove was also a problem; it did not have an automatic pilot light. After a few unsuccessful attempts at cooking. Mrs. Hager was willing to turn this responsibility over to her oldest daughter. "I guess that she is old enough after all," she said.

The Hagers could not afford any extensive changes. Their culture did not support do-it-yourself innovations. The nonhuman environment was one of the only stable things in their lives. There was little energy left to invest in change. □

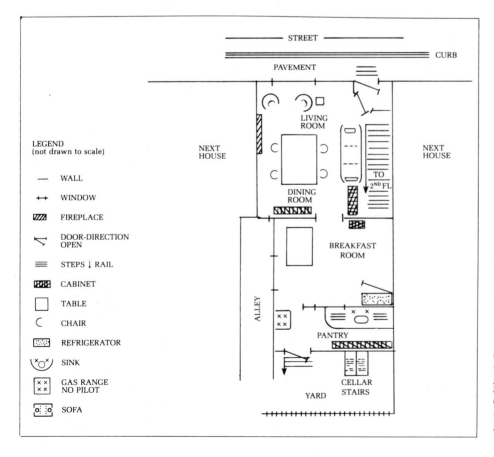

LEGEND
(not drawn to scale)

— WALL
↔ WINDOW
▨ FIREPLACE
⌐ DOOR-DIRECTION OPEN
≡ STEPS ↓ RAIL
▨ CABINET
☐ TABLE
C CHAIR
▥ REFRIGERATOR
⌣O⌣ SINK
x x / x x GAS RANGE NO PILOT
⊙ ⊙ SOFA

Figure 36-3. Floor plan of the first floor of the Hager house. The floor plan depicted here is common in a blue-collar neighborhood near the industrial center of a large city. The houses are over 150 years old. Streets are narrow and barren. Small yards extend for 15 to 20 feet from the back doors. The average income is $18,000 a year for a family of four. This particular neighborhood is close knit and insular. Relatives live "two doors" away or "around the corner."

Body Mechanics and Transfer Techniques

All home care personnel must be skilled in transferring patients under less than ideal circumstances. Caretakers are unfamiliar with the process; they may fear that they will injure the patient or themselves. Also, the occupational therapist must frequently position the patient for activities. This is commonly done without assistance and principles of good body mechanics must be used. Since caretakers and neighbors frequently observe therapy, good technique and an air of competence are essential.

Home Modalities

Modalities and tools must be suited to the home environment. One patient may welcome special equipment and tools while another may refuse to learn new methods to cope with the disability. The lack of material resources may be inconvenient, but this lack should not alter the progress of a rehabilitation program. If equipment is not available, therapists learn to improvise. Commonplace objects can be substituted for "special" equipment. Examples of such improvisations follow:
1. *Weight*—place canned goods in a zippered pocketbook or knotted sock
2. *Stabilizer*—put a damp cloth under the plate or tray
3. *Elastic shoe laces*—use 1/8" elastic and cut to shoe lace size
4. *Skate board*—place a towel under the affected arm, use on a smooth table top
5. *Bathtub transfer seat*—two chairs, one placed inside and one placed outside of the tub

Discharge Planning

The patient's performance in ADL and upper extremity retraining may remain at the same level for several weeks. If this happens, the occupational therapist must prepare the patient and the family for discharge. If the occupational therapist feels that the patient can make further gains, he or she should try to motivate the patient. Few fiscal intermediaries will reimburse agencies for extended maintenance-level treatment.

Discharge plans must be discussed with the patient and the caretakers. At least four visits should be devoted to a home program. Other team members should be informed of your decision to terminate services. The discharge should be gradual and discussed at least two weeks before the date. The patient and family should be weaned from visits. Abrupt changes should be avoided.

After-Care

Home care patients frequently develop a need for service at a later date. Hospitalizations, relapses, and changes in residences may necessitate additional treatment. If so, the patient is referred to a home health agency again, and the delivery cycle is initiated again.

The mechanical aspects of home care delivery were presented in this section. Unfortunately, the fun, excitement, and fascination of home visiting is not easily conveyed in a written narrative. During a home visit the therapist enters the patient's sanctum—his or her home. The therapist becomes privy to confidential information, environmental cues, and emotional displays that are frequently hidden from the professional person's view. This information shapes the quality of care that is offered to the patient and the family.

Outside Issues That Affect Home Care Delivery

There are four factors that directly affect the type of service that is given in the home: funding, documentation, continuing education, and the occupational therapy organization.

Funding

Home health agencies are funded by both public and private sources, including insurance companies, religious groups, charities, endowments, and fees collected for services.

In the United States, most home care programs receive some of their funds from Medicare or Medicaid reimbursement. It therefore seems important to review some aspects of Title XVIII, Title XIX, and Title XX of the Social Security Act. Since Medicare is a national program, guidelines for any national health care program may be based on this legislative package.

Medicare

Title XVIII of the Social Security Act provides legislation for Medicare funding. Medicare provides medical benefits primarily for older Americans, but persons who have been disabled for more than 24 months can also qualify for Medicare benefits. Specific requirements are established for all of the services that Medicare will fund. Not only do these guidelines influence current practice, but they will also affect the future. The importance of Medicare extends beyond funding; it sets national standards for practice. In short, Medicare establishes national priorities regarding the services that will be covered, the quality and nature of those services, and the degree to which the practitioner and the agency will be held accountable for the care they give.

The current Medicare program does not recognize occupational therapy as a primary service. After ten years of work, the medicare law was recently amended during a lame duck session of Congress. Unfortunately, the amendments were rescinded, and confusion reigned for several months. A compromise was negotiated in the Omnibus Reconciliation Act.

The compromise featured one negative point. Occupational therapy is not a primary service. This means that a home care case must be opened by a nurse, physical therapist, or speech pathologist. The positive point is that once a case is opened, the occupational therapist may continue even if there is no further need for other skilled services. This is a welcome change from the previous law.

Another change is also helpful. Formerly there was a limit on the number of home care agency visits that a patient could receive during a calendar year. This limit has been removed. Homecare is thus recognized as an alternative to institutionalization.

Finally, the previous law required a minimum of 3 days of hospitalization in order to receive full benefits. This hospital stay is no longer required.

Medicaid

Medicaid or Medical Assistance, Title XIX of the Social Security Act, is a program for people who have no other means to pay for medical care. The program is based upon a formula for matching federal and state dollars. For example, the state must contribute a percentage of its per capita income. The ratios for the contributions are set by law. Some states do not contribute large sums of money to this program. Their reimbursement rates for home care may not cover half of the actual cost of the services. If services are rendered, the agency must deal with the resulting deficit. If no alternative income is generated, the agency assets will be eaten away. Usually monies from other sources are used to reduce the loss. However, this solution creates a complex and, at times, precarious funding situation. This is one of the reasons for establishment of rigid eligibility criteria. States may also develop their own criteria for eligibility.

Home health may or may not be part of a Medicaid treatment package. Coverage varies from state to state. In some cases Medicaid will pay for 180 days of home care after hospitalization. In other states only a fraction of the cost of home care is reim-

bursed. This situation will strain an agency that wants to serve patients with limited resources.

Other Sources

Other sources of revenue include third party carriers like private insurance companies such as Blue Cross. Coverage varies with the company, the state, and the region of the country. Third party carriers are beginning to recognize the value of home care services. They reduce expensive hospital stays making services less costly. Local communities, through public health departments or grants to private agencies, may commit tax dollars or federal revenue sharing monies to support home care. Hospitals may develop their own home care departments. These groups, like the agencies that provide nonreimbursable services, may use private funds to ease their deficit. Included in this private category are donations, endowments, and contributions from charities like the United Way.

Some organizations offer specific services to patients. Two examples are the loan of adaptive equipment and the purchase of drugs. Religious groups may also contribute to home care assets. Members may volunteer to help with a problem; this may even include human resources that will relieve strained family members for a specific period of time during the day. Hot meals and the purchase of necessary equipment are other examples. Another source of private funds is the collection of fees for services. This may be used on a sliding scale to accommodate for different family incomes.

Another emerging source of referrals and financial support for home care is the federally approved Health Maintenance Organization (HMO). All federally approved HMOs must offer home care services. The HMO is a prepaid group practice. Each subscriber pays a fee which entitles him or her to receive a wide range of health services. Some services that are covered are routine check-ups, eye exams, and prenatal care. All are oriented toward the maintenance of health. When and if a member becomes ill, the HMO provides complete medical care. Therefore, it behooves the HMO to utilize preventative rather than remediation services. If not, all of the practice finances will be absorbed by medical costs.

Documentation

Health care providers sometimes forget that documentation is a form of communication. Home care delivery is not easy to observe because of the number of residences that are served. Documentation, therefore, becomes an important tool to measure the quality of patient care. There is an adage that is frequently repeated by many nursing supervisors—

"if it isn't written, it hasn't been done."[14] This statement reflects the stringent demands of the majority of fiscal intermediaries. Most fiscal intermediaries demand adherence to their guidelines; if not satisfied, a carrier will refuse to reimburse the agency for the visits. Organized, goal-oriented, concise notes that clearly convey the patient's status to the reviewer are essential. Most fiscal intermediaries demand measurable progress in a reasonable period of time.[15] There are few funding sources for extended maintenance–level care.

The majority of fiscal intermediaries rely on Medicare standards for their reimbursement guidelines. The reimbursement guidelines determine the thrust of covered services and the diagnoses and care that will be covered. These guidelines establish the narrowest definition for occupational therapy services. Therefore it seems reasonable to outline this base, although therapists will hopefully be able to deliver broader services. In general, Medicare coverage dictates that the patient must be able to improve significantly in a *reasonable* and generally predictable period of time. Claims for reimbursement for custodial care or maintenance are not accepted by Medicare.

On the first visit of a treatment program to be funded by Medicare, the patient must be evaluated and appropriate goals must be established. Some agencies require a projection of the number of visits that will be needed during the next 60 days. Each visit must move the patient closer to the long-range goals. Every 60 days the case must also be reviewed with other team members. The patient has a limited number of home visits that will be covered (this issue was discussed in the previous section on eligibility criteria); visits must therefore be shared among all of the team members.

At present Medicare defines occupational therapy as a "medically prescribed treatment concerned with improving, or restoring functions which have been impaired by illness or injury or, where function has been permanently lost or reduced by illness or injury, to improve the individual's ability to perform those tasks required for independent functioning."[16] Services may include the following:

1. The evaluation and reevaluation as required of a patient's level of function by administering diagnostic and prognostic tests
2. The selection and teaching of task-oriented therapeutic activities designed to restore physical function . . .
3. The planning, implementing, and supervising of individualized therapeutic activity programs as part of an over-all 'active treatment' program for a patient with a diagnosed psychiatric illness, . . .
4. The planning and implementing of therapeutic tasks and activities to restore sensory-integrative function, . . .
5. The teaching of compensatory techniques to improve the level of independence in the activities of daily living, . . .
6. The designing, fabricating, and fitting of orthotic and self-help devices, . . .
7. Vocational and prevocational assessment and training[17]

There are other restrictions: services must be prescribed by a physician and performed by a qualified occupational therapist or certified occupational therapy assistant who works under the therapist's supervision. The most important clause in the criteria for coverage is that services are considered 'reasonable and necessary" only where the patient's condition indicates that there will be a significant practical improvement in the level of function in a "reasonable" period of time.[18] Occupational therapy must be goal-directed, purposeful activity that can maximize the patient's level of function in a predetermined period of time.

Not all programs are governed by Medicare, but the number of older Americans increases daily and this will in itself expand Medicare services. Also, unfortunately for occupational therapy, Medicare standards are national and therefore influence coverage throughout the country. It is hoped that efforts will be rewarded that seek the expansion of Medicare coverage to include occupational therapy as a primary service.

Programs other than those that are totally dependent on Medicare funds may regard occupational therapy in a different light. In some settings the value of custodial and maintenance services are recognized, and undiagnosed mental illness may also be treated. The boundaries of Medicare coverage are presented here to establish a base for home care practice. Services should not be narrowed further. The home care therapist should define the role of occupational therapy so that the maximum number of patients can be reached. However, if the role were too broadly defined, other services could be duplicated and the unique focus of occupational therapy may be lost. A balanced, well-defined role should be developed and should function within the boundaries of the home care agency's financial resources.

Continuing Education

Home care practitioners function independently. Although they work on patient care teams, they rarely work with other occupational therapists. The practitioner's knowledge and skills can become dated by this isolation. There are few opportunities for discussion regarding new treatment ideas and modalities in the daily home care routine. For this reason, home care practitioners must reach out and create their own educational opportunities. One way to expand learning is to take advantage of continuing education programs. Advertisements appear in occupational therapy journals and newspapers. Active participation in occupational therapy organizations also promotes the sharing of ideas. One should never feel that one works alone, separated from new ideas. Some agencies require that the occupational therapist attend one professional program a year. The future of any specialty practice rests on the continued excellence of the practitioners.

Present Practice

Today therapists work in several different ways. The common practice is for an agency to hire an occupational therapist and to pay a salary. A large agency may even pay for supplies and offer the use of an agency car.

Private Practice

Some therapists are engaged in private practice. They divide their time among several agencies or settings. These practitioners may also receive private referrals. Payment may be a combination of part-time salary and fees-for-service. A fee-for-service is a lump sum of money that is paid to the therapist for each visit. The therapist is not a bona fide member of the agency; no benefits are paid. Note-writing and travel time is included in the fee. At times the agency will pay for attendance at staff meetings and conferences.

One advantage of private practice is the freedom that it affords the therapist. Treatment times and hours and patient-load and demands can be varied. Practice can be carried out in several specialty areas; programs that could not afford occupational therapy can begin to offer the service. This modest beginning does not put the service in a make-it-or-break-it position. Some therapists are combining part-time institutional work with private practice.

Group Practice

Another convenient way to deliver part-time occupational therapy is in a group practice with one therapist acting as coordinator. A registry of local therapists who wish to pursue part-time work is compiled. Once the names are organized, the process is not complex. State laws must be researched for local requirements. This is usually a simple matter for a lawyer to handle. When the group is organized, referrals can be received. Contracts can be signed with several agencies, or single referrals can be accepted.

Individual therapists are assigned to a location near their home or work. Referrals are assigned by location. At least one member must be available during the day for phone calls, referrals, and attendance at meetings.

The benefits of a group practice are numerous. The agency can deal with one coordinator instead of several part-time workers. A broad geographical area can be serviced without wasting time in travel. The group seeks its own members and is better able to evaluate member skills. Service to patients is not interrupted by vacations, illness, and other obligations—the group and not just one person is responsible for the referrals.

The group members benefit because the work is part-time. More therapists can participate in home care delivery. Agencies with small case loads can still provide occupational therapy services. Therapists can join or leave the group without any major disruption of service. The group name becomes familiar to agencies and community centers even if individual therapists have to drop out of the group.

Summary

Practice is the area in which knowledge and skills are put to the test. The essence of home-based occupational therapy is working with people. The therapist is drawn into the family's inner sanctum—its home—to deliver services. Here the family will be taught how to help maximize the patient's level of functional performance.

This chapter can never capture the excitement and fun of the home care treatment process. Every home presents unique problems, new relationships and challenges. After working in the field for a while, therapists begin to wonder whether they might be gaining as much as they are giving.

References

1. Searles, H. F.: *The Nonhuman Environment*, New York: International Universities Press, Inc., 1960, p. 180.
2. Turner, M. M.: *Social Stratification,* Englewood Cliffs, NJ: Prentice-Hall, 1967, p. 12.
3. Ibid.
4. Yerxa, E.: "The Philosophical Base of Occupational Therapy." *Occupational Therapy: 2001.* American Occupational Therapy Association, 1979, p. 26.
5. Brookover, W. B., and Erickson, L. E.: *Society, Schools and Learning.* East Lansing, Michigan: Michigan State University Press, 1969.
6. Boardman, A., Davis, J., and Lloyd, A.: "The determinants of achievement, self-esteem, and the belief in

one's ability to control one's environment," Unpublished paper, 1976.

7. McClelland, D.: *The Achievement Motive*. New York: Appleton-Century-Crofts, Inc., 1953.

8. Florey, L. L.: Intrinsic motivation: The dynamics of occupational therapy theory. Am. J. Occup. Ther. 23:319–322, 1969.

9. Fidler, G. S.: "From Crafts to Competence," Am. J. Occup. Ther. 35:567–573, 1981.

10. Keilhofner, G., Burke, J. P. "Occupational Therapy after 60 Years: An Account of Changing Identity & Knowledge. Am. J. Occup. Ther. 31:675–689, 1977.

11. Florey, p. 320.

12. Mosey, A. C.: *Activities Therapy*, Chapter 3, New York: Raven Press, 1973.

13. Fry, R. E., Lech, B. A., and Rubin, I.: Working with the primary care team: The first intervention. In Wise, H., et al. (eds.): Making Health Teams Work, Cambridge MA: Ballinger Publishing Co., 1974, p. 56.

14. Fischer, P.: Documentation Paper presented with Levine, R. E.: Gerontology Special Interest Symposium, 1977.

15. Home Health Agency Manual for Medicare, 205.2,A. Social Security Administration, Health Information Manual No. 11. Department of Health, Education and Welfare, U.S. Government Printing Office, Washington DC, 1975-210-829:430.

16. Ibid.

17. Ibid.

18. Ibid., 205. 2, B.

CHAPTER 37

Community Home Health Care—In the Rural Setting *Elizabeth B.Devereaux*

Just as each individual patient, each urban setting, and each ghetto has unique characteristics, so does each rural community. To be even minimally effective, the occupational therapist functioning in a rural community must understand the people: their culture, values, and attitudes. Even the therapist who has grown up in a rural community and returns there to practice may find that he or she is considered an "outsider" by virtue of having been away, and even more, having obtained an education while away.

It is natural to assume that, while there are cultural and subcultural differences in this country, we all want pretty much the same things, generally in the form of a "better life"—and a better life demands a better job and a higher income to get there. But these assumptions and the next action—that of the therapist's imposition of his or her own values onto treatment direction—will only lead to frustration in dealing with many of the clients in a rural culture. Actually the characteristics discussed here do not belong exclusively to the rural culture. The distinction should not be made between rural and urban; the distinction should be made between the middle class and a "folk class," which is a working class that seems to fit somewhere between the lower class and lower middle class.[1,2] The folk class appears to exist

wherever people have been limited or defeated by their environment whether this happens in the urban ghettos, the Western plains, or Appalachia.[3]

Most rural areas also have a professional class and a middle class, which are influenced by the culture of the folk class, but usually can be dealt with more nearly as one would deal with such groups anywhere. These two classes generally are seeking the better life. will serve on committees and work for the common good, and want good health care including preventive health care. There is also the lower class, and they would be approached in the rural area as in any other area of the country. They are characterized as a group dealing inadequately with life's problems, with families often having multiple problems that are perpetuated from one generation to another. These people may have aspirations for a better life but are lacking in basic resources such as education, problem-solving ability, work skills, and just plain know-how to work toward the fulfillment of their dreams.

It is not intended that this chapter give an indepth view of the folk class or the folk culture. Rather, the overview given is aimed toward raising the therapist's level of awareness of the attitudes, mores, and values of the culture; the gradations of its influence throughout the various strata of the populations encountered; the lack of results when a therapist works counter to the culture; and some types of approaches and interventions that might work. Much of the material in this chapter is drawn from my own experiences while living and working in West Virginia and Ohio and visiting rural areas in many other parts of the country. This is mentioned to confirm the suspicions of those readers who may detect a strong flavor of Appalachia in these writings. It is true—I have been influenced by the culture.

A Sociocultural Overview

There is men's work and there is women's work in this culture and seldom the I'll-wash-and-you-dry cooperative sharing often seen between husband and wife in the middle class. It's up to the husband to make a living and the wife to take care of the house and children. The wife often does the painting and wall papering, the yardwork and the gardening, although the husband may work in the garden too. Even small children are expected to do their share of helping with the chores.

Frequently the men in this society have fewer years of schooling than the women do. The men have worked outdoors doing physical labor—farming, ranching, lumbering, hunting, fishing, mining where formal education wasn't needed and where social skills weren't particularly needed and there was little opportunity to learn them. Women, though, have learned from each other the skills of cooking and canning, sewing and quilting, and housekeeping and raising children, and have learned a higher level of social skills than the men. Parents, children, aunts, uncles, cousins, and all the other possible relations in an extended family usually live close by. This is particularly true in mining and lumber camps, where houses are often built side by side in a string up the valley until they run into a mountain. This factor makes it easier for women to have social interaction than the men.

Husbands and wives don't seem particularly close to each other and, when groups of people get together, the men congregate in one group and the women in another, and there is little interaction between them. Individuals often seem to lack a feeling of self-worth, gain most of their acceptance and approval from their group, and so tend to avoid taking sides in controversial issues, not wanting to offend members of their group and risk becoming alienated from the security the group represents.

Rural Poverty

The rural poor is composed of the unemployed of any category, including miners, sharecroppers, ranch hands, farm workers, lumbermen, and so forth. The rural poor also includes those whose income falls below the poverty income: migrant farm workers, hired hands, tenant farmers, those who live on the land they own, American Indians, Mexican-Americans, Puerto Ricans, blacks, and whites.[4]

Some who have studied the problems of poverty maintain that the use of a specific subsistence income level to define what is "poor" is less meaningful than a definition that is relative to the society in which the person lives. John Kenneth Galbraith is one who contended that even if people have a subsistence income, if that income is a great deal less than that of the rest of the community, they are poverty-stricken since they do not have a level of existence that is considered decent or acceptable to their community.[5]

Whatever the accustomed level of existence, even that is often in jeopardy. The farmer who is poor generally farms with hand tools on land with poor soil, often on a hillside, and is at the mercy of the weather as well. Miners sometimes lose their jobs with no warning, being told at the end of a shift that the mine is closing. They have been surviving and providing for their families, even though they may live in a company house or a shack on their own land. Every room is usually used for sleeping and there's a television set, but the miners and migrant workers often owe their "whole pay to the company store." When there is no work and no other jobs available, there is no pay and, after trying to exist for a while with no income, even a welfare check (if they are eligible) raises their subsistence level.

With no other marketable skills there's no use moving to the city. The emotional shock that comes with the realization that he can't get a job sometimes causes a man to stop the risk of trying. Feeling controlled by other people and other things and unable to provide for their families, many men just give up. To some outsiders this looks like a loss of interest in work. Eventually it leads to his becoming physically unemployable after a few years. All this results in a fatalistic attitude, summarized, "It ain't no use tryin', nothin's gonna make any difference anyhow. Things is meant to be this way, an' you can't do nothin' to change 'em. It's the Lord's will."

Dependence and Independence

Every culture has its own survival system and one aspect of particular importance in the folk class is the relationship of individuals to their peer groups: men to men, women to women, and each to his or her family. Each is dependent on a peer group and a family for acceptance and security. The family does not seem to know how to nurture its members so they can develop the security to become independent. Being so emotionally dependent only leads to deeper feelings of insecurity.

Some have been able to leave their rural homes and find jobs in the city. These have usually been the younger people with more education and ambition than those left behind who, in turn, have been least capable of changing things for the better.[6] The largest migration at any one time in the United States occurred during World War II. Those who migrated went either to war or to the city to work. They tended to stick together, in living quarters and neighborhoods, and tried to recreate and preserve their culture, returning home frequently to visit "the folks." Many said they would return to their rural area immediately if they could find a job.

With the younger people leaving and birth control methods being used more, the birth rate has been declining and the percentage of elderly increasing in rural communities. This, therefore, means an increase in the group most steeped in tradition with little or no desire or energy to change.

The pioneers and early settlers, ancestors of many of today's folk classes, were noted for their independence, which conveyed a sense of identity, autonomy, self-direction, but did not exclude working cooperatively with neighbors and projects of benefit to all. Weller says that independence has changed to individualism, which has a self-centered focus, so that things are done independently but always with the "what's in it for me?" attitude.[7] Each person's affairs are an individual matter and people are basically against joining anything except one of the political parties. A man may attend a Parent-Teachers Association meeting or go to church occasionally (while many of his wife's activities center around church and school) but, if there's no immediate gratification of his self-interest, he probably won't go back to the next meeting. Living and becoming accustomed to unpredictable rapid changes out of their control, these people see no benefit in planning for the future. There's no concept of committee work or long-term goals or of planning and working for community improvement.

The Children's Place

Family planning is a recent development, and large families have been common in this culture. A high rate of illegitimacy seems accepted. Illegitimate children are seldom given up for adoption, and may be raised by the mother or her parents.

Babies are to be cuddled and played with, but as they begin to assert their individual personalities and become more difficult to control parents play with them less and less, and the children form their own peer groups. The adage that "children are to be seen, not heard" operates in this culture, as opposed to the middle class culture where the children are the center of attention. Children are to behave as "little adults,"

may play if it does not disrupt adult activities, and boys have a lot of freedom where girls are expected to stay close to home.

As contradictory as it seems, child-rearing is permissive, impulsive, and indulgent, yet physical punishment is nearly always used rather than taking away a privilege or scolding. A mother may repeatedly tell a child to "do this" or "don't do that," yet the child keeps right on until the mother spanks, switches, or in some physical way gets the child's attention. But when father speaks or gives a stern look, the child generally obeys immediately. With these kinds of inconsistencies and double messages, children learn to ignore the words and hear the tone and the feeling behind them, and they tend to continue to respond that way as adults.

Sometimes a father's physical discipline is very harsh and a mother will try to stop it or connive with the child so that the father doesn't find out about the child's misbehaving. This makes the child even more dependent on the mother. And just like all children, they can often talk mom into a less severe punishment or none at all. The child develops a fear of punishment because it's aimed at control of the child, and so the child develops resentment toward authority and fears it. This carries over into adult attitudes. These children are threatened with the law, the doctor, with being given away to strangers, all in an effort to keep them in line. Is it any wonder that these children are often sober and sad looking? They lose their spontaneity and playful qualities at an early age.

The "Flying Feds" Syndrome

In planning and developing a program in a rural community, the therapist will be involved with those from the professional class and the middle class. Although they are generally committed to a better life for their community and for themselves, it is well to remember that they have been influenced by the folk culture around them. Often they are not at all conscious of how their behavior has been affected, but a sensitive observer frequently can spot the patterns.

The occupational therapist works with people who are of the folk culture but have moved out of it somewhat. However, under stress, all people tend to revert to old patterns of behavior. Therefore if programs being developed run counter to cultural influences in the rural communities, they simply will never get off the ground. Program planning must accommodate to the cultures involved if it's going to succeed.

All these cultural influences were seemingly ignored by the Flying Feds after the Buffalo Creek, West Virginia, flood in 1972. When mobile homes were assigned, the lowest paid laborer in the mine might find his home situated next to that of the superintendent of the mine. How much easier and quicker would have been the adjustment to the loss if the worker had been surrounded by the familiar cluster of family and friends from his old neighborhood. These people have all too often had things done to them and for them and seldom *with* them.

The flying feds syndrome affects many people in rural communities and occurs in reaction to outsiders' promises to develop programs to meet community needs that (1) never materialize, (2) are superimposed on the community, (3) have criteria so restrictive that, even in the same family, some members may be provided service but others with the same needs may not be, (4) are so general in scope that the particular needs unique to each community are not being served, (5) infringe so much on the rights, freedoms, and dignity of the community and individuals that the community refuses them because the "cost" is too high, (6) duplicate or compete with existing services, or (7) any combination of the above. The flying feds syndrome also makes the people who are affected by it suspicious of anybody who says, "Let's write a federal grant for this program" and of any outsider who comes into the community talking about developing a new program.

The folk culture is suspicious of outsiders and their ideas. It was the outsiders who cheated some of them out of the mineral rights of their land, sometimes because they couldn't read the contract they were signing; who bought their timber for badly needed cash but at a fraction of its worth; who ran railroads and highways over their lands, perhaps paying for them but taking the land whether or not the owners wanted to sell it. The person isolated geographically and culturally, outside of the mainstream of commercial trade, seldom realized the real or potential value of the coal, oil, gas, or timber on the land. Much needed cash and goods were received when the deal was made, but years later he found out that he had also sold land that he wanted to keep in the family. He was lied to and tricked by land agents who told him that they had a prior deed to his land; to avoid going to court he would sign a quit claim which gave the land company mineral and timber rights and, in return, allowed him to continue living on the land. He did not understand the law and courts. He was afraid to speak out in a meeting let alone a courtroom and was afraid that a person like himself would not get a fair deal—he would be the victim again. He didn't have money for a lawyer anyway. The people of this culture, even the children, carry a constant level of fear, uncertainty, and anxiety because much of the control of their lives comes from outside of them—an environment that has defeated them and authority that comes in the form of employer, the law, welfare workers. They do not trust strangers, "experts" in particular.

These are independent people, with a lot of pride and dignity, who are used to taking care of themselves and their neighbors. They really don't like "somebody out there"—some expert—telling them what to do and how to do it. Every so often the leaders of a rural community will refuse to accept federal money rather than accept all the restrictions and the superimposition of control from outside of their community.

Those from the folk class may attend an initial meeting to hear a discussion of a project but probably will not become involved or attend future meetings. However, they will use the service if it is of benefit to them and is suited to them.

There are two reasons, primarily, to include people in planning. First, it is a way to get their support for the program during both its development and its implementation. Second, and this is probably more important, by involving the people for whom the plan is intended, chances are you'll come up with a better plan. They know their real and felt needs better than anyone else. A program specifically tailored to these needs has a better chance of receiving the support of the community and of being used.

Attitude Towards Health Care

People in the folk class are used to taking care of things themselves as much as possible, using folk medicine remedies passed down from generation to generation: herbs; cough medicine made from brown sugar or honey and turpentine, kerosene or whiskey; berries; teas from tree roots; special tonics, brews, and poultices. As a last resort they'll go to a doctor. As a further last resort, they'll go to the hospital, maybe. Hospitals are frightening, impersonal, outside the scope of comprehension; they are where you go to die.

Sickness is feared and health care is mostly sought in crisis situations. Interestingly, Kent and Smith describe similar behavior among ghetto poor (". . . the resistance to involvement and the crisis orientation of the poor . . .") as needing to be considered in developing health programs in the ghettos.[8]

The concept of preventive health care is not understood, and if Johnny cries because the brace hurts his leg, he will not have to wear it even if the purpose is to prevent further deformity. Prenatal care is generally nonexistent. Some babies are born in the hospital, but many are born at home.

If an older person has to hire a neighbor to take him to the doctor where he waits all day to get heart medicine, and the expense of the trip to the doctor and the medicine means the difference between that and money for food for several days, he's likely to choose the latter. His fatalistic attitude may be that

"I'll live 'til my time comes and no medicine will make the difference. It don't matter nohow."

Folk language includes many terms to describe disease and illness that will not be found in a medical dictionary, and it is essential to learn the language in order to communicate. A "bealed toe," "low blood," "bad nerves," "running off," and "the bloody flux" are but a few.

The concept of mental health has no meaning in this culture. Mental illness is little understood and is blamed on "bad nerves" or "poor nerves." If the person becomes violent or causes too much of a disruption, he may be sent to a state hospital, but many are kept at home, particularly in isolated areas.

I once went on a home visit to a 79-year-old woman who lived with her two brothers, one 81 and the other 83. It was a hot summer day and after driving on a dirt road as far as it went, I walked to the creek, took off my shoes and stockings, waded the stream, put shoes and stockings back on, followed the path around the cornfield and up a hollow. There was an old log cabin, very clean and neatly kept, and stepping inside was like stepping into the 1800s. There was no carpeting on the floors, but the cabin was filled with antiques, including a harpsichord against one wall. Sister had "worn-out nerves," played the harpsichord and did beautiful needlework, but was too disoriented and distracted by her voices to do much more. So the "boys" cooked, farmed, did the housework, and took care of her. As the gentlemanly 83-year-old brother escorted me back to the car to show me where to cross the creek on the stepping stones, he confided that his sister's nerves had started "wearing out" about 30 years before, but that the three of them got along just fine. His attitude was one of a completely unquestioned acceptance of responsibility for taking care of his sister, and her "peculiarities" were just something to accommodate to. Their system was in balance and, as a therapist, the best thing I could do was to leave it alone.

THE OCCUPATIONAL THERAPIST IN A RURAL SETTING

Acceptance as a Person, Therapist, and Outsider

Men and women of the folk culture do hard physical work, often for long hours. To endure this, day after day, they have to pace themselves. One of the ways they pace themselves and break into the monotony of their lives is the "come set a spell" approach to business transactions and interaction with neighbors and friends. They have none of the rush-rush-state-your-business-and-leave impersonal encounter of the middle and professional classes. A trip to the store, to buy or sell, includes a "visit," talk about the weather, the family's health, politics, the cow that's about to come fresh.

A visiting therapist needs to build time into the schedule to "visit" with the client and his family, that is, to build a personal relationship along with giving treatment. The therapist may be accustomed to a more structured schedule and a set routine, but he or she can't expect the client to be comfortable or cooperative if the therapist sticks to business only. The therapist plans a schedule, makes it flexible, and keeps it to himself or herself. If the therapist is in the area, he or she should stop and chat even if the purpose is not therapy, because the therapist needs first to be accepted as a person before being effective as a therapist. The therapist is reminded that it took several hundred years for things to get where they are today and no doubt it will take a few years to have things heading in the direction we want them to be. Changes usually occur slowly; perhaps there will be three steps forward and five back and then six forward and only two back. If you know where you're going, you'll eventually get there.

Folk people cannot be hurried or pushed. They will balk just like two-year olds in the negative stage. Passive-aggressiveness is one power of the powerless.

The therapist must talk the language of the people. The folk class person does not understand logic and concepts and the nuances of speech, and he or she generally has a short attention span. If the therapist speaks the language without being condescending toward the client's space- and experience-limited world, communication will begin. This may involve telling a story or using an anecdote to make a point—use the imagery that's within the folk culture's world to get a concept across.

The Therapists's Attitude

It is often difficult for the therapist to separate personal values from those of the client's and to not superimpose expectations onto the client. Using a story (not of the folk class but of the professional class) to illustrate the point, an occupational therapist was working with a handicapped homemaker, and the client was progressing very well with personal grooming skills but very little with cooking and other homemaking skills. This was very frustrating and the therapist couldn't understand it until one day a neighbor of the client's dropped in while the therapist was in the home. After a few minutes chatting about what the client and therapist were doing, the neighbor said, "Huh, why *should* she learn all those things now when it will be twice as hard? Before she got sick she spent all her time playing bridge and her husband did all those things. I wouldn't want to learn either if I was her!" The therapist made an assumption based on her own values and attitudes and her past experiences working with handicapped homemakers: that one of the purposes of therapy and using adaptive equipment should include enabling the handicapped homemaker to achieve maximum functioning ability with home-making skills. In this particular case this was not applicable; the client had a life-style that differed from that which the therapist expected.

While the rural community may be resistant to the influence of outsiders, these same outsiders are needed as models to expose the community members to different methods of doing things. There is opportunity for the stranger to the community to perceive problems from a vantage point that the inhabitants do not have, the latter having been saturated by the cultural traditions and attitude "we've always done it this way." By the same token, because it is a tradition does not mean it is inappropriate and should be discontinued. Many traditions serve a useful purpose and need to be continued, but each tradition should be assessed for its present usefulness. Traditional ways of doing things generally give the individual a sense of place in the world and help to anchor him or her in a world that sometimes changes too quickly. In other words, "don't throw the baby out with the bath water," an expression not infrequently heard in rural communities.

Professional Isolation As a Therapist

Being the only occupational therapist in any community can be a lonely existence professionally. During field work experiences there were occupational therapy supervisors and other occupational therapy students with whom the student could discuss difficult treatment decisions or the relative merits of one splinting material as opposed to another. They could use each other as sounding boards without a lot of explanation because they spoke the same language. They didn't have to redefine the scope of Activities of Daily Living (ADL) first before discussing what was happening with a particular client. Some occupational therapists have had work experience in a clinic setting well-staffed with other occupational therapists prior to moving to a rural setting and, therefore, have a greater depth of practical experience to bring to their new setting. But many occupational therapists in a rural area are newly graduated and are there because of personal reasons. They feel a keen need for professional interaction with other occupational therapists.

Developing Your Own Continuing Education Program

Geographical isolation from occupational therapists does not need to include isolation from their ideas. To keep knowledgeable about the people, issues, and concepts involved in the current practice of occupational therapy, read each issue of *The American Journal of Occupational Therapy,* and the AOTA Newspaper. If an article in the Journal is of particular interest, select additional reading from the references listed. There may not be a library nearby, but many rural areas are served by a bookmobile and the state's interlibrary loan service can provide many books and journals that would not be found on the average community library's shelves. Letters to the editor and to the special information exchange sections of the American Occupational Therapy Association publications can result in much up-to-date information from other therapists. Monographs, thesis copies, and other publications, which may be ordered from the American Occupational Therapy Association national office, are another source of materials.

One of the fringe benefits of working with those trained in disciplines related to occupational therapy is the exchange of reading material. Although they may not relate directly to the practice of occupational therapy, the concerns and theories expressed in such literature are often transferable to the occupational therapy framework and can enrich existing knowledge.

When possible, the therapist should attend state, regional, and national conferences and workshops for the professional stimulation and idea exchange so necessary for continued growth.

State and National Occupational Therapy Associations as Resources

Each of the 50 states has a state occupational therapy association related to the national organization, the American Occupational Therapy Association (AOTA). Both state and national associations are invaluable resources for the isolated therapist. In my experience, a letter or phone call to various members of the state association has resulted in help in presenting a workshop, written material to assist with the treatment of a client, assistance with legislative matters, and newfound friends. Occupational therapists living in the same state generally have specific information about resources and political structures and influences within the state and knowledge of the total health and social systems.

The AOTA may be used in similar ways, although it should not be expected that it would have breadth and depth of information about each state and its organization membership. A list of printed publications and films and other audiovisual material is available from the national office upon request. The AOTA offers a variety of other services.

Demands for Time and When to Say No

As the therapist becomes accepted as both a person and a therapist and as his or her skills and knowledge become apparent, the therapist will be asked to do many things in the community, to speak to various groups, to help plan and lead workshops, and to serve on committees, advisory groups, and boards, to name a few. This is an excellent opportunity to contribute to the community and influence the direction and integration of services. It also provides opportunities to get to know more people in the community and representatives from various agencies with which the therapist will be working. It is the beginning of the development of a lateral network, which will be discussed in greater detail later in this chapter.

When the therapist is the only occupational therapist in a 50-mile or more radius, such demands for time increase to such an extent that the therapist has to become selective. Some therapists make this determination by accepting only those appointments within which they feel they can make a unique contribution. When others can perform a service, the therapist should not do the job.

One therapist was asked to accept the position of Research Chairman on a community board, with the specific assignment to research the literature pertaining to mental retardation. Innovative programming and research being done were of particular interest to this board and, since the therapist had access to this type of information and recognized that reviewing the material would benefit her own continuing education, she accepted the appointment. At the first board meeting she was informed by another board member, "Oh, by the way, you are also in charge of distributing and collecting coin containers." The therapist acknowledged that she *could* do that and do it very well but that she *would* not. She explained that the demands on her time were great, that she had accepted the appointment because she felt she could make a unique contribution here, but that there were any number of people in the community who could perform very well the tasks involved with the coin containers. If the board wished to select someone else to do both tasks, she would be happy to resign so that

they could do that. The chairman asked that the therapist remain as Research Chairman and assured the board that someone else would be found to assume the coin collection tasks.

Program Development

Program development is an art. A variety of skills are required to plan and implement a community program, but it also requires a certain finesse, a flair, to make a plan work.

Some occupational therapists who move into a rural area fill positions in an agency that has an existing occupational therapy program. Others are hired to develop an occupational therapy program. Some are hired by an existing community program that is adding an occupational therapist to the treatment team. Some deal with combinations of the above. But many occupational therapists moving into a rural area are in the position of creating their own jobs. Especially for the latter group, the first step is to work out a definition of occupational therapy that will have meaning in the culture and experience of those with whom the therapist will deal, because he or she will be asked many times "What is it?" and "What does an occupational therapist do?"

Assessment of Needs

Program development should start with an analytical assessment of the needs of the community to be served. What needs are currently filled by existing programs? What are the gaps in service and who is not being served? Can any of the gaps be filled by expanding the scope of an existing program, or does a new program need to be started?

In assessing needs it is helpful to gather comparative statistics for the geographic area the program is to serve. Compared to the rest of the state and nation, is the suicide rate higher or lower here? rate of unemployment? illegitimate birth rates? what percentage of population is over 55? are there many admissions to state psychiatric institutions? what is the number of school drop-outs, their average age, and sex? Problem areas and developing trends can be detected through comparative analysis. Further analysis often suggests when, where, what, and how intervention should occur.

Many states have regional planning agencies whose staff keeps current statistics of this type. Other sources include United States Census Reports, Health Systems Agencies, the State Health Planning and Development Agencies, departments of state government, and local county offices.

Assessment of the data may reveal needs not being met in the community, and yet the local population may deny that this is a problem. On the other hand, these same people may express felt needs that are not supported by the data analysis at all. If this situation exists, chances are that the latter will receive community support no matter how logical the former is. If possible, the therapist should integrate the two needs and emphasize, when selling it to the community, that the "felt" needs are being met.

In assessing needs and developing a program it is important to be aware of the "communities within the community." These may be a particular ethnic or religious group clustered in the same neighborhood, all children under the age of six, all people over the age of 55, or other peer groups. In some communities the folk class might be the "community within." What differences does each subgroup have to which the program could respond, making it more accessible and more used by them? One county with which I am familiar has two rather small towns less than 15 miles apart. During the Civil War the residents of one town sympathized with the Union and the other with the Confederacy. Today, over 100 years later, if a meeting for county residents is held in one of the towns, the people from the other town will not attend.

Programs the Community Will Support

Find out what programs have been started in the community within the past few years. To what extent are they fulfilling their original purpose? Has the program been modified? Why? What financial supports does each have? Who are the people serving on their boards?

Often it is more important to determine which projects were proposed but never developed. What were the blocks that prevented it from happening? What individuals or groups of people kept it from getting started, and why? In other words, who comprises the informal power structure in this community? Once the blocks are identified that might prevent your program from developing, a plan can be formulated to remove or circumvent them.

It may be necessary to define the steps needed to activate the program, although not trying to accomplish them in sequence. For example, sometimes step 6 might be done easily, then step 3, step 11, and so forth, until the entire plan is operational, with minimal resistance having been raised to each step individually, whereas much resistance might be raised to the project in its entirety.

Identifying Personal Interests

Everyone wants something and, whether it is in treating a patient or developing a program, it is in the occupational therapist's self-interest to discover the payoff for each person, group, or agency with which he or she is dealing. A home health care program may be in the personal interest of the state Commission on Aging because many persons receiving the services will be senior citizens; it may be in the president of the local bank's self-interest because his mother had a stroke, is now home from the hospital, and needs rehabilitative services; it may be in the physician's self-interest because he knows his patients need more help than he has the time and energy to provide.

Integration of Services

Every health care professional has an obligation to work toward the integration of services, to make them as visible and as accessible as possible, with continuity of care having one of the highest priorities. In any community there are a number of the same people receiving services from several different health and social welfare agencies, partly because of the fact that they are multiproblem families. It may be because they have problems for which there are no satisfactory solutions but they are still looking. Realistically, it may be because no one agency provides services which deal with every one of their problems. One wonders, how much is due to the fragmentation of services or the widely different approaches to problem resolution from agency to agency with the same family? This pattern of service delivery divides the client into many pieces and results in no one agency being able to use the "whole person" or "whole family" approach. How confusing and frustrating it must be for the client to be dealt with in so many different ways! And how costly in terms of the inefficient use of available resources.

One community's approach toward integration of services and the development of a coordinated plan for clients served by several agencies has been for people offering services to meet every other Saturday morning over coffee and doughnuts for case reviews. Representatives from community agencies, physicians, ministers, teachers, and other community caregivers discuss the clients they have in common and a consistent approach for helping an individual client or a family is developed. This informal evaluation facilitates the delivery of higher quality of service at a lower total cost to the community.

Another approach toward the integration of services is especially practical in a rural community, where duplication of programs for comparatively few clients probably would not occur because of the limits on resources available. Many needs within the community could be met and the health, social services, mental health and education dollar could be stretched by sharing facilities, equipment, staff, transportation, and supplies with day care for the mentally retarded, with partial hospitalization facilities for the emotionally disturbed and the physically handicapped, with the senior citizens program, and with facilities open to community groups, especially youth groups. Separate programs would be required for the groups identified, but activities such as meals, outings, and so forth could often be held jointly. The community will often provide the facilities in the form of church classrooms, empty stores, or areas in city or county buildings for such joint endeavors, and funding can be broad-based by virtue of the funding sources of the groups involved.

The use of health service facilities by community groups would do much to create the image, not of "this is a place for the aged and handicapped," but "this is a place for people." Eventually this supports the awareness that the aged and handicapped are people, first, and people who may have problems, second. Resulting from this interaction should be a synergistic effect having impact on community understanding, education, prevention; a focus on health rather than illness; an emphasis on people's strengths and what they can do rather than what they cannot do; and a concern for their well-being expressed in the strengthening of supports within the community.

Transportation

Transportation is a critical problem in most rural areas, particularly for the disadvantaged. Some places have small buses run by Community Action and a few states now permit the use of school buses for transporting senior citizens and special population groups, but public transportation is often virtually nonexistent. Many people live "up a hollow" or in isolated geographic areas and may have no private means of transportation except walking, if they are able.

The county seat is the center for schools, shopping, doctors, and courthouse services and is usually the location of any clinics and at least the hub for countywide services. It is frustrating and defeating to have facilities, staff, and program in a central area and to know that those in the outlying areas who need the service are unable to get there.

Some programs have been able to include transportation costs in their budgets and have found it works well to hire a driver living at the edge of the geographic area to be served. The driver can pick up people on the way to the center and take them home when going back in the evening.

Another answer is to take the services to the people via a mobile unit. The optimal benefit of some kinds of services is not gained with this method of delivery, but other kinds can be provided very effectively. Taking services to the people of the folk culture

by this method may be the only way to get them to accept the services, at least in the beginning.

Varying levels of success have been achieved by using volunteers to provide transportation. Volunteers often are reluctant, however, to use their own cars to transport clients because of the possible liabilities. For many years the National Therapeutic Recreation Society* has had a service for member agencies through which liability coverage for volunteers can be obtained for a nominal fee.

Providing transportation can be a costly budget item, but service integration in a central area would at least promote maximum benefit for the dollars expended. The bus driver could pick up a senior citizen at one house and the child with cerebral palsy next door, and then stop up the hollow for a mentally retarded teenager.

Community Money Sources

In addition to the usual money sources in any community, such as stores, car dealers, banks, industries, and private citizens, in rural areas there are granges, 4-H Clubs, Future Farmers of America, and Homemaker Clubs. Most of these groups cannot afford to make large contributions, but some may give $25.00 to purchase supplies or buy a piece of equipment, or a church may donate a special Lenten offering to help support the work of the therapy program. Union and union auxiliaries and fraternal organizations are another source. Most of the people living in rural communities are generous in giving what they can, and they are accustomed to helping each other.

If there is a college in the area that the program serves, its various clubs may support the program. National college fraternities and sororities support national and local philanthropic endeavors. Local chapters will often organize and carry out fundraising projects and bring good publicity to your efforts. They are also a good source of volunteers.

Community Linkages— Lateral Networks

There may be formal cooperative agreements between the boards of directors of community agencies, but work between agencies is most often accomplished through an informal lateral network, the linking of one staff member to another. Relationships in an informal lateral network are worth care and nurturing. Red tape can be eliminated much more quickly by staff within an agency than by someone

---

* National Therapeutic Recreation Society, 1601 North Kent Street, Arlington, Virginia 22209.

from without. Processes usually can be set in motion by a phone call. The result is better service performed more rapidly on behalf of the occupational therapist's client and is a vital link in the advocacy role taken by the therapist on the client's behalf. The therapist can then reciprocate when network members request assistance from within the therapist's agency.

Those of us involved in the health care and social service delivery business can be pretty grim at times when we get together to discuss what we are and are not getting done and the lack of resources to meet all the needs. This suggestion is not meant to minimize the seriousness of the job but to suggest a way of freeing the energy to keep going: have fun!

Get together with the caretakers in your informal network for lunch, at a party, or at social affairs. Just as a short-cut language is developed between occupational therapists, the same thing can happen between those who work together in community systems, especially when they take the time to get to know each other as people.

The same type of approach can be used very profitably in joint programming. I was involved for several years in camping programs for residents of state mental hospitals. One part of the program focused on linking the senior citizens of a geographic unit with the area's senior citizens' center, community mental health center, welfare department, county extension agents, and employment security and social security offices in an effort to secure community placement for those from the state hospital who could function in the community with varying levels of assistance. Staff members for the camping program were drawn from all the agencies involved and, in addition to many other positive spin-offs, they had such a good time many were involved year after year. As one staff member said, "I've never worked so hard in my life, nor enjoyed it more!" And there was a definite carry-over during the time between the yearly camping programs in the interaction between the community caretakers involved. They had their own informal lateral network.

Volunteers

The strengths of a volunteer program lie in selection, training, and placement and in helping each to know that time is being spent in a useful, meaningful way rather than in doing busywork. Volunteers should be placed in jobs for which they have the education, training, and demonstrated competence while receiving adequate ongoing supervision. They should be hired and fired just as any paid employee. Volunteers should not perform staff functions but be used to enhance existing programs.

Volunteers often have skills that are useful in ac-

tivity programs, advisory and governing boards, interviewing, and community "buddy" services. While clients are aware of and appreciate the many extras paid staff give, they have a special feeling for volunteers: they are here because they really care and not because they are being paid.

A valuable fringe benefit is that the involvement of volunteers in community programs enables them to tell others about the goals, objectives, and services of the program. Their understanding helps to dispel the prejudice and discrimination which still, unfortunately, often surround mentally and physically handicapped individuals.

The content and extent of training programs the occupational therapist develops for volunteers should be determined by such things as the job they are expected to do, the size of the program, and the number of volunteers. Whatever determinants are factors in training program design, it is essential that training be given. A well-trained volunteer is more confident, becomes involved more quickly at a deeper level, and feels more rewarded. Commitment follows, and involved and committed volunteers who are appreciated for their contribution tend to stay with the program longer.

My approach is to teach empathic listening and responding skills and crisis intervention techniques, using roleplaying to integrate the two, as basic training for all volunteers.[9] Specialized training in the specific task areas assigned to them and information concerning ethics and confidentiality are then given. There is always a psychological component involved when a person is ill or disabled, whether physically or mentally. The combination of empathy and crisis intervention and task-related skills provides each volunteer with tools for interaction with clients in nearly any situation and is useful for building initial and ongoing relationships. Having these skills gives confidence to volunteers and enhances the contributions they can make.

Referrals

The hospital or clinic-based occupational therapy program generally receives many of its treatment referrals from sources in the medical system. Whether in an urban or rural setting, the community-based occupational therapist receives some referrals from medical sources, but frequently receives many more through community contacts, such as those community agencies represented in the therapist's lateral network, the local storekeeper, or law enforcement personnel, to name just a few. The county health nurse and the county extension agent are two particularly good sources, as they visit many homes in the rural area. With referrals originating from so many nonphysician sources, the occupational therapist needs to decide which clients' conditions warrant also securing a physician's referral for occupational therapy. In many states where occupational therapists are licensed, physician referral is required.

The referral may state only "referred for occupational therapy," but that is acceptable as it gives the therapist an opportunity to discuss the client's condition with the physician and to begin the process of physician-education regarding occupational therapy through discussion and reports sent to the physician regarding the occupational therapy treatment plan and the client's progress.

The community-based therapist often spends more time working with groups such as those that focus on the development of work habits or those for the parents of handicapped children than in doing individual treatment. Such groups seldom need a physician referral. However, this decision requires the therapist's determination in relation to each individual situation and to licensing requirements.

The Occupational Therapist as a Consultant in a Rural Community

The occupational therapist may not feel skilled enough yet to function as a consultant, but the chances are that in a rural community the therapist knows more than anybody else about such things as ordering a wheelchair, the kinds of fastenings that make it easier for handicapped children to dress themselves, and many other aspects of helping people to function at their optimal level. The thought of being a consultant can be scary to the therapist who has not realized that he or she has often functioned in such a role in relation to the parents and families of clients and to other members of the health care team as part of his or her daily work as a therapist. Furthermore, most occupational therapists can be a consultant to the architect designing housing for senior citizens and to the teacher of the homebound, as well as other community caregivers and can contribute much to the health and quality of life of people in the community.

If a therapist desires to be a consultant to a particular group or system, for instance, schools, welfare, or ministerial alliance, one way to get their attention is to ask them for consultation concerning a problem. Such a tactic introduces you to personnel within the system, starts a dialogue that shares attitudes, thinking, and skills, and eases the way for their asking for assistance; it may even provide an opportunity for you to offer it.

Extrapolation

The occupational therapist knows the dynamics and process involved in treating the individual client. This same basic model can be extrapolated and built upon in working with groups and in working with the entire community. In other words, assess needs, define goals, specify what needs to be done and the methods to be used, implement the process, and evaluate the results. The following case study is presented as a further illustration of this.

The occupational therapist is functioning as a team member in an interdisciplinary approach to a problem. The role-blurring evident in this situation is a realistic expectation for the occupational therapist working in a rural community. Professionals are few and far between and "one does what one can" to get the job done. As an occupational therapist, one may be uncomfortable losing this much identity and feel that one has lost his or her place; it is essential to have a firm sense of identity in order to role-blur. However, human resources must be used in the most effective and efficient way possible; there is an overlap between many disciplines (occupational therapy, social work, recreation therapy, and so on), and there is a common base shared by these disciplines. We each see the same things when we examine a particular situation, but we see these things from the unique perspective of our own disciplines.

Hotline Expansion Plan for Region X

Hotline, Inc., is a 24-hour, crisis-intervention telephone service staffed by volunteers and based in A County. It accepts collect calls from the eight county catchment area (Region X—A, B, C, D, E, F, G, and H counties) served by the Region X Community Mental Health Center, Inc. (CMHC). A cooperative agreement exists between Hotline and the CMHC. The occupational therapist who developed the plan is being interviewed and questioned as to the purpose of some of the steps detailed in the plan.

What are you trying to accomplish by developing this plan?

"The overall goal for this community organization project is to expand Hotline services throughout these eight counties, with each county's operation having a satellite relationship to the A County unit. The maximum objective is for each county to have its own phone service, trouble teams, and information and referral services with the necessary organizational structure including funding, training, community support, and inter-agency linkages to maintain them. The minimum objective is for each county to have its own trouble teams, information and referral material which will be used by the A County-based phone service to respond to callers' needs, with persons from some of the other counties committed to taking the training and working on the phones in A County and the necessary organizational structure including funding, training, community support, and interagency linkages to support them. Since the 178,000 population of this catchment area breaks down with A County—98,000 and G County—32,000, the other six counties ranging from 15,000 down to 2,000, with eight-party phone lines being prevalent in the smaller counties, the assumption is that no county other than A can reach the maximum objective, but that some of the larger ones may choose to operate somewhere in between the maximum and minimum objectives."

You mentioned maximum and minimum objectives several times and then made the assumption that only County A could reach the maximum. What's the purpose of going through all that?

"Well, this project will be asking an existing organization and a number of volunteers to commit valuable resources—time, energy, and money—and it is important that all involved know not only the *total* of what they want to happen but also what they're willing to settle for. The assumption helps us to be realistic in our expectations. If we did not go through this process of 'thinking through,' we would probably have some people pushing for the maximum objective, wasting energy, and getting frustrated, going right by what realistically could be accomplished, and ending up not accomplishing anything! The minimum objective says that 'this is the bottom line'—if we can't accomplish even that much, then we are better off not using our resources here. It gives us a place to stop without feeling we have failed because we have known all along what the cut-off point was going to be, and why."

There must be a real need for this kind of service for so many people to be so committed to the expansion of it.

"Yes, at the time this plan was developed, Hotline in County A was receiving over 1100 calls each month, and the number climbs steadily. This type of service is based on the theory that crisis intervention at this level by trained volunteers has definite value in the total mental health effort. Our needs assessment included the number of calls being received in County A, including the number received from the outlying counties in Region X, requests for the service from community leaders in each county, requirements of Federal Regulations

for National Institute of Mental Health (NIMH) construction and staffing grants for community mental health services, and requirements of the state's Department of Mental Health licensing regulations for psychiatric programs and facilities.

"The primary target population in each county will be a cross-section of community leaders, including representatives from government, law enforcement, education, health, and social service agencies, industry, news media, churches, ministerial alliance, and so forth, those people who have the power to develop the linkages needed to support this kind of program, whether through funding, direct service, cooperation, or whatever. The individuals in this group may, or may not, wish to be involved in Hotline direct services as a phone worker or trouble team worker. The secondary target will be those persons from the community who wish to be involved in this latter capacity.

"We will be dealing with geographical communities but also the functional communities within the geographical areas. Since the governing board of the CMHC is composed of representatives (community leaders) appointed by the County Court of each of the eight counties, the initial strategy would be to meet with these board members in their county (G County, being the next largest after County A, would be the first county; also the CMHC now has a satellite office there to provide professional back-up services) and discuss the expansion plans with them. The board members are already familiar with the County A Hotline operation and, as a board, have given sanction to the existing Hotline and to expansion of these services. They will be asked to identify and *personally contact* the community leaders in preparation for the first meeting. Past experience has indicated that personal contact by board members is very successful for this type of thing in these smaller counties. Announcement of the meeting to the general community would be by prepared news releases, church bulletins, local radio (if any), and word of mouth. Since none of the counties except A have television stations, it would be necessary to identify the stations watched most in each county for coverage on talk shows, community service announcements, and so forth, and the same process would be used for radio coverage. Periodic checking with the board members prior to the meeting date will provide an indication of any changes needed in this strategy to get key people to attend the meeting.

"A strategy will be to have three or four knowledgeable and experienced A County Hotline members, including the current chairperson and myself, at the organizational meeting to present the concept and purpose and to answer questions. The tactics used will be education, and persuasion through the Hotline representatives' presentations and hand-outs of printed material discussing the organization of, and factors to be considered in developing, a crisis intervention telephone service in rural and semirural areas. Strategy at this meeting will be the selection of a local steering committee with positions paralleling those of the A County Hotline so that A County staff members can work with their G County counterparts (training chairpersons, finances, public relations including a speakers' bureau, scheduling, and so forth). I think it is very important for the *local* people to develop the interagency linkages to support this program, but we would be there to facilitate their assessing the various community power structures and to help them look at the differences in organizational structures of agencies and therefore differences needed in approach.

"Such a service as Hotline provides does not presently exist in these counties, but what we will be taking away from the existing agencies will be any exclusivity of turf, or autonomy, they presently have in dealing with clients in crisis. This may, or may not be, a threat to an individual agency and will need to be dealt with on an individual agency basis, with those needing such to be determined through ongoing analysis and evaluation of progress of the plan toward the stated goal. Tactics for dealing with an agency would probably emphasize education and informing, persuasion, and using existing laws and probably would not include conflict and coercion, though coercion could be used subtly by those in the community power structure if the agency is resistant."

From what you've just said, I'm getting the impression that established agencies might really feel threatened by a new program being organized in the community!

"Yes, this does happen sometimes. You know, agencies, just like individuals, tend to act in their own vital self-interest. In this respect, they are not altruistic! By the same token, agencies are seldom willfully self-destructive, so we need to make cooperation as profitable for them as we possibly can, *or* make noncooperation so painful or costly that they can't afford not to cooperate!

"Anyway, back to the description of the plan. At this point the staff has made the commitment for County G that the A county Hotline will pay expenses and conduct the first training and will also pay travel expenses for A County members to work with them during the initial organizational phase. The same type of commitment to the other counties in the catchment area has been discussed, but since

we are not ready to expand into those counties now, staff has not yet voted on this. The County G people will be involved in every step of setting up and conducting the training, even though they will also be trainees, so that they can learn the process. They may choose phone worker training, trouble team training, or both. We are also giving them the opportunity to tie into an existing program, and sharing knowledge we have gained in developing it. The community is getting a coordinated service to fill some of the present gaps, plus education on the worth of another level of mental health service. The counties will each have members on the staff of the A County Hotline, because it is the parent organization. This type of representation was provided for in the original articles of incorporation and bylaws.

"In developing any plan, it is important to identify negative consequences and the risks involved. We constantly ask the question, 'If we do this, what is going to happen? What are possible negative results from our action?' Once the negative results are identified, we can plan what we will do to counter them *if* they happen.

"Some of the negative consequences and risks which are possible consequences of the strategy and tactics planned have been discussed already, but there are others that also need to be considered. If key agency representatives do not attend the initial meeting in spite of our efforts, then we will assess who in the community has the clout, power, or control to bring pressure to bear on them. For instance, the County Court partially funds many community agencies and the CMHC board members could remind agencies of this; it would be in the agencies' self-interest to cooperate. This is an example of the type of assessment, counter strategy, and tactics which will be employed throughout the process. It is essential to be flexible and do your homework. Then, if the catastrophes occur in spite of your best planning efforts, you are much better prepared to cope with them. In this type of community organization much resistance to being 'overwhelmed' by an outside group (in this case, A County Hotline) can be minimized by the basic view that there are two reasons to involve people in planning: one is to get their support and the other is that, by involving those for whom the plan is intended, chances are you will come up with a better plan because they know their needs, strengths, and weaknesses better than do you as an outsider. People also tend to defend that which they help to create. Watchful inactivity helps in this type of effort. It becomes counterproductive to react defensively to small deviations from the goal and objectives. It is much more productive to give most things time to settle and to know what is *important* to act on immediately.

"A definite time table is difficult to establish for all eight counties. This type of volunteer program needs professional back-up services, and there are few professionals of any discipline with mental health training in the counties other than A, G, and F. Back-up help on the telephone could answer some of the needs, except that the demand for services on all levels already far exceeds the capacity of the small CMHC staff to provide it. So, part of the time table is affected by the amount of funding for additional staff provided by the state legislature and Department of Mental Health. An educated guess is that this will continue to be a problem to community mental health programs for a long while yet. This is an external variable. An internal variable would be the level of service each county selected and training time required to teach necessary skills.

"The time table projected allows that the minimum objective could be accomplished in each county in six to nine months. There is no set deadline, so it is not necessary to set up a calendar chart, working backwards from the deadline date, filling in tasks to be accomplished by specific dates, as I do with projects having a fixed target date. After G County is going, then *they* could organize adjacent F County with consultative assistance and support from A County, while the A County team started with adjacent C County. Then C and F could

organize E and B, two counties adjacent to them, with A and G again providing consultative assistance and support, and so on until each county in the catchment area was organized. Which groups would organize D and H would depend on who had the time and other resources at that point, and that should be determined later. Total time required would probably be two to three years, and a positive spin-off of this type of approach would be the involvement of a number of different leaders, increased commitment, and the reinforcement and up-grading of skills for those involved which will in turn strengthen their local organizations." (See Fig. 37-1).

How will you measure the success of this project?

"Actually, evaluation of the progress of the project will begin along with implementation of the plan and will be ongoing. Success or failure will be evident in the extent of accomplishment of the minimum objectives, any levels above them, and the stated goals. This continuous monitoring of what is happening is crucial in each aspect of the plan so that critical revisions can be made when and where needed to keep things moving, not after the programs are obviously bogged down.

"In this type of service the number of calls tends to increase in direct proportion to the publicizing of service. Therefore, evaluation as to effectiveness of publicity and adequacy of service rendered can be

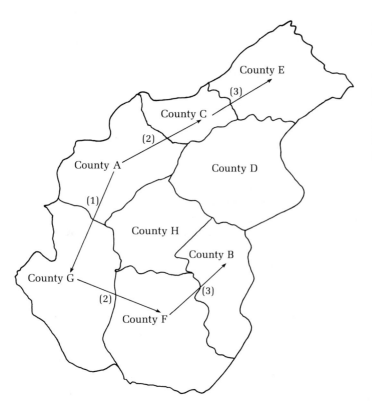

Figure 37-1. Flow chart for Hotline expansion. County A—original Hotline organization. County G—first satellite Hotline. Counties F and C—second and third satellites, organized concurrently by G and A respectively. Counties E and B—fourth and fifth satellites, organized concurrently by C and F respectively. Counties H and D—satellites to be organized last with organizing satellites to be determined later.

monitored by keeping statistics relative to number and type (for example, depression, sexual, dating problems) of calls received each month in each of the local counties or increases in calls received by the A County Hotline from the local counties. The completeness of this type of evaluation is further augmented by feedback from community agencies regarding comments of clients who have used the Hotline service." □

The Future in the Rural Community

As interstate highways have cut through the rural areas and access and secondary roads have been improved, the geographical isolation has become less acute for many. Improved roads have also resulted in less economic isolation and have opened areas to cultural influences from outside the rural communities. In recent years any number of college educated young adults and their older counterpart, the industrial age dropouts, have bought or rented land in rural areas, showing an appreciation for the slower pace and less complicated, less stressful lifestyle found in the rural culture. Television in nearly every house and shack has undoubtedly created an awareness of different cultures, different ways of doing things, and different ways of thinking. Resistance to change is particularly apparent in the men of the folk culture, but the awareness created by television has rather insidiously removed one of the barriers to change: they can now at least "picture" how some of the other folks live.

There is relatively little in the rural areas in the way of community health services. Sieg has indicated that there are more hospitals in rural areas than in urban areas, that rural people are hospitalized more than their city neighbors, and that they tend to stay longer because of the inaccessibility to alternative health care.[10] For years, county health nurses and private physicians have provided the only other health care services in many rural areas.

There are wide gaps in health services available in rural areas. The occupational therapist has more to offer than most other disciplines to the process of filling these gaps because of his or her diversification of skills and knowledge, the whole person treatment approach, and the goal of optimal functioning. The education of an occupational therapist produces a generalist, one who has studied, and usually had direct experience with, the mentally retarded, the physically handicapped, the visually and hearing impaired, the psychiatrically handicapped, the socially and culturally disadvantaged; has taken a wide range of courses from anatomy to weaving, group dynam-

ics to individual evaluation; and has studied aspects of development from conception to senescence, in illness and in health. The generalist occupational therapist can give direct treatment to many as well as screen and refer others to the proper specialists, disciplines, or services. A positive result expected from this type of functioning would be decreased overall health care costs with a higher quality of care provided as more people would receive the type of care needed.

Occupational therapists function within all the levels of prevention in the community defined by Caplan, originally in relation to mental health, but used here to pertain to the very broad area of prevention.[11] Intervention with populations at risk, those who as yet have no symptoms of maladjustment or disease, is defined as primary prevention; intervention in the form of early diagnosis and effective treatment, aimed at shortening the duration of illness of those who are showing symptoms, sometimes in the acute stage, is defined as secondary prevention; and intervention with those who are past the acute stage, needing rehabilitation to reach their optimal level of functioning or to prevent further deterioration, is defined as tertiary prevention.[12,13,14]

The teaching and training offered by an occupational therapist working in the rural community can have tremendous impact on the quality of care given and create an ever-widening area of influence for the fundamental beliefs and practices of occupational therapy. Teaching families of clients, Home Health Aides, Homemaker Aides, nursing home staff and personnel, or adult family care home proprietors when to call the occupational therapist, what to do until the therapist gets there, and what to do between visits enhances the effectiveness of the total treatment process. It will also probably facilitate the referral of many more people in need of the occupational therapist's services.

Several occupational therapists have written of the necessity for the revision of professional curricula to include special skills needed to work in the community, particularly in settings that are not traditional for the occupational therapist.[15,16] This would indeed contribute much to the preparation of the therapists needed to make a difference in the delivery and quality of health care in the rural community.

The Folk Class

The occupational therapist working with the folk class will first have to know these people better than they know themselves. Their patterns of behavior should become more apparent to the therapist than they are to themselves since the therapist is an objective observer. One of the occupational therapist's strengths is the ability to adapt and, when working with people of the folk class, it is crucial to adapt to them—their culture, their world, their way of doing things—if assistance is to be given them towards resolution of some of their problems.

Long-range planning has little meaning to these people. Therefore, it is up to the occupational therapist, perhaps with the involvement of those in the lateral network, to develop the long-range plan and, starting *where they are* in their life and culture, involve the folk class people initially in quick success projects that are steps in the plan and later in those that take longer to complete and are a little more complex, just as in developing an individual treatment plan working toward delay of gratification. The folk class is beginning to be more accessible and *will* tend to get involved in projects that they think will be successful and that will enhance their own self-esteem.

The impetus to change and the solutions to the problems of the folk class must come from within their group, but their resistance to involvement and lack of a concept of the planning process make the former nearly impossible. If the therapist focuses on a situation which needs to be changed and which would *have their support,* whether a real or felt need, and structures their participation to their need for *action,* the therapist will have achieved the first step toward their involvement. Since the people in this class function most of the time from their feelings, structuring the first project around a "felt need" would no doubt enhance the project's chance of success.

The occupational therapist working in the rural community will, of necessity, devote much time and effort to taking an advocacy role on behalf of clients. Taking the "whole person" or "whole family" approach to treatment means that all those factors impinging on the client's ability to function at his optimal level need attention. Mrs. Jones, aged 79 and living alone, may have held things in tenuous balance on a limited income before she broke her hip and was hospitalized; now she is back home, receiving Home Health Care, but really cannot get out to the grocery, nor is she sufficiently mobile to take care of the house, laundry, and cooking. She is afraid that she will have to go to a nursing home and leave her home, afraid she will fall again and no one will be there to help her, worrying in so many ways about her future. Mrs. Jones is in a "situational crisis." The situation that precipitated her present crisis was the fracturing of her hip. As an occupational therapist concerned with restoring physical functioning, it will quickly become apparent that intervention in the situational crisis is needed to prevent Mrs. Jones'

moving into a severe depression, and the intervention must occur before she can regain enough energy to focus on improving her physical condition. As an advocate, the occupational therapist will facilitate Mrs. Jones' securing the temporary services of a homemaker from the county Welfare Department, or a neighbor who will help Mrs. Jones an hour a day, or whatever resources are available to be tapped through the informal lateral network. This, along with the physical restoration, is both secondary and tertiary prevention.

Many of the members of the folk class are quite skilled in the various arts and crafts that have a significant place in their culture. These can usually be adapted to improve or restore functioning, and it is important to utilize them this way to assist clients to keep their "place" in their culture. As clients learn to trust the therapist, the introduction of new experiences and activities may be indicated and possible. In other words, focus is on the use of activities that can be translated into *their* community in both work and play situations. The home visits that are necessary to personalize the therapist's relationship with members of the folk class will also provide the opportunity for observing and finding out what the client needs to function in his or her setting. This enables the therapist to gather the information needed to design an overall treatment and activity plan focusing on total needs. People are judged in their community by what they can do that has meaning in that community. Occupational therapy has a vital role to play in making that doing possible.

With the men in one group, the women in another group, the youth in their group, and the children in yet another group, family activities, except perhaps work projects such as the garden, are practically nonexistent. The occupational therapist who can help a family learn to do something creative together will be breaking into an alienating culture pattern and replacing the alienation with an integrating, constructive activity that moves the members toward the closeness they crave.

To be a change agent in the rural community does not always mean that the therapist is the best person to make the personal contacts. Particularly with the folk class, at least initially, the therapist will be looked upon as an expert. Kent and Smith are among those who have found the use of indigenous (a member of the same subculture) workers, as "bridge" persons or links between the persons being served and those providing the services, particularly effective.[17] This is another approach which probably will be used more in the future, because these workers know the culture and how to work with those within it.

The Rural Community as a Whole

Much of this chapter has dealt with the characteristics of the folk class as a whole. But it is of the utmost importance to be aware that while a total class may have certain characteristics, each member of that class is an individual and one should not attempt to deal with the member in terms of the class, or the class in terms of its members.[18] For instance, within the folk class there are those who want a better life and will respond readily to efforts to help them move closer to middle class values and characteristics as well as those who want to stay with the status quo. Different approaches will be needed with each of these two groups, as well as with the individuals within each group.

The middle class and professional class in the rural areas, and the individuals within them, will require still different approaches. And as the rural areas grow and turn into more commercialized communities and towns, this will lead to less personalization, and will eventually force those in the folk class to change even more.

As the sparsely settled areas reach a greater density of population, the more people available to work for community betterment the greater proportion of the population will get involved.[19] This is another trend that will affect approaches used by occupational therapists working in rural areas of the country. This concept was a definite factor in defining maximum and minimum objectives in the case study of the Hotline expansion. The smaller counties simply could not support the maximum objective.

References

1. Weller, J.: Yesterday's People. Lexington KY: University of Kentucky Press (with the collaboration of the Council of the Southern Mountains, Inc.), 1966, p. 3.
2. Gans, H.: The Urban Villagers. New York: Free Press, 1962, p. 25.
3. Weller: Yesterday's People, p. 5.
4. James, D.: Poverty, Politics and Change. Englewood Cliffs NJ: Prentice-Hall, 1972, pp. 11–12.
5. Galbraith, J.: The Affluent Society, New York: New American Library, 1958, p. 251.
6. James: Poverty, Politics and Change, pp. 11–12.
7. Weller: Yesterday's People, pp. 30–31.
8. Kent, J., and Smith, H.: Involving the Urban Poor in Health Services Through Accommodation—The Employment of Neighborhood Representatives. Foundation for Urban and Neighborhood Development. Denver CO, p. 2. Paper presented before the Maternal and Child Health Section of the American Public Health Association at the Ninety-Fourth Annual Meeting in San Francisco, November 1966. Requests for copies ($2.50) should be addressed to: FUND, Inc. (Foundation for Urban and Neighborhood Development, Inc.), 830 Kipling Street, Suite 304, Denver, Colorado 80215.
9. Carkhuff, R.: Helping and Human Relations, Vols. 1 and 2. New York: Holt, Rinehart and Winston, 1969.
10. Sieg, K.: Rural health and the role of occupational therapy. Am. J. Occup. Ther. 29:76, 1975.
11. Caplan, G.: Principles of Preventive Psychiatry, Vol. 1. New York: Basic Books, 1964.
12. Ibid., p. 26.
13. Ibid., p. 89.
14. Ibid., p. 113.
15. Ethridge, D.: The management view of the future of occupational therapy in mental health. Am. J. Occup. Ther. 30:627, 1976.
16. Cromwell, F., and Kielhofner, G.: An educational strategy for occupational therapy community services. Am. J. Occup. Ther. 30:629–630, 1976.
17. Kent and Smith: Involving the Urban Poor, pp. 1–5.
18. Watzlawick, P., Weakland, J., and Fisch, R.: Change Principles of Problem Formation and Problem Resolution. New York: W. W. Norton & Co., 1974, p. 6.
19. McNeil, H.: Increasing Membership Participation in Voluntary Organization—Some Considerations. Appalachian Center Information Report 4, West Virginia University, Morgantown WV, 1972, p. 6.

Acknowledgment

The author gratefully acknowledges the contributions of friend and colleague Binni M. Bennett, M.S.W., in the preparation of this chapter. Her patience, suggestions, sense of humor and willingness to read, re-read and critique as the chapter was being written, were all invaluable to its development and completion.

PART 7

Managing Occupational Therapy Services

A Systems Perspective— Conceptualizing and Implementing Occupational Therapy in a Complex Environment

Carolyn Manville Baum and Elizabeth B. Devereaux

In order to be effective in implementing occupational therapy services in today's complex environment, the occupational therapist must have an introduction to systems. This chapter is intended to provide a clinically-oriented introduction to systems that can be used by the clinician in implementing occupational therapy service programs in a variety of settings. It is hoped that this basic general introduction will encourage further study of the subject.

The main objective of a general systems approach is to develop a framework for communications between specialists that will allow the entire system to function in an organized fashion to meet its objectives.

"General Systems Theory is the name that has come into use to describe a level of theoretical model building which is somewhere between the highly generalized construction of pure mathematics and the specific theories of the specialized discipline. Each discipline corresponds to a certain segment of the empirical world and each develops theories which have particular application to its own empirical segment."[1] Since the early 1950s it has been felt that there needs to be a process to discuss the general relationship of empirical models; this process is General Systems Theory. General Systems Theory has no specific methodology. It outlines a way of thinking about the relationships of parts and wholes. There are two ways of dealing with complex problems. One is to introduce arbitrary techniques to analyze the system. This is the mathematical approach. The other is to accept the complexities of the system and to search for the structural patterns that will enable us to examine the problem as a whole. This is the systems approach.*

A systems approach allows for the integration of a diversity of programs and values into a unity of action. Each of the components of the system must work in its own way, within its own logic, and according to its own theories in order to be effective. Yet all components must work toward a common goal. Each must accept, understand, and carry out its own function as a part of a whole.

The problem in the systems approach is that it lacks clarity. Communication is a continuing prob-

---

* The "Model" which first made the systems structure visible as a principle of organizational design was NASA, the National Aeronautics and Space Administration, and the development of the United States Space Program in the 1960s.

lem, and a lack of communication causes breakdown in the systems approach. There is a constant need for arbitration of conflicts between various members of the organization. The systems approach demands an absolute clarity of objectives; the objectives for each individual must be derived from the objectives as a whole. Each person must fully understand the missions, objectives, and strategies of the organization. Each person in the system must make an effort to know what goes on throughout the entire system. To implement a systems approach requires a strong manager who takes personal responsibility for relationships and communication, and who functions to integrate the activities and tasks of the personnel to accomplish the goals of the organization.[2]

Systems Theory Terminology

Some key terms to master in the vocabulary of general systems theory include the following:

System: An organized whole consisting of interrelated, interdependent parts.[3]

Open System: The individual and the environment mutually influence one another, and there is an exchange of information, matter, and energy.[4]

Closed System: A closed system is isolated from its environment in that information, matter, and energy are not exchanged.[5]

Patterns of Activities of Energy Exchange[6]

Input: Information taken into a system, through transformation or recognition of energy, matter, or information.

Output: Information flowing from the system.

Feedback Loop: The output is returned to the input, and in the process the system is modified. This process can be positive or negative.[7]

Equafinality: A state of stability in spite of the continuous flow and exchange of information.[8]

One important characteristic to recognize is that if any one part of the system is changed, then all other parts within the system and any related system are changed as a result. The systems approach suggests that looking at only one part of the system in isolation provides a distorted view of the system and any related system. "General Systems Theory has no methodology as do other theories, but it does establish an outline of ways of thinking, of relationships of parts, of wholes, and of inputs and outputs. It furthermore enables the therapist to identify the possibilities among a vast number of variables."[9]

A general systems approach is very valuable to the occupational therapist in viewing patients, pro-

grams, and organizations. It gives a framework for understanding the following:

—Where OT fits into more complex structures

—That change is an element of the whole, and that change has a rippling effect

—The complexity of interaction

—Values that are inherent in a system

—The formal and informal structure of a system

—The personality characteristics of a system

—When you are seeing behaviors that relate to imbalances in the system

System Skills

It is impossible to list all of the skills needed to cope with complex systems. However, some of the most important skills needed by the occupational therapist have been identified. The following list of skills has been adapted from Hall:[10]

1. Recognizing the values of the institution and of other departments within the institution
2. Knowing the future plans of the organization
3. Defining a personal role in the system
4. Contributing to the development of goals for the institution as well as motivating staff members to achieve those goals
5. Analyzing the tasks to be done and delegating the responsibilities, making sure that each is taken care of
6. Distinguishing between myth and the reality of the system
7. Understanding the structure of the institution and recognizing who has authority and power
8. Understanding what knowledge is necessary to implement the full scope of your services within the system

By applying a systems approach, it is possible to exert some control over the environment and to make changes beneficial to clients, the program, and the organization. In addition, the systems approach assists in understanding the consequences of making a change because the change is viewed as it affects the whole. This sort of understanding is a prerequisite to program growth.

Each system has some identifiable characteristics and, although each organizational structure is different, each can be studied from a systems perspective. To demonstrate the systems model, a representation of effective and successful program models of occupational therapy service follows. The models are taken directly from written interviews with the occupational therapy administrator from each facility. Note the values, structure, and personnel requirements of each system. Commentary on each model is also provided to highlight the systems perspective.

Model

Community Psychiatry

Facility

Keystone House, Inc.
Norwalk, Connecticut

Director

Carol A. Nodop, MA, OTR

Objectives of Program

Keystone House, Inc., is a private, nonprofit agency providing transitional living services to adults. Most of the clients served have had multiple hospitalizations for psychiatric illness. The following are the objectives of the facility:

1. To provide intermediate housing to emotionally dysfunctional persons without regard to race, creed, sex, or national origin in order to prevent hospitalization or rehospitalization
2. To provide skill training in activities of daily living necessary for independent community living
3. To provide clients with the opportunity to learn or relearn socialization skills, as appropriate
4. To serve as a facilitator to the client in availing himself or herself of services in the community, for instance, educational, vocational, medical, psychiatric, social.

I believe that the occupational therapist is uniquely trained to provide the services to meet the program objectives. Through my tenure in the position as Executive Director, and resultant participation as a voting member of the Board of Directors, it has been possible to educate the Board about the qualifications and functions of an occupational therapist.

The agency is supported by a grant from the Division of Community Services, Department of Mental Health, State of Connecticut (45% of total budget), resident fees (21%), United Way (6%), private grants and contributions (28%).

Program History

The facility was founded in 1972, incorporated under the laws of Connecticut, and registered as a 501 C 3 nonprofit corporation with the Internal Revenue Service. It was opened to clients in June, 1973, six months after incorporation. Although Keystone House is not a large enough organization to require a formal occupational therapy department, there has been an occupational therapist on staff throughout its history. Currently the agency also employs an occupational therapist with 16 years clinical experience as Coordinator of Residential Services. This O.T.R. is responsible for direct service and supervision of the resident counselor staff. The latter is comprised, as a rule, of graduate students in health professions.

Keystone House has rarely been successful in recruiting either O.T. students or recent graduates to the staff. Since these positions are live-in for full time staff or overnight for relief staff, they seem to conflict with course–work schedules. Student interns have done field work here, not as an exclusive placement, but as part of a placement in the Norwalk Hospital Department of Psychiatry. Since the addition of the Coordinator position is quite recent, preliminary discussions on providing a clinical field work placement have occurred, and such will be offered in the future.

Community and Population Served

Keystone House serves adults receiving outpatient mental health services. This agency will not assume primary responsibility for a resident's treatment. Each resident must have a high enough level of function to assume responsibility for his or her medication regimen. Each must have a daily plan, for instance, work, school, volunteer job, social, vocational, or educational treatment center. The program provided within Keystone House focuses on skills of daily living and is both group and individually oriented. The group sessions address food preparation, housekeeping, budgeting of time and money, vocational issues, and social skills. These sessions are led by an occupational therapist. In addition to the halfway–house program, there are two apartments in the community for residents who are ready for more independent functioning than the group home permits. Staff does not live in the apartments. One group meeting is held each week in this segment of the program, alternating between apartments. This group is also led by an occupational therapist. Individual sessions are held as needed, and include crisis intervention. Both occupational therapists employed by the agency are subject to calls evenings and weekends by the counselor staff, and handle routine and emergency contacts with primary therapists, emergency room staff and others.

Referral Process

Referrals are received from the following sources:
State Hospitals (there are three in the state)
General Hospital Psychiatric Services
Private Psychiatric Hospitals
Private Practitioners
Counseling or Social Service Agencies
City and Town Welfare Departments

Parents or Other Relatives
Clients—Self-referral

Currently there is a waiting list for both men and women. Male referrals have consistently outnumbered female by three to one. The current wait for a male bed is approximately six months, which speaks to the enormous need for this service.

The initial referral is made by telephone. An application form and brochure describing the services provided is forwarded to the referring therapist. The application package must include a psychiatric summary and a physical examination report. An intake interview is conducted by the Coordinator of Residential Services, and the applicant attends a group session and a dinner. If appropriate, a family member is also seen. Following the completion of this process, a decision is made on the acceptance or rejection of the applicant.

Since the wait for admission is lengthy, an orientation group that is both a task group (simple food preparation) and a discussion group has been developed. This is conducted by the Coordinator of Residential Services, and O.T.

Success of the Program

The contributions of the occupational therapist have added to the success of the program.

Environment

The development of a program philosophy and services that address both rehabilitation and prevention provide a professional experience not readily available in a more structured, traditional institution, founded on the medical model. In addition to being an ideal vehicle for using one's skills as an occupational therapist, it has also permitted me to grow and learn as an administrator. Beyond the day-to-day management issues, my role as Executive Director has involved me with legislators, federal grant writing (successful), and external management and advocacy groups, both local and statewide. Since 28% of the total budget is made up of private foundation, corporate, and individual gifts, I am also actively learning the skills of a professional fund raiser. The successful federal grant referred to above is for a Demonstration Program for the Deinstitutionalization of the Chronically Mentally Ill. This approval means that we will substantially renovate the halfway house, adding beds, offices, dining, and recreational areas. The chance to work with staff, Board, Department of Mental Health, and other state and federal officials, other mental health professionals, fund raising experts, AOTA colleagues, clients, and their families makes this a unique opportunity for personal and professional growth. The direct service aspect of the

position is rapidly diminishing, but is not missed, due to the myriad of other challenges presented.

Qualifications of Personnel for the Program

The most important assets for the nonprofessional personnel are level-headedness and common sense. The resident counselor staff is essentially nonprofessional, and therefore, not expected to have the clinical expertise required in other settings. Training is provided here by the Coordinator during formal in-service meetings as well as informal communication. In addition to the above skills, empathy, sensitivity, and intelligence are valuable. This staff and its tenure at Keystone House are comparable to basic professional field work in terms of characteristics and expectations.

The professional staff must possess the same basic assets, but also must have extensive clinical experience in mental health settings, above average oral and written communication skills, and be comfortable in a professional role. Both the Coordinator and the Executive Director represent the agency to professional and lay members of the community, and therefore a strong identity is crucial. In addition to a solid clinical background, the professional O.T. must also know how to grade and structure activities, understand the role of activity in someone's life, and know how to do activities.

Challenging Ongoing Problems as Stated by the Program Manager

1. Keeping the program solvent.
2. Maintaining staff enthusiasm and energy levels until there are better quarters in which to function. This is intense work, and it is my responsibility to the staff to provide an atmosphere conducive to optimum performance.
3. The responsibility which weighs most heavily on each of us, regardless of job title or place in the pecking order, is to be aware of how each resident is faring clinically so that no vital communication is missed. Since this is a residence, it is imperative that standards be maintained, communications always be open, emergency procedures rehearsed. For the Executive Director, as for all staff, it is truly a life and death business. If I think about it for very long, the responsibility is awesome.[11] □

Commentary

Keystone House demonstrates an open system model. The philosophy and values of the system are defined and understood by those people working in it. The structure is clear; staff are responsible to a set of expectations that allow the entire system to operate. The following systems skills, identified earlier in the chapter, are applicable to the manager of this program:

1. Recognizes the values of the institution and of the departments within the institution
2. Knows the future plans of the organization
3. Has defined a personal role for herself in the system as well as assisted staff members in finding their roles
4. Has contributed to the development of goals for the institution and has motivated staff to achieve those goals
5. Has analyzed the tasks and delegated responsibility to be sure that each aspect of the organization is managed
6. Has a clear understanding of the realities of the system
7. Has developed the structure of the institution
8. Understands what knowledge is necessary to implement the full scope of services

As the administrator of this program, Ms. Nodop has exerted control over the environment to make changes beneficial to clients, to the program, and to the organization. Her understanding of the system is a prerequisite, not only to program stability, but to program growth.

Going back to the main objective of General Systems Theory, developing a framework for communication between specialists that will allow the organization to function, it is clear that a general systems model has been implemented within this environment. One important additional systems skill that is demonstrated in this model is that the manager perceives her position as a challenge. Rather than focusing on problems, she focuses on the challenges presented by the system. Thus, she views the demanding position she holds as an opportunity. It is within this framework that the system can most easily stay in balance.

Model

Community Pediatrics

Facility

Occupational Therapy Clinic
Austin, Texas

Director

Patricia A. Ramm, MA, OTR, FAOTA

Objectives of the Program

My independent practice was developed to provide the highest of quality services possible for children with known or suspected developmental problems, especially those related to motor, learning, or adaptive behavior. My previous experience of 10 years in providing children's services through various local agencies, lay the groundwork for developing an independent private service for children.

My professional feelings during those 10 years were ones of dissatisfaction with administrative structure, or other factors that I perceived as limiting my efforts in providing service delivery. This dissatisfaction with service delivery was the key factor in my decision to develop an independently operated clinic.

The decision to open this particular clinic came about only when I felt confident enough to take on the financial responsibility, and when I was secure in my clinical competency to design a program that would be effective and would allow me the opportunity to expand my work through continued study. My philosophy was and is that the ability to learn and to provide better service would result in increasing my financial base and, in effect, provide balance between effort and income.

Program History

The occupational therapy clinic was founded August, 1980. My activity in independent practice began in 1974. Initially, 50% of my work was consultation to related federal, state and local agencies, and 50% was private casework.

Community and Population Served

The population my clinic serves is children and adults aged 0–30 years, though the largest number of clients range from 4–12 years of age. My consultation work with the community infant–parent training program assists in early detection, evaluation, and treatment planning for 0–3 year old children. The community itself is one of interest with a growing population of 300,000; it is a small city with thriving trends. Being the capital of a powerful state, it is the hub of a variety of state activities. Members of the state legislature and staff, along with state agencies and others involved in governmental structure and power, are a key part of this community. Another structure within the community is the statewide university system which is a major power factor as the result of an enormous permanently-endowed financial base. Many special interest groups including health professional organizations have located their headquarters in this community.

State and local agencies make concerted efforts to identify children with developmental disabilities early despite financial limitations. The community houses a regional neonatal intensive care unit (servicing 14 counties) that provides care for hundreds of premature and high risk babies annually.

Clients receiving service at my clinic are from all economic conditions. Parents of mid-economic conditions seem to involve themselves more effectively in the treatment program (see Success of Program section).

Referral Process

Referrals are from the following sources:
—Agencies involved with learning disabilities, including university programs training professionals to address learning disabilities
—Educational personnel—OTs, educational diagnosticians, school nurses, teachers, special educators, principals, psychologists in private and educational programs
—Parents whose children have benefitted from treatment
—Psychiatrists
—Pediatricians
—Neuropsychologists

Success of the Program

Evidence of the success of this clinic is that it has proven to be a financially sound operation that is meeting the original therapeutic goals for quality care. High standards of care and individual programming of chidren are essential factors in the program's success.

Once the evaluation process is completed the following procedure is carried out:
—Parents receive specific information about their child's dysfunction and abilities, based on sound evaluation processes. They are encouraged to provide information and share their concerns about their child's behavior, development, or learning ability. Sometimes concerns are even broader and relate to the overall function of the family.
—Mutually agreed to goals are set, and parent involvement is promoted as vital to the success of the treatment program.
—Parents observe treatment initially, and routinely thereafter.
—Scheduling of treatment is integrated and supportive of the child's overall activities.
—Home programs are designed to strengthen parents' competency with their child, and to avoid encumbering parents with ineffective therapeutic "chores."
—Routine re-evaluation is conducted. Results are used to readjust goals and are reported to parents. This important step keeps the momentum of treatment going. Although this process is ongoing, six-week re-evaluations are considered essential.

I am very goal-structured and oriented basically through autonomy of my work and goal setting. Direction is very pleasurable to me personally. Also, balancing my accounts quarterly tends to make me put a value on my service and incorporate this type of consideration into my services. The balance sheet reflects one's professional competency and effectiveness.

Environment

The treatment setting is situated conveniently for families served. It is close to a major highway artery in the community. The clinic is housed in a business building planned for professional services. It is both clean and open to the outdoors. The clinic has been developed to be attractive and stimulating. The waiting area is comfortable and homey. This environment encourages valuable exchanges between parents.

Challenging Ongoing Problems as Stated by the Program Manager

One challenge is continuing to provide quality programming, which I feel can be an outgrowth of my standards. I continue to study all available information in management and administration. I will be conducting a health–accounting study with the local health department, and will provide data from the study to the American Occupational Therapy Association and the Texas Occupational Therapy Association. I believe that clinical excellence, coupled with administrative creativity, is the key to the advancement of our profession. If we join these two factors, our services can impact any system, given time and energy. O.T. is valuable and under-demonstrated in a broad spectrum of health services.[12] □

Commentary

The Occupational Therapy Clinic demonstrates an open system model. Rather than being a program composed of a large staff, which must be integrated to meet objectives, Mrs. Ramm has integrated her private practice into the community clearly enough to be able to know how she must operate to be an effective and efficient part of that community's health system.

Referring to the systems skills identified earlier in this chapter, Mrs. Ramm has demonstrated the following:
1. Recognized the values of her program and how those values can relate to the values of the community
2. Has a clear plan of her operation and how it fits into the community health need
3. Has developed the program to meet her personal

expectations as a professional occupational therapist
4. Has contributed to the development of the health system in the community
5. Has clearly analyzed the tasks and has developed the resources in the community necessary to support her organization
6. Has a clear understanding of the community and their expectations for health services
7. Has developed her structure to support the community's needs
8. Understands what knowledge is necessary to implement the full scope of her services

As the developer and manager of this program, Mrs. Ramm has developed her understanding of the Austin area to the point that she can control her component of the environment to make changes that are beneficial to clients, to her specific program goals, and to the growth of her organization. Her understanding of the community's system is a prerequisite for maintaining program stability and supporting further growth of her organization.

An additional systems skill, particularly important when an individual is going into a private enterprise, is that she laid the groundwork by demonstrating her competencies and the quality of service that she was able to provide to a broad spectrum of the community. This particular skill has minimized the risks associated with the high degree of autonomy that she enjoys. Because the therapist in private practice does not have as an immediate resource the administrative support system that those in organized facilities may take for granted, working relationships with lawyers, accountants, and insurance companies, as well as with governmental agencies become central to the accomplishment of goals. These relationships require a systems approach.

Model

Community: Gerontology

Facility

Occupational Therapy Consultants, Inc.
Somerville, New Jersey

Director

Cynthia F. Epstein, MA, OTR, FAOTA

Objectives of Program

Historically, occupational therapy (O.T.) practice in long-term care settings has been viewed as providing more "diversional" than restorative treatment programming. The average geriatric O.T. in my geographical area practiced in isolation.

Working in a nursing home setting, the therapist was isolated, overburdened, and unable to broaden O.T. restorative services. Equally important, minimal attempts had been made to expand occupational therapy's influence and approach to care on a facility-wide basis.

Medicare and Medicaid funding for skilled nursing facilities required O.T. availability. Most therapists and their administrators lacked the expertise to develop appropriate and financially sound treatment programs that would meet individual patient needs while engaged in therapy and yet also assure effective carry-over to the total care plan.

Similarly, given the small number of therapists practicing in this specialty area, even less attention was being given to the needs of the frail, "at-risk" elderly still residing in the community.

My initial target population was therefore administrators and therapists of long-term care facilities who were seeking to expand or initiate O.T. restorative services with the realistic expectations of increased reimbursement and an enhanced reputation, which would facilitate patient referral from the health care community and population at large. Education and research are not priorities of the facilities when they initially purchase my services.

My priorities for the majority of my clients, the long-term care facilities, are the following:
1. Service delivery—assuring comprehensive and up-to-date individualized treatment for the patient
2. Education—creating an effective interface program with facility staff to assure that treatment gains are carried over into the care plan
3. Research—developing medical care evaluation studies which demonstrate the effectiveness of O.T. treatment in the facility
4. Community focus—expanding the community's understanding of O.T. services for the elderly both in the facility and the community.

Program History

My private practice began on a part-time basis, as a solo enterprise. It was prompted by a desire to blend roles as wife, mother, and therapist. Self-employment, part-time, with flexible hours and days provided an opportunity to perform all roles. The practice began in 1970. My interest in gerontology and decision to specialize in long-term care was developed over years of working with chronically ill and older people in acute hospitals, rehabilitation centers, and home care settings. From my experience, it was obvious that broader and more sophisticated O.T. services were needed in most long-term care facilities.

In 1978 the State of New Jersey revised its Nursing Home Licensure Code and mandated O.T. services. The O.T. market in long-term care exploded.

In 1979 I formed a corporation (Occupational Therapy Consultants, Inc.) with another OTR, which is geared to providing O.T. restorative treatment, consultation, and education services on a fee for service basis in long-term care facilities. We contract with other O.T.'s and place them in our contracted facilities that are within their geographic area. All our therapists are part-time, and most have small children.

Federal regulations also helped to expand my community consultation role. Increased interest in adult day care evolved with the implementation of Title XX. As a consultant for a community agency interested in day care, I developed their program, established community linkages, wrote their funding grant, hired their staff, and helped get the program on stream.

Community and Population Served

1. Long-Term Care Facilities
   a. Geriatric patient population with some younger chronically ill—program geared to rehabilitation and prevention
   b. Facility staff—program geared to consultation, education and research. Emphasis is placed on "treating the facility along with the patient."
   c. Family or significant others—if patient is returning to community
2. Individual O.T. Departments in Hospitals and Long-Term Care Facilities
   a. Primary emphasis on program development for geriatric caseload
   b. Administrative—providing administrative consultation regarding reimbursement problems
3. Health–Care Personnel Practicing in Long-Term Care Facilities
   a. Educational workshops to improve service delivery and quality care
   b. Publications available in form of guidelines for specific problem areas in service delivery
4. State Health Planners for Long-Term Care Facilities
   a. Volunteer participation on task forces to assure O.T. visibility for long range planning

Referral Process

Primary referral source to obtain facility contacts is other occupational therapists. Second would be

nursing home administrators. Other sources are state surveyors and allied health professionals. Physicians must make patient referrals. We work through nursing initially until the physicians pick up on their own.

Referral sources are initially developed through activity and visibility in local, state, and national O.T. associations. The referral network expanded gradually as the service became known.

Success of the Program

The program's success is due to the high quality of service we deliver and to the forthright approach that we maintain with administrators regarding standards of practice. Our demonstrated success has brought increasing business. Ability to sell, analyze the market, and communicate effectively all contribute to success. Professional manner and dress, combined with good business management, are equally important. Our professional commitment to state and national O.T. organizations, involvement in community volunteer organizations, and membership in related national and state gerontological organizations has also had an impact.

Environment

I enjoy problem solving. Working in a variety of environments with many different people is exciting and rewarding. Since we work in many settings, we can constantly share new information and provide alternate strategies for problems that arise. Our organization provides a natural support network to occupational therapists who otherwise might be working in isolation. It facilitates growth and professional development.

Qualifications of Personnel for the Program

Critical thinking
Good clinical skills
Good communication skills
Professional commitment
Enjoyment of and caring attitude toward the elderly
Ability to work well with other disciplines
Interest in systems development

Challenging Ongoing Problems as Stated by the Program Manager

Maintaining adequate staff
Assuring cash flow and reserves
Expanding service delivery in light of above
Development of more community O.T. placements in adult day care, congregate housing, and so forth, given the current economic climate.[13] □

Commentary

Occupational Therapy Consultants, Inc. demonstrates an open system model. This particular organization has a structure of its own but also must function to meet the values and structures of the facility to which it provides services. Mrs. Epstein has integrated her corporation into a very large community model servicing the states of New Jersey and New York. She has developed a structure for her corporation in such a way that it is possible to clearly identify what it is she is able to offer to the facilities requesting her services. She has maintained a high level of professional standards in providing only those services that are requested that meet the qualifications she has established for her own corporation. Referring to the systems skills identified earlier in this chapter, Mrs. Epstein has demonstrated the following:

1. Identified the values of her program and how those values and the program's structure can relate to the community requiring service
2. Has a clear plan of her operation and how it fits into the health needs of the elderly in her area as well as how it fits in with her personal goals as a wife, mother, and community leader
3. Has contributed to the development of the health delivery system in that area
4. Has clearly analyzed the system in providing geriatric rehabilitation care and has developed the resources to be able to deliver that care to meet the area's needs
5. Has a clear understanding of the community's needs and their expectations for health services
6. Has developed the structure of her corporation to support the community's needs
7. Has developed the knowledge necessary to relate to this service delivery system

The practice was initiated to fill a void in the health delivery system in the New Jersey–New York area. It is recognized that when a vacuum exists, someone will fill that vacuum whether or not it is their ascribed or assumed responsibility. This apparent void in the service delivery system for the geriatric population would have been filled by some other groups or professions, had Mrs. Epstein not organized to provide these services. Another very important systems skill that she used during program development was liaison with her professional organizations, the New Jersey Occupational Therapy Association and the American Occupational Therapy Association. In addition, gerontology organizations were used to gain visibility and resources. She states that all these contacts have contributed to strengthening her position within the system.

Model

Acute Psychiatric Program

Facility

Highland Hospital
Charleston, West Virginia

Director

Suzanne M. Peloquin, OTR

Objectives of Program

Highland Hospital is a private, nonprofit hospital, the only facility of this type in the state of West Virginia. The hospital's primary objective is to provide short-term therapeutic intervention during psychiatric crises. Occupational Therapy services facilitate this process, constantly emphasizing to patients and staff alike the value of engaging, purposefully, in suitable activities that aid the resolution of individual symptomatology and the integration of more adaptive life experiences.

Occupational Therapy's major role as a service provider at Highland is evident upon close examination of inpatient schedules. Patients with open privileges may opt for 7½ hours of O.T. daily; those patients requiring more constant nursing care receive from 2½ to 3½ hours. Only one other kind of session is held daily: a 45 minute verbal interaction group directed by Social Service personnel.

Patient involvement, though ordered on virtually all patients, is optional, with from 75% to 100% participation on any given day, and one flat fee for service for daily involvement. Overall, occupational therapy services over 95% of patients admitted. Activity offerings include crafts, hobby workshops, greenhouse, sports, community outings, relaxation, yoga, and reality orientation, among others. Parallel group types predominate due to brief patient stay.

The Adult Unit services 55 inpatients with a staff of one OTR Director and seven O.T. staff members of varying educational and experiential backgrounds. A newly established Children's Pavilion will serve 15 youngsters with one OTR directing the efforts of childcare worker assistants.

Priorities, then, for occupational therapy at Highland, are the following:

1. Direct and indirect patient services
2. Education—Every attempt is made to clarify the relevance of O.T. and its knowledge base to patients, staff, students, and administration.

Program History

Occupational therapy's development as a service followed a sequence typical of many settings: that of a move from "diversion" to "therapy." Perhaps atypical is that the move has been so recent.

The first patient, admitted in 1955 to what was then the Valley Convalescent Hospital, experienced little by way of structured activity. By 1962, admitting psychiatrists' concerns about patient idleness led to the development of a crafts program, which expanded as the patient census grew. Patients then paid for supplies, but not for service.

With the arrival in 1973 of an OTR who served as part-time consultant, the important concepts of referral, goal-oriented and graded activity, documentation, fees for service, and a balanced schedule of activities were introduced. The service was called Adjunctive Therapy. The staff numbered five by the time the OTR consultant left the area. In her absence, the original craft worker, hired in 1962, attempted to adhere closely to the O.T. recommendations.

From 1979 to the present, as full-time Director of Occupational Therapy, and working alongside this same craft worker, my primary role has been to upgrade the performance, scope, and image of the department while retaining a healthy respect for and sensitivity to the existing structure and staff. My joining the staff was precipitated primarily by Joint Commission on Accreditation of Hospitals and Medicare recommendations, rather than by any hospital-wide canvassing for an OTR.

An overview of the most significant changes effected might clarify some of the sensitive issues that have emerged over the last few years. The existing program had to be assessed and brought into alignment with Standards for Practice and JCAH Guidelines. As a result, direct services were expanded to include weekend and evening coverage; six new O.T. groups were added; and two new staff members were hired. Toward improving the therapeutic aspect and understanding of the program, a daily O.T. meeting was initiated, kardex systems were revised, safety procedures were implemented, and individualized O.T. goals were added to patient care plans. O.T. assessments adapted for groups were devised, numerous written and other communications were developed toward increased patient understanding and participation. Concepts such as activity analysis, activity configuration and the therapeutic use of self were incorporated into weekly staff development meetings on the principles and practice of occupational therapy. After one year the department's name was changed to reflect the service it was now providing: Occupational Therapy.

Community and Population Served

Though the hospital's immediate community is the capital city, we are 15 minutes away from the "hollows" of West Virginia. In this area the negative view of "mental hospitals" is very strong.

Our groups find coal miners working alongside attorneys, self-ordained ministers, housewives, and college students. The most predominant admitting diagnosis over the last two years has been depression.

Referral Process

Eight admitting psychiatrists write orders for O.T. on the patient charts. Referral sheets alert the OTR, who initiates a chart review for each patient toward involvement in the program as of the first day of admission.

Success of the Program

Factors which have contributed to the success of occupational therapy at Highland are the following:
1. Service orientation: O.T. provides the core therapy offered, and has never been challenged in this capacity.
2. The relevance of its offerings: Specific activities introduced years ago during the craft era reflected cultural interests. There has been a sensitivity to this patient population in the introduction of new offerings.
3. Staff: Staff have been enthusiastic and dynamic.
4. Adaptability: Staff have been able to grow, change, and adapt to changing needs and standards, despite the sometimes painful process. Singularly open, the original "craft lady," still with us, has greatly contributed to this.
5. Credibility: O.T. has been acknowledged by administration and other services as a significant department and is included in all meetings relating to treatment and policy.
6. Good fortune: The stamina of the OTRs involved with the facility to date has facilitated growth.

Environment

—Freedom to really direct and implement O.T. Psychiatrists, administrators, and other professionals simply assume professional competence of the OTR, thereby permitting O.T. to function as a strong, independent service.
—On-going opportunity to teach patients and staff the benefits of activity therapeutically applied, a tremendous validation.
—The challenge for the OTR to function in several varied roles: staff therapist, teacher, middle manager, team member, and public relations agent.

Qualifications of Personnel for the Program

—OTR: Flexibility, creativity, stamina, maturity, ability to prioritize

—Aides: Enthusiasm, sensitivity, assertiveness, open-mindedness, sense of humor, eagerness to learn

Challenging Ongoing Problems as Stated by the Program Director

—Facing continued institutional growth with its demands, The Highland O.T. Department is acutely aware of the difficulties involved in securing new OTRs.

—Needing to continually upgrade aides' understanding and execution of therapeutic principles, without the power to reimburse additional effort with any institutional merit raise system.

—Reconciling myself to the fact that my position often necessitates a compromise in the execution of two sets of responsibilities has been difficult. The demands placed on a single OTR involved on a unit, combined with those superimposed by the managerial role are often overwhelming. If never bored by the diversity of the tasks, I must admit to feeling over-extended, often.

—Justifying the rationale for change as well as implementing it at a reasonable pace, and in a sequence which makes sense to those involved, building continually on their previous knowledge. This often means waiting patiently for some ideas to emerge from the group.[14] □

Commentary

The Occupational Therapy Program at Highland Hospital, an open system, has moved into a significant position within the facility in a relatively short period of time. The systems skills employed relate to the following:

1. Recognizing the needs of the institution and of other departments within the institution as well as balancing these needs with the actual needs of the patient
2. Having knowledge of the plans for the organization and being willing to support the development of the institution's goals
3. Clearly defining a personal role for the manager in the system and for the staff members who are able to contribute to that role
4. Contributing to the development of the institution as well as motivating the staff members to achieve those goals also
5. Analyzing and delegating the tasks, allowing some of the changes to emerge from the group rather than forcing the issues and causing conflict which could have compromised the goals of the O.T. program

The position Ms. Peloquin has filled is not unlike those in many facilities across the country where new therapists go into systems where little or no O.T. existed prior to their arrival. She was faced with the task of gaining support from the activities staff, the physicians and other professional staff, and the administration. Her comments indicate that rather than viewing the situation as problem-ridden and hopeless, she viewed it as a challenging opportunity, not only for occupational therapy, but also for her own professional growth. Her perceptions of her skills and her responsibility in relating to the challenges to be faced in this system may, in fact, be energizing for her and have a rippling effect throughout the system.

Model

Rehabilitation Facility

Facility

Rancho Los Amigos Hospital
Downey, California

Director

Dorothy J. Wilson, OTR, FAOTA

Objectives of Program

Rancho Los Amigos Hospital, which is organized into categorical disability services, is capable of providing comprehensive rehabilitative care for physically disabled patients of all ages. Occupational therapy at Rancho Los Amigos Hospital views its functions as the following:

1. To independently evaluate patients from the perspective of identifying residual neuromuscular, physiological, and psychosocial performance components that enable a patient to manage or have potential for managing daily life skills (self-care, work, leisure, or play)
2. To work with a specialized professional team and patient to plan and implement a comprehensive, coordinated care program
3. To provide outpatient care and follow-up to assess effectiveness of the inpatient care plan and to implement any new goals that may be determined
4. To provide patient, family, and community groups with health education that may serve as a preventative measure to development of complications from disease or injury
5. To ensure quality of patient care through education and research
6. To share information about the rehabilitation of the severely disabled.

These functions are performed on a solid base of patient treatment, which takes priority. The unique funding of this county hospital through per-diem billing allows a nice balance of these functions in our department.

Program History

Rancho Los Amigos Hospital is a very old facility. Occupational therapy has been involved since the inception of Rancho Los Amigos Hospital, and has been maintained through its transition from "county poor farm" to acute rehabilitation hospital. Major growth of the department took place at the time of the polio epidemic in the early 1950s, and again with the implementation of Federal Medicaid programs in the early 1960s.

Community and Population Served

The O.T. Department (staff of 80) serves 20 separate categorical medical programs for acute rehabilitation services. All patients at Rancho Los Amigos Hospital have been referred from other acute medical and surgical hospitals. The primary focus is rehabilitation; however, medical and surgical services are provided.

Rancho Los Amigos Hospital is an approximately 400-bed hospital located in Downey, California, a middle-class suburb of Los Angeles. The ethnic composition of the surrounding community is approximately 60% Caucasian, 30% Mexican-American, 18% Black, and 2% other. Our patient population is drawn from all of Los Angeles County. We are also able to accept patients from other states and countries.

The program is primarily restorative in nature. The population consists of children and adults with severe residual functional deficits as a result of injury, disease, or congenital problems.

Referral Process

Patients admitted to Rancho Los Amigos Hospital are admitted primarily for therapy services. The admission orders include an order for routine occupational therapy evaluation, unless there are medical reasons to delay. This process evolved from a "blanket" referral process that is well-known in Rancho's history.

All patients are screened by O.T. within 2 working days of admission. If a therapy program is indicated (and it is for 89% of patients admitted), a complete evaluation is done within 5 working days, and a treatment program implemented.

Success of the Program

O.T. has been successful because of the expectations of the medical leadership. They continually challenge allied health disciplines to be "professionals." Our medical director feels that the people who know most about O.T. are the

occupational therapists and therefore, we have a staff and organization that allow us to develop and grow.

Following the initial order, it is the therapist's responsibility to evaluate and plan a thorough and effective program. The O.T. evaluation summary is routinely countersigned by the physician as the official "prescription." As changes are indicated, the therapist includes them in her or his documentation and the physician again countersigns the order for change. In this way, our physicians have continued to make us responsible for the quality and effectiveness of treatment while meeting the requirements for specific orders.

Our supervisors and instructors constantly monitor treatment outcomes. We have a quality review and audit system to identify problems and work on them. We are encouraged to do research and to take higher education in order to improve our services.

Environment

Rancho is an extremely challenging facility. The physical environment, the O.T. treatment areas, the professional challenge, and the respect for the contributions of occupational therapy make this an extremely satisfying job. We have the problems faced in any large hospital, but we certainly are challenged and expected to work on these problems at all levels.

As Director of O.T., I report directly to the Medical Director and the Hospital Administrator. Occupational therapy is expected to have representation on all the major hospital committees and to do its share in running the hospital.

Qualifications of Personnel for the Program

Sound academic background with emphasis on problem-solving, basic sciences, and O.T. theory is required. Enthusiasm, pride in O.T. as a unique contributing profession, and commitment to the profession are also helpful. Other attributes include the following:
—Written and verbal communication skills, and some degree of assertiveness
—Organization and time–use skills
—Healthy response to stress, as it relates to challenge, pressure, and time constraints
—A variety of other specific skills as needed for vacancies in particular medical programs, such as sensory integration certification for openings in pediatrics

Challenging Ongoing Problems as Stated by the Program Director

The most challenging ongoing problems I face are the ones created by being part of a large, bureaucratic, political system. These include the need for continuous justification of staffing levels, pay increases, and the like, in face of taxpayer revolts such as Proposition 13, which cause budget shortfall. This situation creates a constant threat of drastic reduction of support that could undermine the programs at Rancho.[15] □

Commentary

This O.T. program, an open system, is well-integrated into the values and structure of the facility's other programs. This gives O.T. a very solid position and a responsible role within the facility.

The systems skills that are employed include the following:
1. An understanding of the values of the institution and of the other departments within the institution
2. An understanding of the political and economic conditions that impact on how service is delivered within that institution
3. Mrs. Wilson has defined a role for herself in the system
4. Contribution to the development of the goals of the institution and staff motivation to achieve those goals
5. The tasks necessary to operate the system have been analyzed and delegated to staff to make sure that all responsibilities are fulfilled
6. The realities of the system given the political, economic, and social implications of the community are understood by the program administrator
7. There is an understanding of the structure of the institution and a recognition of who has the authority and power to affect change
8. The program is developed to a level where persons hired in that situation or trained to function within that system have to perform at the knowledge level necessary to implement the full scope of services within the system

Because of the size of this program, a series of never-ending problems is present. Mrs. Wilson, in viewing her position as a challenge, possesses an important systems skill that allows her to focus on strengths and to build the kind of support that minimizes problems, thereby keeping the program geared to the objectives of providing comprehensive rehabilitation services.

Model

Acute Hospital and Outreach Services—Corporate Structure

Facility

Research Health Services, Inc.
Research Medical Center
Clinishare
Kansas City, Missouri

Director

Gloria Scammahorn, OTR

Objectives of Program

Research Health Services, Inc. came into existence in 1981. It consists of several corporations and has much potential for growth. Occupational therapy is currently working in two corporations but has connections for future growth with several others. The occupational therapy department's foundation came through Research Medical Center, an acute-care hospital of 602 beds. Occupational therapy provides services through Clinishare, a corporation that serves the community, schools, long-term care facilities, and rural hospitals. The Research Medical Center and Clinishare are both nonprofit corporations. Direct patient service and consultation on patient services are the main objectives of the department. Research Medical Center also sponsors an active affiliation program (16 to 20 students a year) and currently has several research efforts in progress.

We developed our first Clinishare contract in 1979. We are currently serving 4 school districts, 16 long-term care facilities, and 2 rural hospitals. Future growth in this area is limited only by the capacity of occupational therapy to adjust and to continue to provide quality services.

Community and Population Served

Our starting point is Kansas City, Missouri where the Medical Center is located. The community served encompasses approximately a 100-mile radius from Kansas City.

In the Medical Center, occupational therapy is a member of the rehabilitation and arthritis teams, on the pulmonary team, with pain management, and with orthopedic patients, as well as serving mental health patients. There is also an active outpatient service for hand patients, for all types of pediatric patients, and for patients needing relaxation training (biofeedback). Future program growth includes outpatient pain management and inpatient supportive services to nephrology. Our rehabilitation programs serve all ages.

In the community, we serve all types of pediatric diagnoses. We also serve geriatric patients and the wide variety of diagnoses seen with this population. We do consulting and monitoring in the community.

The therapists in-house have 3½ to 5½ hours of direct patient contact daily, depending on assignment area. Clinishare therapists spend from ½ hour to 4 hours daily traveling and service time proportionate to the distance from the Kansas City base.

Program History

German Hospital was founded in 1886. In 1917 the name was changed to Research Hospital. It was relocated in 1963, and at this time an occupational therapy department limited to psychiatric service was developed. Comprehensive rehabilitation services began in 1967, and a rehabilitation team of occupational therapy, physical therapy, social service and nursing was begun in 1973. This team is headed by the Medical Director. The O.T. space was redesigned and expanded in 1980 to meet the needs of the department. Occupational therapy wrote its first contract with a smaller hospital in 1979 and contractural agreements have expanded since that time. The corporation structure was finalized in 1981, allowing for growth in many areas and giving flexibility to develop programs that would meet the needs of the community.

Referral Process

A physician's referral is required except in schools.

Some services were developed by writing a program proposal to the Hospital Board of Trustees. Other programs were developed because physicians sent so many patients that they grew by themselves. It is easier to develop a program if the physician is the instigator of the need for O.T. service.

Success of the Program

Growth has come because therapists are allowed time to get to know the referring physicians and because an excellent medical director allows freedom of thought in therapists. There is a strong O.T./P.T. team joined by strong members from other areas, such as rehabilitation nurses and social service workers. There is also strong administrative support.

In the community we enjoy the reputation of giving quality service which has meant that our name was shared among facility administrators. We also try to understand how O.T. fits into and has to adapt to the system in which we are working. It has helped to be linked with a major medical center and its resources to begin this growth.

Environment

There is a great deal of administrative support and freedom to develop ideas. Quality care is stressed. People care about their co-workers and about doing a quality job. The administration looks to the future and is well-organized; therefore, O.T. must organize thorough plans for the future.

Qualifications of Personnel for the Program

The need to continue to grow, a belief in O.T., and a well-rounded view of patients are important in the occupational therapy staff. They also need to have a positive attitude and to be self-motivated.

Challenging Ongoing Problems as Stated by the Program Director

These include allowing time for communication with physicians to develop a trust relationship while keeping staffing at a level that allows growth but does not raise costs; keeping staff cross-trained in new programs; keeping advised of government funding and regulations; and pacing growth.[16] □

Commentary

Research Medical Center is an open system, and definitely a model of service for the future, especially for community-based hospitals. This type of programming not only produces revenue for the facility but also establishes referral patterns from the contracted services to the based hospital to fill what could be empty beds.

Mrs. Scammahorn, as the occupational therapy manager, is responsible for a multihospital program. Her management involves being aware and responsive to systems other than her own. The systems skills employed in this environment include the following:

1. Recognizing the values not only of the parent institution but of the other contracted service programs
2. Being aware of the organization and its goals for growth to meet not only the needs of Research Medical Center, but to be responsive to the needs of those facilities under which contract services are provided
3. Defining a personal role for herself in the system that requires an expansion of her basic knowledge of occupational therapy
4. Contributing to the development of goals for the organization and motivating and developing staff members to relate to a more complex organization
5. Understanding the structure of the institution with its component organizations and recognizing who has authority and power over occupational therapy services in the structures
6. Understanding what knowledge is necessary to implement the full scope of the services within the variety of systems requiring service

Because this is a relatively new model for care, communication with physicians and administration as well as with occupational therapy staff providing services to a number of facilities must be consistent. The occupational therapy staff members involved in this type of program must understand and be committed to the values of the institution in which they provide services, as well as to those of the parent organization.

A program of this magnitude must be very strong structurally. Procedures must be clear to all in order to maintain the different levels of programming. The skills and attitudes of personnel are also critical to the program's success. This means that a strong orientation or induction program must exist that clearly spells out the skills and the attitudes necessary to support organizational goals.

Summary

A variety of systems models in which occupational therapists provide services have been presented. Although there are commonalities among systems, it is important to recognize the uniqueness of each institution and of how occupational therapy service can impact on and be a part of each particular organizational structure. The systems skills necessary to identify the values and structure of the organization, and to recognize the knowledge that occupational therapy services bring to that organization, are critical. These systems skills equip the occupational therapist to master the complexities of the organizational environment.

Some Thoughts About Power in the System

The systems skills that have been defined in this chapter assist the occupational therapy manager and the individual clinician in gaining power. Sometimes the person with authority is not the one with power. It is important to realize that both formal and informal power structures exist. According to Kantor "power issues occupy center stage, not because individuals are greedy for more power, but because some people are incapacitated without it."[17]

Authority is defined as the right to give commands or take action,[18] while *power* is influence built through positive carefully planned means[19]. In order to accomplish objectives, it must be determined who has the authority to make necessary decisions and who has the power to influence those decisions.

Power groups may shift, depending on who has the skills to meet current demands of the system. For example, the group with marketing skills may shift to

a position of greater power as hospitals are searching for expanded markets to fill empty beds. Occupational therapy has the potential to be viewed as a power group as the health care field places more emphasis on the functional capabilities of individuals and expects them to be more responsible for their own status.

It is important for the occupational therapy manager to have both authority and power. Authority normally is delegated to the position while power is developed through the ways in which the individual uses that authority. Through developing collaborative relationships, both internal and external to the system, a wide area of influence and, therefore, power is created. If occupational therapists are to accomplish their objectives, they need to gain influence with those persons who have control over services. Examples of those in controlling positions are insurance companies, other third party payers and regulatory agencies, referral services, and the administration.

The manager with power has more opportunity to be creative and to explore, while the manager without power really has no choice but to maintain control over activities within his or her jurisdiction.

"(We) must learn to deal with the subtleties of life and organizations—it comes from practice, learning what your resources are, how you can win support for an issue by changing labels under which you bring it up: or calling in favors that are owed to you—these are skills. How you develop your backing is critical. It is not through independent goal development and education, but through focusing on the organization and sharing with others . . . . successes and failures."[20]

References

1. Boulding, Kenneth E.: General systems theory—The skeleton of science. Management Science 2, No. 3:197–208 April 1956.
2. Gaudinski, M. A.: Intangibles facilitating or inhibiting health care delivery systems. Aviat. Space Environ. Med. 49:1111, 1978.
3. Baker, F.: Paper for Symposium on Systems and Medical Care, Harvard University, Sept. 26–27, 1968, p. 22.
4. Ibid.
5. Ibid.
6. Ibid. p. 10.
7. Ibid. p. 14.
8. Ibid.
9. Grinker, R. R., Sr.: In Memory of Ludwig Von Bertalanffy's contribution to psychiatry. Behavioral Science 21:211, 1976.
10. Hall, B. P.: The Development of Consciousness: A Confluent Theory of Values, New York: Paulist Press, 1976, p. 145.
11. Written interview with Carol Nodop.

12. Written interview with Pat Ramm.
13. Written interview with Cynthia Epstein.
14. Written interview with Suzanne Peloquin.
15. Written interview with Dorothy Wilson.
16. Written interview with Gloria Scammahorn.
17. Kantor, R. M., Men and Women of the corporation, New York: Basic Books, Inc., 1977, p. 205.
18. Thompson, A. M., and Wood, M. D.: Management Strategies for Women or Now That I'm Boss How Do I Run This Place? New York: Simon and Schuster, 1980, p. 44.
19. Ibid. p. 45.
20. Kantor, R. M.: You don't have to play by their rules. Ms. Magazine, Oct. 1979, p. 63.

CHAPTER 39

Management of Finances, Communications, Personnel, with Resources and Documentation *Carolyn Manville Baum*

Management of Occupational Therapy Services

During the last two decades our society has experienced enormous economic growth; these years have also been a period of fast technological change. Social forces and the technological revolution have produced many changes in health care delivery. Because of these forces, governmental regulations, and escalating costs, occupational therapists need to develop basic management skills in order to provide service that is responsive to and anticipatory of society's needs. The leadership required of the occupational therapist to manage a program in a health service system requires what Brian Hall describes as imaginal skills:[1]

1. The ability to create new alternatives
2. The ability to see the consequences of alternatives (negative as well as positive) and to prioritize the more productive ones
3. The ability to criticize and evaluate situations and determine their potential and limitations

These skills, coupled with the systems skills identified in Chapter 38, can support the occupational therapy manager in taking the risks necessary for leading people with the degree of vision and resources needed to accomplish the objectives of the program and the institution. In addition to systems and imaginal skills, there are other areas of management which can assist the occupational therapist in accomplishing objectives.

It is important to recognize that this material is only introductory and that in-depth knowledge should be obtained in order to manage the complexity of the system in which you work.

Financial Management

During the last decade health care facilities have come under firmer governmental regulation and consumer review. Occupational therapists have been given the responsibility of financial management on a day-to-day basis. This responsibility means accountability to the facility's financial officer as he or she develops, interprets, coordinates, and administers the institution's policies on finance, accounting, data processing, insurance, internal controls, admission, and auditing. The financial officer also maintains records and procedures to safeguard the assets of the institution.[2] To relate to the financial officer, the occupational therapist must develop the skills and knowledge of the institution's system and programs that will meet the expectation of the institution. This is critical and relates to the power, or lack of power, that occupational therapists have through financial management. An occupational therapy department that does not meet the financial expectation is a liability to an institution, especially when occupational therapy is one of the departments that is intended to contribute to the financial stability of an institution. There are a number of programs that do not have the potential for producing income. The costs for these programs are distributed through indirect cost allocations to those departments that produce revenue. *Non-revenue producing* departments include administration, maintenance, housekeeping, patient accounts, and admissions; *revenue-producing* programs include the laboratory, radiology, occupational therapy, physical therapy, and respiratory therapy.

Without knowledge of the organization's financial status it is often difficult for occupational therapists to justify charging a patient $40 to $50 an hour for occupational therapy services. The established fee is based on an organizationally defined charge, which creates a stable environment for the institution. In spite of the concern regarding escalating health costs, an occupational therapist who independently determines to charge a patient less than the established fee for service, is compromising the policies of the institution and shows a lack of understanding of the structure and objectives of the institution. The occupational therapist has an obligation to the institution by virtue of an employment agreement to support its established procedures. To compromise these procedures by altering the fee structure is a clue that the therapist may not support the values of the institution and perhaps should consider another system in which to work. In addition, this behavior demonstrates a lack of support for the institution's policies and provides cause for termination of employment.

Budget

The budget is a management tool. Through the budgetary process the occupational therapy manager has the ability to establish programs by obtaining financial support. In planning a projected budget a manager must (1) develop the objectives of the service, and (2) justify the expenses that will be required for implementation. Approval of the budget then allows the manager to carry out the program independently.

A series of questions such as the following must be asked prior to the establishment of a budget:

1. What is the net income of the occupational therapy service per year and does it support the current operation?

2. What is the facility's percentage of reimbursement for occupational therapy from private, federal, and self-pay clients?
3. What costs are considered direct costs?
4. What costs are considered indirect costs?
5. What is the bad–debt percentage?
6. Are capital equipment items to be considered part of the budget or purchased out of a special account and amortized into the indirect costs?

These questions will be answered differently in each setting and are critical to understanding the management function.

The information that may be required for the budgetary process is shown in Table 39-1.

For the purpose of demonstration an example of the budgetary process is given.

Table 39-1 *Budgetary Information*

Direct Costs	Explanation
Salaries	Actual, including merit raises
Payroll taxes	Social Security taxes (currently 6.65%)
Overtime	Usually 2% of total hours
Vacation relief	Self-explanatory
Supplies	Consumable department and clerical services under $300.
Student programs	Stipends or meals
Educational expenses	Tuition and travel to workshops
In-service	Money to pay speakers
Reimbursable supplies	Adaptive equipment and articles to be sold to clients.

Indirect Costs	Explanation
Administrative	Administrative support for personnel, accounting, purchasing functions, and the like.
Housekeeping	Cleaning and maintenance of facility
Laundry	Linens
Plant operation	Maintenance, utilities

Step I. Identifying Direct Costs

Direct costs

Salaries	$100,000
Payroll taxes (6.65%)	6,650
Overtime	2,000
Supplies	6,000
Student programs	1,000
Education	2,000
In-service	750
Reimbursable supplies	12,000
TOTAL	$130,400

Step II. Determining Indirect Costs

Indirect costs are usually delegated by square footage and may be approximated at 40% of the total budget. These indirect costs can be determined by the following formula once the direct costs are established:

$$X = \text{Indirect costs}$$

$$\frac{\text{Direct costs}}{X} = \frac{60\%}{40\%}$$

$$60X = 40\ (\text{Direct costs})$$

$$X = \frac{40\ (\text{Direct costs})}{60}$$

In the example we would find the indirect costs to be:

$$\frac{\$130,400}{X} = \frac{60\%}{40\%}$$

$$60X = 40\ (\$130,400)$$

$$X = 40 \times \frac{\$130,400}{60}$$

$$X = \$86,933$$

Indirect Costs = $86,933

Step III. Determining Bad-Debt Allowance (8% is used for the example)

Direct costs	130,400
Indirect costs	86,933
Total cost	217,333
	× 8%
	$ 17,386
Bad debt-allowance	$ 17,386

Step IV. Determining Total Budget Requirements

Direct costs	$130,400
Indirect cost	86,933
Bad-debt allowance	17,386
Total budget	$234,719

Step V. Determining the Fee for Service

Divide the total budget by the number of procedures projected for the budget period.

Number of procedures for budget period = 20,000
Total budget = $234,719

$$20,000\ \overline{\big)\ 234,719} = 11.735$$

Cost for each procedure = 11.735
Charge for each procedure = 12.00*

*Determine this in consultation with the financial administrator.

Table 39-2 *Planning a Control Budget*

	Procedures		Income	
Month	Planned	Actual	Planned	Actual
January	1666		19992	
February	1666		19992	
March	1666		19992	
April	1666		19992	
May	1666		19992	
June	1666		19992	
July	1666		19992	
August	1666		19992	
September	1666		19992	
October	1666		19992	
November	1666		19992	
December	1666		19992	
TOTAL	20000		240000	

Step VI. Planning a Control Budget

Divide the total budgeted procedures by 12 to determine the number of planned procedures per month. Divide the total budget by 12 to determine the planned income per month.** Record these figures and compute each month the actual with the planned (Table 39-2). Explain any significant differences (.05), either positive or negative, to the administrator in charge of the occupational therapy services.

Managing money is serious business. A skillful occupational therapy manager will be knowledgeable about the financial planning and management of the organization and about the economic environment in which the organization will succeed or fail. The manager must:[3]

1. Understand the source of funding that supports the organization
2. Be knowledgeable about organizational financial policies and procedures, including knowledge of the authority to make financial decisions
3. Be capable of preparing a budget that is correct and has included the departmental plans in the budget requirements so that departmental changes are not delayed by lack of funds
4. Have the reputation for sound financial management, which means that budget variances are not routine, but those administratively responsible for the financial operation trust the manager

** Once data is collected, it is important to vary the monthly proposals according to the variations in caseloads per month. December, for example, may be a light month because of the holidays. The number of work days in the month can serve as a guide.

5. Be responsible for knowing the financial history of the department and understanding the organization's future plans
6. Be familiar with basic accounting principles and terms which includes all cost reports, responding to them, keeping the administrator informed
7. Keep informed by continually reading publications that provide a reliable knowledge of general economic and political trends that will affect the program within the institution.

Being able to function with strong financial accountability is a strong asset to the manager, whose credibility is measured by the ability to function well in this facet of the job.

Communication

Perhaps the most important skill for the manager is communication. Communication is a process by which objectives are established, implemented, and evaluated. Knowledge and skill in interpersonal communication are critical for occupational therapists in the following situations:
Supervising staff, students and volunteers
Cooperating with other professionals
Evaluating programs, treatment, and students
Scheduling, teaching, counseling, consulting, reporting, organizing, planning, directing, and marketing

Perhaps the most basic skill required for communication in a work situation is the ability to recognize an issue, to know where you stand on that issue, and to make recommendations that will lead to a resolution. A process that is helpful in structuring the communication process is found in the *Issue Identification* chart.

This process will provide an objective means for addressing an issue. When an issue is interdepartmental, this process can be used to identify issues and departmental priorities, thus providing for collaboration which will lead to the best solution.

Decision making requires leadership that is forward thinking. A leader must be concerned for the welfare of employees but must be able to confront them and deal with conflict when necessary in order to resolve an issue. Every system needs people who have vision and who are willing to take the risk to institute changes that will strengthen the system.

Effective communication must be mastered by the occupational therapist in order to be successful in any position. There are many resources in a system for support and skill development. A most helpful description of the art of communication is to be found in Ann McKay Thompson's and Marcia Donan Woods' book, *Management Strategies for Women, or Now That I'm Boss How Do I Run This Place?*[2]

Chart

Issue Identification

What do you want to accomplish?

Who is affected by the issue? What is their position on the issue?

What do you have in common to share that will support the issue's being resolved?

List the alternatives:

What will you propose?

In addition to verbal interaction, a manager must be able to communicate through written reports. These may take the form of memoranda, reports justifying expenditures, proposals for expansion and program growth, and business letters. Developing the skill for report writing is important, as these reports comprise the formal communication process used within an organization. A report must be understood at many levels and must be written in a style acceptable within the organization. The following characteristics are essential to various forms of writing.

Report Writing

1. Directness—Get to the point at once; avoid suspense.
2. Summarizing—Begin each section with a summary before going into details.
3. Conciseness—Include only pertinent details.
4. Readability—Use correct grammar and standard spelling.
5. Objectivity—Because a report is a statement of facts, recommendations must be based on facts and not on personal prejudice.
6. Appearance—The appearance contributes greatly to the attention the report is given.

A report justifying additional staff, expansion of services, or requesting program changes may be written in the following sequence:
1. Summary—State the objectives of the report.

2. Introduction—State the problem.
3. Study—Present the data.
4. Conclusions—Present what you expect to occur with the proposed change.
5. Recommendations—State changes requested, including alternatives.
6. Physical facilities—State the effect of change of physical plant.
7. Equipment—List equipment needs.
8. Personnel—Present changes in personnel.
9. Costs—Itemize the cost of the changes.
10. Appendix—Append supporting data.

References are available and should be used in developing a style of management report writing.

Business Letters

Courtesy is more important in a business letter than is brevity. It is important not to be so brief as to seem curt. Present yourself as a friendly, concerned individual, as the letter will build goodwill with those who receive it. If you know the individual with whom you are communicating, it is important to bring some personal items into the letter.[4]

Contractual Letters

Any letter that includes a commitment on the part of a writer or oganization should be written and reviewed with care, because such a letter is a legal contract. It must be complete, accurate, and not ambiguous. The writer must also know that he or she has the authority to make the contract and may need to consult with an administrator before this type of a letter is sent.[5]

Letters Containing Technical Information

When an individual has requested technical information, it may be better to send the requested information in memorandum form.[6]

Managing Personnel
The Staffing Function

The staffing function requires that both the quality and/or the number of persons necessary to accomplish the objectives be identified.

The manager must first analyze the job to determine what qualifications are necessary to perform the job. This will result in a *job description*, which is an organized and factual statement of the duties to be performed, the supervision given and received, the relationship to other jobs, the equipment and materials to be used, and the physical working conditions. The following is an example of a job description for a staff occupational therapist within a physical disabilities treatment setting:

JOB DESCRIPTION

Title: Occupational Therapist, Staff
Reports to: Occupational Therapy Supervisor or Occupational Therapy Senior
Supervises: Occupational Therapy Assistants, Occupational Therapy Students
Provides direction to: Occupational Therapy students, externs, O.T. assistants and aides
General Summary:

Performs evaluations, establishes goals, and plans occupational therapy treatment programs for each patient referred to occupational therapy by the attending physician and provides direct patient care. Directs occupational assistants in providing treatments to patients with outlined treatment programs. Participates in professional responsibilities such as teaching, research, and program development.

Principal Duties and Responsibilities:
    Related to direct service   80%
1. Reviews and evaluates the referral to O.T. services. Obtains physician's signed referral for services; reviews patient's medical records to determine appropriate O.T. treatment.
2. Schedules patients to be seen by O.T. service according to patient's status and in conjunction with other health services.
3. Performs evaluation procedures and records results.
4. Establishes goals based upon all information available from the medical records and evaluation results.
5. Designs treatment programs based upon available data. Administers treatment to the patient or supervises the assistant as direct service is administered.
6. Instructs, motivates and assists patient in achieving maximal potential in the skills basic to living.
7. Supervises the use of specialized equipment for functional activities and endurance training.
8. Trains and assists patients in transfer techniques according to patient's needs and abilities with or without adaptive devices.

9. Recommends splints and adaptive equipment. Fabricates the device with the physician's approval. Evaluates the patient's splint, provides adjustments to insure proper fit. Instructs the patient in the use and care of the splint.
10. Maintains knowledge of task and activity analysis, and performs this function in direct service to the client.
11. Monitors patients during all phases of treatment; adjusts duration and methods of treatment according to the patient and his rehabilitative needs.
12. Exhibits knowledge of principles and application of treatment for success orientation and goal attainment.
13. Assesses and trains patient in basic living skills and in skills basic for vocational training and adaptation to a specific work setting.
14. Confers with other health professionals to coordinate the total rehabilitation program of the individual.
15. Instructs the patient and patient's family in the O.T. program to be continued at home.
16. Recommends or issues necessary adapted equipment to support the patient's functional independence.
17. Maintains records and reports to document service delivered.

Related to indirect service 10%
1. Orients, instructs and directs O.T. assistants and students in patient-related activities.
2. Keeps abreast of current technical and theoretical advances in the field of O.T. Contributes to the ongoing development of programs by providing in-services, sharing expertise and contributing resources.
3. Submits reports of objectives and goals as required. Keeps supervisor informed of progress to reach goals. Keeps the supervisor informed of problem areas and suggests improvements in the service to achieve Institute goals.
4. Maintains the therapeutic work area.
5. Performs other duties as required.

Related to education and research 10%
1. Trains and evaluates clinical students.
2. Plans and presents lectures and special programs on O.T. and related topics.
3. May plan and develop O.T. research, conduct research, and engage in professional writing for publication.

Skills and Abilities:
1. Applies principles of scientific thinking to define problems, collect data, establish facts, and draw conclusions.
2. Interprets a variety of instructions in written, oral, diagramatic or schedule form, including technical instructions.
3. Comprehension and expression of a level to:
Write or edit articles and reports for technical or scientific journals and medical documents.
Prepare and deliver lectures.
Interview, counsel, or advise students and patients.
4. Ability to use tact and to communicate effectively with patients, staff, and other health personnel. Ability to practice confidentiality and professional ethics.

Working Conditions, Physical Demands, Pressures, Hazards:
Standing, walking, kneeling, occasional sharing in medium to heavy lifting, occasional exposure to infection and physical hazards.

Minimum Education, Related Experience:
B.S. in Occupational Therapy from an accredited program and current Certification by the AOTA.

Hiring Process

When it is time to hire an individual to fill the job, a *job specification* (see form) is prepared based on the job description. A job specification identifies the minimum acceptable qualifications for the specific position including experience, education, and specific physical abilities for the job. This form is usually forwarded to the personnel department to initiate the hiring process.

The process described here is one that is supported by each institution's personnel policies and may vary slightly. This sequence reflects the process that is used in hiring a new individual.

1. Recruitment
Recruitment is the process of searching for a possible employee and stimulating a person to apply for the job. Sources include advertising through professional journals, state association recruitment committees, local newspaper ads, schools of occupational therapy, former students, and recommendations of current employees.

2. Application
Applications are received from those persons interested in the position. Applicants are required to complete a formal application that meets the requirements of the hiring institution.

3. Reference Check
References are routinely checked either by the personnel department or the hiring supervisor. Information is sought in the areas of character, education,

(*Text continues on page 822*)

Job Specification

Box # __8062__   Date of request __2/20/81__

Department __Occupational Therapy__   Requested by __Carolyn Baum__   Phone # __2583__

Job Title __Occupational Therapist__   Job code # _____   G-1520 Grade

Replacement for __John Doe__

Vacancy due to: Promotion _____   Resignation __X__   Termination _____   New position _____

Please explain: _____

_____

_____

Working hours __8-5, M-F__	Std work week __40__ Hrs.	Salary range $ __17,000 19,560__ (Hrly, Wkly, Mthly)	Part-time _____ Full-time __X__

__1 Sat. per month__

__Mary Smith/Carolyn Baum__   __227 IWJ__   __ASAP__
Name of supervisor   Room # and location of dept.   Date needed

Education required: B.S. in Occupational Therapy

Special skills required: (i.e., specialized activity, techniques and instrumentation)
            Evaluation and treatment of patients with neurological problems.

ORGANIZATIONAL RELATIONSHIP: i.e., Collaborative effort with other people or positions.
            Collaboration with other OT's, PT's, nurses, speech and social work

DUTIES: (List specific duties of the position in the order of importance,
            and Title of Project, if any)
            Evaluation and treatment of patients
            Participate in teaching and clinical research
            Function as a team member

__Yes, Senior Staff__
ARE THERE PROMOTIONAL POSSIBILITIES? IF SO, NAME THE NEXT HIGHER STEP

__Mary Smith/Carolyn Baum__   __O.T., 227 IWJ__
NAME OF PERSON WHO WILL INTERVIEW   ROOM # AND LOCATION OF DEPARTMENT

_____   STARTING   STARTING
NAME OF CANDIDATE HIRED   DATE _____   SALARY _____

                                JOB
                                TITLE _____

and work performed. The Privacy Act of 1974 limits the information that can be obtained to that which verifies that the employee actually was employed in a certain job for a specific period of time and at a certain level of compensation.

4. Preliminary Interviews

Preliminary interviews are held when there are many applicants for a vacancy, or if they are routine procedure for the hiring institution. These are often conducted by the personnel department.

5. Interview

During the interview process, it is important to discuss the actual job requirements and ascertain if the applicant has the experience, knowledge, and attitude needed to perform the job. It is also important to determine if the applicant's job expectations can be met in the particular position. Questions related to philosophy and values are important to determine if the applicant will fit in with the institutional objectives. Example: If it is the goal of the applicant to perform research and that is not a possible function in the position available, it would be frustrating for both the organization and the individual if the applicant's goals could not be met.

6. Hiring

The actual hiring process may require approval from a supervisor. This would be determined by the personnel procedures of any given institution.

7. Physical Examination

If it is the policy of the institution, a physical examination is performed to determine if the applicant can meet the physical demands of the job. It may also be required to provide a record in order to protect the organization against claims for previously incurred injuries.

8. Induction

When the individual is hired, it is important to provide a structured orientation or induction program. The effort directed toward the timely and comprehensive orientation of the newly hired individual will ensure that the job functions are implemented, and that the desired level of productivity is met, as well as the organizational objectives. The induction program typically includes orientation to policies, administrative and clinical procedures, and, in addition, meeting and being oriented by key persons with whom the employee must collaborate. During the induction period, the newly-hired individual must demonstrate to the supervisor competencies in evaluation, treatment, and communication procedures.

In many organizations, the newly-hired employee is in a probationary period during the induction phase. When this phase is completed (usually after three months), the individual becomes a permanent employee with all personnel benefits and privileges.

During this induction phase it is the employee's responsibility to develop the interpersonal skills necessary to contribute to the organization's objectives. If additional knowledge is necessary to perform the job, the new employee must seek out that knowledge both from the supervisor and through independent study. It is important to concentrate on learning about the organization, not only its history, but its values and its plans for the future. It is at this point that the therapist must develop the systems skills identified in the systems chapter of this book.

If proper attention has been given to recruitment, interview, and induction, at the completion of the induction program the new employee should be able to perform all the job functions as described in the job description.

The Management Function

Once properly introduced, the employee should have ongoing supervision to assist and support his or her professional development. The occupational therapy manager has the responsibility of assuring that the staff functions within the department's established objectives to accomplish the goals of the facility.

A sound performance evaluation for the staff can be an effective management tool. It can help identify when employees are ready for new responsibilities; it can be used to identify problems that can be resolved easily with immediate attention; and it also provides insight into the manager's performance.

Occasionally a staff member may need to be terminated. It is important to be aware of the facility's procedures for termination and to follow them exactly to avoid unnecessary litigation.

Reasons for immediate termination include insubordination, possession of drugs, weapons, or being under the influence of alcohol. When an employee may be terminated, however, it is important to set up a very structured plan for improvement, unless the termination is for a specific behavior that demands immediate termination. A plan for improvement includes the following:
1. Identify the problems observed (have objective information). Examples might be a values conflict, a knowledge deficit, or failure to support procedure.

2. Establish specific objectives or behavioral expectations that can be asked of the employee within a specific time frame.
3. Develop a plan for improvement.
4. Establish a time to reevaluate.
5. Have the employee sign the plan.

This approach will provide feedback to the individual and provide the manager with documentation to eventually terminate the relationship if improvement is not noted. Any action of this type should involve the personnel officer of the facility, and any records in the process should be sent to the official personnel file.

Documentation: Communication and Legal Implications

Occupational therapists working in the health care system are required to collect, disseminate, and protect information about patients' health. The patient's rights must also be protected.

The responsibility of interacting with an individual client requires that the therapist be aware not only of the legal rights of the individual, but also of the implication of the documentation, especially when documentation dramatically affects the individual's right to gainful employment or the right for disability benefits.

Recent court decisions have determined that hospitals and other health care providers maintain records for the benefit of the patient as well as the hospital and the physician. The patient's right to the record is declared to be superior to that of either the hospital or the physician.[7]

The Record

The primary purpose of the patient's record is to document the course of his or her health care and to provide information to all health professionals about current and future care.

In order to accomplish this purpose, data must be well recorded and accessible to the proper persons. The patient must be assured that information shared with health professionals will remain confidential. It is becoming increasingly difficult to maintain confidentiality because so many regulations from the government and insurance companies require that the record accompany reimbursement claims. The sharing of reports between agencies threatens the individual's privacy. It is for these reasons that the American Medical Record Association suggests that

for reasons other than *direct* patient care, if the medical record is released, it must be done with authorization from the patient or the patient's agent.[8] This means that releases are necessary before sending information to insurance companies and attorneys. It is important that each facility have written procedures to regulate the dissemination of information and that these procedures be kept current and enforced.

Description

The record includes information collected about an individual during the course of treatment. It is made up of reports written to document the patient's physical and mental history, and records of previous illness, special factors such as job, marital history, physical findings, treatments ordered, a description of the patient's response to treatment (or lack of it), diagnosis, operations, and plans for follow-up care. This content is collected because many health professionals are working with the patient; the record is their communication tool.

The medical records department of a facility is responsible for designing and implementing the record-keeping system. Normally each facility has an established process for record keeping and for the recording style. The occupational therapy record-keeping procedure should be documented and follow the style utilized by the institution. Information contained in the record is used for many purposes, including research, prospective and retrospective evaluation of quality of patient care, voluntary compliance with standards for accreditation of the institution, demonstrating conformance to government regulations, substantiation of patient claims for health services, surveillance of diseases of epidemiologic significance through statistical analysis, and investigation of disease patterns, to name just a few.[9]

Legality

Medical records may play an important role during litigation. The report may be subpoenaed. If you are called to testify and the record has not been previously subpoenaed, the record must be taken with you and can be introduced and held as exhibit by the court.[10] In some jurisdictions, once the record is introduced, the entire record can be used for evidence. In most jurisdictions, however, only the portion of the record that is pertinent to the issues being litigated can be introduced. These legal implications underscore the importance of documentation. It is critical to be aware of the facility's regulations and procedures in developing your style of documentation and in handling any requests for information.

Style and Frequency of Documentation

Each facility must respond to the agencies that accredit them and, consequently, will have established procedures, and perhaps standards, for documentation. These must be understood and followed in the practice of occupational therapy. The following two publications are recommended for styles of documentation: Occupational Therapy Sequential Client Care Recording System, developed by Lela A. Llorens, Ph.D., OTR and Jonathan J. Shuster, Ph.D., and Medical Records, Medical Evaluation and Patient Care, developed by Lawrence Weed, M.D.[11,12] The weed system is the "problem oriented" medical record better known as the SOAP system. It is a commonly used system throughout facilities in the United States and is often taught in professional schools to physicians, nurses, and many allied health professionals including occupational therapists.

References

1. Hall, B. P.: The Development of Consciousness: A Confluent Theory of Values, New York: Paulistic Press, 1976, p. 173.
2. Thompson, A. M., Wood, M. D.: Management Strategies For Women or Now That I'm Boss How Do I Run This Place? New York: Simon & Schuster, 1980, 129–138.
3. Thompson, et al., pp. 130–133.
4. Ticky, H. J.: Effective Writing for Engineers, Managers and Scientists. New York: John Wiley & Sons, 1966, p. 290.
5. Ibid., p. 293.
6. Ibid., p. 294.
7. Hirsch, H. L.: Legal Implications of Patients Records. South. Med. J., June 1979, Vol. 72, no. 6, p. 728.
8. Medical Record News, "Confidentiality of Patient Health Information: A Position Statement of the American Medical Records Association," April 1978, pg. 10.
9. Medical Records News, April, 1978, pp. 11–14.
10. Hirsch: South. Med. J., June 1979, 72, no. 6, pp. 778–779.
11. Llorens, L. A., and Shuster, J. J.: Occupational Therapy Sequential Client Care Recording System. Am. J. Occup. Ther. 31(6):367–371, July 1977.
12. Weed, L.: Medical Records, Medical Evaluation and Patient Care. Chicago: Chicago Yearbook Medical Publications, 1970.

Resources for Managers

The American Occupational Therapy Association can provide the manager with copies of current standards, model job descriptions, examples of procedures, current laws that affect the manager's performance, and potential resource contacts to assist in problem solving. The manager can contact the federal government either through regional offices or at the federal level for help in interpreting any federal regulations. These contacts and addresses can be obtained from the American Occupational Therapy Association, Government and Legal Affairs Division.

The manager's greatest ally is the administrator, who can provide assistance and support for developing effective management skills. The manager of occupational therapy is an important link in the administrator's management system because it is through these managers that the objectives of the facility are accomplished.

A list of Resources follows:

Managers Bibliography:

Basttistella, R. M., and Rundell, T. G.: Health Care Policy in a Changing Environment. Berkeley: McCutchen, 1978.

Bertalanffy, L. Von: General Systems Theory. New York: George Braziller, 1963.

Brown, M., and McCool, B. P.: Multi Hospital Systems: Strategies for Organization and Management. Germantown, MD: Aspen Systems Corp., 1980.

Brown, J. H. U.: The Health Care Dilemma. New York: Human Sciences Press, 1978.

Cousins, N.: Anatomy of an Illness as Perceived by the Patient. Toronto: W. W. Norton and Co., 1979.

Deutsch, M.: The Resolution of Conflict: Constructive and Instructive Process, New Haven and London: Yale University Press, 1973.

Hall, B. P.: The Development of Consciousness. New York: Paulistic Press, 1976.

Health and United States, U.S. Department of Health, Education and Welfare, Public Health Service, Health Resources Administration, 1978.

Hepner, J., and Hepner, D.: The Health Care Strategy Game. St. Louis: C. V. Mosby, 1973.

Thompson, A. M., and Wood, M. D.: Management: Strategies for Women or Now That I'm Boss How Do I Run This Place? New York: Simon and Schuster, 1980.

Warner, M. D., and Holloway, D. C.: Decision Making and Control for Health Administrators, Ann Arbor: Health Administration Press, 1978.

Other Resources include the following:

Clark, Pat N., "Human Development through Occupation: A Philosophy and Conceptive Model for Practice; Part 1 and 2, Am. J. Occup. Ther. 33 no. 8, 9, August, September, 1979.

Department of Social Services, Your State Comprehensive Annual Social Services Program Plan.

Federal, Digest of Data of persons with disabilities, call your Federal Office Information number.

Federal Report, American Occupational Therapy Association, Government and Legal Affairs, 1383 Piccard Drive, Suite 300, Rockville, Maryland 20850.

Focal Points, U.S. Dept. of Health and Human Services,

Public Health Service Center for Disease Control, Center for Health Promotion and Education. Focal Points, Atlanta, Georgia 30333.

Health & United States, U.S. Department of Health, Education and Welfare, Public Health Service, Office of the Asst. Secretary for Health, National Center for Health Statistics. National Center for Health Services Research,

Center Blvd., 3700 East-West Highway, Hyattsville, Maryland 20782.

Health Resources News, U.S. Dept. Health and Human Services, Public Health Service, Health Resource Administration, Center Blvd. 3700 East-West Highway, Hyattsville, Maryland 20782. Monthly newsletter.

State, Vital Statistics.

CHAPTER 40

Uniform Reporting of Occupational Therapy Data

Sandra J. Malone

History—Background

Although the topic of uniform reporting of health care services goes back a number of years, it received much attention by the government in 1977 with the passage of PL 95-142—the Medicare and Medicaid Fraud and Abuse Amendments. PL 95-142 stipulated that uniform reporting of costs and services be instituted in hospitals certified as Medicare providers. Although the law specified only hospitals, its intent was to include all providers, including home health agencies, skilled nursing, and intermediate care facilities. The purpose of his law was to insure some degree of comparability in the information received from providers in different areas of the country. Medicare and Medicaid officials found that costs reported for the same or similar procedures varied as much as tenfold. Although occupational therapy services were not specifically identified in any of these official reports, it is known from efforts made by the American Occupational Therapy Association (AOTA) to collect samples of occupational therapy fee schedules and treatment costs that much disparity existed throughout the country. Some hospitals reported occupational therapy services at a cost per visit, regardless of the length or nature of the visit. Others charged by the hour or part thereof, and some facilities that were more advanced or sophisticated in their approach charged different fees for different types of services as well as for the time it took to perform them.

To develop guidelines for uniform reporting of services, the Health Care Financing Administration (HCFA) developed a manual entitled *The System for Uniform Hospital Reporting*. However, within the different branches of the federal government, there was controversy over what this system should do. Because it is directly related to the cost of services, some agencies felt a relative value unit system (RVU) should be used for all services to determine fair costs, while others viewed the RVU approach as a form of price fixing. This issue, coupled with the political emphasis on deregulation, has created a holding pattern on the decision related to the use of a relative value unit system in the reporting of services at this time.

Anticipating the development of a system for uniform reporting, the American Occupational Therapy Association appointed a task force through the Commission on Practice to develop a proposal for a national occupational therapy product output reporting system. This proposal was completed in January 1979 and is entitled "Occupational Therapy Product Output Reporting System and Uniform Terminology for Reporting Occupational Therapy Services." (see Appendices D and E) This proposal is a valuable tool for any therapist contemplating the development of a uniform set of terminology for occupational therapy recording. The approach and considerations the task force had taken into account before developing the proposal are sound, given the internal and external demands on the profession itself. In the description of occupational therapy services, emphasis was placed on treatment outcomes rather than treatment procedures and reflects the uniqueness of occupational therapy services in comparison with services from other professions. The section on relative value units discusses the factors and formula used for weighing each service.

Uniform Reporting for Occupational Therapists

All occupational therapy services collect data on patient attendance, treatment schedules, fees for treatment, identification of the type of treatment given, and so forth. However, not all of these services collect the same data in the same manner; therefore, we are unable to compare or combine information that is collected in more than one or two settings. As health dollars become scarce, and as we are asked to describe the impact or outcomes of our intervention in treatment, the importance of comparable data becomes a critical factor.

The benefits of using uniform reporting systems for occupational therapy fall under five general categories important to any occupational therapy service: standards, reimbursement, management, research, and promotion.

As we develop standards for the treatment of specific disabilities, we must also document the types of evaluation and treatment procedures used.

The number of in-hospital days per illness is constantly decreasing owing to attempts to cut costs, and occupational therapy plans of treatment must be modified in order for them to be implemented over shorter periods of time.

Through the development of standards and a uniform way of reporting services, occupational therapists should be able to respond to the following kinds of questions:

"What is the average number of occupational therapy treatments for a stroke patient to achieve independence in ADL activities?"

"How many treatment hours will be required if your case load were to increase by 200 stroke patients next year?"

"If the average number of in-hospital days following stroke were limited to four, what would an occupational therapy plan of treatment include and what would be the anticipated outcomes?"

Occupational therapy treatment is covered by a variety of third party payers. Each third party payer uses guidelines to determine the specific type of occupational therapy covered. In order for us to propose guidelines or modifications to existing guidelines for coverage, we must be able to show evidence that a particular type of treatment is in fact common or the "norm" for a particular disability or problem. The use of standard terminology in clinical reporting systems should help to avoid disparity in the types of coverage for occupational therapy services in different areas of the country.

A uniform clinical reporting system can make program planning and management a much easier task. If the terminology used to describe services is compatible with practice standards, the service manager should be able to project the number of staff needed, number of treatment hours per week or month, budgetary needs compatible with patient load, and amount of income generated. A uniform reporting system can serve as a base from which patient care and administrative audits and peer review activities can be conducted. This information can also be extremely important when planning for the expansion of services or when developing new services.

More clinical research is needed in occupational therapy. The true test of validity for any research is reproducibility of results. Can someone in another setting get the same results? As our treatment and terminology become standardized, the foundation for clinical research grows.

Throughout national, state, and local efforts to promote occupational therapy, we have talked about what occupational therapy is. Through the use of standard terminology and definitions and a uniform way of reporting service, we can now promote what occupational therapists do. Occupational therapy intervention in California should not be unlike what is done in Florida or Michigan. As a profession, we want to have an impact in the public and political arena and on the health care system.

Whenever a new system or a new approach to handling existing functions is considered, there are advantages and disadvantages. Although the advantages of a uniform reporting system with standard terminology outweigh the disadvantages, such a system does impose more regulation, routinization and structure to the clinical operation. Some occupational therapists may perceive infringement on their professional judgement perogatives if there is not a thorough review and understanding of the terminology and definitions. Record-keeping procedures will also become more rigid.

What a Model Uniform Reporting System Might Encompass

In 1977 the Maryland State Department of Health and Mental Hygiene (MSDHMH) instituted a centralized, computerized system of uniform data collection to be utilized by occupational therapists employed in MSDHMH programs and facilities. During the year prior to instituting this system, numerous meetings were held with occupational therapists, administrators, program directors, representatives from county health departments, the Maryland Center for Health Statistics, and the State Division of Reimbursements. These meetings focused on the review of existing statistical recording used locally, identification of common information needs, review of other external systems, review of Federal and private data requirements for reimbursement of occupational therapy services, and exploration of data capabilities of the Maryland Center for Health Statistics.

The initial form design incorporated information from the Prince George's County Health Department Rehabilitation Reporting System (Maryland) and the Washington State Hospital Commission Accounting and Reporting Manual (System of Accounts, Occupational Therapy, Revised 1976). In 1980, modifications were made based on the American Occupational Therapy Association (AOTA) report, "Uniform Terminology System for Reporting Occupational Therapy Services."

The MSDHMH occupational therapy data system in its present state of development is patient-centered, meaning a unique record of service is developed about each individual served by the occupational therapy program. Generally, the individual patient is identified by his or her assigned facility number. No other specific identifiers are entered into the computer tape, although a few facilities may stamp the data form with the patient addressograph if the form is to be inserted into the medical record. Often, the data form is placed in the patient's record to augment occupational therapy evaluation summaries and progress notes and to identify each date service was rendered.

Additionally, the system is designed to produce fiscal and management data through the inclusion of program and project information as part of the basic data set. For example, specific subdivisions of a facility's population (a geographic division, a specific school, a specific budgeted program) can be identified for program planning or fiscal management purposes.

In selecting the system's basic data set, primary consideration was given to the perceived needs of the data users. Experience over time has verified the usefulness of most of the included data elements, although data generated on delivery sites (school, home, kidney dialysis unit, ward, clinic) and by referral sources (physician, family, Division of Vocational Rehabilitation) are of limited use.

The information generated on types of conditions served (for example, arthritis, cerebral palsy, manic depressive syndrome) is currently under review. While the selected condition identifiers are fairly consistent with similar data generated nationally by the American Occupational Therapy Association, the trend locally is toward use of the International Classification of Disease. Another approach to this issue is to identify problems addressed (for example, visual impairment, decreased range of motion, poor work habits) as a mechanism for determining the kinds of services being offered to a given population. Hopefully, the best approach to this issue will become clearer with experience.

Figure 40-1 pictures the front side of the direct service data form with a case history. Figure 40-2 is the back side of the direct service form identifying the coding to be used in completing the front side of the form. Definitions for the assessment and treatment procedures used in the MSDHMH model are contained in Appendix D.

Case History

The patient's identification number is entered in the upper left-hand portion of the form. The patient is male (1) and white (1) and being seen in the outpatient program (03). The first three numbers (123) under primary provider identifies the facility from which the services are rendered; the last two numbers (01) identify the therapist—S. Malone, OTR. The patient's birth date is entered—January 1, 1940. His primary condition is Renal Failure (53). The primary delivery site of service is the operational base O.T. Clinic (01). The patient's admission status to the O.T. service is a "new admission" (01), and his status at the termination of service was due to discharge (05). The referral source was his private M.D. (01) and the county where he resides is Allegany (01).

On January 12, 1981, this patient was initially seen in occupational therapy for an evaluation (005) which took an hour to perform (4 units @ 15 minutes per unit). The evaluation results were documented (945). This documentation required 30 minutes (2 units). The therapist performing those services signs her full name and designation. On the 15th this patient was seen again; his O.T. program

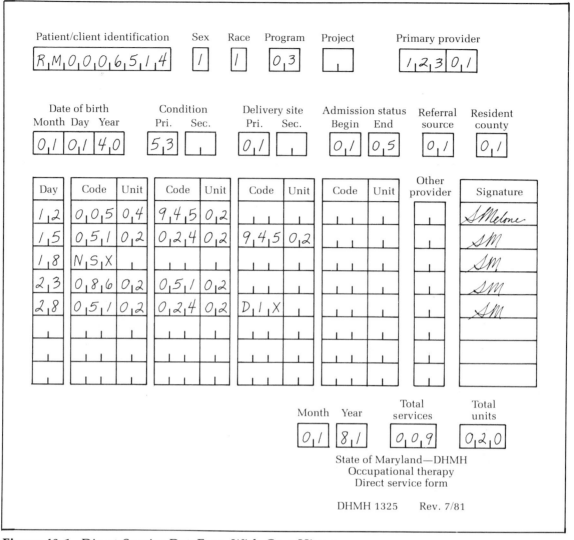

Figure 40-1. Direct Service DataForm With Case History

consisted of Body Mechanics—Energy Conservation (051) and Self Care—Survival Skills (024). Treatment time was 1 hour (2 units per service). The therapist documented the treatment, which required 30 minutes. The therapist, having signed her full name for the initial visit, can now use her initials for subsequent entries for the rest of the month. Refer to Figure 40-2, the back side of the direct service form, and identify the services recorded for January 18, 23 and 28. □

A separate form is completed for each patient seen in occupational therapy on a monthly basis. At the end of each month, the service sends all forms to the Maryland State Department of Health and Mental Hygiene Central Office to be keypunched into the computer (Maryland Center for Health Statistics). The forms are then returned to the service where, in most cases, they are entered into the patient's medical record. In many facilities, copies of the completed

monthly data form and other supplementary information are sent to the patient's health insurance company or other third party payer for reimbursement purposes. Along with the returned forms, each service receives a variety of reports generated from the month's data.

The primary report consists of a listing of all patients by identification number followed by the number of services received and the number of units required to provide those services, for example:

Patient Identification	Total Services	Total Units
RM0006514	9	20

Assessment

001 Screening
002 Patient Related
    Consultation
005 Evaluation
006 Reevaluation
007 Rescreening

Treatment Procedure

Self Care
021 Feeding Skills
022 Grooming/Hygiene
023 Dressing
024 Survival Skills

Cognition
041 Orientation
042 Concept./Comprehen.

Body Mechanics
051 Energy Conserv.
052 Join Protect.
053 Positioning

Therapeutic Adapt.
066 Orthotics
067 Prosthetics
069 Wheelchair
070 Asst./Adapt. Equip.

Psychologic
081 Self Ident./
    Self Concept.
082 Coping Skills

Work
086 Home Management
087 Student/Learner
    Skills
088 Pre-vocational
089 Vocational

090 Infant Stimulation

Play/Leisure
201 Skill/Interest
    Explor.
202 Skill Development
203 Community Resource
    Util.

Sensorimotor
226 Motor
228 Sensory Integration

Social/Interpersonal
251 Diadic Interac.
    Skills
252 Group Interact.
    Skills

800 Other
801 Other
802 Other

915 Patient/Client
    Support Inst.
930 Concurrent Charge
940 Patient/Client
    Related Conf.
945 Documentation
960 Travel
965 Planning
970 Telephone

County of Residence

01 Allegany
02 Anne Arundel
03 Baltimore
04 Calvert
05 Caroline
06 Carroll
07 Cecil
08 Charles
09 Dorchester
10 Frederick
11 Garrett
12 Harford
13 Howard
14 Kent
15 Montgomery
16 Prince George's
17 Queen Anne's
18 St. Mary's
19 Somerset
20 Talbot
21 Washington
22 Wicomico
23 Worcester
30 Baltimore City
40 District of Columbia
41 West Virginia
42 Virginia
43 Delaware
44 Pennsylvania
50 Out of State (other
    than above)
60 Foreign Country
70 Maryland Co. Unknown
90 Unknown

Program
03 Outpatient
04 Inpatient
05 Chronic Obstructive
    Airway Disease
06 Renal Dialysis
07 Mental Retardation
08 Long Term Care
12 Day Care Center
16 Child Health
17 School Health
20 Crippled Children
25 Adult Health
28 Home Health
33 Geriatric Services
96 Other
97 Other
98 Other

Sex

1. Male
2. Female

Race

1. White
2. Black
3. Spanish Surname
4. Oriental
5. American Indian
6. Other

Delivery Site

01 Operational Base
    Clinic
03 Home
04 Community
05 Long Term Care
    Facility
06 School—Public
07 Day Treatment/Care
    Center
08 Kidney Dialysis Unit
10 Ward/Cottage
11 School—Private
12 Other
13 Other

Referral Source

01 Private M.D.
02 Agency Professional
03 Long Term Care Fac.
04 Hospital (other)
05 Community Agency
06 Family or Self
07 Board of Education
08 Other
09 Child Devel. Center
10 Child Health Clinic
11 Diagnostic & Refer-
    ral Clinic
12 Exceptional Child
13 Neurological Clinic
14 Orthopedic Clinic
15 School Health
    Clinic
50 Therapist Initiated
51 Home Health Agency
52 Div. of Vocational
    Rehabilitation
60 Health Department
    (General)
61 Other
62 Other

Admission Status

01 New
02 Continuing
03 Readmission
04 Discontinued
05 Discharged
06 Other

Local Use

A.D.X. New
R.A.X. Readmission
R.R.X. Re-referred
D.I.X. Discharged
D.E.X. Deceased
P.C.X. Program Change
L.O.X. Leave of
    Absence
T.D.X. Temporarily
    Discontinued
N.S.X. No Show
C.D.X. Cancelled
R.E.X. Resumed
M.B.X. Maximum Benefit
O.B.X. Other
O.C.X. Other
O.D.X. Other
O.E.X. Other

Condition

01 Amputee
02 Arthritis
03 Brain Injury
04 Cardiovascular
05 Cerebral Palsy
06 C.V.A.
07 Degenerative Musculoskeletal
08 Developmental Delay
11 Mental Retardation
12 Minimal Brain Dysfunction
13 Orthopedic
14 Perceptual Motor
15 Progressive Neurological
17 Pulmonary
18 Paraplegia
21 Other Neurological
50 Visual Impairment
51 Emotional Problem
52 Hand Surgery
53 Renal Failure
54 Quadriplegia
55 Auditory Loss
56 Burn
57 Medical-Surgical Misc.
59 Malignancy
60 Multiple Anomaly
61 Organic Brain Syndrome
62 Alcoholism
67 Affective Disorder, Bipolar, mixed
68 Affective Disorder, Bipolar, raise
69 Affect. Disorder, Bipolar, depressed
72 Prim. deg. dement., senile onset
73 Dementia assoc. with alcohol
74 Maj. depress., recurrent melancholia
76 Personality Disorder
77 Schizoaffective disorder
78 Conduct disord., undersoc'd non-aggr.
79 Conduct disorder, undersoc'd aggr.
80 Pressure Ulcer
81 Stasis Ulcer
82 General Debilitation
83 Aphasia
84 Other
85 Other
86 Seizure disorder
87 Schiz., disorganized
88 Schiz., catatonic
89 Schiz., paranoid
90 Schiz., undiff.
91 Schiz., residual
92 Substance use disorder
93 Other
94 Att'n deficit disorder
95 Depression
96 Neurosis
97 Character disorder
98 Depressive neurosis

Figure 40-2. Coding for Direct Service DataForm

Occupational Therapy January 1981
Facility 000
Service Codes (1)

Code	Frequency	Percent	Units	Percent
005	11	5.67	46	14.56
007	3	1.55	12	3.80
009	3	1.55	7	2.22
021	1	0.52	1	0.32
022	1	0.52	1	0.32
023	6	3.09	10	3.16
024	7	3.61	17	5.38
042	1	0.52	1	0.32
053	1	0.52	1	0.32
066	6	3.09	13	4.11
070	1	0.52	1	0.32
086	2	1.03	6	1.90
087	34	17.53	42	13.29
090	3	1.55	6	1.90
201	2	1.03	2	0.63
202	4	2.06	8	2.53
226	19	9.79	27	8.54
228	12	6.19	13	4.11
502	1	0.52	0	0.00
915	5	2.58	6	1.90
940	16	8.25	20	6.33
945	21	10.82	33	10.44
960	32	16.49	41	12.97
970	2	1.03	2	0.63
Total	194		316	

Figure 40-3. Samples monthly report. Prepared by the Maryland Center for Health Statistics, March 1981.
Interpretation Notes
This report lists *all* the *Assessment* and *Treatment Procedures* employed by the reporting facility for the specified time frame; *e.g.,* this facility reported six orthotic services (code 066). These represented 3.09% of all services rendered and accounted for 13 units of time or 4.11% of all direct service time.

Occupational Therapy Report January 1981
Facility 000

Program[1]	Patients[2]	Services[3]	Units[4]
07	1	1	1
12	9	39	43
16	9	29	64
17	14	43	61
20	2	8	11
25	1	2	4
28	12	70	132
ALL	48	192	316

	ADMISSION STATUS[5]	
	BEGINNING	ENDING
1	14	0
2	34	43
3	0	0
4	0	2
5	0	3
6	0	0

Figure 40-4. Sample monthly report. Prepared by the Maryland Center for Health Statistics, March 1981.
Interpretation Notes
(1) *Program* refers to Chart of Accounts (*e.g.,* out patients, renal dialysis, home health).
(2) *Patients* refers to total number of patients seen during specified time frame in that particular program.
(3) *Services* indicates total number of services (*e.g.,* screening, self-care, prevocational).
(4) *Units* indicates total time spent by program—1 Unit = 15 Minutes
(5) *Status* refers to admission status both at the beginning and end of the month. During this month for this facility, 14 patients were newly admitted to the Occupational Therapy service, 34 were continued from the previous month, 43 were carried over to February, 2 were discontinued and 3 were discharged.

Figures 40-3 and 40-4 are samples of other reports that can be generated monthly. Refer to Figure 40-2 to decode the report information.

The quarterly reports contain information that is not needed monthly but is needed more frequently than annually. Figures 40-5, 40-6, and 40-7 are samples of quarterly reports. Fluctuations in service and predictable occurrences can be identified through the

		Facility 000			
July 1981 Quarter 7/81–9/81					
Program	Project	Condition[1]	Patients	Services	Units
033	0	2	3	19	36
033	0	3	1	2	5
004	0	5	6	48	79
➡ 004	0	6	8	111	182
004	0	8	15	80	372
003	0	11	5	55	75
003	0	14	2	4	11
003	0	21	2	7	12
➡ 003	1	60	1	1	1
Program Totals			43	327	773

Figure 40-5. Sample quarterly report. Prepared by the Maryland Center for Health Statistics, December 1981.

Interpretation Notes
(1) Condition—a listing of all conditions seen by the Occupational Therapy service during the specified time frame, *e.g.*, during this quarter, eight patients were treated with a primary condition identified as cerebrovascular accident (CVA #6). These patients received 111 services for 182—15 Min. Units of service. All CVA patients were inpatients. Note that a project number (1) was used to indicate that the one patient, with the condition of "Multiple Anomaly" (60) was seen under a federally funded grant program.

Figure 40-6. Sample quarterly report. Prepared by the Maryland Center for Health Statistics, December 1981.

Interpretation Notes
(1) The use of Alpha Codes (Alphabet Letters) was integrated into the system as a mechanism for offering flexibility to local providers in retrieving data elements unique to their facility. Local providers have used Alpha Codes to track patients who did not keep scheduled appointments (*i.e.*, NSX—no shows) and to identify specific dates patient/client was admitted, discharged, or discontinued to/from the service.

Because this system does not include number of visits, only units of time, the SPX has been designated for identifying the number of patient visits.

Some of the alpha codes are not listed on the back side of the data form because they were developed at the facility and are intended for their internal use only.

	Occupational Therapy	Quarter 7/81–9/81		
		Facility 000		
		Local Use Codes[1]		
Code	Frequency	Percent	Units	Percent
ADX	3	0.46	0	0.00
CBX	1	0.15	0	0.00
CDX	3	0.46	0	0.00
DIX	4	0.61	0	0.00
NSX	80	12.27	0	0.00
OBX	380	58.28	0	0.00
OCX	32	4.91	0	0.00
ODX	4	0.61	0	0.00
SPX	144	22.09	261	100.00
TDX	1	0.15	0	0.00
Total	652		261	

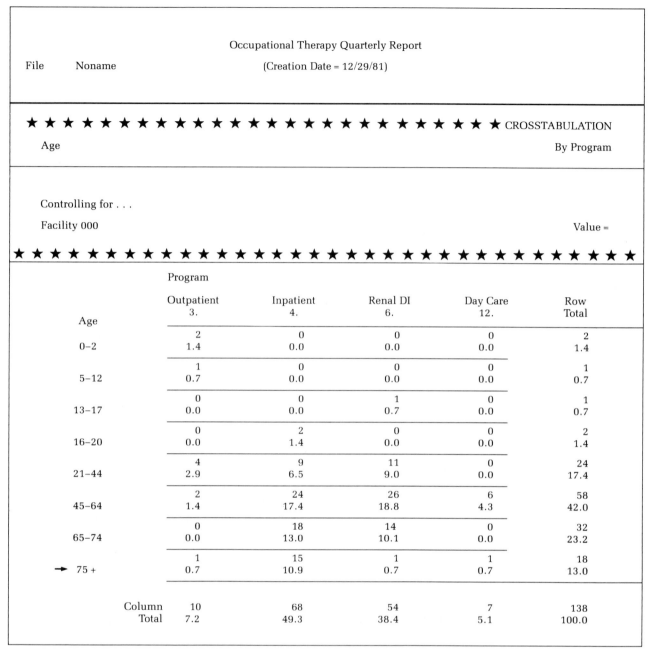

Occupational Therapy Quarterly Report

File   Noname   (Creation Date = 12/29/81)

★ CROSSTABULATION

Age   By Program

Controlling for . . .

Facility 000   Value =

★ ★

	Program				
Age	Outpatient 3.	Inpatient 4.	Renal DI 6.	Day Care 12.	Row Total
0–2	2 1.4	0 0.0	0 0.0	0 0.0	2 1.4
5–12	1 0.7	0 0.0	0 0.0	0 0.0	1 0.7
13–17	0 0.0	0 0.0	1 0.7	0 0.0	1 0.7
16–20	0 0.0	2 1.4	0 0.0	0 0.0	2 1.4
21–44	4 2.9	9 6.5	11 9.0	0 0.0	24 17.4
45–64	2 1.4	24 17.4	26 18.8	6 4.3	58 42.0
65–74	0 0.0	18 13.0	14 10.1	0 0.0	32 23.2
→ 75 +	1 0.7	15 10.9	1 0.7	1 0.7	18 13.0
Column Total	10 7.2	68 49.3	54 38.4	7 5.1	138 100.0

Figure 40-7. Sample quarterly report.

Interpretation Notes

This table is a cross tabulation of age breakdowns by program and by total. For example, 18 patients were reported as being over 75 years of age representing 13% of all patients served. Sixty-eight or 49.3% of all patients served were seen on an inpatient basis.

comparison of monthly and quarterly reports. Quarterly information can also be used to augment grant reporting.

Annual reports for either the fiscal year or calendar year can consist of any combination of information collected on the data form. Special reports such as a listing of all assessment and treatment procedures given to a specific patient population by therapists can be generated on an annual basis. This type of report can be used to develop expected levels of staff performance or to compare actual treatment given with departmental or practice standards. Raw data from monthly, quarterly or annual reports can also be converted into graphic displays as exhibited in Figures 40-8 and 40-9. Graphs and charts are often used to break the monotony of long, narrative reports and enable large amounts of information to be shown quickly. Graphic display of data is frequently

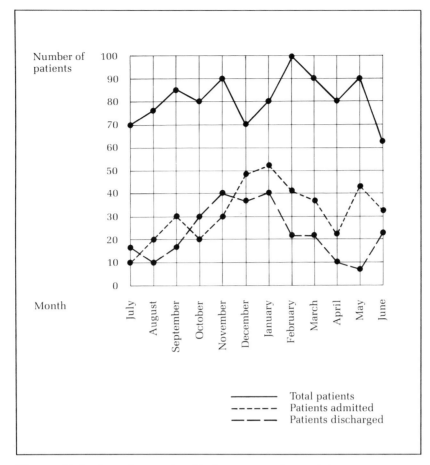

Figure 40-8. Sample graph of information derived from the system of facility Y, July 1980 to June 1981. Rates of admission/discharge to occupational therapy and total monthly census.

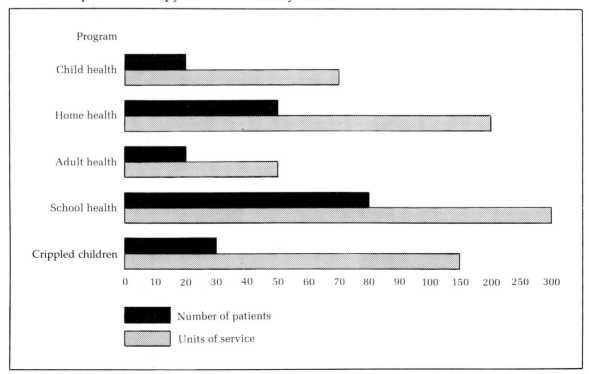

Figure 40-9. Sample graph of information derived from the system of facility B, July 1980 to June 1981. Total number of patients served by program and units of service.

used in the development of reports for accreditation and certification reviews such as "Medicare and The Joint Commission on Accreditation of Hospitals."

The MSDHMH data system has had its growing pains, with many more expected before reaching full maturity. The system does, however, offer some unique features which were unavailable just a few years ago:

—Information can be pulled out and presented in a variety of ways by patient, therapist, program, project, diagnosis, or treatment procedure.
—Large amounts of data can be analyzed for program and planning purposes.
—The occupational therapy manager is provided with a mechanism for identifying trends, therefore predicting occurrences.
—Research on the clinical level can be facilitated.

Although a relative value unit system has not been incorporated to date, this area will no doubt be the major addition to the system in the near future.

Implications for the Future— Data as a Tool for Management

In developing a uniform reporting system it must be recognized that changes will be needed in format, content, and types of reports generated. Current and future changes in Federal and State reporting requirements (for instance, Titles IX and XX) all point to the need to maintain a flexible outlook. Concepts on the desirability of reporting in visits, units, or in actual time spent per service are changing. The development of similar and potentially compatible uniform reporting systems throughout the country encourages innovations worthy of replication. Within the next few years, it may be possible for a unified reporting system to be developed that could accommodate all health professions. Information needed on the patient/client is basic to all involved in developing care. Professional differences lie in the nature of the service delivered. Utilizing a unified approach to data collection would not stifle creativity but could prevent unnecessary repetition of errors, and the data generated would be more generally understood.

Resources

International Classification of Diseases: Manual of the International Statistical Classification of Diseases, Injuries, and Causes of Death, 9th Ed., revised. Geneva, World Health Organization, 1977.

Prince George's County Health Department Rehabilitation Admission & Forms Service. Cheverly, MD, 1977.

The System for Uniform Hospital Reporting: Draft Report—Health Care Financing Administration, [for Public Comment]. Washington, DC, HEW, 1978.

Uniform Terminology System for Reporting Occupational Therapy Services: Commission on Practice Task Force Report. Rockville, MD, The American Occupational Therapy Association, 1979.

Washington State Hospital Commission Accounting & Reporting Manual: System of Accounts, Occupational Therapy, revised. 1976.

CHAPTER 41

Strategic Planning *Sallie Elizabeth Taylor*

In recent years, the practice of formally planning a company's future has become increasingly popular with business managers. The return for the investment of time, energy, and training needed to develop a strategic plan has proven highly satisfactory for companies engaged in this process. As the use of the strategic plan has grown more prevalent in the business world, hospitals and agencies providing health services have begun to recognize the value of this formal planning tool in charting the future of their organizations. Occupational therapy services are often provided by organizations that are critically linked with the political and economic environment. Strategic planning is a concept and a skill that must be included in the efforts of occupational therapists to develop services that benefit the employer organization, the occupational therapy staff, and the consumer.

Purpose of the Strategic Plan

In the management of health-delivery organizations, long-range planning systems respond to environmen-

tal conditions and to the fundamental needs of the organization for survival and risk management. Development of the strategic plan necessitates anticipation of the future and identification of objectives which, when achieved, will tend to assure the long-term viability and optimization of opportunity for the organization. The systematic assessment of risks and opportunities facing an agency is an essential component of the strategic planning process. It enables an organization to develop a series of responses that will tend to ensure the wisest utilization of resources or programs at minimal risk and for maximal benefit of the organization over the long term. Decisions regarding these fundamental areas of survival and risk management fall within the responsibility of the organization's chief executive officer and top management.

Strategic Plan Defined

Peter Drucker, well known for his contributions to contemporary management practices, defines strategic planning as "the continuous process of making present entrepreneurial (risk-taking) decisions systematically and with the greatest knowledge of their futurity; organizing systematically the efforts needed to carry out these decisions; and measuring the results of these decisions against the expectations through organized, systematic feedback."[1] Strategic planning, then, deals not with future decisions but with the futurity of present decisions.

Span of the Strategic Plan

The strategic plan is formulated in three segments: the strategic plan, the developmental plan, and the annual operations plan.

The *strategic plan* is a broad statement of plans for organizational growth and development. It focuses on the range of alternatives available to the organization in addressing questions of survival. It is the portion of the plan in which management anticipates the market and resources 5 to 10 years hence, giving consideration to a variety of factors that influence the viability and competitiveness of the organization's product or service. The actual number of years covered by the strategic plan depends largely upon the product or service offered by the organization. The developmental plan and the operational plan are components of the strategic plan.

The *developmental portion* of the strategic plan is the interim section, which addresses the scope of tasks to be accomplished by the organization in meeting its goals. In this phase of the plan, adjustments of the organization's policies, products, or services are made to accommodate anticipated changes in consumer values and personnel expectations. Generally, the developmental portion of the strategic plan covers a period of 3 to 7 years into the future. It is critical to the optimal management of the occupational therapy service that the department director have both access and input into the formulation of this portion of the agency's plan. In the unfortunate circumstance of managing a department without anticipating at least this much of the organization's future, the occupational therapy director is positioned so that he or she may do little more than react to changes, pressures, and demands placed on the service by the system. Unless the occupational therapy director is privy to the developmental portion of the strategic plan, decisions regarding allocation of financial and human resources in the occupational therapy department can be little more than arbitrary in the overall management of the organization, resulting in wasted staff effort and interest.

The *annual operations plan*, encompassed in the developmental portion of the strategic plan, is the immediate, highly specific phase of the strategic plan framed in a time span of 1 year. Elements of the annual operations plan are stated in definite, measurable terms and have assigned target completion dates.

This plan provides a guide for the manager, supervisor, and staff for day-to-day service to the consumer. This is the planning process with which occupational therapists are most familiar. Effective planning and scheduling of the annual operations of the department are important in assuring that departmental services maintain pace as the total organization moves toward its long range goals. Collaborative planning between staff and manager in this portion of the plan also provides an important opportunity for occupational therapy staff members to plan their professional growth while meeting departmental objectives. Effective planning and scheduling of the annual operations of the organization are essential to the long-term viability of both the occupational therapy department and the total organization.

Establishment of the annual operations plan begins with the organization's goals at the most future point encompassed by the plan and works backwards to the present in order that decisions and actions of the present may provide support to the ultimate accomplishment of the completed plan. While the strategic plan is comprised of three parts, it maintains its integrity as a single plan as long as all parts focus on advancing the organization toward its eventual goal. Change in any given phase of the plan necessitates adjustment in one or both of the other portions of the plan.

Developing the Plan

Strategic planning is an integrated process involving the following eight steps:

1. *Gathering and assessing information on the external environment.*

   This includes information relative to projected change in the political arena, government regulations, capital markets, the industry in which the health provider's services are offered, competitor activity, social changes, supplies, raw materials, and manpower to both provide the services offered to consumers and to manage staff as the plan is administered. Regardless of the soundness of the plan in every aspect, failure to ensure availability of competent manpower ultimately results in failure of the plan.[2]

2. *Gathering and assessing information on the organization's internal environment.*

   The internal assessment identifies the facility's strengths and weaknesses and points out problem areas that may limit future efficiency and growth of the organization.

3. *Establishing corporate objectives.*

   Based on the information gathered, assumptions and predictions are made, and the major problems are identified in the examination of both the external and internal environments.

4. *Determining the gap.* The difference (or gap) between the organization's actual situation at present and its desired situation projected 5 to 10 years into the future is determined.

5. *Developing Strategies.* Action plans are established for achieving the organization's long-term objectives.

6. *Establishing a time table for action.* Check points are assigned target dates toward accomplishment of the plan.

7. *Allocating resources.* Resource's of money and effort are allocated to ensure goal accomplishment.

8. *Annual evaluation.* Evaluation of the organization's strategic plan and progress toward it, followed by a repeat of this cycle, forms the final step in the strategic planning process. As a result of this annual review, adjustments in the strategic plan may become appropriate as new opportunities, changing social purpose, values, customs, and expectations of both consumer and worker are anticipated or become evident.

Other Considerations

Health care agencies and organizations must operate in a social environment of enormous scope. Although managers inevitably look at the operation of their facilities from the inside, the organizational enterprise is actually a creature of society and economy. "Either society or the economy can put any business out of existence overnight," reminds Drucker, who stresses that the organizational objectives must complement social purpose.[3] When health providers fail to offer services which address society's needs and purpose at any point in time, their organizations may lose their competitive edge in the marketplace and take on a higher probability of failure. When the occupational therapy department fails to anticipate and provide treatment appropriate to the needs of the consumer served by the agency with which the occupational therapy department is affiliated, the occupational therapy department loses value to the organization and will ultimately be eliminated.

The strategic plan must include provisions for maintaining viable coalitions among other affiliations with which the organization must cooperate during the years encompassed by the plan. Such cooperative agreement with firms in related fields may occasionally provide means to overcome certain resource shortages. In the same manner, maintenance of viable coalitions with other health services may be helpful to the occupational therapy department within an institution.

Because of the competition with other organiza-

tions for resources, the product or service offered by the organization must have some distinct and obvious advantages, either in the kind of product or service provided or in the methods of creating it.

Boundaries

The parameters of any agency framed by top management's decisions become the boundaries of that organization's business. Decisions and actions of managers are seated in their ideas regarding the kind of business they manage. The strategic plan articulates a relationship between a product or service and the consumer in the marketplace. It is, then, top management that establishes the purpose of the organization in terms of service it will render to society, and defines the boundaries within which the agency will operate.

All elements of the strategic plan must support the realization of the organization's purpose. It is erroneous to select objectives that make no contribution to that purpose or that actually conflict with it. Positive contributions to purpose must be planned if they are to have more than a coincidental effect. Plans for occupational therapy within an organization must be in harmony with the overall organizational plan.

Plans for meeting the institution's long-range objectives may call for substantial growth and development. Such development may involve moving into markets different from those traditionally served by the organization, with services that are different from those currently provided by the facility. Sometimes, however, growth plans may call for serving essentially the same consumers with different or more expanded products and services. The tendency prevails in many organizations toward diversification without thoroughly exploring the possibility of becoming more efficient within the organization's current boundaries. Stewart Thompson warns that "intoxicating enthusiasm for change and new frontiers sometimes leads to neglect of the stable elements which do not change. Anticipation of and planning for change is fruitless unless it is coupled with anticipation of and planning for factors which will remain stable."[4] Occupational therapy services are often caught up in this intoxicating enthusiasm for change. The occupational therapy manager must be particularly careful in planning to give consideration to provision of enough consistency so that the department's service is assigned a role in the minds of both personnel and consumers. Planning and controlling the growth of a changing organization with evolving skills and a growing reputation requires a great deal of managerial skill to avoid dissipation of energy at all levels in the organization's structure.

An important consideration for top management

in formulating the strategic plan, and one which is often overlooked, is examining each product, process, and market in terms of its current relevance to society's purpose and to the organization's goals. This is a critical concept for occupational therapy managers. The occupational therapist must ask the question, "If I weren't already providing this service, would I do so now?" When the answer turns out to be "No," then the inclusion of strategy for abandoning that product or service line should be incorporated into the department's or organization's strategic plan. Drucker calls this "sloughing off yesterday."[5]

Role of Management

The establishment and implementation of a successful organizational plan demands a number of qualities and conditions of managerial personnel. A quality plan presupposes intelligent, experienced, and successful management at the highest level. Personnel in charge must be skilled in supervising people, have a high degree of competence in the specialized requirements of the organization, have general management knowledge or experience, some continuity of tenure, and considerable energy.

Management must answer the questions "What shall we do?" and "Why?" Decisions about risks the institution will take and whether the future of the organization will be staked on existing services or on the development of new services or markets belong to management. Whether or not to make risk-taking decisions is not an option for the manager at the departmental or organizational level; taking risks is part of the job.

Visible commitment on the part of management to the strategic plan and direction the organization will take is essential to the plan's success, for the manager's attitude, as perceived by staff, exerts a decided influence on the functioning of the entire agency.

Implementing the Plan

With the organization's purpose and boundaries set by management, the department head becomes involved with management in addressing the question of how the objectives will be accomplished. Together they scale-down the long term strategies into specific programs and projects to be implemented over the coming 3 to 7 years in the developmental segment of the strategic plan. Costs for accomplishing the objectives are identified and proposed for the budget. A statement of desired outcomes is inherent in this portion of the plan.

Supervisors join department heads in establishing and implementing the annual operations plan. In this phase, goals and targets are set for a one-year time span that will begin the organization's movement toward the accomplishment of its goals. These are highly specific action plans broken down into specific tasks that can be delegated and accomplished by individual therapists in the department and are stated in terms of desired results. A schedule for task accomplishment is part of the operational plan. The operational plan also provides for the measurement and evaluation of results achieved and compares outcomes with the formalized goals of the plan.

Advantages and Disadvantages

The practice of strategic planning has many benefits for occupational therapists. Strategic planning ensures that the organization and its separate departments look ahead to identify constraints and opportunities. Problems for an organization are anticipated long before they become acute. A framework for devising and evaluating alternative futures in the face of uncertainties is established. Strategic planning is invaluable in determining the best allocation of limited resources for accomplishing objectives. The planning process creates a mechanism by which the organization systematically reconsiders previous decisions. Formal planning encourages communication and interaction by management and departmental personnel and maximizes opportunity for better understanding of, and commitment to, overall objectives and goals of the organization. Organizations using strategic planning have experienced superior growth and have a stronger financial base than organizations that do not plan.

The practice of strategic planning also holds advantages for department heads. Department heads are provided with regular opportunities to influence top management. Formal planning aids in winning management's support for activities of strategic significance that otherwise may be masked by day-to-day operations. A further benefit is the clear setting out of results expected from departmental managers, supervisors, and staff as measured by objectives that they have helped to establish. The tendency toward piecemeal solutions to problems is thus prevented.

Formal planning, like anything valuable, has some costs. An investment of time and training is essential to the plan's success. This necessitates diverting significant effort and time from day-to-day operations while the initial plan is formulated. This includes meetings and time for collecting the necessary data to establish the plan.

Conclusion

A carefully conceived and well coordinated strategic plan provides organizations and their separate departments with both distant and interim objectives and a concrete, time-framed system of task accomplishment. These will tend to guide the organization toward attainment of its goals when effectively used. The strategic plan, however, must function as a guide. Neither the organization nor the individual department must place itself in bondage to the plan. Periodic plan review and goal reassessment are useful in assuring the organization's freedom to adjust the plan to changes in its internal and external environments. The strategic planning process provides organizations and their various departments with a valuable tool for planning futures based on well-considered judgments. Health care organizations and the occupational therapy departments within them

will do well to follow the lead of the business community in incorporating the strategic planning process into their practice of management.

References

1. Drucker, P. F.: Management: Tasks, Responsibilities and Practices. New York: Harper & Row, 1974, p. 125.
2. Shearer, R. C.: Developing the Strategic Plan. Unpublished lecture. Dallas, Texas, Southern Methodist University, 1980.
3. Drucker, p. 113.
4. Thompson, S.: What planning involves. In Koontz, H., and O'Donnell, S. (eds.): Management: A Book of Reading, p. 114. New York: McGraw-Hill, 1972.
5. Drucker, p. 126.

CHAPTER 42

Health Care Marketing   *Tina Olson*

Health care marketing emerged in the mid-1970s during a period of escalating concern about increasing regulation of health care, decreasing or maldistributed resources, and changes in reimbursement practices for health care services.

There are three general reasons for an organization's changing from a production orientation to a marketing orientation*: ". . . an internal realization of the value of a true commitment to customer satisfaction, consumerism, and consumerism's growth into government legislation—particularly the Health Systems Agency (HSA) and Health Maintenance Organization (HMO) legislation that brings the consumer into the health planning procedure and recognizes the changing need for alternative delivery systems."[1]

---

* "A production orientation characterizes organizations that spend their major energy on improving the output or reducing the cost of whatever they are producing with little or no regard for the customer's evolving needs."

A sales orientation characterizes organizations that spend their main energy in trying to convince the public to want and buy their current goods. . . . The sales orientation ultimately leads to a consumer credability gap and products that are poorly adapted to market needs."

A market oriented organization "sees its role to be identifying and serving the evolving needs of its customers and publics."[2]

The National Health Planning and Resource Development Act (PL 93-641), which established the Health Systems Agencies (HSAs), created a planning process that determined and established community need for new health services and also reviewed the appropriateness of existing services. Although the original community or area HSAs will not be funded after 1982, the concept remains and is expected to be carried out by state government.

Professional Standards Review Organizations (PSROs) were established by PL 92-603 to examine care provided to clients of Crippled Children's Services and Maternal and Child Health (Title V), Medicare (Title XVIII), and Medicaid (Title XIX) and to assure effective, efficient, and economical delivery of medical care. "Specifically, PSRO's were charged with assessing the necessity of services rendered by physicians to patients, the appropriateness of the facility within which the patient is treated, and the quality of care provided to that patient."[3]

Again, funding for this federal program is in question. However, both HSAs and PSROs provided consumers with an expectation that health care could be accountable to them in measurable ways. This further forced health care institutions to look at the services provided in terms of community need rather than

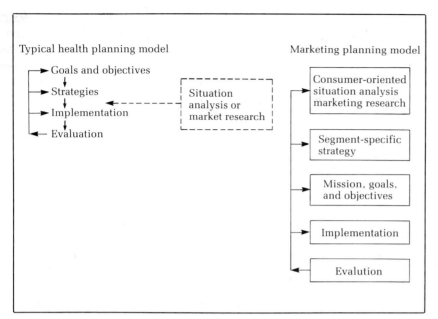

Figure 42-1. A traditional model and a marketing planning model. In the latter, "the consumer of health services (whether viewed as the physician, the patient, the government, or some other purchaser) is recognized as the focal point for making the key choices that dictate the organization's success." Adapted from Berkowitz E. N. and Flexner W. A.[5]

considering only institutional objectives. By refocusing the institution from a production orientation to a marketing orientation, federal legislation has had a role in developing marketing as a tool for health care institutions.

The 1970s also saw the rise of the consumer movement. The greatest criticism of the health care industry was that it was unresponsive to its consumers. The emphasis in health care in the 1960s seemed to be on the complexities of its resources, rather than on the comprehensiveness of its services.[4] When the funding of health care services during the late 1960s and early 1970s are considered, one discovers that the third party payer, in the form of government or private insurance, became the apparent consumer in the health care industry, further removing the health care system's accountability from the patient or community consumer.

Today, in the early 1980s, the economic forecast is quite different. The high costs of federal insurance programs (Medicare and Medicaid) and the enormous cost of health insurance to industry are causing a reassessment of funding for health care. More serious attention is given to alternative delivery systems and to copayment by the consumer as ways of decreasing health care costs. The consumer movement and economic pressures are bringing the recipient of care back into the health care institution's view.

Marketing is a process that focuses the organization on the needs of the consumer. It differs from the traditional health planning model in that it considers the consumer at the beginning of the planning process rather than at some point between the development of strategies and their implementation. Figure 42-1 illustrates conceptually the traditional planning model and a marketing planning model.

Definition of Marketing

By definition marketing involves the planning and management of exchange relationships with important publics.*[6] A common misconception about marketing is that it is the selling of a product. This misconception has made marketing a particularly unacceptable concept for human service professions. Actually, selling or promoting is a visible part of marketing, but it represents only a fragment of a very broad and comprehensive planning and management process. Human service professionals have been using parts of marketing strategy for years as a means of program development, recruitment of personnel, or of encouraging a patient to adhere to a particular treatment program. It is only recently that the marketing process as an integrated concept has been accepted by the human service professions as a viable tool.

A review of several current definitions affirms the concept of marketing as an integrated exchange relationship:

"Marketing is the analysis, planning, implementation and control of carefully formulated programs designed to bring about voluntary exchanges of values with target markets for the purpose of achieving organizational objectives. It relies heavily on designing the or-

---

* "A public is defined as a distinct group of people and/or organizations that have an actual or potential interest and/or impact on an organization."[7]

ganization's offering in terms of the target market's needs and desires, and on using effective pricing, communication, and distribution to inform, motivate, and service the markets."[8]

"Exchange is the central concept underlying marketing. It calls for the offering of value to someone in exchange for value. Through exchanges, various social units—individuals, small groups, organizations, whole nations—attain the inputs they need. By giving up something, they acquire something else normally more valued than that which is given up, which explains the motivation for exchange."[9]

"Marketing is a systematic approach to planning and achieving desired exchange relations with other groups. Marketing is concerned with developing, maintaining, and/or regulating exchange relations involving products, services, organizations, persons, places, or causes."[10] ". . . . the concept of marketing . . . . the design and management of transactions between providers and consumers of goods and/or services so that both are satisfied."[11] "Marketing may also be thought of as the science and art of understanding, predicting, and influencing behavior through the engineering of exchange relationships."[12]

Kotler's "Examples of Early Transaction"[13] have been adapted and applied in Figure 42-2 to the exchanges familiar to the occupational therapist.

Further examples of exchange relationships occur between organizations and their publics. Review of this concept is shown in Figure 42-3, which is, again, adapted from Kotler's work[14] and "classifies organizations in a way that is relevant to marketing."[15]

The reader can identify that there are exchanges of value in all the relationships described in Figure 42-3. The organizations themselves are not marketing organizations, but all can benefit from a marketing approach.

"Marketing is already entrenched in *business concerns* as a widely recognized function. Even here, it should be noted, it first achieved explicit recognition in the consumer goods area, moved later into the industrial goods area, and is now receiving strong attention in the commercial services area. Marketing will become more important in *service organizations'* thinking because of the close analogy between customers-for-profit and clients-for-service. Then it will receive more attention in *mutual benefit associations* as these organizations face

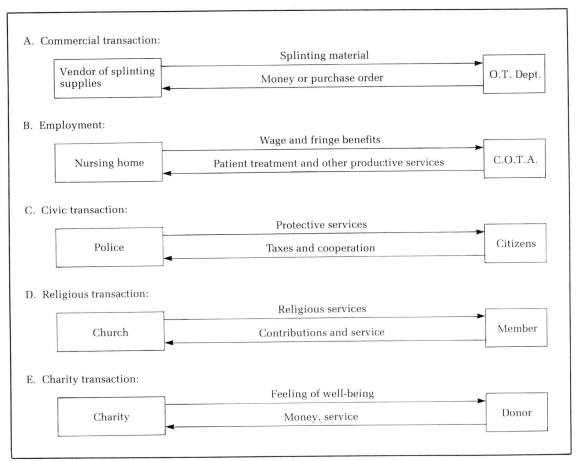

Figure 42-2. Examples of exchange transactions. (Adapted from Kotler P: Marketing for Nonprofit Organizations. Englewood Cliffs, Prentice-Hall, 1975)

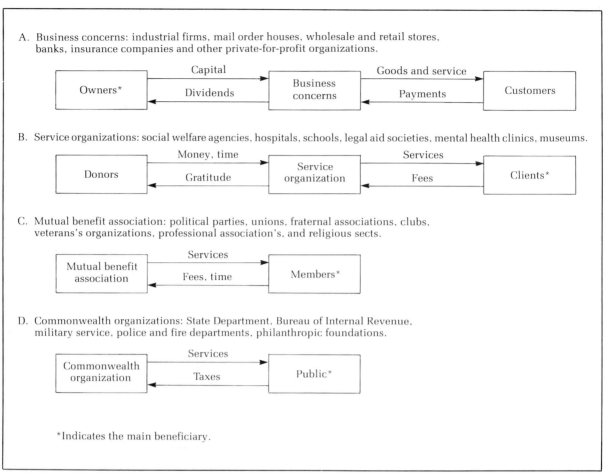

A. Business concerns: industrial firms, mail order houses, wholesale and retail stores, banks, insurance companies and other private-for-profit organizations.

| Owners* | Capital → | Business concerns | Goods and service → | Customers |
| ← Dividends | | | ← Payments | |

B. Service organizations: social welfare agencies, hospitals, schools, legal aid societies, mental health clinics, museums.

| Donors | Money, time → | Service organization | Services → | Clients* |
| ← Gratitude | | | ← Fees | |

C. Mutual benefit association: political parties, unions, fraternal associations, clubs, veterans's organizations, professional association's, and religious sects.

| Mutual benefit association | Services → | Members* |
| ← Fees, time | |

D. Commonwealth organizations: State Department, Bureau of Internal Revenue, military service, police and fire departments, philanthropic foundations.

| Commonwealth organization | Services → | Public* |
| ← Taxes | |

*Indicates the main beneficiary.

Figure 42-3. Exchange relations of four main types of organizations. Adapted from Kotler P.,[14] and Blau and Scott.[16]

increasing problems of attracting and holding members relative to growing competitive uses of member's time and changing values. Finally, marketing is entering the thinking of *commonweal organizations* as they increasingly recognize that the quality of service they render their public affects the amount of public support and the size of their budget."[17]

Marketing Information

A successful approach to marketing depends on reliable and current information. As the process of developing a plan for marketing evolves, the need for information is specific, and the information is often quantifiable. In many ways market planning becomes a process whereby information begets the need for more information, especially from and about the target market or a public that has become valued by the organization.

Market planning information is developed using two general methods, the *market audit* and *market analysis*. Each of these processes focuses on information regarding the needs of the consumer and on the exchange relationship. Each process looks at market-

ing information in a different way and is critical to an integrated marketing approach.

"The market audit examines the organization and its relations with its markets; the market analysis scrutinizes the organization's environment as it does or will affect those relations. The two combined form the marketing data base that leads to understanding, predicting, and influencing the organization's interaction with its markets."[18]

The Market Audit

"A variety of reasons for conducting a marketing audit exists. The dynamic nature of society and the health care industry, in particular, requires up-to-date information for the organization to operate effectively. One must periodically monitor the organization's position and activities to assess their responsiveness to market needs and preferences.

In this dynamic environment, a marketing audit has many purposes:
—it appraises the total marketing operation;
—it centers on the evaluation of objectives and policies and the assumption that underlie them;

—it aims for prognosis as well as diagnosis;

—it searches for opportunities and means for exploiting them as well as for weakness and means for their elimination;

—it practices prevention as well as curative marketing practices."[19]

The three kinds of information that make up a market audit are behavioral, impact-related, and causal factors:

1. *Behavior:* This information reveals the organizational behavioral performance as well as that of the consumer. The behavior of specific homogeneous groups within the consumer group may also be studied in relation to a particular program or service within the organization that serves that segment.*

2. *Impact:* That which happens to the organization or program as a result of the interaction with the market or segment of the market. "Your impacts may be measured in traditional performance terms while theirs may be reflected in health status measures."[21] Traditional means of tracking impact is through measuring such internal information as financial data or numbers of referrals by diagnosis or by physician.

3. *Causal Factors:* "These include both demographic** and psychographic*** characteristics of markets that may aid one in predicting, evaluating, or influencing behavior. One may use such characteristics to identify separable market segments and to forecast their probability of demanding specific services or of preferring one of alternative sources of that service."[23]

External factors significant to the market audit are *environment* and *competition*. Environmental factors include government regulations, the economy, or any factor external to the organization that can change how your market relates to you.

The scope of the market audit procedure is illustrated in Figure 42-4.

"The audit process is represented as a series of circles expanding outward from the consumer. One begins by looking at the size of the consumer market and the various ways that it can be divided or segmented. To this information must be added information concerning one's own health service organization. Often there are internal constraints that must be determined before de-

vising marketing strategies. Beyond the organization, an assessment needs to be made of the competition, its strengths and weaknesses."[24]

Cutting across the concentric circles of the evolving market audit are four variables—price, products and services, channels of distribution, and promotion. These variables can all be controlled by the organization and become the marketing strategy. These will be discussed under *Marketing Mix.*

To illustrate the concept, Mac Stravic's "Suggestions for Market Audit" has been adapted to a typical hospital-based occupational therapy clinical situation (see Sample Market Audit).[26] Before attempting a market audit, the reader is encouraged to pursue further readings.

The sample market audit represents the possible composition of a market audit for an occupational therapy department that wishes to look at strategies for increasing the number of referrals of patients who have had joint–replacement surgery. The items in the audit represent a typical situation, but are not necessarily all the questions that should be asked.

As in any audit process, it is important to have some standard established for the study prior to its inception. In the absence of any published standard, this may have to be the best conjecture of the personnel involved in the particular area to be studied. An example of a published standard for the audit topic in the sample market audit would be a statement by the orthopedic department asserting that every joint–replacement surgery patient will have been referred for an activities of daily living assessment by occupational therapy prior to discharge from the inpatient service.

Market audits and other types of medical audits require full awareness and participation on the part of the personnel involved in the area being studied. Sapienza and Kahn discuss the importance of involving staff members in market research. They point out that "involvement of key staff lends credibility to market research and marketing decisions and gives people a stake in the strategy's success. In short, a manager must pay as much attention to staff involvement as to the marketing project itself."[33] Key areas of staff involvement are in suggesting questions for the composition of the audit, review of drafts of the audit, and discussion of the results as they relate to decision making.

Market Analysis

Mac Stravic indicates that market *analysis* as opposed to the market *audit* described earlier, has three major components, "the market as a whole, environmental factors that affect it, and other organizations provid-

---

* "The sole purpose of segmenting a population is to treat each segment differently either in your analysis, or later, your market strategy—and preferably both."[20]

** Demographic characteristics include such factors as age, sex, religion, income, educational and insurance coverage—much of this information is available within the organization.

*** "Psychographic factors include what people know and believe about health or about your organization."[22]

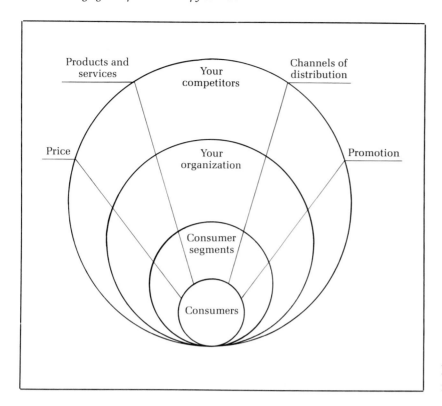

Figure 42-4. The scope of the marketing audit. Berkowitz and Flexner.[25]

STEP 1:	Identification of the market transaction to be audited: In-patient referrals from orthopedic physicians for patients who have had (or will have) joint-replacement surgery.		
STEP 2:	Specific Behavior to be Measured:		
A. Patients		*Time Increments	Source of Data

1. Admitted with diagnosis of joint replacement
 	
  a. Total hip
  b. Total knee
  c. Finger
			Medical Records

2. Length of Stay (LOS)
(average for total population)
 	
  a. (average for each diagnosis)
  b.
  c.
			Medical Records–Diagnostic Index

3. Use of occupational therapy (% of patients with the diagnosis referred to OT to the total population with the diagnosis admitted)			O.T. Department Record
4. Use of physical therapy (% of patients with the diagnosis referred to PT to the total population with the diagnosis admitted)			P.T. Department Record

5. OT Department referrals by diagnosis
  a.
  b.
  c.
			O.T. Department Record

*The time increment may be current year, previous year, and continue for 5 years if data is available. If the volume of surgery warrants, the study may include monthly data as well as yearly data.			

B. Physicians	Source of Data

1. The number of Joint Replacement Patients admitted by orthopedic physicians on staff.
  a. Dr. A
 	
  b. Dr. B
 	
  c. Dr. C
	Figure should = A-1
	
	Patient Origin Study information compiled by Medical Records or Health data available in Medical Records for PSRO Study

2. Length of Stay by physician
  a.
  b.
  c.
	L.O.S. from A-2
	L.O.S. Report from Hospital Administration or Medical Records compiled for PSRO Study

3. Use of OT Services by physician
  a.
  b.
  c.
	A-3
	O.T. Department Records

4. Use of OT Services by type of Joint Replacement, by physician*	O.T. Department Records and B-3

Dr. A. _____

Dr. B. _____

Dr. C. _____
      **increment of time

Total knee	Total hip	Finger

*Once identified, this information could be graphed in order to identify trends.

**This time increment may be by the year or by month—whatever measure is justified by the volume of orthopedic surgery done in the facility.

| 5. Use of Physical Therapy services by physician
  a.
  b.
  c. | A-4

P.T. Department Record |
| 6. Use of Physical Therapy Service by type of surgery, by physician* | Note: Use of physical therapy information may identify areas where the departments could work together for a total program of could assist in identifying orthopedic surgeons whose psychographics include a belief in the usefulness of |

Dr. A. _____

Dr. B. _____

Dr. C. _____
      **increment of time

**increment of time	increment of time	increment of time

*Once identified, this information could be graphed to identify trends.

**The time increment may be by year, or by month—whatever measure is justified by the volume of orthopedic joint replacement surgery done in the facility.

| 7. Comparison of OT and PT use by Physician | A-3/A-4 for each physician. If the volume warrants, this comparison may also be made by diagnosis. |

B. Physicians   Source of Data

Increment of time, i.e./month

STEP 3: Occupational Therapy Department Behavior

A. How does the Occupational Therapy Department behave with
    respect to the orthopedic patient with joint replacement
    surgery (?)

    1. Number of referrals within diagnostic group being
        studied.   O.T. Department Record

    2. Average length of time between referral and
        initial assessment.

    3. Average number of treatments (visits) per
        patient by diagnosis.
        a.
        b.
        c.

    4. Number of treatments not given due to
        therapist unavailability.

    5. Number of treatments not given due to
        patient's unavailability.

                                                                    Data for 3-A4 and 3A5 may have to
                                                                    be projected based on a study of
                                                                    current activity as this type of
                                                                    information is not generally
                                                                    available.

B. How does the Occupational Therapy Department behave
    with respect to the referring physician?

    1. Referral procedure   3B-1 OT Dept. procedure manual
                                                                    exact procedure as communicated
    2. Reporting procedure   to physicians.
                                                                    3B-2, include frequency, location
    3. Percentage of patients for whom there is a   accessibility, content, compre-
        significant delay in implementing treatment   hensiveness. (A chart audit
        (evaluation, splints, adaptive equipment).   would be helpful here.)

                                                                    Review a generous sample of current charts.

B. Physicians   Source of Data

	Increment of time, i.e. current, month, year-to-date	
	current	YTD

STEP 4: Evaluate current behavior and current direction of change in terms of institutional performance.

A. Occupancy Rate

Administrative Records–usually by month. May have to be calculated using nursing or admissions dept. information.

B. Lost patient days because of lack of beds for orthopedic surgery.

C. Lost patient days because of inability of surgeon to get on the surgery schedule.

Department of Surgery

D. Occupational Therapy Dept. revenue from joint replacement surgery patient.

Business Office or calculated from OT Dept. records. May have to project figure if this is a new service.

E. Expenses for occupational therapy dept. for joint replacement surgery patient.

Note: It may be helpful to calculate expense and revenue on a per patient basis, then project a figure for the population of patients within each time period being measured.

    1. Supplies
    2. Direct expense
        a. Salary
        b. Fringe benefits
    3. Indirect expense
        a. Staff education
        b. Allocated indirect expense from Medicare Cost Report
        c. Conference time and charting time
        d. Business office
    4. Total actual expense
    5. Total patient (4E–4 ÷ 3A–1)

STEP 5: Identify patients' demographic and psychographic factors that might explain behavior or be focused on to change it.

A. Demographic

    1. Elderly population that is generally weak and can't tolerate an aggressive program.
    2. The percentage of the population not covered by Medicare or adequate insurance who refuse OT.
    3. The nature of the diagnosis necessitates an aggressive mobilization program by PT, making the patient frequently unavailable for OT.
    4. Elderly are a growing % of total community.

Department Experience

H.S.A. data

B. Psychographic

    1. Patients are fearful of moving previously painful joints and are reluctant to engage in activity.
    2. Patients are fearful of missing their doctors visit, so are reluctant to go to the OT clinic area.
    3. The patient is unable to relate to the importance of ADL training while in the hospital environment because they have not yet experienced a lack of function in their home environment.

B. Physicians	Source of Data

STEP 6: Environmental Analysis[27]

A.   What is the catchment area of the population being served for all diagnoses?

> Patient Origin Study information, by county and HSA information By zip code as well as Medical Record Information

B.   Is the catchment area for this diagnosis different than that of the catchment area for all diagnoses—are gaps apparent?

C.   Are there patients from the catchment area leaving the area to have joint replacement surgery done? (ie., large, urban centers), where? What physicians?

> Patient origin data from state Hosp. Assoc.

STEP 7: Competitor Analysis[28]

A.   What centers that offer joint replacement surgery within the catchment area also offer OT?

> Am. Hosp. Assoc., State OT Assoc., AOTA

B.   What physicians on your medical staff also serve on the staff of:

1.   Centers that offer joint replacement surgery that offer OT.
2.   Centers that offer joint replacement surgery that don't offer OT.
3.   How does the list for 7-B-1 and 7-B-2 compare with 2B-3?

> Local medical society

C.   How does your department rate with competing OT departments in this treatment area? In other treatment areas?

> Subjective assessment

D.   Have your competitors increased in the last 4 years?

E.   Is competition based on a price, promotion, accessibility, or other basis?

STEP 8: Pricing Analysis[29]

A.   What is the basis for charges for OT department services?

1.   Cost
2.   Relative value
3.   Charges for therapist time, only
4.   How are materials marked up?

B.   Physician

B.   How frequently are charges reviewed? (What factors influence an increase or decrease in charges)?

C.   What is the OT charge history over the last 5 years for services included in the treatment of joint replacement patients?

D.   How are your charges viewed by:

1.   Patients
2.   Physicians
3.   3rd party payers
4.   Competitors
5.   Regulators
6.   Your staff

B. Physicians	Source of Data

STEP 9: Product and Service Analysis[30]

A. Describe current and proposed OT Dept. services for the joint replacement patient.

B. What are the outstanding characteristics of each service (current or proposed).

C. What superiority or distinctiveness can be ascribed to your services that exceed the services of competitors.

D. What is the total cost (not revenue) per treatment? Is the service over/under utilized?

E. What services are most heavily used? Why?

    1. Profile of physicians who use each service.
    2. Identify therapists who use some treatment options but disregard others.

F. History of services offered by OT dept. for patients with joint replacement surgery.

    1. Original services offered to population.
    2. Additions or deletions.
    3. What important changes have taken place in the last 10 years in this area?
    4. Has demand for service increased or decreased?
    5. What are the most common complaints about the service?
    6. What services could be added to the department that would make the range of OT services available to this population more attractive to patients, physicians, your staff?
    7. What are the strongest points about your service to patients, physicians, your staff?

STEP 10: Promotion Analysis[31]

A. What is the purpose of the department's present promotional activities?

    1. Protective
    2. Educational
    3. Search out new area of service
    4. Develop all areas of OT
    5. Establishing a new service

B. Has this purpose undergone any change in recent years?

C. To whom have promotion efforts been directed?

    1. Patients
    2. The community
    3. The physician
        a. Current referrers
        b. Potential referrers

D. What methods have been used?

E. How has the effect of promotion efforts been measured?

F. What has been the effect of each method used?

G. What has been the role of the Public Relations Department?

B. Physicians	Source of Data

STEP 11: Distribution Analysis[32]

A. What are the trends in delivery of OT services to the joint replacement surgery patient?

    1. Outpatient
    2. Homebound
    3. Statellite facilities
    4. Inpatient only
       a. Bedside
       b. Clinic

B. What factors have been considered in making treatment location decisions?

C. When did you last evaluate the location of services provided to this population?

D. What vendors do you deal with for supplies?

    1. What has been their performance history?
    2. What would their future performance be if your use of products increased?

E. How large an inventory do you carry?

    1. Can you increase storage space to handle increased volume?
    2. Can you supply outpatients or homebound patients with materials?

ing similar benefits to the market." The analysis examines the same data as the market audit but looks at people who might be future clients.[34] Market analysis looks at the economy, population changes, technology, financing, and regulation of health services that might affect the behavior of the market in the future. Market analysis uses analytical methods for projecting future trends, using data internal and external to the organization.

Kotler approaches market analysis in three broad areas: *market structure analysis, consumer analysis,* and *the marketing mix.*

Market structure analysis is made up of three parts: *market definition, segmentation,* and *position.* Market structure analysis looks at the structure and behavior of the market.

The *market definition* describes the boundaries of a particular market and thus depends on a specific description of the product. Kotler defines product ". . . . to include physical objects, services, persons, places, organizations, and ideas."[35] If the product is described as rehabilitation, then the market would be defined as anyone in need of any number of rehabilitation disciplines. If the product is described more narrowly as pediatric occupational therapy, then the market becomes those individuals less than eighteen years of age who are in need of occupational therapy.

A market consists of those who have an actual or potential interest in a product. Market definition can be further narrowed by differentiating between the *potential market* and the *actual market.* The potential market is made up of those individuals who are ca-

pable of becoming interested in acquiring a product. The actual market is represented by persons who are strongly attracted to the product. Using the pediatric occupational therapy example once again, the potential market would be those pediatric patients admitted to a pediatric unit. The actual market would be those referred to occupational therapy.

Market segmentation, the second component of market structure analysis, determines how complex and specialized a market analysis and plan must be in order to be effective. Market segmentation consists in ". . . dividing the market into fairly homogeneous parts where any part may conceivably by selected as a market target to be reached with a distinct marketing mix."[36]

One of the most common ways of segmenting a market is by using demographics such as age, income, or common need for a particular variation of a product. Each segment of a market will require a different approach once the characteristics that make it different are identified.

Kotler illustrates different approaches to market segmentation, as adapted here in Fig. 42-5.[37]

The segmentation models illustrated in Figure 42-5 could be applied to the population of referrals to an occupational therapy department in a general hospital.

Figure 42-5A illustrates the total population in a given period of time, such as total referrals to occupational therapy in a month's time. This can be treated as homogeneous group.

Figure 42-5B segments the total number of referrals to a program area within the department. Each

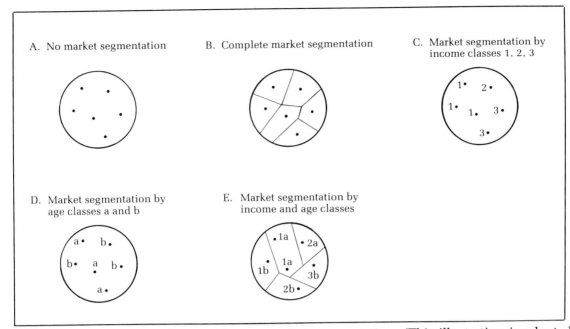

Figure 42-5. A variety of approaches to market segmentation. (This illustration is adapted from Kotler P.[37] for purposes of the example cited.)

member of this market has certain traits in common with the other members of the segment, but each has different needs than members of another segment. For purpose of illustration, the program areas in this department are psychiatry, orthopedics, neurology, pediatrics, oncology, and rehabilitation.

Figure 42-5C shows the total population in terms of income class in which "1" is private insurance, "2" is private pay (no insurance and not eligible for Medicaid) and "3" is Medicare. In this example, for this population, private insurance is the most common means of reimbursement for the department, and private pay is the least common means of reimbursement.

Figure 42-5D demonstrates that many times age is considered an important demographic characteristic. In this example, "a" represents a pediatric population, and "b" represents an adult population.

Figure 42-5E illustrates the combining of characteristics into groups that are sufficiently alike to be treated the same, yet sufficiently different to be treated as distinct groups.[38] Using previously identified traits from this example, the segments would become:

1a: Pediatric patients financed by private insurance with diagnosis of learning disabilities and neurological conditions
2a: Pediatric patients, with an orthopedic diagnosis, financed by the patient's family
1b: Adult patients, with a diagnosis of hip fracture, financed by private insurance
2b: Adult patients seen on the rehabilitation service financed by the patient

3b: Adult patients, with a diagnosis of cancer financed by Medicare

Proper segmentation of the market is crucial to the design of a marketing program that will be attractive to that market. In this approach the patients are identified as the market, but in most cases, the patients do not initiate the request for a service. In the general hospital setting, it is the physician who must be attracted to a program in order for the therapist to have access to the patient. Thus, the medical staff is the most frequent target in a marketing effort in the general hospital setting. In a school setting, the target would most likely be the teacher or school administrator who arranges for service, rather than the ultimate recipient of the service.

These examples used demographic information to segment the market. It is also possible and desirable in many cases to use psychographics, geographics,* or a combination of segmenting variables to define a particular market.

The *marketing position,* a third component of market structure analysis, defines the particular niche an organization occupies. This is generally revealed by market segmentation. In the previous example, the department segmenting its population by program may discover a trend toward increasing specialization in pediatrics. If this is a market segment that is not being covered elsewhere in the community, the department may want to focus its market planning on

* Geographics describe the location where the market may be found, i.e., nursing homes within the county, the pediatric unit of a general hospital, or school districts within a geographic area.

gaining more of the potential pediatric patients. This may involve diverting resources from other programs in order to enhance the position of pediatric services.

Consumer analysis is the component of market planning which focuses on defining consumer wants and needs. It also establishes the values the consumer is willing to exchange for the organization's product. Unfortunately, consumer analysis is the component of market research most often overlooked by the organization. This oversight is the reason most (80%) new marketing ventures fail.[39]

Consumer analysis consists of consumer needs assessment, measurement of consumer perceptions about the organization, measurement of consumer preference among a choice of variables, and level of consumer satisfaction with the product. All four of these areas of measurement require extensive analytical study and impeccable research design. They will be described here in general terms. The reader is encouraged to study Kotler's chapter dealing with Consumer Analysis and the extensive bibliography described therein.[40]

Need: Consumer needs can be measured, but it is difficult because it is hard to differentiate between "need" and "want." People do not clearly express their needs or may have given little thought to them. It is difficult to determine how important a need is to an individual or group of individuals. Needs also change over time, and it is difficult to monitor this.

Perceptions (image): How the consumer sees the organization, or the "sum of the beliefs, ideas and impressions about an object."[41]

Preferences: The value placed on a set of comparable objects.[42] What makes a consumer choose a particular product, given a choice of two products of comparable qualities?

Satisfaction: The measure of how completely a given product served the purpose of meeting a consumer's need. This should be assessed from time to time and can be measured.

The third area of Market Analysis is the *marketing mix* or the actual design of the product. It is in this area that advertising, the most frequently perceived aspect of marketing, is developed. Classically, the marketing mix is described in terms of the four "Ps"—product (or service), price, place (distribution), and promotion. Each of the four "ps" is orchestrated differently for each of the segments of a target market. Again, each aspect of the marketing mix is the result of a series of decisions arrived at through study of the market audit, the structural analysis, the consumer analysis, and those aspects of the target market that make it unique.

Product: ". . . any complex of tangible and intangible attributes that might be offered to a market to satisfy a want or need; it can cover goods, services, organizations, persons, places, and ideas. It is useful

to distinguish between the tangible product, which takes a physical view of the actual product and its attributes, the core product, which represents the essential utility behind the tangible product and all the benefits and costs associated with obtaining and consuming it."[43]

Price: ". . . . includes the understanding people have about how to go about doing business with you and the circumstances under which they can avail themselves of your product. Price is the flip side of product. The financial, physical, and psychological costs to people of doing business with you."[44]

Place (Distribution): ". . . . how the organization plans to make its products and services available and accessible to customers."[45] "The hours, location, eligibility rules, referrals, or admission arrangements that make it possible, easy, or difficult for markets to use your product."[46]

Promotion: ". . . encompasses all the tools in the marketing mix whose major role is persuasive communication."[47] It is ". . . . what and how you inform markets about your product, place, and price."[48]

It is important to differentiate between the types of promotion. Kotler has described five groups of promotional tools:

Advertising: Any paid form of nonpersonal presentation and promotion of ideas, goods, or services by an identified sponsor

Publicity: Nonpersonal stimulation of demand for a product, service, or business unit by planting commercially significant news about it in a published medium or obtaining favorable presentation upon radio, television, or stage that is not paid for by the sponsor

Personal Contact: Oral presentation in a conversation with one or more prospective purchasers for the purpose of making sales or building goodwill.

Incentives: Items of financial values added to an offer to encourage some overt behavioral response

Atmospheric: Efforts to design a place of purchase or consumption in a way calculated to create specific cognition or emotional effects in buyers or consumers.[49]

The promotional tools are well explained in the definitions. One of the tools, advertising, is particularly controversial in the health care environment. Advertising was seldom used in health care fields until the mid-1970s, and in fact was expressly prohibited by the code of ethics of the American Medical Association (AMA). It is currently accessible to occupational therapists as described in the *Principles of Occupational Therapy Ethics*.[50] (See Appendix B).

"Advertising by therapists under their professional title shall be in accordance with propriety and precedent in health professions. Guidelines: Occupational therapists may provide information to the public about available services through procedures established by the employing facility or contracting agency. If an occupational therapist provides an independent service, it is appropriate to advertise those services. The occupational therapist shall not use, or participate in the use of, any form of communication containing a false, fraudulent, misleading, deceptive, self-laudatory or unfair statement or claim. Testimonials or statements which promise a favorable result shall be avoided."

In 1977, *Guidelines on Advertising by Hospitals* were adopted by the American Hospital Association. These guidelines, though very general, represent the code of ethics in the area of advertising. The guidelines called for the following:
—Truthfulness/accuracy, no misleading information
—Avoidance of self-aggrandizement
—No quality comparisons with others
—No claim of prominence, superiority, bigness
—No promotion of individual professionals

It recognized that advertising, bound by such strictures, was perfectly appropriate in such areas as:
—Informing the public about services available, office hours, and so forth
—Educating the public regarding health, including promoting the institution's health education efforts
—Accounting to the community for what you've done with its "trust," for example, annual reports
—Soliciting financial support for capital fund drives, but not political support in lobbying efforts
—Recruiting employees, perhaps even physicians for hospital-based positions.[51]

In 1975, the Federal Trade Commission filed suit against the American Medical Association, challenging the AMA's long-held ethical principle that prevented physicians "from generating business by advertising, price competition and competitive practices resulting in restraint of trade."[52] In 1980, the Federal Court of Appeals ruled that the AMA's "Ethical Constraints had an anticompetitive effect."[53] The Supreme Court upheld this decision in 1982.

Advertising for health care will be closely watched by the Federal Trade Commission as it is an important area of public interest, especially the reporting of tests and surveys.[54]

Marketing and Decisionmaking

Mac Stravic describes three major outputs of market audit or analysis as identification of (1) problem, (2) threat, and (3) opportunities. He defines the outputs as follows:

—"*Problem:* A current situation or trend that, unless changed, will damage the organization's mission or health significantly (if it hasn't already). A problem implies the necessity of taking action to alter deliberately what the future would be without your intervention.
—*Threat:* A potential situation the occurrence of which is by no means certain, but is of sufficient likelihood to justify your concern. A threat implies the necessity of your intervention to *avoid* a change that otherwise might occur.
—*Opportunity:* A potential situation the occurrence of which is by no means certain, but is of sufficient attractiveness to you to justify taking advantage of it. An opportunity implies the desirability of your intervention to achieve a change that will benefit your community, your organization, and it is hoped, both."[55]

The component common to all three outputs is a need to change. A thorough review of the results of market research allows the organization to determine what it is doing well and where there is a need to change. Each of the three outputs requires a different kind of strategy.

Problem. When dealing with a situation where a change is imperative, it is first necessary to thoroughly evaluate the likely causes of the problem. The options for decision making must be carefully studied in order to successfully intervene in a problem situation.

Threat. Three important questions should be answered before developing a strategy to deal with a situation which is to be avoided:
1. What is the likelihood of the threat becoming a reality?
2. What would be the impact of the threat on the organization's mission or viability?
3. Can the organization successfully avoid or accommodate the threatened event if it occurs?

Once these questions have been answered, the next question becomes whether action is necessary at all.

Opportunities: Just as a problem will necessitate change, so too does an opportunity. Mac Stravic describes three types of typical market opportunities:
1. Getting more customers for your present services or opening up new markets for current products
2. Getting current customers to use new services or new products for existing markets
3. Attracting new customers for new services or new products for new markets.[56]

Problems, threats, and opportunities may appear in all five areas of the market audit, or in any combination of the five (impact, behavior, causes, environment, or competition).

Market research clearly points out an organization's strengths and weaknesses. It is then possible by using marketing information to make sound decisions regarding the viability of a program or service—particularly in the assessment of an underutilized service. "Underutilized services represent two sorts of market liabilities. First they indicate that the hospital is not satisfying sufficient numbers of physicians and patients regarding its quality, cost, or accessibility. And inadequate performance in any area is likely to have a halo effect and decrease the acceptance of other programs. Second, whatever resources the hospital is devoting to an unsuccessful program represent opportunity costs because the organization might be using them more effectively elsewhere."[57]

The occupational therapy manager would be wise to include market research as a step in program evaluation in order to assure maximum use of resources. While some aspects of market research are beyond the resources of the occupational therapy manager, access to this information should be available to some degree through the institution or organization.

This chapter is intended to provide a brief overview of a complex system of marketing as a tool for planning, analyzing, and decision making. Marketing in health care is a new and growing discipline in itself, which combines knowledge of health care, its environments, and analytic design, as well as study of their interactions.

References

1. Cooper, P. D., (ed.): Health Care Marketing: Issues and Trends, Aspen Systems Corporation, Germantown, Maryland, 1979, p. 9.
2. Kotler, P.: Marketing for Nonprofit Organizations, Englewood Cliffs, Prentice Hall, Inc., 1975, pp. 52, 53.
3. Cooper, P. D., Ph.D., and Maxwell, R. B. III: Marketing: Entry Points and Pitfalls. Hospital and Health Services Administration, 24(3):34–53, Summer, 1979, p. 38.
4. Cooper, p. 12.
5. Berkowitz, E. N., and Flexner, W. A.: The Marketing Audit: A Tool for Health Service Organizations. Health Care Management Review, 3(4):Fall, 1978, pp. 52, 53.
6. Kotler, P., and Flatman, G.: Social Marketing: An Approach to Planned Social Change. Journal of Marketing, 35(7):3, July, 1971.
7. Kotler, Marketing for Nonprofit Organizations, p. 34.
8. Ibid., p. 5.
9. Ibid., p. 5.
10. Ibid., p. 13.
11. Cooper and Maxwell, p. 34.
12. Mac Stravic, R. E. S., Market Research in Ambulatory Care. Journal Ambulatory Care Management, 4(2):33–40, May, 1981, p. 34.
13. Kotler, Marketing for Nonprofit Organizations, p. 24.
14. Ibid., p. 31.
15. Ibid., p. 31.
16. Blau, P. M., and Scott, W. R.: Formal Organizations, San Francisco: Chandler, 1962.
17. Kotler, Marketing for Nonprofit Organizations, p. 34.
18. Mac Stravic, p. 34.
19. Berkowitz and Flexner, p. 53.
20. Mac Stravic, R. E. S., Marketing by Objectives, Aspen Systems Corporation, Germantown, Md., 1980, p. 8.
21. Ibid., pp. 3, 4.
22. Ibid., p. 10.
23. Ibid., p. 4.
24. Berkowitz and Flexner, p. 53.
25. Ibid., p. 54.
26. Mac Stravic: Objectives, pp. 18, 19.
27. Berkowitz and Flexner, p. 55.
28. Ibid., p. 55.
29. Ibid., p. 56.
30. Ibid., pp. 55.
31. Ibid., p. 56.
32. Ibid., p. 56.
33. Sapienza, A. M., and Kahn, R. A.: Impacting the Product: Staff, Hospital Topics, 58(5):24–7, Sept.–Oct., 1980, p. 24.
34. Mac Stravic, p. 34.
35. Kotler, Marketing for Nonprofit Organizations, p. 95.
36. Ibid., p. 99.
37. Ibid., p. 101.
38. Mac Stravic, Objectives, p. 7.
39. Lauback, P. B., D.B.A., Rand, R. L.A.B.., and Lauback, P.: Marketing Management for Health Care Executives, Seminar of the American College of Hospital Administrators, Wichita, KS, May 19–21, 1980.
40. Kotler, p. 123–159.
41. Ibid., p. 157.
42. Ibid., p. 142.
43. Ibid., p. 174.
44. Mac Stravic, Objectives, p. 11.
45. Kotler, p. 190.
46. Mac Stravic: Objectives, p. 73.
47. Kotler, p. 201.
48. Mac Stravic: Objectives, p. 73.
49. Kotler, p. 201–202.
50. Principles of Occupational Therapy Ethics, adopted April, 1977, Revised, April, 1980, American Occupational Therapy Association, 1383 Piccard Drive, Rockville, Md., 20850.
51. Mac Stravic: Objectives, p. 154.
52. Ibid., p. 154.
53. O'Brien, J. P., Esq.: Council to American Hospital Association, remarks to Academy of Health Care Marketing, Chicago, Ill., April 15, 1981.
54. Ibid.
55. Mac Stravic: Objectives, p. 35.
56. Ibid., p. 41.
57. Ibid., p. 65.

Suggested Readings

Mac Stravic, R. E. S.: The Health Care Market Audit. Hospital Progress, October, 1978.

Reinhardt, V. E.: Table Manners at the Health Care Feast, National Journal, May, 1981, p. 855–61.

Flexner, W. A., Berkowitz, E. N.: Marketing Research in Health Services Planning: A Model. Public Health Rep. 94(6):503–13, Nov., Dec., 1979.

Stuehler, G. Jr., How Hospital Marketing and Planning Relate. Hospitals, 54(9):96–99, 1980.

Galvagni, W.: Hospitals Diversify to Thrive in a Competitive Environment. Hospitals, 55(7):131–2, 134–6, 1981.

Melum, M. M.: Hospitals Must Change, Control is the Issue. Hospitals, 54(5):67–72, 1980.

CHAPTER 43

Quality Assurance— Improving Therapy Outcomes

Patricia C. Ostrow

Patient well-being and the quality of health care are assumed by most to be interrelated. Few people are aware, however, that the viability of the profession is also tied to the quality-of-care issue. This chapter will look at major factors and issues related to quality of health care to see how they influence patient outcomes and professional growth. An overview such as this also lays the foundation for study of specific quality assurance methodologies, detailed elsewhere, such as health accounting and retrospective chart audit, and provides a guide to good quality assurance study topics.[1,2]

Quality Assurance— An Element of Professional Competence

Accreditation of schools, certification of therapists, licensure, and standards for service delivery—are these enough to ensure that a health care practitioner will provide quality care? Some practitioners believe they are, but many assert that a crucial, and often neglected, element in the quest for quality is a process for clinicians to assess actual service delivery and

health care outcomes, be they intermediate or long-range. Quality assurance fills this need. It is a method of studying health care to improve its impact.

Assessing and improving the quality of services are essential components of health care. They should be a part of the treatment process itself. Each therapist carries that responsibility for her or his clients. It is as important as evaluating the individual patient before selecting treatment goals. Occupational therapy is committed to outcome-oriented quality review studies; they are specifically mentioned in the *Standards of Practice* approved by the Representative Assembly of the American Occupational Therapy Association in the Spring of 1978. The evaluation of health care for aggregates of patients with similar problems provides invaluable information to guide a therapist's pursuit of optimal benefits for each client. If, for example, 75% of the patients given ADL training do not successfully use the skills they learned in the hospital, then the treatment approach for individual clients needs modification.

In the last decade, as health care costs became a major social concern, quality assurance was required by law—health care processes and outcomes became the focus of systematic data collection. Legislators, consumers and health care practitioners realized that they must find ways to reduce costs and improve quality. The goals were to eliminate unnecessary or ineffective services, and provide feedback information that would enhance professional growth and refine administrative processes.

Because Congress required it, utilization review came into being. It was conducted to measure the necessity for a service, the efficiency of a service, and whether care was given at the least expensive level commensurate with patient needs (for instance, nursing home vs. acute care). Lengths of hospital stays were averaged for various diagnostic conditions, and patterns of hospital utilization analyzed. Stroke care may be twice as long in one facility as in another. Why? Were the outcomes significantly different? Were the patients significantly different so that one group had more secondary complications? These are the questions for which answers are sought in order to identify under-utilization or over-utilization.

Quality assurance was another type of data collection that became popular in the decade between 1970 and 1980 because it was required by Congress. Quality assurance programs identified problems in health care service delivery and remedied them. Achievable benefits *not* achieved are the focus of quality assurance. Utilization review was initially a separate function from quality assurance. Now both are frequently considered to be part of a quality assurance program.

The basic steps in a quality assurance study are directly comparable to the steps a therapist follows to resolve a patient's problems:

Stage 1, *Identify* significant problems in overall patient care and decide which have the highest priority (comparable to the initial interview of the patient to identify present problems)

Stage 2, *Measure* the problem to confirm and clarify its nature (comparable to specific patient assessments, such as of ADL skills or range of motion, which describe the degree of handicap)

Stage 3, *Improvement planning* (comparable to the treatment plan)

Stage 4, *Improvement action* (parallel to providing treatment)

Stage 5, *Reassessment* (similar to the predischarge assessment to see if the patient treatment plan was effective)

Quality of Care Defined

The quest for quality in health care services is begun by understanding the meaning of quality. Avedis Donabedian, a well-known theorist in health care, has classified the elements of quality care into structure, process, and outcome. He defined the terms as follows:

Structure—the properties of the resources used to provide care, such as physical facilities, equipment, qualified personnel, and the manner in which these resources are organized

Process—the treatment management activities of health care professionals, such as clinical assessment, treatment, and preventive care, as well as documentation, and other related activities

Outcome—the results, to a significant degree, of process and structure in terms of improved health, restored or improved physical and social functioning, and patient satisfaction[3]

A few examples may clarify his terms. One would assess the *structure* of an occupational therapy department by asking questions about the adequacy of space for the number of patients treated, proper certification and licensure of therapists, and the potential hazards equipment may present. *Process* could be evaluated by asking if there was a complete evaluation of the patients' abilities and disabilities as well as patients' goals before a treatment plan was developed, whether the treatment followed the accepted format, and so forth. *Outcome* could be assessed by measuring health care benefits in an aggregate of patients with the same problem or diagnosis when the staff feels that reasonable treatment goals are not being met. There are numerous intermediate outcomes during a hospital stay, as well as discharge outcomes and long-range outcomes to consider.

As a result of this classification system, polarized opinions have developed about the merits of process or outcome elements in quality assurance studies. Donabedian believes that they are both necessary for quality care assessment.[4] From a cost-effective point of view, it seems logical to look at outcomes first. If they do not meet the therapists' standards, then the treatment processes judged to be related to the below-par outcomes must be examined.

The Role of Peers

As early as 1933, it was observed that a decision about quality is based on the standards one has, and that standards may vary from person to person, or place to place. It was agreed that quality of care assessment must rest on the judgement of peers. "Good medical care is the kind of medicine practiced and taught by the recognized leaders of the medical field at a given period of social, cultural and professional development in a community or population group."[5] Perhaps the term "peer review" stemmed from this concept of quality care. Today, peer review is a term with a rich variety of connotations. It is used as an umbrella covering all forms of quality review, which include peer judgements, whether or not the standards for determination of quality are written out before the assessment in an explicit, objective, measurable form. (Quality assurance usually refers to later methodologies that rely on measurable standards.)

Enlarging the Concept

The concept of quality health care was enlarged in 1967 beyond the processes performed by recognized leaders, to emphasize ". . . diagnosis and therapy, both preventative and curative, based on the best knowledge available from science and humanities; and which eventuates in the least morbidity and mortality in the population."[6] In this quote equal emphasis was given to treatment processes and beneficial outcomes. Scientific data as the basis for treatment is an important addition to the understanding of quality.

Another definition of quality, offered in 1975, shows the interplay between technical knowledge or skill and the "art of care", or the ability of the health care practitioner to relate to the client and his or her needs: "Quality of health care is equal to technical care plus the art of care . . ."[7] The art of care here includes patient satisfaction with the milieu, the treatment, communication, and the provider–patient relationship. In this description of quality, random error is also considered.

Balancing Risks and Benefits

A book by Donabedian, published in 1980, is devoted to the definition of quality. He begins his discourse by posing the following: quality of care is ". . . that kind of care which is expected to maximize . . . patient welfare after one has taken account of the balance of gains and losses (health benefits and risks) that attend the process of care in all its parts".[8] The quantity of health care and its monetary costs are inextricably related to quality. Access to care, sufficient care to achieve results, inefficient and unnecessary care all become important, assessable elements of quality. Providing care when there is no expectation of benefit reduces the welfare of both the individual and society itself, because it is an improper use of resources. It deprives the client of time and money, and it robs society of the opportunity to provide care to others who may benefit.

Donabedian suggests the cost of care should be added to the risk as ". . . an unwanted consequence of the provision of care . . ."[9] Considering health care costs in this fashion, he says, allows a more efficient balancing of expected benefits and losses when planning treatment or assessing quality.

Donabedian's description of quality is expanded when he considers how health goals and treatment interventions will be selected. One method is "absolutist": the health care practitioners, as the experts, decide on appropriate health goals and the methods to achieve them. It is a technological decision based on the state of the science and the skill of the professional in applying the science. An "individualistic" alternative for selecting the health goals and treatment plan argues that the client must help select the objectives of care and, by placing his or her values on the benefits and risks of alternate strategies of treatment, share in management decisions. Many clients prefer that these choices be made by the relevant health care practitioner. In that case, the professional is responsible for ascertaining the values of the client. The impact on the client of health care costs thus becomes a necessary consideration in management decisions. Finally, there is a "societal" approach to selection of treatment management decisions. Quality of care in that case could be assessed on the basis of societal health rather than individual welfare. ". . . Quality is the degree to which preventable deaths, preventable functional impairment, and preventable suffering within a defined population are minimized over time."[10]

Efficacy, Effectiveness and Efficiency

Finally, the understanding of quality can be fully rounded out with three terms: efficacy, effectiveness and efficiency. John W. Williamson, professor in Health Services Administration at Johns Hopkins University, calls these the ". . . classic evaluation indicators . . . [they] may well provide the foundation for a more successful approach to developing future quality assurance systems."[11] His definitions for these terms are as follows:

"Efficacy: The extent to which a health care intervention can be shown to be beneficial under optimal conditions of care (such as clinical research).

Effectiveness: The extent to which benefits achievable under optimal conditions of care are actually achieved in clinical practice.

Efficiency: The proportion of total cost (for instance, money, scarce resources, and time) that can be related to actual benefits achieved."[12]

He suggests these definitions because earlier ones have overlapped in meaning and caused confusion. He proposes that quality assurance, as an evaluation study, is a measure of effectiveness; and clinical research, a measure of efficacy. Too often, hazy thinking on these ideas ruins the intent of a quality assurance study when a cause and effect problem (efficacy) will be tackled instead of an effectiveness measure.

Williamson's concept of efficiency echoes Donabedian's concern with cost of care. His definition of efficacy expands the idea of technical knowledge beyond that of the practitioner to the state of the science itself and thus broadens the source of standards for outcomes of care, combining peer judgements with the literature of the field, particularly the hard scientific data on the cause and effect relationship between treatment and outcome. Quality assurance is the interface between clinical research and clinical practice. Williamson and others note the lack of efficacy data, that is, knowledge in the health care field about the causal relationships between treatment variables and patient status.[13,14] In the absence of efficacy data, one can use the consensus opinion of professionals expressed in explicit measurable standards. For Williamson, the assessment of quality care begins with a simple question: In an optimal clinical situation, treatment will accomplish specified results for a particular health problem; are we meeting that achievable goal in this facility?

Application of the Concept of Quality to Health Care

Understanding the issues and factors related to optimal quality in health care assists the professional in two ways:
1. It suggests the areas on which to focus continual review of care for correctable problems
2. It sets forth standards against which to assess care

Applying the idea that cost is one of the risks or losses a practitioner must balance against potential improvements, one approaches current pressures to improve therapists' productivity in a new light. Increasing the number of patients treated without monitoring the outcome raises the likelihood that individuals who do *not* benefit from services will receive them. The therapist should balance productivity drives, which may receive positive reinforcement because they increase hospital income, with her or his knowledge of expected treatment benefits as revealed in research or, in the absence of research, as based on the consensus opinion of professionals. Quality assurance studies can aid the clinician in these judgments by demonstrating that the expected end results are being achieved. Quality assurance studies are a necessary corollary to productivity drives.

A therapist should consider costs when planning treatment. Many practitioners provide services completely unaware of the total bill for the patient. "Insurance pays for it," is a usual attitude, but insurance runs out. A $100,000 policy can be depleted quite easily in eight years. Societal costs must also be taken into account. How to achieve the treatment goal in the most efficient manner is the responsibility of the professional and an excellent quality assurance topic, which can increase therapist productivity in a positive way.

The profession cannot ignore the seriousness of the financial issue. Health care costs have reached crisis proportions: federal expenses, alone, for health care jumped from $4 billion in 1965 to approximately $59 billion in 1980, with total health care costs more than three times as great.[15] These figures are far ahead of inflationary trends. With escalating health expenses seen as fueling an inflation that endangers the society, third party carriers seek to curb utilization of health services. They want to avoid reimbursement of services if the outcomes are questionable or insignificant—or if the treatments are held to be unnecessary. Hysterectomies, tonsillectomies, intermittent positive pressure breathing, and diversional activities are examples of services that have been under scrutiny from third party carriers in the past decade.

To improve the quality of care, it is the responsibility of the profession at the national, state, and individual level to maintain access to occupational therapy services for those patients who significantly benefit from them. Access can be impeded not only by the patient's limited finances, but by limitations in coverage by health insurance programs such as Medicare, Medicaid, Blue Cross, and Blue Shield.

Documentation is an essential weapon in the battle for adequate coverage of occupational therapy. Consider the likelihood of reimbursement, at $50 per hour, for the following treatment described in this way: "Three home visits by the occupational therapist for Mrs. Jones. Potholders were made to improve manual dexterity." Payment for such treatment is likely to be denied. If the therapist says, "Patient participated in an activity providing resistance to finger and thumb flexors to strengthen grasp in both hands. When grasp improves, independent dressing will be achievable," then reimbursement is more likely. The clarity of documentation and the likelihood of coverage would be further served if the therapist noted why this patient was a good candidate for muscle strengthening and how soon results were expected. If the therapist cannot succinctly identify these factors, it is questionable if the patient *should* be making potholders with the therapist at $50 per hour.

Quality assurance studies are of value to help therapists become aware of the outcomes related to a service program. Do stroke patients, for example, achieve the expected improved dexterity, strength, or ADL skill if given potholders to make? That could be assessed in a quality assurance study.

Reimbursement decisions are not always made on a case-by-case assessment unless it is an area under special scrutiny; therefore, the generally held opinion of third party payers and physicians about occupational therapy becomes crucial to insurance coverage. Quality assurance studies reported within the health care facility and in national professional journals build understanding of the positive impact of occupational therapy services, and the professional commitment to quality care. As the health dollar shrinks, reimbursement and utilization will be influenced by the profession's ability to show that significant patient outcomes are reasonably related to that service.

Summary

Many aspects of quality, its assessment, and its improvement have been considered. In the earlier part of the 20th century, quality was thought to be most easily achieved by imitating experts. Standard treatment processes used by recognized leaders and teachers were the guide to quality. A new dimension was later added: beneficial outcomes. The knowledge and skill of the provider and the state of the science, as well as the rapport between provider and client, were recognized as valuable elements of quality. Two names stand out in the quality assurance field in the 1970s: Donabedian and Williamson. Donabedian defined quality care as management reflecting consideration of, and proper balance in, health risks and health benefits.[16] Under-utilization, over-utilization, access to care, management style, and health care costs become critical factors in quality health care. Williamson synthesized his concept of quality into three elements: efficacy, effectiveness and efficiency. The foregoing chapter and the factors related to quality care reveal a wide and varied range of elements essential to optimal health care. Familiarity with these factors and skill in conducting quality assurance studies provide therapists with useful tools to improve the beneficial impact of occupational therapy, enhance their own professional development, and increase appropriate utilization and reimbursement of their services. Step-by-step guides for conducting a quality assurance study are available for both beginners and those with experience.[17,18]

Information about the outcome of treatment for aggregates of patients with similar problems, as measured in quality assurance studies, is probably one of the best ways for a clinician to guide therapeutic efforts that successfully overcome specific handicaps. Quality assurance also provides data that will stimulate the therapists' own selective reach for new information relevant to an improved treatment program.

The three elements of excellence—efficacy, effectiveness and efficiency—summarize the issues in quality care. They are essential if health care professionals are to meet society's needs for improved health as well as society's demand for reduced health care expenditures. Clearly, outcome-oriented quality assurance studies should be an integral part of every clinician's activities.

References

1. Williamson, J. W., Ostrow, P. C., and Braswell, H. R.: Health Accounting for Quality Assurance: A Manual for Assessing and Improving Outcomes of Care. American Occupational Therapy Association, Inc. 1981.
2. Patient Care Evaluation in Action: An Audit Manual for Occupational Therapists. American Occupational Therapy Association, Inc. 1978.
3. Donabedian, A.: A Guide to Medical Care Administration Volume II: Medical Care Appraisal—Quality and Utilization. New York (now Washington, DC), American Public Health Association, 1969, pp. 2–3.
4. Donabedian, A.: The Definition of Quality and Approaches to Its Assessment. Ann Arbor, MI: Health Administration Press, 1980, p. 119.
5. Lee, R. I., and Jones, L. W.: The Fundamentals of Good Medical Care. Publications of the Committee on the Costs of Medical Care, No. 22. Chicago: Chicago University Press, 1933, p. 302.
6. Payne, B. C.: Continued Evolution of a System of Medical Care Appraisal. JAMA, 201:128–130, 1967.
7. Donabedian: The Definition of Quality, p. 28.
8. Ibid., pp. 5–6.
9. Ibid., p. 10.
10. Ellwood, P. M., O'Donoghue, P., McClure, W., Holley, R., Carlson, R. J., and Hoogberg, E.: Assuring the Quality of Health Care. Instudy, Minneapolis, 1974.
11. Williamson, J. W.: Assessing and Improving Health Care Outcomes. Cambridge, MA: Ballinger Publishing, 1978, p. 9.
12. Ibid., p. 10.
13. Williamson, J. W.: Improving Medical Practice and Health Care: A Bibliographic Guide to Information Management in Quality Assurance and Continuing Education. Cambridge, MA: Ballinger Publishing, 1977, p. 9.
14. Brook, R. H.: Quality of Care Assessment: A Comparison of Five Methods of Peer Review. DHEW Publication No. HRA-74-3100, Library of Congress Card No. 73-699243, July 1973, p. 21.
15. Enthoven, A. C.: Health Plan, Reading, MA: Addison-Wesley Publishing, 1980, p. 15.
16. Donabedian: The Definition of Quality and Approaches to Its Assessment, p. 119.
17. Williamson, et al: Health Accounting for Quality Assurance.
18. Ostrow, P. C. and Joe, B. E.: Quality Assurance Primer. American Occupational Therapy Association, Inc., 1982 (in press).

PART 8

Research

CHAPTER 44

The Occupational Therapist as a Researcher

Elizabeth J. Yerxa

A significant characteristic of professional persons is that they are able to work with a considerable degree of autonomy.[1] An example of such professional autonomy is the characteristic of being able to conceptualize, implement, evaluate and report the results of an occupational therapy research study. Occupational therapy researchers possess a high degree of autonomy. Being a researcher is an exciting new role for occupational therapists because it affords such opportunities to make creative and self-directed contributions to the quality of life for persons served by the profession through the generation of new knowledge.

In its quality of autonomy, the researcher role both represents and enhances occupational therapy's progress toward being a more fully developed profession. In exploring the researcher role in occupational therapy this chapter will discuss the nature of research, relationship of research to occupational therapy theory and practice, importance of theory, current status of occupational therapy research, characteristics of researchers who have published their work, content of research, comparison of current and past research efforts, research needs and how they might be met, the model of an occupational

therapy researcher, A. Jean Ayres, and ethical considerations in conducting research.

The Nature of Research

Alfred North Whitehead called research a "welcoming attitude toward change." Kerlinger had a much more formal definition: "Systematic, controlled, empirical and critical investigation of hypothetical propositions about the presumed relationships among natural phenomena."[2] "To see what everyone else has seen and to think what no one else has thought" is the research process according to Wandelt, a nursing researcher.[3] Whatever definition might be proposed, research is the process by which knowledge is developed, tested, and made public.

Relationship of Research to Theory and Practice

Occupational therapy is concerned with helping people. Occupational therapists make decisions which result in a goal being attained for another person, a goal which is perceived as "good" by the person and therapist together. The profession exists for clinical practice. All of occupational therapy knowledge flows from practice. It is generated from what each occupational therapist sees, hears, and feels while working with patients.

As occupational therapists observe, they begin to develop theories. Theories are statements that suggest relationships between the things seen so that they can be controlled, understood, or explained.[4] Making the right things happen in predictable ways is the gift received from theory. When theoretical statements have been formulated, they are tested out in the real world to see if, in fact, they do enable occupational therapists to predict and control phenomena. That phase of the process is *research*, and the goal is to determine to what degree data from the senses confirm or fail to confirm the theoretical statements. Knowledge is developed in this way—knowledge that flows back into practice so that a better job can be done. Practice to theory to research and back to practice is the unending cycle that generates knowledge.

The Importance of Theory

The abstract statements that constitute theories are the source of life for practice and research, for they enable generalizations to be made from direct experience in order to control future events. Imagine a world without theory. Practice would have to be based on trial and error or tradition or intuition. Since there would be no abstract conceptualization, there would be no knowledge. If there were no knowledge, universities could be closed and persons taught all that they need to know by apprenticeship. However, there would be no way to store knowledge or test it or improve upon it. There would be no sense of understanding of how and why things happen, a sense of understanding that can only be conveyed by theory.[5] If there were no sense of understanding, then there would be no way of expanding or improving practice nor any way to assure occupational therapists that what they did for the patients was truly "good."

As has been seen, theories consist of statements that relate concepts. A concept is a way of classifying the world according to some criterion: small, medium, and large are concepts as are play, work, and rest, or apraxia, tactile defensiveness, and form perception. Concepts are the bricks from which theory is constructed. Occupational therapy concepts are often either unclearly defined conceptually or not defined at all. Thus, it is extremely difficult to agree upon their meanings. Occupational therapy knowledge has very few concepts that have operational definitions, that is, definitions that will allow the concept to be

applied or tested in the real world. As one scientist put it, the clearest ideas are the ones that are the easiest to prove false.[6] Occupational therapy needs clear definitions with agreed upon meanings, which can be tested in the real world, in order to determine not only what is true but what is false.

Typologies are classification systems based upon sets of concepts. Ayres' sensory integrative syndromes constitute a sensory integrative dysfunction typology. The few other typologies that have been published are not generally useful for the purposes of science since the concepts employed are often vague and unclear. Typologies allow theoretical statements that relate concepts to be generated. For example, "if a patient has apraxia, then he will have difficulty imitating postures" is a theoretical statement relating the concept of apraxia to the concept of imitating postures, a theoretical statement using the sensory integration typology. A collection of such statements constitutes a theory.

In occupational therapy today, very few theories exist that allow knowledge to be developed and tested. Thus, little basis is available for scientifically predicting, controlling, or even explaining what occurs in practice. Little confidence can be held in the theories that do exist, since very little data support the statements constituting the theory. Occupational therapy practice, for the most part, is based upon tradition and untested hypotheses.

It is proposed that occupational therapy's lack of research activity is directly related to its lack of theory and, paradoxically, that its lack of theory is directly related to the profession's lack of research. What does exist is clinical practice, standing alone, teeming with opportunities to observe, to theorize, and to conduct research in concrete settings.

Current Status of Research in Occupational Therapy

Research in occupational therapy is in its infancy. Many leaders in the profession emphasize that research should have the highest priority in order to develop the knowledge base of the profession.[7] But what, in fact, is being done?

In 1974 a paper was presented at the World Federation of Occupational Therapy Conference in Vancouver. It was titled, "Occupational Therapy Research in 1974: Models of Enlightenment."[8] All papers published in the *American Journal of Occupational Therapy* for the year 1973 were surveyed with the following findings: out of a total of 57 articles, 25 or 44% were concerned with research. Of these 25, 17 employed descriptive research; that is, were concerned with describing selected characteristics of a sample with no attempt to manipulate variables; 1

was philosophical, that is, it discussed the *need* for research; and the remaining 7 were experimental research, that is, involved the systematic and controlled manipulation of variables in order to test hypotheses.

Three of these experimental studies concerned the outcomes or results of occupational therapy and only two of these (or 3% of the total papers) employed statistical tools. The author concluded that "Since the editorial board of the *Journal* is eager to publish research reports which will help substantiate the validity of the profession, we can only conclude that scientific research is rare in occupational therapy at present."[9]

In preparation for writing this chapter, a similar survey was conducted, this time assessing the research content of the *American Journal of Occupational Therapy* for the full calendar year of 1979. In 1979 the *Journal* was published monthly so that this sample was based upon a review of 12 issues, while the 1973 survey contained only 8 issues. Seventy-one papers were published in 1979 (excluding regular feature articles such as "Nationally Speaking"). Of these, 31 or 44% concerned research. Twenty-six or 37% of all the papers reported descriptive research, none was philosophical, one provided education about the research process, and four or 6% were experimental with two of these or 3% of all the papers assessing the effects or outcomes of occupational therapy.

Comparing the quantity and categories of research papers between 1973 and 1979, one is struck by the fact that the percentages of research papers published and the percentages within each category, although six years apart, were almost identical. This finding becomes even more striking when recognizing that only eight issues were published in 1973. If a projection of 3.1 research papers per journal (based upon the average number published per issue in 1973) is extended to a 12-issue year, 1973 would have produced 37.5 research articles compared to only 31 for 1979. In interpreting this result, it is important to realize that six of the 1973 articles were part of the special series on "Research in Sensory-Integrative Development," which might have inflated the research productivity for 1973. However, taking all of these factors into account, based upon the comparison of these two periods, it appears that the quantity and type of research reported in the *Journal* has remained approximately the same with 44% of the papers published being research papers and the majority of these reporting descriptive surveys.

Researcher Characteristics

Author characteristics were assessed in order to determine the source of research productivity. In 1979, 77% of the papers were authored by persons with a Masters degree or above, while in 1973, only 52% of the authors held graduate degrees. The professional roles of authors also demonstrated a dramatic shift. In 1973 only 35% of the authors of research papers were academic faculty members, while in 1979, 58% of the authors came from academia. Thus a trend toward increasing research productivity among those with graduate degrees and faculty appointments might be occurring, perhaps in recognition of the "publish or perish" admonition in academia along with increasing awareness of the vital role of occupational therapy university faculty in generating knowledge.

Research Content

The content of the research papers reported in 1979 will now be looked at more closely. The largest number of papers dealt with characteristics of the disabled, followed by studies concerning occupational therapy education and those focusing on the characteristics of occupational therapy practice. The 12 remaining papers defied categorization, except that two concerned sensory integrative theory. It appears that a majority of research in 1979 was concerned with describing and operationalizing concepts that characterized those aspects of disabled persons that were considered particularly significant to occupational therapy.

The instrumentation, or the measuring tools, employed will now be analyzed. How many 1979 papers employed the use of new instruments designed to operationalize occupational therapy concepts? Seventeen or 24% of the total papers published reported developing a new instrument in order to gather data. Of these 17, only 3 or 18% of the total using new instruments, mentioned procedures designed to estimate their reliability. No papers reported the development of an instrument for use primarily as a research tool, and only one reported the formulation of a new clinical instrument.

Thus, if 1979 is a valid example, it appears that the quantity and type of occupational therapy research have not changed much since 1973. However, more persons with graduate degrees and academic appointments are producing the research. A paucity of papers concerned with the development of research instruments exists. The majority of papers that employed new instruments for data gathering failed to establish reliability for those instruments.

My conclusion about research in occupational therapy since 1973 is different now from what it was then. Occupational therapy research today is highly variable in content, represents a myriad of fragmented theoretical perspectives, is primarily descriptive, and has an urgent need for valid and reliable instruments that operationalize theoretical concepts.

Research Needed

Much of the research that has been done in occupational therapy thus far is descriptive of client characteristics, occupational therapist characteristics, or is concerned with the outcomes of occupational therapy education. Many political and economic pressures are being exerted both from within and outside of the profession for occupational therapy to "prove" its efficacy. Occupational therapy is not alone in experiencing these pressures, since all of the health professions are expected to be accountable in delivering the services they say they are delivering.[10] The current state of research in occupational therapy represents a stage in the normal evolution of professional knowledge which proceeds from the intuitive practice of an untested art to the logically rigorous practice of a science. As will be seen below, *descriptive* rather than experimental research appears to be the appropriate type of research for the development of occupational therapy knowledge at its current state of development. Where should the occupational therapy researcher begin?

Occupational therapists should take a good, hard look at what they are doing. Clinical observation is the beginning of all research. Some scientists suggest that all theory begins with *criticism,* which doesn't stop at criticism but goes on to identify the components of the criticized situation and to suggest solutions or better ways of doing things.[11] Occupational therapy research needs more in-depth case studies, which are carefully described and then published. An individual patient, looked at precisely, can suggest significant variables to be isolated, and generate innumerable questions to be tested in later studies involving groups. The careful observation of individuals can lead researchers to classify important characteristics, give the characteristics names, and define, in words and in operations, what those concepts mean. Later they can be used in typologies to generate questions about whole groups of persons and can then be tested by gathering and analyzing data. *All research begins with giving things names.*

Description is the mother of theory. Unfortunately, occupational therapists sometimes are given the impression that only experimental research is "true" and valuable research (as was my belief in 1974). By "experimental" is meant research that manipulates variables (causes) to produce a predetermined outcome (effect). Such research tests the effects of occupational therapy; for instance, study of the effects of a play intervention program on the developmental skills of children with mental retardation is an example of experimental research.

In my opinion, occupational therapy concepts generally are so nonspecific that the profession needs to give far greater emphasis to descriptive research than to experimental research at this stage of knowledge development. Descriptive research describes what is in the here and now. It enables researchers to objectively catalogue the important characteristics of reality, as seen from the unique perspective of an occupational therapist. Researchers cannot begin to manipulate variables until the important variables in question have been clearly defined and described. Some examples of descriptive research possibilities, which could contribute knowledge development, are the following:

Who are occupational therapy's patients? What characteristics do these patients have that are particularly pertinent to occupational therapy's perspective of human beings as self-directed, active organisms seeking meaning through activity? What is the nature of occupational therapy practice? What sort of intervention is used, with what kinds of patients, under what conditions? For example, Bissell and Mailloux published the results of such a study describing the frequency and extent of the use of crafts by occupational therapists working with patients who have physical disabilities.[12]

How do patients respond to the occupational therapy process and setting? What do they perceive as their need for occupational therapy services? Under what conditions do occupational therapists provide service, that is, one to one, in groups, daily, monthly? Who provides it, OTRs, COTAs? When is it provided in relation to the onset of pathology? Where is it provided? What sorts of evaluation methods are used? What do they show about specific groups of patients? To what extent are patients satisfied with the occupational therapy service they receive? Over time, to what extent do patients maintain the status they had achieved when occupational therapy services were terminated?

What can be learned about so-called "normal" persons? How do happy, productive persons use their time engaging in everyday activity? How much time do "normal" persons spend on self-maintenance, leisure, work? What about retired persons? What is a "balanced" life, and how is it related to other measures of health or healthfulness? These descriptions would contribute knowledge not only to occupational *therapy,* but to a science of human *occupation* and how it relates to health. Both are needed.

Descriptive research enables researchers to isolate variables of interest as abstract concepts, such as community adjustment, independence in self-maintenance activities, and solitary play. Once these concepts have been identified, they need to be operationalized, that is, defined in measurable terms. When that has been done, instruments can be constructed that can be used to measure characteristics of groups of people so that researchers can begin to make comparisons.

There is a pervasive need to develop and test reliable and valid occupational therapy instruments, for the majority of instruments that the profession has are designed for clinical use, not for research. It is not known whether they test what they say they test, nor is it known whether they measure phenomena consistently. Thus they are of little use for knowledge development. Clinical instruments may be refined into research instruments, but instruments that operationalize the concepts constituting occupational therapy theories are also needed. As happened with sensory integrative theory, when standardized tests are available, torrents of research will burst forth utilizing them to evaluate a theory.

Test development and standardization are complex and sophisticated processes, and it is my belief that the profession will not have the instruments it desperately needs until students in occupational therapy doctoral programs produce them. At any rate, until researchers define and measure concepts, the profession will not be able to develop and test occupational therapy knowledge or make it public. Instruments are needed that will accurately measure work behavior, play, leisure pursuits, habits, skills, body scheme, attitudes, precision of motor control, social role behaviors, responses to crafts, goal setting, and successful community adjustment, to name a few.

Once concepts have been defined, conceptually and operationally, on the basis of observation and description, relationships between concepts can be explored. These relationships reflect associations rather than causation and are often expressed as correlations. Some examples of association are such relationships as self-care independence to self-esteem and employment, developmental delays to environmental bleakness, and play behavior to social skill development.

Only after occupational therapy concepts have been defined, operationalized, and related are researchers prepared to conduct studies which manipulate variables to produce both a predictable and "good" result, that is, experimental research which assesses the effects of occupational therapy. Until researchers define treatment as it is generated from a theory and develop valid and reliable ways of measuring outcomes with groups of people, the profession will not be ready to conduct the experimental or quasi-experimental research that it needs.

Meeting Research Needs

How can individual occupational therapists begin to contribute to knowledge development for the prac-

tice of occupational therapy? First, remember that all theory and research are generated from practice and begin with *observation*. Look at your patients and environments, yes, even yourselves with fresh and careful eyes, describing and recording what you see clearly.

Criticize what you see, but don't let yourself stop with criticism. Research and theory are generated when you are dissatisfied with what you are doing and care enough to think of ways to make things better. Theory is generated from events that frustrate and stump people.

Occupational therapy needs to treasure its young people and those who are new to the profession by helping them saturate themselves in its current knowledge, incomplete though it is, and by welcoming their criticism. Considerable evidence exists that the people who invent the truly new ideas or create new theories are usually new to a field and deeply immersed in it, without having preconceptions or vested interest in what is the true or right theory. They have nothing to give up or lose so they invent new theories to explain the same old reality that the rest of the profession has lived with for decades. It is comforting to know that these persons are usually bright people but not necessarily geniuses!

If occupational therapy is to develop and test a unique configuration of knowledge, much hard work needs to be done by dedicated and well-trained people. Think of the road, from observation in practice, to concepts, to definitions, to relational statements, to instruments to experiments. Who is going to do all of these things? Such an effort can best be accomplished by graduate students who work with knowledgeable faculty and clinicians. For this reason, the future potential for knowledge development in the field will only be attained when this profession makes the conscious decision to focus its graduate programs on the development of research competence for students and faculty. A consensus is needed for knowledge generation as well as a willingness to focus all of occupational therapy's graduate educational resources along with the rich intellectual resources of its young people on one goal, *knowledge* that enables occupational therapists to do the best for patients, whether they be persons with chronic schizophrenia, spinal cord injury, or mental retardation.

Occupational therapy researchers need to work closely with the clinicians who have the criticisms and frustrations and who also have access to the patients. This can be accomplished by developing consortia or formalized relationships between academic and clinical programs for the purpose of generating research. Such relationships can provide strong bonds in forging the link from practice to theory to research to practice, generating knowledge and improving the quality of practice simultaneously.

Model of an Occupational Therapy Researcher

Ayres provides a current model of an occupational therapy clinical researcher. In 1963, she published her first papers describing the discovery of a previously unidentified group of perceptual motor syndromes.[13] These syndromes had been identified through a painstaking period of clinical observation followed by conceptualization, descriptions, hypothesis formation, testing of the hypothetical observations in a controlled fashion, careful analysis of the data gathered, and finally the drawing of tentative conclusions about hypotheses. One occupational therapist plans a treatment program for an individual client; Ayres extended the thought process to apply to whole groups of individuals in a scientifically rigorous way. She presented her data for the scrutiny of the disinterested scientific community so that her observations could be tested and evaluated by others. Occupational therapy theory is developed and tested through this process. Isolated and meaningless facts must be interrelated and rendered meaningful in the fabric of a theory, just as isolated threads must be woven into the fabric of a garment to create a design. Each new experiment tests the strength of a theory and either supports its validity or fails to support it. Ayres developed and validated a battery of objective tests in order to evaluate her theory. At present, occupational therapy possesses few such standardized tests for theory testing. This lack of objective instrumentation for the measurement of change constitutes a significant barrier to occupational therapy research productivity.

Ayres serves as an example of an occupational therapist and researcher who was motivated by wanting to improve the lives of children who were handicapped by the inability to process and use sensorimotor information. Her long and sometimes arduous path toward developing theory began with simple clinical observation. Her interest in determining relationships between the clinical facts she discovered, so that they could be organized into a coherent whole, was based upon wanting to do a better job as an occupational therapist. The clinical researcher in occupational therapy obtains the reward of serving patients or clients in numbers far beyond those reached in a one-to-one clinical therapy program. The researcher also enjoys the excitement that comes from the discovery of new knowledge and the

pride that emanates from contributing to the future development of the profession.

Ethical Considerations

The clinical researcher must maintain a high level of consciousness of the ethics involved in protecting the rights of human subjects. All human beings who take part in occupational therapy research have the right to give or withhold their informed consent to participation in the project. Subjects need to know what, if any, risks could accrue to them, as well as any benefits to be obtained for themselves or humanity for participating in the research. They must be informed that they can withdraw from a project at any time without fear of reprisal. They need to be assured that privacy and anonymity will be preserved by the researcher.[14] Signed instruments of informed consent must be retained by the researcher as evidence of the subjects' willingness to participate in the research project.

Conclusion

For those who seek a career that requires a deep personal commitment and provides substantial rewards in the excitement of discovery and the generation of new knowledge, the role of occupational therapy researcher offers a career of unlimited growth along with the opportunity to become self-directed, pioneering, and a leader in determining the future direction of the profession.

References

1. Pavalko, R.: Sociology of Occupations and Professions. Itasca, IL: F.T. Peacock Publications, 1971, pp. 33–36.
2. Kerlinger, F.: Foundations of Behavioral Research. New York: Holt, Rinehart and Winston, 1967. p. 13.
3. Wandelt, M.: Guide for the Beginning Researcher. New York: Appleton-Century Crofts, 1970, p. 8.
4. Reynolds, P. D.: A Primer in Theory Construction. Indianapolis: Bobbs-Merrill, 1971, pp. 3–11.
5. Ibid. p. 7.
6. Ibid. p. 116.
7. Yerxa, E., and Gilfoyle, E.: AOTF Research Seminar. Am. J. Occup. Ther. 30:509–514, 1976.
8. Yerxa, E.: Occupational Therapy Research in 1974: Models of Enlightenment. Proceedings World Federation of Occupational Therapists, pp. 674–680, 1974.
9. Ibid. p. 675.
10. Somers, A.: Health Care in Transition. Hospital Research and Education Trust, Chicago, 1971, pp. 33–36.

11. Wandelt, M.: Guide for the Beginning Researcher. p. 9.
12. Bissell, J., and Mailloux, Z.: The use of crafts in occupational therapy for the physically disabled. Am. J. Occup. Ther. 35:369–374, 1981.
13. Ayres, A. J.: The Development of Perceptual-Motor Abilities: A Theoretical Basis for Treatment of Dysfunction. The Eleanor Clarke Slagle Lectures, American Occupational Therapy Association, Rockville, MD, 1973, pp 127–135.
14. Fox, D.: The Research Process in Education. New York: Holt, Rinehart and Winston, 1969 pp. 384–389.

APPENDICES

APPENDIX **A**
Occupational Therapy Definition for Purposes of Licensure*

Occupational therapy is the use of purposeful activity with individuals who are limited by physical injury or illness, psychosocial dysfunction, developmental or learning disabilities, poverty and cultural differences or aging process in order to maximize independence, prevent disability and maintain health. The practice encompasses evaluation, treatment and consultation. Specific occupational therapy services include: teaching daily living skills; developing perceptual-motor skills and sensory integrative functioning; developing play skills and prevocational and leisure capacities; designing, fabricating, or applying selected orthotic and prosthetic devices or selective adaptive equipment; using specifically designed crafts and exercises to enhance functional performance; administering and interpreting tests such as manual muscle and range of motion; and adapting environments for the handicapped. These services are provided individually, in groups, or through social systems.

* Adopted by the Representative Assembly, American Occupational Therapy Association, March 7, 1981. Published in 1981 Representative Assembly Minutes. Am. J. Occup. Ther. 35:798, 1981. Reprinted with permission of the American Occupational Therapy Association.

all

APPENDIX *B*
Principles of Occupational Therapy Ethics*

Preamble:

The American Occupational Therapy Association (AOTA) and its component members are committed to furthering man's ability to function fully within his total environment. To this end the occupational therapist renders service to clients in all stages of health and illness, to institutions, other professionals, colleagues, students and to the general public.

In furthering this commitment the American Occupational Therapy Association has established the Principles of Occupational Therapy Ethics. The Principles are intended for use by all occupational therapy personnel, including practitioners in all settings, administrators, educators, and students. Licensure laws and regulations should reflect and support these Principles which are intended to be action oriented, guiding and preventive rather than negative or merely disciplinary. The Principles, likewise, should influence the consulting, planning, and teaching of occupational therapists.

It should be noted that these Principles are intended only for internal use by the American Occupational Therapy Association as a guide to appropriate conduct of its members. The Principles are not intended to define a standard of care for patients or clients of a particular community.

Professional maturity will be demonstrated in applying these basic Principles while exercising the large measure of freedom which they provide and which is essential to responsible and creative occupational therapy service.

For the purpose of continuity the following definitions will support information in this document: Occupational therapist includes registered occupational therapists, certified occupational therapy assistants, occupational therapy students; Clients include patients, students, and those to whom occupational therapy services are delivered.

I. *Related to the Recipient of Service*

The occupational therapist demonstrates a beneficent concern for the recipient of services and maintains a goal-directed relationship with the recipient which furthers the objectives for which it is estab-

* Adopted by the Representative Assembly, American Occupational Association, April 1, 1977; revised April, 1980. Am. J. Occup. Ther. 34:896–899, 1980.

881

lished. Services are evaluated against objectives and accountability is maintained therefore. Respect shall be shown for the recipients' rights and the occupational therapist will preserve the confidence of the client relationship.

Guidelines: Recipients of occupational therapy services refer to clients, patients, students and the employers of occupational therapists, i.e., agencies, facilities, institutions, etc.

It is the professional responsibility of occupational therapists to provide services for clients without regard to race, creed, national origin, sex, handicap or religious affiliation. Occupational therapists recognize each client's individuality and worth as a unique person.

Services provided should be planned in concert with clients' involvement in goal-directed activities, in accordance with the overall habilitation or rehabilitation plan. Treatment objectives and the therapeutic process must be measurable to insure professional accountability.

Clients' and students' rights are to be protected as stipulated in the Federal Privacy Act of 1974, in addition to any specified rules, regulations or procedures as may be required by the employer.

The financial gain of occupational therapists should never be paramount to the delivery of services. Those occupational therapists who are compensated by virtue of being a direct service provider or vendor have the right to assess reasonable fees for profit.

Occupational therapists are obligated to provide the highest quality of service to the recipient. If further services would be beneficial to the client, the referring practitioner should be informed. It is also incumbent upon occupational therapists to recommend termination of services when established goals have been met, or when further services would not produce improved recipient performance.

Occupational therapy educators are obligated to provide the highest quality educational services supporting the AOTA "Essentials" and the current theory that supports service delivery.

II. Related to Competence

The occupational therapist shall actively maintain and improve one's professional competence, represent it accurately, and function within its parameters.

Guidelines: Occupational therapists recognize the need for continuing education and where relevant, they obtain training, experience, self-study or counsel to assure competent occupational therapy services.

Occupational therapists accurately represent their competence, education, training, and experience. Occupational therapists must accurately represent their skills and should not provide services or instructions, either for pay or in a voluntary capacity, that are not within their demonstrated competencies.

Occupational therapists must recognize the skills necessary to manage a client or a position. If client needs exist that the therapist cannot effectively manage, the therapist should seek consultation or refer the client to an occupational therapist or another professional who can provide the required service.

III. Related to Records, Reports, Grades and Recommendations

The occupational therapist shall conform to local, state and federal laws and regulations and regulations applicable to records and reports. The occupational therapist abides by the employing institution's rules. Objective data shall govern subjective data in evaluations, grades, recommendations, records and reports.

Guidelines: Occupational therapists realize that reports are a required function of any position. Occupational therapists accurately record information and report information as required by AOTA standards, facility standards and state and national laws.

Occupational therapists fulfilling a teaching role utilize objective data in determining student grades.

All data recorded in permanent files or records should be supported by the occupational therapist's observations or by objective measures of data collection.

Students' records can only be divulged as authorized by law or the students' consent for release of information.

IV. Related to Intra-Professional Colleagues

The occupational therapist shall function with discretion and integrity in relations with other members of the profession and shall be concerned with the quality of their services. Upon becoming aware of objective evidence of a breach of ethics or substandard service, the occupational therapist shall take action according to established procedure.

Guidelines: Information gained or data gathered on a client shall only be divulged as expedient to other professional colleagues, students, referring practitioner, and employer. This includes data used in the course of in-service programs, professional meetings, prepared papers for presentation or publication, and educational materials. Undue invasion of privacy should be of utmost concern. Any reference to quality or service rendered by, or the integrity of a professional colleague will be expressed with due care to protect the reputation of that person.

It is the obligation of occupational therapists with first-hand knowledge of a breach of the ethical principles of this Association, by a colleague or student, to attempt to rectify the situation. If informal attempts fail, such activities or incidents against the ethical principles of this Association should immediately be brought to the attention of the appropriate local, regional or national Association committee/commission on ethical standards. Designated procedures should be followed and at all times the confidentiality of the information must be respected to protect the alleged party.

Practices by an employer that are in conflict with the ethical principles of this Association should also be brought to the immediate attention of the appropriate body(ies).

Information gained in peer review procedures should be held within the realm of confidentiality and be dealt with according to established procedures.

Publication credit for material developed by colleagues must be given. Also, credit for materials used in the classroom, manuals, in-service training, and oral or written reports, for example, should acknowledge the name of the individual or group who developed the material.

V. *Related to Other Personnel*

The occupational therapist shall function with discretion and integrity in relations with personnel and cooperate with them as may be appropriate. Similarly, the occupational therapist expects others to demonstrate a high level of competence. Upon becoming aware of objective evidence of a breach of ethics or substandard service, the occupational therapist shall take action according to established procedure.

Guidelines: Occupational therapists understand the scope of education and practice of related professions, and make full use of all the professional, technical and administrative resources that best serve the interests of consumers.

Occupational therapists do not delegate to other personnel those client related services where the clinical skills and expertise of an occupational therapist is required. Other personnel or students may support treatment or educational goals, but must have demonstrated competency in each aspect of service to the occupational therapist before the responsibility can be delegated.

Occupational therapists who employ or supervise other professionals or technicians, or professionals or

technicians in training, accept the obligation to facilitate their further development by providing suitable working conditions, consultation and experience opportunities.

Occupational therapists protect the privacy of all persons with whom professional collaboration occurs. If, however, an occupational therapist has first-hand knowledge of a colleague's performance which is in conflict with ethical standards, the therapist shall attempt to rectify the situation. Failing an informal solution, the occupational therapist shall utilize procedures established within the facility or agency, or to call the behavior to the attention of management, or utilize procedures established by the profession to handle such situations. Under no circumstances should the occupational therapist remain silent when a client, student or facility's status is in jeopardy.

VI. *Related to Employers and Payers*

The occupational therapist shall render service with discretion and integrity and shall protect the property and property rights of the employers and payers.

Guidelines: Occupational therapists function within the parameter of the job description or the goals established mutually between the employer or agency, and the occupational therapist. Occupational therapists use the utmost integrity in all dealings with the facility, university/college or contracting agency. Established procedures are followed regarding purchasing and bids.

Occupational therapists recommend appropriate fees for services and gain necessary acceptance for fees from the facility, agency and payers. Fees must be based upon cost analysis or a factor that can be justified upon request.

Occupational therapists shall not use the property, such as supplies and equipment, of the employer for their own personal use and aggrandizement.

VII. *Related to Education*

The occupational therapist implements a commitment to the education of society and the consumer of health services as well as to the education of health personnel on matters of health which are within the purview of occupational therapy.

Guidelines: Occupational therapists do not only provide direct service to alleviate specific problems with clients, programs or a community, but in addition, include education of all phases of services which can be provided to the public. This should include education of situations and conditions for which the competency of occupational therapists is recognized to assist in alleviating barriers limiting a person's ability to function socially, emotionally, cognitively, or physically.

The public includes not only individuals concerned with the well-being of a member of their family, but also federal, state and local governmental agencies, educational systems and social agencies dealing with the health and well-being of the public.

VIII. *Related to Evaluation and Research*

Occupational therapists shall accept responsibility for evaluating, developing and refining service and the body of knowledge and skills which underlie the education and practice of occupational therapy and at all times protects the rights of subjects, clients, institutions and collaborators. The work of others shall be acknowledged.

Guidelines: Clients' families have the right to have, and occupational therapists have the responsibility to provide explanations of the nature, the purposes, and results of the occupational therapy services unless, as in some employment or treatment settings, there is an explicit exception to this right agreed upon in advance.

In reporting test results, occupational therapists indicate any reservations regarding validity or reliability resulting from testing circumstances or inappropriateness of the test norms for the person tested.

In performing research and reporting research results, occupational therapists must use accepted scientific methodology.

IX. *Related to the Profession*

The occupational therapist shall be responsible for gaining information and understanding of the principles, policies and standards of the profession. The occupational therapist functions as a representative of the profession.

Guidelines: Occupational therapists should provide accurate information to the public about the profession and the services that can be provided. Occupational therapists should remain informed about changes in the profession and represent the profession accurately to the consumer.

Occupational therapists may provide information to the public about available services through procedures established by the employing facility or contracting agency. When an occupational therapist provides an independent service, it is appropriate to advertise those services in accordance with AOTA established policy.

Occupational therapists should conduct them-

selves in a manner befitting professionals. The profession is judged in part by the conduct of its members as they carry out their functions.

Occupational therapists should show support and loyalty to the Association by cooperating with the Representatives in collecting information regarding proposed Association policy, replying to official requests for information and supporting the policies of the Association. It is the member's duty if he disagrees with an Association policy to work through existing channels to effect change.

Occupational therapists who engage in work or volunteer activities in addition to professional occupational therapy responsibilities, shall not violate the ethical principles of the Association in such activities.

X. *Related to Advertising*

Advertising by therapists under their professional title shall be in accordance with propriety and precedent in health professions.

Guidelines: Occupational therapists may provide information to the public about available services through procedures established by the employing facility or contracting agency. If an occupational therapist provides an independent service, it is appropriate to advertise those services.

The occupational therapist shall not use, or participate in the use of, any form of communication containing a false, fraudulent, misleading, deceptive, self-laudatory or unfair statement or claim. Testimonials or statements which promise a favorable result shall be avoided.

XI. *Related to Law and Regulations*

The occupational therapist shall seek to acquire information about applicable local, state, federal and institutional rules and shall function accordingly thereto.

Guidelines: Occupational therapists are obligated to function professionally as a practitioner within the limits of all laws related to the delivery of health services, and applicable to the practice of occupational therapy. Occupational therapists will not engage in any cruel, inhumane or degrading practices in the treatment of clients or in the education of students, or in supervision of others or in peer relationships.

It is the responsibility of occupational therapists to make known to their employers, employees and colleagues, those laws applicable to the practice of occupational therapy and education of occupational therapists.

XII. *Related to Misconduct*

The occupational therapist shall not appear to act with impropriety nor engage in illegal conduct involving moral turpitude and will not circumvent the principles of occupational therapy ethics through actions of another.

Guidelines: As employees, occupational therapists refuse to participate in practices inconsistent with legal, moral and ethical standards regarding the treatment of employees or the public. For example, occupational therapists will not condone practices that are inhumane, or that result in illegal or otherwise unjustifiable discrimination on the basis of race, age, sex, religion, handicap or national origin in hiring, promotion or training.

In providing occupational therapy services, occupational therapists avoid any action that will violate or diminish the legal and civil rights of clients or of others who may be affected.

As practitioners and educators, occupational therapists keep abreast of relevant federal, state, local and agency regulations and American Occupational Therapy Association Standards of Practice and education essentials concerning the conduct of their practice. They are concerned with developing such legal and quasi-legal regulations that support the interests of the public, students and the profession.

XIII. *Related to Bioethical Issues and Problems of Society*

The occupational therapist seeks information about the major health problems and issues to learn their implications for occupational therapy and for one's own services.

Guidelines: The principle is a philosophical statement that encourages occupational therapists to be global in their views of health in relationship to society.

APPENDIX C
Standards of Practice

Standards of Practice for Occupational Therapy Services for Clients with Physical Disabilities*

Preface

These standards are intended for internal use by the AOTA as guidelines to assist members in the practice of their profession. These standards by themselves cannot be interpreted to constitute a standard of care in any particular locality.

Standard I
A Referral for Occupational Therapy Services Must Be Based Upon the Provisions as Outlined in the Statement on Occupational Therapy Referral.

1. When a referral is received, the therapist shall document:

_____
* Adopted May 1978 by the Representative Assembly, AOTA.

a. the date of receipt and referral source
b. the services requested
c. the above (a & b) within one working day of the receipt of the referral

Standard II
The Occupational Therapist Shall Evaluate the Client's Performance.

1. The therapist shall orient the client, family and/or significant others to the purposes and procedures of the occupational therapy evaluation.
2. An initial evaluation shall be completed at least five working days after acknowledgment of referral receipt.
3. The initial evaluation shall include an initial assessment of the client's goals, and functional abilities and deficits in:
   a. occupational performance (ADL)
      1) self-care skills
      2) home-work-school skills
      3) play/leisure skills
   b. motor skills
   c. sensory integration

887

4. If the results of the above evaluation indicate possible deficits in psychological/social and/or cognitive skills, the therapist should evaluate these areas and document any functional deficits; or should refer the client to the appropriate service.

5. If any of the above evaluation results indicate the client's need for referral to community services or programs, the therapist should determine the availability of such community resources; or should refer the evaluation to the appropriate service.

6. The therapist should obtain information about the client's medical history, education, work history, avocational interest, family, and cultural background. This information may be obtained through client interview, record review, and/or discussion with informed sources.

Standard III

The Therapist Shall Prepare and Document a Program Plan Based Upon an Analysis of the Occupational Therapy Evaluation Data and the Client's Expected Prognosis.

1. The therapist shall document the program plan within six working days after the acknowledgment of the referral receipt.

2. The documented program plan should consist of a statement of:
   a. achievable program goals
   b. methods to achieve the goals

3. The program plan goals and methods should be consistent with:
   a. the evaluative results and expected prognosis
   b. the goals of the client and/or family
   c. the program plans of other health care practitioners

4. The program plan methods may include, but need not be limited to, the use of:
   a. adaptive equipment and techniques
   b. passive, assistive, active and/or resistive activities and exercises
   c. counseling techniques
   d. facilitation/inhibition techniques
   e. joint protection techniques
   f. orthotic and/or prosthetic devices
   g. work simplification techniques

Standard IV

The Therapist Shall Implement the Occupational Therapy Program According to the Program Plan.

1. The therapist shall routinely document the occupational therapy services provided, the frequency of the services, and the client's progress toward goals. The timing of documentation shall be based upon frequency of contact with the patient/client and the significance of change in the client's condition.

2. The therapist shall periodically re-evaluate and document the changes in the client's occupational performance and/or performance component skills.
   a. if the client's program exceeds a three-month period, the client should be re-evaluated at least every two months.
   b. if the client's program is less than three months, the client should be reevaluated at least once per month

3. The therapist shall formulate, document and implement program changes consistent with changes in the client's occupational performance and performance-component-skills.

Standard V

The Therapist Shall Prepare and Document the Occupational Therapy Discharge Plan.

1. The discharge plan shall be consistent with the client's goals, functional abilities and deficits, community resources, and expected prognosis.

2. The discharge plan shall be consistent with the discharge plans of the other health care practitioners.

3. In preparation of the discharge plan, the therapist should allow enough time for coordination, acceptance, and effective implementation of the discharge plan.

4. The therapist shall document within two days following discharge, the client's functional abilities and deficits in occupational performance and performance component skills at time of discharge.

5. The therapist shall recommend discontinuation of occupational therapy services when the client has achieved the program goals and/or has achieved maximum benefit from the services.

Standard VI

The Therapist Should Re-evaluate the Client with Chronic Conditions at an Appropriate Time Interval Following Discharge.

1. The re-evaluation results shall be documented.

2. If the client needs further service, the therapist shall refer the client to the services needed.

Standard VII
The Occupational Therapist Shall Systematically Review the Quality, Including Outcomes, of their Services, Using Predetermined Criteria Reflecting Professional Consensus and Recent Developments in Research and Theory.

1. If actual care does not meet the criteria, it may be justified by peer review.
2. If justification by peer review fails, a program to improve care shall be planned and implemented.
3. Patient care review will be repeated to assess the success of the corrective action.

Standards of Practice for Occupational Therapy Services in a Mental Health Program*

Preface

These standards are intended for internal use by the AOTA as guidelines to assist members in the practice of their profession. These standards by themselves cannot be interpreted to constitute a standard of care in any particular locality.

Standard I
A Referral for Occupational Therapy Services Must Be Based Upon the Provisions as Outlined in the Statement on Occupational Therapy Referral.

1. When a referral is received, the therapist shall:
   a. document the date of receipt and referral source
   b. document the occupational therapy services requested in the referral

Standard II
The Occupational Therapist Shall Evaluate the Client's Performance.

1. The therapist shall evaluate and document the client's goals, functional abilities and deficits in occupational performance (activities of daily living):
   a. self-care skills
   b. work skills
   c. play/leisure skills

---
* Adopted May 1978 by the Representative Assembly, AOTA.

2. The therapist shall evaluate and document the client's goals, functional abilities and deficits in the following performance component areas:
   a. psychological/intrapersonal skills
   b. social/interpersonal skills
   c. cognitive skills
3. If the results of the occupational performance evaluation indicate possible deficits in the client's motor and/or sensory-integrative skills, the therapist should evaluate these areas and document any functional deficits; or should refer the client to another practitioner for evaluation.
4. If any of the above evaluation results indicate the client's need for referral to community services or programs, the therapist should determine the availability of such community resources; or should refer the evaluation to another.

Standard III
The Therapist Shall Prepare and Document a Program Plan Based Upon an Analysis of the Occupational Therapy Evaluation Data and the Client's Expected Prognosis.

1. The documented program plan shall consist of a statement of achievable program goals and the methods to achieve the goals.
2. The program plan goals and methods shall be consistent with the evaluation data on the client's goals, functional abilities and deficits, community resources, and expected prognosis.
3. The program plan goals and methods shall be compatible with the program plans of the other health care practitioners.

Standard IV
The Therapist Shall Implement the Occupational Therapy Program According to the Program Plan.

1. The therapist shall periodically document the occupational therapy services provided and the frequency of the services.
2. The therapist shall periodically re-evaluate and document the changes in the client's occupational performance and performance component skills.
3. The therapist shall formulate, document and implement program changes consistent with changes in the client's occupation, performance and performance component skills.

Standard V
The Therapist Shall Prepare and Document the
Occupational Therapy Discharge Plan.

1. The discharge plan shall be consistent with the client's goals, functional abilities and deficits, community resources, and expected prognosis.
2. The discharge plan shall be consistent with the discharge plans of the other health care practitioners.
3. Sufficient time should be allowed for coordination, acceptance and effective implementation of the discharge plan.
4. The therapist shall document the client's functional abilities and deficits in occupational performance and performance component skills at time of discharge.
5. The therapist shall terminate occupational therapy services when the client has achieved the goals, or when the client has achieved maximum benefit from occupational therapy.

Standard VI
The Therapist Should Re-evaluate the Client
with Chronic Conditions at an Appropriate
Time Interval Following Discharge.

1. The re-evaluation results shall be documented.
2. If the client needs further service, the therapist shall refer the client to the services needed.

Standard VII
The Occupational Therapist Shall
Systematically Review the Quality, Including
Outcomes, of their Services, Using
Predetermined Criteria Reflecting Professional
Consensus and Recent Developments in
Research and Theory.

1. If actual care does not meet the criteria, it may be justified by peer review.
2. If justification by peer review fails, a program to improve care shall be planned and implemented.
3. Patient care review will be repeated to assess the success of the corrective action.

Standards of Practice for
Occupational Therapy Services
for the Developmentally
*Disabled Client**

Preface

These standards are intended for internal use by the AOTA as guidelines to assist members in the practice of their profession. These standards by themselves cannot be interpreted to constitute a standard of care in any particular locality.

Standard I
A Referral for Occupational Therapy Services
Must Be Based Upon the Provisions as Outlined
in the Statement on Occupational Therapy
Referral.

1. A client should be referred to the occupational therapist for evaluation when the client has or appears to have a dysfunction, or has a predisposition towards dysfunction in any of the following areas:
   a. occupational performance (activities of daily living):
      1. self-care activities
      2. home-school-work activities
      3. play/leisure activities
   b. performance components:
      1. neuromuscular development
      2. sensory-integrative development
      3. psychological development
      4. social development
      5. cognitive development
2. When a referral is received, the therapist shall document:
   a. the date of receipt and referral source
   b. services requested in the referral

Standard II
The Occupational Therapist Shall Evaluate the
Client's Performance.

1. The occupational therapy evaluation shall include as assessment of the developmental level, as well as the functional abilities and deficits in the following areas:
   a. occupational performance (activities of daily living):
      1. self-care skills

---

* Adopted May 1978 by the Representative Assembly, AOTA.

2. home-work-school skills
3. play/leisure skills
   b. motor skills
   c. sensory integration
2. If the results of the above evaluation indicate possible deficits in psychological/social and/or cognitive skills, the therapist should evaluate these areas and document any functional deficits; or should refer the client to the appropriate service.
3. If any of the above evaluation results indicate the client's need for referral to community services or programs, the therapist should determine the availability of such community resources; or should refer the evaluation to the appropriate service.
4. All evaluation methods shall be appropriate to the chronological age and functional level of the client. The methods may include, but need not be limited to, observation of activity performance, interview, record review and testing.
5. If standardized evaluative tests are used, the tests should have normative data for the age range of the client. If normative data are not available for the age range of the client, the standardized test results should be expressed in relation to the normative data that are available.
6. The therapist shall document the evaluation results in the client's record. Indicating evaluation tools.

Standard III
The Therapist Shall Prepare and Document a Program Plan Based Upon an Analysis of the Occupational Therapy Evaluation Data and the Client's Expected Prognosis.

1. The documented program plan shall consist of a statement of achievable program goals and the methods to achieve the goals.
2. The program plan goals and methods shall be consistent with:
   a. established principles of normal growth and development
   b. the evaluative results and expected prognosis
   c. the goals of the client, the client's family and significant others
   d. the program plans of the other health care practitioners
3. When the occupational therapy program goal is to prevent or diminish dysfunction in occupational performance (activities of daily living) or to enhance occupational performance, the program plan shall include the use of one or more of the following types of activities:
   a. self-care activities; may also include instruc-

tion in the use of adapted methods and/or equipment
   b. home-work-school activities; may also include instruction in the use of adapted methods and/or equipment
   c. play/leisure activities; may also include instruction of family in play activities appropriate for child's developmental level: instruction in the use of adapted methods and/or equipment
4. When the goal is to prevent or diminish neuromuscular dysfunction or enhance neuromuscular development, the program plan shall include (but need not be limited to) the use of one or more of the following types of activities:
   a. activities which maintain or increase range of motion and/or muscle strength
   b. activities which facilitate integration of developmentally appropriate reflex behavior
   c. activities which provide appropriate sensory stimulation
   d. activities which promote the development of normal movement patterns and motor control
   e. activities which maintain or increase coordination
   f. instruction in use of proper positioning techniques
   g. provision of and instruction in the use of adaptive equipment and/or orthotic devices
5. When the goal is to prevent or diminish sensory-integrative dysfunction or to enhance sensory-integrative development, the program plan shall include (but need not be limited to) the appropriate use of:
   a. sensory input techniques for visual, auditory, gustatory, olfactory, tactile, proprioceptive/kinesthetic, and vestibular stimulation
   b. facilitation techniques
   c. inhibition techniques
   d. activity to promote adaptive motor response
6. When the goal is to prevent or diminish psychological dysfunction or to enhance psychological development, the program plan shall include (but need not be limited to) the use of activities which assist the client in learning to:
   a. experience and cope with competition, frustration, success, failure
   b. identify and respond appropriately to feelings
   c. develop or refine self-esteem; self-identity
7. When the goal is to prevent or diminish social dysfunction or to enhance social development, the program plan shall include (but need not be limited to) the use of activities which assist the client in learning to:
   a. initiate and develop appropriate social behavior

  b. listen and communicate
  c. develop sensitivity to other person's feelings and behavior
8. When the goal is to prevent or diminish cognitive dysfunction or to enhance cognitive development, the program plan shall include (need not be limited to) the use of the following activities which assist the client in developing:
  a. concentration/attention span
  b. memory/recall
  c. decision making and problem-solving skills

Standard IV
The Therapist Small Implement the Program According to the Program Plan.

1. The therapist shall periodically document the occupational therapy services provided and the frequency of the services.
2. The therapist shall periodically re-evaluate and document the changes in the client's occupational performance and performance components.
3. The therapist shall formulate, document and implement program changes consistent with changes in the client's occupational performance and performance components.

Standard V
The Therapist Shall Prepare and Document the Occupational Therapy Discharge Plan.

1. The discharge plan shall be consistent with the client's goals, functional abilities and deficits, expected prognosis, and the goals of the client's family. Consideration should be given to community resources and other environmental factors.
2. The discharge plan shall be consistent with the discharge plans of the other health care practitioners.
3. Sufficient time should be allowed for coordination, acceptance and effective implementation of the discharge plan.
4. The therapist shall document the client's functional abilities and deficits in occupational performance and performance components at time of discharge.
5. The therapist shall terminate occupational therapy services when the client has achieved the goals; or when the client has achieved maximum benefit from occupational therapy.

Standard VI
The Therapist Should Re-evaluate the Client with Chronic Conditions at an Appropriate Time Interval Following Discharge.

1. The re-evaluation results shall be documented.
2. If the client needs further service, the therapist shall refer the client to the services needed.

Standard VII
Occupational Therapist Shall Systematically Review the Quality, Including Outcomes, of Their Services, Using Predetermined Criteria Reflecting Professional Consensus and Recent Developments in Research and Theory.

1. If actual care does not meet the criteria it may be justified by peer review.
2. If justification by peer review fails, a program to improve care shall be planned and implemented.
3. Patient care review will be repeated to assess the success of the corrective action.

Standards of Practice for Occupational Therapy Services in a Home Health Program*

Preface

These standards are intended for internal use by the AOTA as guidelines to assist members in the practice of their profession. These standards themselves cannot be interpreted to constitute a standard of care in any particular locality.

Standard I
A Referral for Occupational Therapy Services Must Be Based Upon the Provisions as Outlined in the Statement on Occupational Therapy Referral.

1. Within one working day of receipt of a referral, the therapist *shall* document:
  a. the date of receipt and referral source
  b. the services requested
2. Within seven working days of receipt of referral, the therapist *shall*:
  a. review client's records

---

* Adopted May 1978 by the Representative Assembly, AOTA.

b. discuss case with other home health team members

c. document the acceptance/rejection of referral or the referral of client to other resources

Standard II
The Occupational Therapist Shall Evaluate the Client's Performance.

1. The therapist *shall* orient the client, family and/or significant others to the purpose and procedures of the occupational therapy evaluation.
2. An initial evaluation *shall* be completed and the results documented within five working days after acceptance of referral.
3. The initial evaluation *shall* include an initial assessment of the client's goals, functional abilities and deficits in:
   a. occupational performance (activities of daily living):
      1) self-care skills
      2) work skills
      3) play/leisure skills
   b. motor skills
4. The initial evaluation *should* include an initial assessment of the client's goals, functional abilities, and deficits in the following performance component skills, if the evaluation of occupational performance (ADL) skills and/or motor skills, or referral indicates possible deficits in these areas.
   a. sensory-integrative skills
   b. psychological/intrapersonal skills
   c. social/interpersonal skills
   d. cognitive skills
5. The therapist *should* evaluate these areas and document any functional deficits; or *should* refer the client to the appropriate service/individual for evaluation if the evaluation is beyond the therapist's expertise.
6. If any of the above evaluation results indicate the client's need for referral to community services or programs, the therapist *should* determine the availability of such community resources and/or *should* refer the evaluation to the appropriate service.
7. If the evaluation results indicate deficits in occupational performance skills, motor skills, sensory-integration, and/or cognitive skills, the therapist *should* evaluate the client's environment in relation to architectural barriers and safety factors. The evaluation results *should* be documented.
8. The therapist *should* obtain information about the client's medical history, education, work history, avocational interests, family, and cultural background. This information may be obtained through client interview, record review and/or discussion with informed sources.
9. The therapist *should* evaluate the ability of the client, family, and/or significant others to implement the home health program.

Standard III
The Therapist Shall Prepare and Document the Program Plan.

1. Seven working days after the acceptance of the referral.
2. The documented program plan *should* consist of a statement of:
   a. client's projected goals
   b. achievable occupational therapy program goals
   c. methods to achieve the goals
   d. frequency of visits
   e. projected length of occupational therapy program
   f. expected need for equipment
3. The program plan goals and methods *should* be consistent with:
   a. the evaluative results and expected prognosis
   b. the goals of the client and/or family
   c. the program plans of other home health team members
   d. client's economic resources and available home health resources
4. The program plan methods *may* include, but need not be limited to the use of:
   a. activities of daily living
   b. assistive, active and or resistive activities and exercises
   c. adaptive equipment and environmental modifications
   d. facilitation/inhibition techniques
   e. joint protection techniques
   f. orthotic and/or prosthetic devices
   g. work simplification techniques
   h. sensory integration techniques
   i. cognitive skill development techniques
   j. counseling techniques

Standard IV
The Therapist Shall Implement the Therapy Program According to the Program Plan.

1. The program should begin within five working days after the documentation of the program plan.
2. The therapist *shall* document for each home visit: the occupational therapy services provided, the length of the service and other pertinent information as required by the home health agency.

3. The therapist *shall* communicate problems or program changes to the physician, client, family and other home health team members.
4. The therapist *shall* document pertinent information obtained through sources other than home visits; e.g., telephone calls.
5. The therapist *shall* re-evaluate and document the changes in the client's occupational performance and performance component skills:
   a. if the client's program exceeds a three-month period, the client *should* be re-evaluated at least every two months.
   b. if the client's program is less than three months, the client *should* be reevaluated at least once per month
6. The therapist *shall* formulate, document and implement program changes consistent with changes in the client's occupational performance/component-skills.
7. When dealing with the medical problem, the therapist shall work in collaboration with the physician managing the case.

Standard V
The Therapist Shall Prepare and Document the Occupational Therapy Discharge Plan.

1. The discharge plan *shall* be consistent with the client's goals, functional abilities and deficits, community resources, and expected prognosis.
2. The discharge plan should be consistent with the discharge plans of the other home health team members.
3. In preparation of the discharge plan, the therapist *should* allow enough time for coordination, acceptance, and effective implementation of the discharge plan.
4. The therapist *shall* document within two days following discharge, the client's functional abilities and deficits in occupational performance and performance component skills at the time of discharge reason for discharge, number and length of treatment.
5. The therapist *shall* recommend discontinuation of occupational therapy services when the client has achieved the program goals and/or has achieved maximum benefit from the services.

Standard VI
The Therapist Should Re-evaluate the Client With Chronic Conditions at an Appropriate Time Interval Following Discharge.

1. The re-evaluation results shall be documented.
2. If the client needs further service, the therapist shall refer the client to the services needed.

Standard VII
The Occupational Therapist Shall Systematically Review the Quality, Including Outcomes, of Their Services, Using Predetermined Criteria Reflecting Professional Consensus and Recent Developments in Research and Theory.

1. If actual care does not meet the criteria, it may be justified by peer review.
2. If justification by peer review fails, a program to improve care shall be planned and implemented.
3. Patient care review will be repeated to assess the success of the corrective action.

Standards of Practice for Occupational Therapy in Schools*

These guidelines are to assist AOTA members and school administrators in the management of occupational therapy in the school systems. These standards by themselves cannot be interpreted to constitute a standard of care in any particular locality.

The occupational therapist shall manage the therapy program in accordance with all available Standards of Practice, as defined by the American Occupational Therapy Association, Inc.

The purpose of the Occupational Therapy program in the school system is to enable the student to gain optimum benefit from the educational program.

Direct Services

Direct services include screening, referral systems, evaluations, program planning, program implementation, re-evaluation and termination of services.

Standard I: Screening
The occupational therapist should be involved in the screening process.

1. The screening process should allow the therapist to identify those students who need further educational and/or related service evaluation.
2. All screening methods shall be appropriate to the chronological, educational and/or functional level of the student, and shall not be racially or culturally discriminatory.
3. The occupational therapist should refer the results and recommendations to the appropriate school educational planning committee.

---

* Adopted April 1980 by the Representative Assembly, AOTA

Standard II: Referral
A referral for occupational therapy must
comply with the AOTA statement on referral.

1. A student should be referred to the occupational therapist for evaluation when the student has or appears to have a dysfunction in any of the following areas:
   a. occupational performance (activities of daily living); self-care activities; home-school-work activities; play/leisure activities; and/or pre-vocational/vocational activities/skills.
   b. performance components: neuromuscular development; sensory integrative development; psychological development; social development; and/or cognitive development.
2. A referral may originate through the individual education plan or educational planning committee (including teachers, other student services staff, parents, physicians, etc.).
3. When a referral is received, the therapist shall document:
   a. the date of receipt and referral source; and
   b. services requested in the referral.
4. If in the therapist's judgment there is the need for medical management of the student, the therapist shall immediately apprise the student's parent/guardian or appropriate person and recommend physician involvement, or the therapist shall, after parental/guardian written permission or release has been obtained, contact the physician.

Standard III: Evaluation
The occupational therapist shall evaluate the student's performance.

1. The initial occupational therapy evaluation shall be completed and results documented according to the time frames established by federal and/or state rules and regulations.
2. The occupational therapy evaluation shall include assessment of the developmental level as well as the functional abilities/capacities and deficits/limitations as related to the student's educational level and needs in the following areas:
   a. occupational performance: self-care activities; home-school-work activities; pre-vocational/vocational activities/skills, and/or play/leisure activities.
   b. performance components: neuromuscular development; sensory integrative development; psychological development; social development and/or cognitive development.
3. If the results of the above evaluation indicate possible deficits in psychological/social, cognitive, physical/medical, speech/language areas, the

therapist should refer the student to the appropriate service and/or request consultation if necessary.
4. All evaluation methods shall be appropriate to the chronological age and/or functional level of the student and identify baseline behaviors. The methods may include, but need not be limited to, observation of activity performance, interview, record review, testing and individual/group screening.
5. If standardized evaluative measurements are used, the tests should have normative data for the age range of the student. If normative data are not available for the age range of the student, the results should be expressed in a descriptive report and standardized scales not used.
6. Tests and other evaluation material used in placing handicapped students will be prepared and administered in such a way as not to be racially or culturally discriminatory, and they will be presented in the child's native tongue.
7. As part of the evaluation process, the therapist may make clinical judgments based on observations and recorded progress during intervention programs.
8. The therapist shall document evaluation results in the student's record, indicating evaluation instruments and procedures and also communicate these findings via written reports, oral conferences, and staffings to the appropriate persons and/or community resources.

Standard IV: Program Planning and/or
Individual Education Plan
The therapist shall prepare and document a
program plan based upon an analysis of the
data from the occupational therapy and other
educational planner's evaluation results.

1. The initial program plan shall be prepared and documented according to the time frames established by federal and/or state rules and regulations.
2. The therapist shall utilize the results of the evaluation process to prepare an occupational therapy program that is:
   a. stated in practical outcomes applicable to the student's needs and educational goals,
   b. consistent with principles and concepts of growth and development; and
   c. consistent with expected behavior/progress for the student's defined educational/health problems and needs.
3. The planning process shall include:
   a. identifying short term and long term (annual) goals;

b. collaborating with child/family/staff to establish appropriate goals to enhance education;

c. participation in staffings to coordinate the occupational therapy program with the other programs within the educational setting;

d. documenting of practical outcomes to be achieved;

e. selecting the media, methods, environment and personnel to accomplish goals; and

f. monitoring and modifying the program to meet the established goals.

4. The documented educational program plan shall consist of a statement of when these services will be provided and how long they will last.

5. When the occupational therapy program goal is to prevent or diminish dysfunction in occupational performance and learning or to enhance occupational performance, the program plan shall include the use of one or more of the following types of activities:

a. self-care activities; may also include instruction in the use of adapted methods and/or equipment, energy conservation, joint protection techniques.

b. home-work-school activities; may also include instruction in the use of adapted methods and/or equipment.

c. pre-vocational/vocational activities/skills may also include improvement of standing or sitting tolerance, general endurance, or awareness and utilization of community resources; and

d. developmental play/leisure activities; may also include instruction of family in activities appropriate for student's developmental level; instruction in the use of adapted methods and/or equipment.

6. When the goal is to prevent or diminish neuromuscular dysfunction or enhance neuromuscular development and learning, the program plan shall include, but need not be limited to, the use of one or more of the following types of activities:

a. activities which maintain or increase range of motion and/or muscle strength;

b. activities which facilitate integration of developmentally appropriate reflex/reaction behavior;

c. activities which provide appropriate sensory stimulation;

d. activities which promote the development of normal postural tone, movement patterns and motor control;

e. instruction in the use of proper positioning and handling techniques;

f. provision of and instruction in the use of adaptive equipment; and/or

g. fabrication/recommendation of splints or orthotic devices/equipment.

7. When the goal is to prevent or diminish sensory integrative dysfunction or to enhance sensory integrative development, the program plan shall include, but need not be limited to, the appropriate use of:

a. sensory facilitation and/or inhibition techniques for vestibular, tactile, proprioceptive/kinesthetic, visual, auditory, gustatory and olfactory stimulation; and/or

b. activities to promote adaptive sensorimotor response.

8. When the interdisciplinary educational evaluation results indicate goals to prevent or diminish psychological or social dysfunction, or enhance psychological or social development, the occupational therapy program shall include, but need not be limited to, the appropriate use of activities which assist the student in learning to:

a. experience and cope with competition, frustration, success and failure;

b. identify and respond appropriately to feelings;

c. develop or refine self-esteem or self-identity;

d. imitate and develop appropriate social behaviors;

e. listen and communicate; and

f. develop sensitivity to other persons' feelings and behaviors (interpersonal relationships).

9. When the interdisciplinary education team evaluation results indicate goals to prevent or diminish cognitive dysfunction or to enhance development in the cognitive areas, the occupational therapy program shall include, but need not be limited to, the appropriate use of activities which assist the student in developing:

a. concentration/attention span;

b. memory/recall;

c. decision making and/or problem solving.

The purposes of the occupational therapy program in the above stated areas, (#8 and #9), are not intended to replace academic or other programming. The purposes are to assist the child to receive maximum benefit from educational programming.

Standard V: Program Implementation
The therapist shall implement the program according to the program plan.

1. The therapist shall periodically and on an ongoing basis document the occupational therapy services

provided (including techniques utilized and the results) and the frequency of the services.

2. The therapist shall periodically re-evaluate and document the changes in the student's occupational performance and performance components.

3. The therapist shall formulate, document and implement program changes consistent with changes in the student's occupational performance and performance components.

Standard VI: Re-Evaluation
The therapist shall re-evaluate the student receiving occupational therapy on a yearly basis.

1. The re-evaluation results shall be documented.
2. If the client needs further service, the therapist shall make appropriate recommendations.
3. A reevaluation does not necessarily constitute a referral for services.

Standard VII: Termination of Services
The therapist shall prepare and document the occupational therapy discharge plan.

1. The discharge plan shall be consistent with the student's goals, functional abilities and deficits, expected prognosis and the goals of the educational planners. Consideration should be given to appropriate community resources for referral and environmental factors/barriers that may need modification.
2. The discharge plan shall be consistent with the discharge plans of the other educational planners and appropriately documented through the individual educational planning process.
3. The therapist shall document the comparison of the initial state of functional abilities and deficits in occupational performance and performance components and the current state of these abilities and deficits at the time of discharge.
4. The therapist shall terminate occupational therapy services when the student has achieved the goals, or has achieved maximum benefits from occupational therapy.
5. Recommendations for follow-up or re-evaluation, if appropriate, shall be documented.

Indirect Services

With the provision of indirect services the occupational therapist in a school-based program performs supervision, consultation and administration/management roles.

Standard VIII: Administration/Management
The occupational therapist shall provide appropriate management and administrative services.

The management and administrative functions for the school-based therapist shall include:
1. Supervision of other personnel as assigned.
   a. informal and formal training of personnel and volunteers assigned to occupational therapy.
   b. reviewing performances (self and others) and providing evaluations.
2. Design of the occupational therapy program with periodic reviews of all aspects of the total occupational therapy program to determine its effectiveness and efficiency.
3. Occupational therapists shall systematically review the quality, including outcomes, of services delivered, using predetermined criteria reflecting professional consensus and recent developments in research and theory.
   a. To determine if actual service may be justified by peer review.
   b. If justification by peer review fails, a program to improve service shall be planned and implemented.
   c. Review will be repeated to assess the success of the corrective action.
4. Maintaining current certification as required by state regulations and AOTA.
5. Maintaining current records and files to meet school requirements and professional standards.
6. Participating in budget planning and is responsible for budget implementation.
7. Responsibility for knowledge, including use of, and utilizing community resources.
8. The therapist shall maintain and update professional knowledge and skills and seek consultation/supervision from others when necessary to assure continued competency.

Standard IX: Consultation
The therapist shall provide consultation services when appropriate.

In the consultation role, the therapist is one member of an interdisciplinary educational team collaborating with a variety of professional personnel to assist students with special needs. The practice of consultation shall include when appropriate:
1. Developing and coordinating occupational therapy programs with the total educational curriculum.

2. Provide consultation for classroom environmental adaptation to enhance the learning potential of students.
3. Provide consultation to teachers and staff regarding the identified special needs of students.
4. Collaborate with the educational team regarding the student's program including the IEP (Individualized Education Program).
5. Provide inservice education.
6. Provide consultation for appropriate programs outside the school program.
7. Provide consultation and education to parents to help them understand the special needs of their child.
8. Provide consultation for home environmental adaptation to enhance independent functioning.
9. Provide consultation to school administrators and staff regarding preventive health education and activities to enhance the educational environment and learning potential of students.

Standard X: Legal/Ethical Components
The occupational therapist shall provide all aspects of direct and indirect services according to legal regulations and ethical standards.

1. The occupational therapist shall practice and manage occupational therapy programs as defined by federal and state laws or legal principles as they apply to issues or situations when relevant to students or themselves in school systems.
2. The therapist shall observe the ethical practices as defined by the American Occupational Therapy Association Standards and Ethics Commission.
3. The therapist should be familiar with and abide by the ethical practices of the specific school district or system in which the therapist serves.

APPENDIX *D*
Uniform Terminology for Reporting Occupational Therapy Services*

Occupational Therapy Function

Occupational Therapy is the application of purposeful, goal-oriented activity in the evaluation, problem identification, and/or treatment of persons whose function is impaired by physical illness or injury, emotional disorder, congenital or developmental disability, or the aging process, in order to achieve optimum functioning, to prevent disability, and to maintain health. Specific occupational therapy services include, but are not limited to the following:

> education and training and evaluation of performance capacity in activities of daily living (ADL); the design, fabrication, and application of orthoses (splints); sensorimotor activities; guidance in selection and use of adaptive equipment; therapeutic use of activities and the *activity process* to develop/restore function performance; prevocational evaluation and training; consultation concerning the adaptation of physical environments for the handicapped; involvement in discharge planning and community re-entry; time/space/role management; and opportunity for self-expression and communication. These services are provided to individuals, groups, and to the community.

_____
* Adopted April 1979 by the Representative Assembly, AOTA.

Description of Occupational Therapy Services

In selecting items and defining terms, the following criteria were taken into consideration:
1. Emphasis on description of treatment outcomes rather than treatment procedures.
2. Reflection of Medicare and Medicaid guidelines in terminology and category selection and definition.
3. Comprehensive description of occupational therapy services/product.
4. Reflection of the uniqueness of occupational therapy services/product in comparison with the services of other professions.
5. Coverage of recognized occupational therapy role in medical practice rather than all possible occupational therapy roles.

I. Occupational Therapy Assessment

> Occupational therapy assessment refers to the process of determining the need for, nature of, and estimated time of treatment, determining the needed coordination with other persons involved, and documenting these activities.

899

A. *Screening*

Screening refers to the review of potential patient's/client's case to determine the need for evaluation and treatment. It includes discussion with other professionals and/or patient advocate, and patient/client interview or administration of screening tool.

B. *Patient-Related Consultation*

Patient-related consultation refers to the sharing of relevant information with other professionals of patients/clients who are not currently referred to occupational therapy. This may include but is not limited to discussion, chart review, treatment recommendation, and documentation.

C. *Evaluation*

Evaluation refers to the process of obtaining and interpreting data necessary for treatment. This includes planning for and documenting the evaluation process and results. This data may be gathered through record review, specific observation, interview, and the administration of data collection procedures. Such procedures include but are not limited to the use of standardized tests, performance checklists, and activities and tasks designed to evaluate specific performance abilities. Categories of occupational therapy evaluation include independent living/daily living skills and performance and their components.

1. Independent Living/Daily Living Skills and Performance (see II A).
2. Sensorimotor Skill and Performance Components (see II B).
3. Cognitive Skill and Performance Components (see II C).
4. Psychosocial Skill and Performance Components (see II D).
5. Therapeutic Adaptations (see II E).
6. Specialized Evaluations.

Specialized evaluations refer to evaluations or tests requiring specialized training and/or advanced education to administer and interpret. Examples of specialized evaluations are employment preparation, evaluation (prevocational testing), sensory integration evaluation, prosthetic evaluation, driver's training evaluation.

D. *Reassessment*

Reassessment refers to the process of obtaining and interpreting data necessary for updating treatment plans and goals. This frequently involves administering only por-

tions of the initial evaluation, documenting results, and/or revising treatment.

II. *Occupational Therapy Treatment*

Occupational therapy treatment refers to the use of specific activities or methods to develop, improve, and/or restore the performance of necessary functions; compensate for dysfunction; and/or minimize debilitation; and the planning for and documenting of treatment performance. The necessary functions treated in occupational therapy are the following.

A. *Independent Living/Daily Living Skills*

Independent living/daily living skills (including self-care) refer to the skill and performance of physical and psychological/emotional self-care, work, and play/leisure activities to a level of independence appropriate to age, life-space, and disability. Life-space refers to an individual's cultural background, value orientation, and physical and social environment.

1. *Physical Daily Living Skills*

Physical daily living skills refer to the skill and performance of daily personal care, with or without adaptive equipment. It includes but is not limited to:

a. *Grooming and Hygiene*

Grooming and hygiene refer to the skill and performance of personal health needs, such as bathing, toileting, hair care, shaving, applying make-up.

b. *Feeding/Eating*

Feeding/eating refers to the skill and performance of sequentially feeding oneself, including sucking, chewing, swallowing, and using appropriate utensils.

c. *Dressing*

Dressing refers to the skill and performance of choosing appropriate clothing, dressing oneself in a sequential fashion, including fastening and adjusting clothing.

d. *Functional Mobility*

Functional mobility refers to the skill and performance in moving oneself from one position or place to another. It includes skills necessary for activities such as bed mobility, wheelchair mobility, transfers (bed, car, tub, toilet, chair), and functional ambulation, with or without adaptive aids. It also includes use of public and private travel systems, such as driving own automobile and using public transportation.

e. *Functional Communication*

Functional communication refers to the skill and performance in using equipment or systems to enhance or provide communication, such as writing equipment, typewriters, letterboards, telephone, braille writers, artificial vocalization systems, and computers.

f. *Object Manipulation*

Object manipulation refers to the skill and performance in handling large and small common objects, such as calculators, keys, money, light switches, doorknobs, and packages.

2. *Psychological/Emotional Daily Living Skills*

Psychological/emotional daily living skills refer to the skill and performance in developing one's self-concept/self-identity, coping with life situations, and participating in one's organizational and community environment. It includes but is not limited to:

a. *Self-concept/Self-identity*

Self-concept/self-identity refers to the cognitive image of one's functional self. This includes but is not limited to:

(1) clearly perceiving one's needs, feelings, conflicts, values, beliefs, expectations, sexuality, and power.

(2) realistically perceiving others' needs, feelings, conflicts, values, beliefs, expectations, sexuality, and power.

(3) knowing one's performance strengths and limitations.

(4) sensing one's competence, achievement, self-esteem, and self-respect.

(5) integrating new experiences with established self-concept/self-identity.

(6) having a sense of psychological safety and security.

(7) perceiving one's goals and directions.

b. *Situational Coping*

Situational coping refers to skill and performance in handling stress and dealing with problems and changes in a manner that is functional for self and others. This includes but is not limited to:

(1) setting goals, selecting, harmonizing, and managing activities of daily living to promote optimal performance.

(2) testing goals and perceptions against reality.

(3) perceiving changes and need for changes in self and environment.

(4) directing and redirecting energy to overcome problems.

(5) initiating, implementing, and following through on decisions.

(6) assuming responsibility for self and consequences of actions.

(7) interacting with others, dyadic and group.

c. *Community Involvement*

Community involvement refers to skill and performance in interacting within one's social system. This includes but is not limited to:

(1) understanding social norms and their impact on society.

(2) planning, organizing, and executing daily life activities in relationship to society, including such activities as budgeting, time management, social role management, arranging for housing, nutritional planning, assessing and using community resources.

(3) recognizing and responding to needs of families, groups, and complex social units.

(4) understanding and responding to organizational/community role expectations as both recipient and contributor.

3. *Work*

Work refers to skill and performance in participating in socially purposeful and productive activities. These activities may take place in the home, employment setting, school, or community. They include but are not limited to:

a. *Homemaking*

Homemaking refers to skill and performance in homemaking and home management tasks, such as meal planning, meal preparation and clean-up, laundry, cleaning, minor household repairs, shopping, and use of household safety principles.

b. *Child Care/Parenting*

Child care/parenting refers to skill and performance in child care activities and management. This includes but is not limited to physical care of children, and use of age-appropriate activities, communication, and behavior to facilitate child development.

c. *Employment Preparation*

Employment preparation refers to skill and performance in precursory job activities (including prevocational activities). This includes but is not limited to:

(1) job acquisition skills and performance.

(2) organizational and team participatory skills and performance.

(3) work process skills and performance.

(4) work product quality.

4. *Play/Leisure*

Play/leisure refers to skill and performance in choosing, performing, and engaging in activities for amusement, relaxation, spontaneous enjoyment, and/or self-expression. This includes but is not limited to:

a. Recognizing one's specific needs, interests, and adaptations necessary for performance.

b. Identifying characteristics of activities and social situations that make them play for the individual.

c. Identifying activities that contain those characteristics.

d. Choosing play activities for participation, such as sports, games, hobbies, music, drama, and other activities.

e. Testing out and adapting activities to enable participation.

f. Identifying and using community resources.

B. *Sensorimotor Components*

Sensorimotor components refer to the skill and performance of patterns of sensory and motor behavior that are prerequisites to self-care, work, and play/leisure performance. The components in this section include neuromuscular and sensory integrative skills, including perceptual motor skills.

1. *Neuromuscular*

Neuromuscular refers to the skill and performance of motor aspects of behavior. This includes but is not limited to:

a. *Reflex Integration*

Reflex integration refers to skill and performance in enhancing and supporting functional neuromuscular development through eliciting and/or inhibiting stereotyped, patterned, and/or involuntary responses coordinated at subcortical and cortical levels.

b. *Range of Motion*

Range of motion refers to skill and performance in using maximum span of joint movement in activities with and without assistance to enhance functional performance. The standard levels of performance include:

(1) active range of motion: movement by patient, unassisted through a complete range of motion.

(2) passive range of motion: movement performed by someone other than patient or by a mechanical device, requiring no muscle contraction on the part of the patient.

(3) active-assistive range of motion: movement performed by the patient to the limit of his/her ability, and then completed with assistance.

c. *Gross and Fine Coordination*

Gross and fine coordination refers to skill and performance in muscle control, coordination, and dexterity while participating in activities.

(1) *muscle control*

Muscle control refers to skill and performance in directing muscle movement.

(2) *coordination*

Coordination refers to skill and performance in gross motor activities using several muscle groups.

(3) *dexterity*

Dexterity refers to skill and performance in tasks using small muscle groups.

d. *Strength and Endurance*

Strength and endurance refers to skill and performance in using muscular force within time periods necessary for purposeful task performance. This involves but is not limited to progressively building strength and cardiac and pulmonary reserve, increasing the length of work periods, and decreasing fatigue and strain.

2. *Sensory Integration*

Sensory integration refers to skill and performance in development and coordination of sensory input, motor output, and sensory feedback. This includes but is not limited to:

a. *Sensory Awareness*

Sensory awareness refers to skill and performance in perceiving and differentiating external and internal stimuli, such as:

(1) tactile awareness: the perception and interpretation of stimuli through skin contact.

(2) stereognosis: the identification of forms and nature of objects through the sense of touch.

(3) kinesthesia: the conscious perception of muscular motion, weight, and position.

(4) proprioceptive awareness: the identification of the positions of body parts in space.

(5) occular control: the localization and visual tracking of stimuli.

(6) vestibular awareness: the detection of motion and gravitational pull as related to one's performance in functional activities, ambulation, and balance.

(7) auditory awareness: the differentiation and identification of sounds.

(8) gustatory awareness: the differentiation and identification of tastes.

(9) olfactory awareness: the differentiation and identification of smells.

b. *Visual-Spatial Awareness*

Visual-spatial awareness refers to skill and performance in perceiving distances between and relationships among objects, including self. This includes but is not limited to:

(1) figure-ground: recognition of forms and objects when presented in a configuration with competing stimuli.

(2) form constancy: recognition of forms and objects as the same when presented in different contexts.

(3) position in space: knowledge of one's position in space relative to other objects.

c. *Body Integration*

Body integration refers to skill and performance in perceiving and regulating the position of various muscles and body parts in relationship to each other during static and movement states. This includes but is not limited to:

(1) *body schema*

Body schema refers to the perception of one's physical self through proprioceptive and interoceptive sensations.

(2) *postural balance*

Postural balance refers to skill and performance in developing and maintaining body posture while sitting, standing, or engaging in activity.

(3) *bilateral motor coordination*

Bilateral motor coordination refers to skill and performance in purposeful movement that requires interaction between both sides of the body in a smooth, refined manner.

(4) *right-left discrimination*

Right-left discrimination refers to skill and performance in differentiating right from left and vice versa.

(5) *visual-motor integration*

Visual-motor integration refers to skill and performance in combining visual input with purposeful voluntary movement of the hand and other body parts involved in an activity. Visual-motor integration includes eye-hand coordination.

(6) *crossing the midline*

Crossing the midline refers to skill and performance in crossing the vertical midline of the body.

(7) *praxis*

Praxis refers to skill and performance of purposeful movement that involves motor planning.

C. *Cognitive Components*
Cognitive components refer to skill and performance of the mental processes necessary to know or apprehend by understanding. This includes but is not limited to:
1. *Orientation*
   Orientation refers to skill and performance in comprehending, defining, and adjusting oneself in an environment with regard to time, place, and person.
2. *Conceptualization/Comprehension*
   Conceptualization/comprehension refers to skill and performance in conceiving and understanding concepts or tasks such as color identification, word recognition, sign concepts, sequencing, matching, association, classification, and abstracting. This includes but is not limited to:
   a. *Concentration*
      Concentration refers to skill and performance in focusing on a designated task or concept.
   b. *Attention Span*
      Attention span refers to skill and performance in focusing on a task or concept for a particular length of time.
   c. *Memory*
      Memory refers to skill and performance in retaining and recalling tasks or concepts from the past.
3. *Cognitive Integration*
   Cognitive integration refers to skill and performance in applying diverse knowledge to environmental situations. This involves but is not limited to:
   a. *Generalization*
      Generalization refers to skill and performance in applying specific concepts to a variety of related situations.
   b. *Problem Solving*
      Problem solving refers to skill and performance in identifying and organizing solutions to difficulties. It includes but is not limited to:
      (1) defining or evaluating the problem.
      (2) organizing a plan.
      (3) making decisions/judgments.
      (4) implementing plan, including following through in logical sequence.
      (5) evaluating decision/judgment and plan.

D. *Psychosocial Components*
Psychosocial components refer to skill and performance in self-management, dyadic and group interaction.
1. *Self-management*
   Self-management refers to skill and performance in expressing and controlling oneself in functional and creative activities.
   a. *Self-expression*
      Self-expression refers to skill and performance in perceiving one's feelings and interpreting and using a variety of communication signs and symbols. This includes but is not limited to:
      (1) experiencing and recognizing a range of emotions.
      (2) having an adequate vocabulary.
      (3) having writing and speaking skills.
      (4) interpreting and using correctly an adequate range of nonverbal signs and symbols.
   b. *Self-control*
      Self-control refers to skill and performance in modulating and modifying present behaviors, and in initiating new behaviors in accordance with situational demands. It includes but is not limited to:
      (1) observing own and others' behavior.
      (2) conceptualizing problems in terms of needed behavioral changes or action.
      (3) imitating new behaviors.
      (4) directing and redirecting energies into stress-reducing activities and behaviors.
2. *Dyadic Interaction*
   Dyadic interaction refers to skill and performance in relating to another person. This includes but is not limited to:
   a. Understanding social/cultural norms of communication and interaction in various activity and social situations.
   b. Setting limits on self and others.
   c. Compromising and negotiating.
   d. Handling competition, frustration, anxiety, success, and failure.
   e. Cooperating and competing with others.
   f. Responsibly relying on self and others.

3. *Group Interaction*

Group interaction refers to skill and performance in relating to groups of three to six persons or larger. This includes but is not limited to:

a. knowing and performing a variety of task and social/emotional role behaviors.

b. understanding common stages of group process.

c. participating in a group in a manner that is mutually beneficial to self and others.

E. *Therapeutic Adaptations*

Therapeutic adaptations refer to the design and/or restructuring of the physical environment to assist self-care, work, and play/leisure performance. This includes selecting, obtaining, fitting, and fabricating equipment, and instructing the client, family, and/or staff in proper use and care of equipment. It also includes minor repair and modification for correct fit, position, or use. Categories of therapeutic adaptations consist of:

1. *Orthotics*

Orthotics refer to the provision of dynamic and static splints, braces, and slings for the purpose of relieving pain, maintaining joint alignment, protecting joint integrity, improving function, and/or decreasing deformity.

2. *Prosthetics*

Prosthetics refer to the training in use of artificial substitutes of missing body parts, which augment performance of function.

3. *Assistive/Adaptive Equipment*

Assistive/adaptive equipment refers to the provision of special devices that assist in performance and/or structural or positional changes such as the installation of ramps, bars, changes in furniture heights, adjustments of traffic patterns, and modifications of wheelchairs.

F. *Prevention*

Prevention refers to skill and performance in minimizing debilitation. It may include programs for persons where predisposition to disability exists, as well as for those who have already incurred a disability. This includes but is not limited to:

1. *Energy Conservation*

Energy conservation refers to skill and performance in applying energy-saving procedures, activity restriction, work simplification, time management, and/or organization of the environment to minimize energy output.

2. *Joint Protection/Body Mechanics*

Joint protection/body mechanics refers to skill and performance in applying principles or procedures to minimize stress on joints. Procedures may include the use of proper body mechanics, avoidance of static or deforming postures, and/or avoidance of excessive weight bearing.

3. *Positioning*

Positioning refers to skill and performance in the placement of a body part in alignment to promote optimal functioning.

4. *Coordination of Daily Living Activities*

Coordination of daily living activities refers to skill and performance in selecting and coordinating activities of self-care, work, play/leisure, and rest to promote optimal performance of daily life tasks.

III. *Patient/Client-Related Conferences*

Patient/client-related conferences include participating in meetings to discuss and identify needs, treatment program, and future plans of referred client, and documenting such participation. Patient/client may or may not be present. Categories of conferences include:

A. *Professional Conferences*

Professional conferences refer to participating in meetings with a group or individual professionals to discuss patient's/client's status, and to advise/consult regarding treatment needs. Synonymous terms for professional conferences include initial conference, interim review, discharge planning, case conference, and others.

B. *Agency Conferences*

Agency conferences refer to participating in meetings with vocational, social, religious, recreational, health, educational, and other community representatives to assess, implement, or coordinate the use of services.

C. *Client-Advocate Conferences*

Client-advocate conferences refer to participating in meetings with client advocate (*e.g.*, family, guardian, or others responsible for patient/client) to assess patient's/client's situation, set goals, plan treatment and/or discharge; and/or to instruct client advocate to support or carry out treatment program.

IV. *Travel: Patient-Treatment Related*

Travel: Patient-treatment related refers to travel by therapists, with or without patient; that is, related to direct patient treatment.

The Following Items Do Not Involve Direct Patient Care

V. *Service Management*

Service management refers to planning, leading, organizing, and controlling the occupational therapy facility and service.

A. *Quality Review/Maintenance of Quality*
Quality review/maintenance of quality refers to those phases of departmental management that serve to assure and document normative standards to occupational therapy service.

1. *Development of Standards of Quality Treatment/Services*
Development of standards of quality treatment/service refers to the development, implementation, evaluation, and documentation of departmental policy and procedures for the purpose of assuring standardized and quality treatment. This policy includes but is not limited to those procedures governing standards of occupational therapy practice, health and safety, infection control, and ethical behavior.

2. *Chart Audit*
Chart audit refers to the evaluation of documentation based on criteria developed within the facility, the profession, Health Systems Agency (Health Planning Act), and/or Professional Standards Review Organizations for a specified geographical area.

3. *Accrediting Reviews*
Accrediting reviews refer to those activities that are necessary to routinely document the meeting of the standards of a recognized accrediting body such as State Department of Health, Joint Committee on the Accreditation of Hospitals, Commission on Accreditation of Rehabilitation Facilities; or other accreditation procedures, voluntary or mandated by state or local law, and/or by the administration of a particular institution.

4. *Occupational Therapy Care Review*
Occupational therapy care review refers to the ongoing evaluation and documentation of the quality of care given. Three review programs may be included in the care review process: pre-admission screening, concurrent review, and retrospective studies.

5. *Inservice Education*
Inservice education refers to the participation on regularly employed occupational therapy personnel (*e.g.,* OTR, COTA, OT Aide, or OT orderly) in regularly scheduled classes, in-house seminars, and special training sessions, either in or outside the facility.

B. *Departmental Maintenance*
Departmental maintenance refers to activities to maintain the physical environment of the occupational therapy department so as to assure the health and safety of patients and staff. Some of these activities are mandated by accrediting agencies, state or local law, or administration of the facility, whereas others may be developed by the occupational therapy service.

C. *Employee Meetings*
Employee meetings refer to meetings of occupational therapy departmental staff for the purpose of disseminating and receiving information, conveying information concerning the administrative policies of the institution and/or conditions of employment, and discussing issues relevant to the management of the program, the development of the department and/or institution, and its relationship to total health care.

D. *Program-Related Conferences*
Program-related conferences refer to interdepartmental meetings for the purpose of disseminating and receiving information and discussing issues relevant to program planning, development, and management.

E. *Supervision*
Supervision refers to activities to enhance the performance of departmental employees through appraisal of their effectiveness, evaluation of their conformance to departmental standards, and/or evaluation of their adherence to specific institutional policies.

VI. Education

Education refers to the dissemination and collection of knowledge pertaining to occupational therapy and health care by means of lecture, demonstration, observation, or direct participation.

A. *Occupational Therapy Clinical Education: Occupational Therapy Students*

Occupational therapy clinical education: occupational therapy students refer to the orientation, instruction, supervision of student involvement in the occupational therapy program. This may include preclinical, fieldwork professional, and/or technical level occupational therapy students.

B. *Occupational Therapy Clinical Education: Others*

Occupational therapy clinical education: others refer to the orientation of nonoccupational therapists to occupational therapy treatment principles and theories and to interprofessional working relationships by occupational therapy departmental staff.

C. *Occupational Therapy Clinical Education: Continuing Education*

Occupational therapy clinical education: continuing education refers to ongoing educational experiences beyond basic education. The purpose of continuing education is to enrich or improve the occupational therapist's knowledge, skills, and attitudes in his/her work performance. Continuing education is designed for therapists interested in maintaining and updating themselves in the field of occupational therapy and in its related aspects such as research, consultation, education, administration, and supervision.

VII. Research

Research refers to formalized investigative activities for the purpose of improving the quality of occupational therapy patient care by means of recognized scientific methodologies and procedures.

Occupational Therapy Product Output Reporting System*

Determination of Relative Value Units

To determine the relative value units which should be assigned to each category of service, five factors which affect cost and productivity levels of occupational therapy services were identified: expertise, equipment and supplies, patient-therapist interaction, facility, and interpretation and analysis. In turn, the four levels were identified for each factor.

A. Factor 1: Expertise

Level 1: omitted

Level 2: performed by an occupational therapist (OTR and COTA) who meets the basic entry levels for the profession of occupational therapy.

Level 3: performed by an Occupational Therapist, Registered, who is experienced in the specific area of occupational therapy practice

Level 4: performed by an Occupational Therapist, Registered, who has specialized training and/or advanced education in the specific area of occupational therapy practice

B. Factor 2: Equipment and Supplies

Level 1: requires no specific equipment and/or less than $5.00 worth of supplies

Level 2: requires equipment valued at $1.00 to $100.00 and/or supplies worth $5.01 to $10.00

Level 3: requires equipment valued at $101.00 to $1,000.00 and/or supplies worth $10.01 to $50.00

Level 4: requires equipment valued in excess of $1,000.00 and/or supplies in excess of $50.01

C. Factor 3: Patient-Therapist Interaction

Level 1: requires preparation, planning, and minimal supervision of a patient, or group supervision of six or more patients

---

* Adopted April 1979 by the Representative Assembly, AOTA.

Level 2: requires preparation, planning, and intermittent supervision of a patient, or group supervision of three to five patients

Level 3: requires preparation, planning, and constant supervision of one to two patients

Level 4: requires one to one interaction between patient and therapist with preparation, planning, and continuous attention and/or supervision

D. Factor 4: Facilities

Level 1: performed in facilities which are not designated specifically to the occupational therapy department (*e.g.,* patient care unit, hospital day room)

Level 2: performed in designated occupational therapy facilities in which concurrent treatments may take place (*e.g.,* general clinic)

Level 3: performed in designated occupational therapy facility in which concurrent treatments do not take place (*e.g.,* occupational therapy evaluation room)

Level 4: performed in specifically designed or specialized facility necessary for carrying out specific occupational therapy evaluation and/or treatment (*e.g.,* wheelchair accessible kitchen)

E. Factor 5: Interpretation and Analysis

Level 1: recording patient performance by daily attendance, census, and/or check-sheet

Level 2: reporting patient performance in the form of daily or weekly progress notation

Level 3: integrating and summarizing evaluation and treatment results in the form of a summary and/or consultation report

Level 4: interpreting test results, analyzing patient performance, and writing a formalized report specifying treatment goals and objectives and results

Each service category was assigned a level on each factor. This was done by consensual agreement of the opinions of the professional experts on the Task Force. An example is shown in the chart on this page.

The numerical values (levels) of the assignments on each factor were summed to give a total score for each category of service. Values across all categories of services were found to range from 8 through 18. These numbers were then multiplied by 10/8 to convert the scale to whole numbers beginning with 10—a scale which was considered to be easier to work with but which preserved the original relative weights between categories. This scale then became the relative value unit assignments for the service categories for individual evaluation and treatment. Readjustment factors were superimposed to bring group evaluation and treatment into a productivity measure realistically proportional to individual evaluation and treatment. Four categories of patient-therapist ratios were designated: 1) one patient per therapist; 2) two to four patients per therapist; 3) five to eight patients per therapist; and 4) nine or more patients per therapist. The readjustment factors were 50% of the individual RVU scale for the two to four patient category, 30% of the individual RVU scale for the five to eight patient category, and 10% of the RVU scale for the nine or more patients category. All RVUs are based on a 15 minute interval of time, or multiples thereof.

Category: Treatment, Independent Living, Work, Homemaking

Levels	Expertise	Equipment & Supplies	Patient-Therapist Interaction	Facility	Interpretation & Analysis
1					
2	X				X
3		X	X		
4				X	

Total Score = 2 + 3 + 3 + 4 + 2 = 14

Relative Value Units = (14) (10/8) = 14 RVUs for first patient category

Description of Accounts—Occupational Therapy

Function

Occupational Therapy is the application of purposeful, goal-oriented activity in the evaluation, diagnosis, and/or treatment of persons whose function is impaired by physical illness or injury, emotional disorder, congenital or developmental disability, or the aging process, in order to achieve optimum functioning, to prevent disability, and to maintain health. Specific occupational therapy services include, but are not limited to, education and training in activities of daily living (ADL); the design, fabrication, and application of orthoses (splints); guidance in the selection and use of adaptive equipment; therapeutic activities to enhance functional performance; prevocational evaluation and training; and consultation concerning the adaptation of physical environments for the handicapped. These services are provided to individuals or groups, and to both inpatients and outpatients.

Description

This cost center contains the direct expenses incurred in maintaining an occupational and patient-therapist ratio categories. Each assigned RVU is measured in 15 minute intervals, or multiples thereof.

Occupational Therapy Relative Values as developed by the American Occupational Therapy Association shall be used to determine the units related to product output of the Occupational Therapy Service Center. Relative Value Units for unlisted procedures or services are reasonably estimated on the basis of other comparable procedures or services.

Count units for all procedures or services rendered.

Data Source

The number of Relative Value Units shall be obtained from an actual count maintained by the Occupational Therapy Service Center.

Occupational Therapy Relative Values

Code Number*	Occupational Therapy Service Category			1 pt.	2–4 pts.	5–8 pts.	9 or more pts.
	I.	Occupational Therapy Assessment					
98001-03		A.	Screening	11	5.5	3.3	—
98004		B.	Patient Related Consultation	14	—	—	—
		C.	Evaluation				
98005-06			1. Independent Living/Daily Living Skills & Performance	18	9.0	—	—
98010-11			2. Sensorimotor Skill & Performance Components	21	10.5	—	—
98015-16			3. Cognitive Skill & Performance Components	20	10.0	—	—
98020-21			4. Psychosocial Skill & Performance Components	18	9.0	—	—
98025-26			5. Therapeutic Adaptations	19	—	—	—
98030-32			6. Specialized Evaluation	23	11.5	6.9	—
98035-36		D.	Reassessment	18	9.0	—	—

The column header "RVUs per 15 minute time interval Patient-Therapist Ratio Categories" spans the four numeric columns.

* Only one code number may be used for a given category. Thus, where a series of code numbers are listed, each code number in the series is to be used for a different patient-therapist ratio category. For example, code numbers 98001 through 98003 are given for Screening. 98001 would be used for screening one to two patients, 98002 for screening a group of three to five patients, and 98003 for screening a group of six to eight patients.

(Continued)

Code Number*	Occupational Therapy Service Category	RVUs per 15 minute time interval Patient-Therapist Ratio Categories			
		1 pt.	2–4 pts.	5–8 pts.	9 or more pts.
	II. Occupational Therapy Treatment				
	A. Independent Living/Daily Living Skills & Performance				
98040-42	1. Physical Daily Living Skills	13	6.5	3.9	—
98045-47	2. Psychosocial/Emotional Daily Living Skills	13	6.5	3.9	—
	3. Work				
98050-52	a. Homemaking	15	7.5	4.5	—
98055-57	b. Child Care/Parenting	18	9.0	5.4	—
98060-62	c. Employment Preparation	19	9.5	5.7	—
98065-67	4. Play/Leisure	14	7.0	4.2	—
	B. Sensorimotor Components				
	1. Neuromuscular				
98070	a. Reflex Integration	18	—	—	—
98075-78	b. Range of Motion	13	6.5	3.9	1.3
98080-83	c. Gross and Fine Coordination	13	6.5	3.9	1.3
98085-88	d. Strength and Endurance	13	6.5	3.9	1.3
98090-92	2. Sensory Integration	16	8.0	4.8	—
	C. Cognitive Components				
98095-98	1. Orientation	10	5.0	3.0	1.0
98100-01	2. Conceptualization/Comprehension	14	7.0	—	—
98105-06	3. Cognitive Integration	14	7.0	—	—
	D. Psychosocial Components				
98110-13	1. Self-Management	14	7.0	4.2	1.4
98115-16	2. Dyadic Interaction	14	7.0	—	—
98120-23	3. Group Interaction	10	5.0	3.0	1.0
	E. Therapeutic Adaptation				
98125	1. Orthotics	20	—	—	—
98130-31	2. Prosthetics	16	8.0	—	—
98135-36	3. Assistive/Adaptive Equipment	16	8.0	—	—
98140-43	F. Prevention	13	6.5	3.9	1.3
98145	III. Patient/Client Related Conferences	14	—	—	—
98150-53	IV. Travel: Patient Treatment Related	12	6.0	3.6	1.2

APPENDIX *F*
Uniform Occupational Therapy
Evaluation Checklist*

Application

The following Uniform Occupational Therapy Evaluation Checklist is designed as a generic occupational therapy guide for baseline data gathering. In order to use this checklist, each therapist will need to select the specific method of evaluation to be utilized. Data may be gathered through such means as suggested in the *Uniform Terminology System for Reporting Occupational Therapy Services;* for example, record, review, specific observation, interview, and the administration of data collecting procedures. Such data collecting procedures include, but are not limited to, use of standardized tests, performance checklists, and activities designed to evaluate specific performance abilities. The occupational therapist should use evaluation procedures that reflect the philosophical base of occupational therapy.

Occupational therapists need to thoroughly understand how to use the Uniform Occupational Therapy Evaluation Checklist. The therapist should:
1. compare/overview the client in all areas,

* Adopted March 1981 by the Representative Assembly, AOTA.

2. determine areas that require specific tests,
3. select specific tests (for example, client may not need Activities of Daily Living, but only tests for sensory integration function; this must be stated in the report),
4. report on all major categories (I A,B,C—II A,B,C,D,E,F) even though all subcategories may not apply,
5. document the type of evaluation used (*i.e.,* record review, standard tests, etc.).

Procedure
I. Demographic Information

    A. Personal Information
        1. Name
        2. Address
        3. Telephone
        4. Date of Birth
        5. Age
        6. Sex
    B. Referral Related Information
        1. Date of Referral
        2. Reason for Referral

3. Referral Source
4. Date client first seen by OT
5. Diagnosis
6. Presenting problems/symptoms
7. Date of onset
8. Medications
9. Precautions/complications
10. Date of evaluation
11. Evaluator

C. Personal History
   1. Developmental History
   2. Educational History
   3. Vocational History
   4. Socio-economic History
   5. Medical History

II. Skills and Performance Areas†

(See the AOTA *Uniform Terminology System for Reporting Occupational Therapy Services,* January, 1979, for definition of categories.)

A. Independent Living/Daily Living Skills and Performance
   1. Physical Daily Living Skills
      a. Grooming and Hygiene
      b. Feeding/Eating
      c. Dressing
      d. Functional Mobility
      e. Functional Communication
      f. Object Manipulation
   2. Psychological/Emotional Daily Living Skills
      a. Self-concept/self-identity
      b. Situational Coping
      c. Community Involvement

3. Work
   a. Homemaking
   b. Child Care/Parenting
   c. Employment Preparation
4. Play/Leisure

B. Sensorimotor Skills and Performance Components
   1. Neuromuscular
      a. Reflex Integration
      b. Range of Motion
      c. Gross and Fine Coordination
      d. Strength and Endurance
   2. Sensory Integration
      a. Sensory Awareness
      b. Visual-Spatial Awareness
      c. Body Integration

C. Cognitive Skill and Performance Components
   1. Orientation
   2. Conceptualization/Comprehension
      a. Concentration
      b. Attention Span
      c. Memory
   3. Cognitive Integration
      a. Generalization
      b. Problem Solving

D. Psychosocial Skills and Performance Components
   1. Self-Management
      a. Self-Expression
      b. Self-Control
   2. Dyadic Interaction
   3. Group Interaction

E. Therapeutic Adaptation
   1. Orthotics
   2. Prosthetics
   3. Assistive/adaptive Equipment

F. Prevention
   1. Energy Conservation
   2. Joint Protection/Body Mechanics
   3. Positioning
   4. Coordination of Daily Living Skills

---

† This outline was taken and adapted from the AOTA Uniform Terminology System for Reporting Occupational Therapy Services, prepared by AOTA Commission on Uniform Reporting System Task Force, Rockville, AOTA, January 7, 1979.

GLOSSARY

A.A.M.D. American Association on Mental Deficiency

Accommodation. the response or the motor process of adjusting the body to react to the incoming stimulation

Achievement motivation. the will to perform or to achieve, using some standard
Low achievement motivation: minimal will to try
High achievement motivation: high level of performance

A.C.L.D. Association of Children with Learning Disabilities: a nonprofit organization, whose purpose is to advance the education and general welfare of children with normal or potentially normal intelligence who have learning disabilities of a perceptual, conceptual, or coordinative nature

Acquisitional. referring to behaviors, attitudes, and ideas that have been learned through experience

Acting out. action rather than verbal response to unconscious drives or impulses; brings temporary relief of tension-situation; may be a substitute for the impulse that originally gave rise to the action.

Active listening. in conversation or interview, attending carefully to what is said by the other—awareness of both verbal and nonverbal communication

Adaptation. any change in structure, form, or habits of an organism to suit a new environment—in reflex action, decline in the frequency of impulses when the sensory nerve is stimulated repeatedly; in psychiatry, those changes experienced by an individual that lead to adjustment

Adaptive behavior. manner with which the individual deals with the cultural, social, physical, and mental demands of the environment

Adaptive skills. learned patterns of behavior that enable the individual to fulfill his/her own needs and the needs of others

Addiction. habit of drug (or alcohol) use, in which the addicted individual has symptoms of distress when deprived of the drug and the irresistible impulse to take the drug

Adolescence. stage of the life cycle lasting from onset of puberty until psychological and biological maturity is reached

Adulthood. stage of the life cycle that begins when the individual attains biological and psychological maturity and ends with the gradual onset of old age

AE. above elbow

Affect. emotional feeling tone-inner feelings and external manifestation-mood

Affiliations. a relationship(s) that helps one to see through the eyes of another and to confirm or reject our own experiences in a warm and accepting way

Aggression. forceful, goal-directed behavior

Agitation. motor restlessness with anxiety

Agnosia. loss of comprehension of auditory, visual, or other sensations although the sensory sphere is intact; inability to recognize an object

Agonist. the muscle directly engaged in contraction as distinguished from muscles that have to relax at the same time

AJOT. American Journal of Occupational Therapy

AK. above knee

Akinesia. absence or diminution of voluntary motion

Alienation. feelings of detachment from self, others, or society in general; avoidance of emotional experiences

Alimentation. giving nourishment

Alloplastic. changing or moving things other than self; the external environment

Amaurosis. partial or total blindness from any cause

Amblyopia. lazy eye; dimness of vision, especially that not caused by refractive errors or organic disease of the eye; may be congenital or acquired

Amnesia, anterograde. loss of memory of events after an injury

Amnesia, retrograde. loss of memory of events immediately preceding injury

Amniocentesis. removal of fluid containing fetal cells from the amniotic sac. The fluid is analyzed relative to metabolic disorders and chromosomal content.

Amphetamine. a central nervous system stimulant

Amputation. cutting off of a limb or part of a limb, the breast, or other projecting part

Amyotrophic lateral sclerosis (ALS). a degenerative disease of the pyramidal tracts and lower motor neurons, characterized by motor weakness and a spastic condition of the limbs associated with muscular atrophy, fibrillary twitching, and final involvement of nuclei in the medulla

Anal phase. second stage of psychosexual development (ages 1-3); interests, activities, and pleasure centered in anal zone

Anastomosis. a natural communication, direct or indirect, between two blood vessels or other tubular structures; an operative union of two hollow or tubular structures, as divided ends of intestine or blood vessels

Anergia. lack of energy, passivity

Aneurysm. circumscribed dilation of an artery or a blood-containing tumor connecting directly with the lumen of an artery

Animism. belief that inanimate objects are alive

Ankylosis. natural fixation of a joint; abnormal immobilization of a joint caused by destruction of articular cartilage enabling bony surfaces to fuse

Anoxia. oxygen deficiency

ANSI. American National Standards Institute

Antagonist. certain muscles opposing or resisting the action of others

Antecedent. refers to that which goes before; preceding circumstance, event, or condition

Anxiety. unpleasurable affect, with physiological and psychological changes; real external danger or threat does not exist; feelings of impending danger, powerlessness, tension, and readiness for expected danger

Apgar test. objective test of newborn's health

Aphasia. impairment or loss in ability to receive or to express verbal symbols or ideas; speech and hearing mechanism may be intact

Apnea. cessation of breathing, usually temporary

Appendicular. relating to the limbs, as opposed to axial, which refers to the trunk and head

Apraxia. inability to perform purposeful voluntary movements, the nature and mechanism of which are understood in the absence of motor or sensory impairment

ARC. The Association of Retarded Citizens: a parent-founded nonprofit association that promotes the general welfare of retarded citizens by encouraging research, advising parents, developing better understanding of retardation by the public, distributing information, and raising funds

Arteriosclerosis. hardening of the arteries

Arthrodesis. fusion of a joint by removing the articular surfaces and securing bony union; operative ankylosis; the surgical fixation of a joint

Arthroplasty. surgical formation of a joint

Artificialism. belief that an action was a result of an outside agent

Art therapy. treatment technique using spontaneous creative work of patients to explore and analyze and express underlying emotional problems

Assimilation. sensory process of "taking in" or receiving information that is external to and/or within the self system

Association. the organized process of relating the sensory information with the motor act and or relating present and past experiences with each other

Astereognosis. loss of the power of judging the form of an object by touch

Asymmetrical. denoting a lack of symmetry between two or more parts

Ataxia. incoordination of voluntary muscle movements, particularly those used in reaching and walking

Atresia. congenital absence or pathological closure of a normal opening, passage, or cavity

Atrophic, atrophy. pertaining to a wasting of tissues, organs, or the entire body

Audiometrist. one who evaluates a person's hearing qualitatively and quantitatively by use of an audiometer

Audit. an official examination and verification of accounts and records

Autition. acoustic ability; hearing

Autogenic. autogenetic; self-producing

Auto-cosmic play. play is centered on infant's body

Autonomic nervous system (A.N.S.). part of nervous system functioning outside of consciousness—directs, for example, breathing, heart rate, and digestion

Autonomy. quality of being self-governing and self-determining (striving toward independence)

Autoplastic. changing or moving one's self

Aversive. causing strong feelings of repugnance, distaste, dislike, or displeasure

Axial. relating to or situated in the central part of the body, in the head or trunk as distinguished from the extremities

Axon. the essential conducting portion of a nerve fiber continuous with the cytoplasm of a nerve cell

Barbiturate. highly addictive CNS depressant (ex. phenobarbital, pentothal)

Basal ganglia. the basal nuclei of the endbrain (telencephalon)

BE. below elbow

Biofeedback. technique in which patient is made aware of unconscious or involuntary physiological processes and learns to control them

BK. below knee

Body image. conscious or unconscious image of one's body (including function); sum of all feelings concerning the body

Body language. system by which a person expresses feelings and thoughts through posture, gesture, and/or movement

Body scheme. refers to the automatic adjustment of skeletal parts and to the tensing and relaxing of muscles necessary to maintain a position

Bolus. a round mass of masticated food that is ready to be swallowed

Boutonnière deformity. PIP flexion with DIP hyperextension

Breech delivery. presentation of the buttocks instead of the head in childbirth

Bruxism. grinding of the teeth, especially during sleep

Carpal tunnel syndrome. compression of the median nerve in the carpal tunnel at the wrist causing thenar atrophy and paralysis as well as trophic changes of the finger tips and sensory disturbance of the first three fingers

Catabolic phase. breaking down in the body of complex chemical compounds into simpler ones, often accompanied by the liberation of energy

Cataracts. partial or complete opacity of the crystalline lens or its capsule

Catchment area. a defined geographical area, representing a specified number of people to be served by a mental health center

Catharsis. release of ideas, thoughts, repressed materials from the unconscious, with emotional responses and release of tension (psychoanalytical term)

Causalgia. a neuralgia distinguished by a burning pain along certain nerves

C.E.C. Council of Exceptional Children: an associated organization of the National Education Association, for the advancement of education of exceptional children and youth, both gifted and handicapped

Centering. ability to focus on only one aspect of situation at a time

Cerebellum. the posterior brain mass; it consists of two lateral hemispheres united by a narrow middle portion

Cerebral contusion. bruising to brain causing diffuse disturbance with edema and hemorrhage and destruction of brain tissue

Cervical. pertaining to the neck and the eight cervical vertebrae

Cesarean section. removal of the fetus by means of an incision into the uterus, usually by way of the abdominal wall

Chaining. in behavior therapy, the process by which behavioral patterns are learned by reinforcements given for behaviors that are associated or related to an established behavior

Childhood. stage of the life cycle lasting from the end of infancy until the onset of puberty

Chorea movements. irregular and uncontrollable movements of muscles of the limbs and face

Chromosomes. the bodies in the cell nucleus that carry the genes

Circ-o-lectric bed. a circular frame containing a bed on which a patient can lie and be passively positioned from supine to prone on an 180 degree axis, by an electric mechanism. The patient can be tilted at any angle on the axis.

CMHC. Community Mental Health Center

C.N.S. central nervous system

Cocontraction. contraction of the agonist and antagonist muscles to provide stability

Cognition. the conscious process of awareness and knowledge of objects through perception, memory, and reasoning; mental process of knowing and understanding; an ego function—thinking, judgment

Cognitive development. the development of a logical method of looking at the world; knowing and understanding

Collagen fibers. protein of the white fibers of connective tissue, cartilage, and bone

Combinational analysis. systematically isolating all the individual variables of a situation, plus all possible combinations of these variables

Compensation. a process in which a tendency for change in a given direction is counteracted by another change so that the original change is not evident; an unconscious mechanism by which an individual tries to make up for fancied or real deficiencies

Competence. quality of adequacy or possession of required skill, knowledge, or capacity

Conceptual. referring to the formation or construct of ideas and thoughts

Conceptual model. an organization of theoretical constructs or of knowledge upon which a frame of reference for action can be based

Concrete operations. the third stage in Piagetian theory during which the 7- to 11-year old begins to think logically although thinking is still limited to what is seen

Conditioning. procedure used to alter behavior
classical: through pairing of stimuli to evoke response
operant: through presentation of reinforcements

Confidentiality. medical ethics, holding secret information that a patient has divulged

Conflict. clash of two opposing emotional forces

Conjugate deviation. forced and persistent turning of the eyes and head toward one side; observed with some lesions of the cerebrum

Conscious. (as a noun) that part of the mind that is experienced in awareness (psychoanalytical)

Consensual validation. comparison of thoughts, feelings, and perceptions with others—results in effective reality testing (Harry Stack Sullivan term)

Conservation. a cognitive ability as described by Piaget as occurring with concrete operations; the time when a child begins to understand physical properties of matter equivalence

Constancy. property of remaining the same, as in perceptual constancy, in which things are perceived as unchanged in form even if position or distance may change

Contract. explicit agreement to a well-defined course of action, as in therapy or in supervision

Contracture. a permanent muscular contraction resulting from tonic spasm or loss of muscular equilibrium, the antagonists being paralyzed

Contralateral. originating in or affecting the opposite side of the body

Coordination. the harmonious working together of several muscles or muscle groups in the execution of complicated movements; the working together of different systems of the body in a given process as the coordination between the system of glands and involuntary muscles in digestion

Cortex. the layer of gray matter that invests the surface of the cerebral hemispheres and the cerebellum

Countertransference. conscious or unconscious responses of therapist to the patient, determined by therapist's need; transferred feelings, not necessarily relevant to the real situation (psychoanalytical)

Creativity. the quality of being productive and imaginative

Crisis intervention. brief therapeutic encounter in time, with limited structure, aimed at amelioration of symptoms

Criterion reference test. oral performance on specifically described skills or knowledge without comparisons between individuals

Crossed diagonal. a highly integrated pattern with flexion of the upper extremities and extension of the lower extremities on the face side with extension of the upper limbs with flexion of the lower limbs on the opposite side (reciprocal)

Crystallized intelligence. cognitive skills such as verbal comprehension and word relationships

Cutaneous. relating to the skin

C.V.A. cerebrovascular accident, a lesion in the brain resulting in paralysis of contralateral side of the body

Cyanosis. a dark-bluish or purplish discoloration of the skin and mucous membrane resulting from deficient oxygenation of the blood

Cytomegalic inclusion disease. caused by the cytomegalovirus, transmitted transplacentally to the fetus from a mother with a latent infection

Dance therapy. technique of using movement and nonverbal communication to aid in rehabilitation; may be group or individual

Debride. to remove (surgically) foreign or devitalized tissue

DB-decibel. a tenth of a bel, a unit frequently used to measure the intensity of sound

Decerebrate rigidity. forceful extension of all joints of the lower extremities, and extension and internal rotation of the upper extremities; caused by brainstem contusion

Decubitus ulcer. a defect of the surface of an organ or tissue caused by prolonged pressure (also known as a bedsore or a pressure sore)

Deductive reasoning. reasoning or thought by hypothesis and adult logic

Defense mechanism. unconscious intrapsychic process (ego defenses) to relieve anxiety and conflict from unconscious drives that are not acceptable; includes conversion, denial, displacement, dissociation, idealization, identification, incorporation, intellectualization, introjection, projection, rationalization, reaction formation, regression, repression, sublimation, substitution, symbolization, transference, and undoing

Deformity. congenital or acquired unnatural distortion or malformation of a part of the body

Degenerative disease. progressive deterioration of tissue, particularly true of diseases of the central nervous system

Degenerative joint disease. a degenerative, noninflammatory, localized form of arthritis that causes breakdown of cartilage and results in limitation of motion and formation of bony outgrowths at the joints affected (osteoarthritis)

Dementia. irreversible, organic brain pathology characterized by a slowly progressive loss of mental capacity including memory, orientation, and ability to do serial tasks. Only a proper diagnosis after other causes are ruled out by adequate history, examination, and lab analyses

Denial. unconscious defense mechanism in which an aspect of external reality is blocked from awareness

Dependency. the state of needing someone or something for support

Depersonalization. sense of unreality about self, others, and environment

Deprivation. a negative reinforcement used to weaken or eliminate an undesired action

Desensitization. reciprocal inhibition (Wolpe); person is conditioned to associate comfortable, supportive surroundings with anxiety-producing stimuli and gradually learns to reduce the adverse effects.

Development. changes in the structure, thought, or behavior of a person that occur as a function of both biological and environmental influences (which may be quantitative or qualitative)

Developmental disability. the result of any condition, trauma, deprivation, or disease that interrupts or delays the sequence and rate of normal growth, development, and maturation

Developmental sequence. an established progression pattern of growth and development

Differentiation. the process of discriminating those essential elements of a specific behavior that are pertinent to a given situation, distinguishing those that are not, and thereby modifying or altering the behavior in some manner

DIP. joint. distal interphalangeal joint

Diplegia. paralysis of similar parts on both sides of the body

Diplopia. perception of two images of a single object (double or binocular vision)

Disability rating. classification of loss of function

Disequilibrium. lack or destruction of equilibrium

Disintegration. psychic disorganization

Dislocation. displacement of a bone from its normal position in the joint

Disorientation. inability to judge time, space, and personal relationships

Displacement. unconscious defense mechanism in which the feeling-laden part of an unacceptable idea or object is transferred to an acceptable one

Dissociation. unconscious defense mechanism in which an idea is separated from its accompanying feeling tone

D.O.T. Dictionary of Occupational Titles

Dramatic play. symbolic play used to display creative ability and physical prowess. It combines reality with magic to fulfill wishes and needs

D.S.M. Diagnostic and Statistical Manual of Mental Disorders of the American Psychiatric Association

Dyadic. refers to relationship, as between two people—one-to-one

Dynamic splint. splint that allows for or provides motion. Motion is provided by transfer of motion from other body parts or by use of outside forces such as springs, rubberbands, carbon dioxide, or electricity

Dysarthria. motor speech deficit

Dysfunction. inability to perform and ineract effectively with the environment; impairment of normal function of a body part or organ

Dyskinesia. impairment of voluntary movement

Dyspnea. shortness of breath

Dyspraxia. difficulty in performing purposeful voluntary movements, the nature and mechanism of which are understood in the absence of motor or sensory impairment.

Echolalia. an involuntary repetition of words; may be accompanied by twitching of muscles

Eclectic. choosing from various sources; not following any single system or frame of reference; selecting and using the best elements of several systems

Edema. a condition in which the body tissues contain an excessive amount of tissue fluid; it may be local or general

Efferent. conducting (fluid or a nerve impulse) outward or centrifugally

Ego. one of three components of psychic structure (with id and superego); mediates between instinctual drives and external reality demands (Freud)

Egocentric. preoccupied with one's own needs; self-centered; lacking interest in others

Ego functions. ego's management of defense mechanisms to meet person's needs—defense mechanisms mediating between id, superego, and reality; reality testing

Ego strength. effectiveness of ego functions. Strong ego can mediate between id, superego, and reality with enough flexibility to retain energy for creativity and other needs

Embolus. clot brought from a larger vessel to a smaller one causing obstruction

Empirical. founded on practical experience but not proved scientifically; based on observable fact or objective experience

Encephalitis. inflammation of the brain

Encopresis. incontinence of feces

Encounter group. a form of sensitivity training, experiencing individual relationships within a group; focuses on present (J. L. Moreno)

Endocept. intrapsychic primitive organization of perceptions, memory traces, and images; preverbal; cannot be shared, experienced vaguely (Arieti)

Engrams. mnemic hypothesis—the theory that stimuli or irritants leave definite traces on neurons

ENT. ears, nose, and throat

Enuresis. bedwetting

Environment. a composite of all external forces and influences affecting the development and maintenance of an individual

Epicritic function. denoting a set or system of sensory nerve fibers, supplying the skin and oral mucosa, enabling one to appreciate the finer degrees of the sensation of touch, pain, and temperature and to localize same; distinguished from protopathic

Epithelium. tissue composed of contiguous cells with a minimum of intercellular substance

Equilibration. process of finding a balance between accommodation and assimilation

Equilibrium. a state of balance or equality between opposing forces; bodily stability or balance

Equilibrium reactions. bodily reactions to retain state of balance in relation to gravity

Erythema. a redness of the skin occurring in patches of variable size and shape

Erythemia. a condition characterized by an increased number of red blood cells; polycythemia

Eschar. a thick coagulated crust or slough that develops following a thermal burn or cauterization of the skin

Escharatomy. an incision in a burn eschar to lessen constriction of a distal part

Etiology. study of causes of a disease

Euphoria. a sense of well-being; the absence of pain or stress that might be exaggerated

Exacerbation. an aggravation of symptoms of a disease

Excitatory. stimulating, increasing the rapidity of the physical or mental processes

Existential psychotherapy. treatment which puts emphasis on here-and-now—confrontation and feeling experiences; based on philosophy that one has responsibility for one's own existence

Exocepts. images (intrapsychic) of actions, movement; kinesthetic-proprioceptive images (Arieti)

Expressive aphasia. impairment of the ability to use speech and to write communicatively

External powered flexor-hinge splint. use of an outside source to provide power for prehension

Exteroceptive. outside the organism, *e.g.*, sense organ of the skin located on the surface of the body

Extrapyramidal. referring to central nervous system control of involuntary motor behavior

Extrinsic motivation. will to act based on external standards or incentives

Extrinsic muscles. muscles whose origin lies outside the part moved

Facilitator. a person who helps to make a process easier, assists progress toward a goal

Family of origin. family into which one is born

Family therapy. treatment of family in conflict; focus is on interactions among all members, not on pathology of one

Fasciotomy. incision through a fascia, used in the treatment of certain vascular disorders when marked swelling is anticipated that could compromise blood flow

Fatigability. susceptibility to fatigue

Fear. unpleasurable feeling with psychological and physical changes in response to realistic threat or danger

Febrile. pertaining to or characterized by fever

Feedback. response to behavior

Festination gait. small-stepped shuffling gait seen in Parkinson's Disease; involuntary increase in momentum to compensate for displaced sense of center of gravity

Fetus. eighth week of gestation to birth

Fibrillation. a small local involuntary contraction of muscle fibers

Fibroblasts. cells that synthesize mucopolysaccharides and collagen fibers necessary for the development of new connective tissue

Fibrotic. pertaining to or characterized by formation of fibrous tissue, usually as a reparative or reactive process

Field dependent. highly motivated to conform to standards or pressures that are external

Flaccid. relaxed, flabby, having defective or absent muscular tone

Flexor hinge. splint or surgery that is used to provide grasp function of the hand through stabilization of the interphalangeal joints of the first two fingers in slight flexion, the thumb in position of opposition, and providing movement at the metacarpophalangeal joint to effect prehension

Fluid intelligence. cognitive capabilities such as associative memory, inductive reasoning, and figural relationship

Forearm orthosis. ballbearing feeder

Formal operations. the fourth and final stage of Piagetian theory beginning at 12 to 15 years and characterized by logical thinking and a grasp of abstract concepts

Formative evaluation. along the way

Frame of reference. belief system based on conceptual models—in therapy, organized basis of theory, delineation of function and dysfunction, evaluation and treatment approaches, postulates regarding change

Froment's sign. flexion of the distal phalanx of the thumb when a sheet of paper is held between the thumb and index finger in ulnar nerve palsy

Functional treatment. relates to a specific function that has been lost and is being relearned or to a function that is being learned for the first time

Gastroschisis. a congenital defect in the abdominal wall, usually with protrusion of the viscera

Gavage feeding. feeding by a stomach tube

Gender identity (core). identification of oneself as male or female

Gender identity. the conviction one has about one's gender and its associated role

Gender orientation. a stable, subjective sense of comfort and liking for one's sex and for those functions that are "sex specific"

Gender preference. the gender role an individual finds most desirable regardless of compatibility with his/her own core gender identity

Gender role. clusters of behaviors or characteristics that are associated with one gender more frequently than the other. A set of cultural prescriptions and prohibitions

Gene. any portion of the chromosome that transmits hereditary characteristics

Generativity. concern with the establishment and guidance of future generations

Genital phase. final stage of psychosexual development, during puberty; pleasure centered on genital to genital contact (Freud)

Geriatrics. physiology and pathology of old age

Gerontology. the study of later maturity and old age

in its biological, psychological, and sociological aspects

Geropsychiatry. branch of psychiatry dealing with problems of the aged

Gestalt. an organized field that has unique properties that cannot be devised merely from the sum of its various component parts; the whole or total quality of the image

Gestalt therapy. psychotherapeutic technique focusing on treatment of person as a whole, focuses on here-and-now experience; use of role playing to promote individual or group growth (Frederick S. Perls)

Gestation. period of fetal development from conception to birth

Glaucoma. disease of the eye marked by heightened intraocular tension; may lead to blindness

Gliosis. proliferation of neurological tissue in the central nervous system

Grand mal. a complete epileptic seizure

Graphesthesia. recognition of the form of a number or letter drawn on the skin

Gray matter. substantia grisea; the ganglionic or cellular portion of the brain and spinal cord

Growth. biological/structural changes of the body; increase in size, function, or complexity up to some optimal point

GTO. Golgi tendon organ

Guillain-Barré syndrome. a spreading paralysis, sometimes reversible, with involvement of nerves, nerve roots, cord, brain and meninges, separately or combined

Gustatory. pertaining to the sense of taste

Habilitate. to educate or train (the mentally or physically handicapped, the disadvantaged) to function better in society

Habituation. the ability to become used to certain stimuli and no longer respond to them

Hallucination. false sensory perception without concrete external stimulus; may be visual, auditory, olfactory, gustatory, or tactile

Haptic. pertaining to touch; tactile

Hematoma. accumulation of blood within a tissue

Hemianopsia. blindness in one half of the visual field; may be bilateral or unilateral; also called hemiopia, hemianopia

Hemiparesis. muscular weakness of one side of the body

Hemiplegia. paralysis of one side of the body

Hemorrhage. bleeding, escape of blood from the vessels

Heuristic. quality that encourages further discovery or investigation

Histologically. dealing with the science of the minute structure of cells, tissues, and organs in relation to their function; microscopic anatomy

HMO. Health Maintenance Organization

Homeostasis. the maintenance of steady states in the organism by coordinated physiologic processes

Homolateral. ipsilateral pattern, with the head, thorax, and pelvis turned toward the flexing upper and lower extremities with extension of the contralateral extremities (camel walk)

Hyaline membrane disease. airlessness of the lungs, seen especially in premature neonates with respiratory distress; pulmonary collapse

Hydrocephalus. a condition marked by an excessive accumulation of fluid dilating the cerebral ventricles, thinning the brain, and causing a separation of cranial bones

Hydroureter nephrosis. distention of the ureter with urine because of blockage from any cause

Hyperactivity. excessive or increased activity

Hyperalimentation (HA). overfeeding, superalimentation, forcing of food upon a patient in excess of the demands of the appetite or of the nutritional needs of a person in health

Hyperesthesia. increased sensitivity to touch

Hyperplasia. rapid growth; abnormal increase of cells without formation of a tumor but with increase in size of an organ or part

Hypertension. tension or tonus above normal; a condition in which patient has a higher blood pressure than normal for his age

Hyperthermia. abnormally high fever; also hyperexia

Hypertonicity. hypertonia; an increased effective osmotic pressure of body fluids

Hypertrophic scarring. enlargement of the scar; excessive growth of the scar

Hypertrophy. the enlargement or growth of an organ or other part of the body; the growth is independent of natural growth and is caused by unnatural increase in the size of cells

Hypoesthesia. dulled sensitivity to touch

Hypotension. decrease of systolic and diastolic blood pressure below normal; deficiency in tonus or tension

Id. one of three components of psychic structure (with ego and superego); unconscious, unorganized, the seat of basic instinctual drives and energy (Freud)

Idealization. unconscious or conscious defense mechanism; person overestimates an attribute or aspect of another person

Ideational apraxia. inability to correlate purpose and accomplishment of tasks

Identification. unconscious defense mechanism in which a person patterns himself/herself after another (distinguished from imitation, which is a conscious process)

Identity. sense of self

Ideomotor apraxia. inability to imitate gestures or perform purposeful activities on command while retaining ability to perform automatic routine activities

Imitation. conscious process of patterning oneself after another

Impotence. inability to perform sexual intercourse; may be erective (inability to achieve erection); ejaculatory (inability to expel seminal fluid); or orgastic (inability to attain full orgasm)

Imprinting. the process by which animals develop a social attachment for a particular object

Incontinence. inability to retain urine or feces through the loss of sphincter control

Inductive reasoning. the ability to use concrete events, objects, perceptions, or representations to solve a problem

Indwelling catheter. a catheter left in place in the bladder

Infancy. stage in the life cycle lasting from birth until approximately 18 to 24 months

Inhibitory. restraining; tending to inhibit

Integration. (1) the organization and incorporation into the personality and functioning of the individual of data and experience gained (2) a reflex is inhibited or excited by higher centers or increasingly complex networks that modify a reflex in such a way that the response is not noticeable; a reflex may work in concert with others to produce movement; primitive reflexes can reappear as a result of brain damage or under stress

Integrative. helping toward wholeness, organization of thoughts, feelings, and actions

Intelligence quotient. a number assigned to express intellectual capacity obtained by multiplying mental age by 100 and dividing by chronological age

Intension tremor. tremor precipitated or increased on attempt to perform a voluntary coordinated movement

Interoceptive. within viscera; inside the organism

Interpersonal thought. the orientation toward the possible and hypothetical; the ability to explore all possibilities by subjecting the problems to a combinational analysis

Interstitial. situated between important parts; occupying the interspaces or interstices of a part

Intimacy. ability to make and abide by commitment to affiliations and partnerships

Intrinsic marriage. marriage based solely on the relationship between two people

Intrinsic motivation. will to act based on personal internal standards, incentives, desires, and needs

Intrinsic muscles. muscles of the extremities whose origin and insertion are both in the same part of the limb (*e.g.,* hand)

Intuitive thought. part of the preoperational period

(approximately 5 to 7 years of age) when a child is able to separate mental from physical reality and to understand multiple points of view

Invariant clauses. segments of thought processes that are unaffected by mathematical or logical operations

Ipsilateral. on the same side; denoting especially paralytic or other symptoms occurring on the same side as the brain lesion causing them

Ischemia. local anemia or diminution in the blood supply resulting from obstruction of inflow of arterial blood or to vasoconstriction

Isolation. a sense of separateness and self-absorption

Jacksonian. spasmodic contractions in certain groups of muscles or paroxysmal paresthesias in certain skin areas as a result of local disease of the cortex

Jargon. unintelligible speech

Jaundice. a condition marked by yellow skin and eye whites, caused by changes in the liver cells or obstructions, which cause the bile pigment, bilirubin, to be diffused into the blood

Job satisfaction. sense of well-being about one's work resulting from a feeling of commitment based on one's personal and interpersonal goals

Job tryout. placement of client on actual job in industry

Kinesthesia. the conscious perception of movement, weight, resistance, and position of a body part; also kinesthesis

Kirshner wire. an apparatus for skeletal traction in long bone fracture

Kyphosis. a convex backward curvature of the spine; humpback

Lability. state of being unstable, changeable, or having lack of emotional control

Laminectomy. surgical removal of the lamina or posterior arch of the vertebrae

Latency. a state of inactivity, where potential is hidden or dormant

Latency phase. stage of psychosexual development (age five to puberty) apparent cessation of sexual preoccupation (Freud)

L.E. lower extremity

Learning. relatively permanent change in behavior or in the capacity for behavior resulting from either experience or practice

Lesion. structural or functional alteration of a part caused by injury or disease

Libido. basic psychological energy inherent in every person; the energy supplies the sexual drive whose goal is to obtain pleasure (Freud)

Life satisfaction. a subjective sense of well-being

Locus of control. the source or origin of direction of events (Rotter)

External locus of control: control of life events from outside oneself

Internal locus of control: control of life events by one's own thoughts, abilities, and actions

Lordosis. hollow back; anteroposterior curvature of the spine

Lower motor neuron lesion (LMN). lesion occurring in the anterior horn cells, nerve roots, or the peripheral nerve system resulting in flaccid paralysis

Ludic. playful, expressing frivolity, excitement, joy, and celebration

Lumbar. pertaining to the lower back and the five lumbar vertebrae

Macrosphere stage. in play a child begins to share with others on a broader scale

Malignancy. condition of being resistant to treatment occurring in severe form and frequently fatal

Mastery. command or grasp of a subject

Maturation. emergence of an organism's genetic potential; includes a series of preprogrammed changes that comprise changes in the organism's structure and form as well as in its complexity, integration, organization, and function

M.B.D. minimal brain dysfunction; diagnostic and descriptive category of neurodevelopmental lags

Menopause. cessation of menses

Microsphere stage. in play a child masters and/or manipulates the world on a small scale

Microthorax. abnormally small chest

Micturition. urination

Milieu. surroundings; social and physical environment

Milieu therapy. treatment using the manipulation of the socioenvironmental setting to benefit the patient

Modeling. setting an example for imitation

Monoplegia. paralysis of one limb

Morality. a sense of what is right and wrong

Morality of reciprocity. parallels the advanced level of abstract thought; the sense of morality enables one to develop a new conscientious, internally sensitive changing of rules (primarily internally monitored value responses)

Morphology. the structure and form of an organism, excluding its functions

MP joint. metacarpophalangeal joint

Multi-infarct dementia. a series of small strokes causing deterioration of personality and intellect; it results in a stepwise deterioration in intellectual function (not uniformly progressive) with some intellectual functions relatively intact early in its course (patchy deterioration)

Multiple sclerosis (disseminated) (MS). patches of demyelination in the white matter of the nervous system, sometimes in the gray matter; progressive disease of the nervous system

Muscular dystrophy (MD). a progressive, familial hereditary disorder, marked by atrophy and stiffness of the muscles and observed when voluntary action is first attempted

Music therapy. use of music as treatment modality

Myasthenia gravis. a disease characterized by an abnormal exhaustibility of the voluntary muscles, manifesting itself in a rapid diminution of contractility, both when the muscle is activated by the will and when stimulated by electric current

Myelination. myelinization; the process of supplying or accumulating myelin during the development or repair of nerves

Myelin sheath. sheath formation of myelin substance that covers axons and nerve fibers

Myelomeningocele (MM). spina bifida with protrusion of both the cord and its membranes

Myoneural junction. the point at which a motor nerve joins with the muscle it innervates

Myopia. defect in vision so that objects can only be seen distinctly when very close to the eyes

NARC. National Association for Retarded Citizens

NASA. National Aeronautic Space Administration

Necrotic eschar. dead scar tissue

Neonate. a newly born individual, especially an infant during his/her first month of life

Neoplasm. a new formation of tissue, abnormally, as a tumor or growth

Nephrostomy. the establishment of an opening between the pelvis of the kidney and the external surface of the body

Neuritis. inflammation of a nerve or nerves, usually associated with degenerative processes

Neurodevelopmental treatment approach. movement as primary modality of treatment (Bobaths)

Neuromuscular spindle. muscle proprioceptor

Neuron. unit of the nervous system, consisting of the nerve cell body and its various processes, the dendrites, axon, and ending

Neurophysiological treatment approach. the activation, facilitation, and inhibition of voluntary and involuntary muscle action through the reflex arc (Rood)

Neurotendinous organ. a proprioceptive sensory nerve ending in which branching nerve fibers are spread over a bundle of encapsulated fibers near their attachment to muscle; Golgi's organ

NIMH. National Institute of Mental Health

NMS. the coordinated actions of the nervous, muscular, and skeletal systems

Nociceptive response. response to stimuli that could cause harm, injury, or pain

Normal development. determined by wide range of data collected for a particular population within a given time and culture, referring to a specific area or segment of development

Normalization. part of the rehabilitation process emphasizing the patient's ability to grow, adapt, and change as he/she moves toward healthfulness, self-directed behavior, and independence of function

Nuclear family. the natural parents and children

Nystagmus. involuntary rapid movement of the eyeball which may be congenital or acquired

Object permanence. the assumption that objects continue to exist when they are out of sight, touch, or some other perceptual contact

Object relations. emotional attachment for another person or object (that which is other than self)

Occiput. occipital area of the skull; the back of the head

Occlusion. act of closing or the state of being closed

Occupational behavior. organization and action based on skills, knowledge, and attitudes to make functioning possible in life roles (Reilly)

Occupational performance skills. those skills required for successful performance of the roles that are assumed by individuals in their lives. Most human roles fall into the categories of play, self-care, and work.

Oedipal conflict. conflict that appears during the phallic stage. It consists of sexual attraction to the parent of the opposite sex and hostility toward the parent of the same sex

Olfaction. sense of smell; the act of smelling

Ontogeny, ontogenetic. relating to the biological development of the individual (distinguished from phylogeny)

Operant conditioning. procedure through which subject is conditioned by use of reinforcement techniques to learn a desired behavior (B. F. Skinner)

Opisthotonic. relating to a tetanic spasm in which the spine and the extremities are bent with convexity forward, the body resting on the head and heels

Optometrist. one who measures the degree of visual powers; a refractionist

Oral phase. earliest stage of psychosexual development (to 18 months); oral zone is pleasure center (Freud)

Orthotics. science that deals with the making and fitting of orthopedic appliances

Osteoarthritis. a degenerative, noninflammatory, localized form of arthritis that causes breakdown of cartilage and results in limitation of motion and formation of bony outgrowths at the joints affected

Osteosclerosis. osteopetrosis; a rare developmental error of unknown cause but of familial tendency, characterized by excessive radiographic density of most or all of the bones

Otologist. one versed in the science of the ear, its anatomy, functions, and diseases

Otosclerosis. characterized by chronic progressive deafness, especially for low tones

Paleo-. prefix meaning older, *e.g.,* paleocortex, the older portion of the cerebral cortex

Paralinguistics. communication through intonation, gestures, and other nonverbal aspects of speech

Paralysis. loss or impairment of motor and/or sensory function of a part caused by injury to nerves or neurons

Paranoid. psychiatric syndrome characterized by delusions

Paraparesis. partial paralysis or weakness in lower extremities

Paraplegia. paralysis of muscles in lower extremities

PARC. Pennsylvania Association for Retarded Citizens

Parkinson's disease. (synonymous with parkinsonism, Parkinson's syndrome) neurological symptom-complex characterized by four major symptoms: rigidity, tremor, akinesia, and loss of spontaneous and automatic movement

Peer. another person of one's own age or status

Perception. mental process by which intellectual, sensory, and emotional data are organized meaningfully; the process of conscious recognition and interpretation of sensory stimuli

Peripatologist. one who teaches a blind person to travel

Peripheral. located or pertaining to an outer portion of the body away from the center, such as the extremities

Petit mal. brief lapse in consciousness

Phallic phase. third stage of psychosexual development (ages 2 to 6); interest, curiosity, and pleasure centered on penis or clitoris. The oedipal conflict is present during this phase (Freud)

Phasic reflexes. observable movements in response to a touch, pressure, or movement of the body or to sight or sound received

Phenomenology. study of consciously-reported experiences

Phenylketonuria (PKU). the presence of a phenylketone in the urine

Phonology. the science of vocal sounds

Phylogeny, phylogenetic. evolutionary development of any plant or animal species; ancestral history of the individual distinguished from ontogeny, the development of the individual

Physical impairment. weakening, damage, or deterioration, *e.g.,* as a result of injury or disease

PIP joint. proximal interphalangeal joint

Plateau. a period or state of relative stability following or preceding fluctuating change

Play. activity voluntarily engaged in for pleasure

Pleasure principle. the notion that a person tries to gain pleasure and avoid pain (psychoanalytical)

PNS. peripheral nervous system

Poliomyelitis. a common virus disease of man that may progress to involve the central nervous system and result in a nonparalytic or paralytic form of the disease, the latter being the classical form of acute anterior poliomyelitis

Polyneuritis. simultaneous inflammation of many nerves that is usually in a symmetrical pattern

POMR. Problem Oriented Medical Record

Postulate. a theoretical proposition assumed without proof

Postural adaptation. righting; midline; stability; equilibrium

Pragmatic. practical; concerned with actual practice

Praxis. the performance of a purposeful movement or group of movments; ability to motor plan

Preconceptual. the first part of the preoperational period lasting from age 2 to 4 in which there is new use of symbols and symbolic play

Prefrontal lobotomy. neurosurgical procedure in which one or more nerve tracts in the prefrontal area of the brain are severed (also called leukotomy)

Prehominids. ancestors of the human species from which humans eventually evolved

Presbyopia. the inability of the eye to focus sharply on nearby objects, resulting from hardening of the crystalline lens with advancing age

Prevocational evaluation. evaluation of activities of daily living (ADL), educational abilities, and physical capabilities and deficits as required for participation in vocational activity

Primary circular reaction. involves an action on the part of the infant that fortuitously leads to an event that has value for him and is centered about his body. The infant learns to repeat the behavior in order to reinstate the event. The culmination of the process is an organized scheme.

Primary degenerative dementia. also called senile dementia Alzheimer type (SDAT); characterized by the same brain pathology as Alzheimer's presenile dementia (senile plaques, neurofibrillary tangles, granulo-vascular degeneration); meets the DSM III criteria for dementia, but has an insidious onset and uniformly progressive deteriorating course; other causes have been eliminated by history, exam, and lab investigation

Prism glasses. for use by the patient lying supine to prevent eye strain by enabling the patient to see in front of him by looking up to the ceiling

PRN. abbreviation of Latin *pro re nata* according to needs, sometimes used in prescriptions or written orders

Prodromal. referring to early or premonitory symptoms of disease

Prognosis. predicted course of an illness over a given period of time

Projection. unconscious defense mechanism. Person

attributes ideas and feelings to another, the ideas, feelings, and impulses that are his/her own but that are unacceptable to him/her

Projective techniques. loosely structured procedures in which the patient reveals feelings, personality, and unconscious material

Prophylactic. preventing disease; an agent (*e.g.*, vaccine) that acts as a preventive against any disease

Proprioception. appreciation of position, balance, and changes in equilibrium of a body part during movement by receiving stimulus within body tissue such as muscles, tendons, and joints

Protopathic function. denoting a set or system of peripheral sensory nerve fibers furnishing a low order of sensibility, enabling one to appreciate pain and temperature but not to a very delicate extent and definitely not localized; distinguished from epicritic

Pseudobulbar paralysis. paralysis resembling bulbar paralysis but caused by lesion of cortical centers

Pseudohypertrophy. increase in size of an organ without increased size of one or more of its components

Pseudostupidity. interpretation of a situation at a more complex level than is warranted

PSNS. parasympathetic nervous system: the craniosacral division of the autonomic nervous system

PSRO. Professional Standards Review Organization

Psychomotor. referring to combination of physical and emotional activity

Psychopharmacology. study of drugs, medications, and their effects on psychological and behavioral processes

Psychotherapy. treatment of mental disorder in which trained person interacts with patient on the basis of a therapeutic contract; treatment is based on communication processes

Ptosis. drooping of the upper eyelid, abnormal prolapse or falling down of an organ or part

Puberty. the period of life when an individual's sexual organs become functional and secondary sex characteristics appear

Pubescence. period of about 2 years prior to puberty; it is a period of physiological change that triggers the emergence of primary and secondary sexual characteristics

Pulmonary stenosis. narrowing of the opening into the pulmonary artery from the right ventricle

Purposeful activity. treatment when directed to a response that enhances neural integration

Quadriparesis. partial paralysis or weakness in all four extremities

Quadriplegia. paralysis of muscles in all four extremities

Qualitative changes. subjective elements; no scale to measure

Quantitative changes. measurable and thus easily understood

Rapport. conscious, harmonious accord or relationship between people

RAS. reticular activating system

Rationalization. unconscious defense mechanism; person uses a feasible, acceptable reason to explain irrational behavior, motives, or feelings

Reactions. complex and inconstant responses developing from integration of simultaneous sensory stimulation such as tactile, vestibular, visual, and auditory

Reality testing. fundamental ego function; objective evaluation of world outside self; testing of real world—human, nonhuman, concrete, ideational

Reality therapy. treatment method in which milieu and therapeutic relationships are based on real and present situations and cause and effect relationships (Glasser)

Recapitulation of ontogenesis. repetition of passage through stages of human development

Receptive aphasia. impairment in interpretation of the meaning of spoken and written words

Reciprocal innervation. contraction in a muscle is accompanied by a loss of tone or by relaxation in the antagonistic muscle

Reenactment. acting out of a past experience as if it were happening in the present—person can feel, perceive, and act as he/she did the first time

Reflex. fetal or neonatal responses that are simple, predictable, resulting from tactile and vestibular stimulation

Reflex action. an immediate unconscious involuntary response of a limb or organ to stimulation of the sensory branch of a reflex arc

Reflex arc. the pathway from the receptor in the skin to the effector organ through which an impulse travels

Reflexes. when a specific event in the environment occurs, the organism automatically responds (Piaget)

Regression. unconscious defense mechanism; person returns to earlier patterns of adaptation

Rehabilitation. the restoration to a disabled individual of maximum independence commensurate with his limitations by developing his residual capacities

Reinforcement. in behavior therapy, strengthening a response by using a stimulus immediately after the response (may be positive or negative)

Reliability. degree to which a test produces the same results on repeated administrations

Remission. an abatement or lessening of symptoms of a disease

Repression. unconscious defense mechanism; removal from consciousness, usually of ideas, impulses, and feelings that are not acceptable (Freud)

Respiratory distress syndrome (RDS). a condition (usually present at birth) formerly known as hyaline membrane disease; clinical signs include delayed onset of respiration; etiology unknown

Reticular formation. a fine network formed by cells or formed of certain structures within cells or of connective tissue fibers between cells

Retinitis pigmentosa. slowly progressing connective tissue and pigment cell proliferation of the entire membrane with wasting of its nerve elements

Retrolental fibroplasia. a blinding disease of the eye affecting premature infants

Reversible dementia. symptomatic dementia, but prompt treatment of its causes will reverse or alleviate the dementia; untreated, it becomes a true dementia

Reward. a positive reinforcement used to strengthen a desired action

RH factor. a potent antigen and its presence or absence in the blood is referred to as RH positive and RH negative

Rheumatoid arthritis. a chronic progressive inflammatory systemic disease that causes pain, swelling, limitation, and deformity in the joints, with accompanying involvement of tendons and sheaths, nerves, and muscles

Righting reactions. reflexes that through various receptors in labyrinth, eyes, muscles, or skin tend to bring an organism's body into its normal position in space and which resists any force acting to put it into a false position, *e.g.*, on its back

Rigidity. inflexible and tonic contraction of muscles giving consistent resistance to passive movement through total range of movement

Role diffusion. identity confusion; discontinuity in both experience and in how others perceive oneself

Rorschach test. projective test in which subject reveals attitudes and emotions through response to inkblot pictures

Rote. habit performance, without meaning; in a mechanical way

Rubella. german measles; an acute, contagious eruptive disease; also called epidemic roseola, French measles

Rural. counties with populations up to 10,000 (additional population begins to be semirural) accompanied by geographic isolation, likely cultural and economic isolation as well

SAR—sexual attitude reassessment. A workshop designed to desensitize and resensitize participants to their sexuality and the sexuality of others, particularly the disabled

Schedule of reinforcement. pattern set up for presentation of reinforcers in behavior therapy

Schemata. Piagetian term that refers to the structure or framework into which one's experiences are integrated

Schwann cell. one of the cells of the neurolemma; a cell that enfolds myelinated and unmyelinated nerve fibers

Sclerosis. hardening of a part with growth of fibrous tissue resulting from atrophy or degeneration of nerve elements

Scoliosis. lateral curvature of the spine

Scotoma. abnormal blind spots

Sealing over. covering up unconscious material

Sebaceous glands. composed of fat, keratohyalin, granules, keratin, and cellular debris

Secondary circular reaction. actions involving events or objects in the external environment; the ability to develop schemes that reproduce interesting events that were initially discovered by chance in the external environment

Secular trend. recent generations tend to be more intelligent, taller, and stronger than previous generations; a generational shift

Sedative. drug that produces calming, relaxing effect—CNS depressant

SEIMC. special education instructional materials centers

Selective inattention. blocking out stimuli that generate anxiety; failing to notice, see, or hear things that the individual may not wish to deal with

Semidomesticated. refers to the situation of wild animals who have an adequate food supply provided artificially and who are relatively free from predators, but who roam a relatively unrestricted territory

Senility. gradual loss of physical and/or mental function and well-being of an aged person resulting in withdrawal, apathy, personal neglect, blunting of memory and cognitive abilities, weakness, poor appetite, and sleep disorders

Sensibility. the ability to perceive, appreciate, and transmit nerve impulses

Sensorimotor stage. the first stage of Piaget's cognitive theory in which the child from birth to 2 years of age seeks to integrate perceptions and bodily motions

Seriation. arranging or organizing in orderly series

Sex typing. process of acquiring the behavior and attitudes regarded by the culture as masculine or feminine

Sexuality. the integration of physical, emotional, intellectual, and social aspects of an individual's personality that expresses maleness or femaleness

Shaping. in behavior therapy, system of establishing desired behavior patterns through reinforcement given for each successive approximation—moving closer to goal

Shearing. distortion of a body by two oppositely directed parallel forces

Shock treatment. psychiatric treatment through use of chemicals or electric current (insulin-ECT or EST)

Significant other(s). human(s) or animal(s) of particular importance to the well-being of another

Situational or simulated job tryout. placement of client in actual work situation in a sheltered workshop or other such institution

SMS. sensory-motor-sensory; sensory feedback integration with the initial sensory input and motor accommodation

SNS. sympathetic nervous system

SOAP. subjective, objective, assessment, plan; used in problem-oriented medical record

Social bond. underlying quality of attachment between two persons

Social interaction. active affectionate reciprocal relationship between two persons

Social-technical evolution. a term referring to changes in human evolution that are not biological in nature. This includes the technology, culture, and social relations that have come about as a function of evolution

Socio-dramatic play. voluntary social play with at least one other child wherein a child imitates the actions and speech of others

Somatosensory. concerning sensation of the body as distinguished from the viscera or mind

Spasm. a sudden involuntary contraction of muscle or group of muscles

Spastic. characterized by spasms and resulting in hypertonia and awkward movements from stiff muscles

Spasticity. state of hypertonicity, involuntary resistance of weak muscle caused by passive range of motion, followed by sudden relaxation of muscle, associated with exaggeration of reflexes and loss of voluntary muscle control; increased muscle tone

Spatial relations. the relationship of the skeletal parts of the body to each other and to objects in the environment

Spatiotemporal adaptation. continuous, ongoing state or act of adjusting those bodily processes required to function within a given space at a given time

Standardized. having established and tested norms

Static splint. splint with no moving parts; maintains a joint in desired position

Stereognosis. the perception and identification of the form and nature of an object through the sense of touch

Stereoscopic. vision in which things have the appearance of solidity and relief as seen in three dimensions

Strabismus. deviation of the eye that the individual cannot overcome

Stress. physical, emotional, or intellectual strain or tension disturbing normal equilibrium

Stroke. a sudden and severe seizure or fit of disease; a popular term for cerebral vascular accident (CVA)

Stryker frame. a bed-turning frame that enables a patient to be rotated from front to back but does not allow tilting

Sublimation. unconscious defense mechanism; replacement of unacceptable wishes, drives, feelings, or goals with those that are acceptable

Subluxation. incomplete or partial dislocation of a joint

Superego. one of three components of psychic structure (with id and ego); (Freud) incorporation of standards, moral attitudes, and conscience

Support system. people, agencies, or institutions that serve to help sustain a person in stress or problems

Supportive. reinforcing the patient's defenses and reassuring him/her (as opposed to probing into conflicts)

Supportive treatment. relates to the psychological and emotional needs and problems

Suppression. conscious act of controlling unacceptable impulses, feelings, or behavior (different from repression, which is unconscious)

Suprapubic catheter. a catheter positioned above the pubic arch

Surrogate mother. someone or something that takes the place of a mother in an organism's life

Symbol. something used for or representing an object, idea, image, or feeling

Symbolization. unconscious defense mechanism; idea or object comes to stand for another, based on similarity or association

Synapse. the point at which an impulse passes from one neuron to another

Synergies. combined or correlated actions of different organs of the body, as of muscles working together

Synoptic. affording or taking a general view of the whole or of the principal parts of a subject

Synovectomy. surgical excision of the synovial membrane

Synovial membrane. connective tissue that lines a synovial joint

Synthesize. to form by combining parts into a single whole

Tactile. pertaining to touch

Tactile defensiveness. the quality of being unable to tolerate touch; resistive and uncomfortable at certain kinds of touch (believed to be a form of sensory integrative dysfunction)

Tactile localization. the ability to determine the location of a cutaneous stimulus

Task-oriented group. group whose focus is on reaching a goal, finding a solution to a problem, or making a product

Tay-Sachs disease. amaurosis; a familial disease occurring almost exclusively in Jewish children characterized by flaccid muscles, convulsions, decerebrate rigidity, and blindness

TD. terminal device in upper extremity prosthetics

Tenodesis splint. functional handsplint that operates on the tenodesis principle of wrist extension and finger flexion

Term infant. infant with gestation period 38–42 weeks

Tertiary circular reaction. the interest in novelty and curiosity about an object; the child no longer relies on previous schemes.

Thematic apperception test. projective psychological test; subject looks at series of ambiguous pictures and interprets what he/she sees; interpretation will be based on subject's own feelings and attitudes

Theory. a set of logically interrelated statements used to explain observed events; a proposed explanation whose status is still conjectural, in contrast to well-established propositions that are regarded as reporting matters of actual fact

Therapeutic recreation. the utilization of recreational experiences for the prevention and/or amelioration of handicapping conditions

Thoracic. pertaining to the chest and ribs and the 12 thoracic vertebrae

Thrombus. a collection of blood or a clot causing vascular obstruction

TIA. transient ischemic attack

TLC. tender loving care

Toxoplasmosis. a disease caused by infection with the protozoa, Toxoplasma gondii; in the congenital form it causes destructive lesions of the central nervous system, jaundice, and anemia

Tracheostomy. surgical formation of an opening into the trachea and suturing of the edges to the skin in the neck for an airway or passage of a tube

Tranquilizer. psychotropic drug inducing calming, soothing effect without clouding consciousness—major tranquilizers, antipsychotic drugs; minor tranquilizers, anti-anxiety drugs

Transaction. interaction between two or more people

Transactional analysis. system centering on study of interactions between people in treatment—four parts: (1) structural analysis of intrapsychic processes; (2) determination of dominant ego state (parent, child, adult); (3) game analysis; and (4) script analysis (finding causes of problems); used in both group and individual psychotherapy (Eric Berne)

Transductive reasoning. refers to the preoperational child's tendency to use associative reasoning rather than inductive or deductive thought (Piaget)

Transference. projection of feelings, thoughts, or wishes on to another who has come to represent someone from the past; inappropriate applied in present context; used in therapeutic process (psychoanalytical)

Trapeze bar. triangular bar attached to a traction frame on the bed so that the patient lying in bed can reach the bar to assist in rolling over, coming to a sitting position, or transferring from the bed to a chair

Trauma. injury as a result of physical or emotional means or insult

Tremor. alternate contraction and relaxation of opposing groups of muscles resulting in involuntary rhythmic and oscillating movements such as quivering or trembling

Trophic changes. changes in function concerned with nourishment of tissues caused by vascular, neurological, nutritional, or endocrine problems or inactivity (disuse)

Trouble team. team composed of two or three people specially trained in crisis intervention, face-to-face counseling skills; usually sent out to meet with the caller when the situation (runaways, attempted suicides, etc.) seems to require more intervention than can be accomplished on the phone

UE. upper extremity

Unconditional positive regard. the quality of accepting another person and communicating that acceptance regardless of what that person says or does (Rogers)

Unconscious. part of the mind in which psychic material—primitive drives, repressed desires, and memories—is not directly accessible to awareness (psychoanalytical)

Underactive. lacking or slow in taking the initiative to act

Underreactive. responding minimally or slowly to stimuli

Upper motor neuron lesion (UMN). lesion occurring in corticospinal or pyramidal tract located in brain or spinal cord resulting in paralysis, increased muscle tone, and pathological reflexes

Utilitarian marriage. marriage not necessarily based on the couple's relationship; purpose of the marriage varies (*i.e.* from pure physical relationship to raising family)

Validity. statistical term; the degree to which a given measure indicates quality or attribute it attempts to measure

Values. ideals, feelings, and beliefs that are acted upon

Vascularity. containing blood vessels

Ventricular septal defect. flaw or defect between ventricles of the heart

Viscera. organs of the digestive, respiratory, urogenital, and endocrine systems as well as the spleen, heart, and great vessels

Visual accommodation. the ability to focus on an object at varying distances

Vocalization. the utterance of sounds

Vocational evaluation. assessment of all factors (medical, psychological, educational, social, environmental, cultural, and vocational) that affect successful employment

Volition. will or purpose

WHO. World Health Organization

Work evaluation. evaluation of vocational strengths and weaknesses through utilization of work (real or simulated)

Work sample evaluation. sample of actual job tasks or a mock-up of actual tasks to determine client's job skills and abilities

Wrist driven flexor hinge splint. use of wrist extension to provide prehension

Index

Numbers followed by an *f* indicate a figure; *t* following a page number indicates tabular material.

Parkinson's disease, 381, 405–407

patient's rights, as societal concern, 277

Peabody Picture Vocabulary Test, 340

Peck, R. C., 723

pediatric occupational therapy, 573–575 *f*, 639
  concepts of, 573–575, 575 *f*, 576 *t*
  evaluation in, 575, 577 *f*, 578
  planning in, 578
  selection of activities in, 225
  theory, spatiotemporal adaptation, 569

pediatric prosthetics, 515–516, 519

pediatrics, community facility for, systems model, 803–805

peer review, 862–863

Pennsylvania Bimanual Work Sample, 370

perception, assessment of, in progressive neurological disorders, 384

perceptual dysfunctions, in hemiplegia, 391–392, 392 *f*

perceptual-motor function, tests for, 341–342, 371

performance testing procedures, in functional restoration process, 360–361, 361 *f*, 370–371, 372 *f*

peripheral nerve injury, 381, 382, 438–440, 468–473
  biofeedback techniques in, 262
  and brachial plexus injury in children, 607, 610, 612 *f*, 613

peripheral nervous system, structure and function, 107, 108

peripheral vascular disease, lower extremity amputation in, 519

personal adjustment training, 253, 254, 255

personnel management, 819–823

phantom limb sensations, 497, 522

phasic reflexes, 176

Philadelphia Jewish Employment and Vocational System, 211

phobia, biofeedback technique in, 263

physical capacities evaluation, 168, 168–173 *f*, 213, 214 *f*

physical therapy, 120, 379

physical training. *See* exercise

physician, role of, 378–379

Piaget, Jean, theories of, 47–48
  adolescence, 68, 70
  adulthood, 73
  circular response concept of, 54, 56, 58
  cognitive development in neonate, 53
  developmental concepts of, 551
  intuitive phase, 62
  play structure, 66, 67 *t*, 68
  pre-school development, 58
  and success motivation, 93

Piagetian concepts of cognitive development, in adult psychosis, 290, 290 *t*

pinch strength measurement, 168

placing, test procedure for, 182–183

planning
  by analysis, 846, 847, 854–857

  by audit, 846–847, 848–854 *f*
  marketing versus traditional, 843–844
  strategic, 837–841

plantar grasp, test procedure for, 182

Plaster of Paris, 455

play. *See also* recreation
  in autism, 628
  behavior, 64
  of children, 64–68
  content and structure, 65–66
  functions, 64–65
  in occupational behavior approach, 33–39, 130, 131
  phases, for learning, 291
  Piaget's evolution of, 67 *t*
  stages of, 65–66
  theories of, 66–68, 547–549

Play History, 131

poliomyelitis, 380, 381, 425–426

Polyform, 455

positioning
  in acute burn management, 483, 484 *f*, 485 *t*
  in cerebral palsy, 662, 674–675

positive support reaction, 176

postural reflex mechanism, 176
  in sensory integrative theory, 125–126

postural strategies, 556

power
  through financial management, 816
  in systems theory, 813

praxia. *See* motor skill

pregnancy, prenatal development and, 50

prehensile reactions, 178–179

premorbid personal development, 357, 358 *f*

prenatal development, 49–51

preprosthetic considerations, 517–518, 519

preschool development, 58–61
  18 months, 58–59
  three years, 60–61
  two years, 59–60

Pre-Speech Assessment Scale, 654

pressure areas, in hand splinting, 457

pressure garment, in burn management, 485–486

pressure stretch techniques, in burn management, 484–487

prevocational activities, selection of, 225

prevocational evaluation, 207, 308

prevocational training, 251–257
  in lower extremity amputation, 521–522
  in upper extremity amputation, 514–515

primary circular response, 54

primary prevention, in mental health, 314

primary standing, test procedure, 182

primary walking, test procedure, 182

prism glasses, 433

private hospital, as psychiatric care facility, 318

private practice, OT, in home care delivery, 776